Nursing Patients with Cancer

For Churchill Livingstone:
Senior Commissioning Editor: Ninette Premdas
Development Editor: Claire Wilson
Project Manager: Derek Robertson; Anne Dickie
Design: Stewart Larking
Illustration Manager: Bruce Hogarth

Nursing Patients With Cancer

Principles and Practice

Edited by

Nora Kearney MSc RGN
Professor of Cancer Care
Director, Cancer Care Research Centre
Department of Nursing and Midwifery
University of Stirling, UK

Alison Richardson PhD MSc BN (Hons) RGN RNT Pg Dip Ed
Professor of Cancer and Palliative Nursing Care
Florence Nightingale School of Nursing and Midwifery
King's College London, UK

Foreword by
Jan Foubert
President, European Oncology Nursing Society

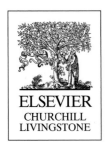

ELSEVIER
CHURCHILL
LIVINGSTONE

EDINBURGH LONDON NEW YORK OXFORD PHILADELPHIA ST LOUIS SYDNEY TORONTO 2006

ELSEVIER
CHURCHILL
LIVINGSTONE
An imprint of Elsevier Limited

First published 2006

ISBN 0 443 07288 4

British Library Cataloguing in Publication Data
A catalogue record for this book is available from the British Library

Library of Congress Cataloging in Publication Data
A catalog record for this book is available from the Library of Congress

NOTE
Knowledge and best practice in this field are constantly changing. As new research and experience broaden our knowledge, changes in practice, treatment and drug therapy may become necessary or appropriate. Readers are advised to check the most current information provided (i) on procedures featured or (ii) by the manufacturer of each product to be administered, to verify the recommended dose or formula, the method and duration of administration, and contraindications. It is the responsibility of the practitioner, relying on their own experience and knowledge of the patient, to make diagnoses, to determine dosages and the best treatment for each individual patient, and to take all appropriate safety precautions. To the fullest extent of the law, neither the publisher nor the Editors assume any liability for any injury and/or damage.

The Publisher

Printed in China

CONTENTS

Contributors . . . . *ix*
Foreword . . . . *xiii*
Preface . . . . *xv*
Abbreviations . . . . *xvii*

SECTION 1: Philosophies of cancer nursing and the context of care
Section Editor: **Yvonne Wengström**

1. Concepts of Health Behaviour 3
    Annie Topping

2. Partnership in Care 21
    Yvonne Wengström, Christina Forsberg

3. The Social and Cultural Context of Cancer Care 37
    Karin Ahlberg

SECTION 2: The scientific basis of cancer care
Section Editors: **Diane Batchelor, Jaqualyn S Moore**

4. Cancer Epidemiology 55
    Helen Evans, Angela Newnham and Henrik Møller

5. Genetic Basis of Cancer 73
    Athena Matakidou, Tim Eisen

6. Pathology 97
    Fred T Bosman

7. The Immunological Basis of Cancer 115
    Jaqualyn S Moore

SECTION 3: Prevention and early detection
Section Editor: **Agnes Glaus**

8. Cancer Prevention 133
    Agnes Glaus, Stella Aguinaga Bialous, Paula Trahan Rieger

9. Early Detection of Cancer 167
    Agnes Glaus, Paula Trahan Rieger

SECTION 4: Treatment and care

Section Editors: **Sara Faithfull, Mary Wells**

10. Decision-Making in Cancer Care 195
    Alastair J Munro

11. The Experience of Cancer Treatment 213
    Deborah Fitzsimmons, Janice M Middleton

12. Surgery 233
    Alastair M Thompson, Mary Wells

13. Radiotherapy 265
    Sara Faithfull

14. Chemotherapy 283
    Melaine Coward, Helen M Coley

15. Biological Therapy 303
    Diane Batchelor

16. Bone Marrow Transplantation 329
    Barry Quinn, Moira Stephens

17. Hormone Therapy 353
    Deborah Fenlon

18. Complementary and Alternative Therapies 381
    Alexander Molassiotis, Anne Cawthorn, Peter A Mackereth

SECTION 5: Symptom management

Section Editors: **Alexander Molassiotis, Gina Copp**

19. Haematological Support .403
    Jacqui Stringer, Jane Collins, Angela Leather

20. Nausea and Vomiting 415
    Alexander Molassiotis, Sussanne Börjeson

21. Pain 439
    Emile Maassen, Elisabeth Patiraki

22. Constipation and Diarrhoea 481
    Tanya Y Andrewes, Christine Norton

23. Breathlessness 507
    Sally Moore, Hilary Plant, Mary Bredin

24. Skin and Wound Care 527
    Wayne A Naylor

25. Lymphoedema 559
    Julie-Ann MacLaren

26. Oral Complications in Patients with Cancer 575
    Karis KF Cheng

27. Alopecia 601
    Diane Batchelor

28. Malignant Effusions 619
Shelley Dolan, Nancy J Preston

29. Anorexia, Cachexia and Malnutrition 633
Alexander Molassiotis, Jan Foubert

30. Cancer-related Fatigue 657
Karin Ahlberg

31. The Impact of Cancer and Cancer Therapy on Sexual and
Reproductive Health 675
Isabel D White

32. Altered Body Image 701
Diana Harcourt, Nichola Rumsey

33. Psychological Care for Patients with Cancer 717
Eileen Furlong, Sinead O'Toole

SECTION 6: Care delivery systems

Section Editors: **Maggie Grundy, Emile Maassen**

34. Cancer Care and Cancer Nursing 741
Maggie Grundy

35. Intensive Nursing Care of the Patient with Cancer 771
Shelley Dolan

36. Rehabilitation and Survivorship 799
Mary Wells, Sheila MacBride

37. Palliative Care 821
Sally Mirando

Index 849

CONTRIBUTORS

Karin Ahlberg RN PhD
Head of Unit, Department of Oncology,
Sahlgrenska University Hospital, Gothenburg
Sweden

Tanya Y Andrewes PGDip BSc(Hons) RGN
Senior Lecturer, Institute of Health and
    Community Studies
Bournemouth University, UK

Diane Batchelor RN MScN NP CON (C)
Advanced Practice Nurse (Oncology)
Patient Care and Consulting in Cancer Care
183 Sydenham Street
Gananoque, Ontario, Canada

Stella Aguinaga Bialous RN MScN DrPH
President, Tobacco Policy
International, San Francisco, CA, USA

Sussanne Börjeson RN PhD
Senior Lecturer
Department of Medicine & Care
Nursing Science
Faculty of Health Sciences
Linköping University
Linköping, Sweden

Fred T Bosman MD PhD
Professor of Pathology
Director of the University Institute of Pathology
Lausanne, Switzerland

Mary Bredin MA RGN PG Dip in Psychotherapeutic
Counselling
23 St John's Terrace
Lewes, East Sussex, UK

Anne Cawthorn RGN MSc
Lecturer/Practitioner
University of Manchester
The Christie Hospital NHS Trust
Withington
Manchester, UK

Karis KF Cheng PhD PGDip Epidemiol & Biostat
Assistant Professor, Nethersole School of
    Nursing,
The Chinese University of Hong Kong
Shatin, Hong Kong

Helen M Coley BSc FIMLS PhD MILT
Senior Research Fellow, Division of
    Oncology
Postgraduate Medical School
School of Biomedical and Molecular
    Sciences,
University of Surrey, Guildford, UK

Jane Collins RGN
Blood Product Specialist Nurse
Christie Hospital NHS Trust
Manchester, UK

Gina Copp PhD MN RGN RCNT
Senior Lecturer, School of Health & Social
    Sciences
Middlesex University, London, UK

Melaine Coward RGN BSc (Hons) Cancer Nursing
PGCHSCE
Lecturer, European Institute of Health and
    Medical Sciences
University of Surrey, UK

CONTRIBUTORS

Shelley Dolan RN BA(Hons) MSc
Nurse Consultant Cancer: Critical Care
Critical Care Unit
The Royal Marsden NHS Foundation Trust
London, UK

Tim Eisen PhD FRCP
Senior Lecturer/Consultant Medical
    Oncologist
The Royal Marsden NHS Foundation Trust
Sutton, Surrey, UK

Helen Evans MSc
Researcher
Thames Cancer Registry
London, UK

Sara Faithfull PhD MSc RGN
Director of Studies
Doctorate of Clinical Practice
European Institute for Health and Medical
    Sciences
Surrey University
Guildford, UK

Deborah Fenlon PhD MSc BSc RGN
Senior Research Fellow
School of Nursing and Midwifery
University of Southampton, UK

Deborah Fitzsimmons PhD BN(Hons) RN
Lecturer, University School of Nursing &
    Midwifery
University of Southampton, UK

Christina Forsberg PhD RN
Senior Lecturer
The Swedish Red Cross University College of
    Nursing
Stockholm, Sweden

Jan Foubert PhD MSc RPN PGDip EdRNT
Senior Lecturer Nursing & Midwifery
Erasmushogeschool Departement
Gelondheidszorg, Jette, Belgium

Eileen Furlong MMedSc(Nursing) HDip Onc RGN
RSCN RCNT
Lecturer, Nursing School of Nursing and
    Midwifery
University College Dublin
Dublin 4, Ireland

Agnes Glaus PhD MSc RN
Nurse Practitioner/Researcher
Center for Tumor Detection and Prevention
St Gallen, Switzerland

Maggie Grundy MSc RGN RM Diploma Nurs
Diploma Nurse Ed (CT) Cert PG Teaching (RNT)
Senior Lecturer, The Robert Gordon
    University School of Nursing and
    Midwifery
Faculty of Health & Social Care
Aberdeen, UK

Diana Harcourt BSc (Hons) MSc PhD
Centre for Appearance Research
Faculty of Applied Sciences
University of the West of England
Bristol, UK

Nora Kearney MSc RGN
Professor of Cancer Care
Director, Cancer Care Research Centre
Department of Nursing and Midwifery
University of Stirling, UK

Angela Leather RGN
Transplant Coordinator, Christie Hospital
    NHS Trust
Manchester, UK

Sheila MacBride MN(Cancer Nursing) BSc(Soc
Sci–Nursing Studies) RGN NDN Onc Cert
Lecturer in Cancer Nursing
School of Nursing and Midwifery
University of Dundee, UK

Julie-Ann MacLaren BSc(Hons) MA DipN (Cancer)
RGN
Lecturer in Cancer Nursing
Royal Marsden School of Cancer Nursing &
    Rehabilitation
Sutton, UK

Emile Maassen RN
Clinical Nurse Specialist, Clinical Research
Nurse, TweeSteden Hospital, Tilburg,
The Netherlands and Nursing Consultant,
Comprehensive Cancer Center 'South',
Eindhoven, The Netherlands

Peter A Mackereth MA RNT Cert Ed Dip Nursing
RGN
Clinical Lead Complementary Therapies
    Christie Hospital & Lecturer
University of Salford, Salford, UK

Athena Matakidou BSc BM
Clinical Research Fellow, Institute of Cancer
    Research, Sutton, Surrey, UK

Janice M Middleton BNSc (Hons) RN RM FETC
Lecturer/Practitioner Oncology Nursing
School of Nursing and Midwifery
University of Southampton, UK

Sally Mirando MSc (Econ) MCGI BSc RGN RM RHV
PgDip Couns
Macmillan Nurse Consultant in Palliative
    Care/Associate Lecturer
Herefordshire Primary Care Trust, Hereford,
    and University College, Worcester, UK

Alexander Molassiotis BSC RN MSc PhD
Reader in Cancer & Supportive Care
University of Manchester School of Nursing,
    Midwifery and Social Work
Manchester, UK

Henrik Møller BA BSc MSc DM FFPH
Director, Thames Cancer Registry,
Professor of Cancer Epidemiology at Guy's,
    King's and St Thomas' School of Medicine
    and London School of Hygiene & Tropical
    Medicine, London, UK

Jaqualyn S Moore RGN RM BSc (Hons) MSc PGCAP
Lecturer, Florence Nightingale School of
    Nursing and Midwifery,
King's College London, UK

Sally Moore MSc BSc(Hons) RGN
Macmillan Lung Cancer Nurse Specialist
Guy's and St Thomas' NHS Foundation
    Trust, London, UK

Alastair J Munro BSc MBChB FRCR FRCP(E)
Professor of Radiation Oncology,
Department of Surgery and Molecular
    Oncology
University of Dundee Ninewells Hospital
    and Medical School Dundee, UK

Wayne A Naylor RN BSc (Hons) Dip Nursing PG
Cert (Palliative Care) Onc Cert
Wound Management Research Nurse
The Royal Marsden NHS Foundation Trust,
    London, UK
Clinical Nurse Educator (Oncology/
Haematology), Wellington Blood and Cancer
    Centre, Wellington, New Zealand

Angela Newnham MA MBBS MFPH
Department of Primary Care and General
    Practice,
The University of Birmingham
Edgbaston, UK

Christine Norton PhD MA RN
Burdett Professor of Gastrointestinal
Nursing Florence Nightingale School of
Nursing and Midwifery, King's College,
London and Nurse
    Consultant (Bowel Control)
St Mark's Hospital, Harrow, Middlesex, UK

Sinead O'Toole RGN Dip App Science (Nursing) BA
MA PG Dip
Lecturer in Nursing, School of Nursing and
Midwifery, University College Dublin
Dublin, Ireland

Elisabeth Patiraki RN BSc PhD
Assistant Professor, Faculty of Nursing,
National and Kapodistrian University of
Athens, Athens, Greece

Hilary Plant PhD BA(Hons) RGN
Lead for Nursing Research and Development
    – Cancer and Haematology,
Guy's and St Thomas' NHS Foundation
    Trust, London, UK

Nancy J Preston PhD BSc (Hons) RGN
Systematic Review Fellow
Royal College of Nursing Institute
Oxford, UK

CONTRIBUTORS

Barry Quinn MSc BD BaccPhil RN
Lecturer Haemato-oncology, Royal Marsden
School of Cancer Nursing and Rehabilitation
London, UK

Alison Richardson PhD MSc BN (Hons) RGN RNT
Pg Dip Ed
Professor of Cancer and Palliative Nursing
    Care
Florence Nightingale School of Nursing and
    Midwifery
King's College London, UK

Paula Trahan Rieger RN MSN CS AOCN FAAN
Director, International Affairs, ASCO
Alexandria, VA, USA

Nichola Rumsey BSc (Hons) MSc PhD
Centre for Appearance Research
Faculty of Applied Sciences
Frenchay Campus
University of the West of England
Bristol, UK

Moira Stephens RN DPSN BSc(Hons) MSc PGC ED
Cert Onc
Clinical Nurse Consultant
Haematology/Oncology, Liverpool Hospital
Southwest Sydney Area Health Service
New South Wales, Australia

Jacqui Stringer RGN BSc (Hons) TIDHA
Clinical Lead in Complementary Therapies
    Christie Hospital NHS Trust
Manchester, UK

Alastair M Thompson ALCM BSc(Hons) MBChB
MD FRCSEd(Gen)
Professor of Surgical Oncology
Department of Surgery & Molecular
    Oncology
Ninewells Hospital & Medical School
University of Dundee, UK

Annie Topping BSc(Hons) PhD PGCE (FE) RGN
Head of Nursing, School of Health Studies
University of Bradford, Bradford, UK

Mary Wells RGN BSc (Hons) MSc
Lecturer and Clinical Research Fellow in
    Cancer Nursing
School of Nursing and Midwifery, University
    of Dundee
Dundee, UK

Yvonne Wengström OCN BSN PhD
Development of Clinical Practice
Division of Nursing Research at Karolinska
    Hospital
Stockholm, Sweden

Isabel D White MSc PGDip BEd(Hons) DipLSc RGN
RSCN RNT Onc Cert Cancer Research UK Nursing
Research Training Fellow, European Institute
    of Health & Medical Sciences (EIHMS)
University of Surrey, Guildford, UK

FOREWORD

Six million nurses comprise the largest group of healthcare workers in Europe. Their realm of activities is far-reaching, including promotion of health, prevention of the severity of disease and the provision of direct care in a variety of settings. The valuable contribution made by nurses is increasingly recognized in the member states of the European Union (EU).

With regard to the European Social Charter, Article 11 and Article 13, we see that nurses are able to identify and develop strategies to improve services in the field of health protection and to ensure that the right to social and medical assistance can be achieved.

Despite increasing recognition, the further development of nursing continues to be affected by many factors. The absence of nurses in policy-making bodies, a shortage of qualified nurses, insufficient resources for education and professional development, inadequate work facilities and an undervaluing of the importance of nursing all negatively impact on the growth potential of the nursing profession in Europe. In addition to these factors, nurses in Europe share characteristics of other female-dominated occupations, which include low pay, low status, poor working conditions, few prospects for promotion and poor education. The fact that Europe is a geographical area encompassing many cultures, languages and forms of government adds to the difficulties in defining, unifying and perhaps even standardizing nursing.

With this background information, the uniqueness of nursing in Europe becomes clearer. Contrastingly, the scope of cancer, including incidence, morbidity and mortality rates, is comparative to most other geographical areas in the world. Research continues to strive to find a cure for cancer, new treatment modalities are being constantly implemented and the ageing population presents a number of challenges for the future. Easier access to information has provided patients with more knowledge and hence greater consumer power and, common to all cancer settings, the cost of providing care is escalating.

It is within this context that *Nursing Patients with Cancer: Principles and Practice*, a comprehensive textbook to meet the specific learning needs of nurses practising in the area of cancer care in Europe, has been developed. The content of this textbook builds on the *Core Curriculum for a Post-registration Course in Cancer Nursing*, 2nd edn, produced by the European Oncology Nursing Society (EONS) in 1999. The curriculum, supported with funding from the EU's Europe Against Cancer Programme, was a product of a consensus with experts involved in education and practice from throughout Europe. To date, the core curriculum has been the most requested and most used piece of educational material produced by EONS. It is estimated that well over 13 countries have utilized the curriculum as the basis for educational development. The fact that the curriculum has found such unprecedented acceptance is not to be treated lightly; the diversity of educational levels, needs and practice environments in Europe makes it extremely difficult to implement any one standard of education for distribution and use in Europe. This textbook will further support the utilization of the curriculum.

Nursing Patients with Cancer: Principles and Practice complements the many other educational resources that EONS has made available to cancer nurses over the past several years. I can proudly and securely state that EONS has been instrumental in advancing knowledge in cancer nursing through educational initiatives in Europe. For example, two of the most recent projects – NOEP (Nutrition Oncology Education Program) and TITAN (Training Initiative Thrombocytopenia, Anaemia and Neutropenia) – used a learning needs analysis as a first phase in the development of educational programmes targeted specifically to fill knowledge deficits. Other EONS-generated surveys have shown that nurses desire to improve their practice through education and that educational courses should be practice-oriented with case studies and evidence-based guidelines. This feedback has provided valuable insight for planning continuing education programmes, including the EONS Spring Convention.

Developing the textbook to complement the core curriculum is important for EONS, which represents around 20,000 nurses across Europe. This partnership approach to education and learning is a key component of EONS' activity and facilitates the potential for widespread dissemination of good practice. The issues addressed within this book are fundamental to cancer nursing practice and EONS, thus addressing the aims of the Society. Over recent years, there has been growing recognition of the need for nurses to deliver increasingly complex cancer care, and knowledge is necessary to competently provide that care. This textbook offers such knowledge and successfully combines the essentials of cancer management within the context of social and cultural factors of relevance to nurses practising in Europe.

On behalf of EONS, I challenge nurses to use the extensive information contained within *Nursing Patients with Cancer: Principles and Practice* to improve the quality of care they deliver to patients and also as a means of contributing to their professional and personal growth through the power of knowledge.

Dr Jan Foubert

PREFACE

Cancer nursing as a specialty continues to develop across Europe, with increasing numbers of education and training opportunities available to nurses to develop their knowledge and skills. This book offers the first comprehensive text to support nurses in Europe in this endeavour. *Nursing Patients with Cancer: Principles and Practice* is the culmination of many debates and reflections on the need to provide a comprehensive textbook that would complement *Core Curriculum for a Post-registration Course in Cancer Nursing*, 2nd edn, published by the European Oncology Nursing Society (EONS) in 1999. This curriculum was prepared by EONS and funded by the EU's Europe Against Cancer Programme. The curriculum is based upon assessment and intervention of patient and family needs, and aims to prepare nurses to work with patients with cancer and their families across a range of settings. The book reflects these basic principles.

This unique edition provides a comprehensive text on adult cancer nursing. It aims to provide European nurses with an understanding of the essential social and scientific basis of contemporary cancer management, and equip them with the key skills and knowledge they will require to work in cancer care teams. While we recognize the availability of North American texts in this area, these are not always useful within a European context, either professionally or culturally. Therefore, we set out to reflect state-of-the-art cancer care across Europe to ensure that nurses wishing to practice across this vast continent would have a key reference text that was not only comprehensive

in relation to cancer care but also acknowledged the diversity of our cultures. The book has contributions from 60 authors from 10 countries, including nurses, basic and social scientists, doctors, allied health professionals and therapists, who have expertise and experience in all aspects of the management of individuals with cancer and their carers, either as practitioners, researchers, teachers or managers. The involvement of so many key individuals has resulted in a text that is a rich resource for cancer nurses and allied health professionals and indeed for other disciplines new to cancer care.

In order to reflect the EONS' *Core Curriculum for a Post-registration Course in Cancer Nursing*, 2nd edn, we have arranged the book into six interrelated sections, each with expert Section Editors. Section 1, edited by Yvonne Wengström, explores the attitudes, values and beliefs of the public, patients with cancer and the professionals who care for them. It examines the key principles of partnership and self-care as well as the social and cultural context of cancer care, particularly relevant to a European audience. Section 2, edited by Jaqualyn Moore and Diane Batchelor, considers in detail the scientific basis of cancer, offering readers in-depth understanding of the genetic processes of cancer and its development. Section 3, edited by Agnes Glaus, addresses the complex issues around prevention and early detection. It explores the concept of health promotion, reviewing the differing strategies adopted in the prevention and early detection of cancer.

Section 4, edited by Sara Faithfull and Mary Wells, examines in some detail the complex treatment strategies utilized in cancer care reflecting on current practice and future trends resulting in a comprehensive overview of cancer therapy. Section 5, edited by Alex Molassiotis and Gina Copp, complements the previous section through consideration of the extensive morbidity experienced by patients with cancer. This section provides a thorough examination of the key issues and identifies optimal supportive care strategies. Section 6, edited by Maggie Grundy and Emile Maassen, debates the diverse care delivery systems that patients access and debates their value in the provision of patient-centred care. It addresses the contribution of cancer nursing to cancer care and explores the concepts of rehabilitation and survivorship.

The above results in an innovative text that provides readers with a valuable resource with which to develop their knowledge of current cancer care while permitting a view of future developments in this area. It is somewhat humbling to see the culmination of our original idea now in its final form and we hope that patients with cancer across Europe will benefit from it as a consequence of improved knowledge.

Such a mammoth task would not have been possible without the commitment, energy and enthusiasm of the Section Editors and the generosity of the authors and we are indebted to them. In particular, we would like to thank all our contributors for their patience, perseverance and belief in our ideas, allowing us to realize what we believe is a most exciting initiative. We would also like to thank EONS for their permission to base this book on their curriculum and for their continued support of this work. Furthermore, we would not have completed this book were it not for the support of individuals at Churchill Livingstone, and later Elsevier, who were closely involved in the book at all stages of planning, writing and production. These include Alex Mathieson, who helped prepare the original outline; Ninette Premdas, who negotiated the commissioning process; and Claire Wilson, for her perseverance and dedication during the production process.

Nursing Patients with Cancer: Principles and Practice is an attempt to produce a text that nurses wishing to build their knowledge and skills might find informative, useful and challenging. We challenge you to put your newly found knowledge to good use, improving the experience and outcome of care for patients who have cancer across Europe.

Nora Kearney
Alison Richardson

ABBREVIATIONS

ABP	arterial blood pressure	CDKs	cyclin-dependent kinases
ABVD	Adriamycin (doxorubicin), bleomycin, vinblastine, dacarbazine	CDT	complex decongestive therapy
		CEA	carcinoembryonic antigen
		CFAM	Calgary Family Assessment Model
ACS	American Cancer Society		
ACTH	adrenocorticotrophic hormone	CI	cumulative incidence
ADCC	antibody-dependent cell-mediated cytotoxicity	CIN	cervical intraepithelial neoplasia
		CINV	chemotherapy-induced nausea and vomiting
AFP	α-fetoprotein		
AHCPR	Agency for Health Care Policy and Research	CLAS	Cancer Linear Analogue Scale
		CMI	cell-mediated immunity
AIE	acute inflammatory episodes	CML	chronic myeloid leukaemia
ANC	absolute neutrophil count	CMV	cytomegalovirus
APC	antigen presenting cell	CO	cardiac output
APS	American Pain Society	CPAP	continuous positive airways pressure
ARDS	acute respiratory distress syndrome		
		CPK	creatinine phosphokinase
ASI	active specific immunity	CRF	cancer-related fatigue
AT	α-tocopherol	CT	computed tomography
ATRA	all-trans-retinoic acid	CTL	cytotoxic T lymphocytes
BCPT	Breast Cancer Prevention Trial	CTV	clinical target volume
BDS	beam directional shell	CVAD	central venous access device
bFGF	basic fibroblast growth factor	CVP	central venous pressure
BIA	bioelectrical impedance analysis	DC	dendritic cell
BMI	body mass index	DCBE	double-contrast barium enema
BMT	bone marrow transplantation	DCIS	ductal carcinoma in situ
BSE	breast self-examination	DHT	dihydrotestosterone
CAB	combined androgen blockade	DIC	disseminated intravascular coagulation
CEA	carcinoembryonic antigen		
CAM	complementary and alternative medicine	DLI	donor lymphocyte infusions
		DLT	dose-limiting toxicity
CBE	clinical breast examination	DMSO	dimethyl sulfoxide
CC	cephalo-caudal	DRE	digital rectal examination
CCU	critical care unit	DSMIV	Diagnostic and Statistical Manual
CD	cluster of differentiation		

DVT	deep vein thrombosis	HAD	Hospital Anxiety and Depression (scale)
EAPS	European Association of Palliative Care	HAMA	human anti-mouse antibody
EBMT	European Group for Bone and Marrow Transplantation	HBM	health belief model
		HDU	high-dependency unit
EBV	Epstein–Barr virus	HIF-1α	hypoxia induced factor-1α
ECG	electrocardiogram	HIV	human immunodeficiency virus
ECM	extracellular matrix	HLA	human leucocyte antigen
ED	erectile dysfunction	HPA	human platelet antigen
EGF	epidermal growth factor	HPV	human papillomavirus
EGFR	epidermal growth factor receptor	HRT	hormone replacement therapy
		HSCT	haemopoietic (haematopoietic) stem cell transplantation
ELCAP	Early Lung Cancer Action Project	hsp	heat shock proteins
EONS	European Oncology Nursing Society	HUS	haemolytic uraemic syndrome
		IARC	International Agency for Research on Cancer
EORTC	European Organization for Research and Treatment of Cancer	IASP	International Association for the Study of Pain
EPA	eicosapentaenoic acid	IBCSN	International Breast Cancer Screening Network
EPO	erythropoietin		
ERSPC	European Randomized Screening for Prostate Cancer	IBIS	International Breast Cancer Intervention Study
		IBMTR	International Bone Marrow Transplant Registry
ET-1	endothelin-1		
FAACT	Functional Assessment of Anorexia/Cachexia Therapy	ICD	International Classification of Diseases
FACT-BMT	Functional Assessment of Cancer Therapy-Bone Marrow Transplant	ICD-O	International Classification of Diseases for Oncology
		ICSI	intracytoplasmic sperm injection
FAP	familial adenomatous polyposis	IFN-γ	interferon-γ
FDA	Food and Drug Administration	IgG	immunoglobulin G
FDT	first-dose toxicity	IL	interleukin; e.g. IL-4
FFP	fresh frozen plasma	IMRT	intensity modulated radiotherapy
FIGO	International Federation of Gynaecology and Obstetrics		
		IR	incidence rate
FNA	fine-needle aspiration	ISHAGE	International Society for Haemopoetic and Graft Engineering
FOBT	faecal occult blood test		
FSH	follicle stimulating hormone		
GCSF	granulocyte colony-stimulating factor		
		ISNCC	International Society of Nurses in Cancer Care
GHRH	gonadotrophic hormone releasing hormone	ITU	intensive therapy unit
		IVF	in vitro fertilization
GI	gastrointestinal	LAK	lymphokine-activated killer
GISTs	gastrointestinal stromal tumours	LASA	Linear Analogue Scale Assessment
		LCIS	lobular carcinoma in situ
GM-CSF	granulocyte–macrophage colony-stimulating factor	LGL	large granular lymphocytes
		LH	luteinizing hormone
GnHRH	gonadotrophin hormone releasing hormone	LHRH	luteinizing hormone releasing hormone
GvHD	graft versus host disease		

LIDCO	injection dilution cardiac output method	OBRMD	optimal biological response modifier dose
LMF	lipid mobilizing factor	OPSI	overwhelming post-splenectomy infection
LMWH	low molecular weight heparins		
LPS	lipopolysaccharide	PA	plasminogen activator
MA	malignant ascites	PAC	pulmonary artery catheter
MAB	maximum androgen blockade	PAI	plasminogen activator inhibitor
MAGE1	melanoma antigen 1	PAN	primary afferent nociceptor
MAP	mean arterial pressure	PAP	pulmonary artery pressure
MART1	melanoma antigen recognized by T cells 1	PAR	plasminogen activator receptor
		PAWP	pulmonary artery wedge pressure
MHC	major histocompatibility complex	PCA	patient-controlled analgesia
MLD	manual lymphatic drainage	PCEA	patient-controlled epidural analgesia
MLLB	multi-layered lymphoedema bandaging	PCPT	Prostate Cancer Prevention Trial
MLO	medio-lateral oblique	PCV	packed cell volume
MMP	matrix metalloproteases	PDGF	platelet-derived growth factor
MoAbs	monoclonal antibodies	PE	pulmonary embolus
MOPP	nitrogen mustard, Oncovin (vincristine), procarbazine, prednisolone	PEG	percutaneous endoscopic gastrostomy
		PET	positron emission tomography
MPE	malignant pleural effusion	PGI	Patient-Generated Index
MQSA	Mammography Quality Standards Act	PG-SGA	Patient-Generated Subjective Global Assessment
MR	mortality rate	PLCO	Prostate, Lung, Colorectal and Ovarian (trial)
MRI	magnetic resonance imaging		
MRSA	methicillin-resistant *Staphyloccus aureus*	PMF	protein mobilizing factor
		PMNs	polymorphonuclear leucocytes (neutrophils)
MUAC	mid-upper arm circumference		
MUD	matched unrelated donor	PMRT	progressive muscle relaxation training
MTD	maximum tolerated dose		
MVD	microvascular density	PNI	psychoneuroimmunology
NCCAM	National Center for Complementary and Alternative Medicine	PONV	postoperative nausea and vomiting
		PSA	prostate-specific antigen
NCCS	National Coalition for Cancer Survivors	PTSD	post-traumatic stress disorder
		PTV	planning target volume
NCI	National Cancer Institute	QALYs	quality-adjusted life years
NfaR	Not For attempted Resuscitation	QOLLTI-P	Quality of Life in Life-Threatening Illness – Patient Version
NHCSPCS	National Council for Hospice and Specialist Palliative Care Services		
		RBCs	red blood cells
NICE	National Institute for Clinical Excellence	RCN	Royal College of Nursing
		RCTs	randomized controlled trials
NIS	newly independent states	rh-tPA	recombinant human tissue plasminogen activator
NK	natural killer		
NSAIDs	non-steroidal anti-inflammatory drugs	SAGM	saline, adenine, glucose, mannitol
NSCLC	non-small cell lung carcinoma	SBS	short bowel syndrome

SERMs	selective oestrogen receptor modulators	TSH	thyroid-stimulating hormone
SIL	squamous intraepithelial lesions	TTO	time-trade-off
SLD	simple lymphatic drainage	TTP	thrombotic thrombocytopenic purpura
SOC	sense of coherence	TURP	transurethral resection of the prostate
SPC	specialist palliative care		
SSRIs	selective serotonin re-uptake inhibitors	Ub	ubiquitin
SVC	superior vena cava	UICC	International Union Against Cancer
SVCO	superior vena cava obstruction	UICC	Union Internationale Contre le Cancer
SVR	systemic vascular resistance		
TAAs	tumour-associated antigens	USPSTF	United States Preventive Services Task Force
TBI	total body irradiation		
T_C	cytotoxic T cell	VAC	vacuum-assisted closure
TCR	T-cell receptor	VAS	visual analogue scales
TENS	transcuntaneous electrical nerve stimulation	VATS	video-assisted thoracoscopic surgery
TGF-β	transforming growth factor-β	vCJD	variant Creutzfeldt–Jakob disease
T_H	helper T cell		
TILs	tumour-infiltrating lymphocytes	VEGF	vascular endothelial growth factor
TLS	tumour lysis syndrome		
TNF-α	tumour necrosis factor alpha	VOD	veno-occlusive disease
tPA	tissue plasminogen activator	VRE	vancomycin-resistant *Enterococcus*
TPC	tunnelled pleural catheter		
TPN	total parenteral nutrition	VTE	venous thromboembolism
TRALI	transfusion-related acute lung injury	WHO	World Health Organization
		WMDA	World Marrow Donor Organization
TRUS	transrectal ultrasound		
TSE	testicular self-examination		

SECTION 1

Philosophies of cancer nursing and the context of care

1. Concepts of Health Behaviour   3

2. Partnership in Care 21

3. The Social and Cultural Context of
   Cancer Care 37

CHAPTER 1

Concepts of Health Behaviour

Annie Topping

CHAPTER CONTENTS

Introduction	3	Limitations of social cognition models	12
The concepts of health and illness	4	Meaning, coping and adaptation	13
Beliefs about cancer causation and threat	5	Health, healthcare professionals and cancer	15
Media, health, communicating risk and the internet	6	Conclusion	16
Health as moral responsibility	8	References	16
Health behaviour and social cognition models of health	9		

INTRODUCTION

WH Auden,[1] in his poem *Miss Gee*, wrote of a doctor talking to his wife, over a meal, about a case. The doctor tells his wife the story of Miss Gee, a women who consulted him about the abdominal pain she was experiencing. The doctor refers her to hospital where an inoperable abdominal sarcoma is found during surgery. The doctor in the poem recounts asking Miss Gee: 'Why didn't you come before?'[1(p215)] No doubt this is a question that has been asked on numerous occasions by many doctors and nurses of their patients and a refrain which crosses the minds of some patients and their families. No doubt it is an issue that confounds and remains, like many associated with human behaviour, unanswered. This chapter sets out to offer some insight into those health behaviours that at times seem to prevent the delivery of effective health care, at others produce poorer outcomes for patients, possibly induce stoicism or an assumed albeit erroneous inevitability about the prognosis of cancer, and ultimately can lead to premature and even unnecessary deaths. Human behaviour is frustratingly complex and is even more bewildering when it is directed towards a disease that is said to be stigmatizing, a modern plague, heroic,[2] arguably in the Western world the most alarming,[3] sinister, 'metaphorically, the barbarian within',[4] or in Auden's words: '... a funny thing'.[1]

This chapter sets out to provide a backcloth against which other dimensions of the cancer experience, from diagnosis to recovery or death, can be examined. Many of the issues raised here will be developed in much greater detail in subsequent chapters of this book. Here a number of themes will be examined that could be loosely brought together under the heading of health behaviour. First, what do people believe causes cancer and why do they hold those beliefs? Secondly, why do people ignore health messages and practise behaviour that puts them at risk? And why do they fail to participate in initiatives that may reduce risk or identify cancer early in the disease trajectory? Thirdly, when they recognize symptoms, why do they not seek help? Or, alternatively, why do they seek attention for symptoms or mistake the significance of signs and symptoms? Lastly, should health-promoting behaviour be encouraged during cancer treatment and are there benefits to positive action?

THE CONCEPTS OF HEALTH AND ILLNESS

Health probably has as many meanings as there are people. Research examining the meaning of health suggests people have little difficulty in judging themselves as healthy or not but cannot articulate what the concept of health means to them.[5] It is said that people talk differently to researchers about health, as they feel governed by perceived expectations and the 'moral pressures of their social and cultural group'.[6 (p366)] This often produces incongruent private and public accounts of health, the latter largely seen through the expression of acceptable or responsible health-related attitudes.[7] Language describing the experience of cancer creates a frame of reference for how we perceive the disease. Indeed, some have argued that the language itself constructs our responses to cancer as well as our experience of it.[2,4] Similarly, there are many different and often competing discourses associated with health.[8] Stainton-Rogers[8] offers a range of different accounts that emerge from understandings of health and illness. These are:

- the body as machine
- the body under siege
- inequalities in access to care
- individual and collective responsibility for health promotion
- individualism and right to chose own lifestyle
- individual will to self-determine
- power of God.

In part, the position of health as an important value in Western societies has led to the emergence of a 'new health consciousness'.[9] This is apparent in many aspects of life, from the messages on product packaging used in advertising and media representations of health to public health policy.

Current thought is that lay understandings of health are derived from not one but many influences that converge to produce explanatory frameworks. These incorporate material, social and bodily features that together allow us to develop a coherent understanding of health at a personal level. This is not necessarily based upon the perception of health as absence of disease. Indeed, there is considerable evidence to suggest that many individuals perceive themselves as healthy during illness and, arguably, wellness within the context of a chronic illness such as cancer may be a more useful conceptualization, particularly as individuals who define health as the presence of wellness are more likely to engage in health-promoting behaviour or activities perceived as health promoting.[10] This caveat is significant, as some behaviours may be misguidedly perceived as beneficial to health and well-being.

Health therefore has at its foundation a confluence of ideas, some of which are passed down through interaction with others, learnt at home, school,[11] work, and frequently are cultural in their origins.[6,12,13] They may be influenced by social and economic factors,[14] family structure,[15] delinquency,[16] gender,[17–19] anxiety,[20] masculinity,[17,21] sexual orientation,[22] femininity and body awareness[23,24] For some, health is correlated with the ability to undertake functional roles such as paid or unpaid work and in some groups manual labour is perceived as synonomous with healthy behaviour.[25] Health is closely associated with lifestyles and these can be health enhancing, such as exercise, or detrimental, such as smoking[26–28] or unprotected exposure to sunlight.[29,30] The evidence related to cancer and stress and stressful life events is more contested.[31–33]

Ill health, however, represents a breakdown in normal expectations, a deviation from what should or usually is. That said, it can be experienced as a chronic state which in itself becomes normalized. An individual may interpret illness very differently from their neighbour and may report illness based on health beliefs.[6] Illness can be perceived as a threat, particularly when it is ostensibly preventing individuals from conducting their normal everyday life. Illness can be construed as liberation from the burden and toil of everyday existence, a legitimate reason for release from responsibilities. Illness can be seen as a form of occupation or career with a trajectory. The career of a cancer patient may involve learning the job and encouragement to undertake the tasks inherent in the role, such as participate in decision-making, comply with treatment regimens, undertake self-care activities that will enhance recovery, minimize or ameliorate symptoms and assist in adapting to change. All these different interpretations can influence how individuals experience a disease such as cancer and, moreover, how they participate in the journey through treatment and beyond. Individuals who view the diagnosis of cancer as segregating them from their social world may well react differently to diagnosis, participation in decision-making and adherence to treatment regimens than someone who sees the disease as an opportunity to absolve themselves from all their normal responsibilities. Likewise, an individual who interprets cancer as a job, a functional role, may interact with health professionals and families and friends with very different motivations and levels of commitment.

BELIEFS ABOUT CANCER CAUSATION AND THREAT

One of the features of the human condition is that we seek to find reason – meaning – for events in our lives such as becoming ill. This process of attributing cause external to ourselves has certain attractions, as it discharges some if not all of the personal responsibility. In Blaxter's seminal work,[34] which examined working class Scottish women's beliefs about disease causation, she found infections – 'bugs and germs '– to be perceived as the main causal agents in disease, closely followed by inherited

susceptibility. The interpretation proposed at that time was that the women held amoral health beliefs in that infections and genetic susceptibility were largely outside the control of the individual. This, when compared with the results from a more recent survey by Blaxter[25] with a similar sample, suggests that health beliefs have changed. The value of personal responsibility for health had been more widely adopted as a belief; further, the majority of women gave behavioural or lifestyle factors as the main unhealthy aspects of their lives. The idea of health as a personal moral value is a theme developed later in this chapter.

But what of other sections of society? Oakley and colleagues[35] collected information from two groups of school-age children (15–16 years old, $n = 226$; 9–10 years old, $n = 100$) about their knowledge of cancers and beliefs about health. They found that children had considerable knowledge about the factors that could be detrimental to health. The children in the study could judge their own health status; nevertheless, the researchers remained less confident that the children could or would translate that knowledge into behaviour. Overall, the children failed to discriminate between behaviours that could be viewed as within their control and adverse factors stemming from their living conditions. In the 15–16-year-old group, most had heard or knew about lung, skin and breast cancer and leukaemia but not other common cancers such as colon or prostate cancer. Young people in the sample from Asian origin were the least likely to know about cancers associated with reproductive organs. In this study young women were more likely to seek information about cancer from their mothers, whereas young men identified teachers as the most likely source of information. Both young men and women participants saw television and other media as their main sources of information. This is an interesting finding in the context of the health images portrayed on television and other popular media, given their utility and efficacy for conveying health messages, and is particularly worrying when smoking may be portrayed or interpreted as a positive image to young people.[36]

In the younger age group (9–10 year olds) the majority ($n = 76$) knew about lung cancer and recognized a relationship between smoking and subsequent cancer development ($n = 78$). The next most frequently identified cancers were skin ($n = 26$), heart ($n = 21$), leukaemia ($n = 24$) and head and brain ($n = 16$). The children were asked to draw anything they knew about cancer and four themes emerged: fires in the body often related to smoking, specific parts of the body particularly associated with hair loss (a common visual image of cancer treatment), cancer as a group of cells and cancer as a monster or unpleasant face. Smoking was identified by the majority of these children ($n = 78$) as causal in the subsequent development of cancer. Other factors the children identified as important in preventing or avoiding cancer included sunburn ($n = 15$), generally keeping healthy ($n = 15$), eating healthily ($n = 12$) and avoiding pollution ($n = 10$).

Moore and Topping[37] investigated English male university students' ($n = 203$) levels of knowledge about testicular cancer and awareness of testicular self-examination (TSE) techniques. Ninety per cent of participants claimed to have heard of testicular cancer but less than half were aware of factors associated with the condition. A small proportion thought the disease was related to sexually transmitted diseases, human immune virus (HIV) or sexual behaviour (13.6%; $n = 26$). Only 43 (22%) of survey participants reported practising TSE and only 13 (6.4%) reported themselves as confident undertaking the technique.

A subset of questionnaires ($n = 218$) from a recent healthcare survey of UK lesbians were analysed to examine explanations for healthcare behaviour of women who had never practised breast self-examination (BSE).[22] The researchers found six different explanations for non-adherence with health advice:

- not knowing what to look for
- not incorporated as a health-protection behaviour
- fear of finding something
- perception of low risk
- uncomfortable with their body
- and partner's responsibility.

For individuals with a high risk of developing cancer, their understanding or experience of living with that threat is an emerging understanding. The scientific advances associated with predictive genetic testing present new challenges for managing health. Much of the rhetoric surrounding genetic testing is focused on freedom to choose, whereas the reality may be more about the constraints imposed by healthcare knowledge, provision and an individual's responsibilities to others.[38-40] In a qualitative study that emerged from interviews with women attending for hereditary breast or ovarian cancer, responsibility was a key theme.[39] The women described responsibilities to kin to determine magnitude of risk to themselves and to other family members, and subsequent to gaining the knowledge to act to modify risk. Murphy[40] talks of uncertainty as the reverse of risk and describes different ways in which individuals deal with a family history of cancer. These include fatalism, denial, anxiety, increased (sometimes inappropriate) demands for surveillance, searching for information and informed (and sometimes in the absence of information) demands for testing. The media attention invoked by genetics as the salvation of illness creates a number of issues. The next section discusses this in the context of risk.

MEDIA, HEALTH, COMMUNICATING RISK AND THE INTERNET

There is a common and arguably appropriate assumption that an individual has the right to information about cancer and, moreover, to be involved in decision-making or choice about treatment. However, the right to know has doubtful utility when what is known is uncertain or incomplete. For example, in rare or unusual cancers the very fact that they have a low incidence makes it difficult to establish any certainty about links between specific factors and causation. Also there is the problem of certainty: i.e. the limits of confidence that a relationship of causation, risk factors, treatment options and likely prognosis are not without caveats. This can and does create problems for decision-makers, whether this is at the level of setting public health policy to the individual patient trying to establish what course of action to choose.

One of the key issues for the public, planners, governments, health professionals and, ultimately, the patient surrounding cancer is the assessment of risk. However, the relationships between available knowledge, volume of evidence – in effect the scientific basis – and public policy is far from linear and even more convoluted when implementation of initiatives have cost implications.[3] Understanding how people – the general public, patients, health professionals – perceive risk and then make use of information to influence their decisions has been the focus of much work over recent decades.[41] It is suggested, unsurprisingly, that the general public are not strictly rational and their decision-making is subject to systematic biases. These biases (heuristics), produced when the decision-making process is short cut, can produce systematic over- or underestimation of risk and therefore have implications for comprehension and assimilation of information and effective informed consent.[42]

Henderson and Kitzinger[43] examined the translation of inherited or genetic breast cancer risk across the media. In the period 1995–1997 they identified 708 breast cancer stories across eight UK newspapers. In one in three of the breast cancer stories, genetic or inherited risk factors formed the focus. This ranged from scientific reporting (21%) to 'human interest stories' (27%). The most prominent storyline throughout the period was prophylactic mastectomy and the experiences of women in 'high-risk families'. The power of the media in representing and forming understandings about health is well known. A review of TV programming for the same period found a similar trend with breast cancer reporting. This frequently focused on family relationships, the dilemmas and drama. Interestingly, genetic stories also featured in TV drama as well as 'true stories'. However, Henderson and Kitzinger[43] followed their analysis with focus group interviews with women ($n = 143$). They found that, in general, participants overestimated inherited (genetic) risk. The majority of the women remembered the human interest stories but with little evidence of understanding the underlying science. This has quite serious implications given the power of soft media formats to influence and inform.

The impact of the 'the avalanche of information'[13(p1099)] about genetics would suggest that the public has a reasonable understanding of the link between genetic causation and diseases such as cancer. Yet, one of the problems for health professionals communicating with at-risk families is they come to consultations with an a priori understanding from knowledge, (mis)information, and the emotional and psychological burden possibly associated with loss and bereavement. Explanations of inheritance underpin much of the communication about risk in hereditary disease, but this is objective information. It comes devoid of the messiness of human life, of family history, and separates the individual from living with the knowledge as divorced from the statistical representation of the risk.[38]

The Internet presents a real challenge to traditional sources of lay information about health and, in particular, impacts upon the monopoly associated with more traditional sources of expertise and knowledge. It has been suggested that the Internet deprofessionalizes medical or expert health knowledge and has the potential to threaten the authority of healthcare professionals as purveyors of expertise.[44] There remains a real digital divide despite the democratic potential of the technology to 'transform the social and economic landscape'.[45 (p178)] Although there are numerous examples of how technology has provided access to previously disadvantaged or alienated groups in societies, there remains a divide between the haves and have nots. That said, trends suggest that women and the elderly (over 65s) are the groups most likely to go online over the next few years. Both are significant groups, as consumers of a higher proportion of health services and, in the case of women, often perceived as the primary decision-makers on health issues in families.[17,18,45]

The challenge presented to governments and health professionals by the global marketplace available through the Internet allows an individual to select information, services and support and potentially transcend local licensing laws relating to drug therapy. It has also been suggested that the Internet, through the proliferation of self-help groups, creates a space for people to open up and to disclose their fears and concerns to strangers within an environment that provides anonymity. According to Giddens,[46] it minimizes the gamble of disclosure inherent in the face-to-face encounter.

From this rather rapid and cursory review, considerable variation can be seen in terms of lay understandings associated with causes of cancer that has implications for health-promoting and/or health-protecting behaviours. Understanding what might inform or produce a particular set of beliefs and consequent behaviour is important not only to better understand the public and patients but also to improve the services provided. This does of course raise the thorny issue of responsibility.

HEALTH AS MORAL RESPONSIBILITY

The responsibility for health and healthiness is somewhat contested ground. In many Western societies with integrated welfare systems, the attempt to provide equitable healthcare provision requires the population, or target population, to participate by taking some responsibility. Social regulation and shared responsibility for health protection through surveillance for disease can be seen as a principle underpinning many successful screening programmes. The notion of a right to screening is an area that is particularly fraught when the evidence in support of introduction of particular screening programmes may itself be weak or contested. There are also concerns associated with the possible ramifications of screening producing unnecessary cancer anxiety.[47] In addition, public confidence in screening is undermined by media reports of poor-quality systems associated with screening tests that have resulted in false results. A screening programme is said to be justified if the test is accurate – has high specificity and sensitivity – and an effective treatment is available,[48,49] as in the case of cervical screening.

In many countries with national screening programmes, participation in breast and cervi-cal cancer screening is presented as responsible health behaviour, with the consequent benefit to participants of early detection producing better outcomes for those found to have cancer. The same benefit is less certain from the introduction of prostate-specific antigen (PSA) testing at this time. A recent study of prostate cancer survivors' attitudes to PSA was undertaken by Chapple and colleagues.[49] They interviewed 52 men and found largely widespread support for both testing and screening, despite most of the respondents reporting having received little or no information about the test and little understanding of what the result would mean. Most of the men gave earlier diagnosis and, accordingly, a better chance of cure as their reasons for advocating the introduction of PSA screening. They also suggested earlier diagnosis would reduce the financial burden on health services. Those few participants ($n = 4$) who disagreed provided an informed evidence-based rationale and recognized that unnecessary anxiety might ensue from testing.

Some commentators, particularly from the social sciences, have become interested in the ways certain categories of disease are used to define boundaries between normal and deviant behaviour and that demarcation carries a moral component.[39,50,51] In a recent study by Bush,[52] who interviewed 35 women aged 20–64 years old living in two communities in South Yorkshire in the UK, two separate but parallel discourses emerged. One theme that emerged indicated that smear tests, Papanicolaou (PAP) smear tests, were a normal part of being a woman and therefore part and parcel of everyday life, although some participants voiced fears of developing cancer and suggested that smear tests were compulsory. A second theme was that to have a smear test was a correct form of behaviour and non-attendance was perceived as a form of deviancy. This moral responsibility to participate in screening has been described as the 'Foucault paradox'[51] in that in return for the provision of greater equity in health care comes regulatory control over populations expressed through health surveillance. There are real benefits associated with surveillance of populations in terms of monitoring trends and efficacy of service provision and this can be seen from the information emerging from cancer registries: nevertheless, this is relatively far removed from the individual deciding to participate.

Much of the discussion thus far in this chapter has concentrated on attitudes and beliefs and the differences that exist between different groups within society. The next section describes some of the social cognition models that offer insight into the different ways in which individuals express their attitudes and beliefs through their health behaviour.

HEALTH BEHAVIOUR AND SOCIAL COGNITION MODELS OF HEALTH

A typical definition of health behaviour is that offered by Kasl and Cobb;[53,54] namely, that it is those actions undertaken by individuals that enhance or maintain their health with the intention of preventing or detecting problems at an asymptomatic stage. This definition fits well with behaviour that is in the domain of the individual to adapt, such as diet modification, or participation in screening, such as asymptomatic breast screening. This definition is limited in the context of the individual with cancer as it does not include behaviour which may impact on disease progression, symptoms, outcomes or prognosis, such as self-management or adopting a healthy lifestyle.[55] This is an issue that will be revisited later in this chapter.

Much of the seminal research, such as that undertaken in Alameda County in the USA, sought to consider the range of health behaviours linked to health outcomes.[56-58] This work demonstrated the significance of a variety of behaviours on health outcomes and identified the seven characteristics of healthy living:

- never smoking
- no or limited alcohol intake
- 7–8 hours sleep every night
- eating breakfast
- rarely eating between meals
- regular exercise
- the maintenance of height-adjusted optimum weight.

At a common-sense level, it would be fair to assume that individuals who practise one of these behaviours would be more likely to practise other healthy behaviours. In fact, researchers have found that there is a low correlation or weak relationship between different types of healthy lifestyle behaviours.[59] A possible explanation is that health behaviour has a number of dimensions, and Vickers and colleagues[60] suggested a four-dimensional model linked to health behaviour. This grouped behaviour into four categories: substance risk taking, accident control, traffic risk taking and wellness behaviour. They suggest this grouping of behaviours allows the relationship between wellness behaviour, say exercise and supplementary vitamin consumption, to remain highly correlated, whereas other dimensions such as smoking (substance risk taking) do not. This provides some clarity and sheds light on why it may be unhelpful to assume that an individual who takes regular exercise would obey traffic regulations to avoid accidents. This conceptualization helps us to better understand and predict the effect of health messages on target populations – and the reverse – to identify those less likely to respond to particular initiatives.

The tendency to judge the focus or object of an attitude positively or negatively is said to be an important determinant of behaviour. Any thing, person, activity or idea can be the object of an attitude, although a classifying division between cognitive reactions towards something, as different from affective reactions and behaviour, has been used to explain different responses. A cognitive attitude to something such as exercise might connect the attitude object to a favourable belief about the benefits of exercise, whereas an affective response would relate to the emotional response engendered by an attitude object such as feeling good about exercise. A behavioural attitude is demonstrated through an overt action to an attitude object such as smoking cessation in response to a relative's diagnosis of lung cancer. There is an assumption that attitudes and beliefs are related.

According to the *expectancy-value model*,[61] an individual's attitude to a possible action is dependent upon the subjective value (belief) attached to the outcome and the perceived

9

likelihood that the outcome will ensue. Hence, individuals' beliefs about low-fat diet and about the possible effect it will have on their body, i.e. weight reduction, will have a direct effect on them adopting the behaviour. Although as an explanation of the relationship between attitudes and beliefs the expectancy-value model may hold currency, the consequence of it in terms of behaviour is less clear or rather more difficult to establish. It is suggested that to confirm a relationship between attitudes and behaviour, the compatibility of the attitude to the behaviour is needed and it is that compatibility which is important for attitude and behaviour change. Hence, campaigns to change specific health behaviours should focus on arguments to convince the target population to change particular, not general, health concerns. For example, to persuade people to use skin protection against the effect of sunlight is likely to be more successful when targeted at holiday times when the public are more likely to be purchasing and using skin-protection products, rather than subsumed in general cancer-prevention messages.

Social cognition is concerned with how individuals make sense of social situations and is based on a premise that behaviour is understood best as a function of an individual's perception of reality rather than an objective description of that reality. So, establishing what cognitions are important in framing and predicting behaviour has been the focus of much research in the area of health.

The *health belief model*[62] emerged to understand why people failed to access disease prevention or asymptomatic screening or failed to comply with or adhere to medical advice or regimens. It is predicated on an assumption that an individual engages in a particular behaviour in response to perceived personal susceptibility to the disease or condition and perceptions of consequences of developing the disease or condition. So, the combination of susceptibility and severity of consequences determines perceived threat to the individual, but it is the likely benefit accrued from action or inaction that may govern behaviour. It has been used as a theoretical framework for health intervention initiatives to improve screening uptake.[63]

In developing the model, Rosenstock[62] proposed that a cue might initiate or trigger an action manifest as a change to, or adoption of, particular health behaviour and that these cues may act to induce participatory intentions. These would be specifically related to when, how and where an action should be initiated and in response to threat. Hence, a woman who develops a vaginal discharge following unprotected sex may henceforth present regularly for cervical screening.[64] By contrast, a young woman taught breast self-examination may fail to perform the technique as she may not perceive breast cancer to be a threat, until a trigger such as a character in a television soap opera finding a lump may precipitate regular adherence with breast awareness advice.

Criticisms of the health belief model focus on the inability to predict the effect or weighting of the different variables on behaviour. For example, HIV is a major health risk, but beliefs held concerning susceptibility might not trigger use of condoms during sexual intercourse. Another criticism is that the positive benefits of particular behaviour such as the pleasure or perceived stress reduction derived from smoking may balance out beliefs about susceptibility.[14,65]

Yarbrough and Braden[66] undertook an integrative review of 16 descriptive studies based on the health belief model relating to breast cancer screening behaviour. The authors concluded that the model failed to consistently predict breast screening behaviour and more work was needed to understand the meaning of breast cancer across populations of women.

An approach with its roots in Rosenstock's health belief model is the work of Pender[67] related to health promotion. Building on the hypothesis that individuals' cognition of health may exert an influence on their participation in health-related behaviours, the desire for positive health (through health-promoting activities) and avoidance of negative health (through health-preventing activities) is likely to influence their motivation to participate. Pender postulated that those who defined health as promoting wellness by emphasizing well-being, balance, stability and adaptation would be more than likely to participate in health-promoting behaviours, whereas those with a clinical conception – absence of disease –

would not. Gasalberti[20] sought to test this hypothesis in a correlational study of women participants ($n = 93$) and frequency of BSE. She found that women who believed health was absence of disease participated significantly less frequently in BSE, and if they were personally worried about threat of breast cancer were less thorough in their use of the technique. This last finding gives some authority to the suggestion 'that there is no convincing evidence that the ritual of monthly breast self examination reduces death from cancer',[68(p442)] if anxiety and personal attribution of meaning of health impact on the ability of the individual to undertake, or interpret the findings from, the intervention.

The health *locus of control* is another model that has been widely used in health practice as explanatory and has its origins in Rotter's social learning theory. It is based on the premise that the likelihood of a behaviour occurring in response to a situation increases when the individual expects a particular reinforcement from the action and values the reinforcement. This was later refined to make a distinction between internal locus of control, i.e. consequences resulting from one's own actions, and external locus, perceived to be unrelated to an individual's personal agency and therefore beyond one's control. Various studies with mixed results have been based upon locus of control theory and it is said to be a weak predictor of health behaviour.[55] More recently, health locus of control has been added to the more general theory of health behaviour – *modified social learning theory*[69,70] – that proposes health behaviour as a function of value, locus of control and self-efficacy. That is: self-efficacy will predict behaviour when an individual values personal health or well-being and has an internal locus of control.

The model of *planned behaviour* examines the influences upon an individual that determines one's decision to adopt a particular behaviour and is based on Fishbein and Ajzen's theory of *reasoned action*.[61] Intentions are an individual's plan or proposal to perform a behaviour. Individuals perceive they have behavioural control to perform the behaviour. Intention is a confluence of three factors – attitudes (individual evaluation of behaviour), subjective norms (beliefs of significant others that consider they should adopt the behaviour) and perceived behavioural control (perception of difficulty or ease associated with performance of behaviour). Each of the three factors have previous determinants:

1 Attitudes:
   - likelihood outcome achievable from performing the behaviour
   - evaluation of the outcome.

2 Subjective norm:
   - perception of significant others' preference that the individual does or does not undertake the behaviour
   - individual's preference to comply with the referent's expectations.

3 Perceived behavioural control:
   - access to resources and opportunities to ensure behaviour is successful
   - weighted by the perceived influence each factor has on ultimate successful execution of the behaviour.

Simply, the likelihood individuals will undertake a specific behaviour will depend on whether they believe they can perform it and the outcome is worth it to them. This is balanced with the views of others they value and the importance they place on those views. All these factors are weighed against the personal resources needed to undertake the behaviour. So, for example, an adolescent girl who perceives herself to have a weight problem, and recognizes that reducing her chocolate and processed food intake might have an effect, will seek confirmation from her friends who she values as to whether she should diet. She will then balance her decision against the likelihood she will be successful with the resources available to facilitate her compliance with a weight-reducing diet. This complex weaving of factors emphasizes the complexity of behaviour and possibly illuminates why so many good intentions never appear to be realized.

Lastly, *self-efficacy theory*[71] offers a slightly different model of health behaviour. This is based on the premise that a perception of degree of personal self-control (self-efficacy) will have a direct influence upon willingness to take a course of action and create a commitment to the outcome.[72] In effect, behavioural change comes from a personal sense of control. Human motivation and action are therefore claimed to be based on three expectancies. These are: situation–outcome, where the individual perceives a threat from a health risk and develops an intention to initiate an action; action–outcome, where the individual considers the risk involved and whether the action is within their capability; and self-efficacy, which is concerned with personal beliefs about level of control.[55] Optimism about the degree of personal control over actions can predict the intention to perform behaviour, and individuals are more likely to undertake behaviour they perceive they have control over the outcome. Likelihood to engage in early detection behaviour such as breast self-examination will be linked to perception of risk and perception of ability to perform BSE effectively: the belief they have the ability to identify a lesion if present or feel confident about not finding an abnormality. Sense of control or self-efficacy has some currency in explaining behaviour which is potentially health damaging and the potential that could be realized from a perception of personal autonomy.[26,73,74]

LIMITATIONS OF SOCIAL COGNITION MODELS

One of the criticisms of social cognition models of health behaviour is that they are divorced from the social context in which people live their lives. For example, the recent World Health Organization press release on the soon to be published expert report on diet and chronic disease[75,76] suggests that it is not only overeating but also an unbalanced diet that underlies much ill health, whereas a study by Devine et al[77] suggests that low status jobs, high workload and lack of autonomy at work are associated with less healthy diets. The negative health effects of exposure to sunlight are well known but the current association of attractiveness with a suntanned skin, looking healthy rather than acting healthily, illustrates the tensions.[29,30] Tobacco is known or is the likely cause of many different diseases and if

current trends continue 450 to 500 million people alive today will be killed over the next 50 years by the effects of tobacco consumption.[78,79] Tobacco control remains a major priority in public health policy across the globe, yet the economic imperatives to grow tobacco and to manufacture, merchandize and sell cigarettes remain significant enough to dissuade governments from moving to total prohibition.

The assumption that attitudes and beliefs are determinants of behaviour underlies the numerous different social cognition models that offer predictive assessment of likely behaviour. However, these models only provide a partial understanding of how health behaviour can be predicted and tend to focus upon attitudes to health care (such as beliefs about quality of provision or likely benefits accrued from treatment), perceptions of threat from a particular disease and influences and norms of an individual's social networks. Other factors that are said to influence health behaviour are accessibility of health services and demographic factors that may be beyond the control of the individual.

Participation rates associated with cancer-detection behaviours vary greatly.[19] An interesting question is whether there is a difference if protection behaviour is self-perpetuated, such as breast self-examination or testicular self-examination, or is something an individual has to actively participate in or passively 'gets done to' as in cervical or breast screening. The responsibility for participation in BSE or TSE rests on those who practise it[20,37] or practise it on behalf of another.[22,80]

Early detection and the promotion of behaviour to encourage early detection is predicated on assumptions that people recognize symptoms as cancer symptoms and then pay attention to them and initiate help-seeking behaviour. de Nooijer et al[19] suggest that health-promotion activity should be two pronged and firstly, focus on emphasizing the advantages of passive detection and differences between symptoms in order to promote appropriate responses and help-seeking behaviour and, secondly, enhancing the likelihood of response to symptoms by increasing knowledge but also emphasizing the moral obligation to participate in health-seeking behaviour and anticipate the regret engendered by failure to seek assistance.

For many cancers the stage at which the patient first presents and enters the healthcare system remains the single most important factor in terms of variation in outcome. Delays may be due to misdiagnosis or delayed diagnosis or failure to recognize symptoms as suggestive of cancer. An individual may delay bringing symptoms to the attention of a healthcare professional due to a myriad of reasons, from denial to not understanding the seriousness of symptoms. Individuals may choose to delay because they feel unable to cope with the implications of a cancer diagnosis at the particular time when they first note the symptom(s). A further complexity is the insidious nature of many cancer symptoms, which can present difficulties for the uninformed reaching a decision that something is wrong. Prior experience may itself discourage attentiveness. For example, a woman with a history of benign breast disease may make an assumption that a new lump will be unproblematic as previously. A woman in her middle years may attribute unusual gynaecological symptoms to menopausal changes rather than cancer. A man who smokes cigarettes may link a troublesome tickly cough to bronchitis, or an unimportant consequence of smoking, rather than malignancy.

Delays in diagnosis and treatment are, according to Kirwan et al, 'deeply ingrained in our psyche'.[81] (p150) Social disadvantage has been proposed as one factor in delay rates. A review of emergency and acute admissions data in North and South Thames for colorectal, lung and breast cancer supports the hypothesis that patients from more deprived areas present at later stages.[100]

Ovarian cancer is a relatively rare disease of insidious onset where the majority of women present with advanced disease. A recent retrospective audit in one UK region[81] showed that most women (78%) self-referred to general practitioners within 4 weeks of noticing symptoms: 73% of women were referred to specialist services within 4 weeks of first presentation to a general practitioner, although only 44% were directly referred to a gynaecology depart-

ment. The main difficulty associated with diagnosis was differentiating symptoms, particularly those more associated with advanced disease such as shortness of breath or abdominal symptoms suggestive of irritable bowel syndrome. Eleven of the women studied ($n = 135$) were referred following routine examination for concurrent illness.

From this discussion it would seem that numerous factors can influence whether an individual (1) is cognisant of the meaning of symptoms, (2) acts upon them by seeking medical attention and (3) is subsequently referred for specialist help. All may ultimately impact upon outcome and present an important agenda for all involved in cancer care. However, in the context of the experience of cancer, health forms an aspect of meaning. In this last part of the chapter, discussion will focus on health in the presence of ill health and health in the context of cancer survivorship.

MEANING, COPING AND ADAPTATION

The terms 'belief' and 'meaning' litter the cancer literature and have been used similarly indiscriminately in this chapter. Richer and Ezer[82] point out that the terms are often used as antecedents to successive aspects of adaptation. Ascertaining beliefs and meaning of illness form a part of any assessment of patients in nursing and form the basis for subsequent work with those individuals and their families. As discussed at some length earlier, what individuals believe to have caused cancer or affected their response will be underpinned by the beliefs they hold. A belief is 'a conviction that something is true'[82] (p1109) and it is learnt, shared, endures and is often supported by social context. Illness can and frequently does challenge beliefs. Ascertaining meaning is more complicated, as there appears to be a distinction between existential meaning –individuals' perception of how they see themselves in the world – and situational meaning – their perception of a new event and their capacity to respond to it – and hence the relationship of meaning to coping. Beliefs and existential meaning will become embedded through life experience and impact upon the way an individual copes through the cancer experience. Nevertheless, that experience is not a given or a fixed thing. The individual will respond dynamically and often resiliently to the challenges presented. Coping is an integral part of everyday life. We face the demands of contemporary life but the diagnosis, treatment and life with cancer can create an additional burden that can threaten an individual's ability to cope and place such a burden that aspects of their life become disintegrated. Coping is complex and the role of the nurse in supporting individuals to cope with cancer and adapt in response to the disease is an important one.[83]

Lazarus and Folkman's[84] theory of stress, appraisal and coping offers one way of explaining this dynamic process. It is predicated on the notion that coping has three aspects: initial appraisal, secondary appraisal and problem-focused coping. The initial appraisal focuses on the meaning of the challenge and the individual interprets the level of threat or potential damage that will be incurred. Following on, secondary appraisal involves the individual estimating their readiness or otherwise to minimize the threat. This is a mode of action characterized by questions such as 'What can I do about this?' Following initial and secondary appraisal, problem-focused coping is targeted on changing the threat, so in the case of cancer information-seeking behaviour may alter the meaning of the diagnosis from imminent death to hope through treatment. By contrast, the direction of emotion-focused responses are inward and focus on the feelings engendered by the diagnosis or disease. A problem-focused approach is viewed as an active response to challenge, whereas an emotion-focused response is a more palliative, albeit reasonable, response when the threat is perceived as beyond the control of the individual, as in the immediate aftermath to the bad news of diagnosis.

Four modes of functioning have been described[83,84] that reflect the dynamic responses inherent in the cancer experience:

- *Information seeking* is a problem-solving approach that provides a basis for subsequent action. By seeking information frequently from multiple sources and by confirming one source against another, the nature of the threat can be better appreciated and responded to.

- *Direct action* is any response to a challenge, such as responding to a physical sign or symptom by seeking attention from a healthcare provider.

- *Inhibition of action* is where the individual may resist the impulse to respond in case the action is inappropriate; this can, of course, result in inaction. In the case of cancer this can explain why some people fail to respond to signs of cancer and/or delay bringing the problem to the attention of a healthcare professional.

- *Intrapsychic processes* is a mode that includes a vast array of cognitive processes – denial, anger, fear, anxiety – that influence emotional response to a situation. These may temporarily bring 'emotional insulation'[83 (p39)] from the overwhelming feelings engendered by the bad news of a diagnosis or recurrence of disease.

How an individual integrates learning to cope in order to adapt is a process in flux, not a single act, and therefore will change over time. This model is useful, as it illustrates how healthcare professionals can facilitate and support individuals to move toward positive ways of coping through initiating treatment, pre-empting and responding to symptoms, through information-giving, by providing support during emotional reactions to the experience and by working with individuals. That said, it is often easy to become focused on delivering efficient and effective services rather than on an individual's coping. A recent contentious systematic review,[85] concerned with psychological coping styles and their relation to survival and cancer recurrence, concluded that, as yet, there is little scientific evidence to support the belief that fighting spirit, denial and avoidance, helplessness and hopelessness are coping styles that impact on outcome. That said, this does not mean that belief in the importance of mind over body is misplaced, just that the current evidence is weak. Social support and social integration do appear to have a positive effect on health-related coping and quality of life.[86,87]

HEALTH, HEALTHCARE PROFESSIONALS AND CANCER

Purandare[88] maintains that it is:

> the attitude a person holds about a certain subject will influence the way that a person behaves when confronted with that subject (p91)

This chapter has concentrated on potential recipients of care rather than providers. That oversight will now be remedied. Nurses, like other health professionals, may not recognize that they hold negative attitudes towards cancer, or may not be aware of the impact those negative attitudes may have on the delivery of care, until they are confronted by patients and their families that challenge their beliefs. The barriers created by negative attitudes to cancer are said to influence the quality of communication and decision-making.

The attitudes that health professionals hold may be linked to their own personal health behaviour and habits and, importantly, their tendency or otherwise to raise health issues with clients.[65] A recent survey of nurses undertaking education in the South of England found some support for that adage but also some discrepancies. For example, nurses recognized exercise was important for health but 61% failed to participate in any exercise themselves. Similarly, 47% of the nurses reported they smoked but all recognized the negative effects to health inherent in this behaviour. BSE and TSE were rated as behaviours less important to health by respondents, a finding that has implications for reinforcing those behaviours in the general public. This could be related to the debate concerning teaching techniques, such as TSE or BSE, that have the potential to become ritualized when undertaken in isolation from more general breast or testicular awareness.[37,68]

Skin cancer incidence has risen in the UK in common with other northern European countries. Amir and colleagues[30] surveyed healthcare workers in one acute hospital setting to ascertain their attitudes and beliefs associated with sunbeds and personal use. They found a strong association between participant's age, gender and smoking behaviour and use of tanning beds. They described the characteristics of a user of sunbeds as a young woman (less than 30 years old) who smokes and clings to the conviction that the use of a sunbed is safer than sunbathing outdoors.

A study of Norwegian female physicians[89] examined their levels of participation in breast self-examination and cervical (PAP smear) screening: 30.6% of the women performed BSE once per month and 54.6% had a PAP smear test once every 3 years. Nevertheless, 19.2% never practised BSE and 16.2% never had routine PAP smears. Interestingly, when a subsample of the physicians were compared with a group of university-educated women in the same age range (35–49 years old), the physicians showed better compliance with recommended BSE advice yet poorer uptake of PAP smears. The researchers suggested that the physicians made a judgement concerning their risk of cervical pathology based on their greater understanding of the disease.

It would appear that nurses and other healthcare workers hold beliefs and behaviour similar to the general public. If there is a relationship between self and professional behaviour, then it warrants further attention. Using the divisions of primary, secondary and tertiary prevention, Cutler[90] presents an overview of the nursing contribution to cancer prevention. The nurse's role in risk reduction is unclear, although political action has been proposed chiefly in relation to tobacco control advocacy.[27] The opportunistic potential present in nursing practice to identify needs and introduce effective interventions associated with primary prevention are considerable. A persuasive argument presented by one commentator[90] is that the personal attitudes or habits of the clinician may deter them from intervening and hence opportunities may be missed. The nurse's role in secondary prevention, particularly in minimizing discomfort, embarrassment and thereby better compliance, may be more effective. There are claims that this might humanize those procedures that can be construed as surveillance: e.g. cervical screening as a monitor of sexual behaviour. Tertiary health prevention is more concerned with preventing or minimizing disability or further disease and complications. It is therefore important in assisting people to make a recovery, to cope and to adapt and participate in rehabilitative activities which positively improve the living experience and the quality of life of the person with cancer.[91]

Lifestyle factors known to increase risks of developing cancer are somewhat of an unknown territory in terms of the impact they may have on disease-free interval, overall survival and preventing or reducing long-term side-effects.[92] There is, nevertheless, an increasing body of evidence which shows the positive effects of healthy lifestyles such as exercise on fatigue, on quality of life in survivors[93–95] and those facing end of life[96] weight gain during treatment,[97] well-being and coping in head and neck cancer,[98] and palliative care.[99] This promotion of health within the patient experience may become an even more significant aspect of the nursing contribution to cancer care in the future.

enhance well-being is enormous. By nurses, I do not just mean those working within the speciality of cancer care that have much to offer, but also include those in the wider community of nursing such as those working in primary care, public health, with children, and older people that can contribute much to changing health beliefs through effective health education and reinforcing health messages. Nurses can of course and do contribute through care delivery but by becoming active agents in health care through informing health policy, service commissioning, contributing to the evidence base that underpins practice, lobbying for resources and tackling health inequalities much more could be achieved. These are challenging agendas for nurses and nursing yet, nevertheless, present real ways for making a difference and impacting on the health burden of cancer.

CONCLUSION

At the beginning of this chapter a number of questions were posed with the intention that they would be explored, if not fully answered, through the theoretical understandings and current evidence presented in the text. As with so much of health care, there are no easy or simple solutions to problems, especially when the individual nature of human attitudes, beliefs and behaviours are involved. Targeting health within the context of cancer requires a keen understanding of the interrelationship between social dimensions, determinants of ill health and the influences of lifestyle on well-being. The first message I hope that has emerged from this chapter is the significance of the context in which health behaviour is enacted and the recognition that human behaviour cannot be stripped of that influence. The complexity of the ways in which we live our lives and the implications at an individual level presents an exciting challenge if effective health care is to be delivered. Secondly, the potential for nurses to contribute to improving health outcomes through working with clients, patients, families, the public and other healthcare providers to

REFERENCES

1. Auden WH. In: Mendelson E, ed. The English Auden poems, essays, and dramatic writings, 1927–1939. London: Faber and Faber; 1977:215.
2. Stacey J. Teratologies: a cultural study of cancer. London: Routledge; 1987.
3. Calman K. Cancer: science and society and communication of risk. BMJ 1996; 313(7068):799–802.
4. Sontag S. Illness as a metaphor. Harmondsworth: Penguin Books; 1988.
5. Miles A. Women, health and medicine. Milton Keynes: Open University Press; 1991.
6. Curtis S, Lawson K. Gender, ethnicity and self reported health: the case of African-Caribbean population in London. Soc Sci Med 1999; 50(3):365–385.
7. Cornwell J. Hard earned lives. Accounts of health and illness from East London. London: Tavistock; 1984.
8. Stainton-Rogers W. Explaining health and illness – an exploration of diversity. London: Harvester Wheatsheaf; 1991.
9. Pierret J. Constructing discourses. In: Radley A, ed. Worlds of illness. London: Routledge; 1993:9–26.
10. Frank-Stromborg M, Pender N, Walker S, Sechrist K. Determinants of health-promoting lifestyles in ambulatory cancer patients. Soc Sci Med 1990; 31(8)1159–1168.
11. Maes L, Lievans J. Can the school make a difference? A multilevel analysis of adolescent risk

and health behaviour. Soc Sci Med 2003; 56(3):517–530.

12. Hyman I, Gurage S. A review of theory and health promotion strategies for new immigrant women. Can J Public Health 2002; 93(3)183–187.

13. Parrott RL, Silk KJ, Condit C. Diversity in lay perceptions of the sources of human traits: genes, environment and personal behaviours. Soc Sci Med 2003; 56(5):1099–1109.

14. Graham H, Blackburn C. The socio-economic patterning of health and smoking behaviour among mothers with young children on income support. Sociol Health Illn 1998; 20(2):215–240.

15. Griesbach D, Amos A, Currie C. Adolescent smoking and family structure. Soc Sci Med 2003; 56(1):41–52.

16. Junger M, Stroebe W, van der Laan AM. Delinquency, health behaviour and health. Br J Health Psychol 2001; 6(2):103–120.

17. White A, Johnson M. The complexities of nursing research with men. Int J Nurs Stud 1998; 35(1/2):41–48.

18. Lockyer L, Bury M. The construction of a modern epidemic: the implications for women of the gendering of coronary heart disease. J Adv Nurs 2002; 39(5):432–440.

19. de Nooijer J, Lechner L, de Vries H. Social psychological correlates of paying attention to cancer symptoms and seeking medical help. Soc Sci Med 2003; 56(5):915–920.

20. Gasalberti D. Early detection of breast cancer by self-examination: the influence of perceived barriers and health conception. Oncol Nurs Forum 2002; 29(2):1341–1346.

21. White A, Johnson M. Men making sense of their chest pain – niggles, doubts and denials. J Clin Nurs 2000; 9(4):534–541.

22. Fish J, Wilkinson S. Understanding lesbians' healthcare behaviour: the case of breast self examination. Soc Sci Med 2003; 56(2):235–245.

23. Bush J. It's just part of being a woman: cervical screening, the body and feminity. Soc Sci Med 2000; 50(3):429–444.

24. Foxall MJ, Barron CR, Houfek JF. Ethnic influences and body awareness, trait anxiety, perceived risk, and breast and gynecologic cancer screening practices. Oncol Nurs Forum 2001; 28(4):727–738.

25. Blaxter M. Why do victims blame themselves? In: Radley A, ed. Worlds of illness. London: Routledge; 1993:124–142.

26. Ho R. Cigarette health warnings – the effects of perceived severity, expectancy of occurrence, and self-efficacy of intentions to give up smoking. Aust Psychol 1992; 27(2):109–113.

27. Sarna L, Brown JK, Lilington L, Wewers ME, Bercht M-L. Tobacco-control attitudes, advocacy and smoking behaviour in oncology nurses. Oncol Nurs Forum 2000; 27(10):1519–1528.

28. McKee L, Laurier E, Taylor RJ, Lennox AS. Eliciting the smoker's agenda: implications for policy and practice. Soc Sci Med 2003; 56(1):83–94.

29. McPhail G. There's no such thing as a healthy glow: cutaneous malignant melanoma – the case against suntanning. Eur J Cancer Care 1997; 6(2):147–153.

30. Amir Z, Wright A, Kernohan EEM, Hart B. Attitudes, beliefs and behaviour regarding the use of sunbeds amongst healthcare workers in Bradford. Eur J Cancer Care 2000; 9(2):76–79.

31. McGee R. Editorials: Does Stress cause cancer? BMJ 1999; 319(7216):1015.

32. Protheroe D, Turvey K, Benson E, Bowers D, House A. Stressful life events and difficulties and onset of breast cancer; case-control study. BMJ 1999; 319 .(7216):1027–1030.

33. Lillberg K, Verkasalo PK, Kaprio J, et al. Stressful life events and risk of breast cancer in 10,808 women: A cohort study. Am J Epidemiol 2003; 157(5):415–423.

34. Blaxter M. The causes of disease. Women talking. Soc Sci Med 1983; 17(2):59–69.

35. Oakley A, Bendelow G, Barnes J, Buchanan M, Nasseem Husain OA. Health and cancer prevention: knowledge and beliefs of children and young people. BMJ 1995; 310(6986):1029–1033.

36. MacFadyen L, Amos A, Hastings G, Parkes E. They look like my kind of people – perceptions of smoking images in youth magazines. Soc Sci Med 2003; 56(3):491–501.

37. Moore R, Topping A. Young men's knowledge of testicular cancer and testicular self-examination: a lost opportunity. Eur J Cancer Care 1999; 8:137–142.

38. Cox SM, McKellin W. There's this thing in our family: predictive testing and the construction of risk for Huntington Disease. Sociol Health Illn 1999; 21(5):622–646.

39. Hallowell N. Doing the right thing: genetic risk and responsibility. Sociol Health Illn 1999; 21(5):597–621.

40. Murphy AE. Dealing with the uncertainty of developing a cancer. Eur J Cancer Care 1999; 8:233–237.

41. Lloyd AJ. The extent of patient's understanding of the risk of treatments. Qual Saf Health Care 2001; 10(1):i14–i18.

42. Doyal L. Informed consent: moral necessity or illusion? Qual Saf Health Care 2001; 10(1):i29–i33.

43. Henderson L, Kitzinger J. The human drama of genetics: 'hard' and 'soft' media representations of inherited breast cancer. Sociol Health Illn 1999; 21(5):560–578.

44. Hardey M. Doctor in the house: the Internet as a source of lay health knowledge and the challenge to expertise. Sociol Health Illn 1999; 21(6):820–835.

45. Pandey SJ, Hart JJ, Tiwary S. Women's health and the internet: understanding emerging trends and implications. Soc Sci Med 2003; 56(2):179–191.

46. Giddens A. Modernity and self-identity. Cambridge: Polity Press; 1991.

47. Wardle J, Taylor T, Sutton S, Atkin W. Does publicity about cancer screening raise fear of cancer? Randomised trial of the psychological effect of information about cancer screening. BMJ 1999; 319(7216):1037–1038.

48. Wilson JMG, Jungner G. The principles and practice of screening for disease. Geneva: World Health Organisation; 1968.

49. Chapple A, Ziebland S, Shepperd S, et al. Why men with prostate cancer want wider access to prostate specific antigen testing: qualitative study BMJ 2002; 325(7367):737–783.

50. Frank AW. Illness as moral occasion: restoring agency to ill people. Health 1997; 1(2):131–148.

51. Howson A. Cervical screening, compliance and moral obligation. Sociol Health Illn 1999; 21(4):401–425.

52. Bush J. It's just part of being a woman: cervical screening, the body and feminity. Soc Sci Med 2000; 50(3):429–444.

53. Kasl SV, Cobb S. Health behaviour, illness behaviour and the sick role behaviour. Arch Environ Health 1966; 12(2):246–266.

54. Kasl SV, Cobb S. Blood pressure changes in men undergoing job loss: a preliminary report. Psychosom Med 1970; 32(1):19–38.

55. Conner M, Norman P. The role of cognition in health behaviours. In: Conner M, Norman P, eds. Predicting health behaviour. Buckingham: Open University Press; 1996:1–22.

56. Belloc NB. Relationship of health practices to mortality. Prev Med 1973; 3(2):67–81.

57. Belloc NB, Breslow L. Relationship of physical health status and health practices. Prev Med 1972; 1(5):409–421.

58. Breslow L, Enstrom JE. Persistence in health habits and their relationship to mortality. Prev Med 1980; 11(1):1–28.

59. Stroebe W. Social psychology and health. 2nd edn. Buckingham: Open University Press; 2000.

60. Vickers RR, Conway TL, Hervig LK. Demonstrations of replicable health behaviours. Prev Med 1990; 19(3):377–401.

61. Fishbein M, Ajzen I. Belief, attitude, intention and behaviour: an introduction to theory and research. Reading, MA: Addison–Wesley; 1975.

62. Rosenstock I. The health belief model and preventative health behavior. Health Educ Monogr 1974; 2(4):354–386.

63. Twinn S. The evaluation of effectiveness of health education interventions in clinical practice: a continuing methodological challenge. J Adv Nurs 2001; 34(2):230–237.

64. Forss A, Tishelman C, Widmark C, et al. I got a letter…' A qualitative study of women's reasoning about attendance in a cervical cancer screening programme in urban Sweden. Psycho-oncology 2001:76–87.

65. Callaghan P. Health beliefs and their influence on United Kingdom nurses' health-related behaviours. J Adv Nurs 1999; 29(1): 28–35.

66. Yarbrough SS, Braden CJ. Utility of health belief model as a guide for explaining or predicting breast cancer screening behaviours. J Adv Nurs 2001; 33(5):677–688.

67. Pender N. Health promotion in nursing practice. 3rd edn. Stamford, CT: Appleton and Lange; 1996.

68. Clayson ME. Breast awareness may reduce mortality. Prof Nurs 1992; (4):321–326.

69. Wallston BS, Wallston KA. Locus of control and health: a review of the literature. Health Educ Monogr 1978; 6(2):107–117.

70. Wallston KA, Wallston BS. Social psychological models of health behavior: an examination and integration. In: Baum A, Taylor S, Singer JE, eds. Handbook of psychology and health. Vol IV, Social aspects of health. Hillsdale, NJ: Lawrence Erlbaum; 1984:25–53.

71. Bandura A. Social foundations of thought and action: a cognitive social theory. Englewood Cliffs, NJ: Prentice Hall; 1986.

72. Schwarzer R, Fuchs R. Self-efficacy and health behaviours. In: Conner M, Norman P, eds. Predicting health behaviour. Buckingham: Open University Press; 1996:196–263.

73. Hervey D, Smith M, McGee HM. Self-efficacy and health behaviour: a review. Irish J Psychol 1998; 19(2–3):248–273.

74. Lesanger A, Kraft P, Roysamb E. Perceived self-efficacy in health behaviour research: conceptualisation, measurement and correlates. Psychol Health 2000; 15(1):51–69.

75. World Health Organization. WHO/FAO release independent Expert Report on diet and chronic disease. Press Release, World Health Organization: http://www.who.int/mediacentre/releases/2003/pr20/en/ 2003a

76. World Health Organization. Executive Summary Joint WHO/FAO Expert Report on diet, nutrition and the prevention of chronic disease. Geneva: WHO; 2003.

77. Devine C , Connors M, Sobal J, Bisogni C. Sandwiching it in: spillover of work onto food choices and family roles in low- and moderate-income urban households. Soc Sci Med 2003; 56(3):617–630.

78. Peto R, Darby S, Deo H, et al. Smoking, smoking cessation, and lung cancer in the UK since 1950: combination of national statistics with two case-control studies. BMJ 2000; 321(7257):323–329.

79. World Health Organisation Fact Sheet No 221 Tobacco – health facts Geneva: World Health Organisation; 1999 http://www.who.int/inf-fs/en/fact221.html

80. Timmermans GM. Using a woman's health perspective to guide decisions made in qualitative research. J Adv Nurs 1999; 30(3)640–645.

81. Kirwan JMJ, Tincello DG, Herod JJO, Frost O, Kingston RE. Effect of delays on survival of women with epithelial ovarian cancer: retrospective audit. BMJ 2002; 324(7330):148–151.

82. Richer MC, Ezer H. Understanding beliefs and meaning in the experience of cancer: a concept analysis. J Adv Nurs 2000; 32(45): 1108–1115.

83. Bush MJ. Coping and adaptation. In: Carroll-Johnson RM, Gorman LM, Bush NJ, eds. Psychosocial nursing care. Pittsburgh, PA: Oncology Nursing Press; 1998:35–52.

84. Lazarus RS, Folkman S. Stress, appraisal and coping. New York: Springer; 1984.

85. Petticrew M, Bell R, Hunter D. Influence of psychological coping on survival and recurrence in people with cancer: systematic review. BMJ 2002; 325(7372):1066–1076.

86. Folkman S, Greer S. Promoting psychological well-being in the face of serious illness: when theory, research and practice inform each other. Psycho-oncology 2000; 9(1):11–19.

87. Michael YL, Berkman LF, Colditz GA, Holmes MD, Kawzchi I. Social networks and health-related quality of life in breast cancer survivors. A prospective study. J Psychosom Res 2002; 52(3):285–293.

88. Purandare L. Attitudes to cancer may create a barrier to communication between patient and caregiver. Eur J Cancer Care 1997; 6(1)92–99.

89. Rosvold EO, Hjartaker A, Bjertness E, Lund E. Breast self-examination and cervical cancer testing among Norwegian female physicians – a nation wide comparative study. Soc Sci Med 2001; 52(2):249–258.

90. Cutler LR. The contribution of nursing to cancer prevention J Adv Nurs 1999; 29(1):169–177.

91. Rutledge DN, Raymon NJ. Changes in well-being of women cancer survivors following a survivor weekend experience. Oncol Nurs Forum 2001; 28(1):85–91.

92. Aziz NM, Rowland J. Cancer survivorship research among ethnic minority or medically underserved groups. Oncol Nurs Forum 2002; 29(5):789–801.

93. Courneya KS, Friedenreich CM, Sela RA, et al. The group psychotherapy and home-based physical exercise (group-hope) trial in cancer survivors: physical fitness and quality of life outcomes. Psychooncology 2003; 12(4):357–374.

94. Burnham TR, Wilcox A. Effects of exercise on physiological and psychological variables in cancer survivors. Med Sci Sports Exerc 2002; 34(12):1863–1867.

95. Schwartz AL .Patterns of exercise and fatigue in physically active cancer survivors. Oncol Nurs Forum 1998; 25(3):485–491.

96. Porock D, Kristjanson LJ, Tinnelly K, Duke T, Blight J. An exercise intervention for advanced cancer patients experiencing fatigue: a pilot study. J Palliat Care 2000; 16(3):30–36.

97. McInnes JA, Knobf MT. Weight gain and quality of life in women treated with adjuvant chemotherapy for early-stage breast cancer. Oncol Nurs Forum 2001; 28(4):675–684.

98. Björklund M, Fridlund B. Cancer patients' experiences of nurses' behavior and health promotion activities: a critical incident analysis. Eur J Cancer Care 1999; 8(4)204–212.

99. Richardson J. Health promotion in palliative care. J Adv Nurs 2002; 40(4):432–440.

100. Pollock AM, Vickers N. Deprivation and emergency admissions for cancers of the colorectum, lung and breast in south east England: ecological study. BMJ 1998; 317(7153):245–252.

CHAPTER 2

Partnership in Care

YVONNE WENGSTRÖM AND CHRISTINA FORSBERG

CHAPTER CONTENTS

Partnership – the starting point for family involvement in care	21
Family caregiving skill – conceptualization of the caregiver role	22
Dimensions of the family caregiver role	22
Experiences of caregiving – the family's point of view	23
The nurse as a mediator in family-centred caregiving – support for family caregivers	24
Assessment	24
Nursing interventions in family-centred care	26
Multicultural aspects and the family	28
Cultural assessment	29
Education based on partnership and empowerment	29
Patient empowerment	30
Strategies to achieve patient empowerment	31
Interventions based on empowerment	33
Self-care – the goal of empowerment	34
Future areas for development for empowerment and family caregiving	35
Conclusion	35
References	35

PARTNERSHIP– THE STARTING POINT FOR FAMILY INVOLVEMENT IN CARE

The care provided by healthcare professionals for the family is a vital part in caring for the person with cancer. The physical effect of the illness is only one part – personal relations are also affected. A good relation with one's family is often a vital source of support for the ill person. This chapter focuses on describing the caregiver role and how nurses in cancer care may support the patient and family. This chapter is divided into two parts: the first part concerns the family's role in cancer care and the second focuses on education based on partnership and empowerment.

Throughout the world the immediate family plays a central role in supporting and providing care for cancer patients.[1,2] Changes in the healthcare system have shifted cancer care from the inpatient arena to ambulatory and home settings. Scientific studies have documented the shortened length of hospital stay and the impact this has had on patients and families.[1,3–5] As a result of changes in society, the level of family involvement in the daily care of the cancer patient has increased. In many European countries these families are being called upon to provide more complex care to ill relatives. This requires a level of knowledge and skill novel to many family members.

Women's role as carers has been deeply anchored in society, in Europe as well as in the USA and England.[6–8] Florence Nightingale proclaimed in *Notes on Nursing*, published in England in 1860, that 'Every woman is a nurse', conveying that in a woman's life caring is an important feature and that women could expect to be providing care for ill and dying people for lengthy periods of time.[9] In today's society, women and caregiving are still synonymous; they predominate over their male counterparts as primary caregivers in every kin category.[10]

Since the concept of family is central in family caregiving, a clear definition is warranted. The literature provides numerous definitions where the focus is on the traditional nuclear family, where the persons included are bonded together by blood relation, marriage or adoption and belonging to the same household. Other definitions are focused on the family as a social system:

> A family is a group of individuals who are bound by strong emotional ties, a sense of belonging and a passion for being involved in one another's lives.[11]

This definition allows for the family as a concept to include more than the traditional nuclear family.

FAMILY CAREGIVING SKILL – CONCEPTUALIZATION OF THE CAREGIVER ROLE

Family caregiving skill is an important nursing concept, with significant clinical and research implications. Concept development of family caregiving is also essential in the present era of health care. Extensive research has been conducted on family caregiving, primarily to identify caregiver burden.[1,2] This has been identified as an important concern; however, other aspects, such as the ability to provide care well, are factors with high clinical relevance for nurses and this concept needs to be further developed.

For families to provide care well, it is important to pay attention to the development of caregiving knowledge, competency and skill.[12] In the work of Schumacher et al,[3] the focus was shifted from the individual caregiver to the behavioural process of caregiving by identifying caregiving (how to) skill rather than caregiver skill.

Schumacher et al define family caregiving skill as the ability to engage effectively and smoothly in nine core caregiving processes. Caregiving is effective when it leads to the best possible outcomes of care, such as optimal symptom management, prevention of injury and early detection of problems. When considering skill development among family caregivers, Schumacher et al[3] conclude the importance of making distinctions between knowing *that* and knowing *how*, as this suggests a need to explore the caregiver's day-to-day caregiving rather than focusing on the caregiver's cognitive knowledge. In other words, to develop caregiver skills requires practise and experience.

DIMENSIONS OF THE FAMILY CAREGIVER ROLE

The dimensions of the caregiving role include interpreting, making decisions, monitoring, making adjustments, taking actions, providing hands on care, working with the ill person, accessing resources and negotiating the health-care system.[3]

The process of making sense of what is observed is defined and *interpreted* by the caregiver. To be a skilful interpreter includes a complex reasoning process to understand changes from normal and the ability to attribute the observation to some cause. For example, a skilful caregiver attributes the care receiver's inability to eat when on chemotherapy to the side-effects (nausea, sore mouth, etc.) caused by the treatment rather than to a lack of will or appreciation of efforts made to prepare meals.

Making decisions is defined as the process of choosing a course of action based on observation and interpretation of a specific situation. This is based on the day-to-day care decision-making process as it is complex and requires priority setting and judgement. If multiple choices exist, the skilful carer makes choices that do not involve unnecessary risk or harm.

Monitoring is defined as keeping an eye on things, observing how the care receiver is doing to ensure that changes in the ill family members condition are noticed. Skilful caregivers take multiple cues into account; this includes verbal and non-verbal behaviour.

Making adjustments is defined as the process of progressively altering caregiving actions until the strategy that works best is found. Skilful adjustment is often related to the amount of something, such as the amount of food or the most effective amount of antiemetic. Skilful caregivers fine-tune the amounts so that the ill family member experiences optimal well-being.

Taking actions is defined as the process of carrying out caregiving instructions and decisions and is characterized by good timing, skilful organization and effective tracking methods by the caregiver.

Providing hands-on care is defined as the process of carrying out medical and nursing procedures. Provision of care from a skilful caregiver is characterized by meticulous attention to both safety and comfort for the ill family member.

Working with the ill person is defined as the process of sharing illness-related care in a way that takes into account the personality of the care receiver and the caregiver. The process to work with the ill person is influenced by the previous history of the relationship but also includes illness-related issues. The skilful caregiver knows when to become more active in the role of illness care, sensing the family member to be too ill to care for herself.

Accessing resources is defined as obtaining the resources needed to provide care, such as information, equipment and supplies for home care and assistance from various community agencies. Skilful accessing involves being able to find 'just the right thing' to fit the need at hand.

Negotiating the healthcare system is defined as the process of making sure the ill family member's needs are met adequately. This responsibility does not rest solely on the caregiver. Knowing when to call the nurse or physician is an issue for many caregivers at home even after instructions to call when any questions arise. With time, caregivers develop a sense of how to best work with healthcare providers by phone.

Family caregiving is a complex role. This knowledge is significant for cancer nursing practice since nurses provide teaching and support to family members as they take on the role as carers. In clinical practice, family members often seek nurses' confirmation and support for the care they are providing and also expect them to help and develop their skills as caregivers. Thus, the fact that nurses will assess caregiving skill and intervene when needed is expected by clients as well as nurses today. Therefore, formal knowledge development around caregiving will give nurses in cancer care new knowledge to implement in practice.

EXPERIENCES OF CAREGIVING – THE FAMILY'S POINT OF VIEW

Cancer is frequently described as a disease affecting the whole family, and general support exists around the notion that needs for care vary as the disease progresses and also as the duration of care increases.[1,3,4] Care responsibilities have been found to be both direct and indirect, since the role of the family's involvement in care has shifted from the strictly custodial to now include symptom management, advanced equipment care, patient advocacy and transportation. People whose usual life roles have no relation to health care undertake many of these tasks with little preparation. Families are deeply committed to their caregiving responsibility and they see what they do as important; the emotional, physical and financial strain can, however, be burdensome.[1]

The relations within the family change as one member encounters a serious illness or dies and another takes on responsibility to care for another member. Research today shows that any illness or change in health status within a family affects the rest of its members.[5]

Variations exist in the demands and responses reported by families, but there is evidence of their involvement throughout the process of adjustment to living with cancer.[6–8] The responses of family members in turn influence patients and the overall family experience. Friesen et al[9] describe an interactive learning process used by families to bring the pieces of the puzzle together to form an integrated picture about how to adjust to the diagnosis of cancer. One of the most accessible learning resources to families was past experience. Families pooled memories of past experiences with cancer and other major illnesses, which helped them to cope with the situation at hand. Positive comparisons were part of reviewing the past; families compared their current experiences to people in worse situations. Role models were also elicited by remembering how others had conducted themselves when they were ill. Families also shared information-gathering, explored medical opinions and learned from the experiences of outside acquaintances. As this was developing, an informed trust was building in relation to the healthcare system. Families also shared their experience of living with someone undergoing treatment for cancer, and patients taught their families about their illness experiences and what constituted effective support.

THE NURSE AS A MEDIATOR IN FAMILY-CENTRED CAREGIVING – SUPPORT FOR FAMILY CAREGIVERS

Increased participation of families in the care of patients with cancer and associated theory development has started to shift and modify the clinical pathway of nursing care. By tradition, nurses have worked mainly with the patient and at times individual family members in providing support and education, without comprehending the entire family as the focus of nursing care.

To increase the family's influence on nursing care demands a change or modification of clinical practice. For nurses in cancer care, this has increased demands for new competencies in relation to assessment and nursing care of families. This not only entails a change of concept but also a paradigm shift in the delivery of nursing care. Knowledge and clinical competencies required should be derived from the family's view on health and illness. This includes the impact of illness on the family and the influence of the family's interaction with the healthcare system. A foundation for interactive clinical care includes an assessment of

interaction between the patient/family and the nurse.

Family-centred nursing care should focus on the *relations* between the different components rather than on the patient, family and nurse as separate entities. The increased focus on interaction between components will lead to a nursing care model that will use available resources and support the entire family system. Every family is unique, with their own resources and problems. Nurses can not only assess the impact of health and illness on the family but also the influence the family has on health and illness.[5]

If a non-hierarchical relationship develops between the nurse and the family where mutual understanding and learning can take place, this may have a therapeutic effect in itself.

ASSESSMENT

The feasibility of maintaining family care of the ill cancer patient is largely based on the willingness, capacity and, last but not least, the availability of the family caregiver to provide care. Nurses need to develop and assess risk profiles to anticipate which members are likely to experience distress and plan support services for them. What resources are needed, how complex is the care? What risk factors predispose caregivers to emotional, physical, social and financial problems? When are structured, formal support and teaching needed? Nurses together with other healthcare professionals in cancer care need to design and work with supportive programmes that will ultimately decrease caregiver distress and burden and thus enhance the quality of life for the ill family member as well as for the family.

The nurse working in partnership with the family caring for the patient needs a structure for assessment of the needs of the family. This will identify problems and resources and enable the planning of interventions needed to minimize problems and allocate resources. A structure or mapping of the family provides a focus for nursing care interventions.

In our society today the family is not yet automatically seen as 'a unit' needing help with specific family-related problems. More commonly, problems are presented as isolated and concerning separate members of the family. It is therefore the nurse's responsibility to assess whether the problem or need should be treated from a family context or not. Family assessment should, however, not be seen as a universal approach or a replacement for individual assessment. Contraindications for family assessment are, for example, if a family member's personal growth will be impeded or if the context of the family situation is impossible to work with.

The Calgary Family Assessment Model (CFAM) is an example of a multidimensional model of assessment. The model comprises three main components: structure of the family, developmental issues and functional issues.[5]

The structure of the family includes assessment of the internal structure of the family, such as which individuals belong to this family. This includes ranking of members: Who takes part and how for example? It is important to consider whom the family themselves consider belongs to the family. The external structure concerns the extended family and other systems of importance, e.g. day care and, overall, the context of the family.

Apart from the structure of the family, it is important for the nurse to consider the developmental life cycle as well. This includes all transactional development processes within a family that concern family growth. When a member encounters a life-threatening illness or change of work and relocation for example, family structure will be affected. Psychological processes such as grief and closeness are also an important part of the family's development.

Functional assessment consists of judging how the individuals in the family actually behave towards each other. The instrumental function concerns routine activities within the family: e.g. cooking, sleeping, giving injections and changing dressings. The expressive function includes emotional and verbal communication and roles within the family and how problems are solved within this family. For the nurse, the focus should be on the interactions between the members.

Each of the main categories consists of several subcategories and should hence be used as a framework, with the nurse responsible for choosing relevant subcategories appropriate for assessment of the specific family at any given point in time. Figure 2.1 gives an overview of the CFAM structure for family assessment.

Structuring assessment using the CFAM means focusing on peoples' beliefs about an illness or how illness and ill health affects the family and vice versa. The researchers who developed the model have, from years of experience with families, come to an understanding that it is beliefs concerning problems that are central. Families that experience problems related to illness or ill health have an attitude

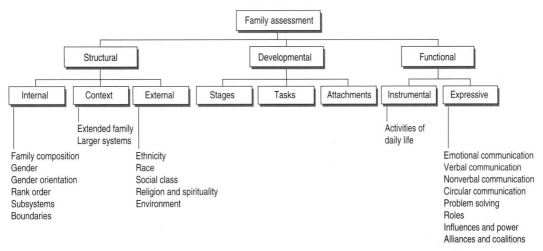

Figure 2.1: Overview of the Calgary Family Assessment Model. (Adapted from Wright & Leahey[10] with permission.)

that hinders or eases a solution to the problem. The therapeutic approach for the nurse is to identify, challenge or try to change the belief that limits or hinders the solution. By lifting the family's beliefs concerning a problem to the surface, the possibilities for change of beliefs and finding alternative solutions increase. During this process the strength and possibilities within the family become focused. This development of the relationship between the family and the nurse demands that there is concordance and a mutual understanding between the nurse's and family's beliefs of the problem. It is also important to understand that the nurse can only offer the family different solutions: whether the family will be open and accept the intervention is dependent on experience of earlier interactions.

A simple yet powerful intervention for nurses to use when working with families with health problems is to ask questions. There are two types of questions to be asked: linear questions and circular questions. Linear questions have a limiting effect, whereas circular questions are generative: they introduce new cognitive contexts and, consequently, make way for new or different behaviours within the family. In other words, linear questions seek relations between cause and effect, whereas circular questions seek a relation or contact between events, persons, beliefs and thoughts.

Using circular questions will allow family members to view their problem from a different angle and, thus, see new solutions.

Box 2.1 is an example of a circular questions relating to intervention within the area of the family's function.

Two other frequently mentioned family assessment models are The Family Assessment and Intervention Model and the Friedman Family Assessment Model.[10] The former model addresses three areas: health promotion, family reactions and restoration of family stability and function. This model provides an assessment instrument, the FS ^{3} I, that provides directions for nurses.

The Friedman Family Assessment Model[10] has a more general approach and views families as subsystems of wider society. The model views the family as an open social system and focuses on the family's structure, functions and rela-

---

Box 2.1

Examples of circular questions for a family member

The nurse assesses what effects one family member's behaviour has on another family member.

Examples of circular questions:

Cognitive: Why do you think your wife doesn't want to visit your daughter at the hospital?

Affective: How do you feel when your daughter cries during her treatment?

Behavioural: What do you do when your wife doesn't visit your son at the hospital?

---

tionship with other social systems. Friedman's assessment model was developed to provide guidelines for the nurse when interviewing families. The model consists of six broad categories of interview questions: identification data; development stage and history; environmental data; family structure; family functions; and family stress and coping. Finally, all three approaches can be used alone or in combination. The advantage with the CFAM is that it includes both assessment and interventions. The model is broad in perspective, although it focuses on internal relations within the family rather than on the interface between the family and the community.

NURSING INTERVENTIONS IN FAMILY-CENTRED CARE

A plethora of concepts, such as treatment, therapy, activity, intervention, action and activity, are used today to label the specific activities conducted by nurses within the treatment part of nursing care. Within this chapter, the word 'intervention' will be used to describe specific nursing care interventions and is defined as:

> any action or response of the nurse which includes the nurses overt therapeutic actions that occur in the context of a nurse-client relationship to affect individual, family or community functioning for which nurses are accountable[11] (p5)

Interventions focused on individual patients in cancer care are found in the literature, but interventions aimed at the family are not very common.[2] What is known is that a nursing care intervention in family-centred care should focus on both the behaviour of the nurse and the reaction of the family. Three important components are included: the nurse's interventions, the family's functional areas and how well the proposed interventions are accepted and fit the family. The purpose of intervention is to offer support and enhance or uphold the family's cognitive, affective and behavioural function.

The nurse invites family members to tell their story in relation to health and illness; every family member's contribution is important. Both the nurse and the family contribute with their expert knowledge and strengths. The nurse can offer the family a new perspective on their experienced problems and acknowledge the resources and strengths within the family to be used for planning care together.

The nurse is often a natural communication partner for family caregivers. She has knowledge of the ill family member as well as the illness and treatment. But mainly the nurse has knowledge of the nursing care interventions that are important, and with a nursing care plan as a basis she can develop a deeper understanding of the effects of the family dynamics on the ill member's well-being. The nurse can develop her role as mediator to ensure structured and conscious family-centred nursing care with a clear goal that is possible to evaluate.

Instead of just offering education and support to individuals, family relations may be developed, lifting nursing care from the individual level to an interactional family level. For families, past experiences with cancer often inform the present. By acknowledging this fact, nurses can help families to identify beliefs that may influence the illness experience. If families are included in teaching sessions, communication between patients, families and healthcare professionals can be facilitated and, by offering learning material to take home, nurses may facilitate the sharing of information-gathering.

To illustrate a specific family intervention using the CFAM, the example shown in Box 2.2 might be helpful. This intervention was aimed at achieving changes within the cognitive area of family function, but also affected the functional area.

For families with an ill family member, information is crucial; from clinical experience, one often comes across family members frustrated from the lack of information available to them from healthcare staff. Nurses are often in a unique position to inform patients and families about how a chronic illness may impact the family. The nurse can also enhance the family's ability to find out what resources are available for them in their unique situation.

Interventions often involve presentation of information and education concerning specific health problems or risks. The treatment goal of the intervention is to change the family's view and belief of the health problem so that new solutions may be found. Harding and Higginson[2] conducted a systematic literature review of interventions aimed at helping caregivers in cancer and palliative care. They identified 22 interventions concerning home care, respite services, social networks and activity enhancement, problem-solving, education and group work. Of these interventions, only a few had been subject to systematic evaluation.

Box 2.2

Example of a specific family intervention using the Calgary Family Assessment Model

For one family with a 26-year-old daughter with advanced cancer the parents had demonstrated engaging support to the point of exhaustion. The parents were at a point where they needed some temporary relief in order to continue supporting the daughter. Together with the daughter, the nurse challenged the view of her perceived helplessness. The daughter looked into what support might be available for her and realized that she qualified for home care. This was arranged, her parents were able to take some time off and reported feeling less strained; the daughter felt in charge of her life and happier. In this example, the nurse aimed at helping the daughter to change her and her parents' cognitive attitudes; but the intervention also had effects on the behaviour of the family.

The authors concluded that the current evidence contributes more to understanding than to effectiveness.

MULTICULTURAL ASPECTS AND THE FAMILY

Galanti[12] concludes that when healthcare personnel work with the patient's beliefs, rather than against them, the outcomes are usually more successful, measured not only in patient satisfaction but also in ease for the medical team in managing the patient and family. The development of cultural competencies requires learning in the affective, cognitive or intellectual, and psychomotor or behavioural domains and assumes skill in critical thinking.

In order to deliver appropriate care, cultural knowledge is needed if nurses are to develop cultural understanding. Papadopoulos, et al[13] have constructed a model for the development of transcultural skills. The model identifies four main concepts: cultural awareness, knowledge, sensitivity and competence. A number of sub-concepts have been identified that need to be considered when attempting to develop transcultural skills. The model should be viewed as a starting tool and, by focusing on the separate concepts, skill development becomes a step-by-step process.

Culture represents a way of perceiving, behaving and evaluating the world. It is of importance for determining people's values, beliefs and practice. Cultural competence may be defined as a process in which the nurse strives to effectively work within the cultural context of an individual, family or community from a diverse cultural background. Box 2.3 provides an overview of the steps involved in developing transcultural skills.[13]

The first step is cultural awareness, and begins with the self and an attempt to examine and understand our own value base. This helps to develop questioning of the traditional health service and social values, such as the power of a profession and the role of medicine in social control. This leads to the exploration of differing views. Empowerment is an impor-

---

Box 2.3

A model for development of transcultural skills

Cultural awareness
Self-awareness
Cultural identity
Heritage adherence
Ethnocentricity

Cultural knowledge
Health beliefs and behaviours
Stereotyping
Ethnohistory
Sociological understanding
Similarities and variations

Cultural sensitivity
Empathy
Interpersonal skills
Trust
Acceptance
Appropriateness
Respect

Cultural competence
Assessment skills
Diagnostic skills
Clinical skills
Challenging and addressing prejudice, discrimination and inequalities

Source: adapted from the model by Papadopoulos et al.[13]

---

tant element in transcultural nursing care, and depends on making links between personal position and structural inequalities. This requires cultural knowledge and understanding. Knowledge is drawn from sociology, but also gained from contact with other people from differing groups, such as patients or colleagues.

Cultural sensitivity may only be achieved when considering our patients and families as true partners. A partnership demands that power relationships are challenged and that real choices are offered. The outcomes of this include a process of facilitation, advocacy and negotiation that may be achieved on a foundation of respect, empathy and trust.

Cultural competence allows the nurse to obtain more specific and complete information to make an appropriate assessment. It facilitates the development of treatment plans that are followed by the patient and supported by the family.

Cultural competence may also reduce delays in seeking care and allows for improved use of health services; it also enhances overall communication and clinical interaction between patient and provider. Cultural competence also enhances compatibility between Western and traditional cultural health practices. Caring for the culturally diverse patient is challenging, since the rules of appropriate behaviour vary in and among cultures.

Guidelines for nurses working with culturally diverse populations include an understanding of one's own personal and cultural values about life, health and illness.[14] As nurses, we need to strive towards facilitating verbal and non-verbal communication with the ill person and family. We also need to accept that an individual's understanding and wishes may be different from that of our own as healthcare professionals, and avoid interpretation of all behaviour as stemming from the patient's illness. For example, there are individual and cultural differences in terms of pain management. Some patients want constant pain medication, whereas others stoically may deny taking pain medication. The role of the nurse is to help individual patients to advocate what feels appropriate for them within their cultural context.

CULTURAL ASSESSMENT

The role of the family differs between different countries and cultures.

Professional caregivers have all had life experiences that influence their beliefs about life, death and the treatment of the patient with a terminal illness. These beliefs stem from their personal beliefs, socioeconomic status, cultural background and religious heritage. The first step in providing a culturally sensitive service to patients is for professionals to recognize and understand their own beliefs about these sensitive issues. In Europe, countries are becoming increasingly culturally diverse and the likelihood of any

nurse treating a cancer patient from another culture has greatly increased. Not only must nurses be aware of their own cultural beliefs about health and illness but they must also seek to understand the beliefs of their patients. Sometimes this information can be sought directly from the patient, at other times families can promote greater cultural understanding.

When assessing individuals and families, the nurse should examine the following factors:

- family roles, particularly communication patterns and decision-making
- health beliefs related to disease and treatment
- patterns of daily living, particularly work and leisure activities
- social networks
- ethnical, cultural or national identity of patient and family
- religious preferences and the impact religion might have on daily living
- culturally appropriate behaviour styles.

Andrews and Boyle[15] have developed a comprehensive transcultural nursing assessment guide. The guide consists of different question themes and examples on basic questions to ask the client. Some examples are given in Box 2.4. This assessment guide could have potential utility when planning for interventions in family-centred care.

EDUCATION BASED ON PARTNERSHIP AND EMPOWERMENT

Nurses can facilitate patient and family learning by considering the interactive manner in which families acquire information. As nurses, we need to take into account the value of learning about illness by experience and also to accept patients and families as experts. By encouraging both the patient's and the relatives' perspectives of the illness, and by giving feedback, coping and support will be enhanced.[9]

An empowerment model can be useful in cancer care.

Box 2.4

A comprehensive transcultural nursing guide
Cultural affiliations Where was the patient born?
Values orientation What are the patient's attitudes, values and beliefs about birth and death, health, illness and health providers?
Communication What language does the patient speak at home? Does the patient need an interpreter? How does the patient prefer to be addressed?
Health-related beliefs and practice To what causes does the patient attribute illness and disease? What does the patient believe promotes health? What is the patient's religious affiliation?
Nutrition What nutritional factors are influenced by the patient's cultural background? What does the patient believe comprises a good versus bad diet? Has the patient chosen a particular nutritional practice?
Socioeconomic considerations Who is the principal wage earner in the patient's family? What insurance coverage does the patient have?
Educational background What is the patient's highest education level obtained? What learning style is most familiar?
Religious affiliation How does the patient's religious affiliation affect health and illness? Are there healing rituals that the patient practises?
Cultural aspects of disease incidence Are there any specific genetic or acquired conditions that are more prevalent for a specific cultural group?
Developmental considerations What factors are of importance in assessing children of various ages? What is the cultural perception of ageing?

PATIENT EMPOWERMENT

The negotiation of a partnership between nurses and patients has been described as the first step in the process of empowerment.[16] Partnership between nurses and patients is often present, but it is the balance in the relationship which is important. A power imbalance between nurses and patients could be an obstruction for partnership in care.[17] Empowerment models are to a large extent based on the assumption that patients have rights and can make their own choices about their health care.

Many definitions of empowerment have been suggested. The World Health Organization (WHO) definition of health promotion is a starting point for some authors, whereby:

health promotion is a process of enabling people to increase control over and to improve their health[18] (p1)

Since then, new definitions of health promotion and empowerment have been published.

Rappaport[19] defined empowerment as a mechanism by which people, organizations and communities gain mastery over their lives, which means that empowerment is something which occurs within an individual and is not a simple transfer of power from one person to another.

According to Mason et al,[20] empowerment generally means enabling people to recognize their strengths, abilities, personal power, power sharing and respect for self and for others. People can only empower themselves through self-awareness and by using available resources that empower. Nurses can facilitate patients in their process of achieving self-care. They can provide patients with the opportunities and resources that they need to be able to influence their health in a positive direction.

Gibson[21] has pointed out four conditions necessary for patient empowerment:

1 The individual has the prime responsibility for his/her own health.

2 The individual's self-determination needs to be respected.

3 Nurses cannot empower people; people can only empower themselves.

4 Nurses have to give up the need to control the patient and focus on cooperating with the patient.

Piper and Brown[22] suggest that the best way forward for nurses is to reflect on their practice and ask questions such as:

• Am I helping patients take control over their own health?

• Am I helping patients to understand the social origins of ill health?

• Am I listening when patients talk about their life situation?

• Am I helping patients to identify their key problems?

• Am I supporting patients to take health action?

Golant et al[23] evaluated a cancer psychoeducational programme aimed at managing cancer side-effects. The programme included clinical information about disease, treatment, information to help improve communication between the patient and caregivers and educational materials. They concluded that the programme was effective in educating patients about side-effects and empowering them to cope more effectively with their illness and treatment.

Patient empowerment is a shift in attitude for both patients and nurses. Patients are seen as the experts on their lives and nurses are seen as experts on nursing care serving as a resource. The goal of patient empowerment is to enable patients to make decisions about their own treatment and care and to be fully responsible members of the health-care team.

Strategies to achieve patient empowerment

Nurse can serve as a resource for patients by explaining, teaching, coaching, supporting, comforting and advocating. There are many guidebooks and brochures on various aspects of cancer and cancer treatment. These are often published by cancer societies throughout the world and are designed to give information to patients and their families. Such information is an example of a one-way communication strategy. To contrast, education is a two-way communicative process where the nurse and patient use different strategies and have different roles. In Table 2.1 can be found an example of different roles adopted by the nurse, the patient and the family in relation to the education process.

The nurse's task is to communicate, motivate and support patients. In using an empowerment model, the nurse must believe in the philosophy of empowerment. This means believing that illness does not involve every aspect of a patient's life and respecting a patient's right to make their own choices. The nurse must also be comfortable with expressions of feeling and encouraging patients to solve their problems.

The patient's task is to pay attention and interpret the message, to acquire new informa-

Table 2.1: The educational task

The nurse	The patient	The family
Communication Assess the patient's need for information by active listening and check for understanding	*Communication* Receive the message and pay attention Interpret the message correctly	*Communication* Receive the message and pay attention Interpret the message correctly
Motivation Explore existing beliefs, attitudes and skills and seek to modify Provide information and new skills Check learning Negotiate and agree contract	*Decision-making* Form appropriate beliefs Acquire skills Agree contract	*Motivation* Discuss existing beliefs Positive feedback Agree contract
Support Help to mobilize social and family support Act as advocate for change Check patient's progress	*Health action* Positive attitude to act Acquire new information and skills Adopt and sustain health Improved well-being	*Support* Daily-based support Encourage health action Positive attitude

Source: modified after Tones in Kendall.[16]

tion and to act in a new way.[16] Patients are recommended to:

- ask questions and articulate their needs
- seek relevant information about disease and treatment
- weigh available options and to reach a decision that is compatible with their values
- learn to react to the stress of cancer
- seek support from their family and friends.

The nurse's contribution in two-way communication involves attending, enabling through coaching and encouraging, interpreting care and patient requirements, responding to the situation and anticipating what will happen to patients. The patient's work involves managing themselves and taking some responsibility for this, surviving the experience, affiliating with healthcare workers and interpreting the experience as it unfolds.

The family also has an important role to motivate and support the patient. It is clear that education and information are essential if family members are to participate effectively in care. Families have reported that they provide much care by trial and error.[4] This creates a sense of uncertainty, that in turn will make caregiving a time-consuming and stressful experience. Information aimed at providing guidance on implementation of care may reduce the stress of caregiving and the associated burdens and feelings of helplessness and inadequacy that come with ambiguity.

The relative's knowledge and support is of great importance when the patient gets a cancer diagnosis. Therefore it is necessary that the patient and a close relative receive information concurrently, especially about the cancer disease and its consequences on the patient's and the family's future life. There is a need for structured and ongoing dialogue with family members concerning treatment goals, plans of care and expectations regarding patient outcomes. Acquiring information and education concerning treatment and illness-related expectations and problems can help caregivers to plan care, anticipate problems and detect changes in the course of the illness.[2] Reasons given by family members for lack of information and education include the inability of family members to ask questions, limited contact with providers, providers who direct attention solely at family members and do not relate to the family and being overwhelmed due to distress.[2]

Interventions based on empowerment

Various theories and models have been used as the conceptual basis for many educational interventions. A common base is to adopt the view that taking action and changing behaviour is dependent on a process of awareness, knowledge, beliefs, attitudes and support.[18] In order to achieve successful results, a variety of different educational interventions may be necessary.

In a meta-analysis of 116 studies, Devine and Westlake[24] evaluated the effects of psychoeducational interventions provided to adults with cancer. They found that psychoeducational care helps adults with cancer in relation to anxiety, depression, mood, nausea, vomiting, pain and knowledge. The most prevalent interventions studied in the review concerned some type of behavioural or cognitive counselling focused on developing skills or changing thoughts and behaviours. They also pointed out that it is important for nurses to know that many different types of psychoeducational interventions can help patients with cancer.

Fawzy[25] showed that a psychoeducational nursing intervention could enhance coping behaviour and the affective state of newly diagnosed malignant melanoma patients. The intervention consisted of health education, stress management and the teaching of coping skills.

Health education

The patients in the experimental group received an educational manual and the content was reviewed with them. The manual was then continually reviewed with the patient during the hospital stay and during follow-up visits at the clinic. Patients also had the opportunity to phone the nurse if they had questions at home. This education process lasted over 3 months.

Stress management

Stress management techniques included teaching the patient the nature of stress, how to assess their own sources and levels of stress and how to relieve stress. Patients were taught how to perform progressive muscle relaxation exercises and requested to practise daily for at least 15 minutes.

Coping skills

Patients were made aware of different ways of coping:

- optimism – or the expectation of positive change
- practicality – options and alternatives are seldom completely exhausted
- flexibility – strategies change to reflect the changing nature of problems
- resourcefulness – referring to one's ability to call upon additional information and support to strengthen how well one copes.

In this intervention the nurse sought to empower patients by directly affecting health-seeking and coping behaviours.

Davidson and Degner[26] evaluated an educational intervention aimed at empowering men with newly diagnosed prostate cancer: 30 men were randomized to receive an intervention programme and 30 men received a written information package alone. The intervention consisted of:

- a written information package with discussion
- a list of questions patients could ask their physician
- an audiotape of the medical consultations.

Results demonstrated that men in the intervention group assumed a significantly more active role in treatment decision-making and had lower levels of anxiety after 6 weeks.

By more frequent use of health promotion models, such as the empowerment model, the nurse can identify and focus on individuals who wish to improve their well-being. The nurse's dilemma lies in applying such models in an individualized way, at the same time as considering the patient's environment and cultural belonging.

Self-care – the goal of empowerment

Self-care is a term representing the range of health-related decision-making and actions undertaken by individuals on their own behalf. Inherent in the concept is the recognition that, whatever factors and processes may determine the behaviour and whether or not self-care is effective and interfaces appropriately with professional care, it is the individual person that acts (or does not act) to perceive health or to respond to symptoms.[27]

Orem has developed a model for self-care, defining the concept of self-care as the power that adult people have to regulate factors that affect their human functioning and human development in that environment where they live their daily life.[28] Self-care when performed effectively may contribute to self-maintenance and to personal health and well-being. When empowerment programmes are related to self-care behaviours they usually address physical, psychosocial and environmental areas. Empowerment means enabling individuals to develop health awareness, develop the skills they need for self-care, which could be to handle radiotherapy successfully, to develop coping strategies and to cope with the effects of a cancer disease.

Patients need skills to maximize their potential for health and well-being related to their disease. Patients themselves should determine what is possible and reasonable to decide about and what kind of health related-behaviour is needed for improving their self-care. Self-care could be seen as a way to cope with one's life situation, not only one's health but also regarding integrity and human development.[17,28] Self-care involves a wide range of strategies that individuals have at their disposal when dealing with well-being, health maintenance and disease-related issues. Focusing the patient's self-care abilities and coping resources and their reaction to the specific diagnosis are of crucial importance when the nurse wants to empower or enable the patient to be co-responsible for their health and well-being.

It should be kept in mind that an individual's ability to engage in self-care is conditioned for instance by age, life experience and sociocultural factors.

Wengström et al[29] investigated whether a nursing intervention using Orem's self-care theory as a framework would affect subject distress, side-effects and quality of life as perceived by breast cancer patients receiving curative radiation therapy. The goal of the nursing intervention was to liberate the patient from dependence on the nurse and to restore self-care to a level sufficient for the patient as soon as possible. The intervention was structured as follows:

- The patient received oral and written cognitive information about simulation and treatment and had the opportunity to talk and ask questions concerning the treatment.

- Individualized education and information based on the patient's needs and preferences. The purpose of this session was to prepare the patient for the possible side-effects of treatment.

- The nurse gave support and guidance and provision of self-care actions pertaining to what the patient herself could do to prevent, alleviate or minimize the side-effects of therapy.

- Psychological support and strategies for coping with emotional reactions were also included.

- Practical advice on how to maintain natural skin integrity during the treatment.

- The patient was encouraged to call the nurse if any problems arose during the treatment period.

The authors found that this nursing care intervention minimized women's subjective distress during treatment. They concluded that this type of nursing intervention should be implemented in the outpatient setting of a radiation therapy clinic. The results have been supported by Faithfull et al.[30]

The patients' insights into their own healthcare needs, the meaning they attach to presenting signs and symptoms and their awareness of the ability or inability to engage in effective required self-care are essential information for nurses to have and use in helping the patients.

Future areas for development for empowerment and family caregiving

There is minimal research concerning patient empowerment. Most published research studies concern patient education programmes, which in some respect are based on empowerment philosophy. There is a need for more randomized studies where the effects of comprehensive interventions are evaluated.

In family caregiving, future areas of development include symptom management strategies, communication, defining patient outcomes and cost-effectiveness. With respect to symptom management, strategies need to be developed towards pharmacological and non-pharmacological approaches and how to monitor unwanted symptoms and side-effects. Research is needed in this area in order to understand key elements that lead to productive patient outcomes. Defining patient outcomes is essential in order to develop standards of family-centred care that link care with outcomes so that knowledge emerges on who is or isn't providing high-quality care, and which patients and families need more skills or information to achieve positive outcomes. If family care is to be included as a part of the healthcare system, research is needed that supports investment of time, information and education, and evidence that working with families leads to better patient outcomes at a lower cost while using less professional time.

CONCLUSION

This chapter provides an introduction to partnership in care from the perspective of the nurse and the patient and family. The families task of caregiver is complex and extensive and requires specific skills. It is necessary for nurses in cancer care to understand the dimensions and experience of caregiving in order to support the care of patients. The value of thorough assessment using structured approaches for mapping the needs of the patient and family with the purpose of offering support, enhancing or upholding the families cognitive, affective and behavioural function, have been described in this chapter. Multicultural aspects of nursing care for families have been illuminated with a model for developing cultural competence, including a model for cultural assessment. This chapter offers strategies for nurses to achieve patient empowerment. An interactive approach to education based on empowerment pedagogy could be of great value in cancer care as this shifts power to the patient and family.

REFERENCES

1. Given BA, Given CW. Family support in advanced cancer. CA Cancer J Clin 2001; 51:213–231.
2. Harding R, Higginson IJ. What is the best way to help caregivers in cancer and palliative care. A systematic literature review of interventions and their effectiveness. Palliat Med 2003; 17:63–74.
3. Shumacher KL, Stewart BJ, Archbold PG, Dodd MJ, Dibble SL. Family caregiving skill: development of the concept. Res Nurs Health 2000; 23:191–203.
4. Aranda AK, Hayman-White K. Home caregivers of the person with advanced cancer. Cancer Nurs 2001; 24(4):300–307.
5. Wright LM, Leahey M. Nurses and families: a guide to family assessment and intervention. 3rd edn. 1999, Philadelphia: FA Lewis; 1999.
6. Hilton BA, Crawford JA, Tarko MA. Men's perspectives on individual and family coping with their wives breast cancer and chemotherapy. West J Nurs Res 2000; 22:438–459.
7. Philips C, Gray RE, Fitch MI, et al. Early postsurgery experience of prostate cancer patients and spouses. Cancer Pract 2000; 8:165–171.
8. Rees CE, Bath PA. Exploring the information flow: partners of women with breast cancer, patients, and health care professionals. Oncol Nurs Forum 2000; 27:1267–1275.
9. Friesen P, Pepler C, Hunter P. Interactive family learning following a cancer diagnosis. Oncol Nurs Forum 2002; 29(6):981–987.
10. Wright LM, Leahey M. Nurses and families: a guide to family assessment and intervention. 3rd edn. Philadelphia: FA Davis; 2000.
11. Bell JM, Wright LM. The future of family nursing: interventions, interventions,

interventions. Jpn J Nurs Res1994; 27(2–3):4–15.

12. Galanti GA. Caring for patients from different cultures: case studies from American hospitals. 2nd edn. Philadelphia, PA: University of Pennsylvania Press; 1997.

13. Papadopoulos I, Tilki M, Taylor G. Transcultural care: a guide for health care professionals. Dinton: Quay Publications; 1998.

14. Congress EP. Clinical work with culturally diverse dying patients. Ethics Network News 1997; 4(3):5–6.

15. Andrews MM, Boyle JS. Transcultural concepts in nursing care. 3rd edn. 1999, Baltimore: Lippincott; 1999.

16. Kendall S, ed. Health and empowerment. Research and practice. London: Arnold; 1998.

17. Henderson S. Power imbalance between nurses and patients: a potential inhibitor of partnership in care. J Clin Nurs 2003; 12:501–508.

18. WHO. Ottawa Charter for Health Promotion. in Conference on Health Promotion. Copenhagen: WHO Regional Office for Europe; 1986.

19. Rappaport J. Studies in empowerment: introduction to the issue. Prevention in Human Services 1984; 3:1–7.

20. Mason DJ, Costello-Nickitas DM, Scanlan JM, Magnuson BA. Empowering nurses for politically astute change in the workplace. J Contin Educ Nurs 1991; 22(1):383–389.

21. Gibson CH. A concept analysis of empowerment. J Adv Nurs 1991; 16:354–361.

22. Piper SM, Brown PA. The theory of practice of health education applied to nursing: a bi-polar approach. J Adv Nurs 1998 27:383–389.

23. Golant M, Altman T, Martin C. Managing cancer side effects to improve quality of life: a cancer psychoeducation program. Cancer Nurs 2003; 26(1):37–44.

24. Devine E, Westlake S. The effects of psychoeducational care provided to adults with cancer: meta-analysis of 116 studies. Oncol Nurs Forum 1995; 22(9):1369–1381.

25. Fawzy NW. A psychoeducational nursing intervention to enhance coping and affective state in newly diagnosed malignant melanoma patients. Cancer Nurs 1995;18:427–438.

26. Davidson BJ, Degner LF. Empowerment of men newly diagnosed with prostate cancer. Cancer Nurs 1997; 20(3):187–196.

27. Dean K, Kickbush I. Health related behaviour in health promotion: utilizing the concept of self-care. Health Promotion International 1995; 10(1):35–40.

28. Orem DE. Nursing: concepts of practice. Chicago: Mosby-Year Book; 1995.

29. Wengström Y, Häggmark C, Strander H, Forsberg C. Effects of nursing intervention on subjective distress, side effects and quality of life of breast cancer patients receiving curative therapy – a randomized study. Acta Oncol 1999; 38(6):763–770.

30. Faithfull S, Corner J, Meyer L, Huddart R, Dearnaley D. Evaluation of a nurse-led follow up for patients undergoing pelvic radiotherapy. Br J Cancer 2001; 85(12):1853–1864.

CHAPTER 3

The Social and Cultural Context of Cancer Care

Karin Ahlberg

CHAPTER CONTENTS

Introduction	37	Coping resources	43	
		The concept of hope	44	
Cancer as a chronic illness	37	Spirituality	45	
The understanding of illness	38			
Recovering from a cancer disease	39	Communication about the subjective		
		experience of illness	46	
Attitudes towards end of life, dying		The patient's story	47	
and death	40			
		Conclusion	48	
Meaning and adaptation in connection				
with cancer	41	References	49	
Social factors that may influence				
meaning and adaptation	43			

INTRODUCTION

The goal of nursing practice is to support the individual's health experience, regardless of medically diagnosed health problems.[1–3] In order to accomplish this goal, nurses need to acknowledge the phenomenon of human responses to various life problems and to help people deal with the problems they experience. The primary idea of caring, defined as the central phenomenon or the essence of nursing,[4] is to alleviate human suffering and to preserve and safeguard life and health.[5,6] Caring represents an essential human need and a fundamental component of the nursing profession. Living with a long-term disease like cancer is a multidimensional phenomenon that may affect every aspect of a person's life. The meaning of living with cancer discloses changes in daily, family, social and working life. This chapter aims to provide a basis for improving the understanding of the patient's experience of living with a cancer disease. The chapter includes a description of cancer as a chronic illness, including its meaning and adaptation to the cancer disease journey. Furthermore, it explores how to use communication as a tool to support patients and their families on their cancer journey, with a particular focus on storytelling.

CANCER AS A CHRONIC ILLNESS

Living with a chronic illness, like cancer, may lead to a variety of changes and consequences for everyday life.[7,8] Chronic illness crashes into a person's life and separates the person in the present from the person in the past.[7] According to Frank,[9(p1)] serious illness is a loss of the 'destination and map' that had previously guided the ill person's life. Illness can be something that is experienced 'internally' or it can be defined 'externally' by somebody other than the individual. With an internal perspective, the basis is the patients' own descriptions of their situation.[10] External perspective disregards the individual's own subjective experience and deals instead with objective and measurable descriptions of disease. The English language differentiates between the concepts of illness and disease. Illness refers to a subjective experience of disease, whereas disease refers to objective changes in the appearance and/or function of the body.[11] A person can experience illness regardless of whether a disease is present or not. Symptoms are seen as an expression of the reality of the patient's world, linked to the stresses and experiences of that person and composed of both cultural and personal meaning. The first stage in treatment is therefore not to explain the disease, but rather to elicit the patient's version of the illness, and areas of most concern to the involved person.[12] Illness is the experience of loss or dysfunction and has more to do with perception, experience and behaviour than with psychological processes.[10,13] Illness is the same as being subjectively ill. Individuals are subjectively ill when they believe or know that they are ill and/or have a mental state resulting from internal causes.[14] Illness arises when the individual subjectively experiences ill health and suffering.

The experience of illness means so much more for the one who is ill compared with how a healthy person will understand the situation. People who are ill can be reminded of their poorly functioning body in everything they do – wherever they are. In order to deal with an afflicted person, it is important that the caregiver understands this, and has insight into the possible problems.

Disease and descriptions of what disease is can look very different in similar societies, depending on culture, and the same applies to different groups of people in each society.[15] The perception of what disease is also differs between various societies and social classes. In some cultures, cases where the experience of a disease can be demonstrated by both patient and caregiver have more legitimacy. Preferably, it should be possible to objectively observe the disease. According to Sachs,[15] a diagnosis fills at least four functions:

1 designation
2 confirmation
3 possibility for treatment and
4 legitimization.

Little is still known about gender differences when it comes to the experience of having a cancer. Variations in men's health may be understood as unfolding within the larger social, cultural and political contexts of gender relations that have emerged historically.[16] Research done in the USA shows that, in general, men suffer more severe chronic conditions, have higher death rates for all 15 leading causes of death, and die nearly 7 years younger than women.[17] Health-related beliefs and behaviours are important contributors to these differences. Men are also more likely than women to adopt beliefs and behaviours that increase their risks, and are less likely to engage in behaviours linked with health and longevity.[17]

The understanding of illness

A holistic viewpoint (including both an internal and external perspective) should be used to understand the situation and needs of a person suffering from cancer. In this manner, attention is paid both to the interaction between body and soul and the social sphere of the individual. From a holistic perspective, continuous attention is paid to interaction with the individuals, their environment and health. Cancer and its treatment have independent effects on the intrusiveness, illness-induced lifestyle disruptions that interfere with continued involvements in valued activities and interests of illness.[18] The provision of skilful psychosocial care to patients suffering from chronic illness starts with an appreciation of what it is like to live with a chronic condition. Definitions of self-esteem may be realigned when patients encounter a prolonged problem, with reliance on professional help. Getting inside the experience of such illness may be the key to understanding patient motivation, non-compliance with therapy and altered patterns of social engagement. Individuals' personal constructs may usefully then be used to explore the extent to which chronic illness sufferers share common problems and needs.[19]

Theories about perceived illness must be developed from the perspective of the patient rather than from the perspective of the caregiver. The discrepancy between the experience of the sick person and the viewpoint of the caregiver can be substantial. Only by eliciting descriptions of a patient's perception of an illness, can one develop an understanding of, and be able to satisfy, a patient's needs.[13] At the same time, Conrad[10] is of the opinion that it is not necessary to study the experience of illness from a patient perspective, but that the focus should be on how people experience and adapt their lives to a disease in daily living. According to Toombs,[11] a medical diagnosis is encumbered with both cultural and personal content and meaning. In Western medicine, disease is often regarded from a biomedical viewpoint, which means that the diagnosis of the patient is made from an external perspective. The body experienced by the patient and the body treated by a professional caregiver is seldom the same. For one individual with pain, the body can be a painful concern; for the caregiver the same body can be viewed as an object that has to be investigated or a problem that must be solved.[20]

Several researchers have attempted to create a model for how experienced illness can be understood. Such a model could lead to better insight for the caregiver as well as the basis for planning and implementing care. The model of Morse and Johnson, 'The Illness Constellation Model',[8] was constructed with the aid of grounded theory. The model is based on six basic assumptions that take into consideration:

1 the entire time during which the feeling of being ill developed

2 that perceptions of illness are dynamic and vary

3 the experiences of patients

4 similarities in perceptions instead of similarities in symptoms

5 a holistic perspective that includes the environment, the context and significant others

6 inductive theory formation.

The model describes various levels, where the initial level is characterized by feelings of uncertainty and the reactions of the patient's own body are observed. These experiences are confirmed when the individual realizes that the disruption is true and demands medical treatment. The next level involves rehabilitating the self. Here, we see an active search for the cause of what has occurred and for information. Thoughts about future consequences take shape. Finally, the individual resumes control over the situation and re-establishes relations with others. The effects of the illness then play a minor role and the trust of the individual in his own body is regained. According to Morse and Johnson,[13] the experience of illness results in a loss of normality. Before a person can experience a sense of well-being, normality must therefore be reconquered and previous roles resumed.

A few decades ago, cancer was a topic shrouded in social silence; today it is explored in television dramas and documentaries, in interviews on radio and in print, and in theatre productions. Stories of cancer have found a place in our culture.[21]

Recovering from a cancer disease

Cancer is not just a single event with a certain end but an enduring condition characterized by ongoing uncertainty, potentially delayed or late effects of the cancer disease or its treatment and concurrent psychosocial issues.[22] Survivors may experience symptoms with long-term effects, such as fatigue, aches and pain, that negatively impact quality of life.[23] Survivorship is a complex term, introduced in the middle of the 1960s, and initially referred to people who lived beyond catastrophic or traumatic events or the living family members of people who have died. Survivorship may be defined as the experience of 'living with, through, or beyond cancer',[24] but any attempt to provide a definition of survivorship remains unrealistic, with all the psychological difficulties that this uncertainty and regular monitoring induce.[25] Cancer survival may be identified as living at any time after diagnosis and treatment have finished, apparently free of cancer.[21] The term has come to represent the state or process of living after a diagnosis of cancer, regardless of how long a person lives.[22] It is a framework used by many healthcare professionals, researchers and cancer survivors to understand not only the physical but also the social, psychological and existential impact of cancer on one one's life and for the remainder of one's life.[22] (See Ch. 36 for a further examination of the concept of survivorship.)

Cancer survivorship is a tumultuous experience of balancing the elation of surviving life-threatening illness with the demands of chronic health concerns and altered life meaning.[26] Increased awareness of the needs of cancer survivors is enhanced by large studies of this growing population, but also by appreciation of individual stories of survivorship. Portraits of survival, in the form of personal narratives, contribute to our understanding of the experience of cancer.[26] The experience of a cancer diagnosis has been reported to occasion changes in patient's values, priorities, activities, relationships and self-perceptions. Research and clinical observations suggest, for example, that there is heightened spiritual awareness among patients surviving cancer.[27] Despite the difficulties with being ill, most patients seem able to adapt to their new life situation and to maintain or restore psychological well-being after an initial adjustment period of 1–2 years. To improve the well-being of cancer survivors, it may be important to continue encouraging them to share concerns and seek information from healthcare providers while strengthening feelings of self-worth.[28]

ATTITUDES TOWARDS END OF LIFE, DYING AND DEATH

Quality end-of-life care is increasingly recognized as an ethical obligation of healthcare providers. The diagnosis of a terminal illness may be seen as a crisis in the fullest sense of the word: an experience of distress or even despair that may in itself offer an opportunity for growth and meaning, as one learns to cope.[29] Measures to address physical, psychological and spiritual domains of end-of-life care have been identified as priorities, both by healthcare professionals and by cancer patients themselves.[29]

Spiritual needs especially – e.g. issues related to maintaining a sense of meaning, peace and hope in the face of advancing cancer – are now in focus.[29] Uncertainty is a common experience for patients living with cancer, particularly when treatment cannot assure disease cure. Some of the domains of quality end-of-life care identified from the professionals' perspective include overall quality of life, physical well-being and functioning, psychosocial well-being and functioning, spiritual well-being, patient perception of care and family well-being and functioning.[30] A study by Singer and colleagues,[31] with the purpose of identifying and describing elements of quality end-of-life care from the patient's perspective, found the following five domains:

- receiving adequate pain and symptom management
- avoiding inappropriate prolongation of dying
- achieving a sense of control
- relieving burden
- strengthening relationships with loved ones.

Singer and colleagues state that these domains, which characterize patients' perspectives on end-of-life care, can serve as focal points for improving the quality of end-of-life care.

Palliative care practitioners themselves have begun to deal with the issue of spirituality and interventions for spiritual suffering.[32,33] Rousseau[33] has outlined an approach for the treatment of spiritual suffering that is composed of the following steps:

1 controlling physical symptoms
2 providing a supportive presence
3 encouraging life review to assist in recognizing purpose, value and meaning
4 exploring guilt, remorse, forgiveness, reconciliation
5 facilitating religious expression
6 reframing goals
7 encouraging meditative practices, focusing on healing rather than cure.

The death of a loved one is acknowledged to be one of the most traumatic of life events. The majority of patients die in hospitals where shortcomings in end-of-life care are endemic and, too often, patients die alone.[34] The quality of care at the end of a patient's life is very important to the family of the patient and can directly affect the way the family deals with the death of their loved ones. There is evidence showing that although nursing staff are aware of medical and physical care needs, they may have insufficient knowledge about the patient as a person, which is a prerequisite for individualized patient-centred care.[35] A study by Sahlberg-Blom and colleagues[36] showed that the possibility of patients participating in decisions about care planning during the final phase of life seemed to be context-dependent. It was affected by many factors, such as the dying patient's personality, the social network, the availability of different forms of care, cultural values and the extent to which nurses and other caregivers of the different forms of care can and want to support the wishes of the patients and relatives in the decision-making process. To provide the best-possible care to dying patients, nurses and other healthcare professionals must attend to their physical, emotional and spiritual needs. They must also be aware of their own feelings towards death and dying.

What is a 'good death'? Despite a recent increase in the attention given to improving end-of-life care, our understanding of what constitutes a good death is surprisingly lacking. Patient involvement in decision-making has been advocated to improve the quality of life at the end of life. Patient and family members may define a 'good' death based on physical comfort, the quality of personal relationships, finding meaning in their life and death, feeling some sense of control in the situation and active preparations for death.[37] Steinhauser and colleagues[38] gathered descriptions of the components of a good death from patients, families and providers through focus group discussions and in-depth interviews. Participants identified six major components of a good death:

- pain and symptom management
- clear decision-making
- preparation for death
- completion
- contributing to others
- affirmation of the whole person.

The six themes are process-oriented attributes of a good death, and each has biomedical, psychological, social and spiritual components.

Patients and healthcare professionals do not adequately discuss patients' preferences for care at the end of life. This is often due to discomfort with talking about death and dying. Also, sometimes, healthcare professionals are afraid that discussing end-of-life care could cause harm. Talking and listening to patients about issues associated with death and dying is both important and difficult. To improve the quality of care at the end of life, we must address the quality of communication about end-of-life care, among other things.

The Swedish philosopher Lars Sandman[39] states that death is generally something bad for us but it can also be something good: i.e. due to us being in a situation that it would be better not to be in. Thus, we have reasons to continue with life to the extent that we can live a life of positive value. Probably, most people would, if it were possible to continue with such a life, desire and choose to do so.

MEANING AND ADAPTATION IN CONNECTION WITH CANCER

One of the most frequent approaches to finding meaning is by attempting to attribute a cause to the cancer. Whereas some patients immediately accept an explanation of cause with complete confidence, others are never certain as to what really caused their cancer.[40] Responsibility and blame may be related to attributing a cause to the cancer. Another aspect of finding meaning is constructing benefit to the negative experience of having cancer.[41]

People often do not see their experience of illness as a disease process, but more in terms of symptoms and how they affect their daily lives.[11] Chronic illness may have significance for the individual's identity and life course, and people with a chronic illness often suffer from identity-loss. Therefore, the illness and its consequences for identity need significantly more attention. It is, for example, important that caregivers, relatives and friends grasp the changes the individual is going through.[42] The perspective of identity after the onset of illness may be influenced by symbolic interactionism, which focuses on the meaning the events hold for people and on the symbols which convey this meaning. Through experience and interaction with others, this meaning is continually developed and modified throughout life. Diagnosis with a life-threatening illness can lead to many changes, called self-transformation, in one's self. These changes are not well understood. People with cancer are likely to encounter a loss of personal control as a result of their illness experience. An empowerment perspective, which emphasizes the possibility of patients 'owning their own lives', is useful for understanding the interpersonal and social dynamics of patients' loss of control and for guiding the development of strategies aimed at maximizing control. Empowerment may be conceptualized as a social process of recognizing, promoting and enhancing people's abilities to meet their own needs, solve their own problems and mobilize the necessary resources in order to feel in control of their own lives. Because the factors influencing an individual's sense of control are multi-levelled, optimal empowerment occurs when strategies are employed at several levels of social organization.[43]

The desire to give life purpose, to actualize values, is called the 'will to meaning' by Frankl,[44] who sees the search for meaning as the primary motivational force in humankind. This meaning is unique and specific to the individual and it must be fulfilled by the individual alone.[44] The period following a cancer diagnosis has been described as a time when concerns about life and death predominate. Park and Folkman[45] describe the concept of meaning as a general life orientation, as personal significance, as causality, as a coping mechanism and as an outcome. The authors also describe two levels of meaning: first, the global meaning, and secondly, the situational meaning. The meaning that individuals with cancer ascribe to their experiences of illness and disease may influence the ways in which they cope with their illness and disease.[46]

A study with the purpose of describing what was involved in the process of the personal search for meaning conducted by patients[47] found six major themes:

- seeking an understanding of the personal significance of the diagnosis
- looking at the consequences of the cancer diagnosis
- reviewing life
- change in outlook toward self, life and others
- living with the cancer
- hope.

Two significant factors were found: faith and social support. With an understanding of the different components in an individual's search for meaning of life, the nurse can facilitate the process by which patients explore what cancer means for their lives.[47] To discover the different meanings of cancer for older women who are long-term survivors of breast cancer, Utley,[48] using a heuristic approach, showed three meanings of cancer:

- cancer as sickness and death
- cancer as an obstacle
- cancer as transforming.

The author concluded that as the women worked through their cancer experience, their perspectives changed. The meaning of cancer after surviving the disease and its treatment centred on positive, insightful experiences and expansive, renewing interactions with their environment. Further research examining the meaning of cancer is needed to broaden the transferability of the findings to other groups. Understanding the meaning of cancer for older women who are long-term breast cancer survivors may enhance nurses' sensitivity to survivors' perspectives. Knowledge of survivors' different meanings of cancer may help to paint a new vision of cancer survivorship comprising potentially positive, transforming experiences.[48] The meaning that patients with cancer ascribe to their disease may well have an impact on the effectiveness of coping strategies used to come to terms with cancer. Healthcare professionals need to know what meanings patients with cancer ascribe to their disease if they are to identify maladaptive coping strategies and ensure that patients receive the support they need in order to promote physical and psychological recovery.[46]

In the past few years it has become increasingly clear that many factors either facilitate or hinder the process of adaptation to a cancer diagnosis; these factors may be either internal to the individual or external.[49] Examples of the internal factors include an individual's sense of coherence,[50] sense of efficacy,[51] perceived control[52] and style of coping.[53] Examples of external factors are the resources that people have at their disposal, including fiscal resources such as income and health insurance, and social resources such as loving and supportive relationships, a network of friends and relatives and a supportive work environment.[49] In the theory of general vulnerability, Cassel[54] highlights the fact that a lack of social support and social network has a negative effect on the individual's physical health. Lazarus[55] stressed that coping is a process, and that coping changes over time and in accordance with the situational contexts in which it occurs. He concluded that the different research approaches of viewing coping as either a style or process are both needed as they address different aspects of the problem.[55] Adaptive coping strategies, such as seeing illness as a challenge, seem to be important in promoting positive feelings about disease and illness.[46]

An experience of cancer can be personally challenging and devastating. Nurses are ideal health professionals to guide patients through this period in their life because they are in the unique position of being an immediate source of support in patient care. It is therefore essential for nurses to understand the challenge that cancer presents to self-concept in order to facilitate coping and adaptation.[56]

Social factors that may influence meaning and adaptation

The extent to which the physical, social, emotional, spiritual or financial concomitants of illness affect well-being may be dependent on the social roles (e.g. spouse, parent or job) in which stressors are experienced.[57,58] Thoits[57] states that stressors arising within certain roles are capable of creating distress because they serve to undermine the identity associated with those roles. Events occurring in specific social roles may be identity-enhancing when individuals are successful at solving role-specific problems caused by a disruption, but are identity-threatening when they cannot.[57,59] Life-changing events are disruptive to the extent that they cause an interruption of the normal process of identity formation and a failure to bring self-perception into line with an underlying identity standard. When individuals perceive themselves as not living up to an expectation or ideal of whom or what they believe they should be, distress is the result.[22] Stress may be explained as the experience of a disruption of meaning, understanding and smooth functioning with possible consequences for the person, in the form of harm, loss or challenge.[60] Stress emotions trigger various coping strategies to enable adjustment.[61] Although all individuals experience stress, people interpret and react differently.

Coping resources

In order to develop and solve problems, one has to have the ability to cope. Coping is generally acknowledged as a complex and multidimensional concept. One of the most accepted definitions is the one proposed by Lazarus and Folkman.[61(p141)] They define coping as 'constantly changing cognitive and behavioural effort to manage specific external and/or internal demands that are appraised as taxing or exceeding the resources of the person', or, more simple stated, 'coping is the effort to manage stress'.[62] Coping is a process concerned with what a person actually thinks and does in a specific context and with the changes in thoughts and actions that occur as the 'situation' proceeds.[61] Weisman[63] states that 'good copers' understand the difference between being hopeless and powerless. 'Poor copers' usually feel powerless, sick or well. Further, the crux dividing 'good copers' and 'bad copers' is the difference between resourcefulness and rigidity. For 'good copers', cancer is a burden, but not crushing.

It is perhaps impossible to experience anything without finding meaning in the experience. Because the act of searching for and finding meaning is such a basic experience, it greatly affects the way people handle events in their lives.[64] Antonowsky[65] has influenced the development of the concept of health in line with the individual's perspective and in the context of wholeness. In 1979, Antonowsky[66] presented a theoretical model designed to advance understanding of the relations among stressors, coping and health. This model later formed the foundation of a salutogenesis orientation called sense of coherence (SOC) (*saluto* = health, *genesis* = the origins of). The concept of SOC is a mirror for the assumption that individuals have to cope with situations of distress. The SOC is defined as:

> a global orientation that expresses the extent to which one has a pervasive, enduring though dynamic feeling of confidence that (1) the stimuli deriving from one's internal and external environments in the course of living are structured, predictable, and explicable; (2) the resources are available to one to meet the demands posed by these stimuli; and (3) these demands are challenges, worthy of investment and engagement.[65 (p19)]

These three components are called comprehensibility, manageability and meaningfulness, respectively. Antonovsky hypothesizes that the stronger the SOC world outlook of a person, the more likely will he be able to cope successfully with life stressor situations. Sense of coherence is applicable to individuals and groups as well as to society at large.

A sense of coherence is important for moving towards the healthy pole of the continuum. The person who experiences the world as comprehensible expects that future stimuli will be predictable or, when they come as a surprise, they will be orderable and explicable. People who experience their world as manageable have the sense, aided by their own resources or by those of trustworthy others, that they will be able to cope. A person who experiences the world as meaningful will not be overcome by unhappy experiences but will experience them as challenges, is determined to seek meaning in them and will do his best to overcome them with dignity. Theoretically, sense of coherence is assumed to be consistent in adult life,[65] and it has been empirically proved that SOC is a relatively stable characteristic.[67] On the other hand, SOC can quickly change in a negative direction, e.g. in connection with a hospital stay.[65] Previous research indicates that relatively disadvantaged sociodemographic groups (women, the poor, the unmarried) are more vulnerable to the impacts of life events. More recently, researchers have hypothesized that the psychological vulnerability of these groups may be due to the joint occurrence of many stress events and few psychological resources with which to cope with such events.[68] Although a sense of personal control and perceived social support influence physical health and mental health both directly and as stress buffers, the theoretical mechanisms through which they do so still require elaboration and testing. New work suggests that coping flexibility and the structural constraints placed on individuals' coping efforts may be important to pursue. Promising new directions in social support research include studies of the negative effects of social relationships and of support giving, mutual-coping and support-giving dynamics, optimal 'matches' between individuals' needs and support received, and properties of groups that can provide a sense of social support.[69]

The concept of hope

Hope is a subtle expectation regarding an abstract but positive aspect of the future, and is an important factor influencing the quality and perhaps the quantity of life for people who have life-threatening or chronic illnesses.[70] The philosopher Marcel has described hope as something very real that transcends all particular objects and is more concerned with a person as a being.[71,72] Marcel states that there must be an interaction between one who gives and one who receives hope and that this intersubjectivity between self and others is essential to hope as an inner force for human survival.

Hope is frequently referred to as important for coping with a disease such as cancer. Hope enables people to cope with difficult and stressful situations and suffering, and is considered to be of great significance for people diagnosed with cancer; thus, it is an important aspect of nursing care.[73] Hope has been conceptualized as an emotion,[73,74] and is an important coping resource for people experiencing difficult situations.[75] Lazarus[74] suggested that hope results from a unique pattern of thoughts and evaluations about a situation and is important for sustaining commitment to desired goals and coping. Koopmeiners and colleagues[76] state that healthcare professionals do influence patients' perceptions of their hope. Although most nursing actions are hope-enhancing, nurses can reduce a patient's sense of hope if information provided or attitude towards the patient is insensitive or disrespectful. Previous studies have shown that social support,[77,78] self-esteem[77,79] and spirituality or support from religious beliefs[80] are important factors for maintaining hope during illness. However, Yates[81] concluded in 1993 that there are many questions about the experience of hope and its impact on the lives of patients with cancer which remain to be answered, and it seems that we still have a lack of knowledge within the area, 20 years later.

A phenomenological study designed to further understanding concerning the concept of hope in a purposive sample of 9 patients with cancer hospitalized for bone marrow transplantation (BMT)[82] showed that participants used six strategies to foster their hope during preparation for BMT:

- feeling connected with God
- affirming relationships
- staying positive
- anticipating survival
- living in the present
- fostering ongoing accomplishment.

Religious practices and family members were the most frequently identified sources of hope. The findings of this study may provide a base for the improvement of nursing practice. The variable that seems to be the one with the single most positive contribution to hope is whether the patient lives alone, particularly when it comes to younger people. Gender, the time elapsed since diagnosis and treatments seem to have no observable effect on the global hope score. However, age, education level and type of cancer can be associated with particular domains of hope.[83]

A frequently heard response from patients and healthcare professionals is 'you can't take away hope'. The line may sometimes be used by healthcare professionals as an excuse for not telling patients the truth. The rationale behind this has often more to do with protecting clinicians from discomfort than protecting the patient.[84] When a patient receives information, the information will become a part of different types of cognitive activities such as analysing, comparing and organizing in a new way in order to make reality comprehensible. The central issue is not whether to tell the truth or not, but how the truth is told. According to Buckman,[85] bad news is information that drastically and negatively alters how the individual views his future. Supporting patients and reinforcing hopes are parts of the foundation of a therapeutic relationship.[84]

Spirituality

Commitment to viewing health care in a holistic manner must include the patient's spiritual concerns.[86] Historically, research on spirituality has focused on religiosity but measures of religious practice are not always reliable indicators of spirituality. Spirituality encompasses man's need to find satisfactory answers to questions about the meaning of life, illness and death.[86] Spirituality may be seen as a belief that relates a person to the world, giving meaning to existence, life, illness and death, and that guides people in the world.[87,88]

A study that was undertaken to describe how Swedish nursing staff characterize spiritual needs in a broad context, including both religious and existential issues, concluded that there was a willingness to pay attention to spiritual and existential needs, but nurses still have difficulty defining what such care should include.[89] The nurses had, for example, some difficulty distinguishing between spiritual and psychosocial care. Taylor and colleagues[90] showed that oncology nurses provide spiritual care in a variety of ways, e.g. praying with patients, referring them to chaplains or clergy, providing them with religious materials, serving as a therapeutic presence and listening and talking to them, yet they do so infrequently and with some discomfort. Integrating patients' spiritual values into health care is important to quality of care.[91] To be able to provide holistic care, including the spiritual dimension, healthcare professionals must dare to use and develop their own skills and possibilities to comfort patients in existential crises struggling with life questions.[92] One study with the purpose of identifying factors that predict nurses' spiritual care perspectives and practices and comparing these between nurses in two subspecialties showed that the hospice nurses used traditional spiritual care interventions more frequently and held more positive perspectives regarding spiritual caregiving than oncology nurses.[93] However, what determined spiritual care practices and perspectives most was the spirituality of the nurse. The authors state that nurses must continue to explore how their personal spirituality contributes to their caregiving.[93] Spiritual care education, including both theoretical and practical aspects, is also needed.[94]

COMMUNICATION ABOUT THE SUBJECTIVE EXPERIENCE OF ILLNESS

Communication is the most important tool we have to support patients and their families on their cancer journey.[95] Communication serves to establish trust and rapport, reduce anxiety and uncertainty, educate, provide support and help establish a treatment plan.[95]

Patients with cancer consistently identify communication as an area of central importance. Communication is a vital component of nursing care that can improve outcomes for patients with cancer and their families in terms of psychological distress.[96] Ineffective communication has negative effects on patient care and causes stress when nurses interact with each other, with medical colleagues and with patients and their relatives. Miscommunication, including inadequate communication and illegible or incomplete documentation, forms a basis for many clinical and interpersonal problems in nursing practice. Patients can be the victims of healthcare professionals' communication difficulties at a time when they are disempowered by their health problems and associated stresses. Wilkinson[97] states that effective communication is achieved when open

two-way communication takes place and patients are informed about the nature of their illness and treatment and encouraged to express their anxieties and emotions.

Listening to what a patient has to say is a general necessity in order to understand the patient's perception of the illness.[98] The subjective experience dimension of illness is difficult to communicate, since its language differs from the medical language.[20] Cancer-related fatigue (CRF) is an example of this. Since CRF is not like the normal tiredness that we sometimes experience, language lacks the ability to describe the experience. Words that are normally used suddenly become insufficient. This can have the result that we do not correctly interpret what the patient tells us.

The subject of cancer is an emotionally charged area and nurses often feel limited in their ability to communicate in an effective way. Nurses often use simple, everyday language that may be said to be informal. According to Bourhis and colleagues,[99] this often replaces medical language, making it easier to communicate with patients and their families. For seriously ill patients, a good relationship with the nurse may be particularly important. Patients who have confidence in their nurse may be glad to allow the nurse to act as their advocate and speak on their behalf if and when they are unable to plead their own case. Conversation is also a means of establishing or strengthening the relationship between patient and nurse, as well as giving emotional support.

The meaning of illness is appreciated when thoughtful communication respects the individual's needs and responses. By encouraging patients to describe their thoughts, hopes and fears about their illness, clinicians will understand what is meaningful in life. Because creating meaning is an individual process, nurses must listen to the patient's personal story and look for the meaning of illness embedded in it.[100] In a phenomenological perspective, it is the body that is the medium that gives us access to the world.[11] All consciousness is embodied, and the body is a prerequisite for understanding human experience. We all experience the world from our own unique position in the world. Madjar and Walton[101] show two fundamental prerequisites for a phenomenological perspective in care:

- the art of contemplation
- the art of formulating one's contemplation.

A phenomenological perspective provides an opportunity to study and reflect on human experiences in the context of a living world and to reflect on the soul of caregiving. Depending on the topic, it may be more or less complicated to communicate, for example, information about death or disease progress than information about symptom management. End-of-life decision-making is often a difficult process and one that many patients and their families will undergo. Providers who are experienced and comfortable are more likely to engage in communication and assessment strategies that facilitate end-of-life decision-making.

The patient's story

We all experience the world from our own unique position in the world. Theories about illness must therefore be developed from the perspective of the patient rather than the healthcare professional.[102] Narrative communication gives access to patients' experiences of an unwanted and painful physiological process leading to forced embodiment of sickness.[103] Narrative practice, in the format of storytelling and listening, leads to ethics-based care that prioritizes the patients' personal meanings, values staff–patient relationships and permits them to define quality care.[104] Individuals' questions about the meaning of their lives can be answered in part by telling life stories. Stories of the past influence human thought and may serve as a vehicle for transmitting beliefs and values, world views and frameworks for making meaning. Stories of the present enable a person to integrate the past with the present in order to find meaning for the future; stories assist people to make the past, present and future meaningful.[105] Taylor[106] believes that storytelling promotes well-being for patients with cancer in several ways. Encouraging people to tell their stories allows them to organize their thoughts and experiences, to further reflect on their past and to make sense of their life. Storytelling also allows them to share and connect with the listener. Finally, storytelling allows the individual to transmit values and leave a legacy.[106]

Many scholars and medical professionals argue over the importance of metaphor in thinking about, and speaking of, cancer and other illnesses. The experience of cancer and cancer therapy obviously involves the patient's body. To comprehend what is happening is a process full of uncertainty and obscurity. Metaphors, such as the cancer 'eating away', are widespread and persistent, whereas the meaning of that metaphor today mirrors new scientific and lay explanations of cancer and cancer treatment. Personal newly created metaphors express threatening experiences in which fear of losing oneself and fear of death are involved. Ambivalent hope in relation to treatment and caregivers is expressed. Creating new metaphors involves imaginatively using the available concepts and metaphors. A study by Gibbs and Franks[107] presents an analysis of the metaphors used by 6 women in their narratives of their experiences with cancer. They claim from their analyses that metaphorical talk about cancer reflects enduring metaphorical patterns of thought. Women used multiple, sometimes contradictory metaphors to conceptualize their complex cancer experiences. Many of their metaphors used to understand cancer are actually based on ordinary embodied experiences such that people still refer to the healthy body in trying to understand cancer even when their own bodies have been disrupted.[107] Majdar and Walton[101] feel that the narrative has an important place, where both narration and listening are important to understand and envision the meaning of caregiving. Benner[108] is of the opinion that narration is important for reflection. Since a narrative is often unsymmetrical and rich in details, openness is of great value. According to Dahlberg and Drew,[109] openness means to enter the world of the patient with curiosity and to let the patient teach us about the phenomenon.

We learn early on to tell our stories in various ways to suit different occasions. The listener or listeners are co-creators of the narrative. There are culturally determined recipes or patterns for how one should arrange one's words and for what kind of language and verbal images one should use. The environment, the context and the participants in a conversation influence our choices of language and phrasing. An individual's experience cannot be communicated directly; it must be transferred through symbols, metaphor and interpretation. According to Ricoeur,[110] understanding must be engendered through explanation. The narrative, Ricoeur says, contains a flow of meaning and can cause a person's lived experience to be seen in a new way. Narratives are found in many different forms: they are heard, seen and read; they are spoken, performed, painted, sculpted and written; and they are international, transhistorical and transcultural.[111] Through conversation, we get to know other people and learn something of their experiences, feelings and hopes and about the world in which they live; the conversation is a fundamental form of human interaction.

A conversation presumes that the listener has sufficient empathy to allow her to enter into the speaker's perceptual world, life world, existential situation or professional world so that an authentic dialogue can arise between them, out of which relevant information can emerge. This requires the listener to be much more than just physically present. Starrin and Renck[112] believe that every conversation is a unique social interaction that contains a negotiation of social roles and frames of reference, primarily between strangers. According to Mishler,[113] every conversation has a dynamic function and triggers narration. Individuals talking to each other can often clarify and understand important events in their lives by talking about them.[114] There is a temporal order that is associated with some form of change. How the narrative is created in the context of illness, for instance, is based on how the narrator experiences her body and is related to the perception of illness, life and culture.[115] The experience is brought back to life through its telling, and this creates a new frame that can contribute to a change in perception, although the new narrative is not necessarily less true than the original. Metaphors are an important part of the narrative. When we encounter something new and strange, we try to find something in the unknown that in some way resembles the known, by which means we insert it into a familiar frame of reference. The narrative may thus be legitimized when a person with cancer, for instance, is meant to understand and explain illness situations and process events.

Narrators must be given time and space to tell their story – to reside in and describe in detail important moments in their lives. It is very important to facilitate and help people who want to talk about important and meaningful events from their lives – the interview will consist of the types of questions that make this facilitation possible. Certain open questions are better than others at eliciting narrative responses. It is preferable to ask questions that open up the subject and allow the respondent/informant to construct responses in collaboration with the listener. Narratives, especially those having to do with critical life events, are often long and full of tangents, comments, retrospection, thoughts about the future and evaluating arguments. It is significant to give respondents the opportunity to answer the questions in a way they find meaningful. An interview is a conversation in which both parties participate, the narrator and the listener/interviewer; they develop the content together. The listener can clear up uncertainty through follow-up questions and an enriching conversation can evolve between the parties. But this often means that the listener must remain silent and allow the narrator time and space to talk about important life events.

CONCLUSION

The knowledge base within cancer nursing is continually expanding, but we also need to build bridges between the patients' perspectives and the healthcare professionals' perspectives. It is important for healthcare professionals to understand the way people with cancer experience the illness. The individual as a whole must be the basis of every contact in health care. Nurses working with severely ill patients need to have time for their own reflections, conversations and supervision to be able to have the strength to carry out their work.

If nurses want to understand what a patient with cancer experiences, a dialogue must be initiated with the patient. The narrative method is being increasingly seen as a valid method of tapping into patients' experiences of their illness. However, the use of narratives is complex, with a diversity of approaches often being presented. Everyday practice provides the context for both patients and healthcare professionals' experience and for the development of expertise from which our patients profit. Narrative, as transformable acts of caring, and the narrative structure of preverbal acts and contexts of care, are naturally connected to the art of nursing and await further research.[116]

REFERENCES

1. Parse RR. Man-living-health. A theory of nursing. Chichester: John Wiley and Sons; 1981.

2. Neuman B. Health as an expanding consciousness. St Louis: C.V. Mosby; 1986.

3. King IM. Health as the goal for nursing. Nurs Sci Q 1990; 3(1):123–128.

4. Leininger MM. Care, the essence of nursing and health. Detroit: Wayne State University Press; 1988.

5. Eriksson K. Understanding the world of the patient, the suffering human being: the new clinical paradigm from nursing to caring. Adv Pract Nurs Q 1997; 3:8–13.

6. Lindholm L, Eriksson K. The dialectic of health and suffering: an ontological perspective of young people's health. Qualitative Health Res 1998; 8:513–525.

7. Corbin J, Strauss AL. Accompaniments of chronic illness. Changes in body, self, biography, and biographical time. Res Sociol Health Care 1987; 6:249–281.

8. Morse JM. Responding to threats to integrity of self. Adv Nurs Sci 1997; 19:21–36.

9. Frank AW. The wounded storyteller. Body, illness, and ethics. Chicago: University of Chicago Press; 1995.

10. Conrad P. The experience of illness: recent and new directions. Res Sociol Health Care 1987; 6:1–31.

11. Toombs K. The meaning of illness: a phenomenological account of the different perspectives of physician and patient. In: Engelhardt HT Jr, Spicker SF, eds. Philosophy and medicine, Vol. 42. Netherlands: Kluwer Academic; 1993:1–161.

12. Tishelman C, Taube A, Sachs L. Self-reported symptom distress in cancer patients: reflections of disease, illness or sickness. Soc Sci Med 1991; 33(11):1229–1240.

13. Morse JM, Johnson JL. The illness experience. Dimensions of suffering. London: Sage Publications; 1991.

14. Nordenfelt L. Quality of life, health and happiness. Aldershot, England: Avebury; 1993.

15. Sachs L. Vårdens etnografi. Malmö: Almqvist & Wiksell Förlag AB; 1992 [in Swedish].

16. Sabo D. Men's health studies: origins and trends. J Am Coll Health 2000; 49(3):133–142.

17. Courtenay WH. Constructions of masculinity and their influence on men's well-being: a theory of gender and health. Soc Sci Med 2000; 50(10):1385–1401.

18. Devins GM, Edworthy SM, Seland TP, et al. Differences in illness intrusiveness across rheumatoid arthritis, end-stage renal disease, and multiple sclerosis. J Nerv Ment Dis 1993; 181(6):377–381.

19. Price B. Illness careers: the chronic illness experience. J Adv Nurs 1996; 24(2):275–279.

20. Gadow S. Body and self: a dialectic. In: Kestenbaum I, ed. V. The humanity of the ill. Phenomenological perspectives. Knoxville: The University of Tennessee Press; 1982.

21. Little M, Paul K, Jordens CF, Sayers EJ. Survivorship and discourses of identity. Psycho-oncology 2002; 11(2):170–178.

22. Zebrack BJ. Cancer survivor identity and quality of life. Cancer Pract 2000; 8(5):238–242.

23. Zebrack BJ, Chesler MA. Quality of life in childhood cancer survivors. Psycho-oncology 2002; 11(2):132–141.

24. Leigh S. Myths, monsters, and magic: personal perspectives and professional challenges of survival. Oncol Nurs Forum 1992; 19(10):1475–1480.

25. Ganz PA. Late effects of cancer and its treatment. Semin Oncol Nurs 2001; 17(4):241–248.

26. Ferrell BR, Dow KH. Portraits of cancer survivorship: a glimpse through the lens of survivors' eyes. Cancer Pract 1996; 4(2): 76–80.

27. Highfield MF. Spiritual health of oncology patients. Nurse and patient perspectives. Cancer Nurs 1992; 15(1):1–8.

28. Dirksen SR, Erickson JR. Well-being in Hispanic and non-Hispanic white survivors of breast cancer. Oncol Nurs Forum 2002; 29(5):820–826.

29. Breitbart W. Spirituality and meaning in supportive care: spirituality- and meaning-centred group psychotherapy interventions in advanced cancer. Supportive Care in Cancer. Published online: 28 August, 2001:1–15.

30. Field MJ, Cassel CK, eds. Approaching death: improving care at the end of life. Institute of

Medicine Report. Washington, DC: National Academy Press; 1997.

31. Singer PA, Martin DK, Kelner M. Quality end-of-life care: patients' perspectives. JAMA 1999; 281(2):163–168.

32. Puchalski C, Romer AL. Taking a spiritual history allows clinicians to understand patients more fully. J Palliat Med 2000; 3:129–137.

33. Rousseau P. Spirituality and the dying patient. J Clin Oncol 2000; 18:2000–2002.

34. Pantilat SZ. End-of-life care for the hospitalized patient. Med Clin N Am 2002; 86(4):749–770.

35. Hermansson AR, Ternestedt BM. What do we know about the dying patient? Awareness as a means to improve palliative care. Med Law 2000; 19(2):335–344.

36. Sahlberg-Blom E, Ternestedt BM, Johansson JE. Patient participation in decision making at the end of life as seen by a close relative. Nurs Ethics 2000; 7(4):296–313.

37. Hanson LC, Danis M, Garrett J. What is wrong with end-of-life care? Opinions of bereaved family members. J Am Geriatr Soc 1997; 45(11):1339–44.

38. Steinhauser KE, Clipp EC, McNeilly M, et al. In search of a good death: observations of patients, families, and providers. Ann Intern Med 2000; 132(10):825–832.

39. Sandman L. A good death. On the value of death and dying. ACTA Universitatis Gothoburgensis, Goteborg, 2002.

40. Taylor Johnston E. Spiritual and ethical end-of-life concerns. In: Yarbro CH, Frogge MH, Goodman M, Groenwald S, eds. Cancer nursing. Principles and practice. 5th edn. Boston: Jones and Bartlett; 2000:1565–1578.

41. Thompson SC, Pitts J. Factors relating to a person ability to find meaning after a diagnosis of cancer. J Psychosoc Oncol 1993; 11:1–21.

42. Asbring P. Chronic illness – a disruption in life: identity-transformation among women with chronic fatigue syndrome and fibromyalgia. J Adv Nurs 2001;34(3):312–319.

43. Gray RE, Doan BD, Church K. Empowerment and persons with cancer: politics in cancer medicine. J Palliat Care 1990; 6(2):33–45.

44. Frankl VE. Man's search for meaning: an introduction to logotherapy. Boston: Beacon; 1959.

45. Park C, Folkman S. Meaning in the context of stress and coping. Rev Gen Psychol 1997; 1:115–144.

46. Luker KA, Beaver K, Leinster SJ, et al. Information needs and sources of information for women with breast cancer: a follow-up study. J Adv Nurs 1996; 23(3):487–495.

47. O'Connor AP, Wicker CA, Germino BB. Understanding the cancer patient's search for meaning. Cancer Nurs 1990; 13(3):167–175.

48. Utley R. The evolving meaning of cancer for long-term survivors of breast cancer. Oncol Nurs Forum 1999; 26(9):1519–1523.

49. Bloom J, Stewart S, Johnston M, et al. Intrusiveness of illness and quality of life in young women with breast cancer. Psycho-oncology 1998; 7:89–100.

50. Antonowsky A. The structure and properties of the Sense of Coherence Scale. Soc Sci Med 1993; 36:725–733.

51. Bandura A. Self-efficacy: towards a unifying theory of behaviour change. Psychol Rev 1977; 84:191–215.

52. Wallston BS, Wallston KA, Kaplan GD, et al. Development and validation of the health locus of control (HLC) scale. J Consult Clin Psychol 1976; 44(4):580–585.

53. Lazarus R. Stress and coping as factors in health and illness. In: Cohen J, Cullen J, Martin RM, eds. Psychosocial aspects of cancer. New York: Raven Press; 1982:163–190.

54. Cassel J. The contribution of the social environment to host resistance. Am J Epidemiol 1976; 104:107–123.

55. Lazarus RS. Coping theory and research: past, present and future. Psychosom Med 1993; 55:234–247.

56. Cook NF. Self-concept and cancer: understanding the nursing role. Br J Nurs 1999; 8(5):318–324.

57. Thoits PA. On merging identity theory and stress research. Soc Psychol Q 1991; 54:101–112.

58. Pearlin LI. The sociological study of stress. J Health Soc Behav 1989; 30(3):241–256.

59. Thoits PA. Stressors and problem-solving: the individual as psychological activist. J Health Soc Behav 1994; 35(2):143–160.

60. Benner P, Wrubel J. The primacy of caring: stress and coping in health and illness. Menlo Park, CA: Addison-Wesley; 1989.

61. Lazarus RS, Folkman S. Stress, appraisal and coping. New York: Springer; 1984.

62. Lazarus RS. Stress and emotion: a new synthesis. New York: Springer; 1999.

63. Weisman A. Coping with cancer. New York: McGraw-Hill; 1979.

64. Steeves RH. Patients who have undergone bone marrow transplantation: their quest for meaning. Oncol Nurs Forum 1992 ;19(6):899–905.

65. Antonowsky A. Unravelling the mystery of health: how people manage stress and stay well. San Francisco: Jossey-Bass; 1987.

66. Antonowsky A. Health, stress and coping. New perspectives on mental and physical well-being. San Francisco: Jossey-Bass; 1979.

67. Langius A, Björvell H, Antonovsky A. The sense of coherence concept and its relation to personality traits in Swedish samples. Scand J Caring Sci 1992; 3:165–171.

68. Thoits PA. Life stress, social support, and psychological vulnerability: epidemiological

considerations. J Community Psychol 1982; 10(4):341–362.

69. Thoits PA. Stress, coping, and social support processes: where are we? What next? J Health Soc Behav 1995; 53–79.

70. Stoner M. Measuring hope. In: Frank-Stromborg M, Olsen J, eds. Instruments for clinical health-care research. London: Jones and Bartlett; 1997;189–201.

71. Marcel G. The mystery of being. Vol 11: Faith and reality. South Bend, IN: Regnery/Gateway; 1951.

72. Marcel G. Desire and hope. In: Lawrence N, O'Connor D, eds. Readings in existential phenomenology. Englewood Cliffs, NJ: Prentice-Hall; 1967:277.

73. Rustoen T. Hope and quality of life, two central issues for cancer patients: a theoretical analysis. Cancer Nurs 1995; 18(5):355–361.

74. Lazarus RS: Emotion and adaptation. New York: Oxford University Press; 1991.

75. Ebright PR, Lyon B. Understanding hope and factors that enhance hope in women with breast cancer. Oncol Nurs Forum 2002; 29(3):561–568.

76. Koopmeiners L, Post-White J, Gutknecht S, et al. How healthcare professionals contribute to hope in patients with cancer. Oncol Nurs Forum 1997;24(9):1507–1513.

77. Foote AW, Piazza D, Holcombe J, Paul P, Daffin P. Hope, self-esteem and social support in persons with multiple sclerosis. J Neurosci Nurs 1990; 22(3):155–159.

78. Gibson PR. Hope in multiple chemical sensitivity: social support and attitude towards healthcare delivery as predictors of hope. J Clin Nurs 1999; 8(3):275–283.

79. Piazza D, Holcombe J, Foote A, et al. Hope, social support and self-esteem of patients with spinal cord injuries. J Neurosci Nurs 1991; 23(4):224–30.

80. Herth KA. The relationship between level of hope and level of coping response and other variables in patients with cancer. Oncol Nurs Forum 1989;16(1):67–72.

81. Yates P. Towards a reconceptualization of hope for patients with a diagnosis of cancer. J Adv Nurs 1993; 18(5):701–706.

82. Saleh US, Brockopp DY. Hope among patients with cancer hospitalized for bone marrow transplantation: a phenomenologic study. Cancer Nurs 2001; 24(4):308–314.

83. Rustoen T, Wiklund I. Hope in newly diagnosed patients with cancer. Cancer Nurs 2000; 23(3):214–219.

84. Buckman R. Communication skills in palliative care: a practical guide. Neurol Clin 2001; 19(4):989–1004.

85. Buckman R. Doctors can improve on way they deliver bad news, MD maintains. Interview by Evelyne Michaels. CMAJ 1992; 146(4):564–566.

86. Ellerhorst-Ryan J. Instruments to measure aspects of spirituality. In: Frank-Stromborg M, Olsen J, eds. Instruments for clinical health-care research. London: Jones and Bartlett; 1997:202–212.

87. Soeken K, Carson V. Responding to the spiritual needs of the chronically ill. Nurs Clin N Am 1987; 22:603–611.

88. Elkins DN, Hedstrom LJ, Hughes LL, et al. Towards a humanistic-phenomenological spirituality: definitions, descriptions and measurement. J Humanistic Psychol 1988; 28:5–18.

89. Strang S, Strang P, Ternestedt BM. Spiritual needs as defined by Swedish nursing staff. J Clin Nurs 2002; 11(1):48–57.

90. Taylor EJ, Amenta M, Highfield M. Spiritual care practices of oncology nurses. Oncol Nurs Forum. 1995; 22(1):31–39.

91. Highfield ME, Osterhues D. Spiritual care rights and quality of care: perspectives of physical therapy students. J Healthcare Qual 2003; 25(1):12–5; quiz 15–16.

92. Eriksson K. Vårdteologi. Institutionen för vårdvetenskap. Åbo akademi, Turku, 1993 (in Swedish).

93. Taylor EJ, Highfield MF, Amenta M. Predictors of oncology and hospice nurses' spiritual care perspectives and practices. Appl Nurs Res 1999; 12(1):30–37.

94. Taylor EJ, Highfield M, Amenta M. Attitudes and beliefs regarding spiritual care. A survey of cancer nurses. Cancer Nurs 1994;17(6):479–487.

95. Radziewicz R, Baile WF. Communication skills: breaking bad news in the clinical setting. Oncol Nurs Forum 2001; 28(6):951–953.

96. Wilkinson S. Schering Plough clinical lecture communication: it makes a difference. Cancer Nurs 1999; 22(1):17–20.

97. Wilkinson S. Good communication in cancer nursing. Nurs Stand 1992; 7(9):35–39.

98. Mattingly C. The concept of therapeutic 'emplotment'. Soc Sci Med 1994; 38(6):811–822.

99. Bourhis RY, Roth S, MacQueen G. Communication in the hospital setting: a survey of medical and everyday language use amongst patients, nurses and doctors. Soc Sci Med 1989; 28(4):339–346.

100. O'Connor AP, Wicker CA. Clinical commentary: promoting meaning in the lives of cancer survivors. Semin Oncol Nurs 1995; 11(1):68–72.

101. Madjar I, Walton JA. Nursing and the experience of illness. Phenomenology in practice. London: Routledge; 1999.

102. Ahlberg K, Gibson F. 'What is the story telling us': using patient experiences to improve practice. Eur J Oncol Nurs 2003; 7(3):149–150.

103. Skott C. Expressive metaphors in cancer narratives. Cancer Nurs 2002; 25(3):230–235.

104. Heliker D. Transformation of story to practice: an innovative approach to long-term care. Issues Ment Health Nurs 1999; 20(6):513–525.

105. Brody H. Stories of sickness. New Haven, CT: Yale University Press; 1987.

106. Taylor EJ. The story behind the story: the use of storytelling in spiritual caregiving. Semin Oncol Nurs 1997 13(4):252–254.

107. Gibbs RW Jr, Franks H. Embodied metaphor in women's narratives about their experiences with cancer. Health Commun 2002; 14(2):139–165.

108. Benner P. From novice to expert. Excellence and power in clinical nursing practice. Menlo Park, California: Addison-Wesley; 1984.

109. Dahlberg K, Drew N. A lifeworld paradigm for nursing research. J Holistic Nurs 1997; 15:303–317.

110. Ricoeur P. Interpretation theory. Discourse and the surplus of meaning. Fort Worth: Christian University Press; 1976.

111. Sadelowski M. Telling stories: narrative approaches in qualitative research. J Nurs Scholarship 1991; 23(3):161–166.

112. Starrin B, Renck. Den kvalitativa intervjun. Ur: Svensson P-G, Starrin B, red. Kvalitativa studier i teori och praktik. Lund: Studentlitteratur; 1996:52–78.

113. Mishler E. Research interviewing: context and narrative. Cambridge, MA: Harvard University Press; 1986.

114. Riessman C. Divorce talk: women and men make sense of personal relationships. New Brunswick: Rutgers University Press; 1990.

115. Kleinman, A. The illness narratives: suffering, healing, and the human condition. New York: Basic Books; 1988.

116. Skott C. Caring narratives and the strategy of presence: narrative communication in nursing practice and research. Nurs Sci Q 2001; 14(3):249–254.

SECTION 2

The scientific basis of cancer care

4. Cancer Epidemiology 55

5. Genetic Basis of Cancer 73

6. Pathology 97

7. The Immunological Basis of Cancer 115

CHAPTER 4

Cancer Epidemiology

HELEN EVANS, ANGELA NEWNHAM AND HENRIK MØLLER

CHAPTER CONTENTS

Introduction	55	Measures of exposure effect	62
		Analytical studies	63
Epidemiology of cancer	55	Issues in epidemiological research	66
Grade	56		
Stage	56	Causes of cancer	67
		Inherited cancer susceptibility	67
Standard classification	56	Polymorphisms and gene–	
Measures of disease frequency	56	environment interactions	67
Drawbacks or limitations to		Tobacco	67
epidemiology	58	Alcohol	68
Factors that affect incidence data	58	Diet	68
Leading causes of death	58	Obesity	68
Incidence and mortality of cancer		Infections	69
worldwide	60		
Cancer in Europe	60	Conclusion	69
Epidemiological studies	62	References	69

INTRODUCTION

This chapter aims to provide a concise overview of the current knowledge in cancer epidemiology and form a strong foundation for further study. Following a definition of epidemiology, the trends in cancer reporting throughout the world are described and finally the major risk factors are discussed.

EPIDEMIOLOGY OF CANCER

Epidemiology is defined as the study of the distribution and determinants of health-related states or events in specified populations, and the application of this study to control of health problems.[1] The purpose of epidemiol-

ogy is to summarize the who, what, when, where and why of the occurrence of a disease. The field of cancer epidemiology has rapidly advanced over recent decades and there are now a number of well-established cancer registries throughout the world, providing data on cancer incidence and survival.[2] Epidemiological studies have identified many risk factors for specific types of cancer, and led to the introduction of prevention and screening programmes. Mortality rates are ascertained from death certificates, which are available in most countries. An increasing knowledge of genetics and molecular biology provides an added dimension to cancer epidemiology research, and will play an increasing role in this field. There are, however, still many areas of uncertainty.

In order to be able to gain a broad understanding of cancer distribution, health-related events and determinants that affect the incidence of certain cancers, universal grading, staging and other measures have been developed.

Grade

The grade of a cancer refers to its differentiation and the degree of anaplasia. A well-differentiated tumour has a lower grade than a poorly differentiated tumour and, in general, patients with higher-grade tumours have a worse prognosis.

This system has been further refined for specific cancers to give a more accurate predictor of prognosis. For example, the Gleason system is commonly used for prostate cancer[3] and uses a system whereby a tumour may be graded from 1 to 5, with grade 1 being well differentiated with uniform gland pattern and grade 5 being very poorly differentiated with no or minimal gland formation. Prostate tumours often display two patterns, in which case they are summed to produce a pattern score ranging from 2 to 10. The lower the score, the lower the grade of the cancer and the better the prognosis.

Stage

The stage of a tumour is a measure of how far it has spread at any particular time. Accurate assessment of the stage of a tumour is important because as well as being used as a prognostic indicator it helps to determine appropriate treatment. In addition to the grade of a tumour, the stage contributes to the severity of the disease.

The most common staging notation is the TNM system. Developed by the International Union Against Cancer (UICC),[4] the TNM system uses the size (and depth of invasion) of the tumour (T), lymph node spread (N) and the presence of distant metastases (M). Although this system is widely used, it is not appropriate for all tumours and other specialist systems have also been developed, such as the FIGO system (International Federation of Gynaecology and Obstetrics) for gynaecological tumours[5] and Dukes' staging for colorectal cancers.[6]

STANDARD CLASSIFICATION

The International Classification of Diseases (ICD), published by the World Health Organization (WHO), is a standard disease classification that is used throughout the world.[7] It is primarily developed for coding causes of death and hospital discharge diagnoses, but is insufficiently detailed for the proper coding of cancer diagnoses.[2] More recently, the International Classification of Diseases for Oncology (ICD-O)[8] has been widely used. This provides morphology and behaviour codes, as well as topography codes. These classifications are periodically revised and updated. Uniform definitions and classifications of cancer are fundamental to epidemiological studies, allowing for meaningful comparisons of morbidity and mortality data to be made.

Measures of disease frequency

Incidence

The incidence of a disease is the number of new cases of disease that develop in a population of individuals at risk during a specified time interval. There are two specific measures of incidence: cumulative incidence and incidence rate. Cumulative incidence (CI) is the proportion of people who become diseased during a specified period of time (e.g. the proportion of people who develop cancer before a defined age) divided by the total population at risk:[9]

$$CI = \frac{\text{Number of new cases of a disease during a given time period}}{\text{Total population at risk}}$$

The incidence rate (IR) measures the rate of development of disease in a population and is the preferred measure of disease occurrence.[2]

$$IR = \frac{\text{Number of new cases of a disease during a given time period}}{\text{Total person years at risk}}$$

When comparing incidence rates from different populations, it is important to remember that the populations may have very different age structures. As cancer incidence rates increase with age, a population with a high proportion of elderly individuals will generally have a higher crude rate of cancer than one with a high proportion of younger people. To make meaningful comparisons between populations, age-standardization is used.[2] An age-standardized rate is calculated by obtaining the rates for individual age groups (age-specific rates) in the population, multiplying them by the relevant standard population proportions and then summing them over all age groups.

This gives an overall incidence rate per 100,000 population, which would occur in the standard reference population, and is a rate that can be compared between populations. There are two standard populations in general use – the 'European standard population' and the 'world standard population',[2] as shown in Table 4.1. The European standard population has a higher proportion of older people and reflects the population structure in developed

Table 4.1: Standard populations

Age group (years)	European Standard Population (proportion of total)	World Standard Population (proportion of total)	England and Wales Population, 2001[a] (proportion of total)
Under 5	8000 (0.08)	12000 (0.12)	3094357 (0.06)
5–9	7000 (0.07)	10000 (0.10)	3307972 (0.06)
10–14	7000 (0.07)	9000 (0.09)	3425075 (0.07)
15–19	7000 (0.07)	9000 (0.09)	3217425 (0.06)
20–24	7000 (0.07)	8000 (0.08)	3122379 (0.06)
25–29	7000 (0.07)	8000 (0.08)	3435108 (0.07)
30–34	7000 (0.07)	6000 (0.06)	3983974 (0.08)
35–39	7000 (0.07)	6000 (0.06)	4093217 (0.08)
40–44	7000 (0.07)	6000 (0.06)	3656335 (0.07)
45–49	7000 (0.07)	6000 (0.06)	3296031 (0.06)
50–54	7000 (0.07)	5000 (0.05)	3590904 (0.07)
55–59	6000 (0.06)	4000 (0.04)	2962130 (0.06)
60–64	5000 (0.05)	4000 (0.04)	2544628 (0.05)
65–69	4000 (0.04)	3000 (0.03)	2292386 (0.04)
70–74	3000 (0.03)	2000 (0.02)	2074462 (0.04)
75–79	2000 (0.02)	1000 (0.01)	1754864 (0.03)
80–84	1000 (0.01)	500 (0.005)	1178269 (0.02)
85 and over	1000 (0.01)	500 (0.005)	1012400 (0.02)
Total	100000 (1.00)	100000 (1.00)	52041916 (1.00)

[a]*Source*: National Statistics website: www.statistics.gov.uk
Crown copyright material is reproduced with permission of the Controller HMSO.

countries more closely than the world population standard. The choice of the standard population to be used largely depends on the populations being compared. For example, if the world population is used, the age-standardized incidence of prostate cancer in the UK, a cancer more common in the elderly, will be relatively lower than if the European standard population is used.

Prevalence

The prevalence of a disease is the proportion of individuals in a population who have the disease at a given point in time.[2] The formula for calculating prevalence (P) is:

$$P = \frac{\text{Number of existing cases of a disease at given point in time}}{\text{Total population}}$$

Prevalence depends on both the incidence and the duration of a disease and will, therefore, be affected by differences in survival. For example, lung cancer has a high incidence but short duration, so the prevalence is quite low, whereas breast cancer has a high incidence and long duration, and so the prevalence is relatively high.[10] Prevalence is important for assessing the total burden of chronic diseases such as cancer and, therefore, it may be useful for planning the use of healthcare resources.[2] The prevalent pool of persons who have had cancer is a mixture of cured persons and persons with latent or active disease who will require treatment.

Mortality rate

The mortality rate (MR) is the incidence of death from a disease during a given time period and is defined as:

$$MR = \frac{\text{Number of deaths from a disease}}{\text{Total population}}$$

A crude incidence, prevalence or mortality rate is one that relates to the population taken as a whole, without subdivision or refinement.

Drawbacks or limitations to epidemiology

In practice, there are many limitations to the use of incidence rates for cancer. There has to be an infrastructure in place to enable the measurement of the size of the population and also the accurate identification of new cases. Reliable estimates of cancer incidence are only available for a small proportion of the world population.[11] Mortality rates are more widely available, because death is an easily defined and obvious event, but they do also have limitations. The causes of death have to be recorded accurately and this is not always possible. Mortality rates approximate to incidence rates for cancers with a poor prognosis, such as lung and pancreatic cancer; however, they give no indication of the burden of cancers with a favourable prognosis, such as endometrial and testicular cancer.[12]

Factors that affect incidence data

Although incidence data are invaluable in the field of cancer epidemiology, there are factors that influence the accuracy of the data. First, reliable incidence data can only be obtained from population-based cancer registries, which depend on accurate diagnosis, coding and reporting. Secondly, changes in diagnostic practices can affect the incidence in several ways. For example, new techniques such as magnetic resonance imaging (MRI) may detect small or slow-growing cancers that would otherwise have been detected at a later stage, if at all. The introduction of screening programmes can lead to an apparent increase in incidence as, for example, when prostate-specific antigen (PSA) testing was introduced in the USA as a screening test for prostate cancer, resulting in a dramatically raised incidence of prostate cancer.[13] Variations in autopsy rates will also affect incidences, particularly of those cancers more often diagnosed at autopsy (such as prostate and stomach cancer). Differing policies across time or between countries need to be considered, therefore, when comparing incidence rates, along with changing risk factors.

Leading causes of death

Due to decreasing birth rates and increasing longevity, the populations of industrialized countries are ageing and, as a result, the major causes of death are changing.[14] Non-communicable diseases are becoming more common in developing countries, where infectious diseases and malnutrition are currently the leading causes of premature death. In addition to ageing, other factors such as smoking patterns also influence trends in cancer. In 1990, trachea, bronchus and lung cancers were the third most common cause of death in developed countries (Table 4.2) and while they did not feature in the 10 leading causes of death in developing counties in 1990, it is predicted that they will be the 15th leading cause of death throughout the world by 2020.[14]

	Table 4.2: The 10 leading causes of death in developed and developing regions of the world in 1990						
	Developed regions			Developing regions			
Rank	Cause	Deaths (thousands)	Cumu- lative %	Cause	Deaths (thousands)	Cumu- lative %
	All causes	10912		All causes	39554	
1	Ischaemic heart disease	2695	24.7	Lower respiratory infections	3915	9.9
2	Cerebrovascular disease	1427	37.8	Ischaemic heart disease	3565	18.9
3	Trachea, bronchus and lung cancer	523	42.6	Cerebrovascular disease	2954	26.4
4	Lower respiratory infections	385	46.1	Diarrhoeal disease	2940	33.8
5	Chronic obstructive pulmonary disease	324	49.1	Conditions arising during the perinatal period	2361	38.7
6	Colon and rectum cancers	277	51.6	Tuberculosis	1922	43.4
7	Stomach cancer	241	53.8	Chronic obstructive pulmonary disease	1887	46.1
8	Road traffic accidents	222	55.8	Measles	1058	48.7
9	Self-inflicted injuries	193	57.6	Malaria	856	50.9
10	Diabetes mellitus	176	59.2	Road traffic accidents	777	52.8

Source: Murray and Lopez.[14]

Incidence and mortality of cancer worldwide

In 2000, there were an estimated 10.1 million new cases of cancer, 6.2 million deaths due to cancer and 22.4 million people living with cancer throughout the world (excluding non-melanoma skin cancer).[11] This represents an increase of around 22% in incidence and mortality since 1990,[11] with both incidence and mortality being higher in men than women. Lung cancer has the highest incidence and mortality in men and in both sexes combined.[11] In women, breast cancer has the highest incidence and mortality.[11] The incidence and mortality of the most common cancers are shown in Tables 4.3 and 4.4.

Cancer in Europe

In common with the global picture, lung cancer is the top cancer for men in Europe, in terms of both incidence and mortality (Table 4.5). Prostate cancer is the second most common cancer, but the mortality rate is lower than that for colorectal cancer, which has the third highest incidence rate in European men. Breast cancer is the most common cancer in European women in terms of both incidence and mortality (Table 4.6). The second and third most common can-

Table 4.3: Cancers with the highest incidence worldwide, 2000

Cancer site	Overall rank	Number of new cases in men[a]	Rank in men	Number of new cases in women[a]	Rank in women
Lung	1	902000	1	337000	4
Breast	2	–	–	1050000	1
Colon/rectum	3	499000	4	446000	3
Stomach	4	558000	2	318000	5
Liver	5	398000	5	166000	8
Prostate	6	543000	3	–	–
Cervix uteri	7	–	–	471000	2
Oesophagus	8	279000	6	133000	9
Bladder	9	260000	7	336000	15
Non-Hodgkin's lymphoma	10	167000	9	121000	10
Oral cavity	11	170000	8	97000	13
Leukaemia	12	144000	10	113000	11
Pancreas	13	116000	13	216000	12
Ovary	14	–	–	192000	6
Kidney	15	118000	12	71000	17

Source: Parkin et al.[11]
[a]To the nearest 1000.

Table 4.4: Cancers with the highest mortality worldwide, 2000

Cancer site	Overall rank	Number of deaths in men[a]	Rank in men	Number of deaths in women[a]	Rank in women
Lung	1	810000	1	293000	2
Stomach	2	405000	2	241000	3
Liver	3	384000	3	165000	6
Colon/rectum	4	255000	4	238000	4
Breast	5	–	–	373000	1
Oesophagus	6	227000	5	111000	8
Cervix uteri	7	–	–	233000	5
Pancreas	8	112000	7	102000	9
Prostate	9	204000	6	–	–
Leukaemia	10	109000	8	86000	10
Non-Hodgkin's lymphoma	11	93000	10	68000	11
Bladder	12	99000	9	33000	16
Oral cavity	13	81000	11	47000	13
Brain, nervous system	14	72000	13	56000	12
Ovary	15	–	–	114000	7

Source: Parkin et al.[11]
[a]To the nearest 1000.

cers in women are colorectal cancer and lung cancer, respectively. Although stomach cancer is a major cause of morbidity and mortality worldwide, it is less common in Europe, with the highest incidence rates for this cancer being reported from Japan and China.[15] Liver cancer also plays a much smaller role in Europe than in the worldwide population as a whole. Although liver cancer is rare in the United States and western Europe, it is very common in eastern Asia and sub-Saharan Africa.[16] The large populations in these areas account for the high worldwide ranking of liver cancer.

Overall cancer mortality is lower for women than men, and the trends for specific cancers also differ between the sexes.[18] Patterns of cancer incidence and mortality vary greatly within and between countries, due to differences in a wide range of factors, including lifestyle habits (smoking, diet, sexual and reproductive behaviour), genetics, environmental factors, diagnostic and screening facilities and accessibility of healthcare facilities and prevention programmes, to name but a few.

Lung cancer has shown some notable trends in recent years and these are evident from European data (Table 4.7).[18] Although different trends are seen in different parts of Europe,[19,20] in general, mortality in men is declining whereas mortality in women is

Table 4.5: Age-standardized incidence and mortality rate per 100,000 population (World Standard) for men in Europe, 1998

Rank	Site	Incidence ASR (W)	Site	Mortality ASR (W)
1	Lung	50.29	Lung	45.56
2	Prostate	42.61	Colon/rectum	17.16
3	Colon/rectum	36.38	Prostate	14.65
4	Bladder	17.87	Stomach	9.68
5	Oral cavity and pharynx	15.92	Pancreas	7.21
6	Stomach	13.33	Liver	7.16
7	Kidney etc.	10.40	Bladder	6.14
8	Non-Hodgkin's lymphoma	10.34	Oral cavity and pharynx	5.77
9	Leukaemia	9.44	Oesophagus	5.71
10	Larynx	7.68	Leukaemia	5.30

Source: Ferlay et al.[17]

increasing. This is thought to be mainly due to changing patterns in smoking habits.[19]

Survival data in Europe

Survival is a key factor for evaluating the effectiveness of cancer care. It can only be calculated if the period of follow-up is known for each patient.[2] The observed survival is the probability of surviving for a specified time period, usually starting at the date of cancer diagnosis, regardless of the cause of death. The cause-specific survival gives a more realistic picture of the excess death rate attributable to a particular cancer.[2] This only counts deaths from the particular cancer in question and patients who die from another cause are 'censored' at the date of death. This does depend, however, on the cause of death being accurately identified and reported. Relative survival compares the observed survival to that expected in the general population with the same age and sex distribution. The calculation of relative survival is less dependent on the accuracy of death certification, but it does need reliable life tables from the population and the patients under study must have the same baseline risk of dying as the general population.[12]

Survival varies throughout the world and Tables 4.8a and 4.8b shows the 5-year relative survival for selected cancer sites in different parts of Europe.[21] Access to adequate healthcare facilities is a key factor in cancer survival, facilitating early diagnosis and effective treatment. Inequality of such access is likely to be a contributing factor for the wide differences in cancer survival across Europe.[22] In general, however, survival has improved over the last 20 years in both Europe and the USA.[22,23]

EPIDEMIOLOGICAL STUDIES

Measures of exposure effect

The main aim for any epidemiological study is to quantify the association between a potential risk factor and an outcome. This may be presented as either a relative measure of effect or an absolute

Table 4.6 Age-standardized incidence and mortality rate per 100,000 population (World Standard) for women in Europe, 1998

Rank	Site	Incidence ASR (W)	Site	Mortality ASR (W)
1	Breast	67.48	Breast	28.28
2	Colon/rectum	23.80	Colon/rectum	17.35
3	Lung	11.97	Lung	15.47
4	Corpus uteri	10.87	Ovary, etc.	8.62
5	Ovary, etc.	10.59	Pancreas	7.43
6	Cervix uteri	8.08	Stomach	7.27
7	Melanoma of skin	7.29	Leukaemia	4.76
8	Non-Hodgkin's lymphoma	6.78	Brain, nervous system	3.02
9	Stomach	6.20	Non-Hodgkin's lymphoma	2.84
10	Leukaemia	5.93	Cervix uteri	2.83

Source: Ferlay et al.[17]

measure.[2] The relative risk (or risk ratio) indicates the likelihood of developing the disease in the exposed group relative to those who are not exposed. It is defined as the ratio of the incidence of disease in the exposed group divided by the corresponding incidence of disease in the non-exposed group.[9] Although this is a useful measure, it does not indicate how many cases are actually involved and so gives little information about the impact of the exposure. The absolute measure, known as the excess risk or attributable risk, is the difference between the risk in the exposed and the risk in the unexposed. This indicates how many extra cases the exposure is responsible for, assuming that the relationship between exposure and disease is causal.[2]

Analytical studies

There are two broad categories of analytical studies used in epidemiology: observational and experimental. Although experimental studies provide more robust evidence, they are

Table 4.7: Age-standardized mortality rates per 100,000 (World Standard Population) from lung cancer in the European Union 1988–1996

Year	Men	Women
1988	52.8	9.4
1990	51.1	9.3
1992	50.3	9.7
1993	49.3	9.8
1994	48.6	10.0
1995	48.2	10.1
1996	47.3	10.1
Change in rate, 1988–1996	−5.5	+ 0.7

Source: Levi et al.[18]

Table 4.8a: Age-standardized 5-year relative survival for men with cancer in Europe, 1985–1989

Country	Age-standardized 5-year relative survival (%)				
	Cancer site				
	Lung	Prostate	Colon	Rectum	Bladder
Austria	10	54	55	47	67
Denmark	6	41	39	38	50
England	7	44	41	40	66
Estonia	5	37	36	34	34
Finland	10	62	48	49	69
France	12	62	52	48	59
Germany	9	68	50	44	75
Iceland	12	66	44	–	67
Italy	9	47	47	43	65
Netherlands	12	55	59	52	65
Poland	6	35	25	21	36
Scotland	6	47	41	36	62
Slovakia	12	60	39	35	60
Slovenia	6	39	33	29	42
Spain	12	54	50	43	69
Sweden	9	65	52	49	73
Switzerland	10	71	52	53	55
Europe	**9**	**56**	**47**	**43**	**65**

Source: Berrino et al.[21]

often not feasible or ethical in the study of cancer aetiology.[24] Epidemiology mainly uses observational methods to elucidate evidence for risk factors in cancer aetiology.

Observational studies

Cohort studies

In a cohort study, a population (cohort) is identified and information obtained as to which members of the cohort are exposed to the factor under investigation. The whole cohort is then followed up over time and the incidence of the disease in the exposed group of individuals is compared with the incidence in the unexposed group. This type of study is useful for studying rare exposures. For rare outcomes, however, large numbers of individuals are needed to detect an association, making the study expensive and time-consuming. A major

Table 4.8b: Age-standardized 5-year relative survival for women with cancer in Europe, 1985–1989

Country	Age-standardized 5-year relative survival (%)				
	Cancer site				
	Breast	Colon	Rectum	Lung	Corpus uteri
Austria	63	44	54	15	81
Denmark	71	43	42	6	76
England	67	41	41	7	73
Estonia	60	38	36	14	65
Finland	78	50	46	11	76
France	80	54	48	16	75
Germany	72	50	44	14	73
Iceland	79	52	52	12	77
Italy	77	47	44	10	73
Netherlands	74	56	54	11	84
Poland	58	23	22	9	66
Scotland	65	41	39	6	70
Slovakia	58	38	37	19	69
Slovenia	64	38	31	7	73
Spain	70	49	43	–	73
Sweden	81	55	52	10	82
Switzerland	80	49	52	10	77
Europe	72	47	43	10	73

Source: Berrino et al.[21]

advantage of cohort studies is the fact that the temporal relationship can be examined, as the exposure is known to precede the outcome.[24]

Case-control studies

In a case-control study, cases with the disease are initially identified along with controls without the disease. The controls must represent the same population that gave rise to the cases. Past exposure to the factor under investigation is then compared in the two groups. Because the study starts with cases, fewer individuals in total are needed to detect an association. Although case-control studies are generally more useful than cohort studies for rare outcomes, they provide less certainty about the relationship between the time of exposure and the development of the disease and information on exposure may be influenced by the presence or absence of disease.[2]

Experimental studies: randomized controlled trials

A randomized controlled trial randomly allocates individuals from a population to two groups – one that was exposed to a factor and one that was not exposed to the factor – and then outcomes are compared. The random allocation allows for similarities between and within groups. The use of such trials in cancer epidemiology is mainly limited to the investigation of exposures that may reduce the risk of cancer, such as dietary modification,[2] as exposing individuals to known carcinogens would clearly not be ethical or acceptable.

Descriptive studies

There are other kinds of study used less often in epidemiology, such as correlational studies, case reports and cross-sectional surveys.[2] These kinds of study are mainly useful for generating hypotheses about potential risk factors. Correlational studies use data from an entire population to compare disease frequencies between different groups during the same period of time or in the same population at different points in time. An example of this is the positive correlation between red meat consumption in different countries and the frequency of colorectal cancer.[25] Countries with low levels of red meat consumption have the lowest levels of colorectal cancer. Although these studies are useful for formulating hypotheses, they cannot link exposures to outcomes in individuals. Case reports provide data about risk factors in individual cases, which can only be suggestive. The presence of a particular risk factor and development of disease may be purely coincidental. Cross-sectional surveys assess the presence or absence of both exposure and outcome in an individual at a particular point in time, which may provide evidence of an association between a risk factor and disease. However, the temporal relationship between exposure and outcome is difficult to establish.

Issues in epidemiological research

Bias, chance and confounding

When evaluating any epidemiological study, it is important to consider whether the results are due to chance, some kind of bias in the way individuals were selected or due to the effect of other differences between the groups that were unmeasured or uncontrolled (confounding).[24] All these factors should be taken into account when designing and interpreting such studies.

The role of bias

Bias is a systematic error that results in an incorrect estimate of the association between an exposure and risk of disease. There are two major types of bias that should be taken into account when designing a study: selection and measurement bias.[2] Selection bias is a problem for case-control studies and occurs when cases and controls are selected according to different criteria. Measurement bias results from systematic differences in the way observations are recorded for cases compared with controls. Recall bias may occur if individuals are asked to describe particular past behaviours, when cases may recall their experiences differently to controls.[24]

The role of chance

Random variability will always exist in the study of human populations. Performing appropriate statistical tests and calculating confidence intervals, however, can assess how likely a result is due to chance. A confidence interval represents the range within which the true magnitude of effect lies with a certain degree of assurance.[2]

The role of confounding

A confounding factor is one that is related to both the exposure and the outcome but is not on the causal pathway. Confounding may lead to the observation of an apparent difference in the two study groups that does not actually exist or it may conceal a true difference.[9] For example, the risk of cancer may have an inverse relationship with the consumption of vegetables rich in beta-carotene because of the beta-carotene itself or it may be due to other differences between consumers and non-consumers of vegetables, such as age or smoking habits.[9] People who eat fewer vegetables may smoke more. The only way to disentangle the role played by a potential confounder such as smoking is to control for it, either at the design stage (include only smokers or non-smokers, or match cases and controls by smoking habits) or at the analysis stage (using statistical techniques such as multivariate analysis).

CAUSES OF CANCER

Epidemiological studies have identified a wide range of factors that increase the risk of cancer. There are endogenous risk factors such as inherited cancer predisposition syndromes and exogenous risk factors such as tobacco, diet and infections. These risk factors are not mutually exclusive, and interactions between genetic and environmental elements may modify cancer risks. The main risk factors for the development of cancer that have been identified through clinical, laboratory and epidemiological studies are summarized below.

Inherited cancer susceptibility

Cancer is essentially a genetic disease, occurring as a result of a mutation or series of mutations in the DNA of genes involved in cellular growth, differentiation, death or DNA repair. Mutations may be present in germline cells, which would result in an inherited predisposition to cancer, or may occur during life as somatic mutations in individual cells.[26] Although a number of highly penetrant inherited cancer predisposition syndromes have been identified, such as familial adenomatous polyposis and Li–Fraumeni syndrome, they only account for a small proportion of the total number of cancer cases worldwide.[27,28] The inherited cancer syndromes result in a strong predisposition to cancer for the affected individual, conferring lifetime risks of cancer up to 50–80%.[28] They are, however, rare in the general population and so constitute no more than 1–2% of all cancers.

From an epidemiological perspective, the moderately increased incidence of more common cancers within families is of greater importance. This may be due to a combination of a small number of genes conferring a moderately strong effect on the risk of cancer and a large number of 'low-penetrance' genes, which have a weaker effect on an individual's lifetime risk of cancer.[27,28] It is likely that there are many more genes to be identified, which together will account for a much higher proportion of cancer overall than the genes involved in the inherited cancer syndromes.

Polymorphisms and gene–environment interactions

The relative importance of genetic and environmental components varies from cancer to cancer.[29] Polymorphisms are mutations that exist in more than 2% of the population and convey a range of biological phenotypes.[26] The prevalence of common polymorphisms in genes involved with metabolism have been compared between patients with cancer and unaffected controls. Although there is evidence that some polymorphisms are associated with an increased or decreased risk of cancer, the results for most polymorphisms are inconclusive.[27] It is possible that people with different polymorphisms of a particular gene will react to a particular risk factor such as smoking in different ways. This is a major area for investigation in current cancer epidemiology.[27]

Tobacco

Tobacco has been used throughout the world for over 400 years, initially for medical purposes, then later for pleasure.[30] It is used in a number of different forms across the world, including chewing tobacco, snuff, smoking pipes and cigarettes. The use of cigarettes spread in the 19th century, and by 1990 an estimated 1 billion people were smoking cigarettes worldwide.[31] The habit started in wealthier countries, but it is becoming an increasing problem in developing countries.[14] The prevalence of smoking increased between 1945 and 1965 in most high-income countries and then stabilized until about 1985, when it began to fall.[32]

An association between smoking and cancer was observed as early as the 18th century,[30] but it was not until 1950 that several well-designed studies were published showing clear evidence for an association between lung cancer and smoking.[30] In 1960, the World Health Organization agreed that cigarette smoking was a cause of lung cancer.[33] At least eight cancer sites have now been definitely associated with tobacco use: lung, larynx, head and neck, oesophagus, pancreas, bladder, kidney and stomach.[34] Other cancers such as liver and cervical cancer have also been associated with smoking, but the evidence is less clear.[34]

The relative importance of tobacco-related cancers varies across countries, depending on the background rate of cancer due to other factors. In the developed world, cigarette smoking is the leading cause of lung cancer, whereas in China tobacco is more important in the development of liver and stomach cancer.[35] The risk of lung and laryngeal cancer conferred by current cigarette smoking is very high, but the risk does decline after smoking cessation. The risk of lung cancers in smokers relative to never-smokers overall is about 8–15 in men and 2–10 in women.[36] There is a strong dose–response pattern, with an increased risk for heavy smokers and for those individuals who have smoked for a longer time. The association is strongest for lung cancers with squamous or small cell histology.[37]

Alcohol

In 1988, the International Agency for Research on Cancer (IARC) of the World Health Organization concluded that there was sufficient evidence to describe alcoholic drinks as carcinogenic in humans.[38] Alcohol intake has been associated with higher risks of cancers of the upper respiratory tract, oesophagus, liver, colorectum and breast.[39,40] There is some evidence that the risk for different cancers varies according to the type of alcoholic beverage being consumed, but this is inconsistent.[41]

Diet

Although it is clear that diet plays a role in the development of some types of cancer, this is a difficult area to investigate.[25] Cancers often take a long time to develop, so the diet of a patient over a number of years has to be considered. It is often difficult for individuals to accurately assess their intake of various dietary components and it is particularly difficult to quantify the intake of micronutrients

such as vitamins and minerals. Biochemical measurements may be made on blood or other tissues to assess the intake of a particular nutrient but this, too, has its drawbacks. Levels may be highly regulated by the body, they may fluctuate over time, and the levels may be affected by the presence of cancer before it is diagnosed.[42]

Some dietary factors have been consistently associated with an increased risk of cancer. The first is a high intake of nitrosamine-rich foods, such as Chinese-style salted fish, which increases the risk of nasopharyngeal cancer.[25] The second is the consumption of foods contaminated with aflatoxins (such as mouldy corn), which increases the risk of liver cancer and is an important risk factor in developing countries.[25,43] The consumption of red and processed meats appears to increase the risk of colorectal cancer and there is some evidence to suggest that high intakes of salted food increase the risk of stomach cancer.[25,44]

The consumption of fruit and vegetables is associated with a reduced risk of several cancers, including mouth, pharynx, lung, oesophagus and stomach.[25,44] Tomatoes, in particular, have consistently been shown to lower the risk of a variety of cancers, including lung, stomach and prostate.[45]

Obesity

Evidence exists for a causal link between obesity and colon cancer, postmenopausal breast cancer, renal cell cancer and cancers in the corpus uteri and oesophagus (adenocarcinoma).[46,47] It is likely that obesity also plays a role in cancers at other sites. About 5% of all incident cancers in the European Union might be prevented if no one had a body mass index above 25 kg/m².[27] It is possible that the effect of obesity on the development of cancer is largely due to changes in the metabolism of hormones such as sex steroids, insulin and insulin-like growth factors.[46,48] Alterations in the levels of these hormones can upset the normal balance between cell proliferation, differentiation and apoptosis. For adenocarcinoma of the oesophagus, there is evidence that obesity increases the risk by increasing gastro-oesophageal reflux.[46]

Infections

The role of infectious pathogens in the development of cancer is becoming increasingly recognized. Viruses have been recognized as having oncogenic potential for many years, but bacteria have only been suspected relatively recently.[49,50]

The bacterium *Helicobacter pylori* (a cause of gastric ulcers) was classified as a human carcinogen in 1994.[51] There is now a wealth of evidence supporting a causal association between *H. pylori* and gastric cancer.[15]

Human herpesviruses, which include the Epstein–Barr virus (EBV), are all potentially oncogenic. EBV has been associated with a number of malignancies, including Burkitt's lymphoma (with malaria as a cofactor), nasopharyngeal carcinoma and Hodgkin's disease.[52] Chronic infection with hepatitis B and hepatitis C viruses are major risk factors for hepatocellular carcinoma, accounting for about 50% and 25%, respectively, of all cases worldwide.[53] In 1995, the IARC concluded that there was sufficient evidence to class human papillomavirus (HPV) type 16 and 18 as human carcinogens.[54] More recently, other types of HPV have also shown to be involved in carcinogenesis.[55] These viruses are the main cause of cervical cancer and are risk factors for other anogenital cancers.[56] Oropharyngeal and non-melanoma skin cancers may also be associated with HPV, but this needs to be explored further. Other viruses that increase the risk of cancer include human T-cell lymphotrophic virus type 1 (some T-cell leukaemias and lymphoma) and human immunodeficiency virus (non-Hodgkin's lymphoma and Kaposi's sarcoma).

Infection with parasites such as schistosomes and liver flukes is associated with an increased risk of cancers, including bladder cancer and liver cancer.[57]

CONCLUSION

Although a number of factors that increase the risk of developing cancer have been identified, the majority of them will only be responsible for causing a small proportion of the total cancer burden. Tobacco is undoubtedly the most important preventable cause of cancer, and up to 90% of all lung cancers can be attributed to smoking.[58] Different risk factors have varying importance in different parts of the world. Alcohol, for instance, accounts for about 4% of breast cancer cases in developed countries but its role in developing countries is negligible.[58] Infections are also a major factor and contribute to about 15% of all cancers worldwide.[27] The role of genetics and the interplay between genes and the environment needs to be further elucidated.

REFERENCES

1. Last JM. A dictionary of epidemiology. 3rd ed. Oxford: Oxford University Press; 1995.
2. dos Santos Silva I. Cancer epidemiology: principles and methods. France: International Agency for Research on Cancer; 1999.
3. Horwich A, Waxman J, Abel P, et al. Tumours of the prostate. In: Souhami RL, Tannock I, Hohenberger P, Horiot J-C, eds. Oxford textbook of oncology. 2nd edn. New York: Oxford University Press; 2002:1939–1972.
4. Werner M, Höfler H. Staging. In: Souhami RL, Tannock I, Hohenberger P, Horiot J-C, eds. Oxford textbook of oncology. 2nd edn. New York: Oxford University Press, 2002:315–322.
5. Neijt JP, Allen DG, Vermorken JB. Epithelial carcinoma of the ovary. In: Souhami RL, Tannock I, Hohenberger P, Horiot J-C, eds. Oxford textbook of oncology. 2nd edn. New York: Oxford University Press; 2002:1789–1807.
6. Northover JMA, Arnott S, Jass JR, Williams NS. Colorectal cancer. In: Souhami RL, Tannock I, Hohenberger P, Horiot J-C, eds. Oxford textbook of oncology. 2nd edn. New York: Oxford University Press; 2002:1545–1589.
7. World Health Organization. International Classification of Diseases and Related Health Problems, 10th revision (ICD-10). Geneva: World Health Organization; 1992.
8 World Health Organization. International Classification of Diseases for Oncology (ICD-O), first edition. Geneva: World Health Organization; 1976.
9. Hennekens CH, Buring JE. Epidemiology in medicine. Boston/Toronto: Little, Brown and Company; 1987.
10. Thames Cancer Registry. Cancer in South East England 2000. London: Thames Cancer Registry, 2003.
11. Parkin DM, Bray F, Ferlay J, Pisani P. Estimating the world cancer burden: GLOBOCAN 2000. Int J Cancer 2001; 94:153–156.
12. Lagiou P, Adami H-O. Burden of cancer. In: Adami H-O, Hunter D, Trichopoulos D, eds.

Textbook of cancer epidemiology. New York: Oxford University Press; 2002:3–28.

13. Hankey BF, Feuer EJ, Clegg LX, et al. Cancer surveillance series: interpreting trends in prostate cancer – Part I: Evidence of the effects of screening in recent prostate cancer incidence, mortality and survival rates. J Natl Cancer Inst 1999; 91:1017–1024.

14. Murray CJL, Lopez AD, eds. The global burden of disease. World Health Organization, Harvard University Press; 1996.

15. Kelley JR, Duggan JM. Gastric cancer epidemiology and risk factors. J Clin Epidemiol 2003; 56:1–9.

16. London WT, McGlynn. Liver cancer. In: Schottenfeld D, Fraumeni JF, eds. Cancer epidemiology and prevention. New York: Oxford University Press; 1996:772–793.

17. Ferlay J, Bray F, Sankila R, Parkin DM. EUCAN: Cancer incidence, mortality and prevalence in the European Union 1998, version 5.0. IARC CancerBase No. 4. Lyon: IARCPress; 1999.

18. Levi F, Lucchini F, Negri E, La Vecchia C. The decline in cancer mortality in the European Union, 1988–1996. Eur J Cancer 2000; 36:1965–1968.

19. Borràs JM, Fernandez E, Gonzalez JR, et al. Lung cancer mortality in European regions (1955–1997). Ann Oncol 2003; 14:159–161.

20. Döbróssy L. Cancer mortality in central-eastern Europe: facts behind the figures. Lancet 2002; 3:374–381.

21. Berrino F, Capocaccia R, Estève J, et al. eds. Survival of cancer patients in Europe: the EUROCARE-2 Study. Lyon: IARC; 1999.

22. Sant M, Capocaccia R, Coleman MP, et al. and the EUROCARE Working Group. Cancer survival increases in Europe, but international differences remain wide. Eur J Cancer 2001; 37:1659–1667.

23. Greenlee RT, Hill-Harmon MB, Murray T, Thun M. Cancer statistics, 2001. CA Cancer J Clin 2001; 51:15–36.

24. Adami H-O, Trichopoulos D. Concepts in cancer epidemiology and etiology. In: Adami H-O, Hunter D, Trichopoulos D, eds. Textbook of cancer epidemiology. New York: Oxford University Press; 2002:87–112.

25. Key TJ, Allen NE, Spencer EA, Travis RC. The effect of diet on risk of cancer. Lancet 2002; 360:861–868.

26. Haiman C, Hunter D. Genetic epidemiology of cancer. In: Adami H-O, Hunter D, Trichopoulos D, eds. Textbook of cancer epidemiology. New York: Oxford University Press; 2002:54–72.

27. Peto J. Cancer epidemiology in the last century and the next decade. Nature 2001; 411:390–395.

28. Ponder BAJ. Cancer genetics. Nature 2001; 411:336–341.

29. Wild CP, Law GR, Roman E. Molecular epidemiology and cancer: promising areas for future research in the post-genomic era. Mutation Res 2002; 499:3–12.

30. Doll R. Uncovering the effects of smoking: historical perspective. Stat Meth Med Res 1998; 7:87–117.

31. Baron JA, Rohan TE. Tobacco. In: Schottenfeld D, Fraumeni JF, eds. Cancer epidemiology and prevention. New York: Oxford University Press; 1996:269–289.

32. Kuper H, Adami H-O, Boffetta P. Tobacco use, cancer causation and public health impact. J Intern Med 2002; 251:455–466.

33. World Health Organization. Epidemiology of cancer of the lung. Report of a study group. World Health Organization technical report series 192. Geneva: World Health Organization; 1960.

34. Kuper H, Boffetta P, Adami H-O. Tobacco use and cancer causation: association by tumour type. J Intern Med 2002; 252:206–224.

35. Proctor RN. Tobacco and the global lung cancer epidemic. Nat Rev Cancer 2001; 1:82–86.

36. Boffetta P, Trichopoulos D. Cancer of the lung, larynx, and pleura. In: Adami H-O, Hunter D, Trichopoulos D, eds. Textbook of cancer epidemiology. New York: Oxford University Press; 2002:248–280.

37. Khuder SA. Effect of cigarette smoking on major histological types of lung cancer: a meta-analysis. Lung Cancer 2001; 31:139–148.

38. International Agency for Research on Cancer. IARC monographs on the evaluation of carcinogenic risks to humans. Alcohol drinking, Vol 44. Lyons: IARC; 1988.

39 Corrao G, Bagnardi V, Zambon A, Arico S. Exploring the dose-response relationship between alcohol consumption and the risk of several alcohol-related conditions: a meta-analysis. Addiction 1999; 94:1551–1573.

40 Collaborative Group on Hormonal Factors in Breast Cancer. Alcohol, tobacco and breast cancer – collaborative reanalysis of individual data from 53 epidemiological studies, including 58515 women with breast cancer and 95067 women without the disease. Br J Cancer 2002; 87:1234–1245.

41. Jensen OM, Paine SL, McMichael AJ, et al, eds. Cancer epidemiology and prevention. New York: Oxford University Press; 1996:290–318.

42. Willett WC. Diet and nutrition. In: Schottenfeld D, Fraumeni JF, eds. Cancer epidemiology and prevention. New York: Oxford University Press; 1996: 438–461.

43. Goldman R, Shields PG. Food mutagens. J Nutr 2003; 133:965S–973S.

44. Riboli E, Norat T. Cancer prevention and diet: opportunities in Europe. Public Health Nutr 2001; 4(2B):475–484.

45. Giovannucci E. Tomatoes, tomato-based products, lycopene, and cancer: review of the

epidemiological literature. J Natl Cancer Inst 1999; 91:317–331.

46. Bianchini F, Kaaks R, Vainio H. Overweight, obesity, and cancer risk. Lancet 2002; 3:565–574.

47. Fogelholm M, Vainio H. Weight control, physical activity and cancer – strong links. Obesity Rev 2002; 3:1–3.

48. Bray GA. The underlying basis for obesity: relationship to cancer. J Nutr 2002; 132:3451S–3455S.

49. Correa P. Bacterial infections as a cause of cancer. JNCI 2003; 95:E3.

50. Montesano R, Hall J. Environmental causes of human cancers. Eur J Cancer 2001; 37:S67–S87.

51. International Agency for Research on Cancer. IARC monographs on the evaluation of carcinogenic risks to humans. Human papillomaviruses, Vol 64. Lyons: IARC; 1994.

52. Mueller NE, Evans AS, London WT. Viruses. In: Schottenfeld D, Fraumeni JF, eds. Cancer epidemiology and prevention. New York: Oxford University Press; 1996:502–531.

53. Montalto G, Cervello M, Giannitrapani L, et al. Epidemiology, risk factors, and natural history of hepatocellular carcinoma. Ann NY Acad Sci 2002; 963:13–20.

54. International Agency for Research on Cancer. IARC monographs on the evaluation of carcinogenic risks to humans. Schistosomes, liver flukes and *Helicobacter pylori*, Vol 61. Lyons: IARC; 1995.

55. Muñoz N. Human papillomavirus and cancer: the epidemiological evidence. J Clin Virol 2000; 19:1–5.

56. Bjørge T, Engeland A, Luostarinen T, et al. Human papillomavirus infection as a risk factor for anal and perianal skin cancer in a prospective study. Br J Cancer 2002; 87:61–64.

57. Abdel-Rahim AY. Parasitic infections and hepatic neoplasia. Dig Dis 2001; 19:288–291.

58. dos Santos Silva I. Alcohol, tobacco and breast cancer: should alcohol be condemned and tobacco acquitted? Br J Cancer 2002; 87:1195–1196.

CHAPTER 5

Genetic Basis of Cancer

ATHENA MATAKIDOU AND TIM EISEN

CHAPTER CONTENTS

Introduction	73	Tumour suppressor genes	83
Normal cell biology: DNA–RNA–protein	74	Process of cancer development	86
DNA structure	74	Hereditary predisposition to cancer	87
The genome	74		
Transcription	75	Carcinogenesis related to exogenous and endogenous factors	88
Regulation of DNA transcription	75	Chemical carcinogenesis	88
RNA processing	75	Physical carcinogenesis	89
Translation	76	Ionizing radiation	89
DNA replication	76	Ultraviolet radiation	91
DNA repair	76	Hormonal influences to carcinogenesis	91
		Infection and inflammation	91
The cell cycle	77		
Cell division	77	Conclusion	92
Regulation of the cell cycle	78		
Withdrawal from the cell cycle	79	References	92
Molecular genetics of cancer	80	Further reading	95
Mutations	80		
Cancer genes	82		
Oncogenes	82		

INTRODUCTION

Cancer arises when a cell escapes the normal constraints placed on its growth and begins to divide in an unregulated fashion. Such escape is facilitated by the accumulation of mutations (alterations in the genetic material) within a cell as a result of the innate and environmental carcinogens to which cellular DNA is subjected.[1] Hence, cancer at a cellular level is a genetic disease.

In order to understand the aetiology and process of cancer development it is essential to comprehend the normal cellular mechanisms that govern cellular growth and replication.

In this chapter we will explore:

- normal cell biology and replication
- normal cell cycle and its control
- mechanisms by which the above are disrupted in carcinogenesis
- mutations, oncogenes and tumour suppressor genes
- the process of cancer development (initiation, promotion, progression)
- carcinogenesis related to hereditary, endogenous and exogenous factors.

NORMAL CELL BIOLOGY: DNA–RNA–PROTEIN

This section discusses the basic principles of DNA structure and its organization into genes, DNA transcription into RNA, the processing of transcribed RNA and protein synthesis and, finally, DNA replication and repair.

DNA structure

Deoxyribonucleic acid (DNA) is a structure composed of individual molecules, called nucleotides, which are arranged in a long chain. Each nucleotide is composed of a sugar (deoxyribose), a phosphate and a nitrogenous base. The DNA molecule is composed of two chains of nucleotides arranged in a double helix. Covalent bonds, called phosphodiester bonds, between adjacent sugars form the backbone of each chain and the two chains are held together by hydrogen bonds between the bases, which point in, towards the centre of the helix. The accompanying four bases can occur in any order and fall into two types, purines (adenine (A) and guanine (G)), and pyrimidines (thymine (T) and cytosine (C)). In general, adenine pairs with thymine and cytosine pairs with guanine, making each chain, or strand, complementary to the other. Each DNA chain has a polarity determined by the orientation of the sugar–phosphate backbone. The chain end terminated by the carbon atom at position 5 of the sugar molecule is referred to as the 5 prime (5′) end, and the end terminated by the carbon atom at position 3 is called the 3 prime (3′) end. In the double-stranded DNA molecule the 5′ end of one strand is opposite to the 3′ end of the other, i.e. they have opposite orientations and are said to be antiparallel. By convention, the DNA sequence is written in the 5′ to 3′ direction and, when a gene is present, the sequence is written such that the DNA coding for the amino terminus of the protein is to the left of the page (the 5′ end of the gene), whereas the carboxy terminus is to the right of the page (the 3′ end of the gene).

The genome

In humans, one copy of the entire double-stranded DNA content is referred to as the haploid genome and contains approximately 3,000,000,000 base pairs, divided in 23 different molecules, each part of a different chromosome. However, virtually all cells are diploid, with two copies of this genome in 46 chromosomes, 22 pairs of autosomes (numbered 1–22) and two sex chromosomes (called X and Y).

The genetic code by which DNA directs the synthesis of the protein constituents of the cell is a series of words (5′ to 3′), each word being a three nucleotide unit (called a codon) which specifies a particular amino acid to be incorporated into the mature protein. There are 64 possible codons (four bases in triplet combinations, $4^3 = 64$), 61 of which specify one of the 20 amino acids and three (TAA, TAG, TGA) are nonsense codons, which terminate the growing polypeptide chain.

Only about 1% of human DNA is decoded into protein sequences. These discrete areas within the genome are referred to as genes. The average size of a gene at the DNA level is about 10,000 base pairs (10 kilobases (10 kb)) and only 2–3 kb of the average gene codes for the eventual protein. Sequences within the gene include coding regions (exons), non-coding regions (introns) and regulatory sequences (Fig. 5.1).

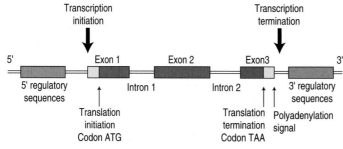

Figure 5.1: Structure of an idealized human gene.

Although the human genome is almost identical from one person to another, there are small variations in DNA sequences between individuals (DNA polymorphisms). These are usually in non-coding DNA, either in the extensive regions of DNA between genes or within introns. These sequence variations have aided the identification of disease-causing genes and are thought to have a role in the inter-individual variation in susceptibility to disease, including cancer development.[2]

Transcription

It is not possible for DNA to be decoded directly into protein. This is because chromosomal DNA remains in the nucleus of a cell and the synthesis of a new protein requires metabolic apparatus associated with ribosomes in the cytoplasm. Instead, a copy of the DNA sequence to be decoded is synthesized in the form of a mobile molecule called messenger RNA (mRNA), which is then used as an intermediary to transfer the genetic information from the nucleus to the cytoplasm. The process whereby genetic information is transmitted from DNA to mRNA is called transcription.

To synthesize RNA the enzyme RNA polymerase II and other associated enzymes distort the chromatin structure to expose the underlying DNA. A section of the double-stranded DNA helix is then unwound and the hydrogen bonds between the bases are disrupted. As a result, a section of DNA can serve as a template for a new polymer. Every base in the new mRNA molecule is complementary to a corresponding base in the DNA of the gene (note that in RNA the base uracil (U) replaces thymine (T) to base-pair with adenine (A)). In any particular gene only one DNA strand of the double helix acts as the so-called template strand. The transcribed mRNA molecule is a copy of the complementary coding ('sense') strand of the DNA double helix. The particular DNA strand used for RNA synthesis appears to vary throughout different regions of the genome.

Regulation of DNA transcription

The activity of RNA polymerase II, and hence the rate of transcription and expression, is tightly controlled. Two major components are involved in this control:

- the presence of specific DNA sequences upstream or downstream of the gene
- proteins that recognize and bind to these specific sequences.

The DNA sequences are called promoter, enhancer or silencer sequences, whereas the proteins that bind to them are called transcription factors.

A promoter consists of a number of short nucleotide sequences (called 'motifs') located within 200 bp upstream (5′) of a gene. The same DNA motif is often found in many different promoter regions. Examples include the TATA box, the GC or GGGCGGG consensus sequence and the CCAAT or CAT box. An enhancer is a DNA sequence that may be positioned from a few hundred bases to tens of kilobases from the start point of transcription of a gene. It can be positioned either upstream (towards the 5′ end) or downstream (towards the 3′ end) of a gene and can affect the transcription of genes in either orientation of the DNA molecule. Promoters and enhancers increase the level of gene transcription. Similarly, other DNA sequences around genes function as negative regulatory elements or silencers, and inhibit transcription. These regulatory elements exhibit a great degree of similarity (homology) among species and are thought to be highly conserved.

Transcription factors are proteins that bind specifically to DNA sequences within DNA regulatory elements and regulate gene expression. Some transcription factors bind to most promoter regions and are essential for transcription, whereas others only bind to promoters and enhancers associated with particular genes and ensure tissue-specific expression of that gene. Transcription factors are frequently mutated in cancer cells as they have an essential role in regulating cellular homeostasis (discussed below).

RNA processing

Before the primary mRNA molecule leaves the nucleus, it undergoes a number of modifications known as post-transcriptional processing

(Fig. 5.2). Immediately after the synthesis of the primary mRNA transcript, nuclear proteins associate with the newly transcribed polymer, which is composed of both introns and exons. It is modified first by the addition of a 5′ CAP structure, and a 3′ polyadenine (polyA) tail, which stabilize the ends of the short single-stranded molecule to protect it against intracellular breakdown. Secondly, highly accurate splicing machinery (an assembly of small nuclear RNAs and proteins called a spliceosome complex) removes introns, joins adjacent exons and creates an exon-only complement. The spliceosome complex coordinates the recognition of splice site consensus sequences, demarcating the exon–intron boundaries, and catalyses the requisite biochemical reactions in order to excise a single intron accurately. Many genes have alternative splicing patterns (where the difference between the processed RNA is the presence or absence of certain exons), which may be exhibited in different tissues, at specific developmental stages or in response to exogenous stimuli.

Translation

The transmission of the genetic information from mRNA to protein is called translation (Fig. 5.3). The processed mRNA migrates out of the nucleus into the cytoplasm, where it becomes associated with the ribosomes (complexes of cytoplasmic rRNA and protein). These contain enzymes, and bind small single-stranded transfer RNAs (tRNA). Each tRNA carries one of the 20 amino acids and the complementary sequence to the corresponding triplet codon (anticodon). The ribosome moves along the mRNA in a zipper-like fashion, the amino acids linking up by the formation of peptide bonds to form a polypeptide chain. When a stop codon is reached, synthesis of the polypeptide chain terminates and the chain is released. The ribosome is then free to associate with another mRNA molecule.

DNA replication

The principle of heredity is the ability of the sequence of DNA bases to be copied faithfully to new daughter DNA polymers, thereby preserving the genetic code in the next generation. Error-proof DNA replication is one of the main cellular processes disrupted during cancer development. During nuclear division enzymes, known as DNA helicase enzymes, cause the unwinding and separation of the two strands of the DNA, and, in a manner somewhat analogous to RNA transcription, the enzyme DNA polymerase initiates two daughter strands, each copied from one of the parental strands.

DNA repair

The maintenance of genetic stability is essential to the viability of multicellular organisms. However, the integrity of the genome is constantly challenged, both by errors occurring

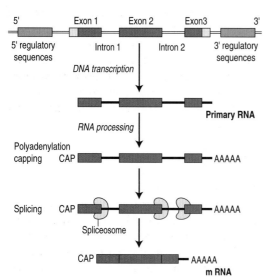

Figure 5.2: Transcription and post-transcriptional processing of RNA.

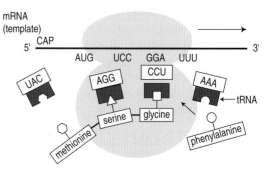

Figure 5.3: Translation of the genetic information carried by mRNA into protein.

during DNA replication and by structural alterations occurring spontaneously or as the result of environmental stimuli (mutagenesis). Organisms have therefore evolved a wide range of molecular mechanisms to remove and repair damaged DNA and hence protect the cell. All DNA repair systems studied so far have been highly conserved during evolution.

The faithful copying of DNA bases during replication is maintained by three processes:

1 Base selection: DNA polymerase discriminates between correct and incorrect nucleotides.

2 Exonucleolytic proofreading: if the wrong nucleotide is incorporated, it is excised by a 3′–5′ exonuclease before the daughter chain is elongated.

3 Mismatch repair: the proteins of mismatch repair can recognize DNA base pair mismatches as well as sites of replication slippage, where the replication machinery has skipped past a few bases at regions of simple repeat sequences. They bind to the DNA in the mispaired region and initiate excision of the mismatched base(s) before synthesizing the repair patch.

Other repair mechanisms have evolved to maintain genomic stability. Some repair proteins are designed to remove specific lesions, e.g. enzymatic reversal of damage by photoreactivation, whereby pyrimidine dimmers induced by short-wavelength UV are snipped apart by enzymes which require absorption of light from the visible light spectrum for their activity.[3] Other repair systems are more versatile and can deal with a number of different DNA lesions. These tend to involve complexes of proteins acting in concert with each other and sometimes with other DNA metabolic processes. The nucleotide excision repair (NER) pathway is perhaps the most versatile and can remove a wide variety of lesions that cause large structural distortions in the DNA.[4] Proteins of the NER pathway operate to monitor the DNA and recognize structural distortions in the helix. The DNA strand carrying the lesion is incised on both sides close to the damaged bases by endonuclease action and the intervening double-helical DNA (with damaged bases) is unwound by a helicase and discarded. Repair synthesis fills the resultant single-strand gap by copying the undamaged complementary strand to form a repair patch, which is then ligated (bound) to the parental DNA by a DNA ligase to complete the process.

The base excision repair pathway reverses damage induced by spontaneous additions of oxygen and hydrogen molecules through a chemical reaction with water (the processes of oxidation and hydrolysis) to the DNA bases, whereas DNA double-strand breaks may be repaired by a variety of ways, including recombination with a homologous duplex (as described above) or simple ligation of the broken ends.

There are a number of rare inherited syndromes with defects in the DNA repair apparatus (e.g. xeroderma pigmentosum, Fanconi's anaemia, ataxia telangiectasia). Each of these confers an excess risk of cancer, directly linking mutations in these genes with carcinogenesis.[5–7] Cancer appears to be the final outcome of unrepaired DNA.

THE CELL CYCLE

A living human cell is both a single entity and part of a multicellular organism. The processes of DNA replication, cellular growth and cell division are strictly regulated to ensure that cells divide at periods appropriate to cellular size and DNA status. Cancer is a genetic disease characterised by uncontrolled cell growth, as a result of multated DNA. In this section the normal cell division cycle and its controls will be described.

Cell division

Mitosis

A resting cell replicates its DNA during a discrete synthetic period (S phase) once it has sufficient nutrients and cellular mass (Fig. 5.4). A further cellular growth phase (G2) is required before the cell can divide into daughter cells. As mitosis (M) commences, chromatin is remodelled to allow the chromosomes to condense; once they have replicated, they appear as a doublet structure of two daughter chromatids joined at the centromere. In the next stage, the nuclear envelope disassembles, and a new subcellular structure, the mitotic spindle, forms by the polymerization of microtubules. Chromosomes attach to the spindle by their centromeres, and migrate to the centre of the spindle. The microtubules then move to opposite ends of the cell, carrying with them the centromeres, which divide to ensure chromatid segregation. At the end of mitosis, the nuclear membrane reforms around the two daughter cells, the chromosomes decondense and a further period of cellular growth (G1) ensues.

Meiosis

Meiosis is the process of nuclear division which occurs during the final stage of gamete (reproductive cell) formation. It differs from mitosis in two respects. First, to ensure that after fertilization a cell with a pair of each type of chromosome (a diploid (2n) cell) is created, a second round of chromatid segregation occurs to reduce the DNA content of each gamete to a single set of chromosomes (haploid (n)). Secondly, at the outset of meiosis, genetic material is exchanged between the paired chromosomes, which form crossover structures known as chiasmata. Several chiasmata may be present per chromosome pair. This process of

DNA recombination is critical in generating the variation that enables species to adapt to their environment.

Normal mammalian cells are only able to undergo a finite number of cell divisions. One explanation for this phenomenon is the failure to repair exogenous damage to important parts of the cell such as the DNA. A further process appears to be of particular importance in limiting the general number of cell divisions, while rendering specific cells (stem cells, germline cells and cancerous cells) capable of dividing an extended number of times as is required. The ends of chromosomes, termed telomeres, are specialized structures that make the chromosome stable by coordinating and positioning chromosomes during mitosis. In this way, chromosomes are prevented from fusing incorrectly, and the cell is, therefore, able to replicate chromosomal ends. Telomeres consist of G-rich sequences (telomeric repeat units), the number of which is reduced at each cell division. Progressive shortening of the telomeres is thought to be responsible for cellular senescence. While cells can counteract the loss of telomeric repeat units during cell division by adding them using the enzyme telomerase and thereby undergo more divisions before becoming senescent, telomerase expression appears to be stringently repressed in normal human somatic tissues. It is, however, reactivated in cancer, suggesting that re-expression of telomerase coincides with immortalization of cells, which is a crucial step in progression to malignancy. Examples of neoplastic cells that have been shown to express telomerase include malignant haematopoietic cells and ovarian carcinoma cells.[8,9]

Regulation of the cell cycle

A series of mechanisms operate to ensure that progression to the next stage of the cell cycle occurs only if the cell is in the appropriate environment, and if the preceding stage of the cell cycle has been completed successfully.[10,11] There are two major decision points within the cell cycle (see Fig. 5.4). The first is called 'Start', and defines the point at which cells are committed to exit from G1 and enter the S phase of the cycle. In mammalian cells this is

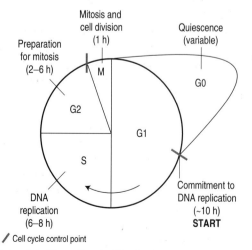

Figure 5.4: The cell cycle. The dashed lines indicate the major checkpoints.

the major transition point in the cell cycle (also known as the restriction point) and it is often described as the point at which cells become committed to a complete cell cycle. This is because cells that are not cycling usually exist in a specialized state referred to as G0 or stationary phase, which they enter from the G1 period of the cycle. Growth-stimulating signals induce passage through 'Start' and growth-inhibitory signals prevent passage through 'Start'.

A second decision point exists prior to the onset of mitosis, at the G2/M border. The function of the G2/M control point seems mainly to ensure that the DNA is free of errors and is ready to be separated at mitosis. Since mitosis is an irreversible act, it is vital that the DNA is completely replicated and undamaged when mitosis occurs. The pathways that ensure that this is the case and act to delay mitosis when problems are detected are known as checkpoints.

Many of the proteins that coordinate and control the cell cycle have been identified. Key regulators of cell cycle progression are the cyclin-dependent kinases (CDKs). Kinases are enzymes that catalyse the transfer of phosphate groups from a high-energy phosphate containing molecule to a molecule on which it is acting. The kinase activity of all CDKs is dependent on their association with cyclins. All cells contain a large number of cyclins, which are groups of proteins that act during the different stages of the cell cycle and fluctuate in level as the cell cycle progresses. The association of CDKs with the different cyclin subunits at each of the different stages of the cell cycle helps to coordinate the cell cycle 'programme'. In order to stop or pause the cell cycle at either of the two major control points, further methods of regulating the activity of these CDK complexes are required, such as phosphorylation (addition of a phosphate) of CDK proteins and specific CDK inhibitors. Two examples serve to illustrate the action of checkpoints:

- If DNA synthesis is interrupted, then cells do not proceed through the G2/M transition into mitosis until the block is removed and DNA synthesis is completed. In yeast cells, mutations in a number of genes have been identified which abolish this checkpoint. In such cells, a block to DNA synthesis results in the catastrophic attempt to segregate the unreplicated chromosomes and subsequent cell death.

- If the DNA is damaged during the cell cycle, this is recognized, and signals are sent that inhibit both the G2/M transition (mitosis) and 'Start' (DNA synthesis). The prevention of passage through 'Start' appears to act through activation of inhibitors of CDK function.

Attempting to either replicate or segregate damaged DNA is likely to lead to the fixation and accumulation of mutations, or genomic instability, both of which are precursors to cancer. Several tumour suppressor genes are involved in the correct operation of the checkpoints, attesting to the important role the checkpoints play in preventing oncogenesis by maintaining the accurate replication of DNA and chromosome segregation.

Withdrawal from the cell cycle

Differentiation

Differentiation is the process by which cells or tissues undergo a change toward a more specialized form or function and it requires a cell to exit the cell cycle, which for some cells occurs when they are deprived of growth factor stimulation. Integration of signals in different cells – some maintained as self-renewing stem cells, others undergoing terminal differentiation – is the essence of development, in which the lineage of a particular cell, as well as the environmental signals that it receives, play a crucial role in shaping its ultimate fate.

Cell differentiation results from differences in gene expression, leading to a distinct cell phenotype. Tumour cells show abnormalities in differentiation (anaplasia) as a direct consequence of the distinct genes they express. The anaplasia of tumours can provide insights into their aetiology, degree of malignancy, prognosis and sensitivity to therapeutic intervention.

Apoptosis

The sculpting or shaping of tissues and organs during development and the maintenance of appropriate cell numbers demands that controlled cell loss occurs alongside proliferative cell gain. The removal of cells which are in excess of appropriate number, or which are aged or damaged, must occur in a manner that avoids the leakage of the contents of the cell in order to prevent the initiation of an inflammatory reaction. Cell death by apoptosis provides the mechanism whereby cells are removed in a regulated way.[12] Apoptosis is a type of cell death which is conceptualized as 'programmed' because it is a death driven from within the cell, essentially a cell suicide. The 'programme' to do this is considered to be intrinsic to all cells and it occurs without breaking the plasma membrane. Cells which depend upon continued growth factor stimulation for survival will undergo apoptosis if they are deprived of growth factors. Additional causes of apoptosis include signals of continued DNA damage, or inflammatory-related stimuli. Programmed cell death occurs in three molecular phases: (1) an initiation event, which is cell type- and stimulus-specific, (2) an effector stage, involving a cascade of enzymes (caspases), leading to (3) the degradation phase. Apoptotic cells are finally engulfed by local macrophages.

In some cell types, particularly certain stem cells, DNA damage readily initiates apoptosis.[13] The deletion of a cell with a damaged genome may be preferable to fixation of the DNA damage and its perpetuation in descendants as a mutation. This might be especially important if these cells give rise to greatly amplified numbers of potentially damaged progeny. Thus, initiation of apoptosis prevents carcinogenesis by removing damaged cells with a potential to undergo malignant transformation. Hence, cancer might be more appropriately conceived as a disease of cell survival, permissive for proliferation.

MOLECULAR GENETICS OF CANCER

Cancer is caused by abnormalities in the genetic mechanisms that control cellular growth, proliferation and survival; hence, at a cellular level, cancer can be designated a genetic disorder. The genetic abnormalities observed in cancer cells are usually acquired (secondary to environmental carcinogens), but in some individuals with a genetic predisposition to cancer they may have been inherited. Almost every human cancer can occur both randomly and as a result of genetic predisposition. Although inherited cancers are uncommon, they are important because it appears that the same genes may be involved in the pathogenesis of both inherited and randomly occurring cancers. Therefore, the identification of the mechanisms of genetic predisposition to cancer should provide an insight into the molecular changes that occur.

Mutations

A mutation is defined as an alteration in the genetic material. Although mutations can occur either in non-coding or coding sequences, it is only in the latter that they are usually of consequence. It is important to note that a mutation arising in a somatic cell cannot be transmitted to offspring, whereas if it occurs in gonadal tissue or a gamete it can be transmitted to future generations.

In the course of a lifetime a variety of mutations accumulate in cells throughout the body. These arise through exposure to chemicals, radiation, viruses and as a consequence of mistakes made by the DNA replicative and repair machinery. Most mutations make no difference to the functioning of the individual cell in which they occur, although some may alter the cell's viability so that it dies. In either case, there are no noticeable ill effects on the well-being of the body as a whole. Occasionally, however, a single cell suffers a series of mutations which, when converted into abnormal cellular machinery, cause the cell and its descendants to proliferate in the unrestrained and uncoordinated fashion characteristic of cancer cells. The following types of mutation are involved in the development of cancer.[14]

Point mutation

This describes the substitution of one base pair of a DNA sequence by another (e.g. substitution of an A:T base pair by a G:C). In the protein which results from this DNA sequence, this single base pair substitution may have a number of effects based on its position:

- The mutation may result in the substitution of one amino acid for another (a missense mutation), resulting in a protein identical to the normal (wild type) except for the single amino acid change. The functional consequences of this change will depend on the nature of the amino acid substitution and the biological activity of the protein.

- If the mutated sequence encodes a signal for the termination of translation (a stop codon), then the protein will be prematurely terminated at this position. As a consequence, a substantial part of the protein may be omitted, rendering it non-functional.

- If a mutation arises in one of the consensus splicing sequences of mRNA, the correct splicing events may not take place and a whole exon may be missed out of the mRNA. When translated into protein, the amino acids encoded by this exon will be absent and a frame shift may be introduced, altering substantially the predicted protein sequence downstream of the mutation.

Translocation

In a translocation, part of one chromosome is joined to another. The outcome is a hybrid chromosome that may be detectable by cytogenetic analysis of tumour cells. At the molecular level, a gene located at or near the breakpoint in one of the two chromosomes is fused to sequences from the other chromosome. This rearrangement of DNA sequences may generate a structurally altered version of the gene and its protein or may place it under new transcriptional control.

Gene amplification

The diploid genome of each human cell normally carries two copies of each gene, one originating from each parent (except for the X and Y chromosomes). Under certain circumstances one copy may be multiplied up to several thousand fold, a phenomenon known as gene amplification. Gene amplification is believed to contribute to tumour development (oncogenesis) by increasing the levels of

mRNA that are transcribed from the gene and, as a consequence, increasing the levels of protein that it encodes. Increased or decreased expression of certain proteins without amplification or any other form of mutation of the DNA encoding them is a common feature of many tumours.

Deletion

A wide range of DNA deletions occur in tumour cells. At one extreme, a single base pair may be removed, whereas larger deletions may encompass part or all of a gene. Finally, a deletion may be large enough to remove a whole chromosome.

Whereas a large deletion will obviously remove from the genome, and hence inactivate, all the genes that are included within it, smaller deletions may also have a number of effects. If the DNA fragment that is deleted results in removal of a segment of the mRNA that is a multiple of three base pairs, then only the amino acid sequence encoded by that segment will be absent from the protein. The consequences of this structural abnormality will depend upon the functional properties of this segment in the normal protein. However, if the deleted segment in the mRNA is not a multiple of three base pairs, then a frame shift will be introduced. The likely consequence is that the amino acid sequence of the protein downstream of the mutation will bear little resemblance to the normal and will often be prematurely terminated because of the presence of a stop codon. The effects of insertions into DNA are subject to the same considerations as deletions but tend to be less common as mutational events in cancer genes.

Epigenetic events

The methylation of DNA (the addition of a methyl group) on specific cytosine residues is believed to contribute to the changes in gene expression that occur during development. Presumably, DNA methylation affects gene expression, because the transcriptional regulatory proteins that bind to methylated DNA differ from those that bind to unmethylated DNA.[15] It has been shown that methylation of regions rich in cytosine–guanine doublets ('CpG islands') in the promoter region in somatic cells is a common mechanism of epigenetic silencing of one or sometimes both copies (alleles) of tumour suppressor genes such as p16[16] and BRCA1.[17] It is not clear whether this silencing of particular genes in cancer occurs through a random process followed by selection, or whether certain promoters are predisposed.[18] It is also unclear what determines whether a particular gene will lose function by an epigenetic or mutational mechanism.

CANCER GENES

A cancer gene is any gene sequence that contributes directly to neoplastic change. Most human cancer genes are generated by mutations in normal (wild-type) cellular genes. Cancer genes that are activated by mutation are referred to as dominant oncogenes. They exert their cellular effects despite the presence of normal gene product from the homologous allele. On the other hand, genes whose cellular functions are inactivated by mutation are called tumour suppressor genes and are described as recessive because they exert their effects only in the absence of normal protein.

Oncogenes

Oncogenes comprise a family of genes that act dominantly to induce or maintain cell transformation. Oncogenes were first demonstrated in RNA tumour viruses,[19] and further research has revealed that they are derived from normal cellular genes that have a potential to transform into an oncogene (called proto-oncogenes).[20] These genes have a role in normal cellular growth and proliferation but, when mutated, may function as oncogenes. More than 60 proto-oncogenes or oncogenes have been reported, and a list of some of those involved in human cancer is shown in Table 5.1. The functions of proto-oncogenes can be classified into four broad groups:

1 growth factors
2 growth factor receptors
3 signal transducers
4 nuclear proto-oncogenes and transcription factors.

Examples of proto-oncogene growth factors include platelet-derived growth factor (*PDGF*), epidermal growth factor (*EGF*), insulin-like growth factors 1 and 2 (*IGF1* and *IGF2*), and transforming growth factor α and β (*TGFα* and *TGFβ*). Overexpression of *IGF2* is a feature of many Wilms' tumours.[21]

Growth factor receptors provide a link between the stimulatory effects of growth factors and the intracellular signalling pathways. Two transmembrane receptors, known as *RET* and *MET*, may be mutated in inherited cancers such as multiple endocrine neoplasia type 2 (MEN2) and familial papillary renal cancer,[22,23] where their mutation results in abnormal activation of the receptor protein.[24,25]

Proto-oncogene signal transducers are components of the intracellular signal transduction systems, responsible for relaying messages from the cell membrane receptors to the nucleus. Examples of such oncogenes include membrane-associated proteins (*RAS*, *ABL*, *SRC*) and cytoplasmic tyrosine kinases (*RAF1*, *MOS*). *RAS* mutations are frequent in human cancers (e.g. colon, pancreas, bladder and lung), although the particular *RAS* gene involved varies between cancer types.[26]

Nuclear proto-oncogenes are DNA-binding proteins, and include transcription factors (*MYC*, *FOS*), which are important in regulating the expression pattern of target genes. Amplification of *MYC* genes has been found in a variety of tumour types, including lung,[27] breast[28] and neuroblastoma.[29]

Mutations in proto-oncogenes are referred to as activating or gain-in-function mutations because they enhance, or confer new properties on the cellular functions of the encoded oncoproteins. Proto-oncogenes may be mutated to promote cell transformation by a variety of mechanisms:

1 *Gene amplification* contributes to the transformed cell by increasing the level of mRNA, and hence protein, that is expressed from a proto-oncogene. However, expression of the amplified gene is sometimes increased out of proportion to the increase in gene copy number, indicating abnormalities of transcriptional regulation.[30] Moreover,

the segment of DNA that is amplified is often large, extending over several hundred kilobases or even megabases. The amplified segment therefore usually stretches well beyond the boundaries of the proto-oncogene and encompasses several other genes. Many types of oncogene are activated by gene amplification. These include the genes for growth factor receptors such as epidermal growth factor receptor (*EGFR*) in malignant gliomas and *ERBB2* in breast cancer,[31,32] and nuclear oncogenes such as *N-MYC* in neuroblastoma.[33] Gene amplification is usually a late, and hence progressive, step in oncogenesis rather than an initiating or early event. Moreover, amplification can sometimes be correlated with poor outcome and late stage, e.g. amplification of the *N-MYC* gene in neuroblastoma is now recognized as an independent clinical indicator of outcome.[33]

2 *Translocations* may activate the proto-oncogene, or result in a 'fusion gene' encoding a novel product. Between 90% and 95% of chronic myeloid leukaemia (CML) carries the translocation between chromosomes 9 and 22, termed the Philadelphia translocation.[34] In the t(9:22) translocation, one allele of the *C-ABL* gene (the human homologue of *V-ABL*, an oncogene carried by the Abelson murine leukaemia virus) is split and joined to a gene on chromosome 22, known as *BCR* (for breakpoint cluster region). The consequence of the rearrangement is that the *ABL* gene loses its most 5′ exon and is joined to an allele of the *BCR* gene which has lost its 3′ region. When the region is transcribed, the resulting mRNA is a hybrid, with the 5′ region composed of *BCR* and the 3′ region of *ABL* sequences. Similarly, the protein is a hybrid of BCR amino acid sequence at the amino terminus and ABL amino acid sequence at the carboxy terminus. A biochemical feature of the ABL protein believed to be of importance both in its normal functions and in oncogenesis is its ability to phosphorylate other proteins on tyrosine residues. The BCR–ABL fusion protein has an elevated tyrosine kinase activity and this may contribute to its oncogenic action.[35]

3 *Point mutations* may alter the function of the gene product and produce a transforming protein. Genes of the *RAS* family provide the best-described examples of oncogene activation by point mutation in human tumours. RAS proteins are signal transduction molecules composed of 188 or 189 amino acid residues which normally undergo a cycle of activation and inactivation. Mutated RAS proteins in human tumours, however, are fixed in the activated conformation, transmitting a continuous growth signal to the nucleus in the absence of growth factor stimulation. The alterations in DNA that result in this change in biochemical activity are almost exclusively point mutations.[26] All are missense, and hence allow translation of a full-length RAS protein. Of particular importance, however, is the restriction of the mutations to certain sites within the gene, namely codons 12, 13 and 61 (that encode amino acids 12, 13 and 61 of the RAS protein). Mutations at other sites are not found in human tumours, nor do most of them result in oncogenic activation in experimental models.[36] Thus it appears that the biological characteristics of RAS proteins place considerable constraints upon the type and location of activating point mutations. Moreover, these structural and biochemical alterations are apparently sufficient for an activated RAS protein to contribute to oncogenesis. Changes in the level of expression of the protein are unnecessary (although occasionally present) and other mutational mechanisms such as translocation or gene amplification are rare.

Tumour suppressor genes

Genes whose cellular functions are inactivated by mutation are called tumour suppressor genes. Tumour suppressor genes are a

Table 5.1: Examples of oncogenes

Proto-oncogene	Tumour	Lesion
Growth factors		
PDGF	Glioma	Amplification
IGF2	Wilms'	Amplification
Growth factor receptors		
MET	Familial papillary renal cancer	Point mutation
RET	Multiple endorine neoplasia type 2	Rearrangement
TRK	Colon carcinoma	Rearrangement
EGFR	Squamous cell carcinoma	Amplification
Signal transducers		
H-RAS	Colon, lung, pancreas carcinoma	Point mutation
K-RAS	Leukaemia, thyroid carcinoma	Point mutation
N-RAS	Carcinoma, melanoma	Point mutation
GSP	Thyroid carcinoma	Point mutation
ABL	Chronic myeloid leukaemia	Translocation
SRC	Colon carcinoma	Point mutation
RAF1	Melanoma	Point mutation
MOS	Sarcoma	Point mutation
Nuclear proteins		
N-MYC	Neuroblastoma, lung carcinoma	Amplification
L-MYC	Lung carcinoma	Amplification
FOS	Osteosarcoma	Unknown
JUN	Sarcoma	Point mutation

class of genes that act in normal cells to inhibit unrestrained cell division. When inactivated (as by mutation) a natural constraint on cell proliferation, cell adhesion or other cellular functions that control cell behaviour is removed. Several human tumour suppressor genes have been isolated and partially characterized in terms of biochemical activities and cellular effects; they are detailed in Table 5.2.

Tumour suppressor genes are described as recessive because they exert their cellular effects only in the absence of normal protein. This usually means that both alleles must be inactivated by mutation for cell behaviour to be neoplastic. Therefore, two independent mutations

Table 5.2: Examples of tumour suppressor genes

Cancer syndrome	Gene	Principal malignancies
Li–Fraumeni	*p53*	Sarcomas, breast, brain tumours
Retinoblastoma	*Rb1*	Retinoblastoma, osteosarcoma
Familial adenomatous polyposis	*APC*	Colon cancer
Familial breast cancer	*BRCA1*	Breast, ovarian cancer
	BRCA2	Breast cancer
Neurofibromatosis type 1	*NF-1*	Neurofibromas, sarcomas, gliomas
Neurofibromatosis type 2	*NF-2*	Schwannomas, meningiomas
Tuberous sclerosis	*TSC2*	Renal and brain tumours
Wilms' tumour	*WT-1*	Nephroblastoma
Von Hippel–Lindau	*VHL*	Renal cell, phaeochromocytomas, haemangiomas

or 'hits' are required.[37] The mutation or hit that inactivates the first allele of a tumour suppressor gene is usually confined to the gene itself or involves the gene and chromosomal DNA that is immediately adjacent to it. In contrast to the dominantly acting genes that are mutated in a consistent manner either by point mutation (*RAS*), translocation (*ABL*) or gene amplification (*N-MYC*), the types of alterations that inactivate a particular tumour suppressor gene such as the retinoblastoma (*Rb*) gene are diverse and include point mutations, deletions and rearrangements. Moreover, these mutations are much less constrained both in their type and position within the gene. For example, the point mutations that inactivate the retinoblastoma or *p53* genes are located at a large number of positions within the gene in contrast to the three codons that are point mutated in activated *RAS* genes. Although they may be missense, they can also be nonsense (encoding translational stop codons) or affect splice sites. Similarly, deletions may affect part or all of the gene and may be in and out of frame. Translocations may occur at virtually any site that will interrupt the production of an intact mRNA.[38]

Although the overall pattern described above is applicable to most tumour suppressor genes, there are differences between them in the predominance of types of mutation. For example, the *APC* (adenomatous polyposis coli) gene, which is responsible for the syndrome of familial polyposis coli and is mutated in a large proportion of colonic tumours, is subject to a preponderance of nonsense mutations such as stop codons, or small deletions and insertions.[39] Translation of the APC protein is usually prematurely terminated, and hence the protein is inactivated. By contrast, in the *p53* gene there is a much higher proportion of missense mutations that result in a full-length protein with just a single amino acid substitution.[38] The reason for this is that some p53 proteins with missense mutations can interact with and functionally inactivate normal p53 protein in the cell without the need for a mutation at the DNA level in the remaining allele.[40]

The mutation that inactivates the second allele of a tumour suppressor gene is, in only a minority of cases, similar in character to the first mutation, i.e. confined to the gene and neighbouring chromosomal DNA. More commonly, it involves loss of a large part and even all of the chromosome upon which the second allele of the tumour suppressor gene is situated. The reason for this difference is probably that the second hit often arises due to errors of mitosis.[41] Such errors, which include non-disjunction (incorrect separation of chromatids during mitosis) or mitotic recombination (exchange of segments of DNA by homologous chromosomes), usually involve large stretches of DNA up to and including a whole chromosome. This phenomenon has been of considerable importance in the detection and localization of tumour suppression genes. By using specific probes it is possible to visualize both parental copies of a particular region independently. If one copy has been lost during oncogenesis, this will manifest itself as loss of heterozygosity (reduction from two bands to one) in the tumour compared to germline DNA. Because the second hit in a tumour suppressor gene is large, the probe can be located several million base pairs away from the gene itself and still detect its presence by loss of heterozygosity. By performing studies in which a set of tumours are examined using at least one probe on each chromosomal arm, it is possible to obtain an approximate picture of the number and genetic locations of the tumour suppressor genes involved in the development of a tumour class.

PROCESS OF CANCER DEVELOPMENT

Carcinogenesis describes the acquisition of those cellular properties that render a cell competent to grow into a tumour. Once tumours have formed, further properties continue to appear in the cells, some carrying selective growth advantage. This evolution of phenotype (the observable physical and biochemical characteristics) within tumours is referred to as tumour progression. Both carcinogenesis and tumour progression represent changes that lead from normality to aggressive tumour growth.

Tumour pathology has often suggested that tumours evolve by a series of discrete transitions. Thus, there are clearly recognizable morphological distinctions between benign and malignant tumours. Similarly, the terms atypical hyperplasia, intraepithelial neoplasia and invasive carcinoma reflect different degrees of deviation from the normal cellular structure and behaviour. Often these lesions occur in isolation, but there are also many observations of, for example, invasive carcinoma existing in the same tumour as intraepithelial carcinoma, of atypical hyperplasia apparently merging with areas of intraepithelial neoplasia, or of carcinoma arising within a pre-existing benign tumour.[42] It appears from these histological patterns that new behaviour is acquired in a sequential, stepwise pattern.

Epidemiological data have shown that the age-related increase in human tumour incidence, with few exceptions, follows a steeply rising curve. The shape of this curve is amenable to mathematical modelling, and one model interprets the slope to indicate the number of separate events involved in carcinogenesis. For the great majority of adult-onset carcinomas, this slope suggests the existence of five or six such independent events.[43] Molecular genetic analysis of human cancers usually demonstrates multiple abnormalities, e.g. activation of two or more oncogenes and loss of tumour suppressor genes. Thus, although a particular genetic alteration may be necessary for carcinogenesis, in most cases a single event is not sufficient. This model is compatible with the concept that the normal cell has multiple independent mechanisms to control growth and differentiation and that aberrations in several distinct pathways or at several sites within a pathway are required to overcome these control mechanisms. For example, if a cell mutates to produce a growth factor to which it already expresses the receptor (autocrine stimulation), that cell will replicate more frequently but will still be subject to cell cycle checkpoints to promote DNA integrity in its progeny. If an additional mutation overriding a cell cycle checkpoint occurs, that cell and its progeny may go on to accumulate further mutations, some of which may allow it to replicate an unlimited number of times by synthesis of telomerase, or to separate from its matrix and cellular attachments without undergoing apoptosis. As deregulated growth continues, cancer cells become increas-

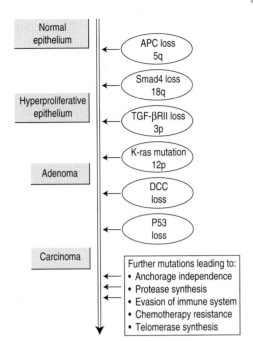

Figure 5.5: Accumulation of genetic changes in the multi-step progression of colorectal carcinogenesis.

ingly unable to differentiate, fail to respond to local signals as in normal tissue and cease to ensure appropriate chromosomal segregation pre-division, generating the classical malignant pathological appearances of disorganized growth, variable levels of differentiation and polyploidy (having more than two sets of chromosomes). This sequence has been very well described for colonic carcinomas[44] and is illustrated in Figure 5.5.

In the majority of patients, there is no inherited defect and somatic cell mutations are solely responsible for the development of disease. It takes years, possibly decades, for the required somatic events to accumulate. Since DNA mutations occur very infrequently, only an occasional cell will go on to acquire a further mutation, but this will be transmitted to the progeny of that cell.

HEREDITARY PREDISPOSITION TO CANCER

Cancer is described as a genetic disease at the cellular level because alterations in genes result in cancer formation. In some individuals, the first genetic alteration is inherited and accounts for an inherited predisposition to cancer. Examples of cancer predisposition syndromes are presented in Table 5.2. This predisposition does not necessarily make cancer inevitable, but it does greatly increase the risk. The risk does not rise to 100% in individuals carrying a predisposition gene because several other independent genetic changes also have to occur. The chance that the disease will develop as the result of inheriting a cancer predisposition is called the penetrance.

In general, inherited predisposition to cancer is likely to be present when cases cluster together in genetically related individuals more often than one would expect by chance. There are two instances when this occurs, the first being when rare cancers cluster in families. If each cancer is a rare event, the chance of two or more cancers representing a random cluster is very low. An example of this is the multiple endocrine neoplasia (MEN) syndrome, in which medullary thyroid cancer clusters with phaeochromocytoma (both are rare tumours in the general population).[45] The second instance is when common cancers cluster in families at a much younger age than in the general population, or where many cases occur in one family. For example, four cases of breast cancer, even at older age of onset, are unlikely to be due to chance alone in the same genetic lineage. Multiple instances of cancer in the same patient are also more common in cancer due to a genetic predisposition (e.g. bilateral breast cancer). Hence, a family is more likely to have a cancer predisposition gene if:

- there are multiple young cases of a common cancer site on one side of the family
- there are clusters of rare-site cancers
- there are clusters of cancers at different sites known to be associated with particular cancer predisposition genes.

However, it is important to note that familial cancer aggregations do not necessarily indicate a genetic basis, and can also be caused by shared environment. The ultimate proof of an inherited cancer syndrome is the demonstration of a germline mutation in the relevant gene.

It has long been recognized that people differ in their susceptibility to cancer. Today, we describe this observation as inter-individual variation in cancer risk manifested as gene–environment interactions, which embodies the concept that heritable traits modify the effects of environmental exposures. The heritable effects of genes in human cancer pathogenesis range from high-penetrance genes, which have a high probability of causing cancer, to low-penetrance genes, which have an increased risk of causing cancer, although this is less likely to occur than with high-penetrance genes. The range from low- to high-penetrance genes is a continuum, and studies in animal models indicate that the effects of high-penetrance genes can be modified by other genes.[46] In humans, high-penetrance genes that cause cancer family syndromes can have substantial impact in affected families, but they affect only a small percentage of the population. In contrast, the manifestations of cancer susceptibility genes with less penetrance contributing to common sporadic cancers will affect a large segment of the population.[47] Thus, the identification and study of low-penetrance genes also has important public health implications. Molecular epidemiology of human cancer risk is the study of inter-individual variation and gene–environment interactions through a multidisciplinary effort (e.g. epidemiology, molecular genetics, cell biology, biochemistry, statistics and bioethics). Recognizing that cancer is a genetic disease involving multiple genes, molecular epidemiology uses biomarkers of cancer risk that will elucidate multiple gene–environment interactions, where several genes and exposures work interactively. Candidate examples of such a model would be inherited variations in the ability to metabolize carcinogens or precarcinogens (e.g. cytochrome P450 polymorphisms and lung cancer in smokers),[48] host factors controlling the immune response to oncogenic viruses (women with the gene *HLA-DQw3* appear to be at increased risk of cervical carcinoma),[49] or defective DNA repair mechanisms.

CARCINOGENESIS RELATED TO EXOGENOUS AND ENDOGENOUS FACTORS

The genetic basis of carcinogenesis has been established through biochemical and molecular analyses of the disease. Many different types of cancer have been attributed to environmental influences (chemical and physical carcinogens, radiation and viruses) and it is becoming increasingly apparent that factors within the organism (hormonal levels, inflammation) play an important role in the process of carcinogenesis. Here we will examine more closely the contribution of these factors to the development of cancer.

Chemical carcinogenesis

A large number of human cancers have been shown to be caused by occupational or environmental exposure to chemical agents.[50] Examples of such cancers are detailed in Table 5.3. Chemical carcinogenesis is a multistep process that begins with exposure, usually to complex mixtures of chemicals that are found in the environment. A chemical carcinogen interacts with DNA and may cause a mutation by modification of the molecular structure of DNA. There are several ways in which the chemical structure of DNA can be altered by a carcinogen, including the formation of adducts, alkylation, oxidation, dimerization and deamination.[51] Chemical carcinogens can also cause epigenetic changes, such as alteration in DNA methylation status. These changes, if not appropriately repaired, may lead to DNA mutation and tumour initiation. Initiated cells are irreversibly altered and at greater risk of malignant conversion than normal cells.[51]

Mutations in oncogenes and tumour suppressor genes may reflect the mutagen that induced them. Evidence for this notion in human tumours has emerged through the study of mutations in the *p53* gene in many types of cancer. A number of tumour types are found to

Table 5.3: Examples of chemical carcinogens implicated in cancer development.[51]

Cancer type	Chemical carcinogen
Lung (small cell, squamous and adenocarcinoma)	Tobacco smoke Arsenic Chromium Nickel Bis ether Diesel exhaust
Oesophagus (squamous cell carcinoma)	Tobacco smoke
Oral cavity (squamous cell carcinoma)	Betel nut Chewing tobacco
Skin (basal cell carcinoma)	Cutting oils Soot Coal tar
Nasal sinuses	Nickel Snuff (tobacco) Isopropyl alcohol
Liver (hepatocellular carcinoma, angioma)	Aflatoxin B_1 Vinyl chloride
Bladder (squamous cell)	Aromatic amines
Acute lymphoblastic leukaemia	Benzene

have a different spectrum of mutations, which in some cases are related to a known mutagen. For example, in smoking-induced lung cancers, the predominant mutation type in the *p53* gene is a G:C to T:A transversion (a transversion mutation is one in which a purine is replaced by a pyrimidine or a pyrimidine by a purine), consistent with the type of mutation induced by mutagens in tobacco smoke.[52] Moreover, in the case of hepatoma, it is believed that exposure to the substance aflatoxin results not just in a par-

ticular type of base change but also in clustering at a particular codon of *p53* around which the DNA sequence may preferentially encourage carcinogen binding.[53]

Most carcinogenic chemicals, once internalized, are subject to competing metabolic pathways of activation and detoxification. Variations among individuals in the metabolism of carcinogens (cytochrome P450 polymorphisms and tobacco), together with differences in DNA repair capacity and response to tumour promoters, govern the relative risk for cancer development of an individual.[54]

Physical carcinogenesis

The term physical carcinogens comprises a wide range of agents, including electromagnetic radiation, alpha and beta radiations, low and high temperatures, mechanical trauma and solid (metals, fibres) and gel (silicone) materials. These agents have the ability to produce cancer mainly, if not exclusively, through their physical properties and physical effects, rather than through their chemical properties and actions, as opposed to the chemical carcinogens.[55] Such physical mechanisms have been regarded as the non-specific irritative effect of hypothetical surface factors on cells that could cause cellular proliferation, the selection of spontaneously occurring transformed clones and the development of neoplasia. However, a possible contribution of chemical mechanisms to the potential of carcinogenesis of these agents remains a possibility that requires further investigation. Examples of physical carcinogens and their associated cancers are detailed in Table 5.4.

Physical carcinogenesis is an important public health, economic and social problem because of the large-scale diffusion of these materials in the workplace, as well as the general and domestic environment, and their increasing use in surgical and dental specialities.

Ionizing radiation

The hazards of exposure to ionizing radiation were recognized shortly after the discovery of the X-ray in 1895.[56] Since then, many experimental and epidemiological studies have

Table 5.4: Examples of physical carcinogens implicated in cancer development.[51]

Physical carcinogen	Cancer type
Metals (gold, platinum, silver, steel) Metallic alloys Polymers (e.g. polyethylene, Teflon, nylon, silicon) Natural organic materials (silk, keratin, ivory)	Sarcomas – fibrosarcomas, rhabdomyosarcomas, osteosarcomas
Asbestos	Lung cancer Mesothelioma (pleural, peritoneal) Pharyngolaryngeal cancer Gastrointestinal cancer Kidney cancer
Erionite Glass wool Talc-containing asbestiform fibres	Mesothelioma Lung cancer
Non-fibrous particulate materials (powered metallic cobalt and nickel, crystalline silica)	Sarcomas Malignant lymphomas Lung cancer

confirmed the oncogenic effects of radiation in many tissues. There are a number of characteristics specific to ionizing radiation that differentiate it from chemical toxic agents or other physical carcinogens. Ionizing radiation has the ability to penetrate cells and to deposit energy within them in a random fashion, unaffected by the cellular barriers presented to chemical agents. All cells in the body are thus susceptible to damage by it, and the amount of damage incurred will be related to the physical parameters that determine the radiation dose received by the particular cells or tissue.

Ionizing radiation results in ionization and excitation of atoms and molecules in the irradiated cells. These molecules are highly unstable and rapidly undergo chemical change, which results in the production of free radicals (atoms or molecules containing unpaired electrons). Free radicals are extremely reactive and may lead to permanent damage of the affected molecule. Chemical damage may be repaired before it is irreversible by the recombination of radicals and dissipation of the associated energy, or it may be modified by agents such as molecular oxygen.[57]

The DNA damage induced by free radicals may result in a variety of cellular and tissue effects. Radiation (1) can kill cells either by inducing apoptosis or by inhibiting mitosis,[58] (2) induce mutagenesis in both somatic and germinal cells,[59] (3) cause chromosomal aberrations (e.g. such as the chromosome 8:14 translocation in Burkitt's lymphoma),[60] and (4) provoke neoplastic transformation.[61]

Ionizing radiation has been called a universal carcinogen in that it will induce cancer in most tissues of all species at all ages. The cancers induced by radiation are of the same histological types as occur naturally, but the distribution of types may differ as follows.

- a higher percentage of small cell carcinomas of the lung occur as a result of exposure to alpha radiation in uranium miners
- radiation induction of follicular and papillary carcinomas of the thyroid but not anaplastic and medullary carcinomas
- chronic lymphocytic leukaemia is apparently not induced by radiation, whereas other common types of leukaemias are.[62]

There is a distinct latent period between exposure to radiation and the clinical appearance of a tumour.[62]

Ultraviolet radiation

Skin tumours in humans account for about 30% of all new cancers reported annually. Epidemiological and laboratory studies provide evidence for a direct causal role of sunlight exposure in the induction of cancer; the high rate of skin carcinogenesis is the direct result of the high dose rate from this causative agent.[63] The target molecule for UV radiation is the DNA itself. The energy absorbed by DNA produces molecular changes, some of which involve single bases (monomeric damage, single-strand breaks), others resulting in interactions between adjacent bases (dimerizations) as well as between non-adjacent bases (inter- or intrastrand cross-links), and others between DNA and its nucleosomal scaffold (DNA–protein cross-links). The DNA damage induced by UV radiation can result in the activation of oncogenes (e.g. *RAS*)[64] and/or inactivation of tumour suppressor genes (e.g. *p53*), and hence initiation of neoplasia.[65] Inter-individual variations in DNA repair mechanisms seem to determine susceptibility to carcinogenesis.[66]

Hormonal influences to carcinogenesis

Hormones play an important role in the aetiology of several human cancers, mainly of the breast, endometrium, prostate, ovary, thyroid, bone and testis.[67] Hormones exert an effect that is independent of outside initiators, such as chemicals and ionizing radiation. Neoplasia appears to be the consequence of excessive hormonal stimulation of the particular target organ, the normal growth and function of which is controlled by one or more hormones. Breast cancer has been widely studied and can be used to illustrate the way hormones affect carcinogenesis. Oestradiol and to a lesser degree other steroid hormones (e.g. progesterone) drive breast cell proliferation, which facilitates mutation, enhances fixation of mutations or facilitates

expression of genetic errors through loss of heterozygosity by defects in DNA repair.[68] Germline mutations in relevant tumour suppressor genes (like *p53* and *BRCA1*, *BRCA2*) further accelerate the transformation to the malignant phenotype.[69–71] Epidemiological studies have shown that the major hormonally related risk factors for breast cancer, all leading to increased exposure to oestrogen and/or progesterone, are early age at menarche, late menopause, late age at first full-term pregnancy, obesity and hormone replacement therapy.[72]

Infection and inflammation

Trauma and chronic inflammation have long been known to be associated with cancer. Their effects may be mediated through increased mitogenesis, which may be associated with increased mutation, or through paracrine effects, e.g. from inflammatory cells.[73] Indeed, *p53* mutations are seen at frequencies similar to those in tumours in chronic inflammatory diseases such as rheumatoid arthritis and inflammatory bowel disease.[74] The strongest association of chronic inflammation with malignant diseases is in colon carcinogenesis, which arises in individuals with inflammatory bowel diseases such as chronic ulcerative colitis and Crohn's disease.[75]

There is a growing body of evidence that many malignancies are initiated by infections. More than 15% of malignancies worldwide can be attributed to infections, a global total of 1.2 million cases per year.[76] Persistent infections within the host may induce chronic inflammation. Leucocytes and other phagocytic cells induce DNA damage in proliferating cells, through the generation of reactive oxygen and nitrogen species that are produced normally by these cells to fight infection. Hence, repeated tissue damage and regeneration of tissue, in the presence of highly reactive oxygen and nitrogen species released from inflammatory cells, interacts with DNA in proliferating epithelium, resulting in permanent genomic alterations such as point mutations, deletions or rearrangements.[77] Examples of the above include hepatitis B and C infection of the liver, which predisposes to liver carcinoma,[78] an increased risk of bladder and colon carcinoma associated with schistosomiasis,[79,80] and chronic *Helicobacter pylori* infection, which is the world's leading cause of stomach cancer.[81]

Infectious viral agents may also directly transform cells by inserting active oncogenes into the host genome. Examples of such viruses include the retroviruses (human T-cell leukaemia virus, human immunodeficiency virus),[82,83] the herpesviruses (Epstein–Barr viruses associated with Burkitt's lymphoma, Hodgkin's disease and nasopharyngeal carcinoma),[84] and human papillomaviruses with cervical neoplasia.[85] It appears that proteins encoded by several DNA tumour viruses, including the human papillomaviruses, can interact with cell proteins such as the retinoblastoma gene product, which normally have tumour suppressor activity.[86] In addition, proteins from these viruses also transactivate expression of cell genes that may be important to initiate or maintain neoplasia.[87] Interestingly, only a subset of individuals infected with these viruses develop virus-associated malignancies.[76] This may reflect immune suppression, the necessity of cofactors necessary for promotion or the fact that a neoplasm can develop only if viral infection has targeted a pluripotent progenitor or stem cell.

CONCLUSION

Although much progress has been made in characterizing human cancer genes and understanding the molecular biology of cancer, there are still many questions to be answered. There are a large number of cancer susceptibility genes that remain to be identified. Recent technological developments have accelerated the search for such genes. The completion of the human genome project has provided a vast amount of information regarding inter-individual variability at the genomic level and is providing an increasing number of candidate susceptibility loci. Susceptibility genes of low penetrance are of particular interest. The aggregate effect of several of these genes and other non-genetic (environmental) predisposing factors may define a spectrum of risk across the population. These factors may then be used to construct 'risk profiles' that would identify either small groups of people at high risk who account for a substantial fraction of cancer incidence, or large groups who are at very low risk. Identification of individuals at high risk of cancer will allow targeted screening, leading to improvements in early diagnosis, intervention strategies for treatment of neoplasia and finally, continued improvements in public health policy. The identification of such susceptibility genes will also allow better characterization of cancer pathogenesis, leading to the discovery of new therapeutic targets and improved prognosis for patients with cancer.

REFERENCES

1. Nowell PC. The clonal evolution of tumour cell populations. Science 1974; 194:23–28.
2. Botstein D, Risch N. Discovering genotypes underlying human phenotypes: past successes for mendelian disease, future approaches for complex disease. Nature Genetics 2003; 33:228–237.
3. Sancar A. Structure and function of DNA photolyase. Biochemistry 1994; 33:2–9.
4. Friedberg EC. How nucleotide excision repair protects against cancer. Nature Rev Cancer 2001; 1:22–33.
5. Kreamer KH, Lee MM, Scotto J. DNA repair protects against cutaneous and internal neoplasia: evidence from xeroderma pigmentosum. Carcinogenesis 1982; 5:511–514.
6. Taylor AMR. Ataxia telangiectasia genes and predisposition to leukaemia, lymphoma and breast cancer. Br J Cancer 1992; 66:5–9.
7. Levine AS. Workshop on molecular, cellular and clinical aspects of Fanconi anaemia. Exp Hematol 1993; 21:703–726.
8. Norrback KF, Roos G. Telomeres and telomerase in normal and malignant haematopoietic cells. Eur J Cancer 1997; 33:774–780.
9. Wan M, Li WZ, Duggan BD, et al. Telomerase activity in benign and malignant epithelial ovarian tumors. J Natl Cancer Inst 1997; 89:437–441.
10. Nurse P. Checkpoint pathways come of age. Cell 1997; 91:865–867.
11. Paulovich AG, Toczyski D, Hartwell LH. When checkpoints fail. Cell 1997; 88:315–321.
12. Lavin M, Watters D, eds. Programmed cell death: the cellular and molecular biology of apoptosis. New York: Harwood Academic Press; 1993.
13. White E. Life, death and the pursuit of apoptosis. Genes Dev 1996; 10:1–15.
14. Stratton MR. Mechanisms of activation and inactivation of dominant oncogenes and tumour suppressor genes. In: Yarnold JR, Stratton MR, McMillan TJ, eds. Molecular biology for

oncologists. London: Chapman and Hall; 1996:16–26.

15. Momparler RL. Cancer epigenetics. Oncogene 2003; 22:6479–6483.

16. Herman JG, Merlo A, Mao L, et al. Inactivation of the *CDKN2/p16/MTS1* gene is frequently associated with aberrant DNA methylation in all common human cancers. Cancer Res 1995; 55:4525–4530.

17. Bianco T, Chenevix-Trench G, Walsh DC, Cooper JE, Dobrovic A. Tumour-specific distribution of *BRCA1* promoter region methylation supports a pathogenetic role in breast and ovarian cancer. Carcinogenesis 2000; 21:147–151.

18. Baylin SB, Herman JG. DNA methylation in tumorigenesis. Trends Genet 2000; 16:168–174.

19. Rous P. A sarcoma of the fowl transmissible by an agent separable from the tumour cells. Nature 1911; 13:397.

20. Stehelin D, Varmus HE, Bishop JM, et al. DNA related to the transforming gene(s) of avian sarcoma viruses is present in normal avian DNA. Nature 1976; 260:170–173.

21. Reeve A, Eccles M, Wilkins R, et al. Expression of insulin-like growth factor-II transcripts in Wilms' tumour. Nature 1985; 317:258–260.

22. Mulligan LM, Kwok JBJ, Healey CS, et al. Germ-line mutations of the *RET* proto-oncogene in multiple endocrine neoplasia type 2A. Nature 1993; 363:458–460.

23. Schmidt L, Duh F, Chen F, et al. Germline and somatic mutations in the tyrosine kinase domain of the *MET* proto-oncogene in papillary renal carcinomas. Nature 1997; 16:68–73.

24. Takahashi M, Ritz J, Cooper GM. Activation of a novel human transforming gene, *RET*, by DNA rearrangement. Cell 1985; 42:581–588.

25. Park M, Dean M, Cooper CS, et al. Mechanism of met oncogene activation. Cell 1986; 45:895–904.

26. Lowy DR, Willumsen BM. Function and regulation of *RAS*. Annu Rev Biochem 1993; 62:851–891.

27. Nau MM, Brooks BJ, Battey J, et al. *L-myc*, a new *myc*-related gene amplified and expressed in human small lung cancer. Nature 1985; 318:69–73.

28. Sinn E, Muller W, Pattengale P, et al. Coexpression of *MMTV/v-Ha-ras* and *MMTV/c-myc* genes in transgenic mice: synergistic action of oncogenes in vivo. Cell 1987; 49:465–475.

29. Schwab M, Varmus HE, Bishop JM, et al. Chromosome localisation in normal cells and neuroblastomas of a gene related to c-myc. Nature 1984; 308:288–291.

30. Sugawa N, Ekstrand AJ, James CD, et al. Identical splicing of aberrant growth factor receptor transcripts from amplified rearranged genes in human glioblastomas. Proc Natl Acad Sci USA 1990; 87:8602–8606.

31. Schimke RT. Gene amplification in cultured animal cells. Cell 1984; 37:705–713.

32. King CR, Kraus MH, Aaronson SA. Amplification of a novel *v-erbB*-related gene in human mammary carcinoma. Science 1985; 229:974–976.

33. Schwab M. Amplification of *N-myc* as a prognostic marker for patients with neuroblastoma (review). Semin Cancer Biol 1993; 4:13–18.

34. Nowell PC, Hungerford DA. A minute chromosome in human chronic granulocytic leukaemia. Science 1960; 32:1497.

35. De Klein A, Van Kessel AG, Grosveld G, et al. Cellular oncogene is translocated to the Philadelphia chromosome in chronic myelocytic leukaemia. Nature 1982; 300:765–767.

36. Bos JL. The ras gene family and human carcinogenesis. Mutation Res 1988; 195: 255–271.

37. Knudson AG Jr. Mutation and cancer: statistical study of retinoblastoma. Proc Natl Acad Sci USA 1971; 68:820–823.

38. Hollstein M, Sidransky D, Vogelstein B, et al. *p53* mutations in human cancers. Science 1991; 253:49–53.

39. Nagase H, Nakamura Y. Mutations of the *APC* (adenomatous polyposis coli) gene. Hum Mutat 1993; 2:425–434.

40. Zambetti GP, Levine AJ. A comparison of the biological activities of wild-type and mutant *p53*. FASEB J 1993; 7:855–865.

41. Cavanee WK, Dryja TP, Phillips RA, et al. Expression of recessive alleles by chromosomal mechanisms in retinoblastoma. Nature 1983; 305:779–784.

42. Wistuba II, Mao L, Gazdar AF. Smoking molecular damage in bronchial epithelium. Oncogene 2002; 21:7298–7306.

43. Peto R, Roe FJC, Lee PN, et al. Cancer and ageing in mice and men. Br J Cancer 1975; 32:411–426.

44. Fearon ER, Vogelstein B. A genetic model for colorectal tumorigenesis. Cell 1990; 61:759–767.

45. Thakker RV. Multiple endocrine neoplasia – syndromes of the twentieth century. J Clin Endocrinol Metab 1998; 83:2617–2620.

46. Halberg RB, Katzung DS, Hoff PD, et al. Tumorigenesis in the multiple intestinal neoplasia mouse: redundancy of negative regulations and specificity of modifiers. Proc Natl Acad Sci USA 2000; 97:3461–3466.

47. Peto J. In: Cairns J, Lyon JL, Skolnick M, eds. Cancer incidence in defined populations, Banbury report 4. New York: Cold Springs Harbor; 1980.

48. McLemore TL, Adelberg S, Liu MC, et al. Expression of *CYP1A 1* gene in patients with

lung cancer. J Natl Cancer Inst 1990;
82:1333–1339.

49. Wank R, Thomseen C. High risk of squamous
cell carcinoma of the cervix for women with
HLA-DQw3. Nature 1991; 352:723–725.

50. International Agency for Research on Cancer.
IARC monographs on the evaluation of
carcinogenic risks to humans. Overall evaluations
of carcinogenicity. Monographs volumes 1–87.
Lyon: IARC; 1971:2004.

51. Yuspa SH, Poirier MC. Chemical carcinogenesis:
from animal models to molecular models in one
decade. Adv Cancer Res 1988; 50:25–70.

52. Greenblatt MS, Bennett WP, Hollstein M, et al.
Mutations in the *p53* tumour suppressor gene:
clues to cancer etiology and molecular
pathogenesis. Cancer Res 1994; 54:4855–4878.

53. Hollestein M, Moeckel G, Hergenhahn M, et al.
On the origins of human mutations in cancer
genes: insights from the *p53* gene. Mutat Res
1998; 405:145–154.

54. Harris CC. Interindividual variation among
humans in carcinogen metabolism, DNA adduct
formation and DNA repair. Carcinogenesis 1989;
10:1563–1566.

55. Infante PF, Schuman LD, Dement J, et al.
Fibrous glass and cancer. Am J Ind Med 1990;
26:559–584.

56. Upton AC. Historical perspectives on radiation
carcinogenesis. In: Upton AC, Albert RE, Burns
FJ, Shore RE, eds. Radiation carcinogenesis.
New York: Elsevier; 1986:1–10.

57. Ward FJ. The yield of DNA double-strand breaks
produced intracellularly by ionising radiation: a
review. Int J Radiat Biol 1990; 57:1141–1150.

58. Little JB. Cellular effects of ionizing radiation. I
& II. N Engl J Med 1968; 273:308–315,
369–376.

59. Grosovsky AJ, Little JB. Evidence for linear
response for the induction of mutations in
human cells by x-ray exposures below
10 rads. Proc Natl Acad Sci USA 1985;
82:2092–2095.

60. Dutrillaux B. Ionizing radiation induced
malignancies in man. Radioprotection 1997;
32:C431–440.

61. Cox R, Little JB. Oncogenic cell transformation
in vitro. In: Nygaard OF, Sinclair WK, Lett JT,
eds. Advances in radiation biology, Vol.15. New
York: Academic Press; 1992:137–158.

62. National Research Council. Committee on the
biological effects of ionising radiation. Health
effects of exposure to low levels of ionising
radiation (BEIR V). Washington, DC: National
Academy Press; 1990:21.

63. Fitzpatrick TB, Sober AJ. Sunlight and skin
cancer. N Engl J Med 1985; 313:818–820.

64. Ananthaswamy HN, Price JE, Goldberg LH,
et al. Detection and identification of activated
oncogenes in human skin cancers occurring on
sun-exposed body sites. Cancer Res 1988;
48:3341–3346.

65. Ziegler A, Jonason AS, Leffell DJ, et al. Sunburn
and p53 in the onset of skin cancer. Nature
1994; 372:773–776.

66. Bootsma D, Kraemer KH, Cleaver JE, et al.
Nucleotide excision repair syndromes: xeroderma
pigmentosum, Cockayne syndrome, and
trichothiodystrophy. In: Vogelstein B, Kinzler
KW, eds. The genetic basis of human cancer.
New York: McGraw-Hill; 1998:245–274.

67. Henderson BE, Ross RK, Pike MC, et al.
Endogenous hormones as a major factor in
human cancer. Cancer Res 1982; 42:
3232–3239.

68. Henderson BE, Ross RK, Bernstein L. Estrogens
as a cause of human cancer: the Richard and
Hilda Rosenthal Foundation award lecture.
Cancer Res 1988; 48:246–253.

69. Malkin D, Li FP, Strong LC, et al. Germ line
p53 mutations in a familial syndrome of breast
cancer, sarcomas, and other neoplasms. Science
1990; 250:1233–1238.

70. Miki Y, Swensen J, Shattuck-Eidens D, et al. A
strong candidate for the breast and ovarian
cancer susceptibility gene *BRCA1*. Science 1994;
266:66–71.

71. Wooster R, Bignell G, Lancaster J, et al.
Identification of the breast cancer susceptibility
gene *BRCA2*. Nature 1995; 378:789–792.

72. Henderson BE, Pike MC, Ross RK.
Epidemiology and risk factors. In: Bonadonna G,
ed. Breast cancer: diagnosis and management.
New York: John Wiley and Sons; 1984:1–17.

73. Friedwald WF, Rous P. The pathogenesis of
deferred cancer. J Exp Med 1941; 73:365.

74. Firestein GS, Echeverri F, Yeo M, Zvaifler NJ,
Green DR. Somatic mutations in the *p53* tumor
suppressor gene in rheumatoid arthritis
synovium. Proc Natl Acad Sci USA 1997;
94:10895–10900.

75. Cohen AM, Shenk B, Friedman MA. Colorectal
cancer. In: DeVita VT, Hellman S, Rosenberg
SA, eds. Cancer: principles and practices of
oncology. Philadelphia: JB Lippincott; 1989:895.

76. Vousden KH, Farrell PJ. Viruses and human
cancer. Br Med Bull 1994; 50:560–581.

77. Nakamato Y, Guidotti LG, Kuhlen CV, et al.
Immune pathogenesis of hepatocellular
carcinogenesis. J Exp Med 1998; 188:
341–350.

78. Nalpas B, Driss F, Pol S, et al. Association
between HCV and HBV infection in
hepatocellular carcinoma and alcoholic liver
disease. J Hepatol 1991; 12:70–74.

79. Cheever AW. Schistosomiasis and neoplasia.
J Natl Cancer Inst 1978; 61:13–18.

80. Chen MC, Chang PY, Chuang CY, et al.
Colorectal cancer and schistosomiasis. Lancet
1981; 1:971–973.

81. Parsonnet J, Friedman G, Vandersteen D, et al.
Helicobacter pylori infection and the risk of
gastric carcinoma. N Engl J Med 1991;
325:1127–1131.

82. Gallo RC, Blattner WA, Reitz MB Jr, et al. The virus of adult T-cell leukaemia in Japan and elsewhere. Lancet 1982; 1:683.

83. Lyter DW, Bryant J, Thackeray R, et al. Incidence of human immunodeficiency virus-related and non-related malignancies in a large cohort of homosexual men. J Clin Oncol 1995; 13:2540–2546.

84. Gaffey MJ, Weiss LM. Association of Epstein–Barr virus with human neoplasia. Pathol Ann 1992; 27:55–74.

85. Meisels A, Morin C. Human papillomavirus and cancer of the uterine cervix. Gynecol Oncol 1981; 12(Suppl):111–123.

86. Dyson N, Howley PM, Monger K, et al. The human papilloma virus-16 E7 oncoprotein is able to bind the retinoblastoma gene product. Science 1989; 243:934–937.

87. Munger K, Phelps WC, Bubb V, et al. The *E6* and *E7* genes of the human papilloma virus type 16 together are necessary and sufficient for transformation of primary human keratinocytes. J Virol 1989; 63:4417–4421.

FURTHER READING

Alberts B, Bray D, Lewis J, et al. Molecular biology of the cell. 3rd edn. New York: Garland; 1994.

Bast RC Jr, Kufe DW, Pollock RE, et al, eds. Cancer medicine. 5th edn. Hamilton: BC Decker; 2000.

Foulkes WD, Hodgson SV, eds. Inherited susceptibility to cancer: clinical, predictive and ethical perspectives. Cambridge: Cambridge University Press; 1998.

Kurzrock R, Talpaz M, eds. Molecular biology in cancer medicine. 2nd edn. London: Martin Dunitz; 1999.

Mendelsohn J, Howley PM, Israel MA, et al, eds. The molecular basis of cancer. Philadelphia: WB Saunders; 2001.

Ponder BAJ, Waring MJ, eds. The genetics of cancer. London: Kluwer Academic Publishers; 1995.

Vogelstein B, Kinzler KW, eds. The genetic basis of human cancer. New York: McGraw-Hill; 1998.

Yarnold JR, Stratton MR, McMillan TJ, eds. Molecular biology for oncologists. 2nd edn. London: Chapman and Hall; 1996.

CHAPTER 6

Pathology

CHAPTER CONTENTS

Introduction	97
General characteristics of tumours	97
Morphological characteristics in relation to tumour behaviour	98
The classification of cancer	99
Tumours composed of epithelial cells	99
Mesenchymal tumours	101
Mixed tumours	101
Other tumours	101
Tumour cells and tumour stroma	102
Clinical relevance	102
Regulation of cell growth	103
Reversible disturbances of cell growth	103

Persistent disturbances of cell growth	103
Regulation of tumour cell growth	105
The stromal response	106
Angiogenesis	106
Tumour stroma	107
Invasion and metastasis	108
Invasive growth	108
Circulating tumour cells	110
Metastasis	111
Conclusion	112
References	113

INTRODUCTION

Cancer is the second most important cause of death in the Western world, after cardiovascular diseases.[1] Cancer is a generic term and encompasses hundreds of different types of malignant tumours that have distinct characteristics according to the organ of origin, the nature of the cells involved and their biological behaviour. Cancer is primarily a disease of advancing age, although certain types of cancer occur predominantly in younger age groups. Men are more prone to develop cancer than women, by a factor of 1:5. Cancer death is higher in men than in women, largely because the most frequent form of cancer in men is lung cancer, which has a particularly poor prognosis. In this chapter, how cancer cells develop and the factors that are responsible for their evolution will be outlined and the factors that are important in the dissemination of cancer will be discussed. The main reasons for high mortality in the most aggressive forms of cancer will be presented.

GENERAL CHARACTERISTICS OF TUMOURS

Based on their morphological characteristics, tumours can be subdivided into two classes, benign and malignant. The morphological characteristics of cancer cell differentiation and tissue architecture are important elements in histopathological tumour classification. Tumours are benign when their growth potential is restricted and are, in general, not life threatening. Tumours are called malignant when they have a strong tendency to grow and invade adjacent structures as well as metastasize to distant sites. This is summarized in Figure 6.1.

Morphological characteristics in relation to tumour behaviour

Benign tumours are composed of well-differentiated cells that strongly resemble the normal cells of the tissue in which they arose. They do not show infiltrative growth but expand: they push aside surrounding tissue and form a pseudocapsule. Cell death, apoptosis or necrosis is unusual in benign tumours.[2] Cell division in benign tumours is limited. In mucous membranes, benign tumours often form pedunculated masses, which are called polyps (Fig. 6.2). Although benign tumours are in general not life threatening, they can lead to significant symptoms due to:

- pressure on the surrounding structures
- narrowing of a blood vessel or a duct, leading to impeded blood flow or secretions
- abnormal production of hormone
- progression into a malignant tumour.

A malignant tumour is usually composed of cells that individually, and in terms of tissue architecture, do not often resemble the cells of the tissues of origin. The shape of the cell and of its nucleus is often irregular and the amount of chromatin (the deeply staining substance of the nucleus and chromosomes of cells) is usually increased (Fig. 6.3). Malignant tumours are rarely encapsulated. Necrosis is frequent

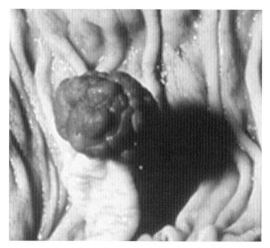

Figure 6.2: Macroscopic image of a pedunculated polyp in the large bowel (arrow). The head of the polyp represents a benign tumour (adenoma), with more vessels which give it a red colour. The stalk is covered with normal mucosa.

because tumour cell growth is often more rapid than the development of its vascular network. This leads to hypoxia and cell death. The determining feature of a malignant tumour is its infiltration into surrounding structures, including blood and lymphatic vessels, which is an element in its capacity to metastasize. Metastasis is the process by which tumour cells detach from the primary tumour, gain access to the blood or lymph circulation, are transported to distant sites in the body, become implanted in another organ and multiply to create a new separate tumour.

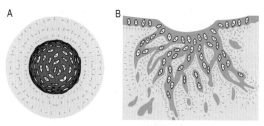

Figure 6.1: Pattern of a benign (A) versus a malignant tumour (B). The benign tumour has pushing borders that tend to form a (pseudo) capsule. In the malignant tumour, infiltrative cells migrate into the surrounding host tissue.

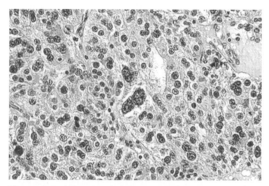

Figure 6.3: Microscopic image of a malignant tumour. The nuclei of the cells vary in size and shape (pleomorphism) and are darkly stained (hyperchromasia). The chromatin is distributed in coarse clumps. The cells are dividing (mitoses).

It is rather difficult to predict behaviour in some tumours that tend to be benign, grow slowly but can invade locally or even metastasize. Tumours with this type of unpredictable behaviour are called borderline tumours. The general characteristics of benign and malignant tumours are summarized in Table 6.1.

THE CLASSIFICATION OF CANCER

In the pathological nomenclature, the suffix -oma is generally used to indicate a neoplasm: adenoma, carcinoma and lymphoma all denote a tumour type.[3] In tumour classification, a number of general rules are applied:

1   Which cell types constitute the tumour?

*   For example, an adenoma is composed of epithelial cells, as is a carcinoma.
    A sarcoma is composed of mesenchymal cells, whereas a lymphoma is composed of lymphocytes.

2   How will the tumour behave?

*   For example, an adenoma is benign but a carcinoma is malignant. A fibroma is benign but a fibrosarcoma is malignant.

3   What are the macroscopic characteristics of a tumour?

*   For example, an adenoma that forms cystic spaces is called a cystadenoma.

4   What is the tissue architecture?

*   For example, if a benign epithelial tumour forms glandular structures, this is called an adenoma. If a benign epithelial tumour forms papillary finger-like structures, this is called a papilloma.

Some tumours are named after people: Ewing's sarcoma, Kaposi's sarcoma, Hodgkin's lymphoma are common examples. The most frequently occurring tumours are listed in Figure 6.4.

Au: Wrong Fig?

Tumours composed of epithelial cells

Benign tumours composed of gland-forming epithelia are called adenoma. Sometimes the cell type is added: a follicular adenoma of the thyroid gland is composed of follicular epithelial cells. Sometimes an architectural characteristic is added: in the colon, tubular adenomas form tubes and villous adenomas form finger-like villi. Benign tumours in stratified epithelia frequently have a papillary architecture and are called papilloma.

Malignant tumours composed of epithelial cells are called carcinoma. The direction of differentiation of the cells can be added: an adenocarcinoma is composed of epithelial cells that are arranged in glandular structures. A squamous cell carcinoma (also called epidermoid carcinoma) is composed of epithelial cells with squamous differentiation. The organ of origin may be included in the name, as in adenocarcinoma of the lung or a squamous cell carcinoma of the skin. For example, mucin-producing adenomas of the ovary are called mucinous cystadenoma; breast cancer is frequently composed of cells with characteristics of mammary ducts and is then called ductal carcinoma. Some microscopic images of cancer are given in Figure 6.5.

Sometimes, tumour cells no longer resemble the normal cells of the tissue in which the cancer developed or have the architectural characteristics of that tissue. When a tumour can be recognized as a carcinoma but the direction of differentiation can no longer be determined, the carcinoma is called undifferentiated or anaplastic. When an epithelial or mesenchymal differentiation of the cancer cells can no longer be

Table 6.1: Characteristics of benign and malignant tumours

Benign	Malignant
Slow growth	Rapid growth
No necrosis	Necrosis
No or few mitoses	Frequent mitoses
Limited cellular atypia	Marked atypia
Well differentiated	Poorly differentiated
Well demarcated	Invasive
No metastatic potential	High metastatic potential

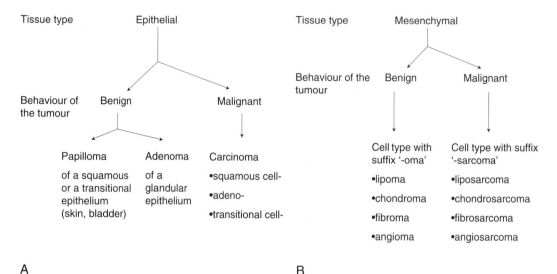

| Tissue type | Epithelial | | | Tissue type | Mesenchymal | |

A

B

Figure 6.4: Classification of epithelial tumours (A) and mesenchymal tumours (B).

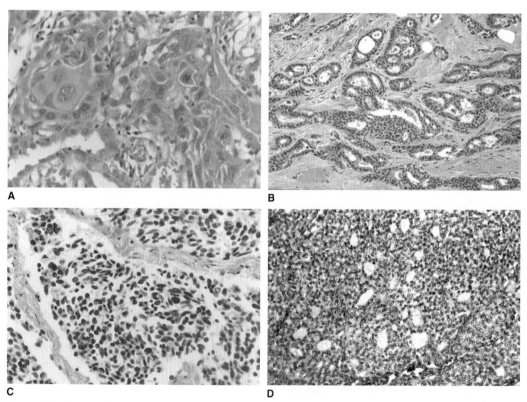

A

B

C

D

Figure 6.5: Characteristic microscopic images of human tumours. A. Squamous cell carcinoma (of the lung). Cells have clear boundaries with bridges (desmosomes) between the cells; the cells tend to keratinize. B. Ductal carcinoma of the breast. The cells form ductular structures, much as in the normal breast. C. Small cell carcinoma of the lung. The cells are small, have dense darkly stained nuclei and do not show any particular architecture. D. Follicular carcinoma of the thyroid. The tumour cells tend to form follicles, much as normal parenchymal cells do in the thyroid.

determined, the diagnosis might not be more specific than undifferentiated malignant tumour.

A carcinoma is by definition malignant. For lesions, which have the morphological characteristics of cancer cells but lack invasive growth, the term *carcinoma in situ* is used. The carcinoma in situ phase is preceded by the development of cells that show some but not all characteristics of cancer cells. In such lesions, proliferation is increased and differentiation incomplete. These lesions are called dysplastic lesions. Commonly, dysplasia is graded according to the degree of cellular atypia in low grade and high grade. High-grade dysplasia has a strong propensity to progress towards carcinoma in situ and invasive cancer.

Mesenchymal tumours

Benign tumours consisting of mesenchymal tissue are classified according to type of the cells that compose the tissue. The suffix -oma is then added: a tumour composed of adipocytes is called a lipoma: a tumour composed of fibrocytes is called a fibroma; a tumour composed of chondrocytes is called a chondroma; and a tumour composed of smooth muscle cells is called a leiomyoma.

Malignant tumours that are composed of mesenchymal cells are called sarcoma and the approach towards classification is similar: liposarcoma, fibrosarcoma, chondrosarcoma and leiomyosarcoma. In classifying these tumours, the nature of the extracellular matrix formed by tumour cells is often important: a chondrosarcoma makes cartilage and an osteosarcoma bone or osteoid. A myxoma shows a loose extracellular matrix containing important quantities of mucopolysaccharides. Also, the site of the tumour might be taken into consideration: e.g. soft tissue sarcoma.

Malignant lymphomas are composed of lymphocytes and might arise anywhere in the body where lymphoid tissue is present and, rarely, even in organs like the brain. Lymphomas are classified as Hodgkin's lymphomas or non-Hodgkin's lymphomas. Non-Hodgkin's lymphomas are further classified according to the direction of differentiation of the neoplastic lymphocytes, B lymphocytes or T lymphocytes. In addition, the stage of maturation of the cells is included: lymphomas are regarded as neoplastic equivalents of the well-defined steps in the differentiation of B or T lymphocytes.

Leukaemias constitute malignant proliferations of bone marrow cells that are shed into the blood. As a consequence, leukaemias are always systemic diseases.

Mixed tumours

Some tumours are composed of epithelial and mesenchymal cells and are therefore called mixed. Well known are mixed tumours of the salivary glands (they are also called pleomorphic adenoma due to the variety in morphology of the cells), in which the tumour cells form glands but also cartilage. Tumours of the synovia (the membrane that lines articular spaces) are mostly composed of cells with epithelial and mesenchymal characteristics. These synovial sarcomas are called biphasic as they comprise two morphologically distinctly cellular components; mesotheliomas, tumours that arise in the pleural or peritoneal membrane, are also biphasic.

Tumours that are derived from germinal cells in the ovary or the testis may be benign or malignant. In these tumours, the cells are derived from more than one germinal layer: e.g. epidermis from the ectoderm, bronchial mucosa from the endoderm and striated muscle from the mesoderm. Such tumours are called teratoma. In women, these ovarian tumours are almost always benign and are therefore called benign teratoma (Fig. 6.6). In the testis, these tumours are usually malignant and are called malignant teratoma. Apart from undifferentiated embryonal cells (tumours composed of such cells are called embryonal carcinoma), these tumours may contain cells that show trophoblastic differentiation, corresponding to cells in the developing placenta, and are then called choriocarcinoma.

Other tumours

Tumours of the pigment-forming cells of the skin, melanocytes, are called melanoma. Tumours of the brain often show glial differentiation and are called glioma. Tumours in infants and children are often composed of tissue with

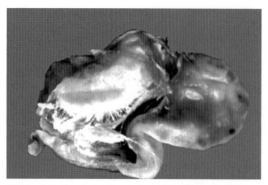

Figure 6.6: Cystic teratoma (epidermoid cyst) of the ovary in a young woman. Hairs and a mass of sebaceous material are indicative of the occurrence of skin in the tumour. Frequently, these benign tumours contain thyroid, nervous tissue, glands or gut mucosa.

strong resemblance to embryonal tissue and are called blastoma. Typical examples are nephroblastoma (in the kidney), hepatoblastoma (in the liver) and retinoblastoma (in the eye).

Some tumour-like lesions are composed of normal tissue components but in an abnormal admixture or architecture. These lesions are called hamartoma. Some hamartomas are genuine neoplasms, others most likely are developmental abnormalities.

Tumour cells and tumour stroma

It is important to realize that almost all tumours consist of a mixture of tumour cells and normal stromal cells. An epithelial tissue, be it normal or cancerous, has a well-composed infrastructure. Epithelial cells stick together through intercellular adhesion. They are supported by connective tissue cells such as fibroblasts and endothelial cells, which form capillaries, bringing nutrients and oxygen to the cells. In a tumour, this connective tissue is called the tumour stroma, and comprises fibroblasts, endothelial cells and an extracellular matrix.[4] This tissue infrastructure is provided to the developing tumour by the host, in response to growth factors – such as epidermal growth factor (EGF), transforming growth factor-β (TGF-β), platelet-derived growth factor (PDGF), basic fibroblast growth factor (bFGF) and vascular endothelial growth factor (VEGF) – released by the cancer

cells. The process of vessel growth in the stromal reaction is called *angiogenesis*. Later in this chapter we will come back to this process, which in recent years has proven to be an essential element in the development of a malignant tumour Occasionally, the stromal response of a tumour is rather voluminous and comprises large quantities of collagen-rich connective tissue. This type of tumour is called desmoplastic. In desmoplastic tumours, the size of the tumour is largely determined by the volume of the stromal component. Cancer cells might even be scarce. Such tumours characteristically have a rather firm consistency due to large numbers of dense collagen fibres. Breast carcinomas typically are desmoplastic.

A stromal reaction is typically evoked by an infiltrative growing tumour. When in doubt, pathologists tend to use the presence of a stromal reaction to tumour cells as an argument in favour of malignancy. Sarcomas and lymphomas also need a stroma, but this is much less defined than in carcinomas.

Clinical relevance

Correct tumour classification is of major clinical importance. The prognosis is usually excellent for a patient with a benign tumour but approximately 50% of malignant tumours will kill the patient, in spite of aggressive treatment.[5] The nature of a tumour can usually be established following morphological criteria in an histopathological examination, a process in which labelled antibodies are used as reagents to histochemically localize immunoreactive substances. The most important histopathological criterium for malignancy is infiltrative growth. Based upon the architecture, the morphology of the tumour cells and the nature of the extracellular matrix, the tumour can be further classified. In addition, the direction and degree of differentiation can be established. For detailed tumour classification, pathologists often use methods developed in cell and molecular biology, such as immunohistochemistry and, lately, also gene expression profiling.[6] Detailed typing of tumours is increasingly important in view of the expanding spectrum of therapeutic options, which allows a certain degree of individualization of treatment, dependent on the cellular or molecular characteristics of the tumour.

REGULATION OF CELL GROWTH

Cancer arises due to a disregulation of the growth and differentiation of cells. In normal tissues, cell turnover is a closely regulated process in which cell loss due to programmed cell death (apoptosis) is in equilibrium with cell renewal by proliferation. When cell loss is insufficiently compensated by proliferation, atrophy will result. When normal cell loss is reduced through disregulation of apoptosis, or cell proliferation exceeds what is necessary to replace lost cells, an abnormal accumulation of cells may ensue. This may be self-limiting and temporary, such as in epithelial hyperplasia. If unlimited cell growth continues, a neoplasm will develop.

Reversible disturbances of cell growth

Prolonged stimulation of cells during their regeneration can lead to local excess: e.g. in a callus that develops on the skin when exposed to prolonged pressure. This is called hyperplasia. When the stimulus is terminated, the situation in principle returns to normal. In practice, two different terms are in use to describe a temporary excess of tissue due to a pathological stimulus. When such a stimulus leads to increased cell volume, this is called hypertrophy. Heart muscle cells will increase in size, for example, in a patient with arterial hypertension because of increased demand: it is not the number of cardiomyocytes that increases but the volume of individual cardiomyocytes, as does their contractile force.

When the number of cells increases, this is called hyperplasia. An example of temporary epithelial hyperplasia is the lactating breast. Once the physiological stimuli that made the cells grow disappears, the tissue resumes its original volume. In some cases hypertrophy and hyperplasia go together, as for example in the enlargement of the prostate in ageing men. Both tend to be diffuse and not lead to a focal accumulation of cells, although there are exceptions; in the prostate, hyperplasia tends

to be nodular (Fig. 6.7). Both are reversible: once the stimulus disappears, the total volume of the cells will return to normal.[7]

Metaplasia is defined as the occurrence of normal differentiated cells at a site where they do not occur normally. The direction of differentiation is what makes this situation pathological. Examples are:

- intestinal metaplasia in the stomach in the context of chronic gastritis
- squamous metaplasia of bronchial epithelium in heavy smokers
- squamous metaplasia in the uterine endocervix.

It is assumed that metaplasia occurs as a response of local stem cells to an altered microenvironment: e.g. chronic inflammation (stomach) or prolonged chemical irritation due to cigarette smoking (bronchus).

Hypertrophy, hyperplasia and metaplasia are all reversible. The cells have a normal morphology and respond normally to the cues that regulate cell growth and cell death.

Persistent disturbances of cell growth

Disturbances of cell growth characterized by significantly increased proliferative activity with incomplete differentiation accompanied by morphological changes similar to those in cancer cells, are called dysplasia.[8] Dysplasia is

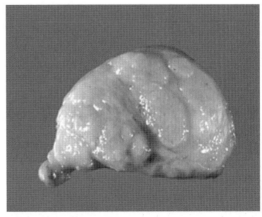

Figure 6.7: Hyperplasia of the prostate. The gland is about twice its normal size and has a nodular structure. The nodules may compress the urethra, causing problems with micturition.

103

an intermediate phase in the development of cancer. Dysplasia persists more often than hyperplasia and the cells look somewhat like cancer cells (Fig.6.8). Microscopically, dysplastic cells show an increased nuclear/cytoplasmic ratio, the nucleus tends to be enlarged and irregular (pleomorphic) and more darkly stained than usual (hyperchromatic). In general, dysplasia consists of a clone of cells that contain abnormalities in their genome, as is characteristically also found in cancer cells. It is therefore appropriate to regard dysplasia as an early step in the development of cancer. The final step in this evolution is a lesion in which the cells look like cancer cells but without infiltrative growth, which is called carcinoma in situ. Usually, a clone of dysplastic cells does not form a cell mass. As dysplasia occurs primarily in mucous membranes, when affected they tend to be slightly thickened or irregular but when viewed during endoscopy may not show consistently recognizable abnormalities.

For diagnostic purposes dysplasia is graded, usually as low grade or high grade. Low-grade lesions have a strong tendency to regress spontaneously. High-grade lesions more often persist or progress. Dysplasia grading is rather subjective and lacks somewhat in reproducibility. There is currently a strong tendency to replace the term dysplasia by intraepithelial neoplasia, the latter comprising all the steps of the evolution of a cancer up to and including carcinoma in situ. In the uterine cervix, this makes for cervical intraepithelial neoplasia, abbreviated to CIN, in the prostate to PIN and in the vulva to VIN. The continuum ranging from normal epithelium to carcinoma in situ is customarily subdivided in three grades (I, II and III). It should be kept in mind that grading is done for practical purposes and that, as yet, there are no unambiguous morphological or molecular abnormalities that establish the three steps as biologically distinct entities.[9]

Most cases of dysplasia, certainly of low grade, are reversible. High-grade dysplasia has a much stronger tendency to progress towards invasive cancer but might still regress spontaneously. Carcinoma in situ has a very strong tendency to progress towards invasive cancer. To this end, the cells that form the lesion need to develop the capacity to dissolve the epithelial basement membrane and actively migrate into the surrounding connective tissue. Through invasion into blood vessels, the cells can enter into the blood or lymph circulation and be transported to distant organs or the regional lymph nodes, where a secondary tumour is formed, a metastasis. Mechanisms involved in invasive growth and metastasis are discussed later in the chapter.

In non-epithelial tumours the sequence of events that leads to invasive cancer is less clearly established. Melanomas can develop from a benign precursor lesion (a mole or nevus), which might become dysplastic and subsequently show an early superficial growth phase and a final deeply invasive growth phase. Some benign mesenchymal tumours tend to develop further towards sarcoma when not treated adequately. This phenomenon is called progression and will be discussed later on in more detail.

When tumours progress, their level of differentiation tends to decrease. Decreased differentiation is usually accompanied by more aggressive behaviour. Some tumour cells are so poorly differentiated that it is impossible to determine their direction of differentiation; these are called anaplastic. Anaplastic tumours are usually highly aggressive: they grow rapidly, are very invasive and metastasize early.

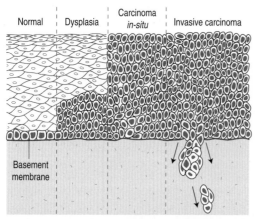

Figure 6.8: Schematic presentation of the pathway of evolution of a cancer in a covering epithelium such as the uterine cervix. Dysplastic cells differentiate incompletely and proliferate more actively than normal cells. When the cells look like cancer cells but are not yet invasive, the lesion is called carcinoma in situ.

Regulation of tumour cell growth

The volume of an organ, a tissue or a tissue component is tightly controlled through close coordination of the loss of cells through programmed cell death or apoptosis and production of new cells through proliferation. The growth of cells is regulated by the cell cycle.

The cell cycle

In all cells, including cancer cells, growth occurs through division in a complex process that is called the cell cycle. Whether or not cells will enter into the cell cycle and whether or not the cycle will progress towards the creation of two daughter cells is controlled by cell cycle regulators. The cell cycle is not extensively discussed here; the reader is referred for further details to Chapter 5. It suffices here to mention that cells pass from a resting phase, which is called G0, into the G1 phase in which they prepare metabolically for the complex procedure of replicating their DNA. In the S phase, which follows the G1 phase, semi-conservative DNA replication ensues. In the subsequent G2 phase, the cells prepare for the final step of cell division, mitosis, in the M phase. The duration of the G1, S and G2/M phases is relatively constant. Cells, also tumour cells, differ in the duration of the G0 phase, which may be days or weeks and sometimes even months.

Regulation of the cell cycle is based upon two important principles:[10]

- Activation, by phosphorylation (the attachment of a phosphate group) of regulating proteins (the so-called cyclins) that control cell cycle progression.

- Cell cycle checkpoints: moments in the cycle at which the cell monitors whether or not the complex molecular machinery functions properly. If not, the cycle is delayed or terminated. In the latter case, the cell usually dies through apoptosis.

Based upon the principle that cancer is a disturbance of the equilibrium between cell loss and cell growth, it is not surprising that cyclins, closely associated regulating proteins (the cyclin-dependent kinases or CDKs) and checkpoint-regulating proteins play a crucial role in the development of cancer (see Ch. 5).

The dynamics of tumour cell growth

The duration of the cell cycle differs significantly from one tumour to another. In leukaemias the cell cycle might not be longer than 20 hours, whereas for solid tumours this might be in the order of months. This difference is not determined by the duration of the S or G2/M phase but mainly by the duration of the G0 phase. The fraction of cancer cells that proliferates actively is called the growth fraction. The growth fraction can be determined by counting mitoses, which is customary for some types of tumour. This, however, underestimates the growth fraction and is somewhat subjective. A more accurate way to do this is to stain tumour cells for the expression of proteins that occur only in cells that actively proliferate. For this purpose in immunohistochemical staining techniques monoclonal antibodies are used, which recognize proteins that occur specifically in the nucleus of cycling cells, such as the Ki-67 antigen (Fig. 6.9). By counting the stained cells a labelling index can be established, which is a reliable parameter of the growth fraction. The growth fraction is often used as a prognostic parameter, tumours with a high growth fraction behaving more aggressively than those with a low growth fraction.[11]

The growth fraction varies for different tumours, from less than 1% to almost 100%. This implies that in some tumours only a limited fraction of the cells will be actively participating in contributing to tumour growth. The cells that do not proliferate might be

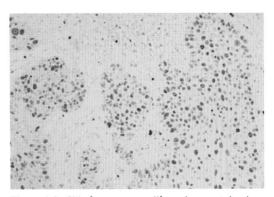

Figure 6.9: Skin (squamous cell) carcinoma stained for Ki-67 antigen, which is only expressed in proliferating cells. In this cancer about 70% of the cells are cycling and participate actively in tumour growth.

programmed to die through apoptosis or they might eventually differentiate. Differentiation tends to be a terminal phase in the life of a cell. Many tumour cells that differentiate will therefore also ultimately die through apoptosis. It is important to keep in mind that the difference between cell loss and cell production determines how fast a tumour will grow. In slow-growing tumours, the growth fraction might not be higher than that in the corresponding normal tissue; decreased apoptosis might be largely responsible for tumour cell growth. Tumours with a high growth fraction might not grow all that fast when most of the produced cells subsequently undergo apoptosis.

Cells in a cancer are almost always monoclonal: i.e. they all developed from a single precursor cell and share the set of genetic abnormalities that has transformed it into a cancer cell.

An important question is how long it takes for one transformed cell to develop into a clinically or radiologically detectable cancer. The lowest threshold of detection using imaging techniques is a mass of about 1 cm^3, which corresponds to about 10^9 cells. For one transformed cell to grow into a mass of 10^9 cells, approximately 30 cell doublings would be required. Chest X-ray studies of patients with lung tumours have shown that the time it takes for a single tumour nodule to double in volume varies from 2 to 3 months to more than a year. If we take as an example a doubling time of 2 months, it would have taken a single transformed cell 30 times 2 months, which is 5 years, to develop into a detectable 1 cm^3 mass of cancer tissue. The time it takes for tumours to develop therefore usually spans several years. However, the tumour can only be detected, e.g. by radiologic screening as for breast cancer, in the last half year. The time line of the development of a tumour is illustrated in Figure 6.10.

THE STROMAL RESPONSE

Angiogenesis

Some time after the transformed cell begins to proliferate, a small cell mass will have formed.

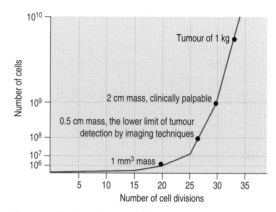

Figure 6.10: Time frame of the development of a cancer from a single transformed cell. The level of detection of a tumour by imaging techniques is about 5 mm, which is attained after about 27 cell doublings. Only seven doublings later, the tumour will have a diameter of about 10 cm and weigh one kilo!

Experiments with cells in culture have shown that a solid mass of cells remains entirely viable up to a diameter of about 1 mm. The innermost cells then are still adequately supplied with oxygen and nutrients, which allows them to survive and proliferate. Once the clump of cells gets bigger, the cells in the centre will become hypoxic. The oxygen supply will become insufficient and the cells might die through necrosis or apoptosis. Transformed cells adapt to this altered environment by switching on the expression of a set of genes that encode growth factors which induce proliferation of stromal cells, including endothelial cells, resulting in the development of a network of new vessels in the tumour. This process is called angiogenesis.[12]

The factors responsible for angiogenesis have been elucidated in recent years. The initial 'master switch' for angiogenesis is a transcription factor (transcription factors are responsible for regulation of DNA transcription in the nucleus) known as Hypoxia Induced Factor-1α (HIF-1α). The expression of HIF-1α is turned on in hypoxic cells.[13] HIF-1α induces the expression of a series of vascular growth factors, of which the most important members are VEGF, bFGF and PDGF. The latter stimulates mostly the proliferation of stromal (myo)fibroblasts. VEGF and bFGF are the main players responsible for endothelial cell proliferation.

It has been discovered recently that there are several forms of VEGF, each with specific characteristics. VEGF-A is mainly responsible for the proliferation of blood vessel endothelium, leading to a capillary network in the developing tumours. VEGF-D on the contrary specifically stimulates endothelial cells of lymphatic vessels to proliferate.[14] It seems that the generation of blood vessels and lymph vessels in a tumour are different events. This gives support to the notion that tumours which metastasize through the blood circulation (hematogenous) and through the lymphatic system (lymphogenous) are biologically different. We will come back to this later on in this chapter.

The ability of the growing tumour to induce the formation of blood vessels largely determines how well the tumour will develop. Conceivably, tumours with a rich vascular network might be able to grow faster and develop hematogenous metastases more efficiently. This idea has been used in histopathology in an attempt to grade the degree of malignancy of different tumours. In several cancer types (including melanoma, breast cancer, lung cancer and colon cancer) the abundance of the tumour microvascular network (microvascular density or MVD) has been correlated with clinical parameters of tumour evolution, such as overall survival or relapse free survival. In general, MVD appears to correlate well with prognosis.[15] This approach has not been sufficiently robust to yield parameters presently useful in the clinical management of patients with cancer. The results do, however, support the importance of angiogenesis in the development of cancer.

Another potentially practical implication of the angiogenesis concept is the possibility of treating cancer through inhibition of angiogenesis.[16] Several proteins have been isolated from experimental cancers, most of them breakdown products of blood coagulation factors such as endostatin and angiostatin, which in the laboratory are capable of halting the further growth of experimental tumours. In spite of great promise, clinical trials using these approaches towards cancer treatment have not fulfilled these great expectations. It is likely, however, that antiangiogenesis drugs will eventually become part of the increasing list of effective new therapeutic modalities, designed on the basis of our current knowledge of tumour development.

Yet another interesting finding in tumour angiogenesis is that blood vessels in tumours are not identical to those in the normal tissue. Tumour vessels appear to be 'leaky': their endothelial lining is incomplete. It has been shown that the vessels that develop in tumours through the effect of VEGF are in this way imperfect. In fact, VEGF was initially isolated as the factor responsible for permeable tumour vessels and was hence called 'vascular permeability factor'. Leaky vessels supply migrating cancer cells easy access to the blood circulation. It has also been shown that the endothelial cell surface proteins of tumour vessels differ from those on normal endothelium. Notably, the expression of the vitronectin receptor, integrin $\alpha_v\beta_3$, is very high in tumour vessels but undetectable on normal endothelium.[17] This finding may have important practical implications. Anti-angiogenic molecules might be specifically targeted to $\alpha_v\beta_3$-expressing endothelial cells, as might chemotherapeutic agents or radiosensitizing drugs. Several studies in experimental cancer have shown that this is potentially feasible.

Tumour stroma

It should be stressed here that, in spite of the high interest gained in recent years by angiogenesis, tumour blood vessel formation is only one part of a stromal reaction to the proliferating tumour cells. As indicated earlier, along with endothelial cells, (myo)fibroblasts proliferate in tumour stroma. PDGF is the growth factor mainly responsible for this. Tumour fibroblasts are contractile, as are their counterparts in wound healing; for this reason, they are called myofibroblasts. In fact, the process of wound healing shows striking similarities with the stromal reaction in tumours. Tumour myofibroblasts deposit collagens in the stroma. As we discussed earlier, in some tumours this is so extensive that there is more stroma than tumour cells (desmoplastic tumours). The factor responsible for the induction of collagen deposition by myofibroblasts is transforming growth factor-1β (TGF-1β).

107

INVASION AND METASTASIS

The key factor which distinguishes a benign from a malignant tumour is the capacity of malignant cells to exit the tissue compartment to which they are normally confined, migrate through the adjacent connective tissue compartment, traverse vessel walls and so gain access to the blood or lymph circulation, survive there and be transported to distant sites to establish a secondary tumour, the metastasis. Most cancer deaths are not due to the primary tumour but to metastatic disease.

Invasive growth

The mechanisms responsible for invasive growth have been most extensively studied in carcinoma or melanoma cells. Sarcomas also invade blood vessels but their architecture is less distinctive than that of carcinomas or melanomas, which makes it more difficult to study their invasive behaviour. We will therefore focus the discussion of the mechanisms responsible for invasion by carcinoma cells.

It is important to realize that although invasion and migration are inappropriate for epithelial cells in the adult, where they are normally confined to their own tissue compartment, epithelial cells do migrate during embryonic development. Also, lymphocytes and phagocytes have a strong capacity to invade into and migrate through epithelia or connective tissue, which is essential for their function in the inflammatory reaction. For cells to invade into and migrate through other tissues is not abnormal. The fact that epithelial cells (in the case of a carcinoma) do this spontaneously, without responding to normal control mechanisms, makes tumour cell invasion such a remarkable phenomenon. For their invasive behaviour, tumour cells use the mechanisms that are also employed by lymphocytes and phagocytes when they invade and migrate.

When carcinoma cells invade surrounding tissues, the following steps can be distinguished in the process:[18]

- intercellular adhesions that normally confine epithelial cells to their compartment are lost

- the invasive cells release proteases that are capable of degrading the extracellular matrix
- the invasive cells migrate through the adjacent connective tissue.

Changes in intercellular adhesion are a result of the altered patterns of expression of adhesion molecules. For epithelial cells to adhere to each other they have adherence junctions, sites of zipper-like connections between the cells. The agent used to create these junctions is E-cadherin. E-cadherin is a protein inserted into the cell membrane but with an extracellular domain and a cytoplasmic domain. The extracellular domain connects with the extracellular domain of E-cadherin molecules on adjacent cells to form strong intercellular bonds. The cytoplasmic domain of E-cadherin connects with proteins called catenins to form what is called the E-cadherin–catenin complex. The catenins, in turn, are connected with the cytoskeleton. In this way, cells in a tissue form part of a molecular architecture that gives, for example, the epidermis of the skin its tensile strength.

In a carcinoma, the number of intercellular junctions is usually strongly reduced. Invasive carcinoma cells show a decreased number of E-cadherin molecules on their cell surface. In some very strongly invasive cancers, such as the diffuse type of gastric carcinoma and invasive lobular carcinoma of the breast, E-cadherin is not at all expressed due to mutations in the E-cadherin gene. In most cancers, however, decreased E-cadherin expression is a result of a temporary reduction in the amount of protein produced by the cell. When metastatic carcinoma cells grow out into a secondary tumour, they reconstruct the tissue architecture by increasing the expression of E-cadherin. In some invasive cancer cells it is the catenins and not E-cadherin that are abnormally expressed. We can therefore conclude that in invading carcinoma cells intercellular adhesion is disturbed due to dysfunction of the E-cadherin–catenin complex.[19]

For cells to connect to the extracellular matrix, they use adhesion molecules known as integrins. Integrins are proteins composed of two different chains (the α and the β chain), both of which may be present in several forms.

This gives rise to a large family of proteins (more than 30 members), all with their specific affinity for one or more of the proteins that make up the extracellular matrix. Like E-cadherin, integrins are transmembranous, with an extracellular domain and a cytoplasmic domain that connects with the cytoskeleton (Fig. 6.11). They contribute to the structural integrity of a tissue by creating a continuum that extends from the extracellular matrix to the cytoskeleton. They also have true receptor functions. When integrins connect with extracellular matrix molecules, intracellular signalling occurs, which leads to changes in cell motility but also the expression of different proteins. Normal epithelial cells adhere to their basement membrane through integrins, notably $\alpha_6\beta_1$ and $\alpha_6\beta_4$, which interact with molecules such as type IV collagen and laminin. When they invade, carcinoma cells detach from their basement membrane

and hook up to type I and III collagen fibres in the interstitial stroma through expression of $\alpha_2\beta_1$ and $\alpha_3\beta_1$ integrins, which allows them to migrate.

In order for the cancer cells to move freely about in the extracellular matrix, the latter is degraded by the tumour cells through extracellular matrix proteases, the most important of which are the matrix metalloproteases (MMP).[20] This is a family comprising more than 20 distinct proteases that are capable of degrading matrix proteins. Some of them have a very specific activity, such as the gelatinases (MMP 2 and 9), which mostly (but not exclusively) degrade type IV collagen, the major structural component of epithelial basement membranes, and consequently the first extracellular matrix structure with which invasive carcinoma cells will be up against. Some MMPs are not secreted but are membrane proteins that concentrate on the invading edge of

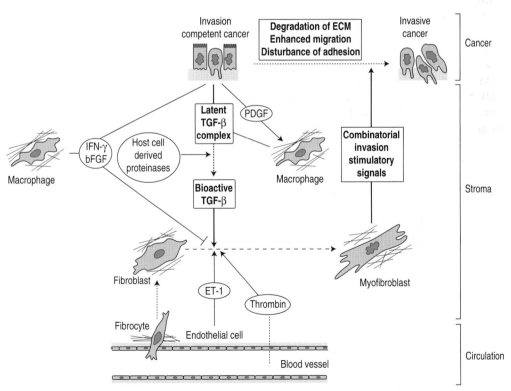

Figure 6.11: Schematic representation of the molecular cross-talk between cancer cells and the host cells in the microenvironment of a primary cancer. Arrows and arcs point to activation and inactivation/blocking, respectively. Lines and dotted lines indicate secretion and diffusion, respectively. Bold type indicates importance of signalling. Abbreviations: bFGF, basic fibroblast growth factor; ECM, extracellular matrix; ET-1, endothelin-1; IFN-γ, interferon-γ; PDGF, platelet-derived growth factor; TGF-β, transforming growth factor-β. (Reproduced with permission from De Wever and Mareel.[4])

a cancer cell. Other MMPs bind to specific receptors on the cell surface. MMPs are not only partly synthesized and released by cancer cells but also many of them are synthesized by stromal cells, such as myofibroblasts and macrophages, when stimulated by proteins released by cancer cells. Receptors on the cancer cells then concentrate the MMPs at sites of active invasion. In addition to degrading the extracellular matrix, MMPs liberate and activate growth factors stored in the matrix. In this way, they provide additional stimuli for the proliferation and migration of the cancer cells. Specific inhibitors, the tissue inhibitors of metalloproteinases or TIMP, counterbalance the activity of MMPs. The key elements of this process are summarized in Figure 6.12.

In addition to MMPs, other proteases such as plasmine play a role in matrix degradation. Plasmine is generated from plasminogen through the activating role of plasminogen activators. Plasminogen activators (PAs) may be generated in the vessel wall (tissue plasminogen activator or tPA) or can be synthesized by tumour cells (urokinase or uPA). PAs are bound to the cell surface by plasminogen activator receptors (PARs). These PARs concentrate PA at the sites of active tumour invasion. Inactivating proteins called plasminogen activator inhibitors (PAIs) specifically inhibit plasminogen activators.

In all, invasion is a complex process in which the cancer cells closely interact with host stromal cells, and in which a large number of proteins play an important role.[20] This complex interaction between cells and matrix proteins results in matrix degradation, where cells actively invade and, in parallel, the liberation of stimuli for proliferation and migration of the cancer cells occurs.

Circulating tumour cells

When tumour cells have invaded vessels, they can enter into the blood circulation or into the lymphatic system. The tumour cells are then passively transported and can lodge downstream, in the first capillary network they encounter, or in a lymph node. When tumour cells are present in the blood circulation, specific adhesion proteins on the cell membrane

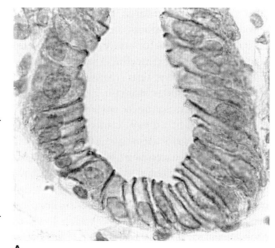

A

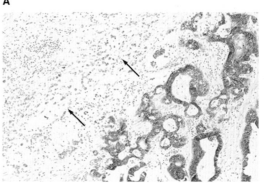

B

Figure 6.12: Immunohistochemical staining of benign colon adenoma (A) and colon carcinoma (B) for E-cadherin. In the adenoma, the cells are well differentiated and form glands requiring the cells to be glued together by E-cadherin, which shows up by immunohistochemistry as a brown line between the cells. In the carcinoma, part of the tissue is well differentiated and still shows E-cadherin; part is poorly differentiated and the cells infiltrate diffusely; they no longer express E-cadherin.

of the cancer cell will interact with adhesion receptors on the endothelial cell surface. This will force tumour cells to adhere. Cancer cells then migrate through the vessel wall and through the perivascular extracellular matrix and subsequently might grow out to form a new tumour – a metastasis. Whether or not tumour cells will multiply at a potential metastatic site will depend on the availability of growth factors locally in the host tissue. One example of this interplay between metastatic cancer cells and the local tissue microenvironment is the bone marrow. Bone marrow cells continuously proliferate in order to meet the demand for new blood cells. This occurs under the stimulus of growth factors, which will also favour the growth of cancer cells. This process offers support to the reason why bone marrow is a favourite metastatic site for many different cancer types. When tumour cells multiply, they will in turn release growth factors that stimulate surrounding stromal cells to proliferate. This is similar to the process of developing a primary tumour. Consequently, when the tumour metastasizes, a stromal reaction accompanies the outgrowth of the cancer cells.

Not every tumour cell that enters into the bloodstream will form a metastasis. The metastatic process appears to be rather inefficient. Experiments have shown that in almost every patient with a clinically detectable cancer, tumour cells circulate in the bloodstream. Most of these, however, will not survive the harsh conditions of this voyage. Others will perish due to an antitumour immune response. DNA derived from cancer cells that have been degraded in the circulation can be detected in the plasma of patients with cancer.[21]

Metastasis

The following phases are commonly distinguished in the process of metastasis:

- transport of tumour cells in the bloodstream and/or lymphatic system
- adhesion of tumour cells to the vessel wall in a capillary network, postcapillary venule or lymph node
- proliferation of the tumour cells at the metastatic site, resulting in a new tumour.

The term metastasis is reserved for cancer cells that have multiplied and form cancer tissue. A single cancer cell in the marginal sinus of a lymph node or in bone marrow does not yet constitute a metastasis. Also, a cluster of cancer cells growing in the lumen of a vessel at some distance from the primary tumour is not a metastasis; this is called a tumour cell embolus. As described in the preceding paragraph, specific interactions between adhesion receptors on the cell surface of endothelial cells (such as selectins and integrins) and adhesion molecules on the cancer cells will determine where a metastasis develops. These specific interactions are responsible for patterns of metastasis, which tend to be characteristic for each type of cancer.

Patterns of metastasis

Invasive tumour cells can grow into an adjacent organ. This is not called metastasizing but tumour invasion by continuity. Tumours that penetrate into a bodily cavity (pleura, pericardium or peritoneum) can migrate in this cavity. This is called transcelomic displacement and it favours tumour cell growth diffusely throughout the cavity, for which the term carcinosis (pleural, peritoneal) is commonly used. When this is accompanied by the retention of fluid in the cavity, the term carcinomatous peritonitis or pleuritis is used.

Sarcomas commonly metastasize through the bloodstream, which is called haematogenous metastasis. Carcinomas tend to disseminate through the lymphatic system, which is called lymphogenous metastasis. Carcinomas also commonly use the haematogenous pathway, but slightly later. The site for development of a haematogenous metastasis depends on a number of factors, notably where the primary tumour is located, whether or not endothelial cells will specifically attract passing cancer cells and whether or not the tissue microenvironment will favour cancer cell growth.

Usually, cancer cells first invade thin-walled vessels such as veins and lymphatic vessels. As a consequence, haematogenous metastases are often found in the first capillary network downstream of the primary site. Haematogenous metastasis of a large bowel cancer, for example, will develop in the liver, because venous blood from the intestines reaches the liver through the portal vein. Lung cancer cells will grow into the wall of pulmonary veins, be transported via the left ventricle into the aorta and will give rise to metastases in peripheral organs, such as the brain, the bone marrow or the adrenal glands. Renal cancer cells will enter the inferior caval vein and, after passing through the right heart, form metastases in the lungs. These patterns, are largely dependent on the site of the primary tumour. The anatomical relationships of the vascular tree are summarized in Figure 6.13.

111

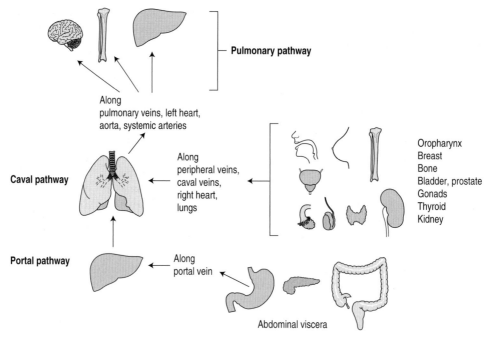

Figure 6.13: Patterns of metastasis of different tumours. Tumours of abdominal organs drain venous blood into the portal vein. Consequently, they tend to form liver metastases (the portal pathway). Liver, breast, renal and many other cancers drain venous blood into the caval veins and migrating tumour cells end up in lung capillaries. These tend to form primarily lung metastases (the caval pathway). Lung cancer drains via the pulmonary veins to the left heart, and the cells then enter the large circulation, targeting a variety of peripheral organs such as bone, the brain and the liver (the pulmonary pathway).

A metastasis can, in turn, give rise to secondary metastases. In the terminal phase of the evolution of cancer, patients will have metastases in many organs and the characteristic patterns described above are no longer found.

Lymphogenous metastases arise when tumour cells grow into lymphatic vessels. In the first lymph node they encounter, tumour cells will grow out in the marginal sinus, the site where they enter. The first lymph node in a regional station reached by tumour cells is called the sentinel node.[22] With a relatively simple procedure, which identifies the lymph node through radioactive tracers or with vital dyes injected into the tumour, surgeons can determine which of the regional lymph nodes is the sentinel node. Once the sentinel node has been identified, it can be biopsied for histopathological analysis to determine whether or not a metastasis exists in this node. This procedure avoids excision of all lymph nodes of a particular station, a procedure which carries a significant risk of secondary effects such as lymphoedema due to interruption of the lymph flow as a result of scarring.

Metastases can become manifest many years after the primary tumour was removed. This is because it takes time for a single metastatic cancer cell to multiply into a clinically manifest or radiologically detectable secondary tumour. For breast cancer, metastases can appear as late as 20 years after the primary tumour was treated. It is assumed that, in this case, the metastatic cells do not proliferate for long periods of time and lie dormant – a phenomenon called dormant metastases.

CONCLUSION

Cancer research has made remarkable progress in the last decade, largely due to the revolution in molecular genetics. We now understand that cancer develops through gene mutations. We also know how abnormalities in different intracellular and intercellular signalling systems involved in the regulation of cell growth, cell death and differentiation interact in carcinogenesis. We know how tumour cells deal with the extracellular matrix when they grow, how they evoke angiogenesis and which factors are involved in the process of invasion and metastasis. It has taken a long time for this knowledge to make its way into the diagnosis, treatment and prevention of cancer. The war on cancer, to use a phrase first pronounced by Richard Nixon, has not yet been won despite enormous progress. New revolutionary methods of analysing cancer cells with DNA chips (genomics and transcriptomics) – which allow detailed study of abnormalities in the genome or gene expression patterns, and by sophisticated protein analysis allow identification of abnormalities in the pattern of proteins synthesized by cancer cells (proteomics) – will lead to new approaches in tumour classification. This will optimize individualized cancer treatment. Improved understanding of the mechanisms involved in carcinogenesis, the stromal reaction, angiogenesis, immunity, as well as invasion and metastasis, will allow the development of new less toxic and more effective drugs and vaccines to help eradicate some forms of cancer. These are exciting times, full of hope.

REFERENCES

1. La Vecchia C, Franceschi S, Levi F. Epidemiological research on cancer with a focus on Europe. Eur J Cancer Prev 2003; 12:5–14.

2. Cotran RS, Kumar V, Collins T, eds. Robbins pathologic basis of disease. 6th edn. Philadelphia: WB Saunders; 1999.

3. Fletcher CDM. Diagnostic histopathology of tumors. Edinburgh: Churchill Livingstone; 2000.

4. De Wever O, Mareel M. Role of tissue stroma in cancer cell invasion. J Pathol 2003; 200:429–447.

5. Levi F, Lucchini F, Negri E, Boyle P, La Vecchia C. Cancer mortality in Europe, 1995–1999, and an overview of trends since 1960. Int J Cancer 2004; 110:155–169.

6. Ramaswamy S. Translating cancer genomics into clinical oncology. N Engl J Med 2004; 350:1814–1816.

7. Guindi M, Riddell RH. Histology of Barrett's esophagus and dysplasia. Gastrointest Endosc Clin N Am 2003; 13:349–368.

8. Baldwin P, Laskey R, Coleman N. Translational approaches to improving cervical screening. Nat Rev Cancer. 2003; 3:217–226.

9. Pucci B, Giordano A. Cell cycle and cancer. Clin Ter 1999; 150:135–141.

10. Sherr CJ: Cancer cell cycle. Science 1996; 274:1672.

11. Pluda JM: Tumor-associated angiogenesis: mechanisms, clinical implications and therapeutic strategies. Semin Oncol 1997; 24:203.

12. Blagosklonny MV. Antiangiogenic therapy and tumor progression. Cancer Cell 2004; 5:13–17.

13. Acker T, Plate KH. Hypoxia and hypoxia inducible factors (HIF) as important regulators of tumor physiology. Cancer Treat Res 2004; 117:219–248.

14. Patan S. Vasculogenesis and angiogenesis. Cancer Treat Res 2004; 117:3–32.

15. Abulafia O, Triest WE, Sherer DM. Angiogenesis in malignancies of the female genital tract.Gynecol Oncol 1999; 72,:220–231.

16. Steeg PS. Angiogenesis inhibitors: motivators of metastasis? Nat Med 2003; 9:822–823.

17. Ruegg C, Dormond O, Foletti A. Suppression of tumor angiogenesis through the inhibition of integrin function and signaling in endothelial cells: which side to target? Endothelium 2002; 9:151–160.

18. Cairns RA, Khokha R, Hill RP. Molecular mechanisms of tumor invasion and metastasis: an integrated view. Curr Mol Med 2003; 3:659–671.

19. Van Roy F, Mareel M. Tumour invasion: effects of cell adhesion and motility. Trends Cell Biol 1992; 2:163–169.

20. Stamenkovic I. Extracellular matrix remodelling: the role of matrix metalloproteinases. J Pathol 2003; 200:448–464.

21. Wong BC, Lo YM. Cell-free DNA and RNA in plasma as new tools for molecular diagnostics. Expert Rev Mol Diagn 2003; 3:785–797.

22. Cafiero F. New fields of application of the sentinel lymph node biopsy in the pathologic staging of solid neoplasms: review of literature and surgical perspectives. J Surg Oncol 2004; 85:171–179.

CHAPTER 7

The Immunological Basis of Cancer

JAQUALYN S MOORE

CHAPTER CONTENTS

Introduction	115	Macrophages	123
		B lymphocytes	123
The nature of immunity	116	Dendritic cells	123
		Antigen presentation	124
Innate immunity	116		
Physical and chemical barriers	116	Lymphocyte memory	124
Inflammation	116		
Phagocytosis	116	Cytokines	124
Complement	117		
Natural killer cells	117	Heat shock proteins	124
Antimicrobial proteins	117		
		Apoptosis	125
Acquired immunity	118		
Antigens and antigenic determinants	118	The immune response	125
The major histocompatibility		The immune system and cancer	126
complex	118	Tumour antigens	126
B lymphocytes	119	Effector cell response to tumour cells	127
Antibodies	119	Mechanisms of tumour tolerance	128
Antibody-mediated immunity	120		
T lymphocytes	121	Conclusion	129
		References	129
Antigen processing and presentation	122		

INTRODUCTION

To examine the relationship between cancer and the immune system is to set out on a journey of discovery. For many, the immune system with its defensive and protective activities appears rather mysterious. However, as an understanding of the immune system is developed it is possible to more fully appreciate its intricacies, complexities and intelligence. An understanding of immunology is important for a number of reasons. First, a greater appreciation of immunological processes will give some answers to the many questions that arise

related to the development and persistence of cancer in the body. Secondly, to know and improve understanding will help in the determination of better treatments and improved strategies for the relief of the multiple symptoms that are consequent on the development of cancer.

In this chapter the role of the immune system in defending the body from infection and disease and in maintaining the internal environment will be described. Following this, an exploration of the role of the immune system in relation to cancer will be made. In particular, the following subjects will be considered:

- cells and molecules of the immune system and their functions
- innate immunity
- acquired immunity
- the immune system response to cancer.

THE NATURE OF IMMUNITY

The immune system is composed of various organs, tissues, cells and molecules whose primary function is to defend the body against pathogenic microorganisms such as bacteria, viruses, fungi and parasites.[1] As well as acting to defend us from such pathogens, the immune system also responds to infected, transformed (cancerous) and transplanted cells (from a blood transfusion, bone marrow or stem cell transplant) and cells which die as a consequence of natural processes.[2] Immunity is defined as the state of protection from infectious diseases[3] and is achieved through the response of the immune system. The immune response has both non-specific and specific components known as innate immunity and acquired immunity, respectively, and their particular roles will now be explored.

INNATE IMMUNITY

Innate immunity, also called natural, native or non-specific immunity, is a mechanism for the disposal of foreign and potentially harmful macromolecules and pathogenic microorganisms (pathogens). Several different mechanisms are involved.

Physical and chemical barriers

The first line of defence against pathogens such as bacteria includes both physical and chemical barriers. The horny layer of the skin on the outer surface of the body and the mucous membranes which line the internal surfaces present mechanical barriers.[4] The substances secreted by mucous membranes provide a variety of chemical barriers such as lysozyme, a natural antibiotic, acid secretions in the stomach, gastric juices and the waxy secretions in the ear, sebum. Sticky mucus secretions will trap particles, while hair-like projections in the respiratory tract sweep dust and bacteria-laden mucus towards the mouth.[5]

Inflammation

An important mechanism in innate immunity is the inflammatory response. The inflammatory response is a complex sequence of events induced by damage to tissues caused by a wound or by invasion by a pathogenic microorganism.[3] Three major events occur during an inflammatory response: (1) vasodilation; (2) increased permeability; and (3) influx of phagocytic cells. These events give rise to what are known as the cardinal signs of inflammation – redness, swelling, heat and pain. As macrophages encounter bacteria in the tissues, they release chemicals that increase the permeability of the blood vessels and, as a result, protein molecules and fluids leak into tissues. In addition, neutrophils and other phagocytic cells adhere to the blood vessel walls and are able to crawl through, a process known as diapedesis or extravasation. The accumulation of fluid and cells at the site of injury or infection causes the characteristic redness, swelling, heat and pain.[1]

Phagocytosis

Probably the most important cells within innate immunity are the phagocytic cells, which destroy pathogens as well as foreign and transformed cells.[1] Polymorphonuclear leucocytes (PMNs), that is neutrophils, are phagocytic white blood cells that circulate in the blood and migrate into tissues should those tissues be invaded by a pathogen.[3] Other groups of phagocytic cells are the monocytes that circulate in the bloodstream and macrophages that reside in body tissues. Large numbers of macrophages are present in different tissues and their various names reflect their tissues locations. For example, Kupffer cells are found lining the blood sinuses in the liver; alveolar macrophages are present in the lungs; histiocytes are found in connective tissues; Langerhans cells in the epidermis; mesangial cells in the kidneys and microglial cells are present in the brain.[3]

The mechanism by which a PMN or macrophage ingests and destroys a bacteria is the process of phagocytosis (Fig. 7.1). In response to chemical stimuli, a polymorph migrates through the blood vessel wall and enters the tissue. The bacterium then adheres to the cell membrane of the macrophage, an attachment which is facilitated by various receptors. In response to the binding of the bacterium to its receptors, the cell membrane of the macrophage invaginates to form a pocket that isolates the bacterium inside a vesicle, called a phagosome, within the cell. The phagosome fuses with a lysosome, which contains toxic chemicals and the bacteria is killed and digested. Bacterial waste is egested from the cell.[1]

Complement

The ability of phagocytes to engulf and destroy certain bacteria is greatly enhanced by a system of plasma proteins known as complement. In a highly regulated cascade, complement facilitates the clearance of pathogens and enhances the inflammatory response.[6] Pathogens coated with complement are more readily phagocytosed by phagocytic cells, whereas the terminal components in the complement cascade generate the membrane attack complex which damages the membrane of the pathogen, causing the cell to die.[1]

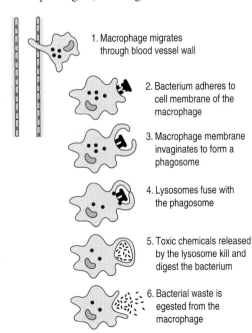

1. Macrophage migrates through blood vessel wall

2. Bacterium adheres to cell membrane of the macrophage

3. Macrophage membrane invaginates to form a phagosome

4. Lysosomes fuse with the phagosome

5. Toxic chemicals released by the lysosome kill and digest the bacterium

6. Bacterial waste is egested from the macrophage

Figure 7.1: The process of phagocytosis. (Adapted from Staines et al.[4])

Natural killer cells

Natural killer (NK) cells are derived from stem cells in the bone marrow and are a population of large granular lymphocytes (LGLs). They can be identified by a surface marker specific for NK cells and, in addition, have receptors for the Fc portion of certain types of antibodies.[7] They are present in the blood and tissues in relatively small numbers. NK cells are able to kill virally infected cells and certain sensitive tumour cells and become activated within a few minutes of encountering these targets.[8] NK cells are generally considered to be part of innate rather than acquired immunity because the mechanism by which NK cells recognize their target cells is not antigen-specific nor do they exhibit other characteristics of acquired immunity. Their mechanism of killing is through a series of enzymes, called granzymes, which are found in the cytoplasmic granules of the NK cells. These granules release perforins, which insert into the membrane of the target cell, inducing lysis.[9] Activated NK cells also synthesize a selection of small protein molecules known as cytokines (described later in the chapter) that rapidly increase the cytolytic, secretory, proliferative and antitumour functions of NK cells. Cytokine-activated NK cells are known as LAK (lymphokine-activated killer) cells.[7]

NK cells tend to accumulate at the site of infection, where the virally stimulated production of interferons enhances NK cell activity, causing them to kill several targets one after the other and to do so more rapidly.[9]

Antimicrobial proteins

Several antimicrobial agents are important in innate immunity, including lysozyme, acute phase proteins and interferons. Lysozyme is a natural antibiotic found in tears and mucus secretions and is an enzyme able to digest bacterial cell walls.[4] Acute phase proteins are produced by the liver during the early phase of an inflammatory response: e.g. C-reactive protein and serum-amyloid.[4] Interferons are a large and diverse family of proteins that inhibit the ability of viruses to replicate inside cells.[10] In addition, interferons are produced by lymphocytes in response to their stimulation by antigen (defined below). These proteins are non-specific, being able to exert their effects against many different types of pathogens.[3]

ACQUIRED IMMUNITY

Acquired immunity, also known as adaptive or specific immunity, demonstrates the immune system's capability of specifically recognizing and selectively eliminating foreign microorganisms and molecules. It is orchestrated by two different classes of lymphocytes that both derive from pluripotent stem cells in the bone marrow. Pluripotency refers to the stem cell's ability to differentiate into a variety of different cell types, depending on the body's requirements. The two classes of lymphocytes responsible for acquired immunity are the B lymphocytes (B cells) and the T lymphocytes (T cells). B cells mediate their destruction of pathogens indirectly through the production of antibodies that can either directly kill the pathogen or will direct other immune system cells to attack them.[11] B-cell mechanisms are often classified as antibody-mediated immunity or humoral immunity. The term 'humoral' is derived from the Latin *humor*, meaning body fluid. Hence, humoral immunity refers to immunity that can be conferred by the antibodies present in serum.[3] T cells attack pathogens more directly and, hence, T-cell immune mechanisms are classified as cell-mediated immunity.

Unlike innate immunity, acquired immunity is characterized by *specificity, diversity, memory* and *self/non-self recognition*.[3] Specificity refers to the ability of immune system cells to detect subtle differences in foreign microorganisms and molecules and the ability to generate enormously diverse populations of B lymphocytes and T lymphocytes.[3] Once the immune system has responded to an antigen, it develops immunological memory, which is the ability to respond more rapidly and more intensely on a second or subsequent exposure to the antigen.[1] Finally, the immune system's ability to respond only to foreign antigens and not to cells of the body indicates that it is able to distinguish self from non-self and, hence, avoid inappropriate response to self-antigens.[6]

Lymphocytes express proteins on their surfaces known as surface markers. B cells and T cells each have unique surface markers that not only distinguish them from each other but also subdivide them into subsets.[11] There is an international system for naming surface markers, which is known as the 'CD' system. CD stands for 'cluster of differentiation' and is followed by a number which refers to a single, defined surface marker molecule.[8] For example, either a CD4 or a CD8 marker will be present on the cell surface of a T cell and indicates that the T cell is either a helper T cell (T_H) or a cytotoxic T cell (T_C), respectively. Both of these are important in determining the role the T cell plays in the immune response and will be discussed in greater detail later in the chapter.

As already indicated, all lymphocytes arise in the bone marrow. They leave the bone marrow via the bloodstream, circulate in the blood, migrate through body tissues and travel in the afferent lymph to lymph nodes, returning to the blood via the afferent vessels.[4] The ability to re-circulate allows the lymphocytes to home to different sites in the body, where they can encounter antigen.

Before proceeding further, it is appropriate to define some of the molecules important in various immune responses.

Antigens and antigenic determinants

Antigens are any molecule that elicits a specific immune response by specifically binding to antibody or T-cell receptors.[4] Most antigens are proteins, peptides or polysaccharides. Some single protein and polysaccharide antigens bear epitopes – which are also known as antigenic determinants. These are regions on the intact antigen molecule which can be recognized by specific antibody. However, T lymphocytes only recognize peptides that derive from processed protein antigen. Antigen processing is discussed later in this chapter.

The major histocompatibility complex

The major histocompatibility complex (MHC) molecules are self-antigens that are found on the cell surface of all body cells.[4] These cell surface proteins are of two types, known as class I and class II MHC molecules. Class I MHC antigens are expressed on the surface membranes of all nucleated cells and their function is to present antigens to those T cells that bear the surface marker CD8. As previously mentioned, these are a subclass of T cells that, generally, are known as cytotoxic T cells. Class II MHC antigens are expressed predominantly on a class of cell called dendritic cells, on B lymphocytes and on macrophages, the antigen presenting cells (which will be discussed later in the chapter), and can be induced on some other cells. Their function is to present antigens to those T cells which possess the CD4 cell surface marker, which are known as helper T cells. Hence, the subset of T cells bearing the CD8 marker (CD8+T cells) are class I MHC restricted T cells and the CD4 marker bearing T cells (CD4+T cells) are class II MHC restricted T cells.[9] In man the MHC is known as the HLA (human leucocyte antigen) system and it is these antigens that are examined in tissue typing. They are highly polymorphic, and, hence, there is a high degree of variation between individuals to the extent that it is unlikely, except in the case of syngeneic (identical) twins, to find individuals with the same MHC.[4]

B lymphocytes

B lymphocytes (B cells) derive from blood cell forming (haematopoietic) stem cells in the bone marrow.[1] They remain in the bone marrow until maturation is almost complete before migrating to secondary lymphoid tissues such as the lymph nodes and spleen.[4] When maturation of the B cell is complete, its surface membrane will contain a number of important molecules which determine the role of the cell in the immune response. For example, the B cell's ability to bind to antigen is through its expression of a unique receptor in the form of an antibody molecule.[3]

In order to become active and exert any immune effect, whether it is the suppression of inflammation or eradication of a foreign antigen, the cells of the immune system must first be able to communicate with and respond to one another and to various stimuli. They do this by means of receptors on their cell surfaces. These receptors act as 'docking points' for antigens and for markers on the surface of other cells. Once the antigen has attached to its receptor, a signal is relayed to the cell nucleus and the cell becomes active. The ensuing sequence of events culminates in the cell becoming responsive to whatever activated it in the first place. Cell surface receptors are embedded in the cell membrane and allow the cell to respond to many influences, including chemicals and hormones as well as foreign antigens. There are a vast number of different receptors on the surface of an individual cell and each will respond specifically to a particular stimulus.

The vast majority of receptors on a B lymphocyte are membrane-bound immunoglobulin (antibody) molecules. Interaction between antigen and the specific membrane-bound antibody on a naive B cell, together with T-cell and macrophage interactions, induce the B cell to divide repeatedly (clonal expansion) and differentiate to form populations of plasma cells and memory cells. Plasma cells are the antibody-secreting cells. Plasma cells from a given B cell will secrete antibody molecules with the same antigen-binding specificity as that of the original B cell.[6] In addition to membrane-bound antibody molecules, a mature B cell will also have other important molecules on its cell membrane. These include CD45, a marker for the B-cell lineage, and class II MHC molecules, which are important in the B cell's role as an antigen-presenting cell (APC), a role which will be discussed later. Receptors for complement and for the Fc portion of a specific type of immunoglobulin molecule, immunoglobulin G (IgG), are also expressed on the surface membrane of the B cell.[9]

Antibodies

Antibodies are a family of structurally related glycoproteins which always initiate their biological effects by binding to antigens and are one of the three classes of molecules used by the immune system to specifically recognize antigens, the others being the MHC molecules and T-cell antigen receptors. As well as being found in serum and body fluids, antibodies are also found on the surface of B cells where they are inserted through the membrane. These membrane-bound forms of antibodies (immunoglobulins) form the B-cell receptor and it is this that mediates the intracellular signals that lead to B-cell activation following interaction with the antigen.[9]

Antibodies are made up of two identical light chains and two identical heavy chains, linked together by disulphide bonds, which loosely fold into what is generally depicted as a 'Y' shape (Fig. 7.2). The heavy chains determine the class of immunoglobulin. Humans have five immunoglobulin (Ig) classes, with μ chains present in IgM, γ chains present in IgG, α chains in IgA, δ chains in IgD and ε chains in IgE. The light chains may be κ or λ type and only one of these distinctly different chains is present in any single antibody molecule. Each of the chains comprises a number of globular regions called domains, which are formed by the folding of the amino acid chain into a three-dimensional shape and the presence of intra-chain disulphide bonds. The amino acid sequences in the 'arms' of the Y-shaped antibody molecule vary widely between different antibody molecules. This variable region is situated at the amino terminal end of both the heavy and light chains and is designated variable light (VL) or variable heavy (VH), depending on the chain being described. The variable region of one light chain and of one heavy chain determine the specificity of the antibody molecule and form one of the antigen-binding sites of the antibody. The number of heavy chain constant regions (CH) in an antibody molecule varies. IgG, IgA and IgD have three constant regions, whereas IgM and IgE both have four constant regions. Light chains have only one constant region (CL).

Antibodies perform a number of important functions that help to eliminate the foreign antigen which first initiated the specific B-cell response. They prevent microbes attaching to cells and invading them. By binding to epitopes on microorganisms and other particles, antibodies mark them as ready for destruction by phagocytes. This coating of the particle with antibodies is known as opsonization

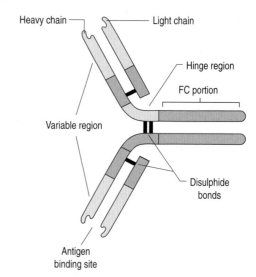

Figure 7.2: Structure of a typical antibody.

and surface membrane receptors on the phagocyte bind to the Fc portion of the antibody, thereby initiating phagocytosis of the particle. Antibody binding to epitopes of microbes at both of its antigen-binding sites clumps small particles or microbes together, thus making them more visible to phagocytic cells. This may also mark microbes as ready for killing by complement, a series of serum and membrane proteins that interact in a complex cascade reaction sequence. The reaction of an antibody with microbe may also set off the complement system, causing inflammation. Antibodies are also able to neutralize toxins released by microbes by adhering to them.[9]

Antibody-mediated immunity

Generation of antibody-mediated immunity occurs primarily in the regional lymph nodes. Here an antigen interacts with and stimulates a particular B cell to undergo mitosis and develop into a clone of cells identical to the original parent cell. Only about 10% of the clone of B cells produced will express membrane-bound antibody with the ability to bind strongly to the antigen. The remaining 90% will be eliminated. Clonal expansion of the selected antigen-reactive B cells leads to a clone of memory B cells and effector cells called plasma cells. The plasma cells secrete antibody reactive with the activating antigen[3] (Fig. 7.3).

Antibody-mediated immunity is characterized by the production of large numbers of antibody molecules specific for antigenic determinants (epitopes) on a foreign pathogen and is uniquely adapted to the elimination of extracellular pathogens.[6] It is estimated that B cells are capable of binding to approximately 10^8–10^{11} different antigens and this is known as the B cell's antigen-binding diversity.[6] During the maturation of the B cell there is gene rearrangment of the immunoglobulin variable-region, resulting in the generation of mature, immunocompetent B cells all expressing IgM and IgD membrane-bound antibody specific for a single epitope. The mature immunocompetent B cells migrate from the bone marrow to the secondary lymphoid organs. If the B cell encounters the antigen for which its membrane-bound IgM and IgD are specific, the cell becomes activated and undergoes clonal proliferation and differentiation. Those B cells which do not encounter antigen for which they are specific die within a few days.

Differentiation of the B cell into plasma cells and memory cells is dependent on either the direct interaction of T_H cells or indirect T_H-cell participation in the form of cytokines.

First contact with an exogenous antigen generates a primary antibody-mediated immune response. This response is characterized by three phases. During the first phase, the lag phase, B cells undergo clonal selection in response to antigen and differentiate into plasma cells and memory cells. A logarithmic increase in serum antibody levels follows this phase until a peak level of serum antibody is reached. This is achieved by eight or nine divisions of the B cell and generates plasma and memory cells. During a primary response, IgM is initially secreted, often followed by IgG. Depending on the persistence of the antigen, a primary response lasts varying periods of time, from a few days to several weeks.[3]

A secondary immune response is generated by activation of memory B cells by antigen and occurs more rapidly than the primary response due in part to the fact that there are more memory cells than there are naive B cells. The antibodies secreted during a secondary immune response also reach a greater magnitude, last for a longer duration and have a higher affinity for antigen than those produced during a primary response to antigen.

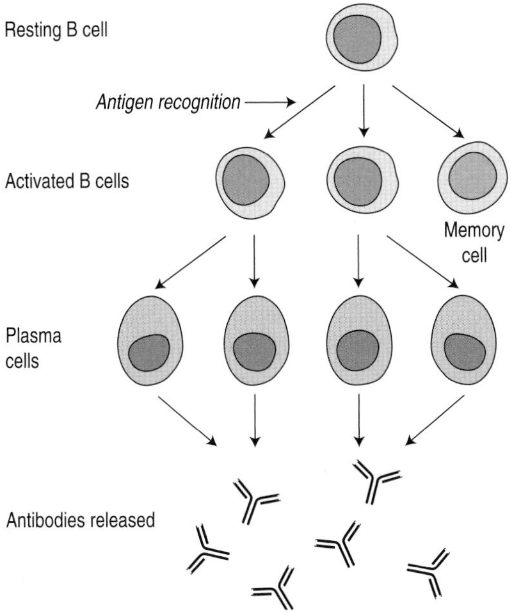

T lymphocytes

T lymphocytes, like B lymphocytes, derive from stem cells in the bone marrow. However, unlike B cells, the T cells migrate to the thymus gland to complete their maturation. Interactions between the maturing T cells, epithelial reticular cells and macrophages within the thymus induce an education and selection process whereby the T cells learn to react in a specific way to the MHC molecules.[4] This is known as MHC restriction. T cells that respond too strongly or too weakly to MHC are destroyed, as are any self-reactive T cells. Hence, many cells entering the thymus die there. T cells must recognize foreign antigens in association with the MHC molecule/antigen and, therefore, self-recognition is important. T cells play a major role as antigen reactive cells, as effector cells in cell-mediated immunity, as well as cooperating with B cells in antibody production.

Resting B cell

Antigen recognition →

Activated B cells

Memory cell

Plasma cells

Antibodies released

Figure 7.3: Antibody production.

121

T-cell receptor

T-cell response to antigen is by recognition via the T-cell receptor (TCR) on its cell surface.[6] The TCR is composed of two polypeptide chains that are linked by disulphide bonds. Most T cells are composed of an α and a β chain, although some are composed of a γ chain and a δ chain. Each chain contains a variable (V) region and a constant (C) region and random rearrangement of the gene sequences gives rise to the formation of innumerable TCRs. The diverse sequences in the variable region of the TCR renders T cells capable of responding to an enormous number of different antigens and ensures that each T cell has a slightly different TCR, giving them a different specificity.[4] The number of different antigens to which the T cells are capable of responding is known as the T-cell repertoire and is estimated to be 10^{17}.[6] The TCR associates on the cell surface with a group of membrane-anchored polypeptides known as the CD3 complex. The TCR–CD3 complex is the defining feature of the T lymphocyte. CD3 is involved in signalling on contact of the TCR with MHC–antigen complex.[3]

Two distinct T-cell populations exist and are denoted by the cell surface markers CD4 and CD8, that are expressed on mutually exclusive subsets of mature T cells. On arrival in the thymus, T cells express neither CD4 nor CD8, but, then, during their early differentiation, the T cells express both CD4 and CD8 on their surface (often called double positivity). The T cells will then lose either the CD4 marker to become CD8+ cytotoxic T cells, or the CD8 marker to become CD4+ helper T cells. The relevance of both of these T cell populations will now be discussed.

Helper T lymphocytes

Helper T lymphocytes are CD4+, class II MHC antigen-restricted, which means that CD4+ T cells can recognize foreign antigen on the surface of a cell only in association with self-antigens of class II MHC. Helper T lymphocytes are necessary for the production of normal levels of antibody by B lymphocytes and also for the normal development of cell-mediated immunity. This 'help' requires the production of the cytokines interleukin-4 (IL-4), IL-5 and either IL-6 or interferon-gamma (IFN-γ). There are two functional T lymphocyte subsets of CD4+ T cells known as T_H1 and T_H2. Cells of the T_H1 subset are characterized by their production of the cytokines IL-2, IFN-γ, tumour necrosis factor alpha (TNF-α) and TNF-β and by their failure to produce IL-4, IL-5 and IL-10. T_H1 subset activity is associated with cell-mediated immunity, including delayed-type hypersensitivity (+++) and T-cell proliferation. The cytokines they produce stimulate macrophages and cytotoxic T cells, which will be discussed later. Cells of the T_H2 subset are characterized by their production of the cytokines IL-4, IL-5 and IL-10 and by their failure to produce IL-2 and IFN-γ. T_H2 cell activation is associated with helper activity for antibody production through the production of cytokines that stimulate B cells to proliferate, differentiate and produce antibody.[3]

Cytotoxic T lymphocytes

Cytotoxic T lymphocytes (CTL) are a T-cell subset, usually CD8+ class I MHC antigen-restricted, which directly lyse target cells. Cytotoxic T lymphocytes kill virus-infected cells and transformed and transplanted cells.[6] Two major mechanisms are used for killing: (1) release of the protein perforin, which inserts into the membrane of the target cell, causing its lysis; (2) binding of a transmembrane protein called Fas ligand on the cytotoxic T lymphocyte to Fas on target cells, inducing apoptosis of the target cell.[6]

T lymphocytes which recognize MHC-bound antigens upon contact with the cells bearing them mediate cell-mediated immunity (CMI). As a result, these antigen-specific T cells proliferate and mature into immunologically functional (effector) T cells. Activated T cells release cytokines which have effects on other cells types so that the effector cell of CMI may be a cell other than a T lymphocyte.[9] CMI is essential against many viral and some bacterial infections as well as being important in allograft rejection.[9]

ANTIGEN PROCESSING AND PRESENTATION

In order for an immune response to take place, antigen must come into contact with lymphocytes, as these are the effector cells of the immune response. Antigens are molecules which elicit an immune response and may be foreign or self.[4] It is, therefore, essential that antigens and lymphocytes come into contact with one another and this is achieved through cells known as antigen-presenting cells (APCs). The three best defined APCs are macrophages, B lymphocytes and dendritic cells.[9]

Macrophages

Macrophages have been described as the professional phagocytes of the body.[12] They originate in the bone marrow and form a part of both the innate and acquired immune responses. During the innate immune response, monocytes are recruited to the site of inflammation through various chemical mediators, including cytokines (whose role and function will be discussed in greater detail later in the chapter). Chemokines, which are a family of cytokines that are able to attract other cells, i.e. they are chemoattractants, as well as other activating properties for various types of immune system cells are also involved. In the presence of specific cytokines such as IFN-γ, monocytes become activated and differentiate into macrophages. Stimulated macrophages bind many different antigens, including foreign particles such as microbes, macromolecules including antigens and also self cells that are injured or dead, with little or no specificity.[6] These antigens are phagocytosed and degraded within the macrophage by lysosomal enzymes. Larger protein antigens are degraded into smaller fragments by the macrophage and it is these smaller particles which are then displayed, together with the MHC molecule, on the surface of the macrophage, so that they can be recognized by antigen-specific CD4+ T lymphocytes. Activated CD4+ T cells secrete IFN-γ, which then activates the macrophages to become more effective killers of microorganisms.

Macrophages phagocytose antibody-coated microbes and cells, release inflammatory mediators such as IFN-γ, and other cytokines, and various chemokines. In addition, they activate secondary immune responses and are involved in tumour killing.[6]

B lymphocytes

During antibody responses, B cells can efficiently present antigens to T-helper (T_H) cells. By doing this, B cells amplify their own secondary antibody responses. The T_H cells synthesize cytokines, which stimulate the B cells to further differentiate into antibody-secreting plasma cells. This mechanism of antigen presentation is only really effective when the numbers of specific B cells are high, as in a secondary immune response.[9]

Dendritic cells

Dendritic cells (DCs) are central to the initiation of the immune response,[13] being competent at presenting protein antigens to T_H cells. It is also thought that DCs are important for inducing T-cell responses to foreign (allogeneic) MHC molecules in tissue allografts.[6] Two types of DCs are evident and have different properties and functions. Interdigitating dendritic cells are present in the interstitium of most organs and are abundant in T-cell rich areas such as the lymph nodes and spleen. They are also found scattered throughout the epidermis of the skin, where they are called Langerhans cells.[6] To induce immune reactivity, Langerhans cells are recruited at the site of antigen, uptake the antigen and migrate from the epidermis into lymphatic vessels, differentiating into potent APCs before they reach the regional lymph nodes.[14] Here, they present protein antigen to T_H, including naive T cells that have not previously been exposed to antigen.[14] The reaction between the lymphocyte and the foreign protein presented by the APC takes place in the microenvironment of the lymph nodes and spleen, where the APCs and reactive lymphocytes come into close contact.[4] The accessibility of antigens to the lymphocytes is facilitated by the DC concentrating antigens on its cell surface. DCs express high levels of class II MHC molecules and other molecules, known as costimulators, which are necessary for an immune response even when they are in the resting state: i.e. without extrinsic stimulation.[6]

Antigen presentation

In order for antigen to be capable of interacting with the TCR, it must first be recognized by the TCR.[6] As previously described, this usually requires that the antigen is presented as a small peptide in the groove of the MHC antigen molecule. Most nucleated cells can present antigen of intracellular origin on class I MHC antigen molecules. Professional APCs are class II MHC antigen-positive and present antigen from extracellular sources on class II molecules. As a general rule, antigen presentation requires that antigens are broken down, by enzymatic degradation, to form small peptides, and antigen processing is the intracellular mechanism by which protein antigens are fragmented into small peptides.[9] There are two major pathways of antigen processing, which are not mutually exclusive but depend partly on whether the antigen is derived from an extracellular source or from intracellular sources.[3] Extracellular proteins are endocytosed and degraded to peptides within APCs. Peptides of 8–9 amino acids in length become anchored to class I MHC molecules and are processed along a different pathway to those peptides of more than 12 amino acids, which bind to class II MHC molecules.[3]

Before looking at the roles of B cells in antibody-mediated immunity and T cells in cell-mediated immunity, the roles of other important cells and molecules will be defined.

LYMPHOCYTE MEMORY

Both T and B lymphocytes mediate immunological memory, and this is reflected in the rapidity of secondary immune responses. Following a relatively short-lived primary response, the majority of the newly generated effector cells are rapidly eliminated, largely through apoptosis. However, a proportion of the antigen-reactive cells become long-lived memory cells. Should re-exposure to the same antigen that triggered the primary immune response occur, a secondary immune response is initiated by memory cells already sensitized to the antigen. Hence, the secondary immune response is faster, more prolonged and more effective than the primary immune response.[5]

CYTOKINES

Cytokines are small protein molecules that can be produced by virtually all nucleated cells in the body. They therefore include lymphocyte-derived factors (lymphokines), monocyte-derived factors (monokines), haematopoietic factors (colony-stimulating factors), connective tissue/growth factors and chemotactic chemokines.[15] Cytokines are regulatory peptides that produce their effects locally, acting on neighbouring cells (paracrine activity) or on the cells that produce them (autocrine activity). Advances in science have allowed the identification and characterization of multiple cytokines (more than 150), many of which have specific and critical functions in the development and maintenance of the immune response.[16] These small protein hormones mediate to a large extent the effector phases of both innate and acquired immunity. Indeed, cytokines can be described as orchestrating the immune response because of the central role that they play.

Cytokines have been classified into two major categories. IL-2, IFN-γ and TNF-α are produced by T_H1 cells, whereas IL-4, IL-10 and transforming growth factor beta (TGF-β), are produced by T_H2 cells. T_H1 cytokines tend to stimulate cell-mediated immunity, whereas T_H2 cytokines enhance the humoral immune response. The ratio between the amount of T_H1 and T_H2 cytokines is considered an indicator of cell-mediated immunity activation or suppression, respectively. There has been wide interest in the effects of the administration of synthetic cytokines on tumour response, and this question will be considered later in the chapter.

HEAT SHOCK PROTEINS

Heat shock proteins (HSP) are a family of intracellular proteins that exhibit a high level of conservation, i.e. the structure of the proteins in humans are extremely similar to those of equivalent molecules found in simpler organisms such as bacteria.[9] Cross-species conservation suggests that a molecule has an important role in the normal functioning of the organism. Heat shock proteins were first discovered following heat stress, although other forms of cellular stress such as severe temperature fluctuations, viral infection, oxidative stress, fever, glucose deprivation and many others may also cause the stressed cells to produce them.[9] In this situation, HSP are produced preferentially and appear to have a protective effect on the stressed cell.

Heat shock proteins are described as molecular chaperones, as they play a critical role in the movement of proteins and peptides from the cytosol to the endoplasmic reticulum within the cell, where they facilitate the assembly of class I MHC molecules with β_2-microglobulin and peptide.[17]

APOPTOSIS

Apoptosis, often called 'programmed cell death', is a phenomenon which is described as the death of cells due to activation of a genetic programme that instructs the cell to commit suicide.[8] Apoptosis is a form of programmed cell death that does not always involve gene expression by the dying cell. It is a non-necrotic cell death in which the cell shrinks, the cell membrane blebs (balloons), cell fragments are released and the organelles and nucleus are rounded up. The chromatin is condensed and the DNA is cleaved into equal-sized fragments. Macrophages, which, as the professional phagocytes of the body, clear cellular corpses, play a key role in the process. Different cell surface receptors on the macrophage recognize signals from the apoptotic cells, and the macrophages speedily engulf them.[12]

The initiation of apoptosis is dependent upon the appropriate signal being delivered to the target cell nucleus. The surface antigen Fas (APO-1 in human cells) has been shown to be involved in the initiation of apoptosis.[9] Apoptosis is an important mechanism for selection in maturation of both T and B cells, as well as the targets of cytotoxic T lymphocytes.[8] Abnormalities of apoptotic cell clearance may contribute to the pathogenesis of chronic inflammatory disease, including autoimmune aetiology.

THE IMMUNE RESPONSE

Having explored some of the major elements of the immune system, such as the physical and chemical barriers and NK cells of the innate immune response and T and B lymphocytes, MHC molecules of the acquired immune response, as well as the roles of cytokines, APCs such as dendritic cells, B cells and macrophages, it may be helpful to further determine what happens during an immune response. This is important because immune system cells and molecules do not work in isolation from each other but, rather, they form part of a complex network where the actions of one component has an effect on another.[3]

The immune system response, then, is a response to antigen and may include both innate and acquired responses. Having breached the physical and chemical defences of the innate defence system, antigens such as bacteria gain entry to the body by adhering to mucosal surfaces, whereas viruses adhere to receptors on target cells, which consequently secrete interferons.[4] Interferons stimulate NK cells, which target the virus-infected cell.

Entry of bacteria into the body initiates several immune mechanisms, including the activation of PMNs and serum proteins such as complement, acute phase proteins, the clotting cascade and kinin system, all of which have a role to play in the attempt to eliminate the bacteria from the body and in the inflammatory response. PMNs such as monocytes and macrophages are involved in phagocytosis of the invader. At the same time, these activated cells produce various cytokines, including IL-1, IL-6 and TNF, often called the pyrogenic cytokines because of their induction of fever. Phagocytic cells may bear Fc receptors and will, therefore, act in an antigen-specific manner through binding antibody. Macrophages, and also NK cells, may be activated by cytokines produced as a result of a specific immune response and, hence, both NK cells and macrophages play a role in both innate and acquired immunity.

When coated with antibodies (opsonized), virus-infected cells and other pathogens may be killed by antibody-dependent cell-mediated cytotoxicity (ADCC).[3] If the invading organism is not eliminated following the inflammatory response, a specific immune response is initiated. Macrophages will engulf the antigen and, by enzymatic processing, degrade the protein antigen into small peptides. These peptides will then be presented on the cell surface of the macrophage in the context of an MHC molecule. A naive T lymphocyte with a TCR specific for the antigen engages with the MHC–antigen complex and, in so doing, becomes activated. Activated T_H cells firstly enlarge, proliferating and maturing to form effector T cells as well as secreting an array of cytokines.[6] Often, both T and B cell responses are generated but the type of response depends on the causative pathogen. For example, intracellular pathogens require a cell-mediated response, whereas antibody is important in controlling disease caused by extracellular organisms.[4] T cells play a central role in the orchestration and amplification of the immune response, secreting cytokines that recruit or augment the activity of various other cells, including NK cells and macrophages. Whereas T cells are vital for the direct elimination of virus-infected cells, B cells are also stimulated, as they are necessary for the termination of the immune response by antigen clearance.[6]

Some of the cytokines produced by the acti-vated T cells are haematopoietic growth factors, such as granulocyte–macrophage colony-stimulating factor (GM-CSF). This stimulates the pluripotent stem cells in the bone marrow to proliferate and release additional blood cells into the bloodstream.[1] Following elimination of antigens, the immune system returns to its preactivated state, but with the addition of B and T memory cells which will enable a speedier secondary response should the same antigen be encountered on a subsequent occasion.

THE IMMUNE SYSTEM AND CANCER

Every advance in understanding of the immune system, and these have been numerous over the last two decades, and of how it functions makes us question why and how tumours are able to develop and, once developed why they are not destroyed.[18 (p293)]

It has long been recognized that a relationship exists between the immune system and cancer.[18] This is evidenced by several factors. Remissions of cancers following bacterial infections were first noted in the late 18th century when a Paris physician injected pus into the leg of a patient with advanced breast cancer and noted that the cancer improved as the infection worsened.[17] During the 19th century German physicians noted that responses in breast cancer and lymphoma occurred in patients who developed erysipelas, a bacterial infection.[19] The work of 19th century American surgeon William Coley is well known. Based on the erysipelas responses, Coley treated over 800 patients with an extract of soluble bacterial toxins and found that approximately half had a good response.[20]

Further evidence of the relationship between the immune system and cancer is seen in the frequent association between cancers and immunosuppression.[18] It is not uncommon for patients with congenital or acquired immunosuppression to develop lymphoreticular malignancies as well as solid tumours, especially gastric cancers.[21] Examples of immunosuppression-associated malignancies include Kaposi's sarcoma, which is associated with human immunodeficiency virus (HIV) and herpes virus infection,[22] skin cancer following solid organ transplantation[23] and lymphoid tumours after stem cell transplantation.[24] Further evidence of the relationship between the immune system and cancer is the presence of immune system cell infiltrates when tumour biopsy material is histologically examined. These cells include T cells (tumour-infiltrating lymphocytes (TILs)), NK cells and macrophages which surround the cell, and indicate that the tumour is immunogenic.[6] In addition, spontaneous regressions of tumours and the regression of metastatic lesions following removal of the primary tumour also indicate that the immune system may be active in the elimination of malignancies.[17]

Tumour antigens

As previously described, in order for any immune response to be mounted the host must first recognize the presence of foreign protein antigens, as it is these molecules that elicit a specific immune response.[3] It was initially assumed unlikely that tumours would express particular antigens, as the cancer cell is derived from a normal self cell. However, abnormal protein antigens such as those that are the result of the complex abnormalities that derive from mutated or viral genes and/or deregulated expression of normal genes can stimulate specific immune responses to tumour cells. In addition, surface proteins peculiar to tumours may serve as targets for effectors of innate immunity such as NK cells.[6] These non-specific tumour antigens may arise by a number of different pathways, such as the expression of viral proteins due to transcription of integrated retroviral genes into the cell.[6] Chemicals may lead to the production of aberrant proteins that initiate surface expression of unique antigens or induce genetic mutations that lead to altered molecular structure. Genetic mutations may also lead to incorrect assembly of complex molecules, resulting in the exposure of normally concealed antigenic determinants.[9] The discovery of α-fetoprotein (AFP) in hepatocellular carcinoma[25] and carcinoembryonic antigen (CEA) in colorectal carcinomas[26] have also confirmed the presence of tumour antigens on some tumours.[17] It is now known that a vast array of cancer antigens exist in addition to oncofetal antigens (CEA and AFP) which are usually only expressed in utero.[17]

Tumour antigens may be found in cancers of the same or different types in different patients: i.e. they may be shared or may be specific for a particular cancer cell in a particular patient.[17,27] Antigens may also be subclassified according to their specificity for particular tissue or tumour types. Some antigens, such as melanocyte antigens Melan-A/MART-1, tyrosinase and gp100, represent differentiation antigens.[28] Although these gene products are expressed in both normal and malignant melanocytes, they are not expressed in tumours derived from other cell types. Some antigens are found only on malignant cells and not normal cells, whereas others are viral in origin, such as cancers that are associated with viral infections, as with the association of cervical cancers with human papillomavirus.[17]

Signals from transformed cells cause activation of antigen-presenting dendritic cells.[18] Such signals may include cytokines or heat shock proteins expressed by cells undergoing damage or death. Once activated, DCs initiate and control a specific immune response that is directed towards tumour-associated antigens (TAAs). For example, TAAs such as melanoma antigen 1 (MAGE1) and melanoma antigen recognized by T cells 1 (MART1), both human melanoma cell TAAs, are taken up by Langerhans cells (DCs in the skin), which then migrate to draining lymph nodes where they stimulate the specific T-cell response.[14] Antigen-specific T- and B-cell responses are initiated by DCs which capture antigens that are secreted or shed by tumour cells or after cell lysis.[18]

Effector cell response to tumour cells

Effector cells of the immune system, including T and B lymphocytes, NK cells and macrophages, as well as being active against infective molecules, have also been found to be active in transformed cells. Recognition of TAAs by appropriate and specific effector cells leads to these cells mediating the killing of tumour cells.[6] However, it is possible that such immune responses are weak, and therefore malignant cells are not prevented from developing into tumours.[29]

T-cell response

Some tumour antigens are molecules that are recognized by T cells. As tumour cells generally express class I rather than class II MHC molecules, T_H cells are unable to recognize the transformed cells themselves but are reliant on macrophage processing and presentation of the tumour-derived proteins as peptide–MHC complexes. These complexes are presented to either CD4+ or CD8+ T lymphocytes. CD4+ T_H cells are unable to kill directly but, once stimulated by antigen, mediate killing through secretion of cytokines that activate T cytotoxic (Tc) cells, macrophages, NK cells (T_H1 cytokines) and B cells (T_H2 cytokines). These cells also produce TNF, which is directly lytic to tumour cells. In contrast to T_H cells, the CD8+ T cells, which are mostly cytotoxic, cause direct lysis of tumour cells by disrupting the cell's membrane and nucleus.[9]

Antibody response

Antibodies may also play a role in the immune system response to tumours, and B-cell lines producing antibodies to TAAs have been derived from the draining lymph nodes of human tumours.[9] These tumour-reactive B cells may also play an important role in the processing and presentation of tumour antigens to T_H cells.[9] Antibodies may cause tumour cell lysis, either by fixing complement to the tumour cell membrane (thereby activating the complement cascade, which ultimately results in cell lysis) or by antibody-dependent cellular cytotoxicity (ADCC) mediated by Fc-receptor-bearing NK cells, killer cells, macrophages and granulocytes.

NK cells response

Natural killer cells, because of their role in innate immunity, are thought to provide initial defence against tumours at both the primary and metastatic sites.[9] The activity of the NK cells is enhanced by cytokines secreted by antigen-stimulated T_H cells. NK cell lysis results from the release of cytotoxic factors, including granzyme, which induce the formation of holes in the membrane of the target cell. Interkeukin-2 and IFN-γ, synthesized by activated T_H cells, enhance this activity. NK cells are not merely direct cytotoxic killers but may also play a critical role in cytokine production, which may be important in controlling cancer.[7]

It has long been recognized that, in vivo, NK cells spontaneously kill MHC class I-deficient tumour cells and their metastases.[18]

Macrophages response

Macrophages also have a role to play in tumour immunity. In particular, they process and present antigen to initiate a specific immune response.[30] However, they are also capable of directly lysing tumour cells. Cytokines such as IFN-γ, TNF, IL-4 and GM-CSF, produced by antigen-stimulated T cells, mediate this cytotoxic activity of macrophages. Thus, the ability of macrophages to affect tumour cell growth is largely dependent upon T-cell immunity.[9] The cytokines that activate the macrophages also influence the mechanism of tumour cell lysis, and hence the precise mechanism by which macrophages destroy the cell will vary.

Cytokines and the immune response

Cytokines play an essential role in the immune response to cancer. They modulate the immune response towards protective antitumour immunity within the tumour microenvironment.[15] The role played by cytokines is both a direct one, through involvement in the cancer cell, and an indirect one, through enhancing the activity of immune cells such as NK cells and macrophages.[9]

Infection, inflammation and carcinogen-induced injury stimulate the release of cytokines, which minimize cellular damage by controlling these cellular stressors. Hence, they suppress the formation of tumours.[31] However, tumour cells can both use host-derived cytokines and synthesize cytokines which can act as tumour cell growth factors.[15,31] Tumour cells may also use host-derived cytokines to increase their resistance to apoptosis and to aid metastasis.[31] Laboratory experiments have shown that a variety of cytokines may be involved in the development or prevention of tumours.[31] It is also suggested that cytokines synthesized by tumour cells may allow tumours to evade immune surveillance.[15]

Mechanisms of tumour tolerance

Despite the many mechanisms possessed by the immune system to eliminate foreign and altered antigens as well as the evidence that the immune system is responsive to cancer cells, tumours frequently grow and become established within the host, evading immune recognition. One area of immunology which looks at the way that tumours are 'sensed' by the immune system and at the properties and mechanisms that affect this process is the field of tumour immunology.[29] The mechanisms by which tumours evade the host immune response are often referred to as tumour escape mechanisms, and a number of such mechanisms have either been identified or proposed.[14]

In some tumour cells there is a reduction in, loss of, or a failure to produce tumour antigens, thus rendering the cell unable to stimulate an antigen-specific response or a meaningful immune response and, therefore, reducing the opportunities for the cell to be recognized and destroyed. Such cells, therefore, possess a selective advantage that allows them to form the dominant population. If the antigen is present, it may not be accessible to the antibodies or expressed in the context of MHC.[17]

In addition to down-regulation of tumour antigens, MHC molecules may also be down-regulated or switched off. Down-regulation of MHC expression may also provide a means of immune escape for the tumour. Class I MHC molecules are usually widely expressed on almost all normal somatic cells and many tumour cells also express these molecules. However, down-regulation of class I MHC molecules on tumours has been reported,[32] and this renders the cell unable to form complexes of the processed tumour antigen peptides and MHC molecules required for CTL recognition. Class II MHC molecules are not normally expressed on human tumour cells and these cells cannot, therefore, directly activate tumour-specific CD4+ T helper cells.[6] As antitumour CTL activity is largely dependent on signals provided by the T_H cell, there is greater reliance on the professional APCs, such as macrophages, infiltrating the tumour in order to take up and present tumour antigens. This ensures the activation of T_H cells, so that maximum antitumour CTL differentiation may occur.

In addition to the recognition of MHC–antigen complex by host T cells, costimulatory molecules must also be present if the T cells are to become activated. Costimulatory molecules are cell surface molecules, other than antigen receptors, that are required for the efficient response of lymphocytes to antigen.[8] Antigen binding without costimulation may lead to unresponsiveness rather than to an immune response. Lack of costimulatory molecules such as B7-1 and B7-2[33] on the tumour cell means that the second signal required for T-cell stimulation is absent. Lack of expression of these costimulatory molecules has been found in many different tumours, and this may give another explanation for the poor or absent T-cell immunity to tumour antigens.[14]

During tumour growth and progression, cancer cells may secrete inhibitory cytokines and many tumours have been shown to express TGF-β, IL-10 and prostaglandin E_2.[34] TGF-β, as well as being a growth factor for many epithelial cells, is immunosupressive, inhibiting a wide variety of lymphocyte and macrophage functions. In particular, it blocks generation of CTL and LAK cells. Interleukin-10 also has potent imunosuppressive effects and may render tumour cells resistant to tumour lysis by T cells.[35,36]

Lastly, tumour cells may actively induce apoptosis in infiltrating immune cells. This is possibly through the expression of Fas ligand on tumour cells, which, when it binds to Fas on T cells and dendritic cells, kills these immune cells.[30] Apoptosis of such cells as TILs will prevent them from lysing the tumour cells.

CONCLUSION

It has not been possible to include everything that is known about the immune system and its role in health and disease in this chapter and the reader is directed to those texts which deal directly with immunity and the immune response. However, key features of the immune system and the immune response have been given consideration. Despite its complexity, the immune system can be seen as possessing active and effective antitumour immunity, achieved through both innate and acquired immune mechanisms. Once described as the 'poor cousin', the innate immune system is now recognized as a critically important component of antitumour immunity.[17 (p188)]

REFERENCES

1. Janeway CA, Travers P. Immunobiology: the immune system in health and disease. 5th edn. Edinburgh: Churchill Livingstone; 2001.
2. Cheng JD, Rieger PT, von Mehren M, Adams GP, Weiner LM. Recent advances in immunotherapy and monoclonal antibody treatment for cancer. Semin Oncol Nurs 2000; 16(4)Suppl 1:2–12.
3. Kuby J. Immunology. 3rd edn. New York: WH Freeman; 1997.
4. Staines N, Brostoff J, James K. Introducing immunology. 2nd edn. London: Mosby; 1993.
5. Marieb EN. Human anatomy and physiology. 5th edn. California: Benjamin Cummings; 2001.
6. Abbas AK, Lichtman AH, Pober JS. Cellular and molecular immunology. 5th edn. London: WB Saunders; 2001.
7. Miller JS. Biology of natural killer cells in cancer and infection. Cancer Invest 2002; 20 (3):405–419.

8. Herbert WJ, Wilkinson PC, Stott DI. The dictionary of immunology. 4th edn. London: Academic Press; 1995.

9. Eales L-J. Immunlogy for life scientists: a basic introduction. Chichester: John Wiley; 1997.

10. Isaacs H, Lindeman J. Virus interference 1: the interferon. Proc Roy Soc Lond (Biol) 1957; 147:257–262.

11. Thibodeau GA, Patton KT. Anatomy and physiology. 5th edn. St Louis: Mosby; 2003.

12. Geske GJ, Monks J, Lehman L, Fadek VA. The role of the macrophage in apoptosis: hunter, gatherer and regulator. Int J Immunol 2002; 76(1):16–26.

13. Vacari AP, Caux C, Trinchieri G. Tumour escape from immune surveillance through dendritic cell inactivation. Semin Cancer Biol 2002; 12(1):33–42.

14. Brinckerhoff LH, Thompson LW, Slingluff CL. Melanoma vaccines. Curr Opin Oncol 2001; 12(2):163–173.

15. Mocellin S, Wang E, Marincola FM. Cytokines and immune response in the tumour microenvironment. J Immunother 2001; 25(5):392–407.

16. Chada S, Ramesh R, Mhshikar AM. Cytokine- and chemokine-based gene therapy for cancer. Curr Opin Molec Therap 2003; 5(5):463–474.

17. Davis ID. An overview of cancer immunotherapy. Immunol Cell Biol 2000; 78:179–195.

18. Smyth MJ, Godfrey DI, Trapani JA. A fresh look at tumour immunosurveillance and immunotherapy. Nature Immunol 2001; 2(4):293–299.

19. Gore ME, Riches P. The history of immunotherapy. In: Gore M, Riches P, eds. Immunotherapy in cancer. Chichester: Wiley; 1996.

20. Coley WB. The treatment of malignant tumours by repeated inoculations of erisipelas: with a report of ten original cases. Am J Med Sci 1893; 105:487–511.

21. McClain KL. Immunodeficiency status and related malignancies. Cancer Treat Res 1997; 92:39–61.

22. Cannon M, Cesarman E. Kaposi's sarcoma-associated herpes virus and acquired immunodeficiency syndrome-related malignancy. Semin Oncol 2000; 27:409–413.

23. Ottley CC, Pittelkow MR. Skin cancer in liver transplant recipients. Liver Transplant 2000; 6:253–262.

24. Aguillar LK, Rooney CM, Heslop HE. Lymphoproliferative disorders involving Epstein–Barr virus after hemopoietic stem cell transplantation. Curr Opin Oncol 1999; 11:96–101.

25. Abelev GI. Alpha-fetoprotein in embryogenesis and its association with malignant tumours. Adv Cancer Res 1971; 14:295–358.

26. Gold P, Freedman SO. Demonstration of tumour-specific antigens in human colonic carcinomata by immunological tolerance and absorption technique. J Exp Med 1965; 121:439–462.

27. de Visser KE, Schumacher TNM, Kruisbeek AM. CD8+ T cell tolerance and cancer immunotherapy. J Immunother 2003; 26(1):1–11.

28. Kawakami Y, Rosenberg SA. Immunobiology of human melanoma antigens MART-1 and gp100 and their use for immuno-gene therapy. Int Rev Immunol 1997; 14:173–192.

29. Todryk S. A sense of tumour for the immune system. Immunology 2002; 107:1–4.

30. Byrne SN, Halliday GM. Dendritic cells: making progress with tumour regression? Immunol Cell Biol 2002; 80:520–530.

31. Dranoff G. Cytokines in cancer pathogenesis and cancer therapy. Nature Rev – Cancer 2004; 4:11–22.

32. Ikeda H, Lethe B, Lehman F, et al. Characterisation of an antigen that is recognised on a melanoma showing partial HLA loss by CTL expressing an NK inhibitory receptor. Immunity 1997; 6:199–208.

33. Dessureault S, Graham F, Gallinger S. B7-1 gene transfer into human cancer cells by infection with an adenovirus-B7 (Ad-B7) expression vector. Ann Surg Onc 1996; 3:317–324.

34. Wojtowicz-Praga S. Reversal of tumor-induced immunosuppression: a new approach to cancer therapy. J Immunother 1997; 20:165–177

35. Petersson M, Charo J, Salazar-Onfray F, et al. Constitutive IL-10 production accounts for the high NK sensitivity, low MHC class I expression, and poor transporter associated with antigen processing (TAP)-1/2 function in the prototype NK target YAC-1. J Immunol 1998; 161:2099–2105.

36. Tanchot C, Guillaume S, Delon J, et al. Modifications of CD8+ T cell function during in vivo memory or tolerance induction. Immunity 1998; 8(5):581–590.

SECTION 3

Prevention and early detection

8. Cancer Prevention. 133

9. Early Detection of Cancer 167

CHAPTER 8

Cancer Prevention

AGNES GLAUS, STELLA AGUINAGA BIALOUS, PAULA TRAHAN RIEGER

CHAPTER CONTENTS

Principles of cancer prevention	134
Primary prevention	134
Secondary prevention	135
Tertiary prevention	136
The fourth level of prevention: prevention of suffering	136
Barriers and opportunities; social and political issues of prevention	136
The role of nurses in health promotion and cancer prevention	138
The tobacco story and its consequences	139
A nursing strategy for the support of smoking cessation	143
The role of nutrition	143
Vegetables, fruits, fibres	145
Vitamins, minerals, nutrients	145
Cooking methods	146
Energy intake, fat, weight, physical exercise, alcohol and related hormonal issues	146
Body weight: its relation to hormones and physical exercise	147
Alcohol	148
Menstrual and reproductive cancer risk factors	148

Other cancer risk factors	148
Cancer risk assessment models	149
Family history: assessing individual risk	150
Screening indications for cancer susceptibility genes	151
Cancer susceptibility genes and genetic counselling in cancer prevention	152
Nature of genetic tests	152
Psychosocial, ethical and legal issues	154
Pre- and post-test counselling	155
Intervention: the role of chemoprevention in cancer control	156
Prophylactic surgical interventions: e.g. prophylactic mastectomy	158
Chemoprevention and other risk-reducing strategies for smokers and ex-smokers	159
Glossary: terms frequently used in cancer prevention	159
References	161

This chapter starts with the principles as well as professional and political issues of cancer prevention. The role of nurses in health promotion and cancer prevention is also discussed. It covers different cancer risk factors and links them to issues of primary prevention. This is followed by an outline of cancer risk assessment methods, including assessment of family history and the role of genetics in the development of cancer, with its significant impact upon the methods used to screen for and ultimately to prevent cancer. The nature of genetic tests and critical issues of genetic counselling are described. Preventative interventions, such as surgery or chemoprevention for high-risk individuals are discussed. Screening methods and strategies for the early detection of breast, ovarian, cervix, colon and prostate cancer as well as the most frequently used diagnostic methods in secondary prevention are outlined.

PRINCIPLES OF CANCER PREVENTION

The World Health Organization (WHO) declared cancer prevention and control as one of the most important scientific and public health challenges of our time.[1] The WHO estimates that there are over 20 million people living with cancer, the majority of whom live in the developing world, and 10 million new cases a year worldwide.[1] Cancer is one of the leading causes of death in Europe and several other developed and developing countries.[2] Its incidence is increasing, with the increase in life expectancy of the world's population and changes in lifestyle factors, such as an increase in the prevalence of tobacco use and changes in dietary patterns. It is estimated that at least one-third of the cases of cancers worldwide could be prevented and another one-third could benefit from early detection and treatment.[1]

Although specific causes for all types of cancers are not known, there are several causal factors and mechanisms that have been identified, many of which can be modified to prevent the occurrence of cancer. The American Cancer Society of the United States estimates that 80% of all cancers are caused by environmental exposures and could potentially be prevented if exposure could be reduced or avoided.[3]

Cancer is a term used to describe many different diseases. They have in common that, at some level of the cell multiplication process, there is a malfunction. In general, cancer causes are classified as endogenous (e.g. associated with genetics, age, gender or ethnicity) or exogenous (e.g. exposure to a carcinogenic agent in the environment such as tobacco, radiation, viruses, etc.). Primary prevention, risk assessment and early detection measures are tailored to address the causation mechanism.

Prevention and early detection are essential components of oncology nursing practice. Although some nurses may believe that taking care of patients already diagnosed with cancer and cancer prevention are separate issues, they are in fact intrinsically related. While conducting screening or early detection for a specific cancer, the nurse should assess risk and recommend screening for any additional type of cancer, as appropriate. For example, assessment of smoking status and referral to cessation services should be part of every nurse–client encounter. Similarly, nurses should support the implementation of tertiary prevention in order to detect secondary cancers and complications at an early stage and develop a plan to prevent suffering as indicated by the patient's condition. Thus, risk assessment is an indispensable component of oncology nursing.

The oncology nurse must be capable of conveying information about risk, i.e. the presence of factors that increase the chances of an individual developing cancer, in a clear manner and stress that the absence of a risk factor is not a guarantee that no cancer will develop. Alternatively, the nurse needs to make sure the client understands that the presence of a risk factor does not lead automatically to the development of cancer. Clarity of message is important in all aspects of screening and detection and has become even more critical with the advances in genetic screening, which often involve explanation of risks associated with genetic concepts that frequently are not part of a client's existing knowledge repertoire. Prevention is commonly classified by four different levels: primary, secondary, tertiary and prevention of suffering.

Primary prevention

The goal of primary prevention is to avoid the development of the disease through the limitation or elimination of carcinogenic exposure. Preventative measures are potentially cost-effective and prevention programmes could greatly contribute to reducing the social burden of cancer. Primary prevention measures are risk-reduction strategies proven effective but do not guarantee that the individual will not later develop cancer, which is always an important message to convey clearly to clients and the media.

Primary prevention is usually divided into medical and behavioural activities. Medical activities include immunization, such as vaccination against hepatitis B to prevent against liver cancer, and reduction in the incidence of human papillomavirus infection for the prevention of cervical cancer. Also included as a medical activity is chemoprevention, the administration of drugs to asymptomatic individuals at high risk for cancer in order to prevent the development of cancer or to arrest the evolution of a precancerous tumor into cancer. Chemoprevention attempts to reverse the natural course of the disease but its utilization for preventing cancer is in its infancy and is discussed in more detail later in this chapter.

Therefore, primary cancer prevention relies mainly on behavioural and cognitive measures anchored in health education, lifestyle and environment modification based on known risk factors. Behaviour modification presents many challenges and is more successful when individual intervention is part of a broader social and political intervention that promotes healthy behaviour as the acceptable social norm. For example, smoke-free environments promote non-smoking as the social norm. Other examples are offering fruits and vegetables at workplaces and school cafeterias or promoting physical activity or smoke-free workplaces. It remains a challenge for oncology nurses to promote cancer prevention behaviours within the political and social context.

The present and future burden of tobacco-related cancers makes tobacco control, including protection against exposure to secondhand smoke and smoking cessation, a high priority for primary prevention. Another behavioural prevention priority is related to diet. Topical behavioural modifications are associated with decreasing the risk of cancer through avoiding excessive sun exposure and wearing protective gear when exposure is necessary to decrease the risk of skin cancer.

Avoiding exposure to environmental contaminants (arsenic in water, radon, etc.), including occupational exposure, and exposure to certain microorganisms, such as hepatitis B and C viruses, human papillomavirus and *Helicobacter pylori*, also represent modern primary prevention measures.

Additional environmental factors associated with a higher incidence of cancer may prove to be more difficult to prevent, as they involve higher levels of policymaking and political will. Such factors include education, living conditions, socioeconomic status and some occupational exposures. Cancer is more prevalent among the less-educated, lower socioeconomic groups and broader social and political changes are necessary before these discrepancies in cancer prevalence will be resolved. It is important to note, however, that many of the primary prevention measures can be included as part of general chronic diseases prevention programmes. Measures related to diet, tobacco use and physical activity, for example, overlap with preventative measures for cardiovascular diseases and it is more cost-effective for many settings to combine and coordinate such prevention strategies. Aspects of primary cancer prevention are described in detail later in the chapter.

Secondary prevention

Many cancer control measures fall into the secondary prevention level. Secondary prevention's goal is to prevent cancer morbidity and mortality; therefore, screening and early detection are the measures associated with secondary prevention. Usually, screening targets at-risk individuals who are asymptomatic and early detection attempts to provide early diagnosis for symptomatic persons. Given that early detection and diagnosis lead to greater chance of successful treatment, it is essential that screening and early detection programmes include a public education component to assist in identifying early signs and symptoms. Such signs are lumps, sores that do not heal, abnormal bleeding, persistent digestive problems and chronic hoarseness.[1] As with primary prevention, it is important for the nurse to clearly communicate to clients that the presence of any of these signs does not imply a diagnosis of cancer, but that they do require immediate medical attention for assessment and further diagnostic tests. Therefore, in addition to health education, secondary prevention measures also include screening through health history, carcinogen exposure assessment, physical examination (including self-examination) and utilization of diagnostic and detection technology, such as Pap smear for the early detection of cervical cancer and mammography for the early detection of breast cancer and, in some cases, genetic testing. Chapter 9 discusses critical issues regarding cancer screening and the most commonly used secondary prevention techniques and trends.

Tertiary prevention

The goal of tertiary prevention is to limit the extent of morbidity and disability and to provide rehabilitation for patients with cancer. Tertiary prevention measures include avoiding complications arising from treatment and from the disease itself, preventing additional morbidity and recurrence and addressing the impact of cancer at the physical, emotional and social level. For example, the provision of rehabilitation care for mastectomized women with lymphoedema could be called tertiary prevention. Another example of tertiary prevention is to assess the risk and monitor the recurrence of cancer in a secondary site through application of appropriate detection and diagnostic methods. It also includes the utilization of chemoprevention agents, when available, to prevent the development of secondary cancers. Other chapters in this book address in depth the issues related to prevention of secondary effects, rehabilitation and secondary cancers.

The fourth level of prevention: prevention of suffering

The World Health Organization has identified prevention of suffering as a determined level of preventative strategies in cancer care. It involves utilizing all available techniques, skills and knowledge to ensure that suffering is avoided or minimized, and that the quality of life of the individuals with cancer and their relatives is supported. It includes the utilization of a combination of therapeutic measures to promote pain control, decrease fatigue, provide nutritional support and identify and respond to psychosocial or spiritual needs. Prevention of suffering and supportive and palliative care are addressed in other chapters in this book.

BARRIERS AND OPPORTUNITIES; SOCIAL AND POLITICAL ISSUES OF PREVENTION

Cancer prevention policies vary widely from country to country and within countries; access to screening and early diagnosis services are unevenly distributed among populations. Even in developed countries with resources and programmes in place, access to these services does not reach equally all segments of the population, with ethnic minorities as well as those in lower socioeconomic strata having less access to services, later-stage diagnosis and higher prevalence of various types of cancer.[7,9,11,12,13,15,18] Barriers may be related to language, cultural perceptions and beliefs associated with disease and health services, finances, including lack of insurance, poor recruitment and lack of health information adequate to the literacy level of different subgroups of the population.[4–6,8,10,14,16,17,19,20] An additional barrier is age, with studies showing that the elderly tend to have lower participation in prevention and early detection programmes.[21,22] There are also barriers associated with healthcare providers and health systems due to a lack of cultural sensitivity, lack of outreach efforts and low priority given to prevention practices and health education.[19,20] Policy changes, including the development of specific nursing roles, are necessary to address these barriers and to increase access to services.

Health policies are determined by the causal model adopted by advocates, policymakers and healthcare professionals. But as Tesh noted:[23] [p155] 'more powerful than vested interests, more subtle than science, political ideology has, in the end, the greatest influence on disease prevention policy'. Politics are an integral part of public health,[24] and political ideology will determine availability and type of services as much, if not more, than epidemiological data and scientific research. Therefore, cancer prevention practices and nurses' involvement in it will mainly be defined at the political level and by nursing involvement with policy development.

Wilson[25] provides a framework for policy analysis that is helpful for nurses assessing cancer prevention policies. He departs from cost and benefit definitions by focusing on determining who benefits and who bears the costs of any given policy and points out that how an issue is framed will largely determine such costs and benefits. Factors to be considered in framing and determining benefits include the level of organization and resources of those affected by the policy (i.e. people tend to organize when effects are concentrated); the number of people affected; and the magnitude of the effect. When benefits are diffuse and costs concentrated, those bearing the costs are certain to organize and mobilize political opposition, and are predicted or expected to win in a political conflict. Therefore, in terms of political influence, the organized, mobilized group opposing a policy could have greater chances of success. For example, it could be the case of large health insurance companies fighting the benefits of prevention strategies that benefit a large, diffuse and often non-organized group of the population. However, issues can be reframed to one's advantage, trying to either diffuse the costs or to concentrate the benefits. The tobacco industry loses revenue when tougher regulatory measures on public smoking are implemented, but the industry may try to diffuse the cost by saying that everyone loses if their rights and freedom to smoke are undermined by regulations. Groups favouring such regulations have then to frame the issue as one of the majority's right to breathe smoke-free air and to highlight that the cost is borne by the concentrated interests of the tobacco industry. Thus, a single policy proposal or programme is not statically in one category of benefits or costs, as these are often relative to the way it is framed.

Also important in the political and policy processes are the definition of the problem and agenda setting. Garvin and Eyles[26] analysed skin cancer prevention policy in Australia, Canada and England and demonstrated how framing of the same problem, i.e. rise in skin cancer incidence, varies based on social, cultural and political circumstances and leads to different health policies and programmes. Problem definition can be changed by advocates, interest groups and policymakers and the 'right' definition helps to move an issue into the political agenda, but other factors influence the setting of both the public and formal agendas. The public agenda is defined as 'issues which have achieved high level of public interest and visibility' and the formal agenda as a 'list of items which decision-makers have formally accepted for serious consideration'.[27] The agenda-building process is dynamic and influenced by several factors, such as whose interests are represented in the definition of the problem, who is involved and mobilized in favour and in opposition to the issue and how the issue is being presented and perceived by the public as well as those affected. Brendtro[28] used the Kingdon agenda-setting model[29] to describe how breast cancer gained its prominence in the formal agenda in the United States, the role of advocates in raising the issue and the potential role for nurses in the political process. Indeed, nurses may play a major role in moving access to cancer prevention into the formal and public agendas.

Cancer issues have a variety of interests involved, from the pharmaceutical and diagnostic technology companies, to patients' advocates and health professionals and, ultimately, the public at large. Although the personal experience of a policymaker is often very important in providing momentum and opportunity for an issue to be placed on the formal agenda, cancer prevention policies may remain largely a product of interest groups politics. Interest groups are an inherent part of the political scene, with few decisions made in governments without the involvement of one or more interest groups.[29–32] Interest groups are often divided into special and public interest groups.

Special interest groups have exclusive, relatively narrow goals. These groups advocate benefits that are shared by few in the community, often to the exclusion or even the adversity of the rest of the community. These dimensions of interest are summarized in Box 8.1.[33]

Public interest groups are defined as groups who advocate for issues that are shared by a substantial number of people, i.e. interests that will benefit a large group (e.g. increased access to cancer screening services), and commonly may be formed by one or more organizations. Cancer prevention advocacy organizations

137

Box 8.1

Four dimensions of conflict between special and public interests

1. Scope
Who is involved, how many and how they become involved. There is tension between privatizing (reducing the number of players) and socializing the conflict (expanding the number of players). Special interests tend to prefer conflict privatization, where they have a better chance of influencing the outcome. In contrast, public interests prefer socialization of the conflict. The more public an issue is made, the better the chances of gathering support for a desired outcome.

2. Visibility
Highly visible issues usually generate more conflict. Again, each side will have a preference to keep an issue with high or low visibility. In general, special interest groups prefer the latter, and public interest groups the former.

3. Intensity
How passionately those involved feel about the issue, which may compensate for lack of financial resources and other organizational drawbacks that public interest groups may experience.

4. Direction
Which is strategically the most important, because it is related to how the conflict is defined, framed. Every change in definition of the problem creates a new division of power and majority position. The challenge is to frame the issue in a way that will become relevant to a large number of people, thus shifting power to one's advantage.

Source: Schattschneider.[33]

often rely on their membership as a tool to gain political leverage, and their strength, independently from funding levels, rests on their ability to mobilize a large number of people to join their 'cause'. Successful advocates are able to expand an issue in order to bring public pressure. It is the grass roots effort that gives public interest groups their power and political leverage.

Cancer prevention is usually described as a public interest and its political aspects do not end at the policymaking level. Indeed, the implementation of prevention and early detection policies may often pose greater challenges. It is at the implementation level that most barriers surface. Part of the problem is that policymakers frequently ignore implementation details while developing policies, despite the fact that implementation should be an integral part of political decision-making.[34] Implementation is different from policy adoption and evaluation. Policy adoption is involved with strategic planning, and implementation is the interpretation of this strategy into operational guidelines and procedures.[34] Evaluation of a policy is usually related to the achievement of desired outcomes.

Nurses are the ones regularly implementing policies that may have been poorly designed; they witness the problems these policies create. At the same time, because nurses are the ones in the front line of implementation, they have great opportunities to influence and improve the policymaking process through increased participation in the political process. It is well documented that access to prevention, screening and early detection services is influenced by race, ethnicity, insurance status, socioeconomic status and educational level.[11,16,19,20] Policies that consider strategies to overcome these barriers at the development stage will have a better chance of a successful outcome.

THE ROLE OF NURSES IN HEALTH PROMOTION AND CANCER PREVENTION

Nurses may represent the largest group of healthcare workers worldwide and, if promotion and prevention practices are incorporated into their daily practice, there is potential for an enormous impact in reducing cancer incidence and prevalence. Health promotion and cancer prevention should not be perceived as tasks only for the nurse working in primary care settings, but for all nurses and at every client contact. However, there are barriers to maximizing nurses' impact. In general, nursing education does not prioritize health promotion topics;[35,38,39] nurses often feel that they lack skills and knowledge to conduct assessments and provide counselling on cancer prevention and, most importantly, the behaviour of nurses themselves has an impact on their willingness and ability to discuss health promotion topics.[36,37] Such barriers are not exclusive to nurses and can also be seen in the health promotion intervention behaviour of other healthcare professionals.[40] Furthermore, cancer-related policymaking tends to emphasize diagnostic testing and treatment, contributing to the low priority given to prevention in the training and practice of healthcare professionals.

At an initial patient assessment, the nurse should collect information about risk factors. This would include, but not be limited to, information regarding family history of cancer, smoking status, dietary habits, physical activity, body mass index, reproductive history (including date of last Pap smear for women), mental health status and exposure to specific and known risk factors, i.e. sun or secondhand smoke exposure. This may be done in addition to, and as part of, the physical assessment and supplementary questions related to physiological functions.

After assessment, nurses should then provide advice as appropriate and refer for additional screening tests if indicated. Unfortunately, there is not a uniform guideline that nurses can follow. Each practising nurse needs to find out what are the standards applicable to his or her setting and community. In general, these recommendations will include protection against sun exposure, moderate but consistent physical activity and a diet rich in fruits, vegetables and whole grains and limited in saturated fat.[1,40–44] There might be genetic factors that can not be modified but can be monitored to facilitate early detection.[1,41,42] Most importantly, if the patient is a smoker, the nurse should provide cessation interventions and refer for additional, intensive assistance as appropriate.[45] A nursing strategy for smoking cessation is outlined in a later section of this chapter.

Nurses should be aware that their role in health promotion and cancer prevention is not limited to healthy or asymptomatic patients. Patients who have a cancer diagnosis, are currently under treatment or are cancer survivors should also receive counselling related to minimization of risks factors, including smoking cessation.[45–47]

Another important role for nurses, previously discussed, is to promote policy and social changes that promote healthier behaviours as the social norm. This includes involvement with nursing organizations to make sure that training and education provide the necessary knowledge and skills for nurses to realize their full potential in the prevention of cancer.

THE TOBACCO STORY AND ITS CONSEQUENCES

Tobacco, a native plant of the Americas, was taken to Europe in the 16th century but it was not until the beginning of the 20th century, with the automation of the cigarette manufacturing process, that its consumption became widespread. Tobacco use has been declared the single most important preventable cause of death and disease by many health authorities.[48]

Currently, over 1 billion people use tobacco worldwide.[48,48a] Approximately half of current smokers will die of a tobacco-related disease, and half of those deaths will occur between the ages of 35 and 69 years.[49] The WHO estimates that 4.2 million people a year die of a tobacco-related cause, and this number will rise to 10 million people a year by 2030 or earlier.[48] Smoking is responsible for 24% of all male deaths and 7% of all female deaths (as high as 40% for men in some central and eastern European countries and 17% for women in the United States).[49]

These statistics should place tobacco control at the highest level on political and healthcare agendas. Unfortunately, health professionals seem not to have given tobacco control its due priority. This may be related to a lack of knowledge about the harmful health effects of tobacco use and the addictive nature of nicotine, lack of skills to help with cessation efforts and a lack of political will. The tobacco industry, by contrast, wields powerful influence in the political process and is a significant barrier to tobacco control.

Tobacco use is declining in several developed countries, but is still climbing in developing countries, mainly among women.[50] Facts about smoking prevalence according to WHO regions are presented in Figure 8.1. Given the lag time between smoking and the development of cancer, it is estimated that the cancer toll in developing countries will increase in the next few decades. Worldwide, tobacco is responsible for 30% of all cancer deaths in developed countries and is rising to similarly troubling levels in developing countries.[1] An estimation of tobacco deaths by World Bank regions for the period 1990–2020 is presented in Figure 8.2.

Tobacco is consumed in many forms (e.g. pipe, cigar, chewing), all of which are harmful.

Cigarette smoking, however, is the most common form of tobacco use. In the past five decades, thousands of studies have demonstrated that tobacco causes a variety of cardiovascular and respiratory diseases, as well as several types of cancer.[51–53] In 2002, the International Agency for Research on Cancer (IARC) released the results of its updated tobacco and cancer monograph,[54] reaffirming that tobacco smoke is a known human carcinogen and, more importantly, confirming that exposure to secondhand tobacco smoke is also carcinogenic in humans.

Cigarettes contain over 60 substances known to be carcinogens. Tobacco smoke produces gene mutations and chromosomal abnormalities in humans. Cigarette smoking is associated with many different types of cancer; an overview is presented in Box 8.2.[54] There is a several-fold increase in the risks for these cancers in the presence of smoking. The increase in risk is as high as 20–30 times for lung

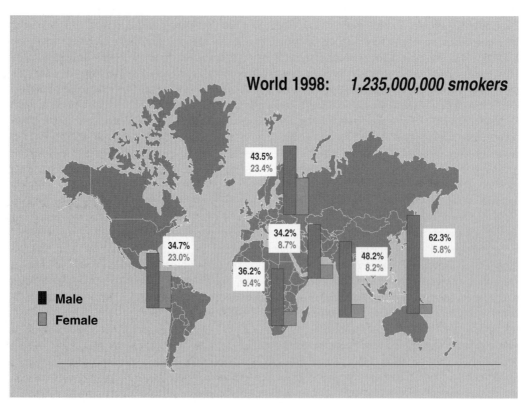

Figure 8.1: Adult smoking prevalence by WHO regions, 1998. (Reproduced with permission from Corrao et al.[48a]).

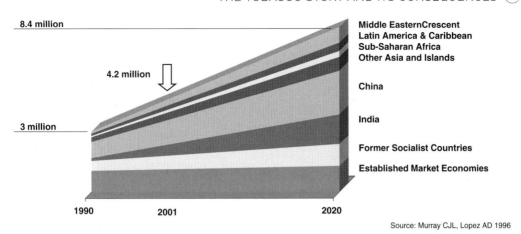

Source: Murray CJL, Lopez AD 1996

World Health Organization

WHO's Research Partners Meeting
for Noncommunicable Diseases
Geneva, December10-12, 2001

Figure 8.2: Tobacco deaths by World Bank Regions estimated for 1990 and 2020. (Reproduced with permission from World Health Organization.[1]).

cancer, but there is a 3–6 times increased risk of developing cancer overall for smokers compared to non-smokers.[1] In addition, a synergistic effect is assumed between smoking and other risk factors for cancer, such as exposure to arsenic, asbestos, radon, plus alcohol consumption and human papillomavirus infection.

The actual exposure to tobacco carcinogens will vary, depending on the amount, intensity and method of individual smoking or tobacco use, as well as length of exposure in terms of years of current smoking and exposure to secondhand tobacco smoke. Stated cigarette package tar and nicotine yields bear no relationship to actual intake. These values are assessed through a machine-smoking test method that does not accurately mimic human smoking.[55] All currently available tobacco products deliver carcinogenic substances when consumed as intended and there are no health benefits in so-called 'light' or 'mild' cigarettes.[56]

Worldwide, lung cancer is the most common cause of cancer death. The IARC estimates that there are 1.2 million cases a year and that number is increasing.[54] The major cause of lung cancer is tobacco smoking, responsible for 80–90% of all cases. Smoking is associated with all histological types of lung cancer and

the risk of lung cancer increases with the duration (length of time) of smoking as well as the number of cigarettes smoked for both men and women. Smoking cessation at any age halts further increase in risks and, after 10 or more years of cessation, the increase in risk is half of that faced by a current smoker.

The risk for other cancers caused by smoking also increases in proportion to the duration and amount smoked. Such dose–response relationships are seen with renal cell, sinonasal, nasopharyngeal, oropharyngeal, hypopharyngeal, oesophageal and laryngeal carcinomas, as well as with cancers of the bladder, ureter, renal pelvis, pancreas and stomach, and with myeloid leukaemia in adults. Tobacco smoke has enough known leukaemogens, including benzene, to account for up to half of the estimated excess of acute myeloid leukaemia.[54]

There is also a causal and a dose-related relationship between smoking and oral cavity cancers (including those of the lip and tongue), and the risk increases when smoking is combined with the use of either smokeless tobacco or alcohol or both.[54] Similarly, a dose–response and a synergistic effect between tobacco use and alcohol consumption is observed in a higher risk for squamous cell carcinoma of the

Box 8.2

Types of cancer caused by cigarette smoking

Lung
Oral cavity
Nasopharynx
Oropharynx
Hypopharynx
Nasal cavity and paranasal sinuses
Larynx
Oesophagus
Stomach
Pancreas
Liver
Kidney (body and pelvis)
Ureter
Urinary bladder
Uterine cervix
Myeloid leukaemia

Source: International Agency for Research on Cancer (IARC).[54]

oesophagus and for laryngeal cancer.[54] For stomach cancer, the causal relationship remains after controlling for other confounding factors such as alcohol consumption, *Helicobacter pylori* infection and diet. Likewise, a causal dose–response association between smoking and liver cancer remains after controlling for alcohol consumption and adjusting for markers of hepatitis B/hepatitis C virus infection. The causal association between squamous cell cervical carcinoma and smoking remains after adjusting for human papillomavirus infection.[54]

Smoking cessation will reduce the risk for several of the cancers mentioned above, with the decrease in risk proportional to the increase in the number of years since successful cessation. A noteworthy exception is oesophageal cancer, for which risks do not seem to decrease significantly after quitting.[54]

IARC[54] stated that the reviewed evidence was not strong enough to declare a causal relationship between smoking and colorectal, prostate, breast and endometrial cancer. In fact, studies have found an inverse relationship between smoking and endometrial cancer. Terry and colleagues[57] offered a possible explanation for this inverse relationship – the antioestrogenic effect of cigarette smoking on oestrogen concentrations in the blood. A similar mechanism is often offered to explain research findings showing a lack of causal association between smoking and breast cancer.[57] However, unlike the inverse association with endometrial cancer, the relationship between smoking and breast cancer remains controversial. Whereas IARC did not find strong evidence to prove causation, other studies have found a causal link and discussed the plausible carcinogenicity of tobacco in breast tissue.[58–60] Terry and colleagues[59] found a 60% increase in breast cancer risk and smoking for women who had smoked 40 years or longer and had started to smoke early in life, compared with those who had never smoked. The authors suggest that smoking might play a role as an initiator, rather than a promoter, in breast cancer development.

The IARC[54] confirmed previous reports[51,53,61,62] of a causal relationship between exposure to secondhand smoke and lung cancer. Secondhand smoke is a mixture of smoke exhaled by the smoker himself as well as smoke released by a lit cigarette (or pipe, cigar, etc.) and diluted in the environment. This mixture contains nicotine and several carcinogens, including benzene, 1,3-butadiene, benzo[a]pyrene and 4-(methylnitrosamino)-1-(3-pyridyl)-1-butanone.[54] The IARC determined that the excess risk for lung cancer is 20% for women and 30% for men exposed to secondhand smoke, the risk rising with increased exposure. The IARC did not find enough evidence to prove a causal relationship between secondhand smoke and breast cancer, despite studies that found a dose–response trend, particularly for premenopausal women.[57]

The WHO describes tobacco use as a communicable disease whose vector is the tobacco industry.[63] For decades, the tobacco industry had known about the carcinogenic effects of cigarette smoking but has not disclosed the relevant data or publicly admitted that tobacco causes cancer.[64,65] The industry continues to deny both the harmful effects of secondhand smoke and the addictive properties of tobacco.[66–68]

The tobacco industry has waged massive public and political campaigns to influence the development of tobacco control policies, including attempts to influence the work of the WHO and IARC.[63,69,70] In addition, the tobacco industry has manipulated the media to confuse the public's understanding of the health effects of tobacco. Worldwide, governmental spending on tobacco control is dwarfed by the tobacco industry's spending on marketing and political strategies. However, tobacco control is a cost-effective measure that alleviates the burden of tobacco-related diseases.[48] The essential elements of a comprehensive tobacco control programme are taxation, regulation of products, restrictions on advertisement and sponsorships, protection of non-smokers, support for cessation, youth access restriction and firm action against cigarette smuggling. Involvement in the political process by health professionals, including nurses, can greatly assist in increasing the power of tobacco control and preventing the growth of tobacco-related cancers for future generations. Tobacco control should be an integral part of oncology nursing practice.

A nursing strategy for the support of smoking cessation

Nursing intervention for smoking cessation has been proven to be an effective way to increase successful quit attempts.[36,71,72] Although smoking is the most common form of tobacco use, the information provided here should also be used to assess other forms of tobacco use (chewing, snuff, etc.) and advice to stop is equally important and applicable. The essential components of smoking cessation interventions include the assessment of tobacco use status, advising smokers to stop smoking, assisting with smoking cessation and follow-up. Details of these components are summarized in Figure 8.3.[73]

THE ROLE OF NUTRITION

Epidemiological and experimental studies on nutrition and cancer have provided evidence that diet can influence the risk of developing different types of cancer. Diet is estimated to contribute to about one-third of cancers, and links have been made with some of the most common cancers such as colon, breast and prostate cancer. Research is primarily based on the idea that some foods or food constituents might have carcinogenic effects and that chemical carcinogenesis would cause actions in the cell and induce genetic changes. However, since the late 1960s the multiplication of population-based cancer registries indicates that there are large variations in incidence of cancers for which the link to exposure has never been clearly identified. It becomes increasingly evident that cancer develops as a result of a complex mix of factors, related to lifestyle issues, such as nutrition, weight, physical activities and smoking, as well as environmental and genetic factors.

Foods may have either protecting or promoting effects on carcinogenesis. The idea that dietary change can alter cancer susceptibility is appealing to people, regardless of cancer risk. Correlation studies in the last decades showed that the incidence of and mortality from cancer of the breast, colorectum and prostate were positively correlated with the food typically consumed in Western societies, such as red meat, animal fat and simple sugars and that it was negatively correlated with the consumption of various vegetables such as grains, cereals and vegetable fibre.[74] However, there remains a lack of consistent scientific evidence and recommendations, which make it difficult to provide nutritional counselling. Three independent expert committees in the late 1990s attempted to summarize principal statements on the basis of available research in the field of cancer prevention through nutrition.[75–77] These evidence-based statements are summarized as follows:

1   The consumption of vegetables and fruit is associated with reduced risk of various cancers, most consistently observed in cancers of the digestive and respiratory tract.

2   Daily consumption of both vegetables and fruit is most strongly associated with a reduction of risk in cancers of the mouth, pharynx, larynx, oesophagus, stomach and lung, whereas consumption of vegetables only (not fruit) is linked to a reduction in risk of colorectal cancer.

143

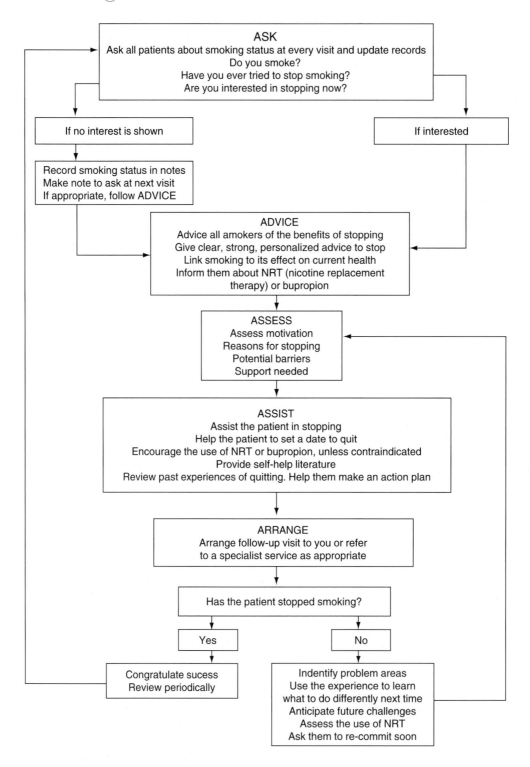

Figure 8.3: Smoking cessation guidelines flow chart. (From Percival[73].)

3 Foods consistently associated with increased risk for colorectal cancer is limited to red meat, mainly beef (but not poultry and fish), and to salted fish for increased risk of nasopharyngeal cancer, mainly in some populations of Asia.

4 The association between fruit, vegetable and meat consumption and various cancers can be considered reasonably established, but there is no definite explanation for the biological mechanisms involved.

Additionally, in 2001, it has been concluded that:[78]

5 The best advice today is to have a well-balanced diet with generous amounts of foods such as fruit and vegetables, which are high in fibre, vitamins and minerals, and go easy on high-fat foods such as dairy products and fatty meat.

The same sort of diet protects against heart disease. While these principles can be used for counselling in daily nursing practice, underlying mechanisms of such a diet remain partially unclear. In the following paragraphs, theories of some selected elements of nutrition-dependent concepts will be explored.

Vegetables, fruits, fibres

A low intake of plant foods is a relatively recent phenomenon. Potential anticarcinogenic agents in plants include fibre, antioxidants and antioxidant enzyme-associated micronutrients and folate. A diet regularly high in plant foods is one to which humans are most adapted and it provides substances, essential nutrients, to which the human metabolism is dependent for good health. Many of these substances can serve to keep enzyme systems 'tuned' to handle occasional intakes of carcinogens, inhibit formation of carcinogens, reduce proliferation of transformed cells and act as antioxidants.[79] Potential anticarcinogenic compounds of plants have complimentary and overlapping mechanisms of action, including the induction of detoxification enzymes, inhibition of nitrosamine formation, provision of substrates for formation of antineoplastic agents, dilution and binding of carcinogens in the digestive tract, alteration of hormone metabolism or antioxidant effects.[80]

The hypothesis that fibres from plant foods decrease the risk of cancer, especially colorectal cancer, is one of the oldest. They can largely be divided into soluble fibres, such as gums, mucilage and pectin, and into insoluble fibres, including cellulose and lignin. Insoluble fibre increases faecal bulk and decreases intestinal transition time. Soluble fibre delays gastric emptying, slows glucose absorption, lowers serum cholesterol and has less effect on bulk and transit time.[81] Fibres are especially related to the prevention of colon cancer but also to hormone-dependent tumours such as breast and prostate cancer. High-fibre foods, such as vegetables and fruits or grains and cereals, appear to show the greatest influence on colorectal cancer, rather than dietary fibre per se. This underlines the fact that it is not clear whether the suggested protective effect is due to fibre or other constituents in the fibre-containing food. Even though epidemiological evidence generally supports a preventative role for fibre in the development of colon and colorectal cancer, conflicting results still challenge future research. The interaction of fat and fibre is a crucial issue, as the protective role of fibre can be seen in populations that consume relatively high levels of fat and also high levels of fibre.[82] Regarding hormone-dependent cancers, it has been observed that women who consume large amounts of fibres also have low levels of circulating oestrogens, which suggests that intestinal reabsorption of hormones is reduced in the presence of fibre but enhanced by fat.[83] A general reduction in the availability of endogenous hormones in individuals consuming a low-fat, fibre-enriched diet may reduce the risk of hormone-dependent cancers and possibly colon cancer.[81] Nurses can draw on this knowledge in cancer prevention counselling and at the same time assure patients and relatives of the potential benefits of fruits and vegetables for the prevention of heart disease.

Vitamins, minerals, nutrients

Patients and relatives are usually very interested to learn about the benefits of micronutrients, as this knowledge allows them to be

145

actively involved in their own health care. *Calcium* may protect against colon cancer. Clinical trials have shown that calcium supplements can reduce colonic cell proliferation in high-risk individuals.[84] It may protect by binding to ionized bile salts and fatty acids in the colon. However, many more complex mechanisms may play a role. *Folate* depletion appears to enhance carcinogenesis in several tissues and folate supplementation conveys a protective effect. Folate is a critical element in DNA metabolism;[85] a depletion of folate is increased in individuals who eat few fruits and vegetables and the regular consumption of alcohol can increase the requirement for folate. It has been observed that a combination of high alcohol intake and a diet low in folate may cause even greater damage in DNA metabolism. It is suggested that diminished folate status is associated with cancer of the cervix, colorectum, lung, oesophagus, brain, pancreas and breast. *Selenium* supplementation was tested in the Nutritional Prevention of Cancer Trial, where a significant 63% reduction of prostate cancer incidence was observed.[86] Further evidence is needed to support its beneficial role. *Soybean constituents* contain several classes of anticarcinogenic agents, such as phytoestrogens and isoflavones, and have been discussed widely in relation to prevention of breast, ovarian and prostate cancer. These substances may competitively counterbalance blood oestrogen levels.

Vitamins are said to have antioxidant activity, especially vitamins E, C and carotenoids, together with other micronutrients like selenium, zinc and manganese. Oxidizing agents from endogenous and exogenous sources are believed to initiate and promote carcinogenesis.[79] Antioxidants appear to be essential to the antioxidant effect of each other; they may also stimulate the immune system. However, a recent study reported an increased risk of lung cancer in smokers receiving beta-carotene in clinical trials, which indicates that the complex interdependence between antioxidants cannot be underestimated[87] and that high doses of vitamins may even be harmful under certain circumstances. For nurses, it is important to know that it has been postulated that sufficient vitamin supply from a well-balanced nutrition may be more effective and probably safer than from high dietary intake of vitamin supplements.

Cooking methods

Information about cancer-enhancing cooking methods is inconsistent. A relationship has been observed in some studies between fried food and cancer risk, whereas in other studies, such as the Nurses Health Study, including 90,000 women, no relationship was found between fried, grilled or well-done meat and colon cancer.[88] Possible human carcinogens are heterocyclic aromatic amines, produced in muscle meat during most cooking methods, and polynuclear aromatic hydrocarbons, formed when fat is burned during open-flame cooking and smoke from burnt fat is produced.[81] Cooking meat in a microwave or choosing methods such as oven roasting or baking rather than high-temperature methods such as frying, boiling or barbecuing, as well as cooking meats 'medium' rather than 'well done', significantly reduces formation of heterocyclic aromatic amines.[81] It appears that these products must be metabolically activated to act as mutagens, and evidence suggests that this process differs among individuals.[89]

ENERGY INTAKE, FAT, WEIGHT, PHYSICAL EXERCISE, ALCOHOL AND RELATED HORMONAL ISSUES

Early laboratory studies in rodents showed that excessive energy intake induced a higher increase in tumour growth than excessive fat intake and that excess fat induced more tumours than excess carbohydrates or protein intake.[90] Epidemiological studies have not yet confirmed the association between total caloric intake and cancer risk in humans. However, in a study involving 30 countries, lower breast cancer mortality was reported in women using calories from vegetable sources in contrast to women consuming calories mainly from animal food sources.[91] Research in this field is scarce, as the adequate assessment of caloric intake and cancer risk is complex, owing to the methodological difficulties of measuring intake, especially on an international level. Furthermore, confounding variables such as body size, caloric balance and physical activity have to be considered. Guidelines for the composition of caloric intake are defined as follows:[92]

- 50% caloric intake from cereals, legumes and tubers
- 10% caloric intake from fruits and vegetables
- 10–15% caloric intake from fish, poultry or meat
- 20–25% caloric intake from fats, preferably mono- and polyunsaturated fatty acids.

Evidence provides support for a direct association between total dietary fat intake, type of fat consumed – such as saturated or animal fat – and increased risk of breast and prostate cancer, as well as colon cancer.[93] The type of fat is believed to be important, and highly polyunsaturated omega-3 fatty acids, found primarily in certain fish oils, may protect against cancer. This fat has been shown to inhibit tumour growth in animals, as does the vegetable oil of olives, even though it largely contains monounsaturated fatty acids. In countries such as Greece, where large quantities of olive oil are consumed, breast cancer risk is lowest within Europe[91] and the incidence of prostate cancer in Mediterranean countries is low as well. However, this does not prove its risk-reducing effect, as other influences, such as protective antioxidants present in olive oil or other factors, may play a more determinant role. Several sources instead support an aetiological role for red meat consumption, specifically within the context of fat consumption and cancer.

It has been postulated that dietary fat may play a role in cancer aetiology by influencing the production or metabolism of circulating hormones. Fatty, unsaturated acids may inhibit the binding of oestradiol by sex hormone-binding globulin, which means that the concentration of bioavailable oestradiol in women and testosterone in men increases.[93] An increase of plasma oestradiol is known to result in increased risk for breast cancer, and this is the case for plasma testosterone and prostate cancer as well.

Body weight: its relation to hormones and physical exercise

Excess body mass or being overweight is associated with increased risk of cancer of the endometrium, breast and colon. Individuals with a body mass index (BMI) of 25–29.9 are considered overweight, whereas individuals with a BMI of 30 or more are considered obese. The type of fat distribution has been discussed, such as the weight-to-hip ratio or abdominal or android obesity. Increased central-to-peripheral body fat distribution may be linked with increased risk for breast cancer, independent of the degree of adiposity.[94] For women, being overweight may increase breast cancer risk in the postmenopausal phase but may slightly reduce the risk in the premenopausal phase, which may be explained by anovulatory cycles or by fewer ovulatory cycles as also determined by pregnancy and lactation.[95] After menopause, obesity may act by enhancing the peripheral production of oestrogen (as opposed to gonodal and cortical).[96] Mortality from various cancers increases progressively with increasing BMI above 25 kg/m^2.[78] Evidence is strongest for endometrial cancer. A possible biological explanation of the association between being overweight and increased risk is that adipose tissue is rich in aromatase, which, for example, converts androstenedione to estrone, thus increasing oestrogenic stimulation of the endometrial mucosa.[96] Variations in the levels of hormones and further factors, such as insulin-like growth factors, may be determined by both environmental and lifestyle factors, as well as by reproductive and inherited genetic characteristics.[96] As body weight is a modifiable risk factor, nurses can take preventative measures in assessing and interpreting the BMI, as well as the distribution of body fat, and can help to support and coordinate weight-regulating activities.

Physical exercise as a cancer preventative measure has become an issue only in recent years and has mostly been discussed in relation to breast, prostate and colon cancer. Studies have found associations between high levels of body fat, a sedentary lifestyle and high blood oestrogen levels. However, it was not excluded that other variables may also have an influence, such as different diets or intake of alcohol, behaviours which also may affect oestrogen levels. It is now known that there is a relationship between high levels of oestrogens and an increased risk for breast cancer in postmenopausal women. Recently, the first randomized clinical trial to assess the effect of exercise on blood oestrogens in postmenopausal women was presented. Exercisers were prescribed 225 minutes exercise per week. Not only was cardiorespiratory fitness increased by 13% after 1 year but also women had a 7% decrease in the level of oestradiol after 3 months, which was not the case in the control group.[97] This indicates that the effect of exercise on oestrogen is probably real, even if started later in life, and supports the evidence that exercise can affect biology related to breast cancer in older women. A protective effect of physical activity was also observed in males for prostate cancer.[98] Considering that evidence, nurses may confidently encourage individuals to be physically active for cancer prevention as well as for cardiovascular prevention.

Alcohol

Alcohol consumption has been related to increased risk for many types of cancer. Evidence has been established for liver cancer[99] and also for oral and pharyngeal cancer.[99] Alcohol may act as a solvent, increasing the potency of other carcinogens. In combination with tobacco, alcohol is seen as the major cause for oral and pharyngeal cancers.[100] Alcohol has also been defined as one of the few modifiable risk factors in breast cancer, and a modest risk increase through moderate alcohol consumption in younger women could not be excluded.[101] It has been suggested that genetic factors influence alcohol metabolism. Alcohol dehydrogenases are a family of enzymes that are rate-limiting in the metabolism of alcohol to acetaldehyde, exposing individuals to higher risk.[102] This illustrates the potential importance of genetic variation in terms of risk associated with exogenous exposures.

MENSTRUAL AND REPRODUCTIVE CANCER RISK FACTORS

Menstrual and reproductive cancer risk factors are the most widely analysed and the best-recognized risk factors for breast cancer. They are generally described as menarche under the age of 12 and menopause after the age of 55, implicating a greater lifetime number of menstrual cycles. In addition, nulliparity predisposes women to greater risk as well as first child birth over the age of 30. Results from studies examining benefits of breast-feeding have been controversial; the Nurses Health Study showed no important link between breast-feeding and breast cancer (n = 89,887).[103] Studies from North America and Italy have indicated that reproductive factors may account for up to 50% of breast cancer on a population level.[104,105] However, most of these factors are hardly modifiable and, consequently, the public health implications are limited. One of the few modifiable hormonal factors is the long-term use of hormone replacement therapy (HRT) (longer than 10 years), which has been associated with a slightly increased risk for breast cancer. However, this implies risk–benefit considerations in the treatment of menopausal symptoms. Further research is needed to provide evidence that HRT with oestrogen alone, as opposed to an oestrogen–progestin combination, is associated with less risk of breast cancer.[106]

OTHER CANCER RISK FACTORS

Many other factors are discussed in the primary prevention of cancer. The health belief model (HBM) (see Ch. 1), frequently used in health education and cancer control, takes into account a person's belief regarding susceptibility of a particular health problem, its severity and the likelihood that a particular behaviour change will be beneficial.[107] Clinical experience from prevention counselling shows that individuals sometimes perceive themselves as predisposed or as resistant against cancer. The role of psychological influences is of public interest. The relationship between emotional disturbances such as depression and cancer aetiology, however, remain unclear. A meta-analytic review of the evidence concerning depression as a risk factor for cancer concluded that depression was a small and marginally statistically significant risk factor.[108] However, diet and physical exercise are possible mediators of the observed relationship between cancer and depression. It can also be argued that the mechanisms responsible for the relationship between depression and cancer are part of a more complex ageing process, producing age-specific vulnerability to disease.

Age, in itself, is one of the major factors that predisposes individuals to cancer. Cancer has been characterized as a disease of old age. This is not true for some diseases, such as for example paediatric cancer or breast cancer in young women, where it is supposed to be largely genetic and related to reproductive factors. Individuals who have survived cancer tend to have a higher risk for a second cancer than those who have never had cancer, which is the reason why they require careful, disease-specific follow-up health care. This includes cancer survivors who have been treated with chemo- and radiotherapy and therefore may be even more susceptible to specific diseases.

Exposure to environmental carcinogens, combined with dietary and smoking habits, exposure to sunlight, radiation, chemicals, pesticides, viruses and other factors can lead to the development of cancer. These may be detected in foods, water, air, buildings and elsewhere. Occupational safety deals with a range of established occupational carcinogens.[109] Florence Nightingale was a pioneer who was very early in identifying the role of clean water and fresh air in healing. Today, nurses have not developed nursing practice strategies to match the emerging science about health effects associated with environmental exposure. It is likely that nurses will have to incorporate such risk factors into their primary prevention work, participate in policymaking activities and engage in environmental research.

Complex interactions between genetic and environmental factors may be important in determining risk of cancer. As an extreme, both genetic and environmental factors may be required to develop cancer. More realistically, persons with certain genotypes (genetic basis for the physical expression) will be much more susceptible to carcinogenic effects of exposure.[110] Lifestyle and environmental factors may also be passed from parent to child, such as dietary habits, alcohol-drinking behaviour or smoking, and this is called cultural inheritance. Familial clustering of environmental factors cannot be seen independent from genetic inheritance. The role of cancer genes and familial clustering of cancer disease will be described in the following section.

CANCER RISK ASSESSMENT MODELS

An important component of cancer prevention is risk assessment. The goals of risk assessment are to understand an individual's perception and concern related to risk for developing cancer, to provide information regarding that risk, to outline recommendations for primary and secondary prevention and to offer psychosocial support so that an individual may better cope with information related to risk and adhere to the recommendations for prevention and screening.[111] The assessment of risk for developing cancer should include obtaining information about risk factors associated with the development of cancer (e.g. exposure to carcinogens), medical history and a detailed family history. When performing risk assessment, it is important that individuals understand that the presence of a particular risk factor or trait does not mean that a person will develop a specific cancer and the absence of a risk factor does not ensure that a person will not develop cancer.

For some cancers, models have been developed for determining risk. The ability to individualize cancer risk assessment will allow targeting screening programmes and prevention strategies more specifically based on personal history than the historical use of generalized recommendations for population screening. This area is most thoroughly developed in breast cancer, for which several tools are currently available for calculating risk. To date, models are not yet available for use in estimating risk for developing other types of cancers such as colorectal or prostate cancer, although statistical information is available on the increase in risk due to family history (e.g. one first-degree relative).

The tools or models used to determine risk for breast cancer use data derived from different epidemiological studies. The most commonly used model was developed by Gail et al from the Breast Cancer Detection Demonstration Project, a large mammography screening programme conducted in the United States in the 1970s.[112] This model incorporates the number of first-degree relatives with breast cancer, age at menarche, age at first live birth and the number of breast biopsies. With respect to breast biopsies, high-risk indicators such as atypical ductal hyperplasia and lobular neoplasia are also factored in. In the United States, the Gail model was used to determine eligibility for participation in the breast cancer prevention trial that led to the approval in 1998 of tamoxifen for chemoprevention in women at increased risk for breast cancer. A software program was developed to facilitate calculation of risk in the clinical setting and is currently being used to determine eligibility for subsequent breast cancer chemoprevention trials. Several studies have evaluated the validity of the Gail model, and it is most accurate as a predictor of risk for Caucasian women undergoing routine mammography screening.[113,114]

The other commonly used prediction model was developed by Claus et al on the basis of data from the Cancer and Steroid Hormone Study, a large, population-based, case-control study of breast cancer in the United States. As compared with the Gail model, the Claus model incorporates more extensive information about family history, but it excludes other risk factors associated with breast cancer. On the basis of knowledge of first- and second-degree relatives with breast cancer and their age at diagnosis, the Claus model provides individual estimates of breast cancer risk according to decade from 29 to 79 years of age.[114,115]

Both models were developed prior to the discovery of specific genes associated with hereditary cancer syndromes. Thus, the models tend to underestimate the risk for individuals from families with hereditary breast cancer, while overestimating the risk in others. The Gail model also fails to factor in the powerful indicator of ovarian cancer in a close relative.

Once genes had been discovered that predispose for a high lifetime risk of developing breast and ovarian cancer – e.g. breast cancer 1 (*BRCA1*) and breast cancer 2 (*BRCA2*) – newer models were needed.

BRCAPRO is a computer program that implements a statistical model for calculating an individual's probability of carrying a deleterious mutation of *BRCA1*, *BRCA2*, neither, or both, on the basis of the the woman's cancer status and the history of breast and ovarian cancer among her first- and second-degree relatives. The process used to validate this model was published in 2002 by Berry et al.[116] Data were analysed from six high-risk genetic counselling clinics and relate to individuals from families for which at least one member was tested for mutations at *BRCA1* and *BRCA2*. The authors concluded that BRCAPRO is an accurate counselling tool for determining the probability of carrying mutations of *BRCA1* and *BRCA2* and can be used in both clinical and research settings. CancerGene is a software tool for running several breast cancer risk assessment models, including BRCAPRO. It may be obtained free at:

http://www.swmed.edu/home_pages/cancergene

FAMILY HISTORY: ASSESSING INDIVIDUAL RISK

Family history is a key determinant of increased risk for developing cancer; hence, it is important to ascertain family history in the clinical setting. Visual representation of the family history in a pedigree is often helpful (see an example presented in Fig. 8.4) to quickly evaluate the cancers present. The accepted standard is to obtain complete information on three generations of the family, both affected (i.e. those with a cancer diagnosis) and unaffected individuals. This is often not realistic in clinical settings outside of specialized high-risk clinics. At minimum, information related to parents, siblings and both maternal and paternal grandparents and aunts and uncles should be obtained. Specific

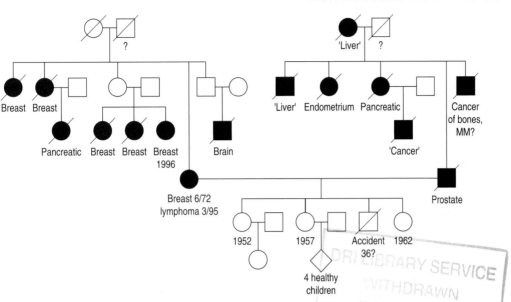

Figure 8.4: Family pedigree showing family with multiple types of cancer (hypothetical example).

details related to cancers present, age at diagnosis, bilateralism of disease (e.g. bilateral breast cancer), presence of more than one primary tumor, preneoplastic lesions and prophylactic surgeries will aid in the identification of individuals at an increased risk for cancer and those who should be referred for cancer genetic counselling because of the potential presence of a hereditary cancer syndrome. In clinics that specialize in the provision of high-risk counselling, confirmation of the cancer diagnoses through pathology reports or death certificates is generally performed for accurate interpretation of risk, as recall of cancer diagnoses by family members may be inaccurate.

SCREENING INDICATIONS FOR CANCER SUSCEPTIBILITY GENES

Patients often tend to overestimate their risk for cancer, and many voice the sentiment that 'everyone in my family has cancer.' Aggregation of cancers in a family may occur because of shared cultural, lifestyle and environmental factors, hereditary influences, chance or a combination of these factors. Today, as a result of

advances in molecular biology and research efforts such as the Human Genome Project, the genes associated with hereditary cancer syndromes are rapidly being identified. To date, numerous cancer-linked genes have been identified.[117] (An online resource for information about genes related to cancer can be found at http://www.ncbi.nlm.nih.gov/Omim/.) It is important that nurses performing cancer risk assessment be able to identify characteristics seen in families with a hereditary cancer syndrome. Common characteristics are:

- the occurrence of multiple cases of cancer, especially cancers of the same type (e.g. melanomas or colorectal cancers) or types related to a specific syndrome (e.g. breast and ovary; bowel and endometrium; leukaemia and sarcoma) within a single lineage (i.e. the maternal side or the paternal side)

- a diagnosis of cancer at an earlier age than is seen in the general population (e.g. breast cancer before 50 years old)

- the occurrence of multiple cancers in one person (e.g. a person with both colon and uterine cancer)

- the presence of rare tumors, such as retinoblastomas or brain tumours

151

- cancer in paired organs (i.e. both breasts or both kidneys)
- non-malignant manifestations of an hereditary cancer syndrome (e.g. hamartomas of the skin and mucous membranes and palmar pits, as seen in Cowden disease).

When any of these conditions is present alone, or in combination, the possibility of an hereditary cancer syndrome should be considered. These criteria can serve as 'flags' during risk assessment to identify individuals who should be referred for more intensive cancer genetic counselling.[118,119]

CANCER SUSCEPTIBILITY GENES AND GENETIC COUNSELLING IN CANCER PREVENTION

Today it is accepted that all cancer is 'genetic,' i.e. cancer occurs because of a series of stepwise mutations in genes that control important cellular processes such as cell growth, differentiation, DNA repair and death. For more details regarding the genetic base of cancer, the reader is referred to Chapter 5. The majority of cancers are sporadic, resulting from a series of mutations in somatic or 'body' cells.[120] It is estimated that only 5–10% of cancers are due to inheritance of a highly penetrant, rare cancer predisposition gene, or cancer susceptibility gene. Mutated genes associated with hereditary cancer syndromes are carried in the germline cells, the cells responsible for reproduction; these genes have the potential to be

passed from generation to generation and confer an inheritable predisposition for cancer development. This means that a person who inherits a mutated gene known to cause cancer has an increased likelihood of developing cancer, although for a cancer to develop, other genetic mutations must also occur. In addition, the effects of environment, lifestyle and other genetic factors on the development of cancer are currently not known.[121] Thus, although cancer susceptibility genes increase the likelihood of developing cancer, cancer is not an inevitable outcome. This concept is especially important for genetic counselling and as an underpinning for cancer prevention. There are many syndromes that include an increased susceptibility to cancer in addition to other abnormalities or diseases. However, the majority of these syndromes, such as Cowden disease, are quite rare. Table 8.1 lists the syndromes most likely to be seen in clinical practice and their other associated clinical features or well-defined hereditary syndromes for which either a positive or negative result will change medical care and for which genetic testing may be considered part of the standard management of affected families. For a more complete review of hereditary cancer syndromes, see Lindor and Greene[117] or the Online Mendelian Inheritance in Man website: (http://www.ncbi.nlm.nih.gov/Omim/).

Nature of genetic tests

Genetic tests may be broadly defined as the analysis of human DNA, RNA, chromosomes,

Table 8.1: Overview of selected hereditary cancer syndromes

Hereditary cancer syndrome	Gene/chromosome locus	Type of gene	Inherited tumour
Breast/ovarian cancer	BRCA1/17q21	Tumour suppressor (potential interactions with RAD51 DNA repair genes)	Early onset breast, ovarian, possibly colon and prostate
	BRCA2/13q12-13	Tumour suppressor (potential interactions with RAD51 DNA repair genes)	Early onset breast, ovarian, male breast cancer, pancreatic cancer, and possibly other cancers

Table 8.1: Overview of selected hereditary cancer syndromes—cont'd

Hereditary cancer syndrome	Gene/chromosome locus	Type of gene	Inherited tumour
Colon cancer Hereditary non-polyposis colorectal cancer (HNPCC)	*hMSH2*/2p16 *hMLH1*/3p21 *hPMS1*/2Q32 *hPMS2*/7p22 *hMSH6*/2p16	DNA damage response genes, also termed mismatch repair genes	Colorectal carcinoma, gastric, endometrial, ovarian carcinoma *hMSH2*: accounts for about 30% of HNPCC *hMLH1*: accounts for about 30% of HNPCC *hPMS1*: accounts for about 5% of HNPCC *hPMS2*: accounts for about 5% of HNPCC Variant: Muir–Torre (*hMSH2*) colon, gastric and larynx tumours Sebaceous skin tumours, keratocanthomata of skin
Colon cancer Familial adenomatous polyposis (FAP)	*APC*/5q21	Tumour suppressor gene	Colorectal cancer Characterized by multiple adenomatous polyps (hundreds) occurring in the colon and rectum Polyps may be found throughout the gastrointestinal tract Non-malignant features include epidermoid cysts, osteomas, desmoid tumours and congenital hypertrophy of the retinal pigment epithelium (CHRPE)
Multiple endocrine neoplasia (MEN) type 2	*RET*/10q11.2	Oncogene	Pheochromocytoma and medullary thyroid carcinomas; parathyroid tumours and neurofibromas in some cases MEN2A: characterized by mutations in exons 10 and 11 of *RET* MEN2B: characterized by a single mutation in codon 918 (exon 16)

proteins or other gene products to detect disease-related genotypes, mutations, phenotypes or karyotypes for clinical purposes. The tests may help to predict those at risk of developing the disease in question, identify carriers, establish diagnosis or prognosis and establish genetic identity.[122] Because genetic testing remains relatively new, at a minimum, the patient must be counselled as to the ramifications of testing and the potential interpretation of test results. Patients must be able to understand what testing can and cannot tell them. A number of different molecular techniques are utilized for genetic testing; however, in most cases, the gold standard remains end-to-end full sequencing of the gene, which is time-consuming and expensive. Unfortunately, even with full-length sequencing, mutations may be missed. Mutations in cancer predisposition genes fall into two major categories, which will determine the difficulty and testing approaches that can be utilized. In many of the cancer predisposition genes, mutations cluster around specific 'hot spots', which allows for testing of specific regions of the cancer predisposition gene. In contrast, mutations are scattered throughout many of the cancer predisposition genes, requiring assessment of the complete regulatory and coding regions of the gene.[123]

Interpretation of testing results can be complex. In general, mutations that are termed deleterious are associated with an increased risk of developing cancer. A term used to describe the degree to which a gene is expressed is penetrance. For a gene such as *BRCA1*, the penetrance would be the risk for developing a breast or ovarian cancer. The degree of penetrance and age of onset of cancer induced by a particular mutation may vary between families and between individuals in a family, and can be influenced by many, as yet undetermined, factors. The risk level should be presented so as to reflect the range of penetrance for abnormalities in the cancer predisposition gene and, where possible, the penetrance for the specific mutation. Where clinical studies have identified appropriate management options, they can be offered to the patient. However, where the appropriate medical approach has not been defined, the alternative options should be described to the patient in a non-directive manner, allowing the patient to make an informed decision.

The interpretation and presentation of test results that do not indicate the presence of a mutation are more complex, particularly if the individual tested does not have cancer. Indeed, it is preferable, but not always possible, to test a family member who is affected with cancer. A failure to detect a mutation could be indicative that mutations in the tested genes are not present in the family. Alternatively, it may suggest that a genetic change is present in the family and was not inherited by the tested individual. A failure to detect a mutation in the cancer predisposition gene may indicate that the mutation is outside of the region tested, not detected by the technique used, or that a mutation is present in an, as yet unidentified, cancer predisposition gene which induces a similar syndrome. In either case, medical management and advice may not change markedly as a consequence of genetic testing. The patient, regardless of test results, may continue to be considered to be at high risk and management options should be reviewed. If a mutation is identified about which insufficient information currently exists to determine whether the changes are deleterious or simply a harmless genetic variation, the result is termed inconclusive. In the United States, after almost 10 years' experience with genetic testing, tests are reliable, commercially available and often partially or fully reimbursed by insurers. This is not the case in many European countries, where commercially available tests, outside of research programmes, are scarce and where insurance companies would reimburse such expensive tests only in very specific hereditary cancer families.

Additional information that is important to review with patients concerning the nature of genetic tests includes potential benefits and risks of testing, other options outside of testing, the costs of testing, how long it will take to obtain results, confidentiality of test results, options for managing risks and potential ethical, legal and social implications.

Psychosocial, ethical and legal issues

There are many potential psychosocial implications associated with cancer predisposition testing. Those that practice in this area know that several factors, such as beliefs about cancer and its prognosis, life history and the level of fear and anxiety present, influence how patients perceive personal risk and their comprehension of risk information. The full spectrum of psychological reactions to the results of genetic testing has not yet been fully elucidated, and thus remains an area of active research. Assessment of family dynamics is important and should be discussed prior to initiation of testing, as results obtained by one family member may have potential impact upon others within the family. Some family members may wish to know their status, whereas others most definitely will not want to know. This can be problematic within the family. Potential negative outcomes that may result from testing include heightened fear and anxiety, depression, changes in family relationship, guilt over transmission of a mutated gene, guilt over not receiving a mutated gene (survivor guilt), changes in functional status and changes in body image and self-perception.

There are also potential benefits that may be obtained from testing. These include relief from the uncertainty of not knowing one's risk status, targeting of aggressive screening measures and prevention strategies to those at the highest risk and to provide information on the potential for children to have inherited a predisposition to develop cancer. Within the context of patients' beliefs about health care and their cultural orientation, the multidisciplinary team must strive to support patients following provision of test results by reinforcing existing coping mechanisms, teaching new ones, providing the necessary information to empower patient decision-making and referral to mental health professionals when warranted. In clinical practice, few patients expressed regret over having received genetic testing results. It is important to reinforce that the presence of a mutated cancer predisposition gene within the family does not mean that every family member will inherit this mutation; the probability is 50% for inheriting a deleterious mutation from a parent.

In the United States, uncertainties regarding the potential for genetic discrimination in insurance or by employers have lessened over time and with the passage of legislation in many states. Efforts continue, however, to pass national legislation that would specifically protect against genetic information. This is only slowly developing in Europe, where in most countries there is no law to protect individuals against potential genetic discrimination, e.g. against rejection of individuals in insurance companies or against non-employment due to a genetic condition. Within the clinical setting, it is important to review with patients how genetic information will be documented in the patient medical record, relevant legislation and any concerns they may have.

Pre- and post-test counselling

It is a generally accepted standard of practice that cancer predisposition genetic testing should not occur without pre- and post-test counselling, irrespective of the setting in which testing occurs (e.g. research vs commercially available testing). Genetic counselling is a risk assessment, communication and educational process by which individuals and family members receive information about the nature and limitations of genetic tests, benefits, risks, costs and meaning of test results. Counselling and support concerning the implications of information gained from testing are a vital component of this process.[124,125] Individuals must receive adequate information to make an informed decision concerning their health and give informed consent to undergo testing. Currently, most cancer genetic counselling is provided in specialty high-risk clinics, and by individuals with specialized training in cancer genetics. Comprehensive services should include determinations of the individual's reasons for seeking cancer risk counselling; data collection that provides an in-depth review of the family history (a minimum of three complete generations) and patterns of transmission of cancers within the family; risk assessment as outlined previously; determination of the client's level of knowledge regarding hereditary cancer syndromes and cancer genetics, self-perception of risk for developing cancer and the motivation for seeking predisposition genetic testing; recommendations for management of risk (i.e. surveillance, chemoprevention, prophylactic surgery); evaluation of the appropriateness of testing; education regarding the testing process and the benefits, risks, limitations, costs and potential outcomes that may result from testing; and disclosure of test results and their implications. All counselling should include an evaluation of the patient's psychosocial status, support systems, ability to receive and cope with test results, and referrals as appropriate for medical or surgical means of early detection or prevention of cancer.

Cancer genetic counselling services are generally provided using a multidisciplinary approach. The majority of counselling is often provided by advanced practice oncology nurses with specialized training in cancer genetics or genetic counsellors with specialized training in the field of oncology in conjunction with oncologists or medical geneticists. Traditionally, the field of genetic counselling has used a non-directive approach, i.e. patients may receive information about available options to manage risk, and then make the ultimate decision on how they wish to manage that risk. While much of cancer genetic counselling does focus on the non-directive approach, as research grows on strategies for managing risk, in the future clinicians may be able to make more definitive, evidence-based recommendations. For some hereditary cancer syndromes, such as familial adenomatous polyposis (FAP), management strategies are well established and a more directive approach is used.

INTERVENTION: THE ROLE OF CHEMOPREVENTION IN CANCER CONTROL

In the first part of this chapter, traditional primary cancer prevention through environmental and lifestyle issues has been described. This was followed by aspects of inheritance and cancer susceptibility. Cultural and genetic inheritance predisposes vulnerable individuals to more or less risk of cancer. Some of the risk factors may be modifiable through lifestyle changes, such as practising a less sedentary lifestyle or decreasing alcohol intake. Some factors, however, may not be modifiable, such as precancerous conditions or familial predisposition to specific cancers, as for example familial breast cancer. These factors, non-modifiable by

lifestyle or change or behaviour, are targets for chemopreventative interventions.

Chemoprevention research efforts started in the early 1980s. It is a promising strategy for cancer prevention and control and is of growing importance, as established prevention and therapeutic modalities have not been fully successful in countering high incidence or low survival rates in many cancers. Chemoprevention is international in application and may be more immediate in worldwide impact than either dietary modification or prevention of exposure to carcinogens.[126] Chemoprevention has been defined as 'the use of specific natural or synthetic chemical agents to reverse, suppress or prevent carcinogenic progression to invasive cancer'.[127] The principles are based on the knowledge of carcinogenesis, the multistep process that involves initiation, promotion and progression of cancer cells. Carcinogens, such as chemicals, viruses or ultraviolet light, are thought to cause changes in the cellular DNA during initiation. These genetic changes can either be reversible or are promoted to malignant cells when exposure to carcinogens continues over time.[127] The opportunity for chemopreventative agents is to intervene and disrupt this initiation process and to halt progression of premalignant cancer cells. Unfortunately, specific initiators have not yet been identified for most cancers and the initiation process may occur long before intervention is considered. Major objectives of current chemopreventative drug development therefore include identification and validation of intermediate biomarkers that are accurate predictors of future cancer incidence and that can serve as surrogate end points for clinical disease.[126]

Clinical prevention trial groups currently test chemopreventative agents in individuals at high risk for cancer due to a genetic predisposition or due to a precancerous condition, for example:

- non-steroidal anti-inflammatory drugs (NSAIDs) (e.g. celecoxib) in individuals with FAP
- tamoxifen in women with a familial history of breast cancer or being identified as carriers of the breast cancer genes *BRCA1* and *BRCA2* (Breast

Cancer Prevention Trial (BCPT), International Breast Cancer Intervention Study (IBIS1)

- finasteride in men age 55 years old or older to inhibit abnormal prostate growth through reduction of dihydrotestosterone (Prostate Cancer Prevention Trial (PCPT), National Cancer Institute).

Currently, approximately 400 compounds are being studied as potential chemopreventative agents, mainly in laboratory research. Over 40 of these compounds are being studied in clinical trials, either as single agents or in combination. These trials look at possible ways to prevent cancer with interventions that include drugs, vitamins, diet, hormones or other agents. The following classes of agents have been defined:[128]

1 Natural retinoids (vitamin A), synthetic retinoids.
2 Other micronutrients (vitamins, calcium, selenium, folic acid and others).
3 NSAIDs such as aspirin and celecoxib.
4 Hormone modulators such as:
   - selective oestrogen receptor modulators (SERMs), such as tamoxifen and other hormonal agents
   - finasteride in men (modulating testosterone levels)
5 Others.

The potential chemopreventative effect and safety of most of these agents needs to be further supported, although some reports are promising. Retinoids have been shown to inhibit carcinogenesis in animal models in epithelial cells in the cervix, lung, breast, colon, pancreas, skin, oral cavity or bladder.[127] Results of studies with vitamins C and E, thought to prevent formation of nitrosamines, remain contradictory. Calcium intake, especially from milk products, has been suggested to lower incidence of colorectal cancer.[129] Reduction of the incidence of prostate cancer was observed by chance in a study testing selenium in squamous cell carcinoma, where it did not prove to be effective,[130] and folic acid appeared to be effective in colorectal cancer.[129] It has been cautioned that a fine line exits between effective and toxic doses of most of these agents.

NSAIDs inhibit prostaglandin synthesis and have been tested widely. It has been concluded that NSAIDs and aspirin can prevent colorectal cancer and precursor adenomas.[131] Further, a 28% reduction of adenomatous colorectal polyps has been observed in patients treated with celecoxib as opposed to 5% reduction of polyps in patients receiving placebo,[132] which prompted the US Food and Drug Administration (FDA) to approve celecoxib in patients with FAP.

Tamoxifen, an SERM, has been known for decades not only to reduce recurrence of breast cancer in the same breast but also to reduce occurrence of breast cancer in the contralateral breast of patients.[133] The preventative effect in the opposite breast of patients and the known reasonable toxicity profile of the drug prompted researchers to study tamoxifen as a preventative agent. Results from the BCPT, involving 13,000 women, showed that tamoxifen reduced the risk of invasive breast cancer by 49% and the risk of non-invasive breast cancer by 50%,[134] clearly indicating benefit in preventing breast cancer. There was an increase of endometrial cancer, however, in the tamoxifen group in women age 50 years old and older, although these were mostly stage 1 and curable. The tamoxifen group also experienced more cases of stroke, pulmonary embolism and deep vein thrombosis, primarily in women aged 50 years old and older. Other symptoms included hot flushes, weight gain, fluid retention, vaginal discharge, nausea and irregular menses.[135] Despite the side-effects, researchers concluded that tamoxifen was considered an appropriate preventative agent for women at increased risk for breast cancer.[133]

A woman's decision regarding breast cancer risk reduction strategies is complex and will depend on her age, agenda of family planning and the importance attributed to information regarding both cancer and non-cancer risks and benefits. Tamoxifen use should be discussed as part of an informed decision-making process, with careful consideration of individually calculated risks and benefits. Oncology nurses may identify women concerned (daughters, sisters of patients) and recommend counselling in specialized settings where experts can offer risk assessment and provide support in decision-making regarding chemoprevention. Experts still recommend to treat women at increased risk in clinical trials only.

Although current research is encouraging and evidence is growing that certain compounds may help prevent cancer in populations at high risk, there is still a long way to go. Large clinical trials, with a duration of many years, including thousands of individuals, are needed to demonstrate whether a compound will reduce the risk of cancer in the general population. Nurses have a role in identifying families at risk (see Cancer risk assessment section). The nurse involved in prevention may be challenged with identifying environmental risk and high-risk populations, recruiting patients for chemopreventative studies, explaining risks and benefits of agents and encouraging patients to comply with preventative regimens.[136]

PROPHYLACTIC SURGICAL INTERVENTIONS: E.G. PROPHYLACTIC MASTECTOMY

The role of cancer susceptibility genes and familial clustering of cancer has been described earlier in this chapter. *BRAC1* and *BRAC2* genes present a topical issue within the context of surgical, prophylactic interventions. Women with known abnormal breast cancer genes know that their risk of developing breast or ovarian cancer is significantly increased by 60–85%. They also have an increased risk of primary peritoneal cancer. This knowledge causes concern and anxiety and preventative measures are often sought. A recent study showed that prophylactic removal of ovaries alone in this subgroup of gene-affected women lowered the risk of breast cancer by 68% and the risk of ovarian cancer by 85% and the combined risk for breast or gynaecological cancer by 75%.[137] These data are promising, but long-term observation is needed.

Should women with *BRAC1* and *BRAC2* be encouraged to have their breasts removed? In a recent Dutch study, it was concluded that prophylactic mastectomy in 73 genetically affected women resulted in complete prevention of breast cancer, as observed over 3 years. In contrast, of the 63 genetically affected women who did not have prophylactic mastectomy, 8 developed breast cancer, as observed

over 3 years. However, as some of these patients also had oophorectomy, definitive conclusions cannot be drawn regarding the value of prophylactic mastectomy and further studies need to separate out the value of each of these procedures.[138]

It is important to know that prophylactic surgery is proposed for women with either known *BRCA1* or *BRCA2* genes or for women with a strong family history, without genetic abnormalites, but with confirmation by a geneticist to confirm the likelihood of an inherited kind of breast cancer. Most breast cancers, however, are not inherited (approximately 10% inherited) and justification for preventative surgery is usually restricted to women with a very high risk of developing breast or ovarian cancer.[138] High-risk populations also can include individuals with ductal carcinoma in situ (DCIS) or lobular carcinoma in situ (LCIS) together with an increased familial risk.

Even after prophylactic oophorectomy, with or without prophylactic mastectomy, women still need to know that careful follow-up care and surveillance is required. Also, surgical options are permanent and irreversible. Surgical risks, self-image issues, sexual functioning and early menopause are to be considered as a balance against the benefits. A psycho-oncological study in 76 women completing prophylactic mastectomy, mostly followed by breast reconstruction, showed, that for the majority of women there was no evidence of significant mental health or body image problems in the first 3 years following bilateral prophylactic mastectomy but women who had complications warranted additional psychological help.[139] Prophylactic mastectomy may help women to relieve psychological distress related to the fear of developing breast cancer.[140]

For women who have had breast cancer in one breast, the risk of developing a new cancer in the other breast is significantly higher compared to women who have never had breast cancer. In addition, having had breast cancer and having a family history of breast or ovarian cancer indicates an even greater risk. In this case, prophylactic mastectomy of the contralateral breast is often discussed and has been shown to reduce risk for a second cancer in the other breast dramatically. However, burdens have to be balanced against benefits and other interventions,

Chemopreventative agents may present an alternative to contralateral mastectomy.

CHEMOPREVENTION AND OTHER RISK-REDUCING STRATEGIES FOR SMOKERS AND EX-SMOKERS

Smoking cessation is the most efficient method of reducing the risk of lung cancer but is often very difficult to achieve.[71,141] Some of the issues to be considered have been described earlier in this chapter. Oncology nurses tend to not promote smoking cessation as frequently and intensely as desired, despite overwhelming clinical and research evidence of the benefits of quitting, even for patients already diagnosed with cancer.[37,142,144] There are numerous resources for helping health professionals who want to help their patients quit smoking and avoid relapse.[143,145] However, new information and technological strategies are being explored with a view to improving the delivery of risk messages in an attempt to improve the success of quit rates. A study by McBride et al[146] discussed the benefits of incorporating information about genetic susceptibility to tobacco-related cancers as part of a smoking cessation intervention. Study participants, all inner-city African-Americans in the United States, were randomly selected to be tested for genotyping the *GST3* gene (*GSTM1*) (genes encoding for the enzyme glutathione-*S*-transferase, related to cancer risk).[146] At the 12 months follow-up, information about genetic susceptibility made no significant difference in the ability to quit smoking. This study provides useful background for discussing the practical implications of genetic screening as a complementary intervention in the promotion of smoking cessation.

Research also continues to improve the results obtained so far with public health and clinical efforts to promote cessation. One such complementary approach is to explore the possibility of *chemoprevention* for lung cancer, mainly for high-risk individuals, i.e. smokers and ex-smokers. Lippman and Spitz[147] reviewed the chemoprevention trials conducted at the primary, secondary and tertiary prevention levels, none of which produced positive results. The authors state that trials have shown that lung cancer was not prevented by alpha-tocopherol, beta-carotene, retinol, retinyl palmitate, *N*-acetylcysteine or isotretinoin in smokers, with only some possible activity of isotretinoin in never having smoked and former smokers. In addition, as pointed out by Hecht,[148] it is unclear if the damage created by exposure to tobacco carcinogens can be overcome by any chemopreventative agent. Lippman and Spitz[147] concluded that

> the future of lung cancer chemoprevention will rely heavily on molecular studies of carcinogenesis and drug mechanisms to develop novel chemopreventive targets and drugs, risk markers, and surrogate end point biomarkers; new preclinical drug-testing models; novel imaging techniques for monitoring agent activity; and molecular epidemiologic risk models for identifying the highest-risk current and former smokers.

It can be concluded that smoking cessation strategies remain a major challenge in health care. Chemopreventative targets and risk markers may support cessation efforts or early detection methods in the future.

Primary prevention of cancer is multifaceted and represents a challenge for nursing. Identification of risk factors and health promotion remain key issues. New roles are evolving for cancer risk assessment and specific genetic counselling. Evidence for cancer preventative strategies for individuals at high risk is growing and nurses may be increasingly involved in aspects of primary cancer chemoprevention or prophylactic surgery. Unfortunately, primary prevention is still limited and secondary prevention through early detection remains a major healthcare issue. Principles of early detection and screening as well as specific screening programmes and diagnostic issues will be discussed in the following chapter.

GLOSSARY: TERMS FREQUENTLY USED IN CANCER PREVENTION

In order to fully participate in prevention efforts, nurses should be familiar with the terms most often used. Some of these terms are summarized below.

absolute risk – the rate of cancer occurring in the general population, often expressed as number of cases per 100,000 population or by stratifying by age group, ethnicity or geographical area, for example. It measures the actual cancer risk or rate in a population and shows how common a disease is.

adjusted rates – rates are adjusted (e.g. age-adjusted rates) to facilitate comparisons. It is important to control (adjust) for certain characteristics for comparisons over time and between countries. For example, rates are adjusted for age distribution of the population; otherwise, with an increase in age and subsequent increase in cancer risk, an increase in rates of cancer could be attributed simply to the ageing of the population, whereas with age adjustment, any increase in rates will imply a true increase in the number of cancers.

attributable risk – the proportion of cancers that can be attributed to a given risk factor, using information about relative risk of cancer given exposure X and the prevalence of exposure X in the population. It estimates what decrease an elimination of the exposure would then lead to a decrease in the number of a specific cancer. It is the case for the tobacco-attributable cancers, which could be reduced by reduction in tobacco consumption.

excess risk – compares the actual cancer rate among at least two groups of people, based on risk factors, by subtracting the risks or rates from one another (e.g. the number of lung cancer cases among smokers minus the number of cases among non-smokers to estimate the excess risk of lung cancer due to smoking).

false negative – normal results for a person who has cancer; i.e. the test failed to detect the cancer. It is problematic since the opportunity for early diagnosis is missed.

false positive – the test identifies a need for additional diagnostic testing which results in no signs or markers for the disease; i.e. the person does not have cancer. It may generate unnecessary psychological stress to the individual, in addition to submitting the person to additional procedures which end up being unnecessary.

incidence – number of new cases of cancer in a given period of time, usually a year.

mortality rate – number of people that die from a specific disease in a given period of time, usually a year.

negative predictive value – the extent to which those given a negative result will not develop the disease.

odds ratios – are used as an estimate of the relative risk. It also indicates the presence of association between exposure and cancer, and compares the odds of an exposure or characteristic among cancer cases with the odds among a comparison group without cancer. Odds ratios are used in case-control studies to identify potential risk factors or protective factors for cancer.

positive predictive value – the extent to which those given a positive result will develop the disease.

prevalence – total number of existing cases of cancer in a given period of time, usually a year, and commonly expressed as number per 100,000 people.

relative risk – compares the chances of developing cancer between exposed and at-risk individuals and non-exposed, not at-risk individuals. If relative risk is greater than 1, than there is an increase in cancer risk associated with exposure. If it is 1 or less than 1, there is no increase in risk or there is lower risk for cancer associated with exposure. It is often used to estimate the reduction in cancer cases that could be associated with prevention programmes.

sensitivity – the extent to which the test can identify individuals who have cancer; i.e. the screening test is positive and the disease is present.

specificity – the extent to which a test is capable of identifying individuals who are disease-free; i.e. screening is negative and the disease is truly absent.

target population – the group of people that have a characteristic that makes them eligible for screening. Such characteristics include gender, family history, exposure to carcinogens and risk factors, age and socioeconomic status. It is determined largely by what is known about the natural development of the disease.

REFERENCES

1. World Health Organization. National cancer control programmes: policies and managerial guidelines. 2nd edn. Geneva: World Health Organization; 2002. http://www5.who.int/cancer/main.cfm?p=0000 000029

2. World Health Organization. The World Health Report 1999. Making a difference. Geneva: World Health Organization; 1999.

3. American Cancer Society. Cancer facts & figures – 2001. Atlanta; American Cancer Society; 2001.

4. Davis TC, Williams MV, Marin E, et al. Health literacy and cancer communication. CA Cancer J Clin 2002; 52(3):134–149.

5. Khanna N, Phillips MD. Adherence to care plan in women with abnormal Papanicolaou smears: a review of barriers and interventions. J Am Board Family Pract 2001; 14(2):123–130.

6. Facione NC, Katapodi M. Culture as an influence on breast cancer screening and early detection. Semin Oncol Nurs 2000; 16(3):238–247.

7. Shinagawa SM. The excess burden of breast carcinoma in minority and medically underserved communities: application, research, and redressing institutional racism. Cancer 2000; 88(5 Suppl):1217–1223.

8. Remennick LI. Breast screening practices among Russian immigrant women in Israel. Women Health 1999; 28(4):29–51.

9. Cooley ME, Jennings-Dozier K. Lung cancer in African Americans. A call for action. Cancer Pract 1998; 6(2):99–106.

10. Hoffman-Goetz L, Mills SL. Cultural barriers to cancer screening among African American women: a critical review of the qualitative literature. Womens Health 1997; 3(3–4):183–220.

11. Segnan N. Socioeconomic status and cancer screening. IARC Sci Publ 1997; 138:369–376.

12. Cava M, Greenberg M, Fitch M, et al. Towards an inclusive cervical cancer screening strategy: approaches for reaching socioeconomically disadvantaged women. Canadian Oncol Nurs J 1997; 7(1):14–18.

13. Pearlman DN, Rakowski W, Ehrich B, et al. Breast cancer screening practices among black, Hispanic, and white women: reassessing differences. Am J Prevent Med 1996; 12(5):327–337.

14. Brown CL. Screening patterns for cervical cancer: how best to reach the unscreened population. J Natl Cancer Inst Monogr 1996; (21):7–11.

15. Breen N, Kessler LG, Brown ML. Breast cancer control among the underserved – an overview. Breast Cancer Res Treat 1996; 40(1):105–115.

16. Womeodu RJ, Bailey JE. Barriers to cancer screening. Med Clin North Am 1996; 80(1):115–133.

17. Wender RC. Barriers to effective skin cancer detection. Cancer 1995; 75(2 Suppl):691–698.

18. Ramirez AG, Villarreal R, Suarez L, et al. The emerging Hispanic population: a foundation for cancer prevention and control. J Natl Cancer Inst Monogr 1995; 18:1–9.

19. Palos G. Cultural heritage: cancer screening and early detection. Semin Oncol Nurs 1994; 10(2):104–113.

20. Iverson DC. Involving providers and patients in cancer control and prevention efforts. Barriers to overcome. Cancer 1993; 72(3 Suppl):1138–1143.

21. Gulitz E, Hernandez MB, Kent EB. Missed cancer screening opportunities among older women: a review. Cancer Pract 1998; 6(5):289–295.

22. Fox SA, Roetzheim RG, Kington RS. Barriers to cancer prevention in the older person. Clin Geriatr Med 1997; 13(1):79–95.

23. Tesh S. Hidden arguments. New Brunswick, NJ: Rutgers University Press; 1988.

24. McKinlay JB, Marceau LD. Upstream healthy public policy: lessons from the battle of tobacco. Int J Health Serv 2000; 30(1):49–69.

25. Wilson J. Political organizations. New York, NY: Basic Books; 1973.

26. Garvin T, Eyles J. Public health responses for skin cancer prevention: the policy framing of Sun Safety in Australia, Canada and England. Social Sci 2001; 53(9):1175–1189.

27. Cobb R, Ross J, Ross M. Agenda building as a comparative political process. Am Polit Sci Rev 1976; 70:126–138.

28. Brendtro MJ. Breast cancer: agenda setting through activism. Adv Pract Nurs Q 1998; 4(1):54–63.

29. Kingdon J. Agendas, alternatives, and public policies. 2nd edn. New York, NY: Harper Collins; 1995.

30. Petracca M, ed. The politics of interests: interest groups transformed. Boulder, CO: Westview Press; 1992.

31. Cigler A, Burdett A, eds. Interest group politics. 3rd edn. Washington, DC: Congressional Quarterly; 1991.

32. Walker J, ed. Mobilizing interest groups in America. Ann Arbor, MI: The University of Michigan Press; 1991.

33. Schattschneider E. The semisovereign people. 2nd edn. Hinsdale, IL: The Dryden Press; 1975.

34. Goggin ML. Policy design and the politics of implementation. Knoxville, TN: The University of Tennessee Press; 1987.

35. Jennings-Dozie, KM. Educational programs in cancer prevention and detection: determining content and quality. Oncology nursing's next frontier. Oncol Nurs Forum 2000; 27(Suppl 9):47–54.

36. Sarna L, Brown LK, Lillington L, Wewers ME, Brecht ML. Tobacco-control attitudes, advocacy,

and smoking behaviors of oncology nurses. Oncol Nurs Forum 2000; 27(10):1519–1528.

37. Sarna LP, Brown JK, Lillington L, et al. Tobacco interventions by oncology nurses in clinical practice. Cancer 2000; 89:881–889.

38. Epstein SS, Ashford NA, Blackwelder B, et al. The crisis in U.S. and international cancer policy. Int J Health Serv 2002; 32(4):669–707.

39. Sarna L, Lillington L. Tobacco: an emerging topic in nursing research. Nurs Res 2002; 51(4):245–253.

40. Sciamanna CN, DePue JD, Goldstein MG, et al. Nutrition counseling in the promoting cancer prevention in primary care study. Prev Med 2002; 35(5):437–446.

41. Carroll-Johnson RM, ed. Cancer prevention and early detection: oncology nursing's next frontier. Oncol Nurs Forum 2000; 27(Suppl. 9):1–61.

42. Mahon SM. Principles of cancer prevention and early detection. Clin J Oncol Nurs 2000; 4(4):169–176.

43. Ishida DN. Making inroads on cancer prevention and control with Asian Americans. Semin Oncol Nurs 2001; 17(3):220–228.

44. American Cancer Society (ACS). Guidelines on nutrition and physical activity for cancer prevention. CA Cancer J Clin March/April 2002. http://www.aafp.org/afp/20021015/practice.html

45. Browning KK, Ahijevych KL, Ross P, Wewers ME. Implementing the Agency for Health Care Policy and Research's Smoking Cessation Guideline in a lung cancer surgery clinic. Oncol Nurs Forum 2000; 27: 1248–1254.

46. Gritz E. Facilitating smoking cessation in cancer patients. Tobacco Control 2000; 9:1950.

47. Bell RM, Tingen MS. The impact of tobacco use in women: exploring smoking cessation strategies. Clin J Oncol Nurs 2001; 5(3):101–104.

48. Jha P, Chaloupka F, eds. Curbing the epidemic: governments and the economics of tobacco control: The World Bank; 1999. URL: http://www1.worldbank.org/tobacco/reports.asp

48a Corrao MA, Guindon GE, Cokkinides V, Sharma N. Building the evidence base for global tobacco control. Bull WHO 2000; 78(7):884–890.

49. Boyle P. Cancer, cigarette smoking and premature death in Europe: a review including the Recommendations of European Cancer Experts Consensus Meeting, Helsinki, October 1996. Lung Cancer 1997; 17(1):1–60.

50. Samet J, Yoon S. Women and the tobacco epidemic: challenges for the 21st century: The World Health Organization/Institute for Global Tobacco Control, Johns Hopkins School of Public Health; 2001. URL: http://tobacco.who.int/repository/tpc49/WomenMonograph.pdf

51. US Department of Health and Human Services. Reducing tobacco use: a report of the Surgeon General. Atlanta, GA: USDHHS Centers for Disease Control and Prevention, National Center for Chronic Disease Prevention and Health Promotion; 2000.

52. US Department of Health and Human Services. 9th Report on Carcinogens. Research Triangle Park, NC: USDHHS, Public Health Service, National Toxicology Program; 2000.

53. Poswillo DC. Report of the Scientific Committee on Tobacco and Health. London, UK: The Stationery Office; 1998. ISBN 011322124x. URL: http://www.doh.gov.uk/public/scoth.htm

54. International Agency for Research on Cancer (IARC). Tobacco smoke and involuntary smoking. Summary of data reported and evaluation. Last updated 24 July 2002; Vol 83. http://monographs.iarc.fr/htdocs/monographs/vol83/01-smoking.html http://monographs.iarc.fr/htdocs/monographs/vol83/02-involuntary.html http://monographs.iarc.fr/htdocs/indexes/vol83index.html

55. Bialous S, Yach D. Whose standard is it, anyway? How the tobacco industry determines the International Organization for Standardization (ISO) standards for tobacco and tobacco products. Tobacco Control 2001;10:96–104.

56. USDHHS National Cancer Institute. Monograph 13: Risks associated with smoking cigarettes with low tar machine-measured yields of tar and nicotine 2001. URL: http://cancercontrol.cancer.gov/tcrb/monographs/13/index.html

57. Terry PD, Rohan TE, Franceschi S, et al. Cigarette smoking and the risk of endometrial cancer. Lancet Oncol 2002; 3(8): 470–480.

58. Johnson KC, Hu J, Mao, Y. Passive and active smoking and breast cancer risk in Canada, 1994–97. Cancer Causes and Control 2000; 11(3):211–221.

59. Terry PD, Miller AB, Rohan TE. Cigarette smoking and breast cancer risk: a long latency period? Int J Cancer 2002; 100(6):723–728.

60. Khuder SA, Mutgi AB, Nugent S. Smoking and breast cancer: a meta-analysis. Rev Environ Health 2001; 16(4):253–261.

61. California Environmental Protection Agency. Health effects of exposure to environmental tobacco smoke: the report of the California Environmental Protection Agency. Bethesda, MD: NIH; 1999. NIH Pub. No. 99-4645. URL: http://www.oehha.org/air/environmental_tobacco/finalets.html

62. US Environmental Protection Agency. Respiratory health effects of passive smoking: lung cancer and other disorders: US Environmental Protection Agency; 1992. USEPA Document No. EPA/600/6-90/006F.

63. Committee of Experts on Tobacco Industry Documents. Tobacco company strategies to

undermine tobacco control activities at the World Health Organization. Geneva: WHO; July 2000. URL: http://filestore.who.int/~who/home/tobacco/tobacco.pdf

64. Hirschhorn N, Bialous S. Second hand smoke and risk assessment: what was in it for the tobacco industry? Tobacco Control 2001; 10(4):375–382.

65. Glantz SA, Slade J, Bera LA, et al. The cigarette papers. Berkeley: University of California Press; 1996.

66. Muggli M, Forster J, Hurt R, et al. The smoke you don't see: uncovering tobacco industry scientific strategies aimed against control of environmental tobacco smoke. Am J Prev Health 2001; 91(9):1419–1423.

67. Drope J, Chapman S. Tobacco industry efforts at discrediting scientific knowledge of environmental tobacco smoke: a review of internal industry documents. J Epidemiol Community Health 2001; 55:588–594.

68. Samet J, Burke T. Turning science into junk: the tobacco industry and passive smoking. Am J Prev Health 2001; 91(11):1742–1744.

69. Ong E, Glantz S. Constructing "sound science" and "good epidemiology": tobacco, lawyers, and public relations firms. Am J Prev Health 2001;91(11):1749–1757.

70. Ong E, Glantz S. Tobacco industry efforts subverting International Agency for Research on Cancer's second-hand smoke study. Lancet 2000; 355:1253–1255.

71. Wewers ME, Ahijavych K, Sarna L. Smoking cessation interventions in nursing practice. Nurs Clin North Am 1998; 33:61–74.

72. Rice VH. Nursing interventions and smoking cessation. A meta analysis. Heart & Lung 2000; 28:438–454.

73. Percival J. Clearing the air 2: smoking and tobacco control – an updated guide for nurses. London: Royal College of Nursing; 2002:40.

74. Amstrong B, Doll R. Environmental factors and cancer incidence and mortality in different countries, with special reference to dietary practices. Int J Cancer 1975; 15:617–631.

75. COMA Working Group on Diet and Cancer. Nutritional aspects of the development of cancer. UK Department of Health Report on Health and Social Subjects No 48. Norwich: HMSO ; 1998.

76. CNERNA, Centre National d'étude et de Recommandation sur la nutrition er l'alimentation. In: Riboli E, Decloitre F, Collet-Ribbing C , eds. Alimentation et cancer: evaluation des données scientifiques. Paris: Lavoisier; 1996.

77. WCRF/AICR. Food, nutrition and prevention of cancer: a global perspective. London/Washington: World Cancer Research Fund/American Institute of Cancer Research; 1997.

78. Peto J. Cancer epidemiology in the last century and the next decade. Nature 2001; 411(6835):390–395.

79. Bostik RM. Diet and nutrition in the etiology and primary prevention of colon cancer. In: Bendich A, Deckelbaum RJ, eds. Preventive nutrition: the comprehensive guide for health professionals. Ottawa: Humana Press; 1997:57–95.

80. Steinmetz KA, Potter JD. Vegetable, fruit and cancer. I Epidemiology. Cancer Causes Control 1991; 2:325–357.

81. Greenwald P, Clifford C. Cooking methods and other diet-related factors. In: Greenwald P, Kramer B, Weed D, eds. Cancer prevention and control. New York: Marcel Dekker; 1995:319.

82. McKeigue PM, Adelstein AM, Marmot MG, et al. Diet and faecal steroid profile in a South Asian population with a low colon cancer rate. Am J Clin Nutr 1989; 50:151–154.

83. Rose DP, Goldman M, Connolly JM, et al. High-fibre diet reduces serum estrogen concentrations in premenopausal women. Am J Clin Nutr 1991; 54:520–525.

84. Appleton GVN, Owen RW, Weeler EE, et al. Effect of dietary calcium on the colonic luminal environment. Gut 1991; 32:1374–1377.

85. Mason JB, Choi S. The mechanisms by which folate depletion enhances colorectal carcinogenesis: a unified scheme. In: Mason JB, Ritenberg G, eds. Cancer and nutrition: prevention and treatment. Nestlé Nutrition Workshop Series Clinical and Performance Program. Karger Basel: Nestlé; 2000; 4:87–101.

86. Clark LC, Combs GF, Turnbull BW, et al. Effects of selenium supplementation for cancer prevention in patients with carcinoma of the skin. J Am Med Assoc 1996; 276:1957–1963.

87. Omenn GS, Goodman G, Thornquist M, et al. The beta-carotene and retinol efficacy trial (CARET) for chemoprevention of lung cancer in high risk populations: smokers and asbestos-exposed workers. Cancer Res 1994; 54(7 Suppl):2038S–2043S.

88. Willett WC, Stamper MJ, Colditz GA, et al. Relation of meat, fat and their fibre intake to the risk of colon cancer in a prospective study among women. N Engl J Med 1990; 323:1664–1672.

89. Deitz A, Zheng W, Leff M, et al. N-Acetyltransferase-2 genetic polymorphism, well-done meat intake and breast cancer risk among postmenopausal women. Cancer Epidemiol Biomarkers & Prev 2000; 9:905–910.

90. Tannenbaum A. The genesis and growth of tumours. Introduction. Effects of caloric restrictions per se. Cancer Res 1942; 2: 460–467.

91. Rose DP, Boyar AP, Wynder EL. International comparisons of mortality rates for cancer of the breast, ovary, prostate and colon and per capita food consumption. Cancer 1986; 58:2363–2371.

92. Munoz de Chavez M, Chavez A. Diet that prevents cancer. Int J Cancer 1998; 54(Suppl 11):85–89.

93. Prentice RL, Thompson DO, Clifford CK, et al. Dietary fat reduction and plasma estradiol in healthy, postmenopausal women. J Natl Cancer Inst 1990; 82:129–134.

94. Ballard-Barbash R, Schatzkin A, Carter CL, et al. Body fat distribution and breast cancer in Framingham Study. J Natl Cancer Inst 1990; 82:286–290.

95. Huang Z, Hankinson SE, Colditz GA, et al. Dual effects of weight and weight gain on breast cancer risk. J Am Med Assoc 1997; 278:1407–1411.

96. Riboli E. The European Prospective Investigation into cancer and nutrition: perspectives for cancer prevention. In: Mason JB, Nitenberg G, eds. Cancer and nutrition: prevention and treatment. Nestlé Nutrition Workshop Series Clinical and Performance Program. Karger Basel: Nestlé; 2000; 4: 117–133.

97. McTiernan A, Irvin M, Ulrich C, et al. Randomised trial of exercise effect on breast cancer biomarkers. Abstract No I 198, Proceedings of the 18th UICC International Cancer Congress, 2002, Oslo.

98. Hartmann TJ, Albanes D, Rautalahti M, et al. Physical activity and prostate cancer in the Alpha-Tocopherol, Beta-Carotene Cancer Prevention Study. Cancer Causes Control 1998; 9(1):11–18.

99. Colombo M, Sangiovanni A. Etiology. In: Livraghi TI, Makuuchi M, Buscarini L, eds. Diagnosis and treatment of hepatocellular carcinoma. London: Greenwich Medical Media; 1991:17–24.

100. Blot WJ, McLauglin JK, Winn DM, et al. Smoking and drinking in relation to oral and pharyngeal cancer. Cancer Res 1988, 48:3282–3287.

101. Russo J, Tay LK, Russo IH. Differentiation of the mammary gland and susceptibility to carcinogenesis. Breast Cancer Res Treat 1982; 2:5–73.

102. Freudenheim JL, Ambrosone CB, Moysich KB, et al. Alcohol dehydrogenase 3 genotype modification of the association of alcohol consumption with breast cancer risk. Cancer Causes Control 1999; 10:369–377.

103. Michels KB, Willett WC, Rosner BA, et al. Prospective assessment of breast feeding and breast cancer incidence among 89,887 women. Lancet 1996; 347:431–436.

104. Madigan MP, Ziegler RG, Benichou J, et al. Proportion of breast cancer cases in the United States explained by well established risk factors. J Natl Cancer Inst 1995; 87:1681–1685.

105. Tavani A, Braga C, La Vecchia C, et al. Attributable risks for breast cancer in Italy: education, family history and reproductive and hormonal factors. Int J Cancer 1997; 70:159–163.

106. Schairer C, Lubin J, Troisi R, et al. Menopausal estrogen and estrogen–progestin replacement therapy and breast cancer risk. J Am Med Assoc 2000; 283(4):285–491.

107. Glanz K, Lewis FM, Rimer BK. Health behaviour and health education: theory, research and practice. 2nd edn. San Francisco: Jossey Bass; 1999.

108. McGee R, Williams S, Elwood M. Depression and the development of cancer: a meta-analysis. Social Sci Med 1994; 38:187–192.

109. International Agency for Research and Cance (IARC). Overall evaluations of carcinogenicity to humans; 2000. Retrieval from the World Wide Web: http://193.51.164.11/monoeval/crhall.html

110. Harris E. Interactions between nature and nurture. In: Greenwald P, Kramer B, Weed D, eds. Cancer prevention and control. New York: Marcel Dekker; 1995:182.

111. Mahon SM. Cancer risk assessment: conceptual considerations for clinical practice. Oncol Nurs Forum 1998; 25:1535–1547.

112. Gail MH, Brinton LA, Byar DP, et al. Projecting individualized probabilities of developing breast cancer for white females who are being examined annually. J Natl Cancer Inst 1989; 81:1879–1886.

113. Vogel VG. Breast cancer risk factors and preventive approaches to breast cancer. In: Kavanagh JJ, Singletary SE, Einhorn N, DePetrillo AD, Malden MA, eds. Cancer in women. Oxford: Blackwell Science; 1998:58–91.

114. Armstrong K, Eisen A, Weber B. Assessing the risk of breast cancer. N Engl J Med 2000; 342:564–571.

115. Claus EB, Risch N, Thompson WD. Autosomal dominant inheritance of early-onset breast cancer: implications for risk prediction. Cancer 1994; 73:643–651.

116. Berry DA, Iversen ES Jr, Gudbjartsson DF, et al: BRCAPRO validation, sensitivity of genetic testing of BRCA1/BRCA2, and prevalence of other breast cancer susceptibility genes. J Clin Oncol 2002; 20(11):2701–2712.

117. Lindor NM, Greene MH. The concise handbook of family cancer syndromes. Mayo Familial Cancer Program. J Natl Cancer Inst 1998; 90:1039–1071.

118. Rieger PT, Tinley ST. Cancer genetics and nursing practice: what every gastroenterology nurse needs to know. Gastroenterol Nurs 2000; 23(1):28–39.

119. Emery J, Lucassen A, Murphy M. Common hereditary cancers and implications for primary care. Lancet 2001; 411(6838):709–713.

120. Hanahan D, Weinberg RA. The hallmarks of cancer. Cell 2000; 100:57–70.

121. Ponder BA. Cancer genetics. Nature 2001; 411(6835):336–341.

122. Task Force on Genetic Testing. Interim Principles of the Task Force on Genetic Testing, 1996. Available at http://www.infonet.welch.jhu.edu/policy/genetics/intro.html.

123. Mills GB, Rieger PT. Genetic predisposition to breast cancer. In: Hunt KK. Robb GL, Strom EA, Ueno N, eds. Breast cancer. New York: Springer-Verlag; 2001:55–92.

124. Offit K. Clinical cancer genetics: risk counseling and management. New York: Wiley-Liss; 1998.

125. International Society of Nurses in Genetics (ISONG), American Nurses Association. Statement on the scope and standards of genetics clinical nursing practice. Washington, DC: American Nurses Publishing; 1998.

126. Greenwald P, Kelloff G. The role of chemoprevention in cancer control. In: Stewart E, McGregor D, Kleihues P, eds. Principles of chemoprevention. IARC Scientific Publications No 139. Lyon: International Agency for Research on Cancer; 1996:13.

127. Lippman S, Benner S, Hong W. Cancer chemoprevention. J Clin Oncol 1994; 12:851–873.

128. NCI Online. Internet. http://cancer.gov retrieved May 2002.

129. Schatzkin A, Kelloff G. Chemo- and dietary prevention of colorectal cancer. Eur J Cancer 1995; 31:1198–1204.

130. Clark L, Dalkin B, Krongrad A, et al. Decreased incidence with prostate cancer with selenium supplatation: results of a double-blind cancer prevention trial. Br J Urol 1998; 81:730–743.

131. Sandler R. Aspirin and other nonsteroidal anti-inflammatory agents in the prevention of colorectal cancer. In: Devita VT, Hellman S, Rosenberg S, eds. Important advances in oncology. Philadelphia; Lippincott-Raven; 1996:123–137.

132. NCI Online. Searle & Co G.D. 1999; Skokie, IL.

133. Fisher B, Costantino J, Wickerham D, et al. Tamoxifen for prevention of breast cancer: report of the national surgical adjuvant breast and bowel project P-1 study. J Natl Cancer Inst 1998; 90:1371–1388.

134. Gail M, Costantino J, Bryant J, et al. Weighing the risks and benefits of tamoxifen treatment for preventing breast cancer. J Natl Cancer Inst 1999; 91:1829–1846.

135. Aikin JL. Tamoxifen in perspective: benefits, side effects and toxicities. In: Dow KH, ed. Contemporary issues in breast cancer. Boston: Jones and Bartlett; 1996:59–68.

136. Jennings K, Mahon S. Cancer prevention, detection and control: a nursing perspective. Pittsburgh: Oncology Nursing Society, 2002:257–275.

137. Offit K, Robinson M, Schrag D. Prophylactic mastectomy in carriers of BRCA mutation. N Engl J Med 2001; 345(20):1498–1499.

138. http://www.breastcancer.org .Internet. Retrieval October 2002.

139. Hopwood P, Lee A, Shenton A, et al. Clincal follow-up after bilateral risk reducing (prophylactic) mastectomy: mental health and body image outcomes. Psychooncology 2000; 9:(6):462–472.

140. Vogel VG. Primary prevention of breast cancer. In: Bland KI, Copeland EM, eds. The breast: comprehensive mangement of benign and malignant diseases. 2nd edn Philadelphia:WB Saunders; 1998:352–369.

141. Rice V. Nursing intervention and smoking cessation: a meta-analysis. Heart Lung 1999; 28(6):438–454.

142. Browning KK, Ahijevych KL, Ross P Jr, et al. Implementing the Agency for Health Care Policy and Research's Smoking Cessation Guideline in a lung cancer surgery clinic. Oncol Nurs Forum 2000; 27(8):1248–1254.

143. Sarna L. Resources for treatment of tobacco dependency. Cancer Pract 2000; 8(5):248–253.

144. Sarna L, Wewers ME, Brown JK, et al. Barriers to tobacco cessation in clinical practice: report from a National Survey of Oncology Nurses. Nurs Outlook 2001; 49(4):166–172.

145. Fiore MC, Bailey WC, Cohen SJ, et al. Treating tobacco use and dependence. A clinical practice guideline. Rockville, Md: US Dept of Health and Human Services; 2000. AHRQ publication No. 00-0032.

146. McBride CM, Bepler G, Lipkus IM, et al. Incorporating genetic susceptibility feedback into a smoking cessation program for African-American smokers with low income. Cancer Epidemiol Biomarkers & Prev June 2002; 11:521–528.

147. Lippman SM, Spitz MR. Lung cancer chemoprevention: an integrated approach. J Clin Oncol 2001;19(18 Suppl):74S–82S.

148. Hecht SS. Cigarette smoking and lung cancer: chemical mechanisms and approaches to prevention. Lancet Oncol 2002; 3(8):461–469.

CHAPTER 9

Early Detection of Cancer

AGNES GLAUS, PAULA TRAHAN RIEGER

CHAPTER CONTENTS

Secondary prevention: cancer screening	167
Screening approaches and principles	168
Opportunistic and mass screening	168
Indicators of effectiveness of screening programmes	168
Critical issues in screening: lead-time and length-time bias	169
Screening and cancer registries	170
Population-related and ethical issues	170
Screening in a high-risk population: cancer surveillance	171
Helping to make the decision: a role for every nurse	171
From recruitment to follow-up	172
Coordination of follow-up	172
Cancer screening recommendations and strategies for specific, frequent types of cancer	172
Breast cancer screening	172
Breast cancer screening through BSE and CBE	173
Breast cancer screening through mammography	174
Ovarian cancer screening	175

Cervix cancer screening	177
The Pap (Papanicolaou) test as cervical screening method	177
Cervical screening recommendations	178
Colon cancer screening	179
Prostate cancer screening	179
Lung cancer screening: future trends	182
Diagnostic methods in secondary cancer prevention /early detection	183
Mammography	183
Cervix cancer screening – diagnostic methods	183
Colorectal cancer screening – diagnostic methods	184
Faecal occult blood test	184
Flexible sigmoidoscopy, colonoscopy, double-contrast barium enema	184
Diagnostic screening methods for prostate cancer	185
Laboratory aspects of screening for cancer: tumour markers	187
The prostate-specific antigen	187
CA 125	187
References	188

SECONDARY PREVENTION: CANCER SCREENING

The previous chapter dealt with primary prevention of cancer with the aim of preventing initiation of carcinogenesis and preventing promotion to premalignant, or progression to malignant cells. This chapter deals with secondary prevention through early detection, with the ultimate goal to improve a patient's prognosis. Effective cancer screening programmes are a way to achieve this goal. Principles, potentials and limits will be discussed.

SCREENING APPROACHES AND PRINCIPLES

Screening for asymptomatic cancer is the most common form of secondary prevention in cancer care. The screening approach can vary from self-examination to professional examination, from opportunistic to mass screening, and also include extensive surveillance programmes or even genetic counselling for identified subgroups (see Ch. 8).

Opportunistic and mass screening

Screening is based on the premise that early diagnosis of the disease at an earlier stage than that at which clinical presentation would otherwise take place leads to reduction of mortality or development of invasive disease.[1] If a patient presents to a physician in order to obtain a medical check-up or a specific screening test, this can be seen as screening; however, it usually does not occur within an established cancer screening programme, neither is it linked with a quality assurance and scientific evaluation programme by a cancer registry. This type of screening is called *opportunistic screening* (or case finding)[2] and it depends very much on the skills and knowledge of the healthcare provider. Opportunistic screening measures may not be covered financially by insurance companies in most countries. By contrast, diagnostic procedures would usually be covered as soon as patients present with a specific health problem. This may be the consequence of a disease-rather than health-oriented medical paradigm.

Mass screening or population-based screening of asymptomatic individuals is usually run as public health policy. This type of screening has a high cost and is only recommended when prevalence of a disease is high, when there is proven effectiveness of the method and where there are resources in place (human, material and financial) to cover at least 70% of the screening target group.[3] In addition, it is important that, before mass screening programmes are undertaken, resources exist for further diagnostic tests, treatment and follow-up of those who receive a diagnosis of cancer. Currently, mass screening is only recommended by the World Health Organization (WHO)[3] for cancers of the uterine, cervix and the breast, with the target population being women 35 years old and older (cervical) and 50 years old and older (breast). However, in some European countries, even those with significant resources such as Switzerland or Denmark, the recommendation for breast cancer screening has not yet been run as a health policy for a variety of reasons.

There is, however, general agreement that screening be directed at cancers with high prevalence and incidence and to which there is treatment available and a reasonable chance of avoiding premature death. It is generally accepted that screening for breast, colorectal, cervical, prostate, testicular, oral cavity and skin cancer have a favourable cost–benefit ratio (the benefit of the screening outweighs the costs), as treatment for these cancers has better success with early detection. Screening for these additional cancers is recommended by cancer and health-related organizations in many developed countries. Such additional screening tests include, for example, faecal occult blood test (FOBT), digital rectal examination (DRE) and sigmoidoscopy to detect colorectal cancer.[2]

INDICATORS OF EFFECTIVENESS OF SCREENING PROGRAMMES

Valid indicators for a screening programme are *reduction of mortality* from cancer, but in some programmes, such as in cervical cancer, it can be the detection of preinvasive disease, and therefore the indicator can also consist of a reduction in the incidence of invasive disease.[4] Accuracy, validity and effectiveness all need to be considered.

A basic measure of validity of a screening test is *accuracy*, usually measured in terms of sensitivity and specificity. *Sensitivity* refers to the ability of the test to detect true cases of the disease, and in screening programmes this is monitored by calculating the incidence of interval cancers according to specific rules. *Specificity* refers to the ability to identify true negatives correctly. Inevitably, in such programmes, some healthy persons may be labelled 'positive' for a short time period. Since the false positives of screening will be identified by subsequent diagnostic procedures, specificity can be calculated as the proportion of all true negatives. Thus, ideally, a screening test goal is to make sure as few as possible individuals with the disease remain undetected (high sensitivity) and that as few as possible without the disease undergo additional testing (high specificity) because this not only causes anxiety but also induces costs. Using a combination of screening tests can increase both sensitivity and specificity, such as the use of two-view mammography as compared with a single view.[1] To be clinically useful, specificity and sensitivity need to be turned into predictive values. As a test cannot be interpreted in a vacuum, the patient's history must be known to make a prediction about the meaning of a test result. Inappropriate testing can yield misleading information and cause unnecessary investigations. Appropriate testing in a high-risk population has a high predictive value. A positive predictive value is the proportion of cancers detected per abnormal examination.[5]

To minimize the inaccuracy of screening, it is essential that quality assurance mechanisms be implemented simultaneously with the implementation of a screening programme. Quality assurance will promote standardization of conduct, both at the clinical as well as at laboratory and radiological levels. Test results should be interpreted the same way by technicians and clinicians.[3,6] However, standardization and quality assurance can minimize, but not eliminate, differences in clinical performance and practice.

Apart from these requirements for a screening test, it is of crucial importance that a diagnostic procedure be *acceptable* to the individual. It should not cause pain or discomfort or create unreasonable or excessive risk. It should also be easily accessible, widely available and cost-effective. However, there are no perfect screening tests yet. Minimum acceptability requirements for screening tests,

---

Box 9.1

Minimum acceptability requirements for cancer screening tests

Disease should be treatable
Treatment for disease should be available
Test must be:
  Clinically relevant
  Able to detect a condition for which intervention at a preclinical stage can improve outcome
  Accurate (acceptable sensitivity and specificity)
  Acceptable to individuals being screened
  Widely available
  Easily accessible
  Cost effective

Source: World Health Organization[3]

---

as defined by the WHO, are summarized in Box 9.1.

CRITICAL ISSUES IN SCREENING: LEAD-TIME AND LENGTH-TIME BIAS

Some critical issues have been raised regarding the usefulness of screening programmes and may be discussed with individuals planning preventative health care. The effectiveness of screening programmes also depends on the natural course of the illness. If the disease cannot be detected at an early stage, or if the treatment available may not be more effective if provided earlier in comparison to the usual time of diagnosis, or if there is no treatment available, this adds to a *lead-time bias*. This means that the disease is diagnosed earlier but, due to the nature of illness and lack of therapeutic possibilities, the end of life is not extended and that time gained as a result of early diagnosis is added to the survival time. Screening tests are considered justifiable only if cancer can be detected before it becomes clinically evident and if effective treatment is available to impact on mortality and morbidity. Another critical concept is *the length-time bias*, considering the fact that some cancers have variable disease patterns. For example, prostate and breast cancers have subsets of both, extremely aggressive and indolent diseases. Aggressive tumours progress rapidly from onset of symptoms to death and indolent cancers may remain localized or in situ for a long time. Because of the rapid growth of aggressive tumours, these are more likely not to be detected in screening programmes. This is referred to as length-time bias and is, as an example, a topical issue in prostate cancer prevention. Proponents of prostate screening programmes maintain that advances in treatment limit morbidity, because treatment initiated at the time of screening may not threaten quality of life as much as delayed treatment.[7] The inability to accurately predict which tumours are indolent and which are aggressive can lead to the rule to treat all prostate cancers when they are found rather than waiting for symptoms. Collecting accurate information regarding family history and defining age categories supposed to be at higher risk can help to outweigh this difficulty to some extent. Risk assessment methods used by nurses and physicians can help to identify individuals at high risk and provide appropriate screening recommendations.

Screening and cancer registries

It has been claimed that such screening programmes have to be linked to cancer registries to identify cancers diagnosed outside the screening programme (interval cancers) and among non-responders to permit completeness of data and to provide the expected incidence and mortality estimates assuming no screening.[8] In some countries, screening programmes are initiated by the cancer registry. Through linkage of the cancer registry database to that of a screening programme, they can contribute to a variety of analyses, such as trends in incidence and mortality and effectiveness of screening. Further, it has been suggested that emphasis must be given to the collection of data on side-effects of screening, going much further than measuring biological or public health outcome, and also issues related to ethics, quality of life, health economics and keeping people up-to-date with relevant information.[9]

POPULATION-RELATED AND ETHICAL ISSUES

Lower and upper age limits for screening programmes in normal risk groups vary greatly between countries and are mainly determined by cost-effectiveness issues. In older women, co-morbidity has to be considered, as severe co-morbidity would for example render mammography screening ineffectual in decreasing mortality in women aged 65 years old and older. McPherson et al[10] in a recent study concluded that mammographic detection would be associated with significantly decreased risk of death for older women of all ages, but for older women with multiple co-morbidity there was no association with improvement in overall survival. Barratt et al[11] concluded that cost-effectiveness estimates for mammographic screening from 69–79 years old compared favourably with extending screening to women aged 40–49 years old. Women aged 70 years old and over may, together with their healthcare provider, want to decide for themselves whether to continue mammography screening or not. Experience shows that the upper age limit may cause feelings of discrimination, especially in countries defining the upper limit at age 64 years old.

The world is becoming progressively more *multicultural* and *population diversity* is characterized by differences in culture, behaviour, beliefs, attitudes, age and socioeconomic status. This diversity also has implications with regard to healthcare access and priority, and limited healthcare resources raise ethical concerns. Accessibility of health care can be more difficult in the preventative environment than in the therapeutic environment for some populations, such as those with low income, limited education, literacy and language barriers. Elderly people, children or women and geographically isolated persons may have limited access and it has been documented that special populations have a higher incidence of cancer and lower survival rates.[12]

The *ethical principles* involved in cancer prevention are, for example, the concepts of justice (fairness), respect for autonomy (self-determination) and non-maleficence (avoiding harm). Autonomy and non-maleficence also refer to characteristics of the screening approach. The only people who really benefit from screening are those who have been diagnosed with cancer by screening and whose death is, as a result, delayed. This implicates that the majority of the mass population being screened does not 'benefit' from screening. However, it can be argued that it is advantageous to be in the group of those who are not diagnosed with cancer and it is a socially accepted means that screening involves large groups and implicates high costs. Offering interventions to healthy subjects is linked to the responsibility of providing full information and to treating screening abnormalities quickly. It has to be made clear that screening is never 100% sensitive and that being screened negative does not mean that either the individual does not have occult cancer or will not develop cancer in the future. False reassurance could lead to subsequently ignoring symptoms.[13] Education therefore remains an important component in screening programmes, such as information about early symptoms. Ethical issues linked to genetic screening are discussed in Chapter 8.

SCREENING IN A HIGH-RISK POPULATION: CANCER SURVEILLANCE

If cancer screening methods are used in subgroups of the population at high risk, this will increase cost-effectiveness, since the yield of cancers detected will be greater.[1] For example, in most countries, the selection by age as a factor for higher risk for breast cancer in women without a family history leads to offering mammography screening between the ages of 50 and 70 years old. This is distinctly different to *screening for known high-risk groups*, where screening may involve much younger women with a strong family history for breast cancer or an occupationally exposed group of individuals. For such groups, a much more individualized approach is needed to develop a *cancer surveillance and risk-reduction plan*. According to Grecco,[14] such a plan can involve the following components:

- information about lifestyle, dietary and environmental factors increasing cancer risk
- frequency and type of examination by healthcare provider
- recommendation of accurate screening test and frequency
- risk and benefits of chemopreventative and surgical prophylactic interventions
- coordination of follow-up care.

Nurses, in general, are ideally positioned to inform and challenge patients and their relatives about screening measures. Specialized healthcare providers, including specially educated nurses, have a pivotal role in caring for individuals referred to such programmes. Health education, instruction for self-examining practices and emotional support and identifying individual fears and needs are major components in such services.

HELPING TO MAKE THE DECISION: A ROLE FOR EVERY NURSE

A number of barriers have been identified that make people hesitant to use preventative measures. These may be linked with the provider, the client or the healthcare system[7] and have been described in Chapter 8. However, the fact that screening recommendations are not uniform worldwide, and within a country may vary from institution to institution, make it more difficult for clients to understand the screening programme and highlights how important it is for the nurse to spend time with the client explaining the need for each screening procedure, the rationale for screening and what can be expected from the results. Oncology nurses must keep in mind that screening guidelines change over time and are used as guidelines to be adapted to each client's needs as appropriate, based on the nurse assessment. Research suggests that a recommendation by a healthcare professional plays a very important role in whether or not a person is screened for cancer, which reinforces the important role nurses play in decreasing cancer morbidity and mortality.[15] When nurses recommend screening to an individual, a far greater chance exists that the individual will actually undergo appropriate screening. This recommendation can easily come in the form of patient education about cancer prevention and early detection.[2,6]

To assist individuals in deciding whether specific cancer screening is beneficial, some principles need to be known and considered. Gordis[16] suggests asking the following key questions:

- Can the cancer in question be detected early?
- What is known about the sensitivity, specificity and predictive value of the screening test?
- How significant is the problem of a false-positive test result?
- What are the costs of early detection (financial, emotional)?
- Can the patient be harmed in any way by early testing?
- Is there a benefit for the individual from having the disease detected early?

Detecting cancer early not only may impact on cancer mortality in the screened population but also morbidity. As an example, early-stage breast cancer may allow for less-invasive surgery, thus preventing women from mastectomy, and this again may decrease the risk for lymphoedema. This means that quality of life of a screened population can also be improved[16] and this may be a good reason in favour of a screening intervention.

FROM RECRUITMENT TO FOLLOW-UP

Recruiting individuals for screening programmes is a challenging issue. Institutions offering screening tests use different approaches to recruit individuals. In opportunistic screening, self-referral may be common. Success of screening programmes may also depend on collegial relationship with referring physicians.[2] Advertising and word of mouth can be effective. Comprehensive cancer screening programmes need a structured referral base of patients and usually depend on referrals from the community, where a prevention programme represents health policy. It has been observed that compliance

with these programmes can be supported by personal invitation, friendly contact and negotiation of acceptable timing of the intervention.

Ways to facilitate screening require good logistics, which can improve recruitment. Opportunistic and mass screening may be offered in different ways, making it more or less easy for those concerned. Work-site programmes are convenient for the employee, large numbers of people can be screened and programmes may be easy to facilitate, but psychological barriers may arise.[2] Free-standing testing services (walk-in facilities) appear to be convenient, but personal patient education is often lacking. From a nursing perspective, it appears desirable to combine easy mass screening methods with a personal provider–client contact, but limited resources make it difficult to strive for this ideal and it remains a future challenge to develop.

Coordination of follow-up

Coordination of follow-up remains a logistic challenge. An important outcome of a cancer detection programme is the assurance that people with abnormal screening tests receive appropriate follow-up. A follow-up strategy must be determined and usually can be accomplished by a letter to patients in case of normal results. Ensuring screening results in a timely fashion can be a challenge. Nurses need to emphasize strength and limits of screening programmes and also to reinforce that negative test results mean that there is no evident cancer disease but that there still is a need for further evaluation and repeated screening.

Some of the most relevant cancer screening programmes and guidelines will now be discussed.

CANCER SCREENING RECOMMENDATIONS AND STRATEGIES FOR SPECIFIC, FREQUENT TYPES OF CANCER

BREAST CANCER SCREENING

Breast cancer is the most common non-skin malignancy among women in all developed countries, apart from Japan. The highest recorded incidence rates are in North America, with an age-standardized rate of 84.0 per 100,000 women. The lowest incidence rates are observed in China, with 14.6 per 100,000. In the northern countries of Europe, incidence is higher than in the southern countries, with the highest incidence rate of 58.0 per 100,000 in England and Wales.[17] In the USA alone, in 2003, it is estimated that over 211,000 new cases of invasive breast cancer will be diagnosed.[18] In addition to invasive breast cancer, over 54,000 cases of in-situ breast cancer are expected to occur, the majority of these being ductal carcinoma in situ (DCIS). The latter is a direct result of mammography screening.

The traditional methods for screening for breast cancer have been breast self-examination (BSE), clinical breast examination (CBE) and mammography.

Breast cancer screening through BSE and CBE

Many health educators and cancer organizations actively encourage women to examine their breasts regularly as a form of self-screening. In fact, in many developing countries, BSE and CBE are the only methods available for breast screening. Despite many studies, it is still not clear whether BSE can reduce the risk of breast cancer death. In a Finnish study involving 28,000 women, it was concluded that there was no difference in stage distribution but that mortality was lower than expected in women practising BSE. However, the authors stated that even though the reduction of mortality was consistent with an effect of BSE, selection bias, inherent in any observational study of screening, could not be ruled out.[19] The Canadian National Breast Screening study compared self-reported BSE frequency before enrollment in the trial with breast cancer mortality and found that women who examined their breasts visually and used their finger pads for palpation, and used their 3 middle fingers, had lower breast cancer mortality.[20] These reports encourage BSE practice. However, other studies, e.g. a large Chinese randomized trial, concluded that BSE had no effect on breast cancer diagnosis and mortality.[21] Nurses are challenged to follow up par-

tially contradictory research in this field and to reflect the value of BSE without providing false reassurance.

Clinical experience shows that too many women still present with large palpable tumours at the time of diagnosis. The reasons for this may be multifaceted. Breast self-awareness may be one concept to influence earlier diagnosis. Through BSE, breast awareness may be supported, and this is one reason to encourage women in the practice of BSE. Sensitivity is influenced by the performance of BSE and also varies according to size, location, shape and composition of a palpable mass but also heavily depends on the size and type of the breast. Empowering women through careful instruction about BSE may increase sensitivity of the method. BSE may also serve as an additional instrument for women who are anxious. Overuse of BSE can occasionally be observed in clinical practice in very anxious women and it is important for nurses to provide women with information regarding frequency of its use (more than once per month may cause more anxiety than benefit) and its limits. Guidelines for BSE practice are summarized in Box 9.2.

Box 9.2
Guidelines for practising breast self-examination
• Perform BSE once monthly, after the age of 20 years old. No upper age limit.
• Perform BSE monthly, after the menstrual period
• (or around the same time each month if not menstruating).
• Combine BSE with visual examination in front of the mirror.
• Report your own observations regarding changes in the breast to the examining physician or nurse to support sensitivity of CBE by professionals.
• Perform BSE as a complementary self-screening method to mammography screening (if available and applicable).

Nurses and clients need to be aware of the possibilities but also the limits of BSE. Some tumours cannot be palpated due to location or size of the breast. Very small tumours rarely can be detected by BSE and are more likely to be detected by mammography. Precancerous lesions, such as DCIS, cannot be detected by palpation either. This makes it clear that BSE can be used as a complementary method in secondary breast cancer prevention but that it cannot replace screening by mammography in specific age populations.

CBE by physicians or nurses, as a screening method alone, has also been studied. Comparison of CBE alone with mammography showed similar outcome regarding diagnosis, stage and mortality.[22] It has been argued, however, that careful training and supervision of the health professionals performing BSE in the study was responsible for this and presented an unusual situation. Detection of tumours by CBE depends very much on the skills of the examiner, and limitations are similar to those associated with BSE. In most European countries, CBE is performed as a screening method by the gynaecologist concurrently when women have their cervical cancer screening test done (see below) but generally is performed complementary to mammography.

Breast cancer screening through mammography

Large-scale research studies have evaluated the efficacy of different methodologies in recent years and have led to changes in screening recommendations. The United States Preventive Services Task Force (USPSTF) recently updated its screening recommendations for breast cancer. The USPSTF is an independent panel of experts in primary care and prevention that systematically reviews the evidence of effectiveness and develops recommendations for clinical preventative services. The USTP-STF recommends screening mammography, with or without CBE, every 1–2 years for women aged 40 years old and older.[23] This recommendation was supported by at least fair evidence that the service improves important health outcomes and concludes that benefits

outweigh harms. Evidence is strongest for women aged 50–69 years old, the age group generally included in screening trials, and grows more favourable with age. At this time, evidence is insufficient to recommend for or against routine CBE alone to screen for breast cancer, or for or against teaching or performing routine BSE. Nearly all North American organizations support mammography screening, although groups vary the recommended age to begin screening (e.g. 40 years old vs 50 years old), the appropriate interval (e.g. every year vs every 2 years) and the role of CBE.

In addition, screening recommendations will be altered and individually adapted for women who are at an increased risk of developing breast cancer through a family history of cancer. There is no definitive information on when screening should be stopped, although the risk for breast cancer continues to increase as women age. The benefits of screening should be weighed against existing co-morbid conditions and the potential that the woman may die from these conditions.

The International Breast Cancer Screening Network (IBCSN) conducted a survey in 1995 in 13 international countries and in 9 countries of the European Network of Pilot Projects for Breast Cancer Screening.[24] The survey collected information on policies and guidelines in use within programmes in 1995. Issues addressed included funding and organization, target population by age and other risk characteristics, screening interval, detection methods, location of service. Eventually, updated information was obtained from 13 members of IBCSN and 9 countries from the European Network. With the exception of France and Luxembourg, the countries involved in the European Network had not begun nationally organized breast cancer screening in 1995 (England, Sweden, Finland and the Netherlands had begun but were included in the international group). Only Ireland planned to expand pilot programmes to allow national coverage of the population. Generally, countries with centralized or at least partially centralized systems for policy, funding and administration appear more likely to have achieved complete coverage of the population. In most countries, dedicated centres for mammography were used rather than existing general radiology departments. This survey from 1995 showed that there had been an increase in the number of countries that had implemented or planned to implement an organized breast cancer screening programme since 1992. A change in guidelines, with age 50 years old being the lower age limit, as well as changes in the detection methods used, were observed, but there were no changes in screening intervals among those countries surveyed.[24] A summary of the guidelines most commonly used in the countries observed is presented in Table 9.1.

There are many clinical considerations that relate to decisions concerning screening. Women are advised to discuss benefits vs potential harms with their healthcare provider. Questions about harm by X-rays and anxiety associated with fear from pain are important issues for nurses to raise when they teach women about mammography because, clinical experience shows that they may have read or heard negative comments about it. These issues are also a challenge to the technicians performing mammography, because a national screening method cannot be successful if it causes fear and pain. A consumer-friendly service and atmosphere may be most helpful in supporting mammography programmes. A central challenge for all professionals involved in mammography screening has been formulated by the British Charity Breakthrough Breast Cancer in 2001 as follows: it is not the question anymore whether we do mammography screening but it is the question how we do it. This challenge involves information, skilled technique, appropriate invitation and follow-up and the development of technical equipment.

In many European countries, the new digital method for mammography is being implemented today. It promises to overcome many of the limitations of conventional film mammography, especially in women with dense breast tissue, because it provides more detailed and specific information about the tissue. Digital data can be used for computer-enhanced image analysis and allows transmission of data as electrical signals by telephone lines (teleradiology) to experts for image interpretation in other places. Digital mammography not only provides better information but also requires slightly reduced doses of X-rays.

OVARIAN CANCER SCREENING

Ovarian cancer is the most common gynaecological malignancy in developed countries, with about twice the incidence of cervical cancer. A 17-fold range in 5-year survival rates between tumours diagnosed when confined to a single ovary (Stage FIGO Ia) and those with distant metastasis (Stage FIGO IV) has been observed.[25] Unfortunately, women remain asymptomatic for a long time, and therefore in most patients ovarian cancer presents at a late clinical stage and is associated with a low 5-year survival of approximately 35%. Screening for early signs remains difficult.

Screening for ovarian cancer, therefore, is not done for the general population due to the lack of inadequate sensitivity and specificity of currently available screening tests.[26] The need is especially acute in high-risk women, e.g. those with a family history of the disease or who are carriers of a deleterious mutation in a cancer predisposition gene that predisposes for the development of ovarian cancer. Current strategies used to screen biannually or annually for ovarian cancer in high risk-populations include measuring the cancer antigen 125 (CA 125), a biomarker for the disease in the serum, in conjunction with transvaginal ultrasound. A National Institutes of Health Consensus Conference on Ovarian Cancer recommended screening for ovarian cancer only in women presumed to be at risk for a hereditary cancer syndrome that predisposes for ovarian cancer.[27] Research continues on new methods to screen for ovarian cancer. In February of 2002, Petricoin and colleagues reported on the use of a new technology, proteomic pattern technology, as a potential screening tool for ovarian cancer.[28,28a] Although very preliminary, this technology was able to discriminate a cluster pattern in a masked test set of 116 serum samples that completely segregated cancer from non-cancer. Further investigation is required to increase the sensitivity and specificity of this or any other new screening technology, to a

Table 9.1: Summary of recommendations for breast cancer screening in 22 countries					
	Age groups		Screening interval		Detection method
	Lower limit	Upper limit	Age 40–49	Age 50+	
International network					
Australia	40	69	2	2	MM
Canada	50	69	1	2	MM BCE BSE
Finland	50	59	NA	2	MM
Hungary	50	64	NA	1	MM CBE
Iceland	40	69	2	2	MM CBE
Israel	50	74	1 high risk	2	MM
Italy	50	69	NA	2	MM
Japan	30	None	1	1	CBE BSE
The Netherlands	50	69	NA	2	MM
Sweden	40–50[a]	64–74	1.5	2	MM
United Kingdom	50	64	NA	3	MM
United States	40-50	None	1	1–2	MM CBE BSE
Uruguay	45	None	1	2	MM CBE BSE
European network					
Belgium	50	69	NA	2	MM
Denmark	50	69	NA	2	MM
France	50	65-69	NA	2–3	MM
Germany[b]	50	None	1 high risk	2	MM
Greece	40	64/none	2	2	MM CBE BSE
Ireland	50	65	NA	2	MM
Luxembourg	50	65	NA	2	MM CBE
Portugal	40	None	[c]	2	MM
Spain	45	64	2	2	MM

NA = not applicable.
[a]Different between countries.
[b]Not implemented 1995.
[c]No recommendation.
Source: from Shapiro et al.[24]

level that is suitable for screening in both the high-risk and the general population.[29,30]

Ovarian cancer screening in high-risk populations is usually linked to breast cancer screening, because genetically associated cancer of the breast can be related to a higher risk for ovarian cancer. Cervical cancer screening should be an integral part of a woman's prevention programme, whether she is at high or at average risk.

CERVIX CANCER SCREENING

Cervical cancer is the most common cancer in women in developing countries and the fourth most common in Europe and North America. Impressive differences were observed in incidence rates, with 9.9 per 100,000 women in North America and 46.8 per 100,000 women in Southern Africa.[31,31a,31b] Mortality rates are high in tropical South America, with age-standardized rates of 17.4 per 100,000, whereas in European areas they are between 3.8 and 5.1 per 100,000 women with the exception of Eastern Europe, with a rate of 8.8 per 100,000.[32] These figures emphasize the impact of sociocultural influences on incidence and mortality of cervical cancer and the need for culturally and socially adapted cancer prevention methods.

Cervix cancer was the first malignancy for which an effective method of screening was introduced and the benefits in terms of reduction of invasive cancer (and subsequent mortality) are generally accepted, although, due to ethical considerations, never subjected to evaluation via a randomized controlled trial.[33] It can be demonstrated that opportunistic screening (see screening principles) does help the individual woman but that it is less effective – in terms of cost and effectiveness – than optimization of a screening programme, which requires a high level of coverage, with regular tests at defined intervals in the age groups at highest risk.[34]

Primary prevention of cervical cancer is linked to the reduction of risk factors, such as early age at first intercourse, a history of multiple sexual partners, smoking, poor nutrition and a history of genital human papillomavirus (HPV) or sexually transmitted disease.[35]

Secondary prevention through screening methods aims at detecting lesions in the precancerous state before the onset of invasive cancer. Rates for carcinoma in situ reach a peak for women between 20 and 30 years of age. Invasive cervical cancer is the final stage of a continuous disease process, in which dysplasia arises in a normal cervical epithelium and progresses through carcinoma in situ to invasive cancer. Early changes are referred to as squamous intraepithelial lesions (SIL) or cervical intraepithelial neoplasia (CIN), and these are divided into low- or high-grade SIL or CIN 1, 2 and 3 that reflect increasingly abnormal changes of the affected epithelium.[36] A total mean duration in the preclinical, non-invasive state of progressive disease has been estimated at 10 years[37] but there is a small subset of rapidly progressive cervical cancers which are diagnosed within 3 years of a confirmed negative Papanicolaou (Pap) test, occurring mainly in younger women.[38] Preinvasive lesions can persist, regress or progress to invasive malignancy.[39] They can be diagnosed with a Pap smear, the Pap test.

The Pap (Papanicolaou) test as cervical screening method

This test was developed in the 1930s by George Papanicolaou who had earlier observed malignant changes in vaginal smears taken from patients with cervical cancers. In the late 1940s it was realized that sampling from the uterine cervix was more efficient than taking a vaginal smear and also that the presence of carcinoma in situ could also be identified in the samples, thus identifying the cervical smear as a potential screening test.[40] The Pap smear has been established as an inexpensive, reliable test. The greater the number of negative tests a women has had, the lower her risk of developing cervical cancer. Sensitivity of the method has been studied in the Netherlands, where it was 83% for carcinoma in situ or invasive cancer.[41]

After inserting the speculum in the vagina, the clinician gently scrapes the entire circumference of the external cervical area to harvest cells. The specimen is then quickly spread on a glass slide and rapidly fixed with a cytofixative to avoid air-drying artefact. It is widely accepted that for a smear to be adequate, endocervical cells must be present, as an indicator that the correct region has been sampled. In many countries, especially developing countries, nurses are involved in taking the smears. Meticulous technique in obtaining a Pap smear is essential in reducing false-negative results.

Specialized cytotechnicians look for abnormalities associated with CIN or dysplasia. A commonly used system of reporting Pap tests is the Bethesda System. The cytological terms used are low- and high-grade squamous intraepithelial lesions (LSIL and HSIL) and they correlate with the histopathological diagnosis of CIN 1 and CIN 2–3, respectively.[36] Quality control is still a major issue and usually involves some form of double reading of a sample of slides.[42]

By instructing women about practical aspects in preparing for a Pap smear, all nurses can help to support sensitivity of the test. The most important issues for women to be aware of when preparing for a Pap test are summarized in Box 9.3.

Alternative tests have been described. The ThinPrep Pap smear cytopathology allows professionals to collect the sample as a cell suspension in a liquid medium, which is credited with decreasing the number of smears that are unsatisfactory because of obscuring artefacts[43]

and offers increased accuracy. Colposcopy is the usual method of evaluating a cervix following the report of an abnormal Pap smear. Other tests – such as the acetic acid test, cervicography or Schiller's test – have also been described but have not been shown to be useful or cost-effective for screening in general.

Cervical screening recommendations

Cervical screening should not only reduce mortality but also reduce the incidence of invasive cancer. It has been shown that the rate of invasive cervix cancer in women aged 35–64 years old could be reduced by 93.5% with screening every year, by 92.5% with screening every second year and by 90.8% with screening every third year.[44] These impressive figures represent safe ground for nurses on which to educate women about the effectiveness of cervical cancer prevention and to actively engage in promoting screening. The theory behind cervical screening recommendations involves the natural history of cervical cancer and the risk factors. Recommendations are summarized in Box 9.4.

The accessibility of the cervix to examination provides a unique opportunity to evaluate disease status and response to intervention.

Box 9.3

Informing women for the Pap test
Women should:
• not be menstruating
• not have a vaginal douche before the test
• not have intercourse a day before the test
• not use tampons or intravaginal medication a day before the test
• document data of last menstrual period
• prepare information about hormonal medication
• report prior disease and treatment.

Box 9.4

Cervical screening recommendations
• Regular gynaecological examination and Pap test for all women at the onset of sexual activity or by the age of 18 years approximately if not sexually active.[36]
• Three-yearly screening has been suggested after two normal Pap tests with little additional benefit associated with more frequent screening.[40]
• Upper age limit at which screening should be discontinued remains unclear and may be subject of personal preferences and financial resources.[52]
• Screening for women above the age of 60 years old who have never been screened before seems to be of value, although the low uptake of screening in older women has led to questions of cost-effectiveness.[53]

Thorough follow-up of women with premalignant lesions is part of the screening programme. Different therapeutic interventions include cryosurgery, loop electrosurgical excision, cold knife conization, laser vaporization. Despite the treatment of intraepithelial lesions, the risk of cancer remains elevated above that of the general population and warrants careful follow-up for at least 8–10 years.[45] Nurses may have a special role in supporting women through periods of anxiety and in fostering hope through information and knowledge about the expected, positive outcome.

COLON CANCER SCREENING

Colorectal cancer is a major cause of illness in North America, Western Europe, Australia and New Zealand.[31a] It is the third most common malignancy in both men and women in the industrialized countries. In 2003, it is estimated that nearly 148,000 new cases will be diagnosed in the USA[18] and it was estimated that in the 18 European member states in 1995 around 198,000 new cases occurred.[46] Colorectal cancer is uncommon before the age of 50 years old but incidence increases rapidly from this age onwards and according to this, the average risk population is defined as individuals over 50 years old.

Colorectal cancer can be cured by detection of early-stage cancer and therefore fulfils the conditions required for mass screening. Screening can prevent the occurrence of colorectal cancer by detection and removing precancerous polyps or can diagnose early disease at a stage when it can be effectively treated. Despite the effectiveness of several existing screening tests, the use of such tests for prevention remains low. An overview of current tests for screening for colorectal cancer and screening recommendations are presented in Table 9.2. The USPSTF recently updated its screening recommendations for colorectal cancer:[23] they strongly recommend that clinicians screen men and women aged 50 years old or older who are at average risk for colorectal cancer. For patients at a higher risk (e.g. those who have a first-degree relative with colorectal cancer), it is proposed to begin screening at a younger age. The European Group for Colorectal Cancer Screening recommends to implement screening in asymptomatic, average-risk adults aged 50 years old and over.[46] The French Consensus Conference on Colorectal Cancer concluded that individuals with an affected first-degree relative under 50 years old, or with two affected first-degree relatives, were at higher risk, and that in this population a screening colonoscopy was advisable.[47]

There are insufficient data to determine which particular screening strategy is best in terms of balance of benefits and harms or cost-effectiveness at this time. The choice of screening strategy should be based on patient preferences, medical contraindications, patient adherence and resources for testing and follow-up.[23] New technology is evolving and virtual colonoscopy, computed tomography (CT) or magnetic resonance imaging (MRI), and colonography have all been reported as promising methods for the future. Acceptability has been suggested to be a potential major advantage; however, sensitivity and specificity as well as cost-effectiveness needs to be further examined before its use in mass screening.[48]

There are many clinical considerations that relate to decisions concerning screening. Patients are advised to discuss benefits vs potential harms with their healthcare provider, including level of risk and recommended age to begin screening. Speaking about your own colon and rectum may, however, be difficult for many, as it may still be perceived as a taboo and nurses need to consider this when teaching about colon cancer prevention.

There is no definitive information on when screening should be stopped, although the risk for colorectal cancer continues to increase as men and women age. The benefits of screening should be weighed against existing co-morbid conditions and the potential that the man or woman may die from these conditions.

PROSTATE CANCER SCREENING

Prostate cancer is the most common malignancy among men in the Western world. International comparison shows that incidence rates were highest in US blacks, with 91.2, and

Table 9.2: Evaluation of colorectal cancer screening

Test	Advantages	Characteristics/limitations	Cost	Screening recommendation
Faecal occult blood test (FOBT)	No bowel preparation Can be performed in the home No direct adverse effects Proven effective in clinical trials	Will miss most polyps and some cancer May produce false-positive test requiring further work-up Pre-test dietary restrictions Must be done annually Most effective when combined with flexible sigmoidoscopy every 5 years	Low	Beginning at age 50, both men and women at average risk, FOBT should be done annually Best used in combination with flexible sigmoidoscopy every 5 years
Flexible sigmoidoscopy	Minimal bowel preparation Done every 5 years Minimal discomfort Does not require a specialist, and can be done by non-physician providers with specialized training Some clinical trials suggest mortality reduction	In general, views only one-third to one-half of the colon Cannot remove all polyps Small risk of infection, bleeding or bowel tears More effective when combined with annual FOBT Additional procedures required if abnormalities detected	Moderate	Beginning at age 50, both men and women at average-risk, flexible sigmoidoscopy should be performed every 5 years Most effective when combined with annual FOBT

| Colonoscopy | Can view the entire colon
Can biopsy and remove polyps
Done every 10 years
Can diagnose other disease
Trials have demonstrated good evidence for detection of adenomas and cancers, some have shown reduction in mortality | Highest complexity
Full bowel preparation required
Requires sedation of some kind
Generally requires specialists
Can miss small polyps
Potential risk of bowel tears, bleeding or infection | Highest costs | Beginning at age 50, both men and women at average-risk colonoscopy should be performed every 10 years |
| Double-contrast barium enema | Can generally view the entire colon
Few complications
Done every 5 years
No sedation required
Reduction in mortality unknown
Sensitivity for cancer or large polyps approximately 48% | Can miss some small polyps and cancer
Full bowel preparation is required
False-positive results may be obtained and will require further testing | Moderate | Beginning at age 50, both men and women at average risk, double-contrast barium enema is recommend every 5 years |

Source: United States Preventive Services Taskforce.[72]

lowest in the Far East, with 1.8 in China and 5.1 in Japan, per 100,000 men.[49] Canada, USA (whites), Switzerland and Sweden are among the countries with the highest rates of incidence, even though they have only about half of the risk of US blacks.[50] In 2003, it is estimated that over 220,900 new cases of prostate cancer will be diagnosed in the USA.[18,49] Incidence rates remain significantly higher in black men than in white men. It is primarily a disease of the elderly, with 73% of new cases in men over the age of 70 years old.[50] It is known that there is a wide range of growth rates in prostate cancer, with subsets of rapidly growing cancers as well as with subsets of relatively slowly growing latent cancers, which adds to the problems of length-time bias for screening interventions (see screening principles). Some major issues in the prostate screening debate are described as a lack of sensitive screening methods, overdiagnosis, side-effects of treatment and costs. However, this major health problem continues to exist, and further research is needed to develop effective screening strategies.

The traditional methods of screening for prostate cancer are digital rectal examination (DRE) and measurement of prostate-specific antigen (PSA) levels in the serum. Large-scale research studies have evaluated the efficacy of these methodologies in recent years, yet screening remains controversial as there is a lack of definitive evidence of benefit, as well as a lack of consensus regarding optimal treatment of localized disease. The American Cancer Society (ACS),[49] in addition to the American Urological Association and the National Comprehensive Cancer Network, continues to recommend that patients be offered screening beginning at 50 years old with the PSA test, together with DRE on an annual basis. ACS specifies that men to be screened should have a life expectancy of at least 10 years, and in men at high risk (e.g. those with a family history in a first-degree relative or who are African-American), screening should begin at 45 years old. All organizations recommend that discussion of benefits and limitations of testing should occur. Many major scientific and medical organizations, such as the USPSTF, American College of Physicians, American Society of Internal Medicine, National Cancer Institute, Centers for Disease Control and Prevention, American Academy of Family Physicians and American College of Preventive Medicine do not advocate routine testing for prostate cancer. The third edition of the USPSTF report was completed on 2003. However, it has also been concluded that recent declines in mortality in the USA, and to a lesser degree in the European Union, are suggestive of the favourable impact of screening and early diagnosis on prostate cancer mortality, and it should be carefully monitored over the next few years.[51]

LUNG CANCER SCREENING: FUTURE TRENDS

Current research focuses mainly on the value of spiral (or helical) CT scanning as a screening tool for lung cancer. Despite advances in therapy, the worldwide survival rate for lung cancer is approximately 14%.[54] Although some studies find promising results and suggest that CT could be employed for lung cancer screening,[55,56,56a,57,57a,58] others disagree with this approach.[59]

CT can detect small-size tumours potentially in early stages of development. Cancers detected at stages I and II hold better prognoses and existing CT technology provides a quick, detailed, low-risk and fairly low discomfort method of early detection. CT provides an early detection rate that is 300–900% greater than chest X-rays.[54] Proponents of CT as a screening tool cite results from the Early Lung Cancer Action Project (ELCAP)[60,61] and studies from Japan.[55,62,63,64] The ELCAP screened 1000 asymptomatic smokers and detected 27 lung cancers, 85% in stage I.[61,65] The ELCAP results led to larger-scale projects with the same protocol: the New York ELCAP (http://www.nyelcap.org/) and the International ELCAP (http://www.ielcap.org/). Nawa et al[55] used low-dose spiral CT during annual health examinations to screen for lung cancer and found primary lung cancer in 40 patients (0.44% of all participants at baseline; 0.07% from repeat screening), 35 of whom had stage I tumours.

Thus, CT screening proponents claim that, with early diagnosis, preservation of lung function is more likely and could potentially be life-saving. Additionally, CT screening protocols include incentives for smoking cessation.[66]

Opponents of CT screening agree with the benefits of early detection, but note that, with currently available information, it is too soon to recommend CT as a routine screening tool for lung cancer. They raise several concerns: no change in disease-specific mortality despite an improvement in 5-year survival rates; potential for lead-time bias (i.e. earlier diagnosis with unchanged time of death); and current CT studies have no control group. Critics are concerned that, in the end, it will be proven that CT can detect tumours at early stages, but this will provide no additional benefit in reducing mortality. Other concerns are the potential for overdiagnosis (detection of tumours that would have remained subclinical), the detection of false-positive tumours and the performance of unnecessary biopsies,[58,59] although supporters argue that overdiagnosis is rare in lung cancer.[56]

Another factor to be considered is cost. Even if screening targets only those at the highest end of the risk continuum – heavy, long-term smokers, etc. – such an approach could still miss many at-risk individuals, and it is questionable if population-level screening would produce cost-beneficial results.[67] Although physicians and clinics could benefit from large-scale screening, governments and health insurers would have to bear the costs. Another concern is that the cost of providing screening for smokers would, in many cases, be greater than the budget allocated to tobacco control initiatives. Screening possibilities have to be weighed against the benefits of a comprehensive, well-funded tobacco control programme that includes prevention and cessation programmes. Therefore, despite the logical appeal of lung cancer screening and early detection, findings are still ambiguous and no policy guidelines have been established. The final investment decision may be a political-ideological one: screening for lung cancer might receive more support under a medical model than it would under a public health model. The latter would favour cessation and prevention as parts of a comprehensive tobacco control programme.

DIAGNOSTIC METHODS IN SECONDARY CANCER PREVENTION /EARLY DETECTION

MAMMOGRAPHY

Mammography is an X-ray examination of the breasts to detect abnormalities that may be breast cancer. Modern mammography is performed on dedicated equipment designed to produce a high-quality image with a low X-ray dose. Two views are generally used in a screening examination: the cephalo-caudal (CC) view and a medio-lateral oblique (MLO) view. The quality of screening examinations has improved over the years through improved equipment that supply a high-quality image with a minimum X-ray dose, training of personnel through professional societies and programmes and legislation requiring minimum standards. In the USA, in 1992, the passage of the Mammography Quality Standards Act (MQSA) required that facilities meet a broad range of technical and personnel standards in order to be certified by the Food and Drug Administration (FDA). The National Cancer Institute provides the public with information about local FDA-certified mammography facilities through the Cancer Information Services hotline at 1–800–4–CANCER (1–800–422–6237). (Also, a list of these facilities is on the FDA's website at http://www.fda.gov/cdrh/mammography/certified.html.)

In October 2001, a report in the scientific literature re-awakened the debate on the value of screening mammography.[68] This analysis, performed by The Cochrane Collaboration and published in *The Lancet* reviewed the large, long-term mammography trials upon which the National Cancer Institute and other groups had based their recommendations and guidelines concerning mammography screening. The review cited possible flaws in the conduct of the trial and methods used to analyse the data. The most serious problems concerned the assembly and maintenance of comparable groups, methods for ascertaining

183

outcomes and generalizability to routine practice. This publication asserted that the studies did not support a benefit from mammography. This publication stirred up much controversy and even had a deleterious impact on screening development in some countries. Numerous breast cancer experts worldwide addressed the publication. It was concluded by many that the article was misleading and scientifically unfounded.[69] The available evidence on breast cancer screening was also evaluated in Lyons by a working group convened by the International Agency for Research on Cancer (IARC) of the World Health Organization in March 2002. This group, consisting of 24 experts from 11 countries, concluded that trials have provided sufficient evidence for the efficacy of mammography screening of women between 50 and 69 years old.[70] The National Cancer Institute (NCI) in the USA, the US Department of Health and Human Services, and the USPSTF all continued to be supportive of the use of screening mammography yet recognized the analysis of the information surrounding mammography is complex, and requires evaluation of new data from studies underway. The NCI is committed to looking beyond the debate over the limitations of current data and to accelerating the development of better screening tools.[71]

Any screening test has limitations. Mammography is estimated to miss approximately 10–15% of cancers, with sensitivity being lower in women less than 50 years old who have denser breasts or who are taking hormone replacement therapy.[72]

Cervix cancer screening – diagnostic methods

For more information about the Papanicolaou test, see previous section.

COLORECTAL CANCER SCREENING – DIAGNOSTIC METHODS

The primary screening methods used for colorectal cancer screening are FOBT, direct visualization of the colon through endoscopy (e.g. proctoscopy, flexible sigmoidoscopy or total colonoscopy) and double-contrast barium enema (DCBE). Table 9.2 reviews each methods, and the advantages and disadvantages of each. The goal of screening is to detect cancers at the earliest stages, when it is most curable, or to remove polyps, especially adenomatous polyps, which are considered precursors of cancer.

Faecal occult blood test

The least sensitive of colorectal screening methods is FOBT, with an estimated sensitivity ranging from 50% to 90% for a one-time test.[73] Factors that impact on sensitivity and specificity are the type of occult blood test used, whether or not the specimen is rehydrated with a drop of water prior to testing, how the specimen was collected, the number of samples collected per test and the quality of interpretation. Dietary and medication restrictions are generally recommended (e.g. no red meats, poultry, fish, raw vegetables, vitamin C, aspirin or other non-steroidal anti-inflammatory drugs (NSAIDs) to optimize results with FOBT. Randomized trials in both Europe and the USA have shown reductions in the risk of death from colorectal cancer from a low of 15% to a high of 33%.[72]

Flexible sigmoidoscopy, colonoscopy, double-contrast barium enema

Endoscopy allows for direct visualization of the colon and the removal and pathological evaluation of polyps. Flexible sigmoidoscopy allows for only partial visualization of the colon, but requires less preparation prior to the examination and generally no patient sedation. Colonoscopy yields a total colon examination, yet requires thorough bowel preparation and patient sedation. It is also considerably more costly than sigmoidoscopy. An issue related to the use of endoscopy as a screening method for colorectal cancer is the expanding need for this service and a lack of qualified, trained personnel to perform the service. The competent performance of flexible sigmoidoscopy requires both cognitive and technical skills such as knowledge of anatomy, physiology and pathology of the colon and abdomen and indications/contraindications for screening flexible sigmoidoscopy. In many settings, highly trained nurses, generally advanced practice nurses, are used to perform this procedure, and current research and practice publications illustrate the safety, accuracy and support for the performance of routine screening flexible sigmoidoscopy by registered nurses.[74]

DCBE is an X-ray examination of the bowel that uses a combination of barium contrast and instilled air. This test is preferred over the single-contrast (no air) study because of its better ability to detect smaller lesions and polyps. It requires a thorough bowel prep, which is critical to test sensitivity and specificity – which have been reported in the range of 85–95% and 95–99%, repectively.[75] Most studies of DCBE to determine accuracy have important limitations, and to date, no trial has examined the ability of DCBE to reduce mortality from colorectal cancer.

Research continues to determine new methods of screening for colorectal cancer. One method currently being advertised to the public is the use of CT holography, or 'virtual colonoscopy'. The procedure is appealing because it is non-invasive, yet produces images of the colon lumen, can be performed in about 10–15 minutes and currently requires preparation similar to that used for colonoscopy. Early reports have demonstrated sensitivity and specificity in the range of 85–90% in the research setting; studies have not yet examined clinical outcomes with CT holography screening.[76,77] Another non-invasive approach being investigated is the use of molecular techniques to screen faecal DNA for mutations that may signal an increased risk for developing cancer or the presence of cancer. There is a compelling biological rationale to target DNA alterations exfoliated from cancers into stool, and multiple DNA markers would need to be assayed because of the genetic heterogeneity of colorectal neoplasia. Early clinical studies assessing multiple markers suggest high sensitivity for both colorectal cancer and premalignant adenomatous polyps while maintaining high specificity; however, large-scale clinical studies are clearly warranted to corroborate the early results.[78]

DIAGNOSTIC SCREENING METHODS FOR PROSTATE CANCER

Three main methods currently in use for prostate cancer screening are DRE, transrectal ultrasound (TRUS) and PSA testing. Table 9.3 outlines the advantages and disadvantages of each of these screening methodologies. Prior to the 1990s, DRE was the test traditionally used for screening; however, currently, it is generally used in combination with PSA testing. Imaging with TRUS is generally used for diagnostic work-up of an abnormal screening test only due to its low sensitivity and specificity.[79] To date, screening remains controversial due to a lack of definitive evidence of benefit. Variables that remain under consideration are the PSA cutoff level, where biopsy would be indicated and the frequency of screening.

Two large trials are currently in progress to determine whether screening can reduce mortality from prostate cancer. The Prostate, Lung, Colorectal and Ovarian (PLCO) cancer screening trial is in progress by the Division of Cancer Prevention, National Cancer Institute, Bethesda, Maryland, USA. One objective of the PLCO trial is to determine whether screening men aged 55–74 years old with DRE and PSA can reduce mortality from prostate cancer. A secondary objective is to assess screening variables other than mortality for each of the interventions, including sensitivity, specificity and positive predictive value. The design is a multicenter, two-armed, randomized trial. More than 12,000 participants were enrolled in the pilot phase (concluded in September 1994). Changes in eligibility criteria followed and the trial closed accrual in September 2001 with nearly 155,000 men and women. Although the recruitment phase is complete, PLCO will continue to collect and analyse essential health data from participants to determine if certain cancer screening practices reduce the number of deaths from prostate, lung, colorectal and ovarian cancer. In the intervention arm, the PSA test is performed at entry, then annually for 5 years. The DRE is performed at entry and annually for 3 years. Patients will be followed for a total of 13 years.

Table 9.3: Advantages/disadvantages of prostate cancer screening methods

Tests	Advantages	Limitations	Costs	Screening recommendations
Digital rectal examination (DRE)	Inexpensive Relatively non-invasive Can be taught to a variety of healthcare professionals Non-morbid	Effectiveness depends on the skill and experience of the examiner Reduction in cancer mortality has yet to be determined Abnormal results may require further work-up, biopsy for potentially benign conditions May miss cancers in non-palpable areas of the prostate or smaller, earlier cancers	Low	Offered annually beginning at age 50 to men who have a life expectancy of 50 years. Men at higher risk should begin testing at age 45 years
Prostate-specific antigen (PSA)	Simple Objective Reproducible Relative lack of invasiveness Can detect early cancers Strong sensitivity Clinical trials have demonstrated effectiveness, trials in progress assessing reductions in mortality	False-positive results require further work-up and potential biopsy Imperfect specificity (benign conditions may cause abnormal readings)	Relatively low	Offered annually beginning at age 50 to men who have a life expectancy of 50 years. Men at higher risk should begin testing at age 45 years
Transrectal ultrasound (TRUS)	Primary role as a diagnostic tool Useful for directing prostate needle biopsy Useful for measuring gland dimensions and volume	Low sensitivity and specificity for use as a screening tool	Moderate	No recommendation for use as a screening tool

Source: National Cancer Institute.[49]

The European Randomized Screening for Prostate Cancer (ERSPC) trial is also currently under way, and is aimed as assessing whether screening reduces prostate cancer mortality. Seven European countries are participating in this trial. The principal screening method is DRE, but some centres are also using PSA. As of January 2002, recruitment had reached 163,126 men aged 55–69 years old at entry. It is expected that the trials will have the power to show definitive results in 2005–2008.[80,81] More information about the PSA test can be found in the next section on laboratory aspects of screening for cancer.

LABORATORY ASPECTS OF SCREENING FOR CANCER: TUMOUR MARKERS

Anatomical pathology involves cytology and histology laboratories for the investigation of biopsies: needle aspirates or resection specimens are required for a definitive diagnosis of the disease process (i.e. to label it with an exact name and to classify it according to internationally agreed systems). Laboratory tests, involving tests on blood, urine or other body substances, are used to screen for disease risk, for early detection or confirming a disease and monitoring disease remission or progression. This section focuses on tumour markers as a method of early detection.

Tumour markers are substances secreted by the malignant cells into the peripheral blood. Only some type of cancer cells secrete such markers and this determines and limits their use in cancer screening and treatment. Specific markers are generally used in association with breast and ovarian cancer and colon and prostate cancer. However, the use of tumour markers for screening and early detection in asymptomatic individuals is generally still limited to the PSA in prostate cancer and ovarian cancer, where it is considered to have potential screening utility.

The prostate-specific antigen

Serum PSA exists in both free form and complexed to a number of protease inhibitors. Assays for total PSA measure both free and complexed forms. Several studies have addressed whether complexed PSA or per cent free PSA (ratio of free to total) might be more sensitive and specific than total PSA. This may be especially useful in evaluating the 'gray zone' of total PSA, the range from 2.5 to 10 ng/ml. The use of PSA density is another strategy. Reports have suggested indexing PSA to gland volume by using a measure known as PSA density (i.e. serum PSA divided by gland volume). This approach requires ultrasound to measure the gland volume. Another type of adjustment that may be used is PSA density of the transition zone. These two tests would hopefully adjust for benign sources of PSA increase and may lead to a decrease in biopsies that ultimately prove benign. PSA levels increase with age, and some series have evaluated whether age-adjusted PSA might be useful to reduce the false-positive screenings.

CA 125

Serum CA 125 is a widely used tumour marker in clinical practice with the aim of revealing the presence of a recurrence of ovarian cancer before it is clinically apparent. CA 125 was developed by raising a monoclonal antibody in an ovarian cancer cell line. The antibody reacts with a cell surface antigen on many histological types of non-mucinous epithelial ovarian tumours. In women with a diagnosis of ovarian cancer, CA 125 levels are elevated above 35 U/ml in over 80%[82] and there is a clear correlation between the CA 125 level and the stage of the disease, indicating that sensitivity will be lower in less advanced tumours. This leads to the question whether the marker is sensitive enough for screening asymptomatic women. The answer is that studies have suggested that CA 125 would be a sensitive screening test for women with ovarian cancer at a treatable stage.[83] However, to be clinically useful, CA 125 needs to be turned into predictive values; the likelihood that the test will be positive needs to be considered. Elevated CA 125 levels are more likely to be associated with ovarian cancer in postmenopausal women or in younger women with a strong family history of ovarian cancer, as disease prevalence in these two groups is higher that in women generally. This is the reason why the test is used as a screening method in defined groups, especially in women with first-degree relatives with ovarian cancer because they are at higher risk of developing the cancer. In this situation, the test is usually performed together with endovaginal ultrasound, biannually or annually, according to the risk status of the women.

Only few unaffected women (less than 5%) have elevated CA 125 levels (false positive).[83] This can be observed in the presence of benign disease of the reproductive and digestive tract as well as cancers at various other sites. Benign ovarian tumours, endometriosis and liver cirrhosis are benign conditions, seldomly associated with raised levels of CA 125.

This chapter has dealt with principles of secondary prevention, early detection, screening and some technologies involved in such programmes. If pathological findings require further attention, specific diagnostic procedures are warranted and, if cancer is diagnosed, cancer staging follows.

REFERENCES

1. Moss S. General principles of cancer screening. In: Chamberlain J, Moss S, eds. Evaluation of cancer screening. London: Springer Verlag; 1996:1–13.

2. Mahon SM. Principles of cancer prevention and early detection. Clin J Oncol Nurs 2000; 4(4):169–176.

3. World Health Organization. National cancer control programmes: policies and managerial guidelines. 2nd ed. Geneva: World Health Organization; 2002.

4. Hakama M. Planning and designing of screening programmes. In: Sankila R, Démaret E, Hakama M et al, eds. Evaluation and monitoring of screening programmes. European Commission, Luxembourg: Office for Official Publications of the European Communities; 2001:13–28.

5. Trapkin L. Pathology and the clinical laboratory in cancer control. In: Jennings J, Mahon S, eds. Cancer prevention, detection and control: a nursing perspective. Pittsburgh: Oncology Nursing Society; 2002:143–172.

6. Carroll-Johnson RM, ed. Cancer prevention and early detection: oncology nursing's next frontier. Oncol Nurs Forum 2000; 27(Suppl. 9):1–61.

7. Foltz A. Issues in determining cancer screening recommendations: who, what and when. Oncol Nurs Forum 2000; 27(Suppl 9):13–17.

8. Sankila R, Démaret E, Hakama M et al, eds. Evaluation and monitoring of screening programmes. European Commission, Luxembourg: Office for Official Publications of the European Communities; 2001:233–241.

9. Sankila R. Lessions learned from neuroblastoma screening. In: Sankila R, Démaret E, Hakama M, et al. Evaluation and monitoring of screening programmes. European Commission, Luxembourg: Office for Official Publications of the European Communities; 2001:233–243.

10. McPherson CP, Swenson KK, Lee MW. The effects of mammographic detection and comorbidity on the survival of older women with breast cancer. J Geriatr Soc 2002; 50(6): 1061–1068.

11. Barratt AL, Les Irwig M, Glasziou PP, Salkeld GP, Houssami N. Benefits, harms and costs of screening mammography in women 70 years and over: a systematic review. Med J Aust 2002; 176(6):266–271.

12. National Cancer Institute. Clinical trials and insurance coverage: a resource guide. Retrieved August 1999.
http://www.cancertrials.nci.nih.gov/ NCI_CANCER_TRIALS/zones/TrialInfo/ Deciding/insurance.html.

13. Chamberlaine J, Moss S. Evaluation of cancer screening. London: Springer Verlag; 1996:11.

14. Grecco K. Genetic counselling and screening. In: Jennings K, Mahon S, eds. Cancer prevention, detection and control: a nursing perspective. Pittsburgh: Oncology Nursing Society; 2002:762.

15. Smith RA, Mettlin CJ, Davis KJ, Eyre H. American Cancer Society guidelines for the early detection of cancer. CA Cancer J Clin 2000; 50:34–49.

16. Gordis L. Epidemiology. 2nd edn. Philadelphia: WB Saunders; 2000.

17. Office of Population Censuses and Surveys. 1987 cancer statistics registrations. Series MB1 No 20. London: HMSO; 1993.

18. American Cancer Society 2003: Cancer facts and figures.
http://www.cancer.org/ (see statistics). Retrieved August 2003.

19. Gastrin G, Miller AB, To T, et al. Incidence and mortality from breast cancer in the Mama Program for breast screening in Finland 1973–1986. Cancer 1994; 73:2168–2174.

20. Harvey BJ, Miller AB, Baines CJ, et al. Effect of breast self examination techniques on the risk of death from breast cancer. Can Med Assoc J 1997; 157(9):1205–1212.

21. Thomas DB, Gao DL, Self SG, et al. Randomised trial of breast self-examination in Shanghai: methodology and preliminary results. J Natl Cancer Inst 1997; 89(5):355–365.

22. Bobo JK, Lee NC, Thames SF. Findings from 752,081 clinical breast examinations reported to

a national screening program from 1995 through 1998. J Natl Cancer Inst 2000; 92(12):971–976.

23. United States Preventive Services Task force – http://www.ahrq.gov/clinic/uspstfix.htm Retrieved 08/2003.

24. Shapiro S, Coleman EA, Broeders M, et al. Breast cancer screening programmes in 22 countries: current policies, administration and guidelines. Int J Epidemiol 1998; 27:735–742.

25. Folke P. Annual report on the results of treatment in gynaecological cancer. 20th Volume International Federation of Gynaecology and Obstetrics; 1998.

26. Skates SJ, XuF-J, Yu Y-H, et al. Toward an optimal algorithm for ovarian cancer screening with longitudinal tumor markers. Cancer 1995; 76:2004–2010.

27. Carlson KJ, Skates SJ, Singer DE. Screening for ovarian cacner. Ann Intern Med 1994; 121: 124–132.

28. Petricoin III EF, Ardekani AM, Hitt BA, et al. Use of proteomic patterns in serum to identify ovarian cancer. Lancet 2002; 359:572–577.

28a. Petricoin EF, Mills GB, Kohn EC, et al. Proteomic patterns in serum and identification of ovarian cancer – authors reply. Lancet 2002; 360:170–171.

29. Rockhill B. Proteomic patterns in serum and identification of ovarian cancer – letter. Lancet 2002; 360:169–170.

30. Diamandis EP. Proteomic patterns in serum and identification of ovarian cancer –letter. Lancet 2002; 360:170.

31. Parkin DM, Pisani P Ferley J. Estimates of the world wide incidence of eighteen major cancers in 1985. Int J Cancer 1993; 54:594–606.

31a. Parkin DM, Whelan SL, Ferley J, et al. Cancer incidence in five continents. Vol. VII (IARC Scientific Publications No 143). Lyons: International Agency for Research on Cancer; 1997.

31b. Parkin DM, Whelan SL, Ferlay J, et al. Cancer incidence in five continents. Vol VII (IARC Scientific Publications No 143). Lyons: International Agency for Research on Cancer; 1999.

32. Pisani P, Parkin DM, Ferley J. Estimates of the world wide mortality from eighteen major cancers in 1985. Implications for prevention and projection of future burden. Int J Cancer 1993; 55:981–993.

33. Smith J, Parkin DM. Evaluation and monitoring of screening for cervix cancer: time trends. In: Evaluation and monitoring of screening programmes. Brussels: European Commission; 2001:59–76.

34. Parkin DM. A computer simulation model for the practical planning of cervical cancer screening programmes. Br J Cancer 1985; 51:551–568.

35. Kjaer SK, de Villiers EM, Dahl C, et al. Case control study of risk factors for cervical neoplasia

in Denmark. I: role of the male factor in women with one lifetime sexual partner. Int J Cancer 1991; 48(1):39–44.

36. National Cancer Institute. Screening for cervical screening. Retrieved November 2002. http://www.nci.nih.gov

37. Habbem JDF, Lubbe JTN, van Oortmarssen GJ, et al. A simulation approach to cost-effectiveness and cost-benefit calculations for early detection of disease. Eur J Op Res 1987; 29:159–166.

38. Schwartz PE, Hadjimichael O, Lowell DM, et al. Rapidly progressive cervical cancer: the Connecticut experience. Am J Obstetr Gynecol 1996; 175(4):1105–1109.

39. Barron BA, Richart RM. Statistical model of the natural history of cervical carcinoma. II: estimates of the transition time from dysplasia to carcinoma in situ. J Natl Cancer Inst 1970; 45(5):1025–1030.

40. Chamberlain J, Moss S, eds. Evaluation of cancer screening. Berlin: Springer; 1996:23.

41. Van der Graaf Y, Zielhuis G, Peer P, et al. The effectiveness of cervix screening: a population based case-control study. J Clin Epidemiol 1988; 41:21–26.

42. Moss S. Screening for cancer of the cervix. In: Chamberlain J, Moss S, eds. Evaluation of cancer screening. Berlin: Springer; 1996:15–32.

43. Farley Omerod K. Cervical cancer. In: Jennings K, Mahon S, eds. Cancer prevention, detection and control: a nursing perspective. Pittsburg; Oncology Nursing Society; 2002:539–551.

44. IARC Working Group on Evaluation of Cervical Cancer Screening. Screening for squamous cervical cancer – the duration of low risk following negative results in cervical cytology tests: introduction. In: Hakama M, Miller AB, Day NE, eds. Screening for cancer of the uterine cervix (IARC Scientific Publications No 76). Lyons: International Agency for Research on Cancer; 1986:15–24.

45. Soutter WP, De Barros Lopes A, Fletcher A, et al. Invasive cervical cancer after conservative therapy for cervical intraepithelial neoplasia. Lancet 1997; 349 (9057):978–980.

46. European Group for Colorectal Cancer Screening. Recommendation to include colorectal cancer screening in public health policy. J Med Screening 1999; 6:80–81.

47. Conférence de connsencus. Prévention, dépistage et prise en charge des cancers du colon. Gastroenterol Clin Biol 1998; 22:S275–S288.

48. Fenlon HM, Nunes DP, Schroy PC, et al. A comparison of virtual and conventional colonoscopy for the detection of colorectal polyps. N Engl J Med 1999; 341:1496–1503.

49. National Cancer Institute – Cancer.gov Prostate Cancer (PDQ®): Screening health professional version. http://www.nic.nih.gov/

50. Chamberlain J, Melia J. Screening for prostate cancer. In: Chamberlain J, Moss S, eds. Evaluation of cancer screening. Berlin: Springer; 1996:117.

51. Levi F, Lucchini F, Negri E, et al. Recent trends in prostate cancer mortality in the European Union. Epidemiology 2000; 11:612.

52. Van Wijngaarden WJ, Duncan ID. Rational for stopping cervical screening in women over 50. BMJ 1993; 306:967–991.

53. Fletcher A. Screening for cancer of the cervix in elderly women. Lancet 1990; 335:97–99.

54. Giarelli E. To screen or not to screen: using spiral computerized tomography in the early detection of lung cancer. Clin J Oncol Nurs 2002; 6(4):223–224.

55. Nawa T, Nakagawa T, Kusano S, et al. Lung cancer screening using low-dose spiral CT. Results of baseline and 1-year follow-up studies. Chest 2002; 122:15–20.

56. Grannis FW Jr. Lung cancer screening: conundrum or contumacy? Chest 2002; 122:1–2.

56a. Grannis FW Jr. Lung cancer screening. Who will pick up the tab? Chest 2002; 121(5): 1388–1390.

57. Henschke CI, McCauley DI, Yankelevitz DF, et al. Early lung cancer action project: a summary of the findings on baseline screening. Oncologist 2001; 6(2):147–152.

57a. Henschke CI, Naidich DP, Yankelevitz DF, et al. Early lung cancer action project: initial findings on repeat screenings. Cancer 2001; 92(1):- 153–159.

58. Reich JM. Improved survival and higher mortality: the conundrum of lung cancer screening. Chest 2002; 122:329–337.

59. Woloshin S, Schwartz LM, Gilbert Welch H. Tobacco money: up in smoke? Lancet 2002; 359:2108–2111.

60. Henschke CI, Yankelevitz DF, Mirtcheva R, et al. CT screening for lung cancer: frequency and significance of part-solid and nonsolid nodules. Am J Roentgenol 2002;178(5): 1053–1057.

61. Henschke CI, Yankelevitz DF, Libby DM, et al. Early lung cancer action project: annual screening using single-slice helical CT. Ann NY Acad Sci 2001; 952:124–134.

62. Sone S, LI F, Yang Z, et al. Results of three-year mass screening programme for lung cancer using mobile low-dose spiral computed tomography scanner. Br J Cancer 2001; 84:25–32.

63. Sone S, Li F, Yang Z, et al. Characteristics of small lung cancers invisible on conventional chest radiography and detected by population based screening using spiral CT. Br J Radiol 2000; 73:137–145.

64. Sone S, Takashima S, Li F, et al. Mass screening for lung cancer with mobile spiral computed tomography scanner. Lancet 1998; 351: 1242–1245.

65. Henschke CI, McCauley DI, Yankelevitz DF, et al. Early Lung Cancer Action Project: overall design and findings from baseline screening. Lancet 1999; 354(9173):99–105.

66. Ostroff JS, Buckshee N, Mancuso CA, et al. Smoking cessation following CT screening for early detection of lung cancer. Prev Med 2001; 33(6):613–621.

67. Marshall D, Simpson KN, Earle CC, et al. Economic decision analysis model of screening for lung cancer. Eur J Cancer 2001; 37(14):1759–1767.

68. Gotzsche PC, Olsen O. Is screening for breast cancer with mammography justifiable? Lancet 2000; 355:129–134.

69. Nyström L, Andersson I, Bjurstam N, et al. Long-term effects of mammography screening: updated overview of the Swedish randomised trials. Lancet 2002; 359:909–919.

70. IARC Press Release (19 March 2002) From: http://www.iarc.fr

71. National Cancer Institute – Cancer.gov Breast Cancer (PDQ): Screening health professional version. http://www.nci.nih.gov/cancerinfo/pdq/screening/breast/

72. United States Preventive Services Task force – Updated 7/15/02http://www.ahrq.gov/clinic/3rduspstf/colorectal/

73. Pignone M, Rich M, Teutsch SM, Berg AO, Lohr KN. Screening for colorectal cancer in adults at average risk: a summary of the evidence for the U.S. Preventive Services Task Force. Ann Intern Med 2002; 137(2):132–141.

74. Society of Gastroenterology Nurses and Associates. Performance of flexible sigmoidoscopy by registered nurses for the purpose of colorectal screening. Position statement. 1999. http:// www.sgna.org

75. Connolly DJ, Traill ZC, Reid HS, Copley SJ, Nolan DJ. The double contrast barium enema: a retrospective single centre audit of the detection of colorectal carcinomas. Clin Radiol 2002; 57(1):29–32.

76. Ota A. Virtual endoscopy. Eur J Radiol 2002; 42(3):2231–2239.

77. Fenlon HM, Nunes DP, Schroy PC, et al. A comparison of virtual and conventional colonoscopy for the detection of colorectal polyps. N Engl J Med 1999; 341:1496–1503.

78. Ahlquist DA, Shuber AP. Stool screening for colorectal cancer: evolution from occult blood to molecular marker. Clin Chem Acta 2002; 315(1–2):157–168.

79. National Cancer Institute – Cancer.gov Prostate Cancer (PDQ): screening health professional version. http://www.nic.nih.gov/

80. De Koning HJ, Auvinen A, Berenguer Sanchez A, et al. Large-scale randomized prostate cancer screening trials: program performances in the European Randomized

Screening for Prostate Cancer trial and the Prostate, Lung, Colorectal and Ovary cancer trial. Int J Cancer 2002; 97(2):237–244.

81. Prorok PC, Andriole GL, Bresalier RS, et al. 2000. Design of the Prostate, Lung, Colorectal and Ovarian (PLCO) Canner Screening Trial. Contr Clin Trials 2000; 21(6 Suppl):273S–309S.

82. Cuckle H, Wald N. Screening for ovarian cancer. In: Miller AB, Chamberlain J, Day NE, et al, eds. Cancer screening. Cambridge: Cambridge University Press; 1991:228–239.

83. Zurawski VR, Sjovall K, Schoenfeld DA, et al. Prospective evaluation of serum CA 125 levels in a normal population, phase 1: the specificities of single and serial determinations in testing for ovarian cancer. Gynecol Oncol 1990; 36:299–305.

SECTION 4

Treatment and care

10. Decision-Making in Cancer Care 195

11. The Experience of Cancer Treatment . . 213

12. Surgery 233

13. Radiotherapy. 265

14. Chemotherapy 283

15. Biological Therapy 303

16. Bone Marrow Transplantation 329

17. Hormone Therapy 353

18. Complementary and Alternative
    Therapies. 381

CHAPTER 10

Decision-Making in Cancer Care

ALASTAIR J MUNRO

CHAPTER CONTENTS

Introduction	195
What is a decision?	195
What clinicians do	196
A simple classification for decisions in cancer care and control	196
Psychological approaches to decision-making	196
The logical, or deductive, approach to clinical decision-making	198
Decision analysis	198
The evidence-based approach	199
Computers are no panacea	201
Ethical perspectives on decision-making in oncology	202
Pragmatic or empirical approaches to decision-making	202

A decision can be regarded as a process with three components	202
Inputs	202
Assessing the quality of the decision-making process	205
Problems with assessing the outcomes of decisions	207
What actually happens?	207
Models for decision making by nurses	207
Why did nurses not use findings from research to inform their clinical decisions?	208
Decision aids	208
Nursing in no-man's-land	209
Decision making in cancer care – the future	210
Conclusion	210
References	211

INTRODUCTION

Decision-making is something we all take for granted. It is simply a part of our professional duties and, as such, is not a process that we scrutinize too carefully. However, our decisions have important consequences, not just for ourselves but also for many other people (our patients and their families, our colleagues, future patients and their families, those who pay for health care). These consequences bring with them responsibilities, one of which is to try both to understand and to improve the decision-making process. We have a duty to become more self-aware of how and why we make the decisions we make. This chapter aims to shine light into some of the darker areas of our professional lives: to demonstrate that decision-making is too important, and too all-pervasive, to be taken for granted.

WHAT IS A DECISION?

A decision is something that terminates a process of cogitation; it is the point at which thought moves into action. Ideally, decisions should be informed. An informed decision has been defined as:

> one where a reasoned choice is made by a reasonable individual, using relevant information about the advantages and disadvantages of all the possible courses of action, in accord with the individual's beliefs.[1] (p1)

The problem here is the possible conflict between 'the individual's beliefs' and the 'reasoned choice'.

WHAT CLINICIANS DO

As clinicians, we spend much of our time making decisions. We picture ourselves as people of action: giving chemotherapy; removing tumours; and prescribing radiotherapy. In fact, we probably spend more time thinking about whether and how to do these things than we spend actually doing them. Even a busy cancer surgeon will spend less than 20% of his or her working time actually operating on people.

A SIMPLE CLASSIFICATION FOR DECISIONS IN CANCER CARE AND CONTROL

Decisions can be placed along a spectrum that extends from the prevention of cancer at one extreme to the care of the dying patient at the other. Another perspective would look at the scale upon which decision-making is taking place: from decisions made by individuals to choices made by society as a whole. These two aspects can be combined, as in Figure 10.1, to provide a matrix within which decisions related to cancer might be classified. This schema accommodates virtually all possible decisions: from an individual's decision to stop smoking (top left) to the World Health Organization's decision that opiates, rather than radiotherapy, are the intervention of choice for patients in the developing world with cancer-related pain (bottom right). This scheme illustrates the complexity of decision-making, with the clear implication that there can be no single approach to decision-making that will be sufficient for every circumstance. Perhaps the best way of trying to understand decision-making is through a systematic consideration of the difficulties involved in trying to make sense of the topic.

Each cell in the matrix (Fig. 10.1) can be considered from a variety of perspectives. These viewpoints can be summarized as psychological, logical, ethical and empirical.

PSYCHOLOGICAL APPROACHES TO DECISION-MAKING

Psychologists who examine decision-making can be (crudely) divided into two schools: normative and descriptive. The normative approach implies that there is a correct way to make decisions, that we have this knowledge and, in order to improve decision-making, all we have to do is apply it. The descriptive approach is far less rigid. As a result of observations on how decisions are made we may, or may not, make suggestions as to how matters might be improved. This dichotomy, between normative and descriptive, is artificial. Most psychological approaches to decision-making combine elements of both.

Almost by stealth, the approach to decision-making developed by Tversky and Kahneman[2] has come to dominate the literature on clinical decision-making. The Tversky and Kahneman approach is succinctly summarized as 'heuristics and biases'. Although their approach is mainly descriptive, there is – as witnessed by their use of the term biases – an underlying prescriptive element. Kahneman and Tversky[3] describe 'judgmental heuristics' as a small number of distinct mental processes which are used to mediate intuitive prediction and judgement. Their use of the term 'heuristic' presumably implies that these processes have developed through a process of trial and error. They point out that, on the basis of these 'heuristics', we make decisions: if a politician has an upright and dignified bearing, we decide that he is probably honest. However, our heuristics may be biased and this can lead to problems: not all handsome politicians are honest (e.g. Jeffrey Archer). Much of Kahneman and Tversky's work concerns these biases – where they come from and how to avoid them.

Scale \ time	well	worried well	symptoms	investigation	diagnosis	staging	treatment	follow-up	rehab.	terminal care
individual										
team										
department										
hospital										
trust										
region										
nation										
international										

Figure 10.1: A matrix for classifying decisions in oncology.

We may make decisions based not on how we feel about things at the moment but on how we might feel in the future. I could explain to a patient that, given the low risk of residual disease, adjuvant chemotherapy is unlikely to be of benefit. The patient might still demand chemotherapy saying, 'But what if the disease did come back, I would feel that by chickening out now I had blown my chance of cure'. This is the phenomenon of anticipated regret (sometimes termed the chagrin factor[4]).

Our memories are fallible; our ability to recall is prone to bias. In childhood, it never rains. Our recollections of pain associated with medical procedures such as colonoscopy are dictated by any peak in discomfort and our sensations during the last few moments of the procedure. The overall duration of the experience is only poorly recalled.[5] This knowledge could, potentially, be exploited in order to manipulate decision-making based on patients' recollections of previous clinical experiences. Biases involving memory and recall can be a potent influence on clinical decisions.

THE LOGICAL, OR DEDUCTIVE, APPROACH TO CLINICAL DECISION-MAKING

Put simply, this approach involves applying the scientific method to clinical decision-making. It is, fundamentally, normative. Its most recent incarnation is in the concept of evidence-based practice. Its fullest and most florid expression is found in that repertoire of techniques known as decision analysis.[6]

Decision analysis

Decision analysis is a highly structured approach to decision-making. The construction of a decision tree is the key to a decision analysis. The initial choice is defined and, thereafter, the problem is structured as a series of points (chance nodes) at which mutually exclusive outcomes can be defined. It is simpler to explain the concept graphically. Figure 10.2 shows a decision tree for a simple clinical choice: should a patient with a cancer of the larynx be treated with primary radiotherapy (with surgery reserved for failure of treatment), or should they be treated immediately by laryngectomy? The initial choice is represented by a square (a decision node); the round nodes are chance nodes. Probabilities govern the outcomes at each of the chance (round) nodes. The rule is that, at each of the nodes, the probabilities should add up to 1.0: i.e. they should be mutually exclusive. For example, after surgery there are 4 possibilities and we could assign each a probability: die from complication (0.001); die from disease (0.10); cured (0.85); or die from unrelated cause (0.049). The outcomes are defined at the terminal nodes (triangular in the decision tree shown in Fig. 10.2). Each outcome has a value associated with it. In economic analyses the values are usually monetary; in clinical decision analyses, values are usually expressed in life-years, or quality-adjusted life years (QALYs). In Figure 10.2 only the quality adjustment factors are shown: 0.8 for life without larynx, 0 for death and 0.95 for life with an irradiated larynx. The anticipated value at each node can be calculated by multiplying the value associated with each branch by its probability. The value of the surgery node would be, assuming a normal life-expectancy of 10 years, 6.8 QALYs (Fig.10.3).

The calculations (Fig. 10.3) start at the terminal nodes and proceed backwards to the branches of the decision node, a process known as 'folding back'. Putting probability values into the tree consistent with the results of radiotherapy for early laryngeal cancer produces a value for radiotherapy of 8.0 QALYs. The rational decision-maker chooses radiotherapy (since 8.0 is greater than 6.8). This grossly oversimplified example tells us nothing we did not already know: radiotherapy is a better treatment than laryngectomy for early laryngeal cancer. The great power of decision analysis is its ability to ask, simultaneously, a variety of 'what if' questions. What if we lowered the cure rate with radiotherapy (as might apply to a more advanced tumour) and increased the quality factor for life after laryngectomy to 0.85? How might this affect the balance of the decision? This approach enables us to identify the key variables that influence the decision and, if these variables happen to

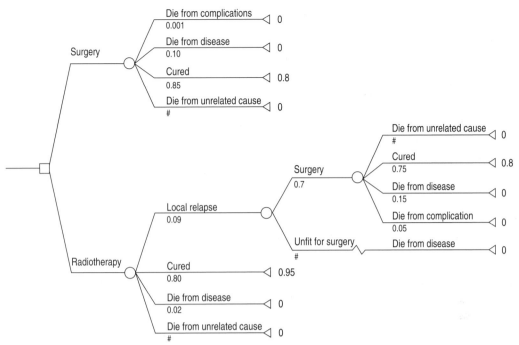

Figure 10.2: A simple decision analysis for the management of laryngeal cancer. Square, the original decision node; circles, chance nodes; triangles, the outcomes. The numbers along the branches of each node indicate the probability of that particular route being followed; the numbers beside the triangles indicate utilities for that particular outcome (on a scale from 0 = dead to 1.0 = perfectly normal life).

be ones about which we know very little, tells us the research questions we should be asking.

The real challenge posed by decision analysis is that we need, in order to make the best decision for each individual patient, to have a very clear numerical estimate of the value that the individual patient, personally, would assign to the possible outcomes covered in the analysis. These values vary between subjects[7] and it is this variation that hinders the application of decision analysis to groups of patients. Decision analysis is time-consuming and has not been widely adopted in clinical practice. Evidence-based practice is, in a sense, a poor person's decision analysis. It shares many of the advantages, and disadvantages, of formal decision analysis – but at least it does not take so long.

The evidence-based approach

The evidence-based approach has been applied both to medicine and to nursing. In essence, it is a reaction against uninformed dogma and demands that decisions be based upon data, rather than habit, opinion or prejudice.

Evidence-based medicine[8] (and, by extension, evidence-based nursing[9] and evidence-based oncology[10]) can be defined as 'as the conscientious, explicit, and judicious use of current best evidence in making decisions about the care of individual patients'.[11] The repertoire of techniques that have been used in evidence-based medicine do not straightforwardly translate into nursing.[12] There are differences in both primary focus and in methodology. Doctors are primarily concerned with interventions and their effects on disease. Nurses are more concerned with patients as individuals and their responses to illness in general. Medical research places heavy emphasis on quantitative methods and the quest for statistical significance. Nursing research makes greater use of qualitative methods and is more concerned with personal significance. These distinctions are not new:

in these and many other similar diseases the exact value of particular remedies and modes of treatment is by no means ascertained, while there is

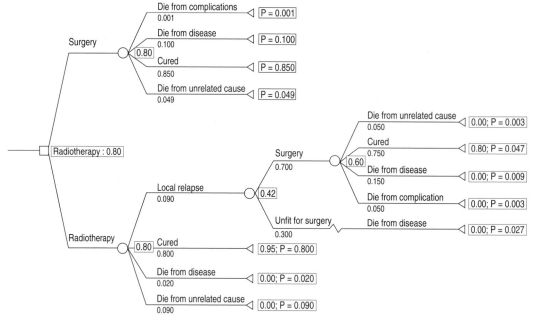

Figure 10.3: Figure 10.2 with the calculations performed. The numbers within the rectangles indicate the multiplied probability × utility values at each point in the tree.

universal experience as to the extreme importance of careful nursing in determining the issue of the disease.[13]

The precise criteria for a process to be granted the soubriquet 'evidence-based' have evolved over the years. A recent review[14] recognizes five main steps in the process:

1 Convert information needs into answerable questions.

2 Track down the best evidence with which to answer these questions.

3 Critically appraise the evidence for its validity and importance.

4 Integrate this appraisal with clinical expertise and patient values to apply the results in clinical practice.

5 Evaluate performance.

This position represents a retreat from a much harder line: in its original form, evidence-based medicine would only accept data from randomized controlled trials. There was little place for 'integration with clinical expertise and patient values'. The expanded definition is not particularly precise – indeed it would be

hard to identify many clinical practices that fell outwith the current definition.

The first step is to ask the right question. The question should be focused enough to be relevant, but not so tightly framed that there is no available evidence: 'Is chemotherapy of benefit to women with breast cancer?' is too general; 'Will a 35-year-old woman with a 15 mm G2 tumour and 0/25 axillary nodes positively benefit from adjuvant chemotherapy with CMF?' is, perhaps, too specific. Web-based systems, using analysis of matching patients, may be of some help in providing support for decisions in specific circumstances.[15] There are, however, problems with matching and obsolescence. Ten-year survival data can only be accurately based on results from patients treated a decade ago. Investigations and treatment have changed since then and so direct extrapolation is not entirely justified. Matching is also a problem. For the example of the 35-year-old woman, there are only 4 matching patients in the Finnish database – the 95% confidence interval on the 3-year survival rate extends from 1% to 99%. In order to support precise matching, databases need to be very large. The acquisition and maintenance of such databases requires considerable investment of time and resources. The costs are immediate, but the benefits, in terms of accurate individualized information, will be deferred. The approach is quite clearly a sensible way forward but, in order to be successful, will require both enthusiasm and several acts of political will. In the meantime we can only ask less-specific questions: 'Is adjuvant chemotherapy beneficial for women under 40 years old with node positive breast cancer?'.

Once an answerable question has been posed, the next step is to track down all the relevant evidence – particularly that from randomized controlled trials. The Cochrane Collaboration[16] has evolved in parallel with evidence-based medicine and provides, in a systematic form, a considerable body of evidence upon which to base decision concerning health care. The Collaboration seeks, edits, collates and publishes (via the Cochrane Library) systematic reviews of randomized controlled trials. So far, there are over 120 systematic reviews of relevance to the management of cancer in the Cochrane Library. If there is no reliable systematic review published, then an evidence-based approach would demand that the decision-maker should perform such a review. This is no trivial task and would certainly be beyond the resources (in both time and expertise) of most of us. Sometimes, particularly for rare tumours, there simply are no relevant trials and we have to rely on non-randomized data – with all their inherent biases.[17] A study in haematological malignancy[18] showed that evidence from randomized trials was available for only 24% of potential decisions; 55% of decisions would have to be made on the basis of anecdotal evidence. The remaining 21% of decisions could be supported by data from non-randomized observational studies. The analysis was applied prospectively to 255 patients: 78% of initial decisions could be based upon results from randomized trials; overall, however, 52% of decisions had to made in the absence of any high-level evidence.

Not all evidence is equal. Once the available evidence has been assembled, it must be appraised. The criteria for appraisal include:

- Relevance: Did the patients studied resemble my patient?

- Methodological rigour, best assessed using the CONSORT checklists:[19] Was this a randomized trial? If so, was randomization robust, were exclusions accounted for, was blinding used appropriately, were results reported according to intention-to-treat, etc.?

- Feasibility: Do I have the skills and resources to manage my patient with this particular intervention?

The decision is made using appropriately weighted evidence taken in conjunction with the patient's preferences and the experience and expertise of the clinicians involved.

The loop should be closed. Once a decision has been made, and acted upon, then the decision-makers should follow up the consequences of that decision. If the outcome is unfavourable, then there should be a reappraisal of the whole process. Was crucial evidence missed? Was the correct intervention chosen, but implemented incompetently?

In one sense, the evidence-based approach simply describes what good practitioners have always done. Its important contribution has been to highlight sloth and inertia in decision-making and to provide a framework whereby the worst can move in the direction of the best.

Computers are no panacea

One consequence of the rational analytical approach to decision-making is that it can easily be encoded into a computer's instructions. The computer can help with decisions, either by acting in the clinician's stead (an expert system) or by providing timely and relevant information (a decision support system).

The availability of a system is not just a question of how far it is to the nearest terminal: although, in some clinical circumstances, this can, itself, be an important issue. It is also a question of how quickly and efficiently the system responds to requests. How long are you prepared to spend typing in user names and passwords as you percolate through different levels of security for each different database? When you eventually reach the point at which you can type in your question, how long should you have to wait for a response? The computer systems used in health care are almost entirely static: terminals located in nursing stations, receptionists' desks and consulting rooms. Clinical practice is not static: clinicians move between consulting rooms, patients' homes, procedure rooms, treatment machines, imaging facilities and patients' bedsides. If computers are to have any wide application in clinical decision-making, then we need to move on from the concept of the static terminal and harness the new technology, such as wireless networks and web-based systems, to make decision support available instantly at point of use.

ETHICAL PERSPECTIVES ON DECISION-MAKING IN ONCOLOGY

Any clinical decision should be based on the four cardinal principles of medical ethics: beneficence, non-maleficence, autonomy and distributive justice.

Beneficence implies that good should be done; non-maleficence dictates that harm should not be done; autonomy indicates that the patient's right to make their own decisions should be respected; and the principle of distributive justice demands that there is equality of access and entitlement – there must be fair shares for all.

The rule of double effect implies that we should be judged by the intention of our decisions, not by their consequences. The most vivid illustration of this dilemma in clinical practice is the question of whether or not to give an opiate to a dying patient who is in pain. Giving the drug will shorten life (which is wrong); not giving the drug will fail to relieve suffering (which is also wrong). Our intention is to relieve pain and, therefore, according to the rule of double effect, we will be judged according to our ability to relieve pain, not by the fact that our intervention may have hastened death.

PRAGMATIC OR EMPIRICAL APPROACHES TO DECISION-MAKING

This is a straightforward approach: from our own experience, or that of others, we think we know what works, and so we keep on doing it. This is, I suspect, how the majority of decisions in clinical practice are made. It is a defensible approach provided we occasionally take time to revise our practices. We need to reflect on what we have achieved (and not achieved); we need to incorporate any new information that has come to light since we last established our practice. We need to be continually testing and refining our approach; otherwise, decision-making stagnates and progress becomes impossible.

A DECISION CAN BE REGARDED AS A PROCESS WITH THREE COMPONENTS

One simple way of parsing a decision is to divide it into three compartments: inputs, process and outcome. Each of these components can be assessed separately. The main input into a decision is information. The decision-making process itself can be rated according to the quality of the procedures used: the important caveat here is that it is not always easy to achieve consensus on the criteria to be used to define quality. The outcome of the decision can be assessed in two ways: Was the outcome favourable? Was the overall process performed satisfactorily? There may be a dichotomy between process and outcome. Extreme views are sometimes taken:

> We argue, however, that the actual treatment decision may not be relevant, because an optimal decision does not depend on the actual choice but on how that decision is reached.[20] (p512)

Inputs

Input information can be divided into:

- that which is available (and relevant)
- that which is available (and irrelevant)
- that which is actually used.

Information has to be communicated and so language is an important aspect of input into the decision-making process.

Only rarely do we have all the information we need in order to make a decision. Typically, this would include information about the patient, the illness and the risks and benefits associated with specific interventions. We imagine that this, in the era of evidence-based, guideline-driven, oncology, is a process that is both rigorous and straightforward. But it is not. How do we assess the patient, and how do we assess the extent to which the patient in the clinic resembles patients for whom we have evidence? The answer is: fairly crudely. We rely on simple measures such as age, gender, histology of tumour, performance status and clinical stage as factors in any matching that takes place. We ignore more subtle features that may be of relevance such as long-term illness, drug treatment, social background and support, individual psychology and preferences.

The problem of language

For a decision to be successful, all involved need to be speaking the same language. The meanings of words should, throughout the dialogue, be consistent. If I mean one thing when I speak, and you hear another thing when you listen, then our communication will, at best, lack clarity and, at worst, lead to catastrophic misunderstandings. Examples of words causing confusion are: remission (used by clinicians to indicate a temporary respite, taken by patients to mean cure) and chronic (used by patients to describe a pain that is severe, understood by clinicians to mean that the pain has been present for quite some time).

Language can be considered in a broader sense. The formats chosen to communicate numerical or statistical data are a type of language. The expressions used in Box 10.1 are examples of framing effects. The underlying data are the same, but the expressions are different and the potential for manipulating decisions is self-evident. If you want someone to have chemotherapy, tell them that they will increase their chances of cure by more than 15%; if you want someone to refuse chemotherapy, explain the disruption and tox-

icity to them and then point out that, for every 25 patients treated, only 1 patient achieves personal benefit. Framing effects[21] can be far less subtle: a 50% chance of surviving is, after all, a 50% chance of dying. This is merely the oncological version of pointing out that a glass that is half full is also half empty.

Appropriate and precise communication between participants is an important part of the decision-making process. If there are problems with language and understanding, or with the honesty of disclosure, then, as mentioned above, there will be problems with reaching a decision that serves the interests of all involved parties. What doctors say, and what patients hear, are often very different. Conversely, what patients are able to say, when they get the chance, might not entirely agree with what their doctors seem to hear. In an investigation of patients' decision-making concerning participation in phase I trials, Meropol et al[22] found that physicians claimed that they had discussed quality of life issues with 73% of patients. Only 28% of patients indicated that the topic had been discussed: same consultation, different recollection.

Box 10.1
Framing effects
Polychemotherapy produced, overall, a highly significant 15.7% (SD 2.4) reduction in the annual hazard ($2p < 0.00001$)
Survival rate with chemotherapy 65.4%; without chemotherapy 61.4%
Odds ratio 0.843 (from whence the 15.7% is derived; 100−84.3 = 15.7)
Relative risk = 0.896
Absolute rate difference = 4%
NNT = number of patients needed to treat with chemotherapy to prevent one death = 100/4 = 25
It is a long way from a '15.7% reduction' to 'in order to save one life 25 women are given chemotherapy without personal benefit' – and yet both statements are compatible with the same data

Even in discussions about palliative treatment, physicians appear to dodge psychosocial issues. Emotional functioning was, in one study, only discussed in 35% of consultations; if discussed, the topic was raised by patients (79% of the time) rather than by physicians (21% of the time).[23] The decision to steer clear of such issues is, perhaps, driven by the clinicians' fear that such discussions will take up too much time. When clinics were running late, emotional problems were less likely to be discussed than in clinics that were running to time. This study, in common with others, shows that, contrary to clinicians' apparent beliefs, discussion of emotional problems did not have a significant effect on the overall length of the consultation. There was a clear communication mismatch: patients talked about health-related quality of life 48% of time; physicians spent only 23% of their time on such issues.

Sometimes it is hard to tell the truth. Hope may be all that a patient has left. To tell such a person that they will surely die, and die soon, will remove their final defence. However, autonomy is an ethical imperative and to withhold truth is to compromise autonomy. How can patients make an informed decisions if they only have information that is distorted or incomplete? Honesty is usually the best policy: but will we recruit successfully to clinical trials if we are completely honest with patients about why we want them to enter randomized trials? And if we are not honest, what has happened to the ethical principle of autonomy?

It is not just the clinicians who fail fully to disclose. Patients may not choose spontaneously to disclose all their symptoms, all their concerns, all those many personal factors that will ultimately and importantly affect any decision that they might make. In a study of patients with colorectal cancer 46% of symptoms experienced by patients were not spontaneously reported to the doctor.[24]

The critical issue is to ensure that patients have the information they need, at the rate at which they can assimilate it, so that they can, in their own time, make a decision that is right for them. Nurses have a crucial role to play here. They can facilitate the process whereby patients and carers navigate through the complex array of available material. Unlike physicians, nurses are less likely to be perceived, or to behave, as if they are more concerned with issues of control rather than with justice and individual choice. The nurse, in this view, is not a passive conduit channelling information between the two key players (doctor and patient). The nurse is a facilitator and translator, interpreting the world of medicine for the patient, and helping the doctor appreciate the patient's view of the world. The nurse also plays a permissive role, indicating that it is not wrong to ask questions of medical and nursing staff, that it is perfectly reasonable, if it helps, to involve partners and relatives in decision-making and that it may take time to resolve an important decision.

The problem of preferences

How do we know what people really want? In order to incorporate patients' hopes, fears and expectations into a decision, we need to know how they set and rank their priorities. There are two key areas here: how to elicit preferences and the stability of the preferences that we have elicited. It is not just whether, today, you would trade off 6 months of survival to avoid a colostomy. It is the question of whether or not you would make the same judgement 6 weeks or 6 years from now.

Problems with eliciting preferences

There are two widely used techniques for assessing preferences: the standard gamble and the time-trade-off (TTO) methods. In the standard gamble the patient is asked to choose between a guaranteed period of survival, with impaired health, and a gamble in which there are only two possible outcomes: perfect health and immediate death. The probabilities within the gamble are systematically altered until the patient is unable to choose between the certainty and the gamble (Fig. 10.4). The value of the gamble, at this indifference point, can be used to derive a utility for the health state under consideration.[25,26] The standard gamble is not easily understood by patients and so a simpler approach has been devised. The TTO method simply uses a graded series of questions to ascertain how much time in impaired health a patient would relinquish in order to enjoy perfect health. The time period, expressed as a proportion of expected survival in impaired health, is used as a proxy measure of utility.

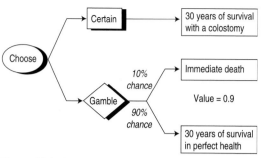

Figure 10.4: Standard gamble.

By obtaining a series of utilities for different health states, it is possible to obtain a rank order for patients' preferences. This approach has been widely applied in oncology.[27–32] Even the simple TTO procedure is not understood by all patients: those who are less numerate have problems both with the standard gamble and with TTO.[33]

Pascal's wager[34] is an important influence on decision-making for patients who regard themselves as terminally ill. Pascal recommended backing a belief in God in any gamble concerning the existence of a deity: if you believe, and He exists, you win all; if you believe, and He does not exist, you have lost nothing. If there is a treatment, such as tamoxifen, that is simple and relatively non-toxic, then it is worth trying, even if the chances of success are very small. If it works, you have gained an unexpected bonus; if it does not work, then you have lost very little.

The instability of preferences

We all change our minds from time to time. If preferences are unstable (if I change my mind) how can any decision ever be either consistent or rational. Under pressure, we base our decisions on what we want. Once we have had time to reflect, decisions are more likely to be based on what we feel we ought to do.[35] Decisions made on the spot, in clinic, are more likely to be 'want' decisions. Those made at home, after consultation with family members, are more likely to be 'should' decisions. Viewed against this background it is easy to see why patients might seem to be so fickle, changing their minds from week to week.

Response shift is the jargon term for something more understandably expressed as: 'If I'd known then, what I know now'. As our circumstances change, then so do our priorities. Cancer changes peoples' lives, and their priorities. There is therefore no reason to suppose that preferences are stable as people move from well, through diagnosis and treatment and, for some, towards relapse and facing up to death. If our priorities change, then so might our decisions. It is completely rational for decisions to be inconstant over time.

Assessing the quality of the decision-making process

We make decisions for a variety of reasons and the parties to the decisions have a variety of perspectives, only some of which may be shared. It is impossible, therefore, to devise a single metric for assessing the quality of a decision. The answer you get will depend upon whom you ask. One recent approach has been to assess decision-making according to the extent to which decision-making has been shared between patient and clinician.[36,37] As outlined previously, there are various normative approaches: psychological, analytical, ethical and so on. Sometimes, these schools of thought agree, sometimes they do not. The strenuous debate about the ethics of using QALYs to guide decisions affecting public health is an excellent example of two cultures

Box 10.2
Time-trade-off (TTO) method
If you were offered 30 years of survival with a colostomy or 25 years of perfect health, which would you choose?
Answer: colostomy
If you were offered 30 years of survival with a colostomy or 27 years of perfect health, which would you choose?
Answer: I couldn't choose between these options
The patient is prepared to trade 3 years of survival in order to avoid a colostomy; their utility for life with a colostomy is therefore 27/30 = 0.9 that of perfect health

(ethicists and decision analysts) in collision. An ethically just decision may be economically unacceptable, and vice versa. There can be no uniform mechanical process for decision-making in oncology: different processes will suit different contexts and, in this regard, a wide variety of choice is a blessing, not a curse.

The problem of the clinical environment

It is not easy to make good decisions in the clinic or ward. We do not ever seem to have enough time, the information we need is never to hand and we are constrained by the institutional environment and the hidden pressures exerted by our peers. Our patients may feel inarticulate and stripped of power.

The more pressure you apply to a tired and uncomfortable person, the more likely it is that they will guess, rather than decide. There are no insoluble problems here: it is the will to recognize and solve the difficulties that is lacking. We pay lip service to the concept of patient-centred care but, in reality, the institution can only really cope with patients by regarding them as a commodity to be shuffled and traded. Until such time as hospitals choose to organize themselves for the benefit of their patients, clinical decision-making will be unnecessarily compromised. Nursing has a great deal to offer here. Patients spend far more time with their nurses than with their doctors. The care that nurses provide should

---

Box 10.3

Example of decision-making for chemotherapy treatment

Consider the levels and perspectives, which apply to a decision as to whether or not an 80-year-old man with Dukes' C carcinoma of the rectum should be treated with adjuvant chemotherapy. Suppose this man is hypertensive, but otherwise medically fit, and has recovered well from his surgery. He lives a 2-hour drive away from the cancer centre and is the main carer for his wife who has Altzheimer's disease. On the grounds of his age, it might be considered inappropriate to give him chemotherapy, but on the basis of his performance status, chemotherapy would be a reasonable option. What are the other issues?

Psychological perspective
If he doesn't have chemotherapy and his disease returns, how will he and the medical team feel about the decision not to treat him? What does he perceive are the advantages and disadvantages of having chemotherapy? What is his attitude to risk? How will his family, who have visited all the appropriate websites, feel if a decision is made not to give chemotherapy? Will they feel he is being cheated because he is old? How bitter may they feel if he were to develop recurrence?

Logical perspective
Only a full-blown decision analysis will help us here.

Evidence-based perspective
Evidence suggests that adjuvant chemotherapy should be given to all patients with Dukes' C carcinoma of the rectum who are under 75 years old. How does this evidence apply to this particular 80-year-old patient? How can we apply evidence in the absence of any evidence, always remembering that absence of evidence is not evidence of absence? Given that he is hypertensive, is there a risk to using 5FU (5-fluorouracil) chemotherapy?

Ethical perspective
Whose decision is this anyway? Does he know enough, can he know enough, to make an informed decision? Does this man have the right to use resources that, in pure health economic terms would be better used to treat younger patients? He's had a good innings, why not let nature run its course? Will chemotherapy add any benefit? How will the chemotherapy affect this man's ability to care for his wife? Does he want to travel to and from the hospital for 2 days every 2 weeks for the next 3 months? If he lived closer and did not have a dependent wife, would he be offered chemotherapy?

Pragmatic perspective
Have any other 80-year-old patients been treated recently with adjuvant chemotherapy? What happened? How does this man feel about the potential side-effects of chemotherapy?

include support for patients facing difficult decisions – as ever, the problem is time. There is an intrinsic conflict for nurses on a busy oncology unit: they have to cope with both the technical and the human aspects of caring. It is easier to judge the former than the latter, and so performance review is often based on technical competence rather than human warmth. And yet it is that very warmth that is so important to those patients who feel cold and isolated as they wrestle with the complexities of decision-making.

Problems with assessing the outcomes of decisions

It is unusual for decisions to please everyone: one person's gain may be another person's loss. This creates tension, particularly for clinicians. If a nurse decides to spend time with the relatives of a dying patient, then he may not be able to give sufficient care to the other patients for whom he is responsible. If one consultant decides to treat all her patients as inpatients, regardless of their clinical needs, then this will create pressure on inpatient beds for the unit as a whole. It could, for example, mean that the unit was accommodating hotel guests while being unable to admit genuine emergencies. This concept, whereby a decision that is of benefit in one area but causes disadvantage in another, is called 'opportunity cost'. The decreased care for the other patients was the opportunity cost of the nurse's decision to spend time with the dying patient; the lack of emergency beds was the opportunity cost of the consultant's decision to admit all her patients for treatment, regardless. The concept of opportunity cost can be broadened considerably: the opportunity cost of futile treatment is the loss of time that could have been better spent with family and friends.[38]

Perspective is crucial

An economist or manager may only be concerned with whether or not a decision saved money: well-being and happiness, in this view, are only secondary consequences. A clinician may be interested in whether or not a tumour has shrunk or not, regardless of expense. A patient primarily is concerned with whether or not they can be cured (or at least have their distress relieved): the cost should not matter to them and mere shrinkage of tumour is insufficient.

We should learn from the consequences of our decisions. When we achieve success, we should try to repeat it: if we fail, we should try something different next time.

WHAT ACTUALLY HAPPENS?

Most published research on decision-making has dealt with one category of decision, the strategic, and considered only two classes of decision-maker, patients and doctors. This overlooks the fact that living with cancer is not just about the strategic decisions: it is a series of daily skirmishes, each demanding its own tactical decision.

A recent NHS R&D study[39] looked at nurses' roles in clinical decision-making. The report was based on observation and interviews with 120 nurses working in the acute setting: surgical wards medical wards and coronary care unit. The authors identified four key areas:

1 Choices concerning intervention:
   • Which intervention, for which patient, at which time?
2 Communication:
   • Imparting and receiving information (patients, relatives, colleagues).
3 Organization of services:
   • How best to deliver and manage a clinical service.
4 Interpretation:
   • How is this experience affecting this particular individual at this particular time?

Models for decision making by nurses

Thompson and colleagues[39] defined three main models for decision-making, as it applies to nursing:

1 Classically rational model (approximates to an evidence-based approach, objective)

Define the problem   then
Define what you need to know   then
Gather the evidence   then
Evaluate the evidence   then
Assign values to outcomes   then
Incorporate evidence and values
into a structured analysis   then
Evaluate the overall value associated
with each possible choice   then
Choose that option associated with
the highest expected value

2 Experience and intuition (subjective)

Make the decision on the basis of what you can remember and what you feel to be right

3 The spectrum model

All our decisions can be classified along a spectrum extending between the two extremes defined above: from completely subjective (model 2) to completely objective (model 1). The precise location of an appropriate decision along this spectrum will depend upon the individuals facing the decision and the clinical circumstances. A heavily subjective model would be entirely appropriate (and a totally objective model completely inappropriate) for a patient with terminal lung cancer deciding whether or not they should make a pilgrimage to Lourdes. Conversely, it would be totally inappropriate to adopt a wholly subjective approach to a decision concerning whether or not to implement a national screening programme for colorectal cancer.

Why did nurses not use findings from research to inform their clinical decisions?

The R&D report[39] identified four main barriers to the nurses' use of research information to inform their clinical decisions. These may be caricatured as follows:

Fear of numbers and the words they trail behind them

Statistical analyses use a difficult and intimidating vocabulary to summarize and interpret numerical data. The words, and the underlying mathematical concepts, are hard to understand. As a result, nurses fail to read or to understand that which they would like to read and understand.

Rage against the machine

Nurses who would like to use data to make decisions, and have the confidence to do so, feel that the system is against them. The culture, organization and working environment conspire to make it difficult for them to put their skills into practice.

The ambassadors from cloud-cuckoo-land don't impress me

Nurses who advocate the use of research findings in clinical decision-making are perceived as airy-fairy academics who, by virtue of their merely fleeting contacts with the hurly-burly of daily nursing practice, lack clinical credibility. There is deep suspicion concerning whether or not the nostrums they peddle have any relevance for the real world of clinical nursing.

Won't somebody help me? Is there anybody out there?

Nurses who lack self-confidence in their own abilities but appreciate the need for decisions to be, whenever possible, evidence-based, would like help from more confident colleagues. They would use research findings in their clinical practice if these findings could be put into a form that is both accessible and understandable. Despite the extensive range of support materials available, both written and electronic, they prefer to have their advice from people, rather than books, protocols or computers.

It is clear, from this report, that we have some distance to travel before we can be complacent about decision-making.

DECISION AIDS

Decision aids (or tools) are designed to improve the quality of decisions. One immediate problem is the definition of quality. The argument may become circular. We decide, perhaps arbitrarily, on a set of quality standards. We design a decision aid to improve the extent to which these standards are achieved. We test our decision aid against these standards and find that decision 'quality' has been improved. By our own standards, things have improved – but were our standards necessarily the most relevant ones? One proposed definition of an effective decision is that it is 'informed, consistent with personal values, and acted upon'.[40] Other outcome measures, such as anxiety or retrospective regret, may also be relevant.

Another problem lies with the definition of what exactly are decision aids: One definition is:

> Decision aids are interventions designed to help people make specific and deliberative choices among options by providing information about the options and outcomes that is relevant to a person's health status.[41]

This is a fairly broad definition, which would include many straightforward clinical interactions. When a patient attends for their first course of chemotherapy their nurse will almost certainly provide information about options and outcomes relevant to their health status. In a practical sense, decision aids attempt to present information specific to an individual's predicament in a form that is readily understood and which enables patients to explore their personal preferences. Techniques that have been used include printed material, decision boards, video films and workbooks with supportive audiocassettes. Future developments will include web-based materials and access to call centres (the latter, it would appear, to be staffed by nurses).

A systematic review of randomized trials of decision aids[41] shows that, overall, these aids improved subjects' knowledge and decreased decisional conflict. If subjects had been exposed to a decision aid, they were less likely to choose surgery over a more conservative approach. Decision aids appeared to have no effect on subjects' satisfaction with their decisions. There is no evidence that oncologists felt threatened by the introduction of decision aids, quite the reverse. Only 6% of oncologists in Ontario asked about the use of a decision aid to facilitate decision-making by women with node-negative breast cancer felt that decision aids had no place in clinical practice.[40] Fifty per cent of oncologists faced with a clinical scenario in which adjuvant therapy was only of uncertain benefit felt that a decision aid would be extremely helpful. This study may, however, overestimate the acceptability of decision aids since the clinicians were dealing with a hypothetical, as opposed to an actual, decision aid. Acceptability to clinicians will be influenced by actual decisions. If the decision that is supported by the decision aid differs from that which the oncologist would recommend, then this would be a potential source of conflict which might influence the practical acceptance of decision aids by clinicians.

NURSING IN NO-MAN'S-LAND

The balance of power in clinical practice is shifting. Twenty years ago, power and control lay almost exclusively with medical staff and, inevitably, doctor knew best. Nowadays, there is an increasing emphasis on the autonomy of the individual patient. These are uncertain times: boundaries are being redrawn; unwritten contracts are being codified; written contracts are being renegotiated; professional distinctions are blurring; and the delivery of health care is, increasingly, being managed by people with little experience of what it is actually like to deliver care.

The transition from physician-centred medicine to patient-centred medicine will not be accomplished abruptly. Change will be gradual and, for different individuals, at different places, and at different times, will occur at different rates. For many clinical encounters, this is likely to leave a no-man's-land in which the physician has relinquished power, or is trying to do so, but the patient feels unable or unwilling to take on full responsibility for decision-making (Fig. 10.5). The nursing profession is ideally placed to occupy this vacant territory. The role of nurses as patients' advocates has been well rehearsed.[42,43] At the same time, the professional role of the nurse has expanded: nurse prescribing; nurse-led chemotherapy units; nurse-led follow-up; and nurse-led diagnostic and screening programmes. The profession works both sides of the street and is uniquely placed to understand and to resolve potential conflicts.

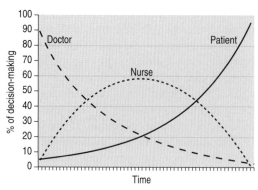

Figure 10.5: Like a bridge over troubled water: as, over the next few years, doctors disengage from involvement in decision-making, there will be a lag period before patients are able fully to engage in the decision-making process. During this transitional period it is almost inevitable that nurses will be required to step into the breach.

DECISION MAKING IN CANCER CARE – THE FUTURE

We have a wealth of theory but a scarcity of facts. Decision-making is an important aspect of cancer management and has not received the attention it deserves. This neglect stems partly from the complexity of the subject and partly from the fact that there has been no uniform approach to the study of decision-making. Research on the subject is jargon-ridden and factional. The psychologists take one view, the ethicists another, and both are viewed askance by analysts using maximum utility as a yardstick. The literature is, as a consequence, opaque and contradictory.

The next generation of researchers will need to take a far more integrated approach using information from all the relevant disciplines. Decisions should be considered within a framework such as that outlined in Figure 10.1. We need to recognize that different circumstances require different decision-making techniques, and different criteria for defining the 'good' decision. Most good decisions may, ultimately, be no more than the judicious application of some relevant wisdom governed by respect for the rights of the individual. Given the trust placed in them both by the public and by other clinicians, nurses are in a

unique position to study, and to improve, decision-making in cancer care.

CONCLUSION

A decision is the point at which thought moves into action. Decision-making in oncology must be considered in context, and context applies not just to the nature of the decision but also to its scale (from individual to international). The literature on decision-making is confusing. This is mainly because the issue has been approached from a variety of different perspectives and disciplines. The main approaches have been: psychological; logical/analytical; ethical; and empirical/pragmatic. Evidence-based nursing is a variant of the logical/analytical approach. There are important differences between evidence-based nursing and evidence-based medicine and, if these differences are ignored, then cancer nursing will be doing itself a disservice. Nursing and doctoring are distinct activities and demand different research methods and should be judged by different criteria.

Given the importance of context and scale, it is impossible to devise a set of quality standards for judging decision-making in cancer care. One approach would be simply to look at the inherent problems, and judge a decision-making process on the extent to which these difficulties had been successfully resolved.

A decision can be reduced to a simple three component model: input/process/output. Evidence-based medicine/nursing concentrates attention on the quality of the inputs. Process is also important, in particular adherence to the cardinal ethical principles of autonomy and equality.

Language is important. Decisions may be corrupted by framing effects: the way in which propositions are put may have an unwarranted influence on an individual's choice. The assessment of outcomes is not easy. Professional perspective will influence interpretation: a decision that is ideal to an ethicist may be unacceptable to an economist. Amidst these turf battles we run the risk of losing sight of the most important participant of all – the patient. Patients are sometimes accused of being irrational. Once again, perspective is crucial. As professionals, we have no right to impose our own value systems upon those who come to us for help.

Clinical decision-making occurs within an environment that is far from ideal: too pressured, too busy and too noisy. For a variety of reasons, nurses have problems making research-based decisions. Most decisions are based on a mixture of intuition and remembered facts and are coated with a veneer of rationality. In part, this is due to a lack of self-confidence, both personal and professional. Nurses know more than they think they know and they are wiser than they believe themselves to be. By appreciating their own strengths and by acquiring the ability to use evidence more effectively, cancer nurses have the opportunity to improve not only decision-making but also their own professional standing. Nurses have a crucial role to play in supporting people through some of the most difficult decisions they will ever have had to make.

REFERENCES

1. Bekker H, Thornton JG, Airey CM, et al. Informed decision making: an annotated bibiography and systematic review. Winchester, England: Health Technology Assessment; 1999; 3(1):1–168.

2. Tversky A, Kahneman D. Judgment under uncertainty: heuristics and biases. Science 1974;185(4157):1124–1131.

3. Kahneman D, Tversky A. On the reality of cognitive illusions. Psycholog Rev 1996; 103(3):582–591.

4. Feinstein AR. The 'chagrin factor' and qualitative decision analysis. Arch Intern Med 1985; 145(7):1257–1259.

5. Redelmeier DA, Kahneman D. Patients' memories of painful medical treatments: real-time and retrospective evaluations of two minimally invasive procedures. Pain 1996; 66(1):3–8.

6. Munro AJ. Decision analysis in oncology: panacea or chimera? Clin Oncol 1992; 4(5):306–312.

7. McNeil BJ, Weichselbaum R, Pauker SG. Speech and survival: tradeoffs between quality and quantity of life in laryngeal cancer. N Engl J Med 1981; 305(17):982–987.

8. Sackett DL, Rosenberg WMC, Muir Gray JA, Haynes RB, Richardson WS. Evidence based medicine: what it is and what it isn't. BMJ 1996; 312:71–72.

9. Pape TM. Evidence-based nursing practice: to infinity and beyond. J Cont Educ Nurs 2003; 34(4):154–161; quiz 189–190.

10. Bentzen SM. Towards evidence based radiation oncology: improving the design, analysis, and reporting of clinical outcome studies in radiotherapy. Radiother Oncol 1998; 46(1):5–18.

11. Sackett DL. Evidence-based medicine and treatment choices. Lancet 1997; 349(9051):570; discussion 572–573.

12. Lavin MA, Meyer G, Krieger M, et al. Essential differences between evidence-based nursing and evidence-based medicine. Int J Nurs Terminol Classif 2002; 13(3):101–106.

13. Nightingale F. Notes on nursing: what it is, and what it is not. Boston: Lippincott, Williams and Wilkins; 1859:1992.

14. Straus SE, McAlister FA. Evidence-based medicine: a commentary on common criticisms. Can Med Assoc J 2000; 163(7):837–841.

15. Lundin J, Lundin M, Isola J, Joensuu H. Infopoints: a web-based system for individualised survival estimation in breast cancer. BMJ 2003; 326(7379):29.

16. Munro AJ. Systematic reviews and the Cochrane Collaboration. Eur J Cancer Care 2003; 12:286–296.

17. Sackett DL. Bias in analytic research. J Chronic Dis 1979; 32(1–2):51–63.

18. Djulbegovic B, Loughran TP Jr, Hornung CA, et al. The quality of medical evidence in hematology-oncology. Am J Med 1999; 106(2):198–205.

19. Altman DG, Schulz KF, Moher D, et al. The revised CONSORT statement for reporting randomized trials: explanation and elaboration. Ann Intern Med 2001; 134(8):663–694.

20. Gattellari M, Voigt KJ, Butow PN, Tattersall MH. When the treatment goal is not cure: are cancer patients equipped to make informed decisions? J Clin Oncol 2002; 20(2):503–513.

21. Edwards A, Elwyn G, Covey J, Matthews E, Pill R. Presenting risk information – a review of the effects of "framing" and other manipulations on patient outcomes. J Health Comm 2001; 6(1):61–82.

22. Meropol NJ, Weinfurt KP, Burnett CB, et al. Perceptions of patients and physicians regarding phase I cancer clinical trials: implications for physician-patient communication. J Clin Oncol 2003; 21(13):2589–2596.

23. Detmar SB, Muller MJ, Wever LD, Schornagel JH, Aaronson NK. The patient–physician relationship. Patient–physician communication during outpatient palliative treatment visits: an observational study. JAMA 2001; 285(10):1351–1357.

24. Funch DP. Predictors and consequences of symptom reporting behaviors in colorectal cancer patients. Med Care 1988; 26(10):1000–1008.

25. Boyd NF, Sutherland HJ, Heasman KZ, Tritchler DL, Cummings BJ. Whose utilities for decision analysis? Med Decis Making 1990; 10(1):58–67.

26. Jansen SJ, Kievit J, Nooij MA, Stiggelbout AM. Stability of patients' preferences for chemotherapy: the impact of experience. Med Decis Making 2001; 21(4):295–306.

27. Llewellyn-Thomas HA, Sutherland HJ, Thiel EC. Do patients' evaluations of a future health state change when they actually enter that state? Med Care 1993; 31(11):1002–1012.

28. Ortega A, Dranitsaris G, Sturgeon J, Sutherland H, Oza A. Cost-utility analysis of paclitaxel in combination with cisplatin for patients with advanced ovarian cancer. Gynecol Oncol 1997; 66(3):454–463.

29. Grann VR, Panageas KS, Whang W, Antman KH, Neugut AI. Decision analysis of prophylactic mastectomy and oophorectomy in BRCA1-positive or BRCA2-positive patients. J Clin Oncol 1998; 16(3):979–985.

30. Grann VR, Sundararajan V, Jacobson JS, et al. Decision analysis of tamoxifen for the prevention of invasive breast cancer. Cancer J Sci Am 2002; 6(32617):169–178.

31. Ringash J, Redelmeier DA, O'Sullivan B, Bezjak A. Quality of life and utility in irradiated laryngeal cancer patients. Int J Rad Oncol Biol Phys 2000; 47(4):875–881.

32. Unic I, Stalmeier PF, Verhoef LC, van Daal WA. Assessment of the time-tradeoff values for prophylactic mastectomy of women with a suspected genetic predisposition to breast cancer. Med Decis Making 1998; 18(3):268–277.

33. Woloshin S, Schwartz LM, Moncur M, Gabriel S, Tosteson AN. Assessing values for health: numeracy matters. Med Decis Making 2001; 21(5):382–390.

34. Pascal B. Pensees. London: Dent; 1932.

35. Bazerman MH, Tenbrunsel AE, Wade-Benzoni K. Negotiating with yourself and losing: making decisions with competing internal preferences. Acad Manage Rev 1998; 23(2):225–241.

36. Elwyn G, Edwards A, Wensing M, et al. Shared decision making: developing the OPTION scale for measuring patient involvement. Qual Saf Health Care 2003; 12(2):93–99.

37. Elwyn G, Edwards A, Mowle S, et al. Measuring the involvement of patients in shared decision-making: a systematic review of instruments. Patient Educ Counsel 2001;43(1):5–22.

38. Munro AJ, Sebag-Montefiore D. Opportunity cost – a neglected aspect of cancer treatment. Br J Cancer 1992; 65(3):309–310.

39. Thompson C, McCaughan D, Cullum N, et al. Nurses' use of research information in clinical decision making: a descriptive and analytical study. Report presented to the NHS R & D programme in evaluating methods to promote the implementation of R & D. University of York; 2003.

40. O'Connor AM, Llewellyn-Thomas HA, Sawka C, et al. Physicians' opinions about decision aids for patients considering systemic adjuvant therapy for axillary-node negative breast cancer. Patient Educ Counsel 1997; 30(2):143–153.

41. O'Connor AM, Stacey D, Entwistle V, et al. Decision aids for people facing health treatment or screening decisions. Cochrane Database of Systematic Reviews (Online: Update Software), 2003; 2:CD001431.

42. Morra ME. New opportunities for nurses as patient advocates. Semin Oncol Nurs 2000;16(1):57–64.

43. Crockford EA, Holloway IM, Walker JM. Nurses' perceptions of patients' feelings about breast surgery. J Adv Nurs 1993; 18(11):1710–1718.

CHAPTER 11

The Experience of Cancer Treatment

DEBORAH FITZSIMMONS AND JANICE M MIDDLETON

CHAPTER CONTENTS

Introduction	213	After treatment	225
		Follow-up	226
Approaches to understanding the		Recurrence of cancer	226
treatment experience	214	Palliative care	226
The biomedical perspective	214		
A psycho-oncology perspective	214	Reconfiguring cancer nursing	
A quality of life perspective	215	services – are nurse-led models of	
		care feasible?	226
Negotiating the treatment experience	217		
Deciding upon treatment options	218	Methods to assess treatment	
		experience	227
Undergoing treatment	220		
The cancer treatment environment	221	Conclusion	227
The language of cancer treatment	221		
The impact of treatment on patients'		References	229
quality of life	222		

INTRODUCTION

Increasingly, the focus of cancer care delivery is centred on improving patient experience, particularly with regard to cancer treatments. Much of the focus of nursing care at this time is supporting patients and their families through their treatment experience and optimizing their quality of life. In order to facilitate this process, the cancer nurse requires knowledge and understanding of the actual and potential impact of cancer treatments on patients and their families, in order to deliver effective care, based on identified patient needs.

The cancer treatment journey is often referred to as one part of the disease continuum,[1] with the potential expected outcome of cure, control and/or palliation. However, cancer treatment is rarely a one-off event; a whole range of treat-ments may be experienced during the course of the disease.[2] The course of treatment will be variable, according to the disease; e.g. treatment pathways for haematological malignancies will differ substantially from treatments for solid malignancies. Traditionally, the experience of cancer treatment has often been depicted as a series of discrete steps in an overall treatment pathway, such as tests and investigations that lead to diagnosis, primary treatment, adjuvant treatments, followed by a period of remission, with long-term survival or recurrence, palliative treatment, terminal illness and death. Today, with the ambiguities of cancer being viewed as both a life-threatening yet chronic disease,[3] the cancer treatment journey cannot be viewed in such a simplistic manner. For many of our patients, this journey is confusing, difficult, and involves a variety of complex treatments, some of which extend over days, weeks, months, years or the rest of a person's life span. A plethora of treatments may be experienced by the patient, including conventional treatments, clinical trials and innovative treatment approaches. For the patient, there may never be a time where there is a treatment-free phase. Patients may receive long-term hormonal treatments, require control of their disease symptoms (or indeed symptoms or side-effects resulting from their actual treatment) or be faced with periodic episodes of further treatment when faced with disease recurrence and/or metastatic disease.

Therefore, there is no 'typical' cancer treatment experience and, as such, it is difficult to exactly define what the experience of cancer treatment is, or how it impacts on a person's quality of life. Although there may be common features, such as disease site and stage, treatment plan or place where treatment is delivered, each person with cancer will have a very individual treatment experience, according to his or her own personal circumstances. Furthermore, there are a number of approaches that can be taken to understanding the treatment experience. The focus of this chapter is therefore not to approach the experience of cancer treatment as a series of discrete treatment interventions but to focus on understanding what factors contribute to, and impact upon, the treatment experience throughout.

In this chapter, we review the following key themes:

- approaches to understanding patients' experiences of their cancer treatment
- a review of the key milestones in patients' treatment experience
- the importance of understanding the context of patients' experiences during their treatment journey.

To illustrate these themes, excerpts of patients' narrative accounts from two studies undertaken by the authors will be used. The first study was an in-depth qualitative study of 21 patients' quality of life during their illness and treatment experience for pancreatic cancer.[4,5] The second study was an in-depth qualitative study of 26 patients' experiences of chemotherapy services.[6]

APPROACHES TO UNDERSTANDING THE TREATMENT EXPERIENCE

Before we can begin to understand what influences and impacts upon the cancer treatment experience, there is a need to understand the perspectives that we draw upon in order to understand the complexities of patients' experiences.

The biomedical perspective

From a biomedical perspective, the impact of cancer treatment is often concerned with the measurement of clinical outcomes. These include toxicity and treatment side-effects, changes in performance status and objective disease response, to name but a few. Much of the medical literature on cancer treatments has been devoted to assessing the impact of cancer treatments from this perspective. Language such as '5-year survival' and 'treatment response' is commonplace in our clinical vocabulary, and is often used to portray the success or otherwise of cancer treatments.

Some of this information can be gathered through review of studies (e.g. reviewing the evidence of large multicentre randomized clinical trials) or epidemiological data (e.g. national 5-year survival rates from each country). The value of these approaches is that they are purported to be objective, utilize valid and reliable measures and direct comparisons can be made across groups. However, one of the fundamental limitations of this approach is that it neglects the individual experience of cancer treatment, and focuses solely on clinical indicators rather than actual 'real-life' experiences. Often, one of the difficulties is translating this evidence (e.g. from clinical trials), and interpreting what this means for our individual patient. Therefore, new approaches to understanding the impact of cancer treatment from the patients' perspective have been required.

A psycho-oncology perspective

The emergence of the field of psycho-oncology has provided a theoretical basis on which to understand the process of coping, adapting and adjustment to cancer and its treatments. This has centred upon understanding the cognitive, emotional and behavioural aspects of cancer.

The psychological consequences of cancer treatments are diverse, both in type and degree. Earlier work in breast cancer patients has suggested that psychological morbidity can impact upon treatment experience and may be associated with long-term outcome.[7] Other factors that have been suggested to influence and impact upon cancer experiences include stressful life events, younger age, personality type and past response to loss and illness.[8] A number of common themes are proposed in patients' reactions to cancer treatment. These include uncertainty, vulnerability, loss of control, helplessness and feelings of loss, grief and despair.

A number of coping styles have been proposed for coming to terms with, and adjusting to, cancer and its treatment. These include having a fighting spirit, helplessness, stoic acceptance and denial and anxious preoccupation, fatalism and cognitive avoidance.[7] With regard to adaptation, patients are often faced with trying to come to terms with cancer itself and the impact of treatment while also coming to terms with alterations to one's life which have been brought about by the disease.[9]

Although this work has provided a considerable basis on which to look at the impact of cancer and its treatments on the patient's psychological well-being, the limitations of this approach are the focus on measuring psychological attributes and their consequences, and that many of these factors remain stable over time, or that there is a predictive pattern of coping and adjustment to cancer. These theories suggest that these reactions are experienced by all cancer patients and move forward in a series of stages, emphasizing an overly constrained notion of what is normal and healthy adjustment.[2] There is also a lack of exploration of the contribution of other factors, such as social support, in influencing the type of coping strategies employed.[4]

A quality of life perspective

One of the significant approaches over the past two decades to gain an understanding of the impact of cancer and its treatments is the assessment of the quality of life of patients during their cancer treatments. There is little doubt of the importance of exploring the impact of cancer treatments on the quality of life of patients. This has resulted in considerable interest and activity in developing optimum methods of assessing the impact of cancer treatments on patients' quality of life and evaluating the success or otherwise of new treatments from this perspective.

What do we mean by 'quality of life' in relation to the cancer treatment experience?

It is well recognized that cancer treatments can have a significant impact on patients' psychological and social well-being and, consequently, the quality of life of these patients.[10,11] However, despite consensus within the literature that quality of life is subjective (can only be rated by the individual concerned), multidimensional (composed of a number of key areas or domains of a person's life) and contextual (can change according to a variety of circumstances), there is still considerable variety in the way quality of life has been defined for the person with cancer[12] (see Box 11.1 for examples). Indeed, despite the wealth of literature pertaining to examine quality of life, for most of us the concept remains vague.[13,14]

Much of this confusion has been due to the variety of methodological approaches that have been taken in attempting to understand quality of life, ranging from phenomenological studies of patients' quality of life through to the development of standardized assessments (typically, patient self-completed questionnaires). It is this

---

Box 11.1

Some definitions of quality of life
'Quality of life measures the difference, or gap, at a particular period of time between the hopes and expectations of the individual and the individual's experiences.'[15]
'Quality of life refers to patients' appraisal of and satisfaction with their current level of functioning as compared to what they perceive as ideal.'[16]
'Quality of life is an individual's perception of their position in life in the context of the culture and value systems in which they live and in relation to their goals, expectations, standards and concerns.'[17]

215

latter approach which has been reported most widely to date within the cancer literature. The reported value of this approach has been the ability to capture patient-based outcomes in a standardized manner that allows direct comparisons to be made, the rigorous development of many of these measures, evidence of their reliability and validity in a number of cancer patient populations and their widespread use in clinical trials and studies.

This measurement-orientated approach has focused predominantly on viewing quality of life from a functional perspective. Typically, the most popular measures currently used to assess quality of life of patients undergoing cancer treatments (e.g. EORTC QLQ-C30[18] and FACIT[19]) focus upon specific domains. These are usually assessing disease symptoms, treatment side-effects, physical functioning (e.g. mobility, self-care activities), psychological functioning (e.g. anxiety and depression), cognitive functioning (e.g. concentration), health status and to a lesser extent, occupational and social functioning[5] (Table 11.1).

Table 11.1: Common domains of health-related quality of life (QoL) assessments

Domain	Examples
Physical functioning	Mobility Self-care activities (e.g. washing/dressing) Activities of daily living (e.g. household chores, meal preparation) Physical activity Disease symptoms (e.g. pain, appetite, dyspnoea, fatigue) Treatment side-effects (e.g. nausea, constipation, infection)
Psychological, emotional	Depression Anxiety Adjustment to illness Coping Fear Self-esteem Body image Life satisfaction
Cognitive	Confusion Memory loss Concentration
Social	Personal relationships Ability to carry out hobbies and interests Sexuality Social isolation
Occupational	Work activities Financial status
Satisfaction with care	Information and communication Support from health professionals
Global assessments	Global health Global QoL

There is an increasing amount of literature available that explores the impact of cancer treatment from this approach, and this work has been an important move forward to considering the outcome of cancer treatment from the patients' perspective. Nevertheless, there are limitations that are increasingly being acknowledged. First, the focus on a functional perspective has neglected the consideration of the wider consequences of cancer treatment on a patient's life, such as sexuality, hope and expectations, social support, value and beliefs and the family. Secondly, there is again emphasis on understanding the impact of cancer treatments on groups of patients rather than on the individual. One of the present difficulties is using these popular measures of quality of life, which were designed originally as research tools, in clinical practice.[12]

Therefore, although these two latter approaches do have significant value in contributing to understanding the treatment experience, they are limited because they do not attempt to understand the social-cultural context of this nor the day-to-day realities of living through this experience. There is therefore a need to consider other approaches to explore the context of the cancer treatment experience.

The cultural and social experience of cancer treatment

In order to understand the context of patients' experiences, the social and cultural construction of illness, treatment and care should be considered. One approach has been through in-depth personal accounts of individuals' experiences such as Stacey[20] that provide insight and allow understanding of treatment in relation to personal, familial and social contexts.[21]

Research studies have also explored the contextual nature of treatment. This has been undertaken using qualitative methodologies such as phenomenological approaches to gain understanding of the 'lived experience' of cancer treatment. Some of these studies are generic, focusing on mixed groups of cancer patients[22] or looked at specific treatments such as radiotherapy,[23] bone marrow transplantation[24] or at the longer-term consequences of cancer treatments, such as survivorship.[25]

Many of these studies describe the treatment experience through the use of narrative accounts. These are a form of storytelling and their value in cancer nursing practice has been suggested to allow us to explore the experiences of people living with cancer and listen to the issues that are important to them.[26] This approach allows insight into how experiences change throughout the course of treatment.[22,27]

The value of these approaches is that they not only describe the outcomes of treatment experience on the individual and family but also explore the context and process of this experience, often providing in-depth accounts of what it is like on a day-to-day basis to live through the treatment journey. However, the main limitation of these approaches is that gathering this information can be lengthy and time-consuming, and that the generalisability of findings from patients' individual accounts is questioned.

Therefore, to understand the complexities of the treatment, experience all perspectives should be considered. We will now focus on reviewing the treatment experience and potential factors that impact upon this experience.

NEGOTIATING THE TREATMENT EXPERIENCE

Alongside the need to make sense of the diagnosis of cancer, perceived expectations of cancer treatment and actual daily realities of the treatment experience are also important in defining patients' experiences.

An in-depth study[28] has explored the treatment experience as a social process, through framing the cancer treatment journey as a treatment calendar, providing both supporting experiences and challenges. Once diagnosis is made (often complicated by surgery), patients embark on adjusting to daily life to accommodate the proposed treatment calendar (plan), which the authors refer to as preparing for life in the treatment calendar. This is described as a difficult process, influenced by factors such as resource availability, time to set up treatment plans, coordination of treatment schedules and dates, coordination of the different health professionals involved in the delivery of treatment and transfer of information between different departments and institutions. Once treatment plans are established, patients move into being treated and navigating their way through their treatment calendar. Each treatment calendar for the individual will often be several discrete calendars at once, some lasting longer than others. The experience is depicted as challenging in terms of the time and energy required to navigate a way through this process, dealing with side-effects and often managing several modes of treatment at once with a direct impact on patients' quality of life.

Central to this view is that the treatment experience is not static, but changes according to timing, circumstances and context. The experience of treatment will be constantly challenged and redefined as patients progress through their treatment journey. One of the ways that experience of treatment challenges or threatens patients is with regard to their self-identity. Treatment can result in a number of 'threats' to the patients' identity. One of the biggest struggles for patients is to interpret the meaning of their treatment and the changes that occur as a consequence of this, renegotiating their identity through their treatment experience, and to try and 'normalize' the treatment experience within daily life.[29,30]

It is impossible to try and distinguish what influences the experiences of cancer treatment from the experiences of cancer or indeed daily life per se; all influence and impact upon each other. It is essential that the experiences of treatment be placed in context with patients' overall illness experience and also in context with their daily life during this part of their cancer journey.

Deciding upon treatment options

Before we can understand what may influence our individual patients during their treatment journey, it is imperative that we explore their cancer experience to date. Two key factors in understanding are:

1 The prior experiences and perceptions of cancer treatment.

2 Their cancer journey up to this point in relation to accessing treatment.

Prior experiences and impact on treatment

Each individual will have a very different perception of what cancer treatment is and how it impacts on a person's life. Much of this perception will be influenced by past experience of cancer treatment (e.g. own or experiences of family, friends or colleagues), past values and beliefs about cancer treatment (e.g. cultural or religious beliefs about cancer) and also through media and literature on the subject.

There has been a considerable move within the popular media in recent years to capture in-depth experiences of cancer and its treatments. This has been portrayed through a number of mediums, including 'fly-on-the-wall' television documentaries, diaries of popular media personalities with cancer published in newspapers and biographies of peoples' experiences in magazines. One of the most significant advances has been the growth of the Internet. This has facilitated a wealth of information to be made available to individuals about cancer treatment, but the quality of much of this information is questionable, with regard to its evidence base. It is difficult for health professionals with considerable experience and knowledge in this area of health care to navigate through this maze; never mind for the patient, who at a time of significant upheaval, is faced with this complex and often conflicting information and advice.

Accessing treatment

Before a diagnosis of cancer is given, patients may have already embarked on their treatment journey. Investigations and tests for suspected malignancy may occur simultaneously with treatment (e.g. removal of polyps during a colonoscopy); often, confirmation of the diagnosis of cancer and early treatment (typically surgery) can occur at the same time. Waiting for histological confirmation of the diagnosis of cancer and embarking on treatment can result in anxiety for patients and their families. What is often common at this time for patients is a significant amount of disruption and uncertainty which surrounds making decisions about treatment for the individual, often when they are still coming to terms with the actual diagnosis of cancer itself. The complexity of this period (e.g. different investigations may result in different healthcare professionals seen or visits to different hospitals) can have an impact on patients' subsequent perceptions of treatment. Perceptions of the quality of care received at this time can also shape this experience, particularly with regard to communication between patient and health professional, support received, confidence in doctors and satisfaction with care.[31] This is illustrated by the quote in Box 11.2 from Philip, a 54-year-old builder, who was asked to recall his experiences of investigations and consultation prior to being informed that his pancreatic adenocarcinoma was inoperable[5]

The older person with cancer – Does age impact upon treatment experience?

Recent analysis of patients recruited into a variety of trials showed a substantial under-representation of patients of 65 years old or older.[32,33] Although epidemiological evidence shows that older patients have shorter survival than their younger counterparts,[34] age alone should not be used in deciding cancer treatment options.[35]

However, it is difficult to formally determine if there are differences in quality of life and treatment experience between younger and older patients with cancer. At present, the evidence is inconsistent. Studies have shown that older patients with cancer have better scores in some aspects of quality of life.[36,37] However, increasing age has been associated with decreasing quality of life[38] and diminishing

expectations of quality of life.[39] Severe long-standing illness and disability, which are common in the elderly, may affect quality of life.[40,41] Clearly, more understanding of the impact of treatment from the viewpoint of the older person with cancer is required.

Deciding on treatment pathways

There is considerable demand to include patients throughout the decision-making process, regarding their treatment and care. This demand has come from patients themselves,[42] and is reflected in national cancer policies and guidelines. In the UK, for example, the NHS Cancer Plan[43] is based on optimizing the patient experience and access to treatment, including incorporating patients' views when making decisions about treatment. As discussed in the previous chapter, there are a number of models of decision-making. From a clinical perspective, many of the decisions regarding treatment pathways will be determined beforehand, based on information such as site, stage and spread, gathered through a variety of data such as clinical, radiological and histological examination. Furthermore, other important factors such as patient fitness or significant co-morbidity will play an important role in this decision-making process. Inherent in this, should be an understanding of the costs and benefits of treatment from the perspective of the patient and family.

Costs and benefits of treatment

Weighing up the proposed benefits against the anticipated costs of treatment in terms of its outcome is one of the key factors in deciding on an individual treatment journey. However, this is often defined from the viewpoints of health professionals, through a biomedical perspective, rather than from patients themselves.

The benefits of treatment are usually defined in terms such as improvements in disease-free survival, symptom relief, improved functioning and improvements in quality of life. Conversely, the costs of treatment are typically presented in terms of side-effects, toxicity, deterioration in functioning and decline in quality of life. Much of the literature in this area has investigated patients' preferences in trading off costs against benefits, which is usually defined, as survival

---

Box 11.2

Perceptions of early treatment

'Well, I've found the actual care side of it wonderful. The administration side I find difficult to describe, but I think it's terrible chaos; the administration side … well it seems that one person doesn't know what another is doing. Difficult to explain it, but I was asked the same question by about five different people. Is there any need for that really? On the surgical side of it one doctor said, "Yes, we can operate". I went a fortnight later and, "No, we can't operate". I mean, surely that's devastating that is. Surely they could get it together and tell you one way or another before they make, commit themselves to a statement.'

benefit.[44,45] Although there is disparity in the findings from such studies, there is a suggestion that patients will accept relatively small survival benefits at the cost of mild toxicity. What is difficult to draw any definitive answers to is the influence of factors such as socioeconomic status, age, past experience and coping mechanisms on these decisions. Also, what these studies fail to explore is the real-life experience that individual patients with similar diagnoses and clinical characteristics will have markedly different preferences for treatment outcomes,[46] or indeed, the type of involvement that patients wish to have in this process.[47] As highlighted by Corner and Kelly,[48] there is increasing evidence to suggest that whereas the majority of people within the general population would wish for an active role in their treatment, this may not be the case when diagnosed with a life-threatening illness such as cancer.

Again, the biomedical emphasis fails to look at the wider costs and benefits of cancer treatments for the individual patient. These have been described in terms of:

- emotional (e.g. uncertainty, anxiety, loss of control)
- social (e.g. disruption to daily life, role changes, disruption to family life, stigma, disruption of employment);
- physical (e.g. loss of functioning, symptoms such as fatigue)
- economic (e.g. costs of travelling, prescription charges, loss of earning for individual and/or caregiver, extra support services).[49]

This may also include the cultural and spiritual costs of treatment. The biomedical emphasis continues to be on the negative aspects of cancer as an illness. However, for some patients, there may well be positive benefits associated with this experience, such as allowing re-prioritization of life events and lifestyle, and greater family cohesiveness. For many patients, these are somewhat difficult to articulate, but can be an inherent part of their treatment experience. Michael, a 56-year-old, when asked to comment on any positive experiences of his chemotherapy treatment (Box 11.3) summarized this feeling.[5]

Box 11.3

Positive experiences of treatment

'It takes something like this for some people, strangely enough, doesn't it? It sort of shows a family's true colours I think. Pretty marvellous, isn't it? They've been great.'

Clinical trials

Clinical trials are the standard route for evaluating the efficacy of new treatments. With recent initiatives to increase access for patients into clinical trials, more patients will be faced with decisions whether to participate. Often, this decision is made when there is little information on the benefits of treatment.[50]

Again, much of the focus of understanding the experience of clinical trials has been from a biomedical perspective rather than understanding the experience from the patients themselves. A qualitative study[51] has explored the experience of 55 patients recruited into early-phase clinical trials. This study illustrated key themes shaping patients' experience as hope offered by treatment, participants' desires to help others, not having choice and that burden of trial participation with regard to frequent hospital visits, travelling, side-effects, completing lengthy questionnaires, uncertainty of outcome and the sense of disappointment at the end of the trial. In a review of the literature, Kelly et al[52] discuss the actual and potential problems of participation such as increased anxiety and depression on the psychological well-being of patients. A review of the literature on the value of incorporating users' experiences,[53] emphasizes the importance of incorporating the user perspective into the design and conduct of cancer clinical trials in the future. Better understanding of patients' experiences in this context may contribute to improved recruitment and attrition, two significant problems in many cancer clinical trials.

UNDERGOING TREATMENT

For many patients and their families, embarking upon the cancer treatment pathway brings with it considerable disruption and anxiety as they enter this part of their cancer experience. For some, before definitive treatment, interventions such as establishing central venous access to receive chemotherapy, stem cell harvesting or complex planning prior to receiving radiotherapy may be required. They are faced with a number of different health professionals, a new environment and language, as well as trying to come to terms with the day-to-day realities of the impact of treatment on their lives. Often the realities of having cancer are often only fully realized at the point of starting treatment, as shown by Susan's (a 46-year-old woman with breast cancer) view of chemotherapy treatment for the first time[6] (Box 11.4).

The cancer treatment environment

There have been tremendous changes to the delivery and organization of cancer services in recent years, all of which will impact on patients' experiences. Advances in the way that cancer treatments are delivered have resulted in significant changes to where patients undergo their cancer treatment. Some patients may spend a large part of their treatment experience in an acute hospital environment. For others, most of their experience will fall outside these traditional 'institutional' settings. One of the significant advances has been in the growth of ambulatory cancer care, mainly through day care treatment. However, many hurdles remain, which can be illustrated when trying to understand the experiences of

chemotherapy. Although few data have been collected on how long patients wait to commence chemotherapy treatment, or the length of waiting time at each chemotherapy treatment appointment, there is evidence to suggest that patients experience delays in commencing treatment.[54] There are often problems in the way treatment systems are organized, so that delay and cancellation of treatment sessions can occur, and this is frustrating and worrying for patients.[55-57]

Practical difficulties can occur, such as travelling – frequently, treatments are based in regional centres, often requiring patients to travel long distances on a daily basis. Although evidence is inconclusive, travelling is often inconvenient to patients and may be a possible barrier to treatment.[58] Access to direct transportation to the place of care is sometimes unavailable, which can result in even more disruption to normal life routines. Some may spend a significant proportion of their day travelling back and forwards to treatment. Others may have to move temporarily from family/friends (e.g. to patient hotels or other accommodation) or be admitted as an inpatient due to difficulties in getting to treatment. Having arrived for treatment, there may be significant waiting times for actual treatment, again compromised by availability of resources, waiting to see the relevant healthcare professional and actual time for treatment to be delivered.

Patients' perceptions and expectations of the environment with which they are confronted can be crucial in shaping their experiences, particularly when it is their first visit. Even if there have been attempts to prepare patients for this milestone, it can still be one of tremendous shock and isolation as they enter this new and unfamiliar 'world'. This is illustrated by John and Kathy's accounts of entering their first chemotherapy outpatient clinic and their perceptions of this experience[6] (Box 11.5).

The language of cancer treatment

Much of the language of cancer treatment is often perceived in terms of 'battle talk', such as waging battles against cancer through the use of chemical or biological weapons.[59] Treatments

---

Box 11.4

The realities of treatment

'I don't think I really acknowledged that I had cancer until I saw the drugs ... and the thing is, I think, I mean, when I was diagnosed everything happens so quickly, you go into hospital, everything, like on an escalator, a roller coaster you know. And well, I don't think you have time to absorb it you know, cause you're given these dates for surgery, you go to pre-clerking, you have your surgery, come home, you know, district nurse comes in, bla, bla, bla, back to the clinic, you don't have time to think and I think I didn't. And it doesn't sink in and I don't think it sunk in until I saw this tray of drugs coming along, you know.'

Box 11.5

The treatment environment

John's account
'Well – I just want to say this actually, on my very first chemo I was absolutely petrified. I was. I froze in the corridor on the way down to the ward, I was like no, I don't want it, I don't want to go through with it. I wanted to go home but my wife was with me and she talked me round and one of the nurses, the one with the glasses, she came up and she said, "Come on then, off we go", sort of thing, you know, not having none of this sort of thing, took me down to the waiting room and I was just sat in the little area there. I was in tears, I don't want to do this, I want to go home. It's the unknown you know you didn't know, you don't know what to expect and everything and when you think of chemo you see like the pictures of it, all the adults and children like with no hair and in isolation tanks and all this sort of thing, and it's like oh my god what's going to happen to me. I felt then and I said this to the nurse a little while ago. I said: "It would have been so much nicer if one of the patients had come up to me and said: Look, it's going to be alright", but they didn't.

Kathy's account
'I had already decided in my mind I was going in on my own, I wanted to cope with it on my own. I walked through the door and I've never been down to the Chemotherapy department. I knew to a certain degree what to expect, there was going to be lots of people in there without hair or wigs on or looking slightly iller than normal but I walked round the corner, sure enough, it was a room full of people just like that and I sat down, and I found it very, very (big sigh). I wanted to burst into tears to be honest, and at that particular time, I thought, it might have been quite nice if somebody had come up to me and said something, explained. They haven't got time to do that I suppose but it would have been nice maybe if somebody could come and said to me, "Oh, this your first time", because they would have seen that from my card, and said this is what is going to happen, but I sat there for ages and felt very apprehensive about the whole thing.'

are often seen as leaving the person mutilated or scarred and the outcomes seen as either winning the war or being 'cured' or losing the battle and failure of treatment through cancer recurrence. Patients often use language to describe their experiences as a 'roller coaster' or 'conveyer belt'.[60] Often, language can reinforce the 'cancer label', as patients are treated in areas which are often identified by treatment intention, e.g. radiotherapy unit or breast cancer clinic. Daniel, a 54-year-old engineer, illustrates the potential impact of this language on patients' experiences with pancreatic cancer on his perception of his chemotherapy clinic[5] (Box 11.6).

The impact of treatment on patients' quality of life

Although there is considerable evidence of the toxicity and symptoms experienced as a result of treatment, there is relatively little written on the daily disruption brought about by symptoms and treatment-related side-effects.[48] There is increasing emphasis within the nursing literature on the documentation of these issues.[61–63] The treatment-related problems of common treatments will be discussed in depth in the following chapters.

From a biomedical perspective, the emphasis has usually been on measuring symptoms such as vomiting or weight loss, as these can be objectively rated, rather than the understanding of symptoms such as fatigue, which have a subjective basis of interpretation,[64] and how patients cope with managing these symptoms on a daily basis.[65] Also the focus is often on measuring these symptoms at discrete one-off time points rather than understanding the cumulative effect of symptom and treatment problems and their consequences on all aspects of a person's life.

The interplay between different symptoms has been identified as important in shaping experience.[66] For example, patients experiencing nausea and vomiting may also experience loss of appetite, taste changes, fatigue, weight

Box 11.6

The language of the cancer treatment environment

'I think the only thing I found, I found the hospital depressing. With the word cancer written everywhere, everywhere I went. I think, you don't want to be reminded of it. You know you've got it, or you've had it, whatever the case is, but you don't want the constant reminder and I think when you walk into the hospital you're constantly reminded what you're there for.'

loss and muscle weakness, which affect their functioning in terms of ability to carry out daily activities. This may also have an indirect effect on other aspects such as social functioning, self-esteem and satisfaction with life and, consequently, impact on patients' experiences. It is now well established that quality of life during treatment is much more than just the impact of symptom experience or patients' functional status.

The importance of understanding the context of treatment experience is fundamental in evaluating the impact of treatments on quality of life. There is evidence to suggest that, in cancer patients, factors such as perceived social support, existential issues and satisfaction with care can assume the same or greater importance as issues related to symptoms or physical functioning.[67-72] Other important considerations in the process of quality of life perception is the perceived gap between hope, expectations and realities of the treatment experience in patients,[15] cultural value systems[17] and appraisal of current health status against an ideal.[16] From our previous work,[4,5] we suggested some of the factors that influence quality of life perception during the experience of treatment (Fig. 11.1).

From a nursing perspective, there has been considerable activity in assessing the nature of cancer symptoms and problems that result from treatment[73] and towards evaluating interventions for these.[48] However, for the individual patient, it is very difficult to understand what it is like to experience the treatment journey on a day-to-day basis. Although treatment-induced problems are well established for individual treatment modalities, what is central to understanding this from a patient perspective is gaining an insight throughout the entire treatment experience and how the patient copes (or does not cope) and manages the treatment experience as part of daily life. Clearly more attention is needed towards strategies for preventing or minimizing these problems or facilitating their management once they arrive.[48]

Does quality of life change during the treatment experience?

One of the increasing areas of research is exploring the impact of cancer treatments over time and whether there is any predictive value in quality of life scores. Some studies have shown that some domains of patients' quality of life scores can distinguish treatment outcome,[74,75] and so may be able to provide useful information when evaluating whether to continue treatment pathways.

One of the difficulties in understanding the impact of treatment over time is the fluctuation in quality of life perception, depending on timing and circumstances. However, this change in quality of life is somewhat inconsistent, and often it is difficult to judge what are meaningful changes to patients' quality of life

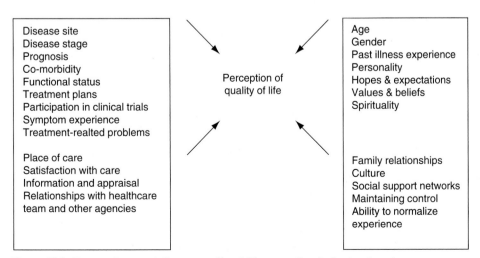

Figure 11.1: Factors that may influence quality of life perception during treatment.

over the treatment journey. For example, although this fluctuation can be dramatic over a short-term basis, there is increasing evidence to suggest that when examined over a longer period these changes appear to be much more stable than expected. There is empirical evidence to suggest[76,77] that even with apparently life-threatening illness, patients report either stable quality of life throughout their illness trajectory or that their quality of life is not inferior to patients with less severe disease.

One of the factors that may be important in exploring relatively long-term stability in quality of life is the impact of a response shift.[78] This phenomenon relates to the fact that as patients progress through their treatment and illness experience, their values and priorities change in addition to changes in their actual health state. The importance of this phenomenon in relation to evaluating the outcome of treatment has been highlighted,[79] as it may exaggerate patients' perception of treatment effects as they adapt to treatment toxicities or disease progression over time.

The difficulties in understanding the impact of treatment over time on patients' quality of life has been reported for a number of cancer diagnoses and treatments. A study of 58 patients receiving radiotherapy for head and neck cancer[80] showed that within relatively short time points (first week of treatment, last week of treatment and 1-month following treatment), there were increased levels of physical and functional symptoms and depression between the first and last week of treatment, with some improvement between the last week and 1-month follow-up. However, with regard to emotional functioning, there were no changes in emotional and social well-being over time. Similarly, a study of the quality of life of 5 different treatment groups of prostate cancer patients over an 18-month period[81] demonstrated that, although there were no significant differences between groups in health status or quality of life, different treatments produced different symptom profiles, such as radiotherapy producing more gastrointestinal symptoms and surgery more sexual functioning symptoms. In a study to examine predictors of health-related quality of life in 227 women with early-stage breast cancer at 1 year,[82] most women reported high levels of functioning and quality of life with no relationship between type of surgery and quality of life.

This picture can become even more ambiguous over a long-term period. In a follow-up study of 277 testicular cancer survivors 3–13 years after treatment, the findings demonstrated that when compared to an 122 age- and sex-matched group within the general population, their health-related quality of life was as good as, or even better than, that of the men in the general population.[83] In a study to evaluate the quality of life of adult survivors 2–4 years after allogeneic stem cell transplantation,[84] although impairments in functional status were found, such as cough, sexual problems, tiredness and anxiety, when compared to population norms, the general health and quality of life was described as quite good or excellent by 80% of the patients. Further work is required to understand the impact of the treatment experience over time, and one of the disparities that should be recognized is in the approach taken to evaluate quality of life over time. The importance of experience should be acknowledged and appears to be important in interpreting patients' preferences for treatment and also impact on treatment outcomes.[85]

Quality of care and its impact on quality of life

In their construct of patients' experiences of navigating the treatment calendar, Schou and Hewison[28] highlight the importance of the quality of care perceived by patients in terms of how patients deal with their quality of life concerns and interpret their treatment experience. Factors which have been crucial in shaping this perception are understanding the rationale when treatment changes occur, or when inconsistencies in the 'system' have a direct bearing on the individual patient's treatment, as illustrated by David, a 52-year-old college lecturer receiving adjuvant chemotherapy for colorectal cancer (Box 11.7)

Consistency in the treatment process can help to facilitate patients' experiences, particularly in consistency in the health professionals seen, management of their treatment and also in information received about their progress. In a study of six cancer narratives, Van Der

Box 11.7

Patients' perceptions of changes in treatment systems

'Well, yeah, that (the system) frustrates me because if I made an appointment with a student for 1:30, I'd expect him to be there at 1:30 and I would be there, but here it's normally a half to three-quarters of an hour wait to see the doctor. If you're coming in for just a bottle change it can be anything from a few minutes to about an hour or, I have the 1:30 appointment so I'm already 15 minutes late, but of course there's people off ill. But the big frustrating thing is – it got me quite annoyed, well a couple of things – once they'd forgotten to order my 5FU, but they'd ordered my bottle; another time they'd forgotten to order my drugs but they'd ordered the bottle … . Another time my bottle didn't work after I came in on a Thursday; there's no one here over the weekend; rang them Monday morning and they said come in we'll give you another bottle, we'll order one from pharmacy, I spoke to the sister. So I said: "I don't want to hang around for hours"; so she said: "Well come in, in a couple of hours". Came in, in a couple of hours; the pharmacy had rejected the order because I wasn't due until Thursday – this was Monday. They then sent down to pharmacy again and pharmacy had lost my chart!'

Molen[86] illustrates the importance of information provision in allowing patients to cope through their treatment, and that information needs change over time and vary from person to person. However, the concept of information was related to medical aspects of patients' lives rather than other areas. Also, the ability to process information could only be undertaken when respondents identified themselves as living with cancer. Therefore, although information may be readily available to patients, the ability of patients to process and utilize this will be influenced by context: Jenny, a mother of four children in her forties, undergoing treatment for colorectal cancer, illustrates this:

It wasn't really until I came out of hospital even though I knew I had cancer that I wanted to identify myself as being part of a community of people living with cancer. I was prepared to identify myself as a single mother, a health professional … but I wasn't at that stage ready, prepared to identify myself as someone living with cancer.[86(p45)]

However, preparedness to receive information may well be down to the individual. In a study of information needs of patients receiving day-case chemotherapy, most patients wanted to receive all possible information at the beginning of their treatment, and the amount actually received was perceived as about right. However, over half of the respondents commented on the lack of information about the impact of treatment on family relationships.[57]

An important component in the communication of information is assessing patients' ability to articulate their health needs. A study of the perceived met and unmet needs of 11 patients with prostate cancer highlighted that, although patients' functional health needs were met by health professionals, issues related to their existential needs were mostly not met. This was linked to whether patients were seen as passive or active receivers of care. Passive receivers were contradictory with regard to explicitly stating their satisfaction with care but at the same time implicitly referring to their needs as unimportant and not met, whereas active receivers talked about their needs explicitly with staff.[87] This work highlights the importance of nurses being sensitive to patients' accounts and to actively seeking what are their individual needs.

AFTER TREATMENT

The point of departure from treatment can bring with it new uncertainties and disruption to the lives of patients and their families. This point is often expected to be a significant milestone in the cancer journey. However, for many, this may not be the reality; even with patients who face the prospect of cure, it may be difficult, indeed unfeasible, for them to return to their pre-illness identity.

Often, one of the most ambiguous times is the period when 'definitive' treatment (e.g. course of chemotherapy or radiotherapy) is completed yet the problems of treatment continue. The time taken to overcome these problems will vary again, according to the patient's circumstances. For some treatments such as radiotherapy, problems may not occur until the end or once completed. For other treatments, patients will be faced with the consequences of treatment for the rest of their lives: for example, loss of a breast or limb or the need to continue on long-term treatment (e.g. tamoxifen for breast cancer). Loss of function, such as sexual functioning and/or fertility, may continue indefinitely. The impact of the treatment experience on family and on social and occupational roles may also be difficult to readjust to.

Follow-up

There is debate as to the value of routine follow-up for patients, focusing on the effectiveness of follow-up in surveillance and detecting local recurrence or metastatic disease. However, this debate should be discussed from a broader perspective, rather than solely an emphasis on the purported clinical benefit of these services, and should consider the meaning of follow-up to the individual patient and the purpose of follow-up in meeting the emotional and social needs of patients. The biomedical viewpoint of 5 years as indication of long-term survival,[88] means that patients are still faced with returning to the cancer environment at regular intervals, and makes assumptions that there is a cut-off point for when the cancer label ceases; however, for many patients, the identification as a cancer patient continues to persist regardless of time since treatment or recurrent disease.[27]

Corner[89] sees this as opportunity for specialist nursing to transform this area of care, reorienting care to assisting people to monitor themselves, and providing open access to support, information and investigations of symptoms. With many patients now surviving long term with cancer, or living with cancer, this area requires careful consideration, particularly in patients' willingness to accept such changes to care. A recent randomized study[90] assessed the effectiveness of specialist nurse-led follow-up and conventional medical follow-up in patients with lung cancer. This study demonstrated high patient acceptability of the service with improvements in dyspnoea at 3 months, emotional functioning and satisfaction with care. No differences were recorded in survival or disease progression. This model of follow-up care was shown to be safe, acceptable and cost-effective. However, further work is needed before these findings can be generalized, particularly for other cancer diagnoses and care settings.

Recurrence of cancer

One of the greatest fears for patients is that the cancer will return or, for patients receiving palliative treatment, that this is no longer controlling the disease and/or symptoms. This stage is often seen as one of shock, despair and considerable threat to the patient and their family. Individuals may feel angry, frustrated and despondent with a need to regain control.[91] This time may result in patients re-entering or modifying their treatment journey. Understanding the context of this will be fundamental in optimizing patients' experience at this difficult and vulnerable time.

Palliative care

Understanding the treatment needs of patients and their families during the palliative phase of their cancer experience is an important aspect of nursing practice. It is beyond the scope of this chapter to give an in-depth account of the treatment experience within palliative care, and work by Lawton[92] gives an insight into the complexities from the perspectives of patients receiving palliative care. For some patients this may occur after a significant period of remission; for others, palliative care will commence at the same time as their diagnosis of cancer. Here, the focus of treatment is on improving symptoms and optimizing quality of life. In deciding treatment options, the patient, family and healthcare team must weigh up the costs and benefits of treatment on these outcomes rather than improved survival or improved disease response. The ethical dilemmas of whether to offer further treatment or when to stop treatment should be carefully considered during this time.

RECONFIGURING CANCER NURSING SERVICES – ARE NURSE-LED MODELS OF CARE FEASIBLE?

There is increasing consensus that there is a need to re-frame services around meeting the needs of patients during their treatment experience. One of the potential areas for remodelling the treatment experience for patients is through nurse-led models of care delivery, as outlined above. A diverse range of settings for nurse-led activities have been reported in the literature, including symptom management,[93] follow-up clinics in specific diseases,[94,95] delivering a psychological intervention,[96,97] rehabilitation post-treatment completion,[98] radiotherapy follow-up[99,100] and chemotherapy.[101]

In a review of the therapeutic benefits of nurse-led models of care delivery,[6] the evidence suggests that there are benefits to such models in improving patient experience with regard to satisfaction with care and improved quality of life. Other potential benefits include improved communication and better organization and efficiency of care, including savings in time and resources. There is considerable scope for nursing innovation in this context. However, this should be undertaken in parallel with rigorous evaluation on outcomes that reflect patient experience.

METHODS TO ASSESS TREATMENT EXPERIENCE

As there are a variety of perspectives in understanding the treatment experience: there are a number of methods that can be used to assess treatment experience, all with their advantages and disadvantages when it comes to use within the clinical setting (Table 11.2). Nevertheless, assessing the impact of treatment and the evaluation of strategies to optimize patient experience should be undertaken at all stages of the cancer treatment journey. One of the most important issues that requires critical debate is whether the use of quality of life instruments, patient satisfaction scales and measures of patient functioning truly capture the most important and relevant aspects of treatment experience for patients. With the need to ensure evaluation of new services and interventions from a user perspective,[43] there is a demand for robust patient outcomes that reflect this perspective. To date, there is little work on developing user-generated measures of outcomes for cancer patients, or the potential application of measures which are appro-

priate for use in studies which evaluate clinical service models or interventions. Within this context, broad areas such as symptom perception and self-management may be the most relevant areas of treatment experience for cancer patients.

With regard to who should assess experience, there is consensus that, whenever possible, this should be patients themselves. However, the value of proxy responders has been debated. In summarizing the evidence, Addington-Hall and Kalra[78] report some of the advantages of proxy responders (e.g. caregivers or health professionals) are that there is usually moderate agreement between patients and proxies, and that proxies are almost as good at detecting changes over time, and can provide useful information on the more concrete, observable aspects of quality of life. The disadvantages reported include the overestimation of some aspects of quality of life and the changing priorities of patients over time. Also, the importance of understanding the context of patients' experiences should be acknowledged when making any interpretations from such assessment.

CONCLUSION

The cancer treatment experience is often long, complex and impacts on all aspects of patients' lives. With the increasing emergence of new interventions and therapies, treatment should be viewed as an ongoing process throughout the cancer patient journey. Although there are significant milestones reported within the literature that are common to many of our patients, each experience will be unique to the individual concerned, according to his or her own circumstances.

Understanding the complexities of cancer treatment requires understanding from a variety of perspectives in order to facilitate and support patients through their treatment experience and optimize their quality of life. A summary of the implications for cancer nursing practice is given in Box 11.8.

Further evidence is needed to fully explore the role of the nurse within this context, particularly with regard to innovating new models of nursing care delivery. The care of the patient

Table 11.2: Review of some of the methods to assess treatment experience

Method	Advantages	Disadvantages
Performance status (e.g. Karnofsky scale[102])	Widely used Allow comparisons across different patients Quick and simple to use Provide a single score	Focus upon physical performance only Objectively rated by professional rather than patient Lack of validity
Toxicity scales/criteria	Widely used Rates toxicity Provides information across broad spectrum of treatment-related problems Allow comparisons across different patients	Focus upon symptom toxicity only Objectively rated by professional rather than patient Lack of data on reliability and validity
Structured symptom assessments (e.g. C-SAS[73])	Rates a range of symptoms/treatment-related problems Often provide information on severity/bother of symptom experience Developed for use in clinical practice	Focus upon symptom experience only Responsiveness to change over time not assessed Lack of comparison across different treatments
Cancer-specific quality of life instruments (e.g. EORTC QLQ-C30[18])	Cover important issues for cancer patients Relevant to problems across cancer patients Often have diagnosis/treatment specific modules available	Lack of cross-study comparisons Often emphasis on functional status and symptom experience Lack of information of use in clinical practice/individual patients
Structured diaries	Consider subjectivity of patients' experience Allows experience to be captured throughout treatment Captures individual perception	Often lengthy and time-consuming to complete Compliance may be a problem Reliability and validity require further assessment
Individualized structured assessments of quality of life (e.g. SEIQOL[103])	Capture individual perception Responsive to changes in individuals across time	Trained-interviewer administered Not tested in many patient populations Validity and reliability require further assessment
Interviews	Capture individual perception and context of experience	Trained-interviewer administered Lengthy and time-consuming Generalizability of information questioned

Box 11.8

Summary of implications for cancer nursing practice

1. A variety of perspectives contribute to understanding the complexities of the cancer treatment experience in order to assess patient and family needs.

2. Patients' perceptions of their treatment experience are shaped by a number of factors: understanding these experiences and patients' expectations of their treatment is required in order to plan and implement effective nursing care.

3. Nursing assessment should focus on understanding the impact of treatment from the viewpoint of the individual patient and family.

4. Patients' experiences are contextual, and may fluctuate according to timing and circumstances during their treatment journey: nurses must ensure that patients' needs are continually assessed, and the outcomes of care delivery re-evaluated.

5. Providing support, information and coordination of the patient's treatment journey is integral to the delivery of care.

6. The treatment experience does not end with the cessation of active treatment: further work is needed to develop effective patient-centred models of follow-up.

7. There is tremendous potential for innovation of nurse-led models of care, based around meeting the needs of patients during their cancer treatment experience: it is imperative that service development should be undertaken alongside rigorous evaluation.

8. There is scope for the use of structured measures to inform nursing assessment, although further work is needed to ensure appropriateness for the clinical setting.

should not end once treatment is completed; the therapeutic role of the nurse in follow-up and surveillance should be further examined. The following chapters will examine in depth the specific experiences of patients in relation to the major treatment modalities and more recent treatment developments, and the role of the nurse in caring for the patient during this experience.

REFERENCES

1. Corner, J. The scope of cancer nursing. In: Horwich A, ed. Oncology: a multidisciplinary textbook. London: Chapman and Hall; 1995.

2. Wells, M. The impact of cancer. In: Corner J, Bailey C, eds. Cancer nursing care in context. London: Blackwell Science; 2001:3–85.

3. Tritter, JQ. Cancer as a chronic illness? Reconsidering categorization and exploring experience. Eur J Cancer Care 2002; 11:161–165.

4. Fitzsimmons D, George S, Payne S et al. Quality of life in pancreatic cancer: differences in perception between health professionals and patients. Psycho-Oncology 1999; 35:939–941.

5. Fitzsimmons D. Quality of life in pancreatic diseases. Unpublished PhD thesis, University of Southampton; 2000.

6. Fitzsimmons D, Hawker SE, Johnson CD, et al. Phase 1 Exploratory study of a nurse specialist managed chemotherapy service. Final Report to NHS South East Research and Development Directorate: University of Southampton; 2002

7. Greer S, Morris T, Pettingale PW. Psychological responses to breast cancer: effect on outcome. Lancet 1979; ii:785–787.

8. Burton M, Watson M. Counselling people with cancer. Chichester: Wiley Press; 1998.

9. Guex P. An introduction to psycho-oncology. London: Routledge; 1989.

10. Maguire P, Selby P. Assessing quality of life in cancer patients. Br J Cancer 1989; 60: 437–440.

11. Fallowfield L. The quality of life: the missing measurement in health care. London: Souvenir; 1990.

12. Carr AJ, Higginson IJ. Are quality of life measures patient centred? BMJ 2001; 322:1357–1360.

13. Aaronson NK. Quality of life in cancer clinical trials: a need for common rules and language. Oncology 1990; 4:59–66.

14. Gill TM. Quality of life assessment values and pitfall. J Roy Soc Med 1995; 88:680–682.

15. Calman KC. Quality of life in cancer patients – a hypothesis. J Med Ethics 1984; 10:124–127.

16. Cella DF, Tulsky DS. Measuring quality of life today: methodological aspects. Oncology (Huntingt) 1990; 4:29–38.

17. WHOQOL Group. The World Health Organisation Quality of Life Assessment (WHOQOL): Position Paper from the World Health Organisation. Soc Sci Med 1995; 46:1569–1585.

18. Aaronson, NK, Ahmedzai S, Bergman B, et al. The European Organisation for Research and Treatment of Cancer QLQ-C30: a quality of life instrument for use in international clinical trials in oncology. J Natl Cancer Inst 1993; 85:365–376.

19. Cella DF, Tulsky DS, Gray G, et al. The functional assessment of cancer therapy scale: development and validation of the general measure. J Clin Oncol 1993; 11:570–579.

20. Stacey J. Tetatologies; a cultural study of cancer. London: Routledge; 1997.

21. Taylor K. Researching the experience of kidney cancer patients. Eur J Cancer Care 2002; 11:200–204.

22. Matheson CM, Stam HJ. Renegotiating identity: cancer narratives. Sociology of Health and Illness 1995; 17:283–306.

23. Wells M. The hidden experience of radiotherapy to the head and neck: a qualitative study of patients after completion of treatment. J Adv Nurs 1998; 28:840–848.

24. Gaskill D, Henderson A, Fraser M. Exploring the everyday world of the patient in isolation. Oncol Nurs Forum 1997; 24:695–700.

25. Breaden K. Cancer and beyond: the question of survivorship. J Adv Nurs 1997; 26:978–984.

26. Van Der Molan B. Using cancer narratives to influence practice. Eur J Cancer Care 2001; 10:284–289.

27. Little M, Jordens FC, Paul K, et al. Liminality: a major category of the experience of cancer illness. Soc Sci Med 1998; 47:1485–1494.

28. Schou KC, Hewison J. Experiencing cancer: quality of life in treatment. Buckingham: Open University Press; 1999.

29. Muzzin LJ, Anderson NJ, Figueredo AT, Gudelis SO. The experience of cancer. Soc Sci Med 1994; 38:1201–1208.

30. Cowley L, Heyman B, Stanton M, et al. How women receiving adjuvant chemotherapy for breast cancer cope with their treatment: a risk management perspective. J Adv Nurs 2000; 31:314–321.

31. Henman MJ, Butow PN, Brown RF, et al. Lay constructions of decision making in cancer. Psycho-Oncology 2002; 11:295–306.

32. Hutchins LF, Under JM, Crowley JJ et al. Under-representation of patients 65 years of age or older in cancer treatment trials. N Eng J Med 1999; 341:2061–2067.

33. Simmonds PC. Palliative chemotherapy for advanced colorectal cancer: systematic review and meta analysis. Colorectal Cancer Collaborative Group. BMJ 2000; 321:531–535.

34. Office for National Statistics. Cancer survival data: five year-relative survival by age at diagnosis and sex, England and Wales; adults diagnosed 1986–1999. London: HMSO; 1999.

35. Balducci J. Perspectives on quality of life of older patients with cancer. Drugs Aging 1994; 4:313–324.

36. Rustooen T, Moum T, Wikllund I. Quality of life in newly diagnosed cancer patients. J Adv Nurs 1999; 29:490–498.

37. Lakusta CM, Atkinson MJ, Robinson JW. Quality of life in ovarian cancer patients receiving chemotherapy. Gynecol Oncol 2001; 81:490–495.

38. Farquhar M. Elderly people's definitions of quality of life. Soc Sci Med 1995; 41:1439–1446.

39. Staats SR, Stassen MA. Age and present and future perceived quality of life. Int J Aging Hum Dev 1987; 25:167–176.

40. Grimby A, Svanborg A. Morbidity and health-related quality of life among ambulant elderly citizens. Aging (Milano) 1997; 9:356–364.

41. Kempen GI, Ormel J Brilman EL, et al. Adaptive responses among Dutch elderly: the impact of eight chronic medical conditions on health related quality of life. Am J Pub Health 1997; 87:38–44.

42. Department of Health National Survey of NHS Patients Cancer National Overview 1999/2000. London: Department of Health; 2002.

43. Department of Health. The NHS Cancer Plan. London: Department of Health; 2000.

44. Silvestri G, Prithcard R, Welch HG. Preferences for chemotherapy in patients with advanced non-small lung cancer: descriptive study based on scripted interviews. BMJ 1998; 317: 771–775.

45. Jansen SJ, Kievit J, Nooij MA, et al. Stability of patients' preferences for chemotherapy: the impact of experience. Med Decis Making 2001; 21:295–306.

46. Lubeck D, Grossfeld G, Carroll P. A review of measurement of patient preferences for treatment outcomes after prostate cancer. Urology 2002; 60(Suppl 1):72.

47. Beaver K, Luker K, Glynn Owens R, et al. Treatment decision making in women newly diagnosed with breast cancer. Cancer Nurs 1996; 19:8–19.

48. Corner J, Kelly D. The experience of treatment. In: Corner J, Bailey C, eds. Cancer nursing care in context. London: Blackwell Science, 2001:143–155.

49. Pearce S, Kelly D, Stevens W. 'More than just money'– widening the understanding of the costs involved in cancer care. J Adv Nurs 2001; 33:371–379.

50. Cox K. Informed consent and decision-making: patients' experiences of the process of recruitment to phase I and II anti-cancer drug trials. Patient Educ Couns 2002; 46:31–38.

51. Cox K. Enhancing cancer clinical trial management: recommendations from a qualitative study of trial participants' experiences. Psycho-Oncology 2002; 9: 314–322.

52. Kelly C, Ghazi F, Caldwell K. Psychological distress of cancer and clinical trial participation: a review of the literature. Eur J Cancer Care 2002; 11:6–15.

53. Donovan JL, Brindle L, Mills N. Capturing users' experiences of participating in clinical trials. Eur J Cancer Care 2002; 11:210–214.

54. Commission for Health Improvement National Service Framework No.1. NHS Cancer Care in England & Wales. London: HMSO; 2001.

55. Sitza J, Wood N. Patient satisfaction with cancer chemotherapy nursing: a review of the literature. Int J Nurs Stud 1998; 35:1–12.

56. Topham C, Moore J. Patient preferences for chemotherapy schedules used in the treatment of advanced colorectal cancer – a pilot study. Eur J Cancer Care 1997; 6:291–294.

57. McCaughan EM, Thompson KA. Information needs of cancer patients receiving chemotherapy at a day case unit in Northern Ireland. J Clin Nurs 2000; 9:851–858.

58. Payne S, Jarrett N, Jeffs D. The impact of travel on cancer patients' experiences of treatment: a literature review. Eur J Cancer Care 2000; 9:197–203.

59. Bailey C. Cancer, care and society. In: Corner J, Bailey C, eds. Cancer nursing care in context. London: Blackwell Science; 2001:26–45.

60. Van Der Molen B. Relating information needs to the cancer experience. 2. Themes from six cancer narratives. Eur J Cancer Care 2000; 9:48–54.

61. Sitza J, Hughes J, Sobrido L. A study of patients' experiences of side-effects associated with chemotherapy: pilot stage report. Int J Nurs Stud 1995: 32:580–600.

62. Dikken C, Sitza J. Patients' experiences of chemotherapy: side-effects associated with 5-fluorouracil and folinic acid in the treatment of colorectal cancer. J Clin Nurs 1998; 7:371–379.

63. Williams PD, Ducey KA, Sears AM, et al. Treatment type and symptom severity among oncology patients by self-report. Int J Nurs Stud 2001; 38:359–367.

64. Raber MN. A patients' perspective on cancer-related fatigue. Cancer 2001; 92:1662–1663.

65. Richardson A, Ream EK. Self-care behaviours initiated by chemotherapy patients in response to fatigue. Int J Nurs Stud 1997; 34:35–43.

66. Newell S, Sanson-Fisher RW, Girgis A, et al. The physical and psycho-social experiences of patients attending an out-patient medical oncology department: a cross-sectional study. Eur J Cancer Care 2002; 8:73–82.

67. Cohen SR, Mount BM, Tomas JJ, Mount LF. Existential well-being is an important determinant of quality of life: evidence from the McGill Quality of Life Questionnaire. Cancer 1996; 77:576–586.

68. Koller M, Kussman J, Lorenz W, et al. Symptom reporting in cancer patients. The role of negative affect and experienced social stigma. Cancer 1996; 77:983–995.

69. Magnusson K, Moller A, Ekman T, et al. A qualitative study to explore the experience of fatigue in cancer patients. Eur J Cancer Care (Engl) 1999; 8:224–232.

70. Sahey TB, Gray RE, Fitch M. A qualitative study of patient perspectives on colorectal cancer. Cancer Pract 2000; 8:38–44.

71. Wan GJ, Counte MA, Cella DF. The influence of personal expectations on cancer patients' reports on health-related quality of life. Psycho-Oncology 1997; 6:1–11.

72. Velji K, Fitch M. The experience of women receiving brachytherapy for gynecologic cancer. Oncol Nurs Forum 2001; 28:743–751.

73. Brown V, Sitza J, Richardson A, et al. The development of the Chemotherapy Symptom Assessment Scale (C-SAS): a scale for the routine clinical assessment of symptom experiences of patients receiving cytotoxic chemotherapy. Int J Nurs Stud 2001; 38:497–510.

74. Tamburini M, Brunelli C, Rosso S, Ventafridda V. Prognostic value of quality of life scores in terminal cancer patients. J Pain Sym Management 1996; 11: 32-41.

75. Ringdal GI, Ringdal K, Kvinnsland S, Gotestam KG. Quality of life of cancer patients with different prognoses. Quality of Life Research 1994; 3:143–154.

76. Breetvelt IS, Van Dam FSAM. Underreporting by cancer patients: the case of response shift. Soc Sci Med 1991; 32:981–987.

77. Wisloff F, Eika S, Hippe E, et al. Measurement of health-related quality of life in multiple myeloma. Br J Haematol 1997; 92:604–613.

78. Addington-Hall J, Kalra L. Who should measure quality of life? BMJ 2001;322:1417–1420.

79. Schwartz CE, Sprangers MAG. Methodological approaches for assessing response shift in longitudinal health-related quality of life research. Soc Sci Med 1999; 48:1531–1548.

80. Rose P, Yates P. Quality of life experienced by patients receiving radiation treatment for cancers of the head and neck. Cancer Nurs 2001; 24:255–263.

81. Galbraith ME, Ramirez JM, Pedro LM. Quality of life, health outcomes and identity for patients with prostate cancer in five different treatment groups. Oncol Nurs Forum 2001; 28:551–560.

82. Shimozuma K, Ganz PA, Petersen L, et al. Quality of life in the first year after breast cancer surgery: rehabilitation needs and patterns of recovery. Breast Cancer Res Treat 1999; 56:45–57.

83. Rudberg L, Carlsson M, Nilsson S, et al. Self-perceived physical, psychological and general symptoms in survivors of testicular cancer 3 to 13 years after treatment. Cancer Nurs 2002; 25:187–195.

84. Edman L, Larsen J, Hagglund H, Gardulf A. Health-related quality of life, symptom distress and sense of coherence in adult survivors of allogenic stem-cell transplantation. Eur J Cancer Care 2001; 10:124–130.

85. Stigglebout AM, de Haes JC. Patient preference for cancer therapy: an overview of measurement approaches. J Clin Oncol 2001; 19:220–230.

86. Van Der Molen B. Relating information needs to the cancer experience. 1 Jenny's story: a cancer narrative. Eur J Cancer Care 2000; 9:41–47.

87. Jakobsson L, Hallberg IR, Loven L. Met and unmet nursing care needs in men with prostate cancer. An explorative study. Part II. Eur J Cancer Care 1997: 6:117–123.

88. Frauman, JF, Devessa SS, Hoover RN, et al. Epidemiology of cancer. In: De Vita VT, Hellman S, Rosenberg SA, eds. Cancer principles and practice of oncology. Philadelphia: JB Lippincott; 1993.

89. Corner J. Cancer nursing: a leading force for health care. J Adv Nurs 1999; 29:275–276.

90. Moore S, Corner J, Haviland J, et al. Nurse led follow up and conventional medical follow up in management of patients with lung cancer: randomised trial. BMJ 2002; 325:1145–1153.

91. Watson M, Greer S, Rowden L, et al. Relationships between emotional control, adjustment to cancer and depression and anxiety in breast cancer patients. Psychol Med 1991; 21:51–57.

92. Lawton J. The Dying process. Patients' experiences of palliative care. London; Routledge; 2000.

93. Bredin M, Corner J, Krishnasamy M, et al. Multicentre randomised controlled trial of nursing intervention for breathlessness in patients with lung cancer. BMJ 1999; 318:901–904.

94. Helgesen F, Andersson SO, Gustafsson O, et al. Follow-up of prostate cancer patients by on-demand contacts with a specialist nurse: a randomized study. Scand J Urol Nephrol 2000; 34:55–61.

95. Sardell S, Sharpe G, Ashley S, et al. Evaluation of a nurse-led telephone clinic in the follow-up of patients with malignant glioma. Clin Oncol (R Coll Radiol) 2000; 12:36–41.

96. McArdle JM, George WD, McArdle CS, et al. Psychological support for patients undergoing breast cancer surgery: a randomised study. BMJ 1996; 312:813–816.

97. Maughan K, Clarke C. The effect of a clinical nurse specialist in gynaecological oncology on quality of life and sexuality. J Clin.Nurs 2001; 10:221–229.

98. Berglund G, Bolund C, Gustafsson UL, et al. A randomized study of a rehabilitation program for cancer patients: the 'Starting Again' group. Psycho-Oncology 1994; 3:109–120.

99. Campbell J, German L, Lane C, et al. Radiotherapy outpatient review: a nurse-led clinic. Clin Oncol (R Coll Radiol) 2000; 12:104–107.

100. Faithfull S, Corner J, Meyer L, et al. Evaluation of nurse-led follow up for patients undergoing pelvic radiotherapy. Br J Cancer 2001; 85:1853–1864.

101. Porter HB. The effect of ambulatory oncology nursing practice models on health resource utilization. Part 1, Collaboration or compliance? J Nurs Adm 1995; 25:21–29.

102. Karnofsky DA, Abelman WH, Craver LF, et al. The use of nitrogen mustards in the palliative treatment of carcinoma. Cancer 1948; 1:634–656.

103. O'Boyle CA, McGee HM, Hickey A, et al. The schedule for the evaluation of individual quality of life (SEIQoL): administration manual. Dublin: Royal College of Surgeons in Ireland; 1993.

CHAPTER 12

Surgery

ALASTAIR M THOMPSON AND MARY WELLS

CHAPTER CONTENTS

Introduction	233
The role of surgery	233
Changing practice	234
Prophylactic surgery	235
Reconstructive surgery	235
Pain control	235
Surgical specialization	235
Preoperative, intraoperative and postoperative care and the role of the nurse	236
Preoperative care	236
Intraoperative care	237
Postoperative care	238
Principles of surgical management of patients with cancer	239
Breast cancer	241
Principles	241
Diagnosis	241
Staging	241
Decision-making process (multidisciplinary team)	242
Neoadjuvant downstaging	242

Breast cancer surgery	243
Oesophageal/gastric cancers	247
Introduction	247
Presentation	247
Diagnosis	247
Staging	247
The multidisciplinary meeting	249
Neoadjuvant therapy	249
Resection of upper gastrointestinal cancer	249
Recovery and rehabilitation	253
Colorectal cancer	254
Principles	254
Diagnosis	254
Staging	255
Multidisciplinary meeting	255
Surgery and reconstruction	256
Recovery and rehabilitation	260
Innovations in surgery for cancer	260
Conclusion	261
References	261

INTRODUCTION

Surgery has historically been the main treatment for most types of cancer. Today it is usually combined with other modalities to treat cancer, including radiation, chemotherapy and, more recently, novel approaches using light (photo-dynamic therapy) and targeted biological thera-pies aimed at specific genes (*HER2*, *c-kit*) or deposits of tumour cells in bone (bisphospho-nates). This chapter considers the role of sur-gery and some general principles in the management of patients with cancer, including the role of nurses in the supportive care of patients undergoing surgery. Then using breast, oesophageal, gastric and colorectal cancer as examples, the surgical management of patients with these diseases is described.

The role of surgery

In general, the place of surgery in the treat-ment of an individual patient should be deter-mined by a multidisciplinary team; the surgery should be linked in with other modalities and based, where possible, on scientific evidence, including randomized trials. This approach is increasingly used in the treatment of patients with many solid cancer types.

The role of surgery encompasses diagnosis (particularly tissue biopsy), staging (which may or may not require surgery) to determine the extent of disease, primary excision of the cancer, regional metastatic and even distant metastatic disease with the intention of cure, debulking tumour burden and/or surgical treatment of metastatic disease (Box 12.1). Like all cancer treatments, surgery occurs within the context of the individual's social, psychological and illness experience, and therefore the meaning and impact of surgery will vary greatly depending on the individual's characteristics, stage of cancer and functional and psychological consequences of the surgical procedure.[1]

Surgery alone may be curative (e.g. excision of a small colonic cancer polyp), without the need for further therapies. Alternatively, surgery may be used as local treatment (e.g. wide excision of a small breast cancer), in combination with adjuvant therapy (e.g. radiotherapy), to secure local disease control.

An operation may achieve staging, provide prognostic information and attain local control in a single procedure, such as axillary clearance for breast cancer. Surgery may also be appropriate as a curative procedure in some patients with metastatic disease: patients with colorectal cancer in the right lobe of the liver can achieve 40% 5-year survival after resection of the metastasis.

Supportive surgical techniques include the insertion of central venous catheters such as Hickman lines for the safe administration of cytotoxic drugs and blood products during chemotherapy, and feeding tubes such as percutaneous endoscopic gastrostomy (PEG) tubes to ensure adequate nutritional support for patients undergoing head and neck or upper gastrointestinal surgery.

As a palliative procedure, surgery can reduce pain, maintain mobility and improve quality of life in patients with, for example, femoral shaft metastases threatening bone integrity. Surgery is also the best option in the treatment of spinal cord compression, if the patient has a single metastasis and is otherwise fit. In some cases, surgery can be helpful in relieving obstruction or debulking advanced disease, therefore reducing symptoms such as pain, discharge or haemorrhage. Thus, surgery has a role in the cure, palliation, and treatment of primary cancer and can have a role in the treatment of metastatic disease.

Changing practice

Just as the role of surgery has changed to become integrated with other modalities, the nature and extent of surgery has also changed over the years. These changes in practice are exemplified by the history of breast cancer surgery, where radical mastectomy (resecting the breast and all pectoral muscles) gave way to modified radical mastectomy (leaving pectoralis major), then wide local excision (of the breast tissue bearing the cancer) which, combined with breast radiotherapy, has equivalent results to mastectomy in appropriately selected women.[2] Similarly, the approach to regional lymph nodes has moved from complete node dissection (with associated morbidity) to node sampling, preferably directed by radio-labelled colloid and blue dye, for melanoma and small breast cancers.

Box 12.1
The role of surgery in the management of cancer
Role: Diagnosis   Staging   Treatment of primary   Treatment of metastasis
Intent: Prophylactic   Curative   Supportive   Palliative
Approach: Endoscopic   Laparoscopic   Open (resectional)   Reconstruction

Minimally invasive approaches to the abdomen (laparoscopy, endoscopy) and thorax (thoracoscopy) have greatly improved patient care both for staging disease and for resectional treatment. Laparoscopy, endoscopy and laparoscopic/endoscopic ultrasound via these routes can prevent inappropriate major surgery (e.g. for gastric, pancreatic or oesophageal cancer) and can be used to resect superficial early-stage urological (particularly of the bladder) or gastrointestinal cancers (e.g. colonoscopy), without the need for conventional surgery.

Prophylactic surgery

More recently, surgery for prophylaxis, such as the excision of individual colonic polyps, colectomy for familial adenomatous polyposis (FAP) and bilateral mastectomy for *BRCA1* or *BRCA2* gene carriers, has become established. Optimal restoration of function and appearance is clearly particularly important after prophylactic surgery, so as to ensure that the quality of the patient's life is minimally impaired.

Reconstructive surgery

Restoring intestinal continuity at the time of oesophageal, gastric, pancreatic or colorectal resection is clearly desirable in helping a patient return to normal life. As disruption to gastrointestinal anastomoses may be life threatening, integrity of the join is vital. Sometimes the risks of anastomosis are too great, and hence a stoma is required. For example, following resection of the bladder, a conduit is reconstructed (usually from the ileum; see Fig. 12.14) to communicate between the ureters and the abdominal surface.

While all types of surgery can impair a patient's body image, surgery to the breast or head and neck is particularly visible, and reconstructive surgery plays a vital role in reconstructing skin, muscle and bone following removal of the tumour (see below).

Pain control

Whereas some surgical procedures for cancer such as colonic polypectomy may be painless, most surgery for cancer involves somatic nerve damage. Optimal pain control is thus a significant consideration. Prophylactic blockade (by local, regional or epidural anaesthetic), anxiolytics and adequate postoperative pain management are essential for wound healing (see below). Many other preoperative, intraoperative and postoperative factors, outlined below, can influence the speed and evolution of postoperative rehabilitation and hence both directly or indirectly affect the patient's quality of life. Nurses are largely responsible for the assessment of postoperative pain, and thus are uniquely positioned to ensure that patients' pain is adequately managed. Evidence suggests, however, that many surgical staff have fundamental misconceptions about the use of opiates in patients with cancer[3] and that doctors differ considerably in their decision-making about acute postoperative and cancer pain management.[4] Continuous educational and professional development of staff is essential, as is an integrated approach to pain management, involving information, strategies to reduce anxiety, detailed pain assessment, regular analgesia and psychological support.

Surgical specialization

The role of specialist surgical units and the relationship between surgeon or hospital volume and patient outcomes has been topical over the past decade. While it makes sense that some degree of specialization and familiarity by repetition must have some effect, the evidence is not compelling for many tumour types. The beneficial effects of multidisciplinary team working and the provision of adequate back-up services must also be taken into account. However, specialist training in a given technique can improve outcome, for example, in rectal cancer.[5] If there is a volume effect, it is that occasional operators or very low volume hospitals (<5 patients undergoing resection per year) should not be conducting gastrointestinal cancer surgery.

In this chapter, general considerations of the operative pathway and the principles of surgical management will be discussed, then illustrated using cancers of the breast and GI tracts, with particular emphasis on integrating the issues facing nurses involved in treating and caring for surgical patients with cancer.

PREOPERATIVE, INTRAOPERATIVE AND POSTOPERATIVE CARE AND THE ROLE OF THE NURSE

The preoperative preparation (Box 12.2) intra-operative care (Box 12.3) and postoperative management (Box 12.4) of patients with cancer involves teamwork between ward and outpatient nurses, specialist cancer nurses, allied health professionals, anaesthetists and surgeons.

Preoperative care

The preoperative preparation of patients includes assessment of features relevant to all patients undergoing surgery (Box 12.2). Nurses are increasingly involved in preoperative assessment, and in preparing patients for surgery. It is important to reassess knowledge and understanding and reinforce preoperative information throughout the surgical period, as qualitative studies have shown that patients have difficulty processing all the information they are given prior to surgery. Despite receiving information about the possible effects of surgery, men who had undergone radical prostatectomy were ill-prepared for the complications they experienced and felt that some of the risks had been underplayed.[6]

For patients with cancer, particular consideration needs to be paid to the physical and psychological impact of the disease and its surgical ablation. Some patients are attracted to the concept of 'cutting out' the cancer with the cleansing connotations and finality of this action. However, the anticipation associated with a surgical operation, which is likely to dramatically change a patient's life, can be very frightening and it is probably impossible to prepare someone fully for what they will experience. As the writer and broadcaster John Diamond said,

> The problem with major surgery – any surgery – is that there is no real way of anyone telling you how it will be when you come round. I'd had conversations with various of the medical people and although nobody goes into any great detail about the tubes and the bed, I had some idea of the wreckage that my physical form would suffer – that I'd be cut, and bandaged, and scarred. And I'd guessed that I'd feel pretty miserable, although misery wasn't really the term to describe the mixture of drug-dampened pain, irritation and physical constraint. But nobody can tell you how it feels to be that post-operative person, the person who is lying there waiting for the new chapter to start and with no idea of how that chapter will read. I knew that everything that had been done to me would have a permanent effect, but I couldn't say what that effect – on my constitution, my looks, my voice, my career, my persona – would be.[7 (p158)]

Nurses have a vital role to play in discussing how patients feel about impending surgery, minimizing misconceptions, and providing verbal and visual information about possible bodily changes, including what any drains or tubes might look like. Patients undergoing gynaecological surgery or the removal of sexual organs need particular support to enable them to come

Box 12.2

Preoperative factors	
Assessment:	**Information and education:**
Functional assessment	Discussion of therapeutic options; verbal and written information
Psychosocial assessment	Informed consent
Co-morbidities	Preoperative education:
Cognitive and mental status assessment	– pulmonary exercises
	– physiotherapy
Skin assessment	– mobilization
Medication	– stoma care etc.
Nutritional assessment	
Fluid and electrolyte balance	Discussion of body image issues and potential functional changes
Pain assessment	Referral to specialist nurse or therapist as appropriate

to terms with the loss of fertility, as well as of feelings of femininity or masculinity. Patients undergoing major head and neck surgery may also suffer considerable psychological morbidity in coping with dramatic changes in facial appearance. Preoperative assessments by a speech therapist and a dietitian are also extremely important in this patient group.

The physical impact of surgery is particularly apparent in patients with gastrointestinal cancer. Nutritional status (e.g. oesophageal cancer causing dysphagia), fluid and electrolyte balance (e.g. gastric cancer causing outflow obstruction and vomiting, rectal cancer causing the loss of potassium-rich mucus) and the possible need for a stoma merit particular attention. Preoperative instruction in breathing exercises to promote postoperative pulmonary function (for thoracic and abdominal surgery and where there is a history of pulmonary disease) and physiotherapy instruction (for mobilization of the upper limb following axillary surgery for breast cancer, shoulder mobility following radical neck dissection) demonstrably improve postoperative recovery.

Nurses are particularly well placed to advise on the preparation and placement of stomas (which should be marked preoperatively, allowing for the patient's clothing and body shape). Prior to theatre, many institutions now have checklists to ensure patients have been consented, the correct side (where relevant) marked and the patient adequately prepared for theatre. Preoperative assessment, education and psychological support are as important as physical preparation for surgery, if successful postoperative rehabilitation is to be achieved.

Intraoperative care

Intraoperative (in theatre) nursing (Box 12.3) is a highly specialized field where good communication between nursing and anaesthetic and surgical staff is paramount.

The choice of local, regional or general anaesthetic can significantly improve postoperative outcome. Measures to reduce and replace heat and fluid, and positioning the patient to ensure skin, joints and peripheral nerves are protected are needed. The site of

---

Box 12.3

Intraoperative factors

Communication – between surgeon and scrub nurse, between nurses and between the surgical and anaesthetic teams

Choice of anaesthesia – local, regional, general

Site of operation

Hypothermia

Fluid loss

Skin care, joint care, peripheral nerves

Recovery

---

operative access (Fig. 12.1) can also influence postoperative outcome, as some incisions (upper midline, thoracolaparotomy) may be more painful than others (infraumbilical laparoscopic incision). Prophylactic blockade with, for example, an epidural, can be particularly helpful in elderly patients with cardiorespiratory disease. Recovering the patient from the anaesthetized state to consciousness is an important prelude to postoperative care. A recent Finnish study of perioperative nursing care revealed that patients were extremely happy with the physical care received during this period, but that they felt less satisfied with

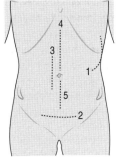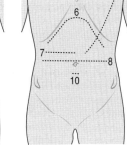

1. Nephrectomy (extraperitoneal)
2. Pfannensteil (gynaecology)
3. Paramedian
4. Upper midline
5. Lower midline
6. Roof-top (pancreatobiliary, gastric)
7. Transverse (colectomy)
8. Transverse (vascular surgery)
9. Thoracoabdominal (extending over left thorax: gastro-oesophageal surgery)
10. Laparoscopic port site

Figure 12.1: Operative approaches to the torso. (After Thompson AM, Park KGM. Finals in surgery. 2nd edn. Edinburgh: Churchill Livingstone; 2001.)

the information they were given and the extent to which they were involved in or able to influence their care.[8]

Postoperative care

The range of postoperative issues facing a surgically treated patient with cancer is extensive (Box 12.4).

Probably the single most important issue is to maintain tissue oxygenation. This should allow wound healing, including gastrointestinal and vascular (e.g. tissue flap) anastomoses, to proceed. Adequate tissue oxygenation requires sufficient pulmonary and cardiovascular function; impairment of these (e.g. by drugs, electrolyte disturbance, inadequate pain control) can result in an increasingly difficult situation. Thus, a patient who is confused (perhaps due to drugs) will try to remove his oxygen mask, reducing cerebral oxygenation and resulting in worsening confusion. This hypoxia may adversely affect wound healing. The patient may pull out intravenous and even central venous access,

---

Box 12.4

Postoperative factors

Immediately postoperatively (to first 72 hours)
Analgesia
Restoring body temperature
Respiratory function
Cardiovascular function
Tissue perfusion (including flaps)
Fluid/electrolyte balance
Cognitive function – postoperative confusional states due to hypoxia (many causes – hypovolaemia, reduced oxygen exchange in lungs, anaemia, etc.), drugs, alcohol withdrawal, metabolic (including electrolyte imbalance)

Longer-term issues (after the first 3 days)
Early ambulation/mobilization
Deep vein thrombosis (DVT) /pulmonary embolus (PE)
Wound healing
Wound infections – intrinsic vs extrinsic factors; classification as clean, clean-contaminated, contaminated, dirty
Nutrition
Body image
Discharge planning

---

resulting in deranged fluid and electrolyte balance, and since early mobilization is less likely, the risk of deep vein thrombosis (DVT) and pulmonary embolism increases.

For major resectional surgery for cancer, e.g. of the gastrointestinal (GI) or genitourinary tracts, high dependency (HDU) or intensive therapy (ITU) units offer enhanced nursing and medical care to ensure a smooth postoperative outcome. Careful monitoring of respiratory, cardiovascular, electrolyte and haematological indices can be combined with regional anaesthetic techniques (e.g. epidural anaesthesia) and regular chest physiotherapy.

Patients with cancer generally have less reserve and slower healing processes than non-cancer patients. A proportion of cancer surgery is performed on structures that contain substantial bacterial loads (e.g. mouth, colon) and may result in contaminated or dirty wounds, whereas neurosurgical resection of a tumour should be a clean procedure. Compounded with the co-morbidity (particularly cardiorespiratory) present in many patients, wound healing may be prolonged or, rarely, dehisce (fall apart) – applicable to any wound on the surface or within the body. Nutritional support is thus particularly important.

In addition to these crucial aspects of physiological recovery, nurses also play a major role in supportive care to promote psychosocial adjustment and a return to as normal a life as possible. As hospital stays decrease, there may be an increasing role for nurses in the support of patients in the early postoperative period. A study of 63 men in the first few months after radical prostatectomy revealed many areas of concern, including not knowing what to expect, problems with pain and infection, how to manage unexpected levels of urinary incontinence and coping with erectile dysfunction.[6] Patients who had received support from nurses at home expressed fewer concerns, and the authors suggest that home visits and telephone calls play an important part in supporting postoperative recovery. A study of nurse-led early discharge following axillary clearance surgery[9] suggested the immediate postoperative needs of patients recovering from breast cancer surgery can be effectively managed by a combination of home visits by breast care nurses, telephone assessment and rapid communication with the primary care team.

The transition from hospital to home and the associated loss of immediate advice and support can be difficult for some patients. Liaison with primary care staff and clear follow-up arrangements are important so as to reduce the uncertainty associated with the end of each stage of treatment. Multidisciplinary assessment involving social workers, occupational therapists, dietitians, stoma nurses, speech therapists and district nurses can ensure that patients who have undergone major surgery are adequately supported in their recovery. Adapting to changes in physical function and body image can be a long and complex process, and requires the input of a multidisciplinary team skilled in rehabilitation (see Ch. 36).

PRINCIPLES OF SURGICAL MANAGEMENT OF PATIENTS WITH CANCER

The surgical management of patients with cancer revolves around an accurate diagnosis. The history and clinical examination may point to the likely diagnosis but more definitive diagnostic tests are required before proceeding to surgery (Table 12.1).

Tissue diagnosis may include cytology (often via fine needle aspiration or microscopic examination of urine or sputum), biopsy (core biopsy of accessible tumours such as breast; forceps biopsy of intraluminal tumours of the GI tract, genitourinary tract) or a resected specimen.

Other cancers may have pathognomonic features on imaging, e.g. intracranial neoplasms, hepatic primary and secondary cancers, which

Table 12.1: Key symptoms, radiological imaging and diagnostic tests for common cancers

Cancer	Symptoms	Radiological imaging	Common diagnostic tests
Bone	Pain	MRI scan	Biopsy
Melanoma	Skin lesion	CT scan	Biopsy
Head and neck	Lump	CT scan	FNA cytology
Breast	Lump	Mammogram	FNA cytology
CNS	Pain/epileptic fit	MRI scan	
Bladder	Haematuria	–	Cystoscopy
Prostate	Usually nil	CT scan	PSA
Lung	Cough/breathlessness	Chest X-ray, CT scan	Sputum cytology/ biopsy
Oesophageal/stomach	Dysphagia/pain	CT scan	Endoscopy/biopsy
Colon/rectal	Change in bowel habit/PR blood	CT scan	Colonoscopy/biopsy
Ovary	Abdominal swelling	CT scan	Biopsy

CNS, central nervous system; CT, computed tomography; FNA, fine needle aspiration; MRI, magnetic resonance imaging; PR, per rectum; PSA, prostate-specific antigen.

because of their anatomical site (intracranial) or likelihood of intraperitoneal dissemination or bleeding (hepatoma), may make biopsy less desirable prior to definitive surgery.

Wherever the tumour site, staging of the tumour size and local invasiveness (T), nodal status (N) and the presence or absence of metastasis (M) can give a clinical, radiological or pathological guide as to the most appropriate treatment plan. For many healthcare systems, tumour (e.g. breast) or system-specific (e.g. gastrointestinal) multidisciplinary teams help in this decision-making process.

It may be appropriate to 'downstage' advanced cancers using neoadjuvant, non-surgical approaches, followed by surgery to excise the residual tumour. This is particularly beneficial for more advanced rectal cancer, breast cancer and oesophageal cancer. Patients may benefit by no longer requiring surgery (e.g. following chemoradiotherapy for anal cancer), show improved disease control (rectal cancer treated preoperatively with radiotherapy),[10] need less radical surgery (lumpectomy rather than mastectomy for breast cancer)[2] and even improved survival (with preoperative chemotherapy for oesophageal cancer).[11]

The methods for measuring the effectiveness of the downstaging often involve radiological imaging such as computed tomography (CT), magnetic resonance imaging (MRI), ultrasound or positron emission tomography (PET) scanning rather than simple clinical measurement.

For most patients, surgical removal of the primary cancer (often with regional lymph nodes) follows the diagnosis, staging and consideration of all the therapeutic options. Surgery should combine radical excision (removing all the macroscopic and microscopic primary tumour) with reconstruction of the tissues to minimize the detrimental effects of organ removal on the patient. Supportive care, such as HDU for patients requiring support for (potentially) single organ failure and those with significant co-morbidity, may be sufficient. However, ITU care may be required following extensive surgery (e.g. thoracotomy for oesophagectomy and node dissection), particularly if the patient has cardiorespiratory co-morbidity.

Although most surgery for cancer should be aimed at cure, and conducted electively after appropriate staging, some patients present as an emergency requiring relief of symptoms. Obstructing cancers of the oesophagus, pancreas and colon are particularly common examples of emergency presentation, requiring urgent intervention to relieve the obstruction and hence buy time to ensure staging may proceed to definitive treatment. Not infrequently, patients present with surgically incurable disease, but (as outlined above) in order to improve the quality of life, appropriate surgical intervention to resect, bypass or reinforce the site of metastasis can be beneficial. Ovarian cancer is one case in point where resecting the bulk of disease before proceeding to chemotherapy can have a substantial impact on survival. Indeed, there is evidence that gynaecology oncologists may be more rigorous than generalists and also contribute to improved survival.[12] Specialist surgeons, either surgical oncologists (specializing in cancer surgery) or organ-specific surgeons (e.g. breast surgeons) and the potential benefits they bring remain controversial. Similarly, the role of specialist units and the number of operations each surgeon should do each year to maintain his or her skills is still openly debated.

The surgical management of patients with cancer may be best exemplified by considering:

1 breast cancer, where the non-surgical options are many but surgery plays a key role in diagnosis and local disease control, and

2 common cancers of the gastrointestinal tract (oesophageal, stomach, colon and rectum), where surgical intervention remains the mainstay of treatment.

Rather than consider individual patient scenarios, these sections attempt to follow the patient pathway, outlining the options for patients with each type of these particularly common cancers:

Symptoms or Screening

↓

Presentation

↓

Diagnosis

↓

Staging

↓

Multidisciplinary preoperative assessment

↓

(Downstaging – neoadjuvant therapy)

↓

Surgery

↓

Pathology

↓

Multidisciplinary team meetings

↓

Adjuvant therapy

↓

Follow-up

↓

Survival or death

BREAST CANCER

Principles

Breast cancer is increasing worldwide[13,14] and remains a major surgical and oncological challenge. Surgery for breast cancer aims to excise, with a margin of normal tissue, the cancer in the breast and thus, in combination with other therapies (radiotherapy, chemotherapy, endocrine therapy), achieve local control of the disease. In addition, sampling or excision of the lymph nodes in the axilla is usually performed to ensure local disease control, stage the disease and provide prognostic information which will direct therapy.

Breast cancer is a good example of the role of surgery in cancer therapy, given that it is such a common disease, can dramatically affect body image and usually requires a combined modality approach to treatment and follow-up.

Diagnosis

The diagnosis is established by a process of triple assessment, whereby clinical history and examination (Table 12.2), radiology (mammography, Fig. 12.2 and/or ultrasound) and pathology (cytology, core or diagnostic biopsy) are combined to determine whether there is a cancerous process going on in the breast. Many women worried about cancer will turn out to have benign changes only; hence, using triple assessment to exclude a cancer in such women is also important.

Staging

Breast cancer is staged using the TNM system based on the clinical size of the cancer, palpation of axillary and supraclavicular lymph nodes and the presence or absence of clinically detectable metastases. Evidence-based staging comprises bilateral mammography, chest radiograph, haematology and biochemistry (including liver function tests). For T3 (>5 cm in size) or T4 (cancers involving the skin or chest wall), where detectable metastases are more likely, it is important to include a liver ultrasound or CT scan for liver metastases and an isotope bone scan supplemented by plain radiographs if abnormalities are detected. The reason for seeking such distant metastases is to target treatment approximately. For example,

Table 12.2: Clinical features of breast cancer

Feature	Description
Lump	Usually painless
Skin dimpling	May be accentuated by raising arms
Nipple indrawing	May be accentuated by raising arms
Bleeding nipple	Usually from a single duct
Nipple eczema	Non-healing
Skin redness	May be painful and confused with infection

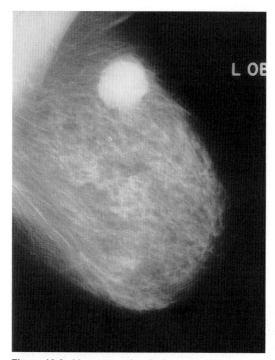

Figure 12.2: Mammography of a breast containing a cancer. (From Thompson AM. General surgical anatomy and examination. Edinburgh: Churchill Livingstone; 2001.)

mastectomy may be avoided if there is already evidence of liver metastases, there being little advantage to the woman of undergoing mutilating surgery when the liver metastases are likely to shorten her survival.

Decision-making process (multidisciplinary team)

Historically, the decision on what operation to perform was left to the surgeon; it was only postoperatively that an oncologist might be involved in the decision-making with regard to adjuvant therapy. Preoperative multidisciplinary review of the diagnostic and staging information, coupled with the social and other clinical features of each individual patient, is useful to decide what therapy is most suitable for an individual patient. This will determine whether neoadjuvant therapy or surgery (of whatever type), followed by adjuvant therapy, is most appropriate.

In general, adjuvant therapy is aimed at reducing the risks of recurrence, either locally in the breast or chest wall or at distant metastatic sites. The choice of therapy for breast cancer for local disease control comprises adequate surgical clearance of the cancer with local radiotherapy to reduce the incidence of local disease recurrence. Thus, the local recurrence rate following wide excision of a cancer plus radiotherapy to the breast approaches that of mastectomy alone.[15] Chemotherapy, endocrine therapy (whether oophorectomy or tamoxifen for premenopausal women or tamoxifen or aromatase inhibitors for postmenopausal women), and to some extent radiotherapy, all protect against systemic recurrence and reduce the incidence of contralateral breast cancer.

There are many complex factors involved in decision-making (see Ch. 14), but multidisciplinary input ensures that an appropriate clinical decision is made for the patient. Breast care specialist nurses have a particularly important role in supporting the patient (and her relatives) in the decision-making process and in the coordination of the clinical team.

Neoadjuvant downstaging

For cancers over 4 cm in size, or those invading the skin or chest wall (T4 cancers), preoperative shrinkage is now considered appropriate. For cancers which on pathological examination of the biopsy contain oestrogen or progesterone receptors, endocrine therapy (tamoxifen or aromatase inhibitor for postmenopausal women, tamoxifen or ovarian suppression for premenopausal women) is employed; for receptor negative cancers, preoperative chemotherapy usually containing an anthracycline is used. Over a 3- to 6-month period, the cancer can be monitored for a change in size using clinical, ultrasound and/or mammographic measurement.

In breast cancer, the aim of this approach is to render inoperable disease (e.g. T4 cancer) operable to achieve local disease control or to allow a large cancer (e.g. 4 cm in size) to shrink and thus provide patients with the choice between breast conservation (wide local excision) and mastectomy, where previously only mastectomy would have been considered.[2] At one time, elderly women relatively unfit for surgery (for example, with a history of previous myocardial infarction) were given tamoxifen as sole long-term therapy with the aim of avoiding surgery. While the cancer would usually shrink or even disappear, in time (usually 24–36 months) the tumour would escape tamoxifen control and require resection in, by then, an even more elderly and unfit individual.[16] This approach has now fallen into much less frequent use with more consideration of the individual circumstances of each patient.

Breast cancer surgery

Surgery to the primary cancer

Surgery for breast cancer aims to excise, with a margin of normal tissue, the cancer in the breast and thus, in combination with other therapies (radiotherapy, chemotherapy, endocrine therapy), achieve local control of the disease. In addition, sampling or excision of the lymph nodes in the axilla is usually performed to stage the disease, provide prognostic information (Fig. 12.3), which will direct postoperative systemic therapy and ensure local disease control. Reconstruction, either at the time of mastectomy or as a delayed procedure, should be offered (Box 12.5).

There are currently four options for local control of a breast cancer:

1 Primary medical therapy: i.e. no surgery (reserved for the medically unfit for surgery).[16]

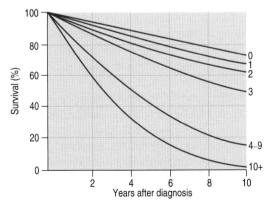

Figure 12.3: Relationship between number of axillary lymph nodes involved with breast cancer and survival.

Box 12.5
Surgical options for breast cancer
Breast: Wide excision Quadrantectomy Mastectomy
Axilla: Sentinel node biopsy 4 node sample Axillary clearance
Reconstruction: Implant Tissue expander Myocutaneous flap Contralateral adjustment

2 Wide local excision: excision of the cancer, aiming for a 1 cm rim of normal tissue around it; the tissues are closed to minimize the defect in the breast shape and the skin scar placed in the skin lines of the breast. Clearly, this conservation approach is only suitable for comparatively small cancers (up to 4 cm) in a breast sufficiently large to allow a reasonable cosmetic result (Fig. 12.4).

3 Quadrantectomy: a wider rim of normal tissue around the cancer than wide excision, usually taking the whole quadrant of the breast.

4 Mastectomy: excising the breast tissue down to but not including pectoralis major muscle (which was removed by the radical mastectomy now of historical interest only) and the skin overlying the cancer together with the nipple areolar complex. At the time of surgery, a vacuum drain is inserted to remove serosanguinous fluid, which otherwise collects. The skin is closed, resulting in a transverse scar (Fig. 12.5). At the time of mastectomy (or if a major tissue defect results from quadrantectomy), reconstructive surgery may be performed (see below).

In many centres about 50% of patients with breast cancer undergo mastectomy, although this figure may be lower where larger numbers

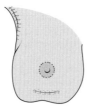

Figure 12.4: Breast conservation scars. (From Thompson AM, Park KGM. Finals in surgery. 2nd edn. Edinburgh: Churchill Livingstone; 2001.)

of small (e.g. screen detected) cancers are treated. However, even where the cancer is small and could be treated by local excision, some women choose to undergo mastectomy as they 'feel safer' having the whole breast removed.

Surgery to regional nodes

Sampling or excision of the lymph nodes in the axilla is usually performed to stage the disease and provide prognostic information, which will direct therapy and ensure local disease control (see Fig. 12.3).

There are three options (see Box 12.5):

1 Sentinel node biopsy selectively excises the first one or two nodes draining the breast cancer. These nodes are identified by injecting radioisotope-labelled colloid prior to surgery and subsequently blue dye at the time of surgery at the site of the cancer; the combination identifies over 95% of sentinel nodes accurately.[17] A similar technique is favoured for regional lymph node detection in melanoma, where it is very successful, and

is under investigation in gastrointestinal cancer surgery, where its usefulness has yet to be demonstrated.

2 Axillary node sample aims to excise 4 representative lymph nodes from the lower axilla. Evidence suggests that this too can accurately stage the axilla without the morbidity of axillary clearance.[18] If subsequent examination of the lymph nodes shows tumour deposits, either axillary radiotherapy or an axillary clearance is required for disease control.

3 Axillary node clearance excises the axillary contents, including the lymph nodes (ranging between 10 and 50 in number), thus emptying the axilla bounded by the axillary vein, first rib, pectoralis major, latissimus dorsi and subscapularis and the chest wall.[19] This provides excellent local control of disease (and generally prevents local recurrent disease in the axilla), but can damage the intercostal brachial nerve, reducing sensation in the axilla and upper arm. Postoperative upper limb lymphoedema is a recognized complication of axillary clearance in 5% of patients but can be minimized by attention to detail intraoperatively and by avoiding postoperative radiotherapy of the axilla after a clearance.

Breast reconstruction

Ideally, breast reconstruction would be unnecessary if all cancers were detected at a small size (and hence suitable for breast conservation). Mobilization of the remaining breast tissues and taking sufficient but not excessive excision of normal tissue around the cancer should give a reasonable cosmetic result (Box 12.6). However, mastectomy remains a mainstay for larger cancers.

At the time of mastectomy or quadrantectomy, it may be possible to insert a silicone- or saline-filled implant. For bilateral mastectomy for prophylaxis (sometimes nipple and areolar preserving), this approach may be sufficient. However, after mastectomy, there is often a need to expand the skin (+ deeper tissues) to allow placement of a correctly positioned and sized implant with adequate ptosis. This can be

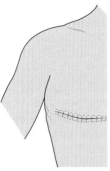

Figure 12.5: Mastectomy scar. (From Thompson AM, Park KGM. Finals in surgery. 2nd edn. Edinburgh: Churchill Livingstone; 2001.)

Box 12.6

Methods of breast reconstruction

With breast conservation	With mastectomy
Mobilization of breast tissues	Implant
Latissimus dorsi miniflap	Tissue expander, then implant
	Latissimus dorsi flap ± implant
	Transverse rectus abdominis muscle (TRAM) flap
	Deep inferior epigastric perforator (DIEP) flap

accomplished by inserting a tissue expander deep in the pectoral (+ upper abdominal) muscles with a port into which saline is injected on a weekly basis over several months to inflate the expander to greater than the size actually needed. Subsequently, the expander can be partly deflated or replaced with a silicone implant to ensure symmetry with the contralateral side. Capsule (fibrotic) reaction around the implant, implant migration or implant leakage are all recognized long-term sequelae of this approach. The consensus of evidence is against any association between silicone breast implants and connective tissue disorders.

Autologous myocutaneous flaps offer the advantages of using the patient's own tissue with a 'feel' that is akin to normal breast. Two flaps are in common use – the latissimus dorsi and overlying skin (which can be swung round at the time of quadrantectomy or mastectomy and can be combined with an implant) and the rectus abdominis muscle flaps – either the transverse (TRAM) flap or a flap based on perforating vessels (deep inferior epigastric perforator or DIEP). The abdominal flaps generally contain sufficient tissue in themselves but are even larger operations than the latissimus dorsi approach.

Subsequent minor modifications to the reconstructed breast size and shape may be required and may be combined with tattooing or surgically creating a nipple/areolar structure (alternatively a stick-on version can be used). Contralateral breast surgery (reduction, mastopexy or enlargement) may be offered to ensure an adequate cosmetic result.

For many women, reconstructive surgery is an important factor in being able to get on with normal life, but not all women wish to have reconstruction either immediately (at the time of initial mastectomy) or delayed (at any time thereafter). Interestingly, there is some evidence to suggest that quality of life may be adversely affected by some types of reconstruction. Reconstructive surgery may improve body image, but it seems not to diminish the fear of recurrence, which, for many women, is the most difficult aspect of life after cancer.[20]

For those who do not opt for reconstruction, a prosthesis (soft, immediately postoperative; shaped silicone, longer term) should be offered and correctly fitted to allow each woman to wear the clothing (including swimwear) she chooses with confidence. However, it must not be assumed that all patients want to wear a prosthesis. One woman described how unsupported she was in her decision not to do so:

> A figure slides up to me as I stride down the ward towards the exit. 'Have you been fitted?' she asks, while looking at my left breast. 'No' I tell her. 'You're going to come back?' This is a cross between a question and a statement. 'No' I reply, 'I am not going to wear a prosthesis.' 'Oh dear' she exclaims. 'You'll have to, otherwise you'll make people feel uncomfortable'. I don't feel angry. I feel sad. I HAVE JUST HAD A BREAST CUT OFF AND...OTHER PEOPLE MIGHT FEEL UNCOMFORTABLE WITH THIS. I smile. Hold my head high and walk.[21]

Patient choice, in discussion with the breast care nurse, relatives and clinical team, is important in selecting how best to minimize the impact of surgical treatment and support psychological adjustment to bodily change.

Supportive care and recovery from surgery

Surgery for breast cancer requires both physical and psychological support,[22] including addressing fears about additional treatments and concerns for the future. The impact of surgery on aspects such as body image remains considerable, even despite the increased use of breast conservation and reconstruction. Support from the patient's partner, family and multidisciplinary team is key to her confidence throughout surgery and adjuvant therapy. Specialist breast care nurses play a major role in supporting patients throughout their treatment and there is evidence to suggest that such support can significantly reduce psychological morbidity.[23]

Although the analgesic requirements following breast conservation or mastectomy may be less than one might expect, the axillary surgery (particularly axillary clearance) can cause increasing discomfort and shoulder stiffness. Non-steroidal anti-inflammatory drugs (NSAIDs) and analgesics are usually sufficient and, combined with preoperative education and postoperative practise of shoulder mobility exercises (internal and external rotation are particularly affected), should allow full upper limb function to be regained.

Vacuum drains left in the axilla and deep to the mastectomy flaps can be removed once drainage is less than 50 ml/day. Subsequent seroma formation is not uncommon and seromas can be aspirated if uncomfortable for the patient.

Lymphoedema is a complication of breast cancer surgery and radiotherapy for which the aetiology and pathogenesis is poorly understood.[24] At the time of axillary surgery, preventing damage to those lymphatic channels which do not need to be excised as part of the axillary clearance can substantially reduce postoperative lymphoedema. The combination of axillary clearance and axillary radiotherapy, no longer routinely practised, was particularly prone to causing upper limb lymphoedema. Preventing skin damage (e.g. wearing gloves when doing housework or gardening) can reduce the chance and progression of lymphoedema. Should it occur, skin care, massage, bandaging and compression hosiery may all have a role to play. Early identification and intervention may prevent worsening lymphoedema, but treatment can be complex and continue for many years.[25]

Pathology

The pathology describes the size and type of breast cancer, whether in situ or invasive (commonly ductal carcinoma, but special types have a better prognosis), the histological grade of the cancer (high grade, poorer prognosis), the presence of cancer at the resection margins (incomplete excision results in a higher incidence of local disease recurrence) and the presence of lymphatic or vascular channel invasion or lymph node metastases. Some of these factors are combined in the Nottingham Prognostic Index (NPI) which groups patients according to their likelihood of disease recurrence (Box 12.7).

Additional histological sections can be stained to detect the oestrogen receptor, progesterone receptor and HER2 receptor. Sections of cancer staining highly for oestrogen of progesterone receptor suggest that the tumour may have been dependent on oestrogen for growth and so adjuvant endocrine therapy is likely to be useful. Cancers that express high levels of HER2 may be treated with a humanized antibody to HER2, either in the adjuvant setting or more commonly for advanced disease. This pathology data, together with the patient's views and suitability for further treatment, are important in determining the postoperative (adjuvant) treatment.

Prophylactic or adjuvant surgery

Prophylactic mastectomy for women with a familial breast cancer gene mutation (*BRCA1*, *BRCA2*) has been established as improving the outlook for such women[26] and so bilateral mastectomy, often sparing the nipple areolar

---

Box 12.7

Nottingham Prognostic Index (NPI)

Nottingham Prognostic Index (NPI)
=
0.2 × histological size in cm
+
grade
(score 1 for grade 1; 2 for grade 2; 3 for grade 3)
+
axillary nodal metastases
(score 1 for no nodes involved; 2 for 1–3 nodes involved; 3 for 4 or more nodes involved)

complex, combined with breast reconstruction, is the method of choice.

Bilateral oophorectomy, now usually carried out laparoscopically, can reduce the recurrence of breast cancer in gene carriers.[27] It is used as adjuvant therapy for women who are pre-menopausal and had an oestrogen receptor-positive primary cancer. Alternatively, monthly injections of LHRH (luteinizing hormone releasing hormone) agonists produce a medical, reversible oophorectomy or a radiation-induced menopause may be considered.

Palliative surgery

Local resection of fungating chest wall disease may help establish local disease control and may be combined with local radiotherapy and chemotherapy.

The role of surgery to visceral secondaries such as liver, pleura, lung or brain is confined to single operable metastases. Given the frequently multiple nature of such metastases in breast cancer, surgery is rarely an option. However, in combination with postoperative radiotherapy, additional palliation lasting a few months may be possible in some patients.

Orthopaedic intervention to resect/stabilize bones such as the femur which contain metastatic deposits liable to pathological fracture should be actively considered, preferably as prophylaxis before the limb fractures.

Prognosis

Surgery for breast cancer may by itself be curative for smaller cancers. However, by the addition of radiotherapy to improve local disease control and endocrine therapy, chemotherapy, bisphosphonates and/or biological therapy, survival for breast cancer now approaches 80% at 5 years and 60% at 10 years.

OESOPHAGEAL/GASTRIC CANCERS

Introduction

Oesophageal and oesophagogastric junction cancers are increasing in incidence,[28] balancing the reduction worldwide in gastric cancers.[14] The usual ideals of early diagnosis, complete resection with regional nodes removed and reconstruction to allow restoration of normal life are rarely met in surgery for upper gastrointestinal cancer in the Western world.

Presentation

Most upper gastrointestinal cancers present late (only one-third undergo resection) and curative resection is unusual, with 10–16% 5-year survival figures quoted.[28] Late presentation is associated with poor nutrition (due to narrowing of the oesophagus or junction), anaemia (from the cancer bleeding into the lumen) and electrolyte disturbance (from vomiting due to gastric cancer paralysing the stomach and/or gastric outflow obstruction).

Diagnosis

The diagnosis of oesophageal or gastric cancer is increasingly made by upper gastrointestinal endoscopy, usually performed for symptoms of dysphagia, heartburn or epigastric pain; at endoscopy, small biopsies can be taken for pathology examination, including a search for *Helicobacter pylori* infection, which is strongly associated with distal gastric cancers and lymphoma of the stomach. Upper gastrointestinal contrast studies, usually with barium-based examinations, can successfully outline the oesophagus or oesophageal gastric junction (a barium swallow, Fig. 12.6) and the stomach (a barium meal) but cannot be used to establish a tissue diagnosis. Endoscopy, particularly using video equipment, is now the gold standard.

Staging

Staging these diseases (Table 12.3) includes CT scan of the chest and abdomen in an attempt to gauge the depth of penetration of the cancer through the wall of the oesophagus or stomach, invasion into adjacent structures, node metastasis and more distant (liver, lung) metastasis (Fig. 12.7).

Endoscopic or laparoscopic ultrasound have both been used to assess tumour penetration and node status, and may turn out to be more effective than CT scanning, particularly when combined with staging laparoscopy, which may

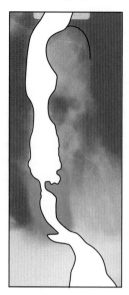

Figure 12.6: Barium swallow, showing a distal oesophageal cancer. (From Thompson AM. General surgical anatomy and examination. Edinburgh: Churchill Livingstone; 2001.)

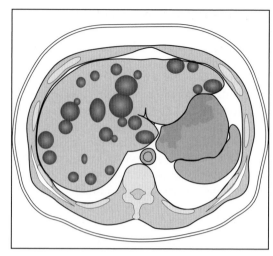

Figure 12.7: CT scan of the liver and stomach, demonstrating primary gastric cancer with liver metastases. (From Thompson AM. General surgical anatomy and examination. Edinburgh: Churchill Livingstone; 2001.)

identify peritoneal seedlings or other indications of metastatic/local disease invasion in up to 40% of patients. Haematology (for anaemia which may be corrected by transfusion prior to surgery), biochemistry (for correctable electrolyte disturbances) and physiological assessment of the patient's cardiovascular and respiratory systems are routinely performed. The latter is particularly important, as oesophageal and gastric cancer often affects patients over 65 years old with concurrent cardiorespiratory morbidity who usually require major surgery and a high level of postoperative care. Thus an electrocardiogram (ECG), echo (ultrasound) assessment of cardiac function and pulmonary function tests are desirable as part of the preoperative work-up, particularly where thoracic surgery is planned.

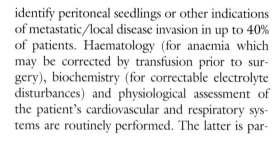

Table 12.3: Staging investigations for oesophageal and gastric cancer

Investigation	Purpose
Full blood count	To check for anaemia
Urea and electrolytes	To look for low sodium, dehydration
Liver function tests	To seek evidence of liver metastases
Arterial blood gases	To assess respiratory function
Pulmonary function tests	To assess respiratory function
CT scan chest/abdomen	To look for local invasion and metastases
Endoscopic ultrasound	To look for local invasion and nodal metastases
Laparoscopy	To look for local invasion, peritoneal/ liver metastases

The multidisciplinary meeting

Increasingly, multidisciplinary teams are being established to discuss the management of patients with upper gastrointestinal cancer, similar to the way in which breast cancer is managed. For oesophageal and gastric cancer this is particularly important in assessing which patients are suitable for resection, both in terms of disease stage and fitness-for-operation. For the majority (two-thirds) who are not suitable for curative surgery, neoadjuvant downstaging, surgical bypass (of gastric outflow obstruction), stent placement to restore a channel through the cancer, laser ablation of intraluminal tumour and enteral or parenteral feeding are alternatives carried out by surgical teams. Radiotherapy, chemotherapy and chemo-radiotherapy can provide equivalent levels of palliation and, indeed, cure, compared with surgery in selected patients. Overall, in population-based studies in western Europe,[31] only a third of cancers are operable at the time of presentation and only half of those patients have long-term survival after surgery.

Neoadjuvant therapy

Neoadjuvant downstaging may not only improve the chances of resection but may also increase the survival of patients with oesophageal cancer.[12] Although there is conflicting evidence to this effect, some countries have adopted this perioperative chemotherapy approach as a routine standard of care for already operable disease. The evidence for similar benefits for gastric cancer is not yet mature, but proponents suggest operable gastric cancer too may be best treated by chemotherapy prior to surgery. If the neoadjuvant approach is pursued for an individual patient, then restaging may be advisable before major resectional surgery goes ahead.

Resection of upper gastrointestinal cancer

Surgery for oesophageal and gastric cancer falls into four categories: localized resection of the primary (e.g. endoscopic mucosal resection), conventional excision of the tumour-bearing organs and resection of the regional nodes (with any metastases therein), reconstruction of intestinal continuity and supportive measures (Table 12.4).

Surgery with curative intent

For the rare, small, superficial (polypoidal) cancers of the oesophagus or stomach or large gastric polps with malignant potential, local resection of the lesion may suffice. This may be achieved endoscopically by cutting through

---

Table 12.4: Surgical therapy for oesophageal and gastric cancer

	Curative intent	Surgical palliation
Oesophagus	Endoscopic mucosal resection Oesophagectomy – Transhiatal – Thoracoabdominal – 2 or 3 stage – Thoracoscopic	Stent placement Laser therapy Alcohol injection
Stomach	Polypectomy – Endoscopic – Open Total gastrectomy Subtotal gastrectomy Distal gastrectomy	Laser therapy Palliative resection Gastroenterostomy

the mucosa wide and deep to the lesion and retrieving the specimen in a manner analogous to a colonic polypectomy. Alternatively, a gastrotomy may be performed to locally excise the lesion. This is only possible for very early lesions and hence in Western practice is applicable to <5% of patients undergoing resection.

For all other resectable cancers (T1, T2, T3 stage), oesophagectomy (for mid/lower oesophageal cancers, oesophagogastrectomy (for lower/OG junction cancers), gastrectomy (for cardia, body cancers) or distal gastrectomy (for antral/prepyloric cancers) are performed (Table 12.5).

The surgical approach to each procedure differs and has possible variations. For example, an oesophagectomy (Fig. 12.8) can be performed via a single incision (left thoracoabdominal), abdominal and right thoracic incisions, or abdominal with transhiatal mobilization and a left neck anastomosis or thoracoscopically assisted (with abdominal and neck incisions). There appears to be little difference in the morbidity, node dissection yield or survival with any particular approach and so each has its proponents. The draining nodes (coeliac and mediastinal) should be resected and current, Western, practice is to perform reconstruction of the oesophagus using a gastric tube or (for junctional cancers) small bowel.

Gastrectomy, whether total[29] (Fig. 12.9), subtotal (leaving a small rim of proximal stomach) or distal (for antral cancers)(Fig. 12.10), is performed through a midline or inverted V (roof top) abdominal incision. Current practice is to leave the spleen and tail of pancreas in situ, as resection of these organs is associated with increased morbidity and mortality.[30] Small bowel is used to reconstruct the following gastrectomy, either as a Roux-en-Y reconstruction (Fig. 12.9) or pouch, although the latter has few functional advantages. If the spleen is sacrificed, vaccination against *Pneumococcus*, *Meningococcus* and *Haemophilus* is recommended and the patient should take penicillin long term to avoid OPSI (overwhelming post splenectomy infection) with such capsulated organisms.

Regional node dissection of the first tier of nodes to which the cancer may have spread is routine. This may include mediastinal, coeliac, perigastric or peripancreatic nodes. In most European centres, the extensive node dissection practised in the Orient is rarely performed due to the increased morbidity and mortality of such procedures in Western patients, cancelling out any advantage from resecting involved nodes at these sites.

Supportive care

Supportive care in the perioperative period for oesophagectomy or gastrectomy includes oxygen, intravenous fluids, analgesia (ideally an epidural for the first few days), chest physiotherapy and enteral (nasoenteral or jejunal feeding tube) or parenteral nutrition (via a central line).

Patients undergoing upper gastrointestinal cancer surgery are at particular risk of thromboembolic disease and postoperative wound infection; therefore, DVT prophylaxis (using

Table 12.5: Surgical reconstruction following resection of oesophageal or gastric cancer

Tumour site	Resection	Reconstruction
Middle third oesophagus Lower third oesophagus	Oesophagectomy	Gastric tube (Fig. 12.8)
Oesophagogastric junction Gastric cardia	Oesophagogastrectomy	Roux-en-Y (Fig. 12.9)
Body of stomach	Gastrectomy	Roux-en-Y (Fig. 12.9)
Gastric antrum	Distal gastrectomy	Polya reconstruction (Fig. 12.10)

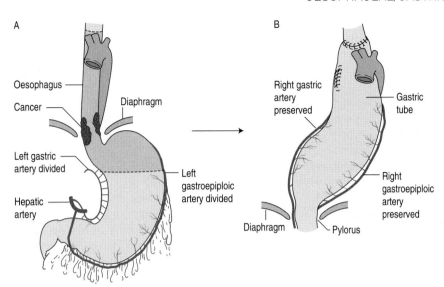

Figure 12.8: Oesophagectomy (A) with gastric tube reconstruction (B). (From Garden OJ, Bradbury AW, Forsythe JLR. Principles and practice of surgery. 4th edn. Edinburgh: Churchill Livingstone; 2002.)

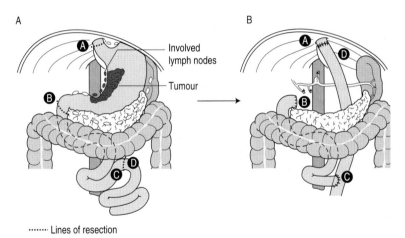

Figure 12.9: Total gastrectomy with Roux-en-Y reconstruction. Letters A–D identify preresection (Fig. 12.9A) and postreconstruction and anastomotic anatomy (Fig. 12.9B) (From Garden OJ, Bradbury AW, Forsythe JLR. Principles and practice of surgery. 4th edn. Edinburgh: Churchill Livingstone; 2002.)

mechanical and pharmacological methods) and antibiotic prophylaxis should be commenced prior to surgery. Heparin may need to be withheld until an epidural has been placed immediately preoperatively to avoid problems with bleeding into the epidural space.

Respiratory complications, then cardiovascular events (myocardial infarction, dysrhythmias), are the most frequent early postoperative problems occurring in some 40% of patients.[31] Anastomotic leakage occurs in 6.5% of patients, particularly following total gastrectomy, where leakage of the jejunal/oesophageal anastomosis may be identified by contrast swallow (conducted routinely by some units at day 5 before the patient resumes oral intake), and necrosis of the gastric tube, although rare, may be catastrophic post oesophagectomy.

Usually, patients undergoing oesophagectomy or gastrectomy are cared for in high-dependency or intensive therapy beds for the first 24–48 hours, then if postoperative care proceeds smoothly, returned to a ward with patient-controlled analgesia for pain relief.

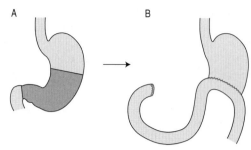

Figure 12.10: Partial (distal) gastrectomy (A) with gastroenterostomy reconstruction (B). (From Garden OJ, Bradbury AW, Forsythe JLR. Principles and practice of surgery. 4th edn. Edinburgh: Churchill Livingstone; 2002.)

Chest physiotherapy is important throughout this time, and careful nursing care is a vital part of minimizing complications.

Surgical palliation

Palliative surgery for distal gastric cancer involves a gastroenterostomy through a small midline or left transverse incision or can be performed laparoscopically to bypass the gastric outflow obstruction. It is important that non-cancer bearing stomach is used for the anastomosis and a wide gastroenterostomy is fashioned to allow passage of food.

Palliative resection of advanced oesophageal, junctional or gastric cancer is currently frowned on – the patients do not usually live long enough for a full recovery from the operation. Occasionally, where the patient has presented an as emergency with bleeding or perforation, patients under 70 years old (without too great a disease burden) may benefit from a palliative gastrectomy.[32] However, placement of a stent (an expandable metal mesh has largely taken over from plastic tubes) endoscopically or under radiological guidance can effectively maintain swallowing through obstructing oesophageal and gastric-oesophageal cancers.[33] Reflux of gastric contents (with possible aspiration) can occur, so patients are advised to sleep propped upright and to take a proton pump inhibitor or an H_2 antagonist. Alternatively, or in combination with stent placement, laser therapy can cauterize the oesophageal or gastric-oesophageal junction cancer and restore the ability to swallow.

Ferrell et al's[34] descriptive study illustrates the importance of considering social and psychological factors in decision-making regarding surgery for advanced cancer. They suggest that although the physical impact of uncontrolled symptoms is the primary motivation for palliative surgery, the social impact of symptoms and the need to maintain hope are also relevant.

Prophylactic surgery

There remains ongoing debate about the role of prophylactic surgery in the upper gastrointestinal tract. There is little doubt that a proportion of patients with Barrett's oesophagus showing a high cytological grade of dysplasia will progress to invasive cancer. Resection of the lower oesophagus carries a mortality, and hence other means of prevention, including chemoprevention with NSAIDs or argon beam ablation of the Barrett's mucosa, are in development.[35] At present, high-grade dysplasia in an otherwise fit patient should be resected.

Postoperative multidisciplinary team meeting

Where surgical resection with the intent of cure is not possible, a combination of stent, laser, chemotherapy and radiotherapy may be used effectively to palliate oesophageal or gastric cancer and to prolong survival. Postoperative chemotherapy or radiotherapy, or a combination, may also improve survival following gastric cancer[36] or oesophageal cancer resection. This choice of which therapies to use may be decided by the multidisciplinary team on the basis of the pathology.

Pathology

Adenocarcinoma of the lower oesophagus, oesophago-gastric junction or stomach is the most frequent indication for surgery, but squamous oesophageal cancer (particularly in the middle third) and rarer histological types occur. With a recognition that Barrett's oesophagus (a metaplastic change in the epithelial lining of the lower oesophagus from squamous to columnar epithelium) may progress to adenocarcinoma, Barrett's oesophagus showing features of high-grade dysplasia may also be resected.

Generally, the pathology of oesophageal and gastric cancer identifies tumour infiltration (submucosal and/or through the wall) deeper than clinical or radiological examination had suggested. Circumferential, distal or proximal resection margins are very poor prognostic features: signet ring appearance on histology is a poor prognostic feature, whereas the presence of eosinophils in gastric cancer is a marker of relatively good prognosis.

Recovery and rehabilitation

Since surgical resection or palliation can carry a substantial morbidity, with over 40% of patients suffering respiratory or cardiovascular complications following resection,[31] postoperative recovery and rehabilitation for the patient require substantial input from nurses and allied health professionals (Table 12.6). Increasingly, upper gastrointestinal cancer specialist nurses are employed to support patients both pre- and postoperatively. They may have a particularly important role in the assessment and management of postoperative symptoms[37] and in the provision of information and education.[38]

Physically, support including encouragement of breathing exercises (instruction for which

should begin preoperatively), dressings of wounds, drain and feeding line sites and early mobilization postoperatively aid recovery. Psychologically, the impact of major surgery, waking up in a intensive or high-dependency unit with multiple lines and tubes attached and gradual recovery thereafter, requires continued support.[7]

Given that the stomach acts as a reservoir for food, following surgery for oesophageal or gastric cancer, patients have to learn to eat small quantities of food frequently and gradually increase the amount of food they can take in at any one time over a 3- to 6-month period. Taking in too much food at one time, at least until the gut adapts, can result in feelings of bloating, fullness or 'dumping', where the sudden intake of food results in fluid shifts into the gut and/or changes in insulin dynamics in the bloodstream with consequent sympathetic symptoms including sweating, pallor and dizziness.[39]

For the patients undergoing palliation, e.g. with a stent, nutritional advice is important. In particular, more semisolid foods and liquids are less likely to impact and stick on the stent and, particularly for plastic stents, drinking a fizzy drink after food intake will help to keep the stent clear. Oral supplements, whether milk based or fruit flavour based, can be useful in maintaining an adequate balanced calorific intake.

Patients who have had a gastrectomy, will no longer manage to absorb vitamin B_{12} (since they no longer produce intrinsic factor to allow the absorption of vitamin B_{12}) and will require injections of vitamin B_{12} every 3 months. If a splenectomy has been performed at the time of surgery, inoculation against *Meningococcus*, *Haemophilus* and *Pneumococcus* is required and additional long-term low-dose penicillin is also recommended.

Quality of life after resection of an oesophageal cancer[40] may be severely disrupted. During the first few months after resection of oesophageal or gastric cancer, the patient may require sustained encouragement with adapting his diet and trying to restore weight; it is usual for such patients to lose weight around the time of their surgery and unusual for them to gain much weight in the

Table 12.6: Recovery from oesophageal and gastric cancer surgery

System	Therapy
Respiratory function	Oxygen, physiotherapy, antibiotics
Cardiovascular function	Accurate fluid and electrolyte balance
Nutrition	Enteral, parenteral feed, dietetics advice Vitamin B_{12} (postgastrectomy)
Mobility	Physiotherapy and nursing staff
Psychological	Patients, relatives, multidisciplinary team

long term. Some patients develop difficulties in swallowing due to stricturing at the site of the anastomosis (whether the anastomosis is performed by suturing or stapling) and so patients should be warned that this may require dilation (usually performed endoscopically under sedation using a balloon dilator) on more than one occasion.

Follow-up of patients who have had a curative resection should include annual endoscopy of the upper gastrointestinal tract to examine the mucosa for disease recurrence, which might be amenable to further therapy (e.g. radiotherapy, laser treatment). Some centres also undertake annual CT scanning to examine for systemic metastasis, although the evidence as to whether this is of benefit to the patients is lacking.

In most European population-based studies, two-thirds of patients present too late to undergo curative resection of oesophageal or gastric cancer;[31] for the minority of patients in whom surgical resection is appropriate, surgical removal of the cancer and management within a multidisciplinary team (with additional therapies where appropriate) offers the best chance of cure.

COLORECTAL CANCER

Principles

For what is one of the most common cancers,[14,41] surgery offers the only opportunity of cure and also provides the mainstay of treatment for more advanced disease, including metastatic deposits.

Diagnosis

The majority of patients with carcinoma of the colon and rectum present either with abdominal symptoms (abdominal discomfort, bloating or change in bowel habit, particularly looser stools or increased frequency) or symptoms of anaemia (fatigue, breathlessness), rectal bleeding (blood mixed in with the stool or on the stool) or mucus discharge per rectum. Clearly, some of these symptoms are not specific to colorectal cancer and so in many European countries a quarter to a third of patients present as a surgi-

cal emergency. Emergency presentation is typically with large bowel obstruction (Fig. 12.11): abdominal pain, abdominal swelling, vomiting and constipation for stool or even flatus. Such patients should ideally have a preoperative water-soluble contrast enema to confirm the diagnosis of colorectal cancer (Fig. 12.12) and to exclude the diagnosis of pseudo obstruction which may

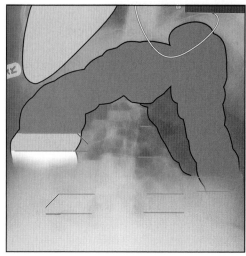

Figure 12.11: Erect abdominal radiograph of large bowel obstruction. (From Thompson AM. General surgical anatomy and examination. Edinburgh: Churchill Livingstone; 2001.)

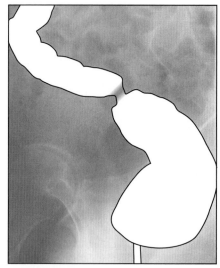

Figure 12.12: Single contrast barium enema of rectosigmoid cancer. (From Thompson AM. General surgical anatomy and examination. Edinburgh: Churchill Livingstone; 2001.)

mimic true obstruction but does not require colonic resection. Bleeding or prolapse of a rectal cancer through the anus may also lead to emergency presentation.

Increasingly, patients may present via a screening programme, usually from faecal occult blood testing of successive stool samples. Confirmed positive testing requires follow-up colonoscopy. Identification of polyps (which with increasing size are more likely to be cancerous) by colonoscopy and snaring any polyps can effectively treat precancerous or early cancerous change. Providing the polyp has clear margins without evidence of submucosal spread of tumour and is not a high histological grade, endoscopic resection alone may be sufficient to both diagnose and treat the cancer. Colonoscopy may also identify cancers requiring surgical therapy.

Colonoscopy is equally effective as a combination of flexible sigmoidoscopy and barium enema in the diagnosis of colorectal cancer,[42] so the local availability of the two approaches may dictate which type of investigation is most commonly used. More recently, radiological techniques such as computed tomography pneumocolon or magnetic resonance colography, which have the advantage of allowing staging of the disease at the same time (particularly to detect local invasion and liver metastases), have shown promise, but are not widely available.

Where a lesion has been identified, an endoscopic biopsy prior to definitive surgery provides histological proof of the malignant process. Clearly this may be easier for a rectal cancer or on endoscopic examination of the rest of the colon, and some think this approach is preferable to the non-invasive radiological methods where biopsy cannot be performed.

Staging

For elective colorectal cancer, the opportunity to stage the disease (Table 12.7) is essential unless it will not materially change the management plan. CT or MRI scanning of the abdomen (for liver metastasis) is more sensitive than transabdominal liver ultrasound, although intraoperative ultrasound and palpation by a surgeon's hand may be even more accurate.[43] For rectal

cancer, endoanal ultrasound may also be useful.[44] A chest X-ray (or CT scan) should be performed to rule out lung metastasis, and any anaemia and electrolyte abnormalities should be corrected. In addition, serum CEA (carcinoembryonic antigen) may be measured: it is typically at a high level in the presence of metastatic colorectal cancer; preoperative measurement may act as a baseline for future follow-up.

Since synchronous cancers occur in 5% of patients, and these may not be easily detectable at the time of surgery, complete colonic examination, as for the diagnosis (above), is necessary before elective colorectal cancer resection.

Multidisciplinary meeting

Increasingly, colorectal cancer patients are discussed at a multidisciplinary meeting preoperatively (for elective patients) and particularly postoperatively (for all patients) with regard to adjuvant chemotherapy or radiotherapy. Multidisciplinary discussion including specialist colorectal nurses, radiologists, surgeons, oncologists and allied health professionals may also identify patients with rec-

Table 12.7: Staging investigations for colorectal cancer	
Test	**Purpose**
Full blood count	To look for anaemia
Urea and electrolytes	To look for low potassium, dehydration
Liver function tests	To look for liver metastases
Colonoscopy	To look for additional polyps or cancers
CT scan of abdomen and chest	To look for metastatic disease
CT/MRI of pelvis	To assess invasion of rectal cancer
Endoanal ultrasound	To assess penetration of rectal cancer

tal cancer for whom neoadjuvant therapy (see below) can be effective in downstaging the cancer prior to definitive surgery.[10] In such meetings, review of the radiological and pathological findings by the relevant specialists can be put in the context of the patient's personal and social circumstances and then used in discussion with the patient and relatives of the optimal management plan. It is rare not to offer surgical resection, even to frail patients, as the consequences of future lumenal occlusion by a cancer usually result in emergency admission at a later date. The patient's operative course, pathology report and personal and social context can be brought together to help the patient to decide what adjuvant therapy may be appropriate and whether there are clinical trials available. This individualized approach is particularly important in the elderly, as there is evidence that treatment decisions are affected by age alone, rather than considering functional and social status.[45]

Surgery and reconstruction

Precancerous and small cancerous polyps may be excised by colonoscopic snaring; further surgery is then only required if there is tumour within 1 mm of the resection margin, there is lymphovascular invasion or the cancer is poorly differentiated.[46] Nonetheless, many colorectal

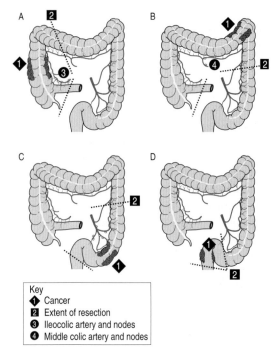

Key
1 Cancer
2 Extent of resection
3 Ileocolic artery and nodes
4 Middle colic artery and nodes

Figure 12.13: Surgical resections dependent on the position of the colonic or rectal cancer demonstrating the arterial anatomy: (a) right hemicolectomy; (b) extended right hemicolectomy; (c) anterior resection; and (d) abdominoperineal resection. (From Thompson AM. General surgical anatomy and examination. Edinburgh: Churchill Livingstone; 2001.)

cancers without evidence of distant metastasis by preoperative staging require formal surgical resection (Table 12.8).

Table 12.8: Surgical options for colorectal cancer	
Site of cancer	**Surgical method**
Colonic polyp Rectal polyp	Snare polypectomy or localized excision
Superficial rectal cancer	Transanal resection
Caecal cancer Ascending colon cancer Transverse colon cancer Descending colon cancer Sigmoid cancer	Colectomy (Fig. 12.13)
Rectal cancer	Anterior resection with coloanal anastomosis or abdominoperineal resection

Since patients undergoing colorectal cancer surgery are particularly at risk of thromboembolic disease and postoperative wound infection, deep venous thrombosis prophylaxis and antibiotic prophylaxis[47] should be commenced prior to surgery. DVT prophylaxis may include mechanical methods such as stockings and anticoagulants such as heparins, although the latter may need to be withheld until an epidural has been placed immediately preoperatively. Antibiotic prophylaxis should cover both aerobic and anaerobic organisms and should commence within 30 minutes of anaesthesia.

While it is conventional to administer preoperative bowel preparation to reduce the faecal load in the colon, at least for elective patients, the evidence that this confers a patient benefit is not strong. Administering oral sodium picosulfate or other oral agents in the 24 hours prior to surgery reduces the faecal load and thus may facilitate the operative procedure, but in elderly patients may also result in fluid and electrolyte depletion and is not possible where the colon is obstructed.

Surgery for colorectal cancer traditionally requires a laparotomy through a vertical midline or transverse incision (Fig. 12.1). The tumour-bearing colon is resected bearing in mind its vascular supply (Fig. 12.13). In elective colonic surgery, the ends of the bowel are anastomosed, restoring intestinal continuity. However, for emergency surgery or where the blood supply (a prerequisite for safe wound healing) may be compromised, bringing the proximal end of the bowel to the surface as an end stoma may be necessary (Fig. 12.14). The end of the remaining distal bowel can be brought out as a mucous fistula or oversewn and left closed within the peritoneal cavity. Even where an anastomosis is possible, a covering ileostomy or colostomy diverting the faecal stream from particularly a low rectal or coloanal anastomosis may be required. In general, male sex, increasing age, obesity and an anastomosis within 5 cm of the anal margin are risk factors for anastomotic leakage.[48]

For rectal cancers, excision of the rectum and surrounding mesorectal tissue (mesorectal excision) reduces the risk of local recurrence and improves local disease control by achieving

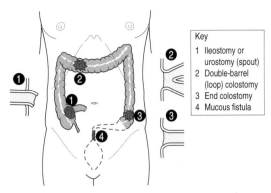

Figure 12.14: Abdominal stoma types and sites. (From Thompson AM. General surgical anatomy and examination. Edinburgh: Churchill Livingstone; 2001.)

Key
1 Ileostomy or urostomy (spout)
2 Double-barrel (loop) colostomy
3 End colostomy
4 Mucous fistula

good circumferential clearance around the tumour.[5] An important principle of the technique is to preserve the pelvic nerves to minimize disruption to bladder and sexual organ function, particularly in men. For rectal cancers in the mid and lower rectum, a coloanal anastomosis can be fashioned. There is now good evidence to suggest that a J-shaped pouch constructed from the colon to replace the excised rectum may improve bowel function towards normal.[49]

For low rectal cancers, resection of the anus and adjacent tissue may be required, an abdominoperineal resection; as a consequence, the perineum is closed and an end colostomy brought out into the left iliac fossa.

Historically, staged procedures were performed: a defunctioning loop colostomy (Fig. 12.14) with resection at a later date and rejoining the bowel ends as a third procedure. This sequence of events is now unusual. Indeed the trend now is to perform a single procedure (even as an emergency and including removal of organs involved by direct invasion of the colorectal cancer where that is possible) and to use a temporary stoma to protect or divert the faecal stream from the anastomosis.[50] For patients who present with malignant bowel obstruction from a colorectal cancer, removal of the cancer by primary resection with immediate anastomosis may be possible if there is sufficient surgical expertise.

More recently, laparoscopic-assisted colectomy, where the colon is mobilized laparoscopically, may be used to reduce the size of surgical incisions, with the anastomosis being done on the surface. Hand-assisted laparoscopic resection is a more recent development whereby a hand can be inserted through a port into the abdominal cavity. At present, the oncological equivalence of laparoscopic resection compared with open resection remains unproven, but the laparosopic approach can reduce postoperative pain, analgesia use, hospital stay and blood loss.[51]

For superficial rectal cancers, transanal resection using a resectoscope (analogous to the use of a cystoscope for superficial bladder cancer) may be an option which does not require formal bowel resection. This has the advantage of less morbidity than radical surgery but is associated with higher rates of local recurrence, and hence should be restricted to patients with cancers that have not yet involved the submucosa and hence where involvement of the regional lymph nodes is low.

Whichever resectional approach is used (with the exception of polypectomy and transanal resection), the regional lymph nodes draining the cancer are also resected. Thus, the vessels feeding a colon cancer and the venous and lymphatic drainage are divided close to the aorta.

The anastomosis between ends of bowel may be by conventional sutures, in one or two layers, individual sutures or continuous sutures or, alternatively, use a staple device to appose the ends. Drainage of the pelvis is required after abdominoperineal resection and should remain in place for about 5 days.

Surgery for metastatic disease

There is good evidence that hepatic resection for technically suitable metastatic colorectal cancer can improve survival,[52] to around 40% 5-year survival following liver metastasis resection, with some evidence that similar results can be obtained for resection of appropriately selected lung metastases from colorectal cancer. This is in contrast to resection of liver metastases from upper gastrointestinal cancers or breast cancer, where hepatic resection of metastases is rarely of benefit. In-situ ablation of liver metastases using modalities such as cryotherapy may also be of benefit (in terms of survival) to patients with liver metastases that are not amenable to resection.

Perioperative management

The support and advice of a stoma nurse specialist is acknowledged to be of great value, so all patients who are likely to require a stoma (whether permanent of temporary) should be assessed by a stoma nurse specialist preoperatively, and for elective surgery, prior to admission to hospital. This reflects the importance of marking the stoma site on the skin in a position that will be least awkward for the patient: avoiding where the patient's belt will press on the abdominal wall for example.

Perioperative management of the patient includes advice on stoma care (where a stoma is likely), DVT prophylaxis, antibody prophylaxis, epidural anaesthesia, oxygen therapy, fluid and electrolyte balance, postoperative advice on what to expect and dietary advice. Postoperative oral intake was traditionally restricted until bowel function returns (flatus then stool); more recently, oral intake as tolerated by the patient has become more widely practised. Potential complications include respiratory atelectasis/chest infections through to anastomotic leakage or even death. As already outlined, the maintenance of a pain-free, adequately hydrated patient who may be optimally nursed with invasive monitoring such as a CVP (central venous pressure) line where appropriate on a high-dependency ward will allow postoperative recovery to progress speedily.

Concern regarding perioperative blood transfusion and the suggestion that this might increase the risk of postoperative recurrence (presumably through an immunological suppression-mediated mechanism) has not been substantiated[53] and so blood transfusion should not be withheld from patients undergoing colorectal cancer resection.

The perioperative mortality of colorectal cancer surgery ranges from about 4% for elective surgery up to over 20% for emergency surgery for colorectal cancer.

Pathology

The pathological review of a resected colorectal cancer and its associated tissues is central to the decision-making process after surgical resection. As for breast cancer and now upper gastrointestinal cancers, the colorectal cancer specimen should be received fresh by the pathologist so that the proximity of the cancer to the resection margins and the lymph nodes can be assessed. Histologically, tumour differentiation, vascular invasion, assessment of the resection margin and presence of lymph node metastasis influence further treatment and outcome. The Dukes' staging system (Table 12.9) and the TNM system are both widely used to document the extent of local invasion and the extent of metastatic spread to the regional and even distant tissues.

Adjuvant therapy

Adjuvant chemotherapy following colorectal cancer should be considered for Dukes' C tumours. The evidence for patient benefit with adjuvant chemotherapy for Dukes' B cancer is lacking but may be offered to patients with poor prognostic features. Similarly, infusion of chemotherapy via a portal vein catheter or hepatic artery infusion for colorectal metastases should only be conducted in specialist centres as part of clinical trials.

Adjuvant radiotherapy for rectal cancer,[54] and for that matter, preoperative neoadjuvant radiotherapy[10] for rectal cancer, improves local disease control but has not been shown to have a definite survival advantage. Indeed, the toxicity of the radiotherapy to the remaining bowel may significantly hinder the patient's quality of life.[55]

Emerging evidence suggests that adding synchronous chemotherapy to local radiotherapy increases the response rate of rectal cancer and may convert inoperable rectal cancer into operable disease.

Prophylactic surgery

Surgery to prevent the development of colorectal cancer is usually confined to patients from adenomatous polyposis (FAP) families. Individuals at risk of developing colorectal cancer due to inheriting the autosomal dominant gene which causes FAP require regular endoscopic screening and, when adenomas have developed in the colon, should undergo surgery.[56] The surgical options are proctocolectomy with an ileostomy, proctocolectomy with an ileoanal pouch reconstruction or colectomy without removing the rectum and an ileorectal anastomosis. The last of these carries a lower operative morbidity and better functional results (particularly fewer episodes of defecation per day and more solid stool), but patients require sigmoidoscopic surveillance of the rectum postoperatively because of the risk of developing cancer in the retained rectum.

Endoscopic surveillance of the upper gastrointestinal tract, particularly for duodenal adenomas and ampullary cancer, is needed for patients who have required surgery for FAP, as cancers of the upper gastrointestinal tract may develop and kill patients in whom the lower gastrointestinal tract has been removed. Similarly, individuals with an hereditary predisposition to colorectal cancer, such as those from hereditary non-polyposis colorectal cancer (HNPCC) families, require

Table 12.9: Dukes' stage for colorectal cancer (modified)

Dukes' stage	Pathology findings
A	Limited to the submucosa
B1	Tumour invades into but not through muscularis propria, no nodes involved
B2	Tumour invades through muscularis propria, no nodes involved
B3	Tumour invades other organs or structures
C1	Regional lymph nodes involved
C2	Metastases present in nodes at mesenteric artery ligature (apical nodes)
D	Distant spread

regular endoscopic surveillance of the upper and lower gastrointestinal tracts and may come under surgical care either for polypectomy or if they develop a colorectal cancer.

Palliative surgery

Palliation of colorectal cancer usually comprises overcoming intestinal obstruction where curative resection is not possible (Table 12.10). This may be performed effectively by placing a colonic stent through the cancer either under radiological or endoscopic control, in a way analogous to oesophageal cancer stenting. This may either be used as palliation in itself or to facilitate improvements in the patient's general condition before proceeding to a formal resection.[57] Alternatively, the use of laser to ablate tumour accessible in the rectum or sigmoid colon can be used to maintain the lumen.

Alternatively, creating a loop colostomy or loop ileostomy (either as an open procedure or laparoscopically assisted) may provide relief of distal obstruction that is irresectable. This may be appropriate prior to neoadjuvant radiotherapy to a rectal cancer. Similarly, performing an enteral bypass (for example an ileo transverse colon anatomosis) either as an open or laparoscopic procedure can bypass an obstructing irresectable proximal colonic cancer (e.g. caecal cancer).

Recovery and rehabilitation

Surgery to treat colorectal cancer can result in physical changes, including bowel dysfunction, living with a stoma, urinary disorders, erectile dysfunction and altered body image. Residual pain and constipation can have an adverse impact on quality of life, even 2 years after diagnosis and curative treatment.[58] Together with the uncertainty of having had colorectal cancer, substantial psychological and rehabilitative support may be required from family members and the multidisciplinary team. Specialist colorectal nurses are increasingly involved in the continuing care of patients after colorectal surgery, and have a role to play in symptom management, psychological care, support for lifestyle change and follow-up. Recent research suggests that interventions such as progressive muscle relaxation training can have a beneficial effect on anxiety and quality of life in patients who have recovered from stoma surgery, and that nurses should incorporate such techniques into their practice.[59]

INNOVATIONS IN SURGERY FOR CANCER

Although surgery has been established as the major modality for the treatment and cure of solid cancers for over a century, over the past decade, several innovations have developed.

Minimal access/minimally invasive approaches are established for the endoscopic investigation and therapy of early cancers of the stomach and colon. This now includes endoscopic ultrasound, particularly for upper gastrointestinal cancers and rectal cancer. Laparoscopic staging of upper gastrointestinal cancer (including laparoscopic ultrasound) also has advantages in

Table 12.10: Palliative surgery for colorectal cancer	
Obstruction	**Technique**
Colon and/or small bowel with normal bowel distal	Surgical bypass: enteroenterostomy to bypass obstruction(s)
Colonic or rectal obstruction	Proximal stoma formation – loop colostomy – end colostomy (Fig. 12.14)
Distal colonic or upper rectal obstruction	Stent placement

preventing laparotomy for irresectable or disseminated intraperitoneal disease.

Laparascopic resection of colorectal cancer, gastric cancer and pancreatic cancer and thoracoscopically assisted oesophageal cancer resections have all been reported. Colorectal resection has perhaps the widest application, but even when 'hand assisted', its long-term potential as an anticancer operation remains uncertain.

Innovative therapies delivered with minimally invasive approaches are under development. Using photodynamic therapy (light source activation of chemicals preferentially taken up into cancer cells) to treat precancerous Barrett's oesophagus and in established biliary tree carcinoma is the subject of clinical trials. Cryotherapy to liver metastases not suitable for resection can be applied laparoscopically to slow disease progression. As novel biological therapies become available, these too may be delivered by minimal access techniques.

CONCLUSION

Surgery remains the principal therapy with potential for cure for most solid adult malignancies. Multidisciplinary team working and advances in perioperative and holistic patient care have improved in the last two decades. Good nursing care has been and will remain central to continued advances in the outlook and survival for patients with cancer.

Acknowledgements
The authors thank the specialist cancer nurses Gillian Little, Caroline Ackland and Jackie Kerrigan for their helpful suggestions in preparing this chapter.

REFERENCES

1. Downing, J. Surgery. In: Corner J, Bailey C, eds. Cancer nursing. Care in context. Oxford: Blackwell Scientific; 2001.
2. Fisher B, Brown A, Mamounas E, et al. Effect of preoperative chemotherapy on local-regional disease in women with operable breast cancer: findings from National Surgical Adjuvant Breast and Bowel Project B-18. J Clin Oncol 1997; 15:2483–2493.
3. Wells M, Dryden H, Guild P, et al. The knowledge and attitudes of surgical staff towards the use of opioids in cancer pain management: can the Hospital Palliative Care Team make a difference? Eur J Cancer Care 2001; 10:210–211.
4. Green CR, Wheeler JRC. Physician variablity in the management of acute postoperative and cancer pain: a quantitative analysis of the Michigan Experiment. Pain Med 2003; 4:8–20.
5. Martling AL, Holm T, Rutqvist LE, et al. Effect of a surgical training programme on outcome of rectal cancer in the County of Stockholm. Stockholm Colorectal Cancer Study Group, Basingstoke Bowel Cancer Research Project. Lancet 2000; 356:93–96.
6. Moore KN, Estey A. The early post-operative concerns of men after radical prostatectomy. J Adv Nurs 1999; 29:1121–1129.
7. Diamond J. Because cowards get cancer too. London: Vermillion; 1998.
8. Leinonen T, Leino-Kilpi H, Stahlberg M-R, Lertola K. The quality of perioperative care: development of a tool for the perceptions of patients. Meth Issues Nurs Res 2001; 35:294–296.
9. Wells M, Harrow A, Donnan P, et al. Patient, carer and health service outcomes of nurse-led early discharge after breast cancer surgery: a randomised controlled trial. Br J Cancer 2004; 91(4):651–658.
10. Munro AJ, Bentley AHM. Adjuvant radiotherapy in operable rectal cancer: a systematic review. Semin Colon Rectal Surg 2002; 13:31–42.
11. Medical Research Council Oesophageal Cancer Working Group. Surgical resection with or without preoperative chemotherapy in oesophageal cancer: a randomised controlled trial. Lancet 2002; 359(9319):1727–1733.
12. Junor EJ, Hole DJ, McNulty L, Mason M, Young J. Specialist gynaecologists and survival outcome in ovarian cancer: a Scottish national study of 1866 patients. Br J Obstet Gynaecol 1999; 106(11):1130–1136.
13. Chetty U. In: Black R, Stockton D, eds. Scottish Executive Health Department cancer scenarios: an aid to planning cancer services in Scotland in the next decade. Edinburgh: The Scottish Executive; 2001.
14. Stewart BW, Kleihues P, eds. World Cancer Report. Lyons: IARC Press; 2003: oesophagus pp 223–227, gastric pp 194–197, colon pp 198–202, breast pp 188–193.
15. Fisher B, Anderson S, Redmond CK, et al. Reanalysis and results after 12 years of follow-up in a randomised clinical trial comparing total mastectomy with lumpectomy with or without irradiation in the treatment of breast cancer. N Engl J Med 1995; 333:1456–1461.

16. Bates T, Riley DL, Houghton J, Fallowfield L, Baum M. Breast cancer in elderly women: a Cancer Research Campaign trial comparing treatment with tamoxifen and optimal surgery with tamoxifen alone. Br J Surg 1991; 78:591–594.

17. McIntosh SA, Purushotham AD. Lymphatic mapping and sentinel node biopsy in breast cancer. Br J Surg 2000; 85:1347–1356.

18. Steele RJ, Forrest AP, Gibson T, Stewart HJ, Chetty U. The efficacy of lower axillary sampling in obtaining lymph node status in breast cancer: a controlled randomised trial. Br J Surg 1985; 72:368–369.

19. Thompson AM. Axillary node clearance for breast cancer. J R Coll Surg Edinb 1999; 44:111–117.

20. Nissen MJ, Swenson KK, Kind EA. Quality of life after postmastectomy breast reconstruction. Oncol Nurs Forum 2002; 29:547–553.

21. Miller J. An experience of breast cancer: a patient's personal view. In: Macfarlane S, Sheeran J, eds. A picture of health: paintings and drawings of breast cancer care. Hebden Bridge: Sheeran Lock Fine Art Consultants; 1995: 48–57.

22. Fallowfield LJ, Hall A, Maguire GP, Baum M. Psychological outcomes of different treatment policies in women with early breast cancer outside a clinical trial. BMJ 1990; 301:575–580.

23. McArdle JM, George WD, McArdle CS, et al. Psychological support for patients undergoing breast cancer surgery: a randomised study. BMJ 1996; 312(7034):813–816.

24. Pain SJ, Purushotham AB. Lymphoedema following surgery for breast cancer. Br J Surg 2000; 87:1128–1141.

25. Williams A. Lymphoedema. In: Faithfull S, Wells M, eds. Supportive care in radiotherapy. Edinburgh: Churchill Livingstone; 2003.

26. Hartmann LC, Schaid DJ, Woods JE. Efficacy of bilateral prophylactic mastectomy in women with a family history of breast cancer. N Engl J Med 1999; 340:77–84.

27. Moller P, Borg A, Evans GD, et al. Survival in prospectively ascertained familial breast cancer: analysis of a series stratified by tumour characteristics, *BRCA* mutations and oophorectomy. Int J Cancer 2002; 101:555–559.

28. Thompson AM. In: Black R, Stockton D, eds. Scottish Executive Health Department. Cancer scenarios: an aid to planning cancer services in Scotland in the next decade. Edinburgh: The Scottish Executive; 2001.

29. Qadir A, Trotter C, Park KG. D2 gastrectomy for an antral stomach tumour. J R Coll Surg Edinb 2000; 45:242–251.

30. Bonenkamp JJ, Songun I, Hermans J, et al. Randomised comparison of morbidity after D1 and D2 dissection for gastric cancer in 996 Dutch patients. Lancet 1995; 345:745–748.

31. Gilbert FJ, Park KGM, Thompson AM, eds. Scottish audit of gastric and oesophageal cancer. Edinburgh: Scottish Executive Health Department; 2002.

32. Hartgrink HH, Putter H, Klein Kranenbarg E, Bonenkamp JJ, van de Velde (for the Dutch Gastric Cancer Group). Value of palliative resection in gastric cancer. Br J Surg 2002; 89:1438–1443.

33. Cowling MG, Hale H, Grundy A. Management of malignant oesophageal obstruction with self expanding metal stents. Br J Surg 1998; 85:264–266.

34. Ferrell BR, Chu DZJ, Wagman L, et al. Patient and surgeon decision making regarding surgery for advanced cancer. Oncol Nurs Forum 2003; 30:E106–E114.

35. Morris CD, Byrne JP, Armstrong GRA, Attwood SEA. Prevention of the neoplastic progression of Barrett's oesophagus by endoscopic argon beam plasma ablation. Br J Surg 2001; 88:1357–1362.

36. Macdonald JS, Smalley SR, Benedetti J, et al, St Vincent's Comprehensive Cancer Centre, New York, USA. Chemotherapy after surgery compared with surgery alone for adenocarcinoma of the stomach or gastroesophageal junction. N Engl J Med 2001; 345(10):725–730.

37. Sweed MR, Scheich L, Barsevick A, Babb J, Goldberg M. Quality of life after esophagectomy for cancer. Res Briefs 2002; 29:1127–1131.

38. Mills ME, Sullivan K. Patients with operable oesophageal cancer: their experience of information-giving in a regional thoracic unit. J Clin Nurs 2000; 9:236–246.

39. Anderson ID, MacIntyre IMC. Symptomatic outcome following resection of gastric cancer. Surg Oncol 1995; 4:35–40.

40. Zieren HU, Jacobi CA, Zieren J, Muller JM. Quality of life following resection of oesophageal carcinoma. Br J Surg 1996; 83:1772–1775.

41. Dunlop MG. In: Black R, Stockton D, eds. Scottish Executive Health Department. Cancer scenarios: an aid to planning cancer services in Scotland in the next decade. Edinburgh: The Scottish Executive; 2001.

42. Rex DK, Weddle RA, Lehman GA , et al. Flexible sigmoidoscopy plus air contrast barium enema versus colonoscopy for suspected lower gastrointestinal bleeding. Gastroenterology 1990; 98:855–861.

43. Knol JA, Marn CS, Francis IR, et al. Comparisons of dynamic infusion and delayed computed tomography, intraoperative ultrasound and palpation in the diagnosis of liver metastases. Am J Surg 1993; 165:81–87.

44. Kwok H, Bissett IP, Hill GL. Preoperative staging of rectal cancer. Int J Colorectal Dis 2000; 15:9–20.

45. Bailey C, Corner J. Care and the older person with cancer. Eur J Cancer Care 2000; 12:176–182.

46. Chapman MAS, Scholefield JH, Hardcastle JD. Management and outcome of patients with malignant colonic polyps identified from the Nottingham Colorectal Screening Study. Colorectal Dis 2000; 2:8–12.

47. Glenny AM, Song F. Antimicrobial prophylaxis in colorectal surgery. Qual Health Care 1999; 8:132–136.

48. Rullier E, Laurent C, Garrelon JL, et al. Risk factors for anastomotic leakage after resection of rectal cancer. Br J Surg 1998; 85:355–358.

49. Sailer M, Fuchs KH, Fein M, Thiede A. Randomized clinical trial comparing quality of life after straight and pouch coloanal reconstruction. Br J Surg 2002; 89(9):1108–1117.

50. Dehni N, Schlegel RD, Cunningham C, et al. Influence of a defunctioning stoma on leakage rates after low colorectal anastomosis and colonic J pouch-anal anastomosis. Br J Surg 1998; 85:1114–1117.

51. Maxwell-Armstrong CA, Robinson MH, Scholefield JH. Laparoscopic colorectal cancer surgery. Am J Surg 2000; 179:500–507.

52. Scheele J, Stang R, Altendorf-Hofmann A, Paul M. Resection of colorectal liver metastases. World J Surg 1995; 19:59–71.

53. McAlister FA, Clark HD, Wells PS, Laupacis A. Perioperative allogeneic blood transfusion does not cause adverse sequelae in patients with cancer: a meta-analysis of unconfounded studies. Br J Surg 1998; 85:171–178.

54. Camma C, Giunta M, Fiorica F, et al. Preoperative radiotherapy for respectable rectal cancer: a meta-analysis. JAMA 2000; 284:1008–1015.

55. Dahlberg M, Glimelius B, Graf W, Pahlman L. Preoperative irradiation affects functional results after surgery for rectal cancer: results from a randomised study. Dis Colon Rectum 1998; 41:543–549.

56. Rhodes M, Bradburn DM. Overview of screening and management of familial adenomatous polyposis. Gut 1992; 33: 125–131.

57. Camunez F, Echenagusia A, Simo G, et al. Malignant colorectal obstruction treated by means of self-expanding metallic stents: effectiveness before surgery and in palliation. Radiology 2000; 216:492–497.

58. Rauch P, Conroy T, Miny J, Neyton L, Guillemin F. Quality of life among disease-free survivors of rectal cancer. J Clin Oncol 2004; 22:354–360.

59. Cheung YL, Molassiotis A, Chang A. The effect of progressive muscle relaxation training on anxiety and quality of life after stoma surgery in colorectal cancer patients. Pyscho-Oncology 2002; 12:254–266.

CHAPTER 13

Radiotherapy

SARA FAITHFULL

CHAPTER CONTENTS

Introduction	265	What happens before treatment can begin?	272
What is radiotherapy and why is it used for cancer?	266	What information is needed to prepare patients for radiotherapy?	274
How is radiotherapy administered?	266	The treatment process	274
How does radiotherapy work?	268	What side effects does radiotherapy cause?	276
Repair of radiation damage	269		
Repopulation of the irradiated cells	270	What are the common problems experienced as a result of radiotherapy?	276
Redistribution of the cells within the cell reproductive cycle	271		
Reoxygentation of the tumour	271	Conclusion	279
How long is a course of radiotherapy?	272	References	280

INTRODUCTION

Radiotherapy plays a key role in the treatment of patients with cancer in Europe. After surgery, it is the most effective curative treatment for cancer,[1] and it is also used extensively for palliating symptoms and as an adjunct to other cancer treatments such as chemotherapy, surgery and hormone therapy. The value of radiotherapy lies mainly in its local application, whereby defined areas, which might otherwise be inoperable, can be treated successfully. Radiation causes damage to both normal and malignant cells, but damage is confined to the area of treatment delivery. Recent developments in radiotherapy, such as new brachytherapy techniques, intensity modulated and conformal therapies, exploit the potential for radiotherapy to induce maximum cell damage where it is most desired, at the same time as minimizing long-term side effects. Despite the huge growth in radiation technology and technique, our understanding of side effects and supportive care is still limited, and there is relatively little evidence on which to base our efforts.

Oncology nurses often lack awareness of the effects of radiotherapy and its impact on individuals and their family members. In addition, as over half of people with cancer receive radiation therapy at some time in the course of their disease, often alongside other therapies, it is imperative that healthcare professionals have an understanding of radiotherapy in order to effectively support patients through the cancer journey. Knowledge is important not only to understand the side effects of radiotherapy but also to answer questions such as:

- What is radiotherapy?
- How does the treatment work?
- Why do I have to have treatment every day?

- What happens during treatment and what effects will it have on me?

Many people have little understanding of what radiotherapy is, and hold fundamental misconceptions about its dangers, often believing that external beam treatment will render them radioactive. Many of these perceptions arise as a result of media coverage or historical knowledge about nuclear power stations and atomic bombs. Compared with the media interest in new drugs, molecular discoveries and gene therapies, radiotherapy tends to gather little interest, despite many exciting new developments. The fact that radiotherapy kills cancer cells is often understood but many patients are very conscious of the damage it also causes.[2]

To understand how people are affected by radiation therapy we need to understand why different doses and schedules are used and what their implications are for side-effect occurrence and symptom management. Radiotherapy is essentially an outpatient therapy, and patients are often not referred for nursing support unless they require a specific nursing procedure during treatment, which might occur as a result of side effects. Individual assessment and effective teamwork are vital to the management of acute side effects experienced during treatment, and nurses have a great deal to offer here. After treatment is completed, symptoms may continue for many weeks, and late radiotherapy effects can occur months to years later. Patients often develop problems outside the normal working hours of a radiotherapy centre; thus, it is important that nurses in both the hospital and the community are skilled in the assessment and management of radiation side effects. This chapter focuses on the principles and practice of radiotherapy treatment delivery, explaining the underlying radiobiology and the experience of patients throughout their treatment journey, as well as providing an overview of some common acute and late side effects.

sciences of physics, molecular biology and mathematics have enhanced our understanding of how radiotherapy works, resulting in the development of better treatment delivery techniques, and new technologies that enhance the action of radiotherapy.[3]

Radiotherapy is the use of ionizing radiation. The process of ionization damages deoxyribonucleic acid (DNA) and, consequently, causes cell death, especially when the cell attempts to replicate. Radiation may take several forms. It may consist of particles (bits of atoms) such as neutrons, protons or electrons or, in the case of electromagnetic radiation, both X-rays and gamma rays. The commonest form of radiotherapy is that of X-ray photon therapy, which has properties similar to that produced by radio waves, microwaves and visible light.[3] Ionizing radiation, by definition, produces ionization of atoms and molecules when it comes into contact with them.[4]

A simple understanding of atomic structure can help explain the nature of these changes. Atoms are part of the chemical elements that make up the cells of the body. Ionizing radiation has sufficient energy to cause atoms of cells in its path to lose orbiting electrons. When an electron is dislodged from its orbit, the atom fragments acquire a positive electrical charge. These energetic electrons are called 'recoil' electrons and, themselves, interact with neighbouring atoms, and hence these atom fragments acquire a negative electrical charge. When electrons are released from their orbit, energy in the form of free electrons is released at high speed and dislodges more electrons from neighbouring atoms, which in turn release energy, and continue further ionizations, until all the energy is dissipated.[3] The electrically charged particles are called ions, and the process of their development is called ionization (Fig. 13.1). This ionization is responsible for the chemical and biological changes that occur to tissues in the form of radiotherapy.

WHAT IS RADIOTHERAPY AND WHY IS IT USED FOR CANCER?

Radiation therapy is one of the oldest cancer treatments and has been used over the last 100 years for treating cancer. In the last decade the

HOW IS RADIOTHERAPY ADMINISTERED?

Most radiotherapy treatment is delivered using external beam radiotherapy (teletherapy) equipment, which produces photons or elec-

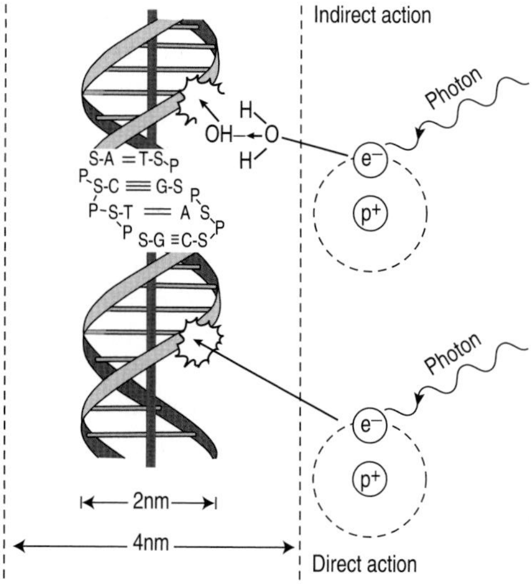

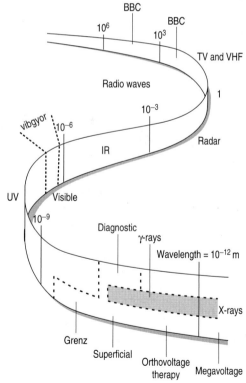

Figure 13.1: The process of ionization and DNA damage. Radiation causes damage by photons, resulting in direct action where the secondary electron resulting from absorption of the X-ray photon interacts with the DNA. The indirect action is where the electron interacts with molecules to produce free radicals, which in turn damage the DNA. (Reproduced with permission from Hall 2000: see Faithfull S, Wells M, eds. Supportive care in radiotherapy. Edinburgh: Churchill Livingstone; 2003:77.)

tant, as increased energy of radiation produces a greater penetration of tissues. These different energy levels are often used for differing sites for radiotherapy treatments. Electrons travel only short distances, so are often limited in their therapeutic use, but are appropriate for superficial treatments such as basal cell skin cancers.

Radiation dose is defined as the amount of energy absorbed per unit mass of tissue. This is measured in gray (Gy), where 1 gray = 1 joule/kg. For a conventional curative course of external beam radiotherapy, the dose ranges from 55 to 75 Gy and is given in daily treatment of 1.6–2.5 Gy over 4–6 weeks. This splitting of the overall dose is termed fractionation. External beam radiotherapy utilizes a beam from which the patient is placed at a defined distance (usually 100 mm). The 'iso' dose is

trons. The rays occur when speeding electrons hit high atomic weight targets such as tantalum, situated within the machine. Modern megavoltage machines, known as linear accelerators (LA) (Fig. 13.2), use a radio-wave guide to further accelerate electrons produced in this way. These electrons bombard the target at high energy, producing X-rays in the range of 6–25 MV (megavolts). The radiation beams are directed at the tumour in such a way that they deposit a dose of ionizing radiation at a specific depth in the tissues. At low energies, the X-rays produced are absorbed to varying degrees by different tissues and result in a clear distinction between bone, soft tissue and air interface, which is visible on diagnostic radiographs (X-ray films). Superficial irradiation occurs with photon energies of 150 keV and orthovoltage at 300 keV (Fig. 13.2). At megavoltage energies (6–25 MV), photons penetrate the deeper tissues. Linear accelerators have sophisticated computerized systems that deliver a range of radiation doses and volumes. These differences in energy levels are impor-

Figure 13.2: The electromagnetic spectrum: this demonstrates the differences in energy of treatment radiation to that of radiowaves and diagnostic techniques. (Reproduced with permission from Bomford & Kunkler 2002: see Faithfull S, Wells M, eds. Supportive care in radiotherapy. Edinburgh: Churchill Livingstone; 2003:76.).

the distribution of absorption of radiation in the tissues and varies at any point within the tissue, depending on the distance from the X-ray source. These distributions often look like contours on a map and reflect changes in radiation dose (Fig. 13.3). The clinical target volume (CTV) is extended to delineate a planning target volume (PTV), which accounts for any spread of disease or movement while the person is receiving treatment.[5] High-energy X-rays produced by the linear accelerator deposit most of their energy at some distance from the skin surface. This is known as a 'skin sparing' effect and can diminish skin damage.

Alternative radiation sources include naturally occurring radioisotopes such as cobalt, which is housed in a treatment machine. These elements have unstable nuclei that release energy in the process of spontaneous disintegration, either in the form of gamma rays, high-speed electrons or other particles. A variety of other radioactive isotopes are administered orally or intravenously to treat specific cancers. Such isotopes are used systemically, and are sometimes known as unsealed sources. Localization of the isotope around a tumour occurs when the radioactive chemical is metabolized. An example of this is where radioactive iodine (I^{131}) is taken up selectively by the thyroid gland, and is thus able to administer radiation specifically to a cancer of the thyroid.

Brachytherapy, or the use of sealed sources, is another method of delivering radiotherapy internally. It involves the placing of radioactive sources close to the tumour, using an applicator to position the sources. Over 4% of new cancers in the UK are now treated with brachytherapy;[6] however, this varies across the world, with 12% of new cancers being treated in this way in the USA, where more brachytherapy facilities tend to be available. Because the dose of radiation decreases at a rate equal to the square of the distance from the source, the tumour receives a higher dose, with little radiation reaching the surrounding normal tissues. The most common example of brachytherapy is the insertion of radioactive caesium for the treatment of uterine or cervical carcinomas. The technique of placing the source in small catheters that can be safely inserted and withdrawn – termed 'after loading' – is designed to provide maximum radiation protection for staff[7] and has revolutionized the delivery and safety of this treatment.

HOW DOES RADIOTHERAPY WORK?

Radiation interacts either directly or indirectly with tissues to produce short-lived ion radicals. These are associated with damage to the DNA

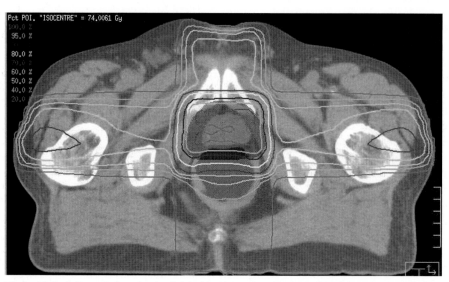

Figure 13.3: Contours of treatment field with clinical target volume (CTV) and planning target volume (PTV) outlined.

and result in single- or double-strand breaks. The DNA controls all cellular functions and any damage to it may lead either to the cell not functioning properly or to cell death (Fig. 13.4). The cell may subsequently repair this damage, as do normal tissues, which have a greater ability to repair themselves than cancer cells.[8] Differences in how cells respond to irradiation explain some of the reasons for the differences seen in the radiosensitivity of different cancers. The response to radiation is affected by other factors, including oxygenation, the number of cells actively dividing and the rate the cells grow within the tumour. These parameters are often termed the 4 R's and are important principles in understanding the rationale behind radiotherapy treatment delivery: they influence the impact of radiation therapy on both cancer and normal tissues.[9] Application of these principles guides clinical practice to maximize damage to the cancer cells, but also to minimize normal tissue damage. The 4 R's are:

1 Repair of radiation-induced damage.

2 Repopulation of the irradiated area by remaining cancer cells.

3 Redistribution of the cells within the cell reproductive cycle.

4 Reoxygentation of the tumour.

Repair of radiation damage

Ionizing radiation interacts directly or indirectly with the tissues and induces cell damage. Direct damage occurs in the nucleus of the cell and affects the DNA through single- or double-strand breaks that may be temporary or permanent. The cell is either unable to repair itself or does so inaccurately, resulting in cell death after several cell divisions. Indirect effects involve interaction of free radicals within the cells. The indirect damage does not damage DNA initially; instead, it acts particularly on the water molecules in the presence of oxygen to create pairs of ions that are unstable, called 'free radicals', within the cell. These are very reactive chemicals that cause damage to DNA production. This disturbance of DNA synthesis leads to abnormal mitosis (Fig. 13.5).

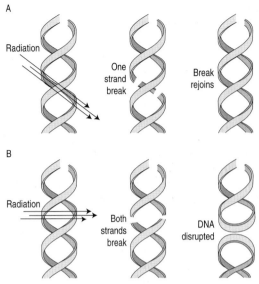

Figure 13.4: Radiobiological effect of damage to DNA: damage to DNA may be (A) temporary and reparable or (B) may be serious and have long-lasting effects. (Reproduced with permission from Wootton 1993; see Faithfull S, Wells M, eds. Supportive care in radiotherapy. Edinburgh: Churchill Livingstone; 2003:78.)

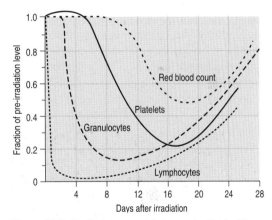

Figure 13.5: Radiation repopulation and mitosis. The pattern of loss of cells and recovery of cells are dependent on the radiosensitivity of the tissues affected and the lifetime of mature functional cells. This graph illustrates the pattern of recovery of components of circulating blood. (Produced with permission from Hall 2000; see Faithfull S, Wells M, eds. Supportive care in radiotherapy. Edinburgh: Churchill Livingstone; 2003:80.)

Only a few cells (e.g. lymphocytes and germs cells) die immediately after radiation damage; that is why the gonads are so sensitive to radiation and side effects such as infertility occur at very low doses of radiation. Cells that have a short mitosis (e.g. blood and mucosa) will show signs of radiation damage more quickly than those whose cell cycle is longer. Damage to slow-dividing cells may be responsible for many of the late complications of radiation.[10] This is also why a slow-growing cancer may take many months to shrink following radiotherapy. Normal tissues that may surround the cancer also show different degrees of sensitivity, both to the extent of damage and the timing of the effect of this damage.[11] Differences in this repair capacity between cancers may be part of the explanation for the differential responses of tumours to fractionation regimens, especially when using low doses of radiation.[12] By giving radiotherapy in a way that impacts most effectively on the cancer cell type and nature of the patient's tumour, the treatment will be more effective. A series of fractionated doses increases this difference in repair ability between normal tissue and tumour (Fig. 13.6).

The dose–response curves for both normal tissues and cancer cells are similar. A relatively small change in the dose can have major impli-

cations for both tumour control and the side effects of treatment. In clinical practice the optimum dose is often weighed up against possible complications; however, some individuals appear to be more sensitive than others.[13] Certain tissues are very sensitive to radiotherapy (e.g. eyes, lung, ovaries and testes) and the dose that can be given to these areas is very limited. Radiosensitivity is also related to the wide variation in how people respond to radiotherapy. This tolerance to treatment is often the factor that limits the dose of radiation. There is a threshold dose below which tumours are controlled but above which control increases steeply (Fig. 13.7). The success of treatment depends in part on whether the normal tissues can repair themselves faster and more fully than cancer cells. The greater the difference between the two curves, the greater the therapeutic ratio.[9] This makes it difficult to choose an optimal dose and, inevitably, some people are on the boundary either above or below this threshold of cell repair and subsequently experience side effects of radiotherapy.[14] Acute effects tend to occur during treatment and are related to the total dose of radiotherapy and the length of time over which the treatment is delivered. Late effects occur 6 months after treatment and are also dependent on dose but are more related to the dose per fraction. Late tissue changes may be related to damage to blood vessels and the connective tissues within the treatment field, causing abnormalities such as fibrosis, and are not necessarily related to the extent of acute effects experienced.

Repopulation of the irradiated cells

Once irradiation has been given, those cells not dividing, i.e. not damaged by the radiation, start to divide and replace the cells that have been damaged. Cancers that grow very fast show accelerated regrowth, especially at the beginning of therapy, and can outpace the delivery of radiotherapy so that the potential for a cure is reduced. Tumours that show accelerated repopulation will not be cured if the cancer cells continue to grow faster than they can be destroyed. It is this factor that is recognized as important in limiting the effectiveness of radiotherapy. Treatment delay therefore can

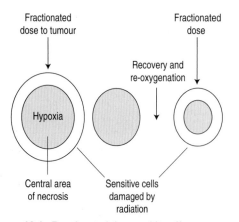

Figure 13.6: Fractionated dose and its effect on cancer cells. Dose fractionation allows the recovery of normal tissues as well as optimizing destruction of cancer cells. Cancers have an initial rapid death, which then slows, i.e. a biphasic decay. This is because tumours have a central area of necrosis or relative hypoxia, which is thus less resistant to the effects of ionizing radiation. One dose of radiation kills the sensitive cells in the periphery, allowing aeration of the hypoxic centre. These can be killed by the next dose, i.e. there is a chance for the tumour to oxygenate between each fraction.

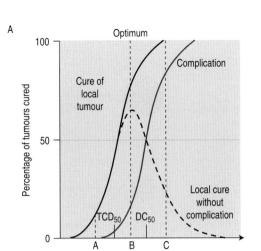

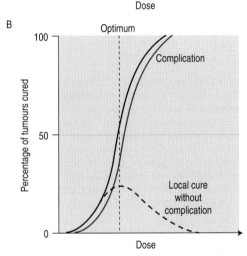

Figure 13.7: Threshold dose–response curve. The theoretical dose–response relationship for the percentage of local control of the cancer and the appearance of complications is illustrated by the S-shaped curve: (A) cure achieved without complications; (B) the optimal dose; and (C) cure of all the cancer cells but with the consequence of complications. The radiosensitivity of the normal tissues included in the field determines how many complications arise from treatment and this can widen or reduce the threshold of the dose-response curve. (Reproduced with permission from Tubiana et al 1990; see Faithfull S, Wells M, eds. Supportive care in radiotherapy. Edinburgh: Churchill Livingstone; 2003:90.)

have disastrous consequences if repopulation has been encouraged but subsequent treatment delivery is insufficient to keep up with new growth of the tumour. This is why even a small gap in radiotherapy is discouraged. It has been estimated that extending a planned course of radiotherapy by 1 week may decrease the cure

rate by 13%.[15] Worldwide, only about a third of patients complete their radiotherapy in the prescribed time, the remainder taking longer because of breaks in treatment.[1]

Patients may feel that they need a rest in the arduous schedule of treatment; however, the consequences of such a break could be disastrous. Repopulation also explains why different treatment schedules have been developed to improve fractionation time. Accelerated treatment, where radiation is delivered twice daily, aims to overcome the problem of tumour cells repopulating as rapidly as the normal tissues.[16] Treatment is given twice per day, so as to reduce the overall treatment time. Hyperfractionated treatment aims to improve the therapeutic ratio by reducing the dose given in each fraction but also increasing the frequency of treatment delivery to two or more times a day.[17] This is to reduce late side effects and permits an increased total dose to the tumour. Hyperfractionated regimens have been used successfully in the treatment of head and neck cancer.[17] Hypofractionated regimens are often used for palliative treatments, where the patient has a shorter treatment time and receives a higher dose of radiotherapy per fraction.[18]

Redistribution of the cells within the cell reproductive cycle

When cells are damaged by radiation, it is the cells that are not dividing that enter the cell cycle at G0 to replace the cells destroyed by treatment; hence the term redistribution. Prolonged fractionation means that cells have a greater chance of being in a sensitive phase of the cell cycle. Cells are more resistant to radiation in the S phase and more responsive in M and late G2.

Reoxygenation of the tumour

Many tumours have a poor blood supply and have areas of hypoxia, which are relatively resistant to radiotherapy. The oxygen levels in the tissues depend on several factors, such as blood supply to the tissue and whether the person is anaemic. Studies have found that there is a correlation between poor response to radiotherapy and anaemia; therefore, it is important to check the full blood count prior to radiotherapy, especially if bleeding has been experienced. Normal tissues have a delicate network of capillaries that supply oxygen to the area; however, tumours often outgrow their blood supply and are poorly diffused. The lack of oxygen to the tissues affects the indirect radiation damage. Increasing the treatment time using a fractionated schedule allows hypoxic cells to reoxygenate themselves, so that areas of previously hypoxic cells become more responsive to treatment (Fig. 13.8). New developments, such as drugs that augment radiotherapy, have been used to reduce hypoxia and sensitize cells to radiotherapy effects.[19] An example of this is in the treatment of locally advanced head and neck cancer, where a synergy has been demonstrated between low-dose fractionated radiotherapy and chemopotentiator drugs (paclitaxel and carboplatin) in experimental studies. However, the longer-term impact of chemoradiation on survival and toxicity has not yet been identified.[20]

HOW LONG IS A COURSE OF RADIOTHERAPY?

Many people who are told they need to receive radiotherapy are surprised at the length of time that a course of treatment takes. Often they compare notes with others who have also received treatment and realize that the regimens are very different across different treatment centres and between different clinical oncologists. Some people interpret a short course as not so good or a long course of treatment as meaning that their cancer is worse than they had been led to believe. For example, regimens for the treatment of bone metastasis include a 10 Gy single fraction, 20 Gy in five fractions over 1 week and 20 Gy in 10 fractions over 2 weeks. It might appear that the shortest regimen delivers only one-third of the treatment of the longest one. However, the effect of radiotherapy is dependent not just on the total dose but also on the time over which it is given.[3] Often, the effects are similar and the radiotherapy regimen chosen may be based on local resource issues. For the palliative treatment of bone metastasis many treatment centres have adopted the shorter regimen, to deliver radiotherapy more effec-

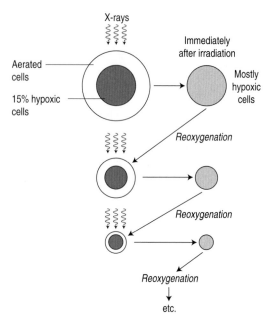

Figure 13.8: Oxygenation and its effects. Cancers contain a mixture of aerated and hypoxic cells. Radiation kills a greater proportion of aerated than hypoxic cells because they are more radiosensitive. Immediately after irradiation there are more hypoxic cells, but this rapidly changes as the previously hypoxic cells reoxygenate. (Reproduced with permission from Hall 2000; see Faithfull S, Wells M, eds. Supportive care in radiotherapy. Edinburgh: Churchill Livingstone; 2003:83.).

tively and reduce the time the patient has to be in hospital. Radical treatments also vary considerably and it can be quite confusing for patients to understand that radiation treatment may be given in different ways. There is huge variety across Europe in both the dose delivered per fraction and the nature of fractionation schedules.[14]

WHAT HAPPENS BEFORE TREATMENT CAN BEGIN?

It is only natural that once individuals have been diagnosed with cancer, they want treatment to start straight away. However, with radiotherapy there are several stages to treatment, and the planning stage can take several weeks. Most radiotherapy is delivered via a rectangular field, shaped by thick collimators on the machine head, which, once set, determine the size of each field being given. To define exactly where the treatment should be given, it is important to determine accurately the shape and extent of the tumour. The volume of the tissue to be treated is determined by findings from diagnostic computed tomography (CT) or magnetic resonance imaging (MRI) and knowledge of the usual patterns of spread of the cancer. The reproducibility of daily treatment is an important factor in delivering accurate radiotherapy. Most radiotherapy is planned in two dimensions, but more sophisticated computer programs are used for shaping complex field arrangements for three-dimensional planned treatment. This type of planning requires reconstruction of tumour and target volumes from CT or MRI images, so that the treatment volume can be localized and defined accurately for deep internal structures (Fig. 13.9). During these procedures, localization of the target volume is achieved with reference to the patient's contours as well as indelible skin markers such as tattoos or ink. Structures that may be at risk from toxicity of treatment can also be identified and the field sizes and beam arrangements modified if appropriate. When sensitive tissues are adjacent to the treatment fields, fixation devices such as moulds or plastic casts are used to keep the patient as still as possible. The radiotherapy dose prescription and fractionation regimen is then defined, detailing the dose to be delivered to target volume from each beam during radiotherapy. The standard dose that the patient receives is defined at the isocentre, the point where the beams intersect. Once this plan of therapy has been devised, the patient is simulated to verify the size, shape and placing of the proposed beams.

Some people interpret delays in starting treatment as a sign that their cancer is not as serious or that they have been forgotten in the system. Of course this is not true, but people make assumptions based on common sense and the lack of activity or lack of knowledge about the planning process can heighten anxiety.[21] Although radiotherapy is given daily, there are different stages of treatment, each producing differing anxieties and fears. This process of undergoing radiotherapy is very much a treatment trajectory (Box 13.1).

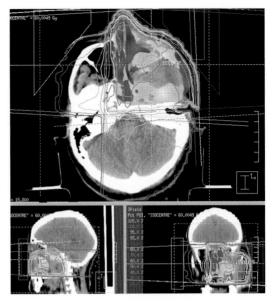

Figure 13.9: CT/MRI planning. Accurate localization and staging of the tumour using CT or MRI scanning is crucial to accurately plan modern radiotherapy. By identifying structures that are more sensitive to radiotherapy, it is possible to plan dose and volume of radiation treating the tumour but avoiding potential damage and late effects.

The prospect of radiotherapy adds considerable anxiety to fears, which already exist as a result of the diagnosis of cancer, changes in body image, physical effects of treatment or worries about travelling to the treatment centre. Many patients fear and misunderstand the use of radiation treatment and have negative attitudes to its effectiveness in cancer treatment.[22–24] A study of women with breast cancer who were faced with making a decision between mastectomy or lumpectomy with radiotherapy found that patients were concerned about the efficacy of radiation and its side effects and this significantly influenced their decisions.[25] Koller et al's study[26] also found that inpatients asked about their perceptions of palliative radiotherapy after they had completed treatment had misconceptions as to the purpose of their treatment. Radiotherapy can, however, be extremely effective – in early cancers of the larynx the cure rate is over 90% and in palliative situations radiotherapy can significantly reduce or eliminate pain from bone metastases.[27]

For a large proportion of patients, radiotherapy is not an isolated event. Many people have

Box 13.1

Planning

Planning can make many patients feel anxious, especially if they require a mould or beam directional shell (BDS) made before treatment of a head and neck cancer. The making of the BDS usually occurs in two stages. First, an impression is made where the patient's face and neck are partially covered in plaster of Paris. Impressions of the plaster cast are made to make a Perspex shell that is individually moulded. At simulation, this Perspex shell is fitted over the patient's face and secured to stop movement during treatment. Patients often dislike the feeling of being pinned down during planning and treatment. John Diamond, a journalist who had radiotherapy for tongue cancer, described this experience as the worse element of receiving his treatment. He says: ' Had you told me that I would spend 15 minutes a day thus constrained I'd have told you about my small claustrophobia problem and tried not to vomit in your lap at the thought. But even claustrophobia becomes routine.' (Diamond J. Because cowards get cancer too. London: Vermillion; 1998:106.)

already undergone neoadjuvant chemotherapy and surgery, and feel that radiation treatment is the final insult. They may still be suffering from side effects of other treatments, and therefore it is important that the entirety of that experience is recognized. Costain Schou and Hewison[28] found that some patients receiving adjuvant radiotherapy were told that their 4–5-week course of radiotherapy was just a precaution. Although this could be seen as reassuring, the authors point out that it may also underestimate the impact radiotherapy can have and may make it more difficult for patients to express their anxieties and concerns.

WHAT INFORMATION IS NEEDED TO PREPARE PATIENTS FOR RADIOTHERAPY?

Misapprehensions about radiotherapy may be due to the lack of information prior to the planning session. One of the problems at this stage of treatment is that other physicians refer patients for radiotherapy and so there are often assumptions made about how much people know. Vague explanations are more frightening than information aimed at answering the practicalities of: 'What can I expect?'.[29] McNamara,[30] in a postal questionnaire of a patients a week before they started radiotherapy, found that although 80% had been given information about their treatment, there were discrepancies in the degree of information and support provided. Nearly a third indicated they would have liked more support at home and the level of information provided depended on their age and diagnosis. Patients who were younger had more information than those who were older. Women with breast cancer were also more likely to have seen a nurse than other patient groups. Although it is now recognized that providing patient information can affect perceptions of radiotherapy side effects[31] and reduce anxiety,[32] clearly, radiotherapy information provision requires more effort. Because radiation cannot be seen, providing sensory information about the environment in which radiotherapy takes place can reduce anxiety.[33] Video or photographs of the radiotherapy centre and machines as well as information as to the sounds that might be heard during the course of treatment can help reduce patient's initial anxiety. Alternatively, providing an orientation to the radiotherapy machines and an initial interview prior to radiotherapy can also be helpful.[34]

THE TREATMENT PROCESS

A course of radiotherapy may last for several weeks, during which time daily visits to the hospital become part of a patient's routine (Box 13.2). Once radiotherapy has started, many patients do feel less anxious about treatment. The daily routine and practicalities of travel to the hospital can, however, be an additional burden for those who may be feeling unwell or frail due to their disease. The experience of radiotherapy is emotionally and physically demanding and levels of distress or anxiety may change over the treatment trajectory. Wells,[35] in a study of head and neck patients, found that the treatment environment can inhibit patients from revealing their concerns and that the perception that staff are busy or preoccupied can prevent patients from asking for help when they need it. She quotes a patient as saying:

> The people you get having radiotherapy would all be people who are trying to make the best of the situation … you want to be positive … you want to feel fine so you play down how you really feel … anyway everybody knows that when you have radiotherapy you don't feel well.

Wells's study uncovered a number of other factors that appeared to affect the degree to which patients admitted how they really felt. She identified that patients had difficulty in legitimizing the side effects of treatment, in comparison to the diagnosis of cancer. Patients described the insidious onset of symptoms and the tendency to compare themselves with other patients who seemed 'worse' and therefore had more to complain about. Wells concluded that these perceptions also played a part in deterring patients from reporting problems.

The completion of radiotherapy treatment can also be an extremely difficult time for patients. The transition from the daily certainty of receiving therapy to the unknown period of surveillance and follow-up creates its own anxieties. The support and reassurance of seeing fellow patients, radiographers and nurses on a day-to-day basis, is to some extent, withdrawn

at the end of treatment. Although some patients may be referred for community support, not all healthcare professionals in the community may be equipped with either the knowledge or the information they need to manage radiation side effects. Holland et al[36] found that as women neared the end of their treatment, they were more depressed and were less hopeful about their treatment. Ward et al,[25] in their study of women's reactions to completion of treatment, acknowledged that the end of treatment was not always one of relief. Out of the 38 women interviewed, a third found termination of treatment upsetting, and this was frequently connected to a worsening of side effects rather than just a withdrawal of treatment. Women who were most anxious or depressed at the beginning of treatment were those who were most upset at treatment completion. Graydon,[37] and work by Anderson and Tewfik,[38] identifies that emotional distress at the, beginning of treatment is predictive of post-treatment functioning. It is important that healthcare professionals do not make the erroneous assumption that the end of treatment will always come as a relief (Box 13.3).

Understanding the whole cancer experience is essential if nurses are to provide seamless supportive care during radiotherapy. Hinds and Moyer[39] described the experiences of 12 patients and 5 family caregivers to ascertain their support needs during radiotherapy. They identified that patients found family and

---

Box 13.2

Travelling

Travelling to and from the radiotherapy department each day can be difficult, and it is important to remember that many patients are newly diagnosed and may be struggling with the impact of their diagnosis as well as having to deal with the treatment itself. One man having radiotherapy for prostate cancer described the fatigue he felt travelling each day for treatment: 'Prior to the radiotherapy I was just exhausted. I think it was mental exhaustion. I didn't really have any energy for anything … while the radiotherapy was on I was probably a bit more tired and also travelling up and down every day 5 days for 7 weeks. It was suggested that a reason why I shouldn't do radiotherapy because of all that hassle of having to come every day and that was never a factor as far as I was concerned although I did meet some people when I was talking to other patients in the waiting room some of them had endless journeys'.[81]

Box 13.3

End of treatment

Finishing treatment can be quite an anticlimax after the day-to-day focus of getting through the radiotherapy and coping with side effects. The completion of therapy is often a time of transition where patients moving from a stage of action to one of waiting. One man with bladder cancer described his fears: 'The chances are that the radiotherapy will have blasted it sufficiently for them to say it's gone. Well the thing that I'm worrying about is they are going to say it hasn't worked and you've now got to have the operation but I'm hoping that's not going to be the case … . I try not to think about it basically, I mean here I am with things going on, I try to push it to the back of my mind'.[81]

friends to be their main sources of support and that supportive behaviours consisted of those of 'being there', 'giving help' and 'giving information and advice'. It was the way in which support was provided that was important. Clearly, patients need different types of support at different times during radiotherapy treatment and it is often the continuity of contact and support that patients most value.[40]

WHAT SIDE EFFECTS DOES RADIOTHERAPY CAUSE?

Side effects from radiotherapy vary, but are mainly localized to the area being treated. Obviously, certain symptoms that occur during or after treatment may be a result of the disease process, rather than the radiotherapy. Identification of the treatment area and underlying tissues is important, and careful assessment is required to identify patient needs and establish causal factors for symptoms. Adverse effects of treatment can be very debilitating and can have a substantial impact on quality of life.

Acute effects are those that occur during and immediately after radiotherapy and as a result of damage to functional cells that are lost as part of the normal tissue turnover but are not replaced because of damage to the stem cells.[41] In tissues such as the skin and gut, there is often a compensatory growth mechanism within the stem cells, and subsequent cell replacement means that symptoms often diminish near the end of treatment. Late effects can develop many months to years after treatment. Late effects tend to occur in tissues with a slow cell turnover such as the subcutaneous, muscle and fatty tissues. Changes include those of fibrosis, necrosis, atrophy and vascular damage.[41] Late effects develop through a complex process related to the immune response to radiation damage. Some of the changes are linked to cytokines that are normally released as part of an inflammatory process caused by tissue damage. In radiotherapy, the continuing damage to cells leads to an adaptive response in surrounding tissue, which can produce late effects. Damage to the vasculature enables cytokines to be released into the tissues, which promotes collagen deposition. This is rather similar to wound healing, where waves of cytokines are produced to promote healing.

Radiotherapy can also exacerbate symptoms already existing as a result of the cancer or chemotherapy. Symptoms such as urinary frequency or breathlessness can get worse as treatment progresses due to oedema and initial repopulation of the tumour. Increased late effects are being observed because of the introduction of new aggressive adjuvant therapies and the interaction between these treatment modalities. Tissues particularly susceptible are the urinary tract, intestinal mucosa and skin.

In many respects, the simple classification of acute or late effects under-represents the complexity of the normal tissue response to radiation injury (Fig. 13.10). Increased knowledge of the molecular mechanisms of radiation injury and radiobiology has provided greater understanding of the interaction between these early and late effects. In some patients acute reactions fail to heal completely and effects persist into late side effects. Distinguishing different mechanisms between these two reactions is difficult when damage is ongoing.[42] Understanding potential side effects is, therefore, important for nurses not only in terms of monitoring and assessing needs but also in supporting patients through symptom management.

WHAT ARE THE COMMON PROBLEMS EXPERIENCED AS A RESULT OF RADIOTHERAPY?

As already explained, symptoms caused by radiotherapy are usually related to the area which is being treated. There are, however, a number of generalized effects, which are not related to a particular area but are extremely common. Many patients complain, for instance, of extreme fatigue during and after radiotherapy treatment and the incidence of this symptom has been reported to be as high as 75%.[43] The aetiology of fatigue is uncertain, but the pattern of occurrence is that it is cumulative and increases over the course of treatment. Travelling to the radiation centre, other

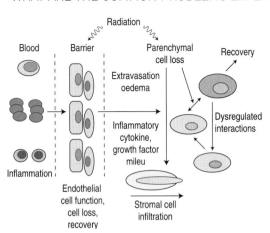

Figure 13.10: Radiation damage to normal tissues and late effects.

symptoms that disturb sleep, such as nocturia or diarrhoea, can exacerbate fatigue and it is often difficult to determine the real cause of the problem. The management of fatigue is often limited during radiotherapy, with an undue focus on anaemia-related problems rather than on providing wider strategies for support,[44] as described in Chapter 30. Radiation side effects vary from site to site and a comprehensive discussion is beyond the scope of this chapter. For each area chosen for discussion – the chest (lung and breast cancers), head and neck and pelvis (prostate and cervical cancers) – a description of associated symptoms and their management is briefly explored.

Radiation to the *chest* may include treatment of the lung, oesophagus or breast, all of which can cover areas of lung tissue, which are very radiosensitive. Clinical oncologists try to avoid irradiating areas of lung as part of a treatment field. Little research addresses the immediate side effects of radiotherapy to the chest, but such treatment can exacerbate existing breathing problems or cause chest pain.[45] Early effects can become apparent during and up to 3 months after radiotherapy. Devereux et al,[46] in a large survey of patients following palliative lung radiotherapy, found that 58.5% of patients reported symptoms within the first 24 hours of radiotherapy. These were most commonly chest pain (46%) and fever (36%). Patients reported that these symptoms were short-lived. However, other patient groups – e.g. those who have received irradiation prior to bone marrow transplantation – are especially at risk of radiation pneumonitis, a very dangerous and debilitating consequence of treatment.[47] Risk factors for its occurrence include poor performance status, co-morbid lung disease, poor pulmonary function and smoking. Treatment factors such as prior chemotherapy and chemoradiotherapy have also been indicated as potential risk factors.[48]

Current treatment approaches for radiation pneumonitis rely heavily on the administration of corticosteroids and antibiotics and of oxygen.[49] Wider non-pharmacological approaches can also be of benefit to patients experiencing these symptoms (see Chs 30 and 33). Cardiac complications as a result of radiotherapy can be a serious complication of chest irradiation; shielding and conformal treatment are the main strategies for prevention. If damage does occur, the symptoms of chest and pleuritic pain, dizziness, fatigue and breathlessness can be very distressing. Pericarditis has been reported in up to 30% of patients with Hodgkin's disease in those that had received a mean cardiac dose of 46 Gy and in only 2.5% of patients that had received a smaller dose. Treatment is aimed at reducing symptoms with aspirin or non-steroidal anti-inflammatory drugs (NSAIDs).[50]

Radiation to the *head and neck* can cause a whole range of problems to skin, salivary glands, mucosa and bone. Skin changes develop from the first few days of radiotherapy and are described by patients as a feeling of heat and soreness, known as erythema, or dry and moist desquamation, as skin layers diminish. These changes occur when the basal cell layers of the epidermis fail to proliferate and the normal replacement of functional cells is lost.[51,52] Mild skin reactions are common to all sites of radiation therapy (80–90% erythema); however, more serious problems such as moist desquamation are less common (10–15%). However, from clinical experience, patients with head and neck cancer may experience more skin problems than other groups, possibly because of the skin folds, moisture and visibility of any skin reactions. Although skin reactions are relatively short-lived, they can be painful, itchy and are sometimes dose-limiting.[53] A number of risk factors have been found to affect the severity, onset and duration of skin reactions. Intrinsic factors such as general skin condition, nutrition, smoking and general health play a part,[54,55] and extrinsic factors include dose energy and fractionation regimen. The increasing use of chemoradiotherapy also affects the severity of skin reactions. A radiation recall phenomenon can occur several months after radiotherapy, where the radiation field turns red and can become itchy during chemotherapy.[56]

There is often a great deal of controversy and lack of consistency on best practice approaches for managing radiation skin reactions.[57] There are relatively few published guidelines or protocols; however, this is partly because the evidence base is limited.[58,59] Those guidelines that have been published advocate gentle washing, garments that reduce friction, use of simple moisturizers such as aqueous cream, avoidance of perfumed products and protecting the skin from wind and extreme weather. For broken skin, moist wound healing principles have been advocated through recourse to hydrocolloids, hydrogels and alginates. Non-adherent dressings and tulles can stick and cause pain and trauma when dressings are removed before radiotherapy, so some of the new atraumatic wound dressings may be useful. Research also highlights the importance of intrinsic factors such as smoking and body mass index (BMI) in any analysis of radiation skin reactions.[54,55]

Mucositis is a frequent symptom of head and neck radiotherapy, with the incidence of this side effect being as high as 60% with standard radiotherapy and more than 90% in patients receiving chemoradiotherapy.[60] Patients often describe a dry mouth, eating difficulties related to swallowing or taste changes and pain.[61,62] The aetiology of mucositis is similar to skin changes, where there is a lack of replacement cells from the proliferating tissues. The damage becomes progressively worse over the course of treatment and may take several weeks to heal after completion of treatment.[63] If the salivary glands, specifically the parotid glands, are irradiated, dry mouth can be a particular problem. Damage occurs primarily in the parenchyma of the salivary gland rather than in the ducts, but inflammation, vascular changes and oedema can still result in functional loss. Swelling of the glands and tenderness can occur with the first few radiotherapy treatments – saliva is reduced, becomes sticky and viscous. It makes eating, speech and wearing dentures difficult and contributes to the pain of mucositis. Recovery of the salivary glands, if it occurs at all, may take months to years, and late effects such as mucosal fibrosis, atrophy, dental carries, osteoradionecrosis and taste dysfunction cause long-term disability.[64] The combination of side effects can have a tremendous impact on basic activities of life, including eating, drinking, speaking, breathing, communicating and kissing.[65] It is important that careful assessment prior to radiotherapy is undertaken with inclusion of the multidisciplinary team to address potential problems such as nutrition and dental hygiene prior to the start of radiotherapy.[66] Management of mucositis, pain and nutrition can be found in Chapters 21, 26 and 29.

Radiation to any site within the pelvis can cause damage to many adjacent structures. Although some such damage is intentional in order to treat the cancer, it also occurs unintentionally when treating prostate, rectal and gynaecological cancers. Because pelvic tumours commonly sit close to or invade surrounding organs, incidental irradiation of bladder tissues is often inevitable. *Urinary symptoms*, such as pain or burning on micturition, increased frequency and urgency of passing urine, incontinence or leakage and nocturia, are a common complaint following pelvic irradiation. The reported incidence of such symptoms varies widely, from 23% to 80%.[67,68] This wide variance partly reflects the different time–dose–volume factors inherent in different treatment regimens, but also the hidden and embarrassing nature of such symptoms and possible under-reporting.[69] These symptoms can continue for many weeks to months, and the resulting effects are uncomfortable and can influence quality of life. There is little consensus around the management of radiation-induced urinary problems. Clear assessment of the nature of symptoms and whether they were a problem before treatment can help in providing a management strategy that incorporates both pharmacological and behavioural interventions.

Gastrointestinal effects such as nausea, diarrhoea and proctitis can occur as a result of a range of radiotherapy treatments, especially where the abdomen is included in the radiation field. The incidence of acute gastrointestinal symptoms is high, particularly in patients receiving total body irradiation (89–100%)[70] or upper abdominal irradiation (50–80%),[71,72] with studies of general treatment groups suggesting that as many as 40% of patients experience some nausea and vomiting with radiotherapy treatment.[73,74] In pelvic treatments, the incidence is lower, with 56% of men following prostate irradiation[75] and 86% of women receiving pelvic radiotherapy complaining of symptoms. Such symptoms can cause fatigue, distress, be socially isolating and can influence nutrition and sexuality.[76] Poor assessment of these symptoms has, in the past, led to an underestimation of the extent of bowel toxicity. Patient self-report data suggest that 13% of men continue to have diarrhoea several times a day, up to 3 months after completing radiotherapy for prostate cancer.[77] Chronic radiation enteritis has also been described in women up to 1 year after completion of pelvic radiotherapy.[78] Treatments for nausea as a result of radiotherapy are described in Chapter 20. Treatments for rectal complications include oral anti-inflammatory agents, pain management, intrarectal steroids and dilation of strictures. The dietary management of acute and chronic symptoms is controversial, as the evidence base for best-practice approaches has not been tested.[79]

Sexuality and fertility problems frequently affect men and women following pelvic radiotherapy. As survival prospects increase for patients who have undergone treatment, the risk of infertility and the impact of tissue damage on sexual function can have implications on an individual's rehabilitation and quality of life. Depending on the field of radiotherapy, damage can occur in several areas of the reproductive system. It is advised that patients should not try to have children within 12–18 months of any radiation to the gonads, as genetic damage may still be present. Ovarian effects can result in early menopause for women, and these effects may be associated with feelings of reduced femininity and sexuality. Where a woman has had a therapeutic dose of radiation to the uterus and vagina, there may be detrimental effects such as reduced uterine volume, decreased elasticity, impaired endometrial blood flow, reduced vaginal lubrication and strictures and fibrosis.[80] Further information on how to assess and manage problems as a result of radiotherapy damage to the sexual organs is described in Chapter 31.

CONCLUSION

Radiotherapy is one of the oldest and most established cancer treatments and is relatively cheap compared to other treatment modalities. Many exciting developments, new technologies and scientific achievements are currently influencing the use of radiotherapy in the management of cancer. Radiotherapy today is increasingly sophisticated, as technical advances such as intensity modulated radiotherapy (IMRT) improve the accuracy and delivery of treatment. However, in many countries these new techniques are unavailable: some 22 countries in Africa and Asia do not have any radiotherapy machines. On average, the developed world has just one radiotherapy machine per several million people compared with one machine per 250,000 in many developed countries. The problems of treatment delivery are compounded by a lack of trained staff, a problem not just reserved for the developing countries.

The delivery of radiotherapy has also gone through major change, with transformations in working practice, multidisciplinary team working and service configurations. Many health services have suffered from a lack of strategic planning, failing to take into account increases in cancer incidence and the increasingly ageing population. In many European countries, e.g Sweden, specially trained nurses rather than radiographers deliver radiotherapy. It is also important for those nurses not involved in the direct delivery of radiotherapy to have an awareness of how radiotherapy works and the potential problems patients may experience. In many countries, such as the UK and Ireland, nurses are not involved in the delivery of treatment, as therapeutic radiographers are wholly responsible for providing both the treatment and ongoing care and support of patients. Radiotherapy effects can, however, be long lasting, and supportive care must take into account not only the radiotherapy but also the combined effects of cancer treatment modalities. The growing delivery of chemoradiation and combination therapies requires a wide knowledge of treatment effects and how to manage subsequent adverse effects; thus, nurses are in a unique position to provide supportive care. The success of such care requires effective working practices, in particular multidisciplinary working, in order to manage the complex issues that can result from combined therapies and increasingly complex radiation treatments.

REFERENCES

1. Burnet N, Benson R, Williams M. Improving cancer outcomes through radiotherapy. BMJ 2000; 320:198–199.

2. Hammick M, Tutt A, Tait D. Knowledge and perception regarding radiotherapy and radiation in patients receiving radiotherapy: a qualitative study. Eur J Cancer Care 1998; 7(2):103–112.

3. Adamson D. The radiobiological basis of radiation side effects. In: Faithfull S, Wells M, eds. Supportive care in radiotherapy. Edinburgh: Churchill Livingstone; 2003.

4. Hall E. Time, dose and fractionation in radiotherapy. In: Hall E, ed. Radiobiology for the radiologist. 3 edn. Philadelphia: Lippincott; 1988; 239–259.

5. Dodd J, Barrett A, Ash D. Practical radiotherapy planning. 2nd edn. London: Edward Arnold; 1992.

6. Fieler V. Side effects and quality of life in patients receiving high-dose rate brachytherapy. Oncol Nurs Forum 1997; 24(3):545–553.

7. Ahmad A, Jingram A. New radiation techniques in gynecological cancer. Int J Gynecol Cancer 2004; 14:569-579

8. Powell S, McMillan T. DNA damage and repair following treatment with ionizing radiation. Radiother Oncol 1990; 19:95–108.

9. Withers R. Biological basis of radiation therapy for cancer. Lancet 1992; 339:156–159.

10. Hopewell J, Calvo W, Reinhold H. Radiation effects on blood vessels: role in late normal tissue damage. In: Steel C, Adams G, Horwich A, eds. The biological basis of radiotherapy. 2 edn. Amsterdam: Elsevier; 1989:101–112.

11. Hill R, Rodemann H, Hendry J, Roberts S, Anscher M. Normal tissue radiobiology: from the laboratory to the clinic. Int J Radiat Oncol Biol Phys 2001; 49(2):353–365.

12. McMillan T. The molecular basis of radiosensitivity. In: Steel C, Adams G, Horwich A, eds. The biological basis of radiotherapy. 2 edn. Amsterdam: Elsevier; 1989:29–44.

13. Burnet N, Nyman J, Turesson I. Prediction of normal-tissue tolerance to radiotherapy from in-vitro cellular radiation sensitivity. Lancet 1992; 399:1570–1571.

14. Munro A. Challenges to radiotherapy today. In: Faithfull S, Wells M, eds. Supportive care in radiotherapy. Edinburgh: Churchill Livingstone; 2003.

15. Dische S. Clinical radiobiology. In: Price P, Sikora K, eds. Treatment of cancer. 3rd edn. London: Chapman and Hall; 1995.

16. Trott K, Kummermehr J. What is known about tumour proliferation rates to choose between accelerated fractionation or hyperfractionation? Radiother Oncol 1985; 3:1–9.

17. Saunders M, Dische S. Continuous hyperfractionated accelerated radiotherapy (CHART) in non small cell carcinoma of the bronchus. Int J Radiat Oncol Biol Phys 1990; 19:1211–1215.

18. Price P, Hoskin P, Easton D, et al. Prospective randomized trial of single and multi-fraction schedules in the treatment of painful bone metastasis. Radiother Oncol 1986; 6:247–255.

19. Denny W. The role of hypoxia activated prodrugs in cancer therapy. Lancet Oncol 2000; 1(1):25–29.

20. Arnold S, Regine W, Ahmed M, et al. Low dose fractionated radiation as a chempotentiator of neoadjuvant paclitaxel and carboplatin for locally advanced squamous cell carcinoma of the head and neck: results of a new treatment paradigm. Int J Radiat Oncol Biol Phys 2004; 58(5):1411–1417.

21. Nicolaou N. Radiation therapy treatment planning and delivery. Semin Oncol Nurs 1999; 15(4):260–269.

22. Eardley A. Expectations of recovery. Nurs Times 1986(April 23):53–54.

23. Forester BM, Kornfield D, Fleiss J. Psychiatric aspects of radiotherapy. Am J Psychiatry 1985; 142:22–27.

24. Peck A, Boland J. Emotional reactions to radiation treatment. Cancer 1977; 40:180–184.

25. Ward S, Goldberg N, McCauley V, et al. Patient-related barriers to management of cancer pain. Pain 1993; 52:319–24.

26. Koller M, Lorenz W, Wagner K, et al. Expectations and quality of life of cancer patients undergoing radiotherapy. J R Soc Med 2000; 93:621–628.

27. Symonds R. Recent advances in radiotherapy. BMJ 2001; 323:1107–1110.

28. Costain Schou K, Hewison J. Experiencing cancer. Buckingham: Open University Press; 1999.

29. Kagan A, Levitt P, Arnold T, Hattem J. Honesty is the best policy: a radiation therapist's perspective on caring for terminal cancer patients. Clin Oncol 1984; 7:381–383.

30. McNamara S. Information and support: a descriptive study of the needs of patients with cancer before their first experience of radiotherapy. Eur J Oncol Nurs 1999; 3(1):31–37.

31. Kim Y, Roscoe J, Morrow G. The effects of information and negative affect on severity of side effects from radiation therapy for prostate cancer. Support Care Cancer 2002; 10(5):416–421.

32. Porock D. The effect of preparatory patient education on the anxiety and satisfaction of cancer patients receiving radiotherapy. Cancer Nurs 1995; 18(3):206–214.

33. Frith B. Giving information to radiotherapy patients. Nurs Stand 1991; 5(34):33–35.

34. Holland J, Tross S. Psychological sequelae in cancer survivors. In: Holland J, Rowland J, eds. Handbook of psychooncology. Oxford: Oxford University Press; 1989.

35. Wells M. The impact of radiotherapy to the head and neck: a qualitative study of patients after completion of treatment [MSc Cancer Care]. London: Institute of Cancer Research; 1995.

36. Holland J, Rowland A, Lebovitz A, Rusalem R. Reactions to cancer treatment: assessment of emotional response to adjuvant radiotherapy as a guide to planned intervention. Psychiatr Clin N Am 1979; 2:347–358.

37. Graydon J. Factors that predict patients' functioning following treatment for cancer. Int J Nurs Stud 1988; 25(2):117–124.

38. Anderson B, Tewfik H. Psychological reactions to radiation therapy: reconsideration of the adaptive aspects of anxiety. J Personality Soc Psychol 1985; 48(4):1024–1032.

39. Hinds C, Moyer A. Support as experienced by patients with cancer during radiotherapy treatments. J Adv Nurs 1997; 26:371–379.

40. Faithfull S, Corner J, Myer L, Huddart R, Dearnaley D. Evaluation of nurse-led care for men undergoing pelvic radiotherapy. Br J Cancer 2001; 18(12):1853–1864.

41. Stone H, Coleman C, Ansher M, McBride W. Effects of radiation on normal tissue: consequences and mechanisms. Lancet Oncol 2003; 4:529–536.

42. Denham J, Hauer-Jensen M, Peters L. Is it time for a new formalism to categorize normal tissue radiation injury? Int J Radiat Oncol Biol Phys 2001; 50(5):1105–1106.

43. Vogelzang N, Breitbart W, Cella D, et al. Patient, caregiver, and oncologist perceptions of cancer-related fatigue: results of a tripart assessment survey. Semin Haematol 1997; 34(3(suppl 2)):4–12.

44. Faithfull S. Fatigue and radiotherapy. In: Faithful S, Wells M, eds. Supportive care in radiotherapy. Edinburgh: Churchill Livingstone; 2003.

45. Wells M. Pain and breathing problems. In: Faithfull S, Wells M, eds. Supportive care in radiotherapy. Edinburgh: Churchill Livingstone; 2003.

46. Devereux S, Hatton M, Macbeth F. Immediate side effects of large fraction radiotherapy. Clin Oncol (Royal College of Radiologists) 1997; 9:96–99.

47. McBride W, Vegesna V. The role of T cells in radiation pneumonitis after bone marrow transplantation. Int J Radiat Oncol Biol Phys 2000; 47:277–290.

48. Molls M, Herrmann T, Steinberg F, Feldmann H. Radiopathology of the lung: experimental and clinical observations. In: Hinkedbein W, Bruggmoser G, Rommhold H, Wannenmacher W, eds. Recent results in cancer research. Vol. 130. Berlin: Springer-Verlag; 1993.

49. Inoue A, Kunitoh H, Sekine I, et al. Radiation pneumonitis in lung cancer patients: a retrospective study of risk factors and the long-term prognosis. Int J Radiat Oncol Biol Phys 2001; 49(3):649–655.

50. Khoo V. Other late effects. In: Faithfull S, Wells M, eds. Supportive care in radiotherapy. Edinburgh: Churchill Livingstone; 2003.

51. Hopewell J. The skin its structure and response to ionizing radiation. Int J Radiat Biol 1990; 57(4):751–773.

52. Archambeau J, Pezner R, Wasserman T. Pathophysiology of irradiated skin and breast. Int J Radiat Oncol Biol Phys 1995; 31: 1171–1185.

53. Campbell I, Illingworth M. Can patients wash during radiotherapy to the breast or chest wall? A randomized controlled trial. Clin Oncol 1992; 4:78–82.

54. Porock D, Kristjanson L. Skin reactions during radiotherapy for breast cancer: the use and impact of topical agents and dressings. Eur J Cancer Care 1999; 8:143–153.

55. Porock D, Nikoletti S, Cameron F. The relationship between factors that impair wound healing: severity of acute radiation skin mucosal toxicities in head and neck cancer. Cancer Nurs 2004; 27(1):71–78.

56. Sitton E. Early and late radiation induced skin alterations: Part 1 Mechanisms of skin changes. Oncology Nurs Forum 1992; 19(5):801–807.

57. Wells M, MacBride S. Radiation skin reactions. In: Faithfull S, Wells M, eds. Suportive care in radiation therapy. Edinburgh: Churchill Livingstone; 2003.

58. Glean E, Edwards S, Faithfull S. Intervention for acute radiotherapy induced skin reactions in cancer patients: the development of a clinical guideline recommended for use by the College

of Radiographers. J Radiother Pract 2001; 2:75–84.

59. Mallett J, Mullholland J, Laverty D. An integrated approach to wound management. Int J Palliat Care 1999; 5:124–132.

60. Sutherland S, Browman G. Prophylaxis of oral mucositis in irradiated head and neck cancer patients: a proposed classification scheme of interventions and meta-analysis of randomised controlled trials. Int J Radiat Oncol Biol Phys 2001; 49(4):917–930.

61. Epstein J, Emerton S, Kolbinson DA, et al. Quality of life and oral function following radiotherapy for head and neck cancer. Head Neck 1999; 21(1):1–11.

62. Bjordal K, Hammerlid E, Ahlner-Elmqvist M, et al. Quality of life in head and neck cancer patients: validation of the European Organization for Research and Treatment of Cancer Quality of Life Questionnaire-H&N35. J Clin Oncol 1999; 17(3):1008–1019.

63. Dorr W, Hamilton C, Boyd T, et al. Radiation-induced changes in cellularity and proliferation in human and oral mucosa. Int J Radiat Oncol Biol Phys 2002; 52:911–917.

64. Cooper J, Fu K, Marks J, Silverman S. Late effects of radiation therapy in the head and neck region. Int J Radiat Oncol Biol Phys 1995; 31:1141–1164.

65. Wells M. Oropharyngeal effects of radiotherapy. In: Faithfull S, Wells M, eds. Suuportive care in radiotherapy. Edinburgh: Churchill Livingstone; 2003.

66. Biron P, Sebban C, Gourmet R, et al. Research controversies in management of oral mucositis. Support Care Cancer 2000; 8:68–71.

67. Klee M, Thranov I, Machin D. The patients' perspective on physical symptoms after radiotherapy for cervical cancer. Gynaecol Oncol 2000; 76:14–23.

68. Marks L, Carroll P, Dugan T, Anscher M. The response of the urinary bladder, urethra, and ureter to radiation and chemotherapy. Int J Radiat Oncol Biol Phys 1995; 31(5):1257–1280.

69. Faithfull S. Urinary symptoms and radiotherapy. In: Faithfull S, Wells M, eds. Supportive care in radiotherapy. Edinburgh: Churchill Livingstone; 2003.

70. Buchali A, Feyer P, Groll J, et al. Immediate toxicity during fractionated total body irradiation as conditioning for bone marrow transplantation. Radiother Oncol 2000; 54:157–162.

71. Aass N, Fossa S, Host H. Acute and subacute side effects due to infra-diaphragmatic radiotherapy for testicular cancer: a prospective study. Int J Radiat Oncol Biol Phys 1992; 5:358–363.

72. Roberts J, Priestman T. A review of ondansetron in the management of radiotherapy-induced emesis. Oncology 1993; 50:173–179.

73. Feyer P, Stewart A, Titlbach O. Aetiology and prevention of emesis induced by radiotherapy. Support Care Cancer 1998; 6:253–260.

74. The Italian Group Farir. Radiation induced emesis: a prospective observational multicentre Italian trial. Care 1999; 44(3):619–625.

75. Yeoh E, Botten R, Russo A, et al. Chronic effects of therapeutic irradiation for localized prostatic carcinoma on anorectal function. Int J Radiat Oncol Biol Phys 2000; 47(4):915–924.

76. Klee M, Thranov I, Machin D. Life after radiotherapy: the psychological and social effects experienced by women treated for advanced stages of cervical cancer. Gynaecol Oncol 1999; 76(5–13).

77. Beard C, Propert K, Rieker P, et al. Complications after treatment with external beam irradiation in early stage prostate cancer patients: a prospective multiinstitutional outcomes study. J Clin Oncol 1997; 15(1):223–229.

78. Yeoh E, Lui D, Lee N. The mechanism of diarrhoea resulting from pelvic and abdominal radiotherapy; a prospective study using selenium-75 labelled conjugated bile acid and cobalt-58 labelled cyanocobalamin. Br J Radiol 1984; 57(684):1131–1136.

79. Faithfull S. Gastrointestinal effects of radiotherapy. In: Faithfull S, Wells M, eds. Supportive care in radiotherapy. Edinburgh: Churchill Livingstone; 2003.

80. White I, Faithfull S. Sexuality and fertility. In: Faithfull S, Wells M, eds. Supportive care in radiotherapy. Edinburgh: Churchill Livingstone; 2003.

81. Faithfull S. Supportive care in radiotherapy: evaluating the potential contribution of nursing. Ph D. London: London University; 2000.

CHAPTER 14

Chemotherapy

MELAINE COWARD AND HELEN M COLEY

CHAPTER CONTENTS

Introduction	283	Intra-arterial administration	291
		Oral chemotherapy	291
Goals of chemotherapy treatment	284		
		Assessment of patients receiving	
Pharmacology and mechanisms of		chemotherapy	291
chemotherapy action	284		
Mitosis and cell division	284	The nursing role within chemotherapy	292
Classification of cytotoxic drugs	285	Administration and safety	292
		Patient education and information	293
Assessing risk prior to chemotherapy	287	Side-effect management	293
Routes of chemotherapy		Ongoing support for chemotherapy	
administration	287	patients	297
Intravenous route	290		
Intramuscular and subcutaneous		Innovations in chemotherapy treatment	298
injection	290	New and forthcoming treatments	298
Intrathecal administration	290		
Intrapleural administration	291	Conclusion	300
Intravesical administration	291		
Intraperitoneal administration	291	References	300

INTRODUCTION

In the past 30 years there have been major improvements in the use of chemotherapy, and this has subsequently affected survival of cancer patients. With respect to the use of cytotoxic drugs, developments are largely due to the increasing use of clinical trials to produce reliable and relevant data.[1] This has resulted in more information about drug toxicity and incidence of adverse effects and also provided comparative data with which to make clinical decisions. Additionally, advances in techniques of delivery such as oral chemotherapy and portable infusion devices have changed the way that patients experience chemotherapy,

with future delivery increasingly moving to outpatient and home-care settings. There has also been the development of supportive agents, such as the colony-stimulating factors, which reduce chemotherapy side-effects and inpatient stays and can enhance patient's quality of life.

The primary aim of chemotherapy is to have a systemic effect on cancer cells and therefore prevent cell replication and halt cell division.[2] Consequently, healthy cells as well as malignant cells will be affected, meaning that the patient can anticipate certain side-effects of their treatment in areas of high cell division, such as bone marrow depression, gastrointestinal disturbance and alopecia.[3] These side-effects are usually reversible, depending on the drug type and total dose given as well as the client's existing health. Chemotherapy can be used in a number of ways and also in conjunction with other anticancer treatments.[4] It can be used prior to surgery to reduce the size of a tumour and therefore minimize the amount of surgical intervention required (neoadjuvant). It can also be used as an adjunct to surgery and radiotherapy, reducing the risk of microscopic disease and metastatic invasion. Finally, chemotherapy may be administered in the palliative care setting as a means of minimizing or alleviating the symptoms of advanced disease.

This chapter provides an overview and explores:

- the mechanisms and rationale for chemotherapy
- delivery techniques
- practice issues surrounding routes of administration.

Patient satisfaction with chemotherapy is very dependent on the environment of provision, technical aspects of care including side-effect management, communication and patient education as well as the nurse's interpersonal skills.[5] Many patients (15–20%) refuse or drop out during chemotherapy treatment, and this is often attributed to cancer patients' misperceptions of chemotherapy which are often contrary to the actual benefits patients might achieve.[6] Nurses, therefore, play an important part in how patients experience chemotherapy, whether they administer the drugs or provide ongoing support. Innovations within chemotherapy are occurring constantly, with clinical services reacting to such developments by implementing new chemotherapy nursing roles, clinical trials and new protocols.

GOALS OF CHEMOTHERAPY TREATMENT

The goals of chemotherapy are diverse and it can be used as a curative agent or for palliation. The aims of chemotherapy could be to achieve a cure, to control disease or to relieve symptoms of the cancer, such as pain or breathlessness. Its use within cancer treatment is increasingly being used as a combination therapy in conjunction with surgery, hormone therapy and radiotherapy. Adjuvant chemotherapy refers to the use of chemotherapy after removal of the primary cancer to eliminate microscopic remaining cells. Neoadjuvant chemotherapy refers to the use of chemotherapy to reduce in size the tumour before surgery or radiotherapy to preserve function or reduce potential toxicity. Chemotherapy is therefore a systemic treatment in that it treats the whole body to prevent cancer cells from multiplying, invading adjacent tissues or developing metastases.[7]

PHARMACOLOGY AND MECHANISMS OF CHEMOTHERAPY ACTION

The word cytotoxic describes the overall action of this group of drugs: 'cyto' meaning cell and 'toxic' meaning harmful. The end-point of treatment is to either increase the amount of cell loss that occurs or to decrease cell production, both of which have an effect on tumour size by interfering with the normal mechanisms of cell division. Chemotherapy has a direct action on the cell cycle and, therefore, reproductive activity.[8] but is therefore unable to select malignant cells from normal healthy cells.

Mitosis and cell division

Cells that are reproducing go through a five-stage process in order to produce daughter cells. Figure 14.1 shows these phases and the order in which they occur. Understanding the changes in cell growth is important to understanding the action and targets of chemotherapy agents. The majority of cells at a given time can be described as laying in a dormant state or resting phase. This means that they are not actively reproducing but they may, however, be conducting normal cellular functions, depending on their type and role within the body. Within the cell cycle, this rest time is demonstrated as stage G0, although some cells may be permanently in this state, as is the case of those within the central nervous system.[8] The amount of time that cells spend in the G0 phase is dependent upon their function and also the individual demand at that time.[8]

The first growth phase that occurs within cell division is represented on Figure 14.1 as G1. During this phase, synthesis of ribonucleic acid (RNA) and proteins occurs in preparation for deoxyribonucleic acid (DNA) synthesis.[9] This leads on to the synthesis (S) phase, where DNA is synthesized and also doubled in preparation for cell division.[10,11] The synthesis phase can last from 10 to 30 hours,[8,9] although it appears that normal cells spend less time synthesizing than malignant cells do.[8] The penultimate phase in cell division, shown as G2 on Figure 14.1, is described as either the second growth,[8] or premitotic phase.[9,10] During this time, a mitotic spindle forms within the cell in preparation for division while also undertaking further synthesis of RNA.[9,10] This phase lasts for 1–12 hours.[8,9]

The final and most productive phase of the cell cycle is also the shortest. The mitosis phase, when actual cell division will occur, can last from 30 minutes to 1 hour.[8] After mitosis, a new identical daughter cell will have been produced and will be able to fall into its own cell cycle to continue reproduction. Mitosis can be subdivided into four phases, which take place in order for division to succeed.

The first of these four phases is prophase. During this phase, the chromosomes become visible and split to form two chromatids and the nucleus and nuclear membrane completely disappear. This then leads into metaphase, when the chromatids arrange themselves along the centre of the cell. The chromatids carefully lay over the mitotic spindle, which runs from each of the poles of the cell. The chromatids then separate in anaphase and move to opposite sides of the cell. The final stage of mitosis is telophase, where the nuclear membrane starts to reform and the mitotic spindle disappears. The cell cytoplasm then starts to divide while forming a new plasma membrane to enclose two new identical daughter cells.

Classification of cytotoxic drugs

Cytotoxic drugs can be classified into groups depending on their specific cell action and also the phase of the cell cycle in which they are active (Table 14.1).[2] This first step in drug classification will signify whether drugs are said to be cell cycle phase specific or cell cycle phase non-specific. In simple terms, drugs which are cell cycle phase specific are known to be active in a particular area or areas of cell division, whereas drugs that are cell cycle phase non-specific are active at any point of the cell cycle including resting phase (G0). Therefore, drugs which are cell cycle phase non-specific are often considered more useful in having cellular effects, as they do not require division to be actively occurring to disrupt DNA synthesis.[8] Conversely, this means that the cell cycle phase non-specific drugs will also have a greater cell kill effect on normal cells such as those of the peripheral blood, causing greater toxicity and potential danger to the patient. The importance of drug activity is dependant upon tumour type. Histopathology provides information on the type of cancer and from this the clinician can make judgements as to where the most cellular activity is occurring in that particualr type of cancer. This allows for drugs to be selected that are known to have activity within the specific area of the cell cycle where cancer cell proliferation has its greatest activity.

Alkylating agents

Alkylating agents are a group of compounds which interact with intracellular DNA.[9] They interfere through cross-linking strands of DNA that are subsequently unable to separate, leading to inhibition or erroneous replication of

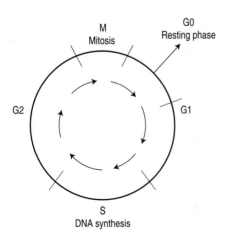

Figure 14.1: Cells that are reproducing go through a five-stage process.

285

Table 14.1: Classification of cytotoxic drugs

Drug group	Examples of drugs
Alkylating agents	Busulfan, carboplatin, cisplatin, cyclophosphamide, ifosfamide, melphalan, procarbazine
Antimetabolites	Cytarabine, 5-fluorouracil, hydroxycarbine (hydroxycarbamide), methotrexate
Cytotoxic antibiotics and anthracyclines	Bleomycin, daunorubicin, doxorubicin
Mitotic inhibitors	Docetaxel, paclitaxel, vinblastine, vincristine, vinorelbine
Topoisomerase inhibitors	VP16/etoposide, topotecan

the cell, which ultimately leads to mutation or cell death. As alkylating agents are active in this vital part of cell division, which includes the resting phase, they are commonly used to debulk rapidly growing tumours with good effect.[9] These drugs are commonly seen to cause nausea and vomiting when given intravenously. Also, due to their effects on rapidly dividing cells, they affect normal functioning of the gastrointestinal tract, haemopoietic ability and reproductive functioning.

Antimetabolites

Antimetabolites, which are structural analogues of intracellular metabolites required for cell function and replication, are used to disorder cellular metabolism.[9] They prevent synthesis of DNA and lead to cell death. As they are more active in the synthesis phase of the cell cycle, they are active against rapidly dividing tumours. Side-effects for this group are generally similar to those for alkylating agents.

Cytotoxic antibiotics and anthracyclines

Cytotoxic antibiotics and anthracyclines act by binding to DNA, preventing its synthesis and replication.[9] They are active in all phases of the cell cycle. This group of cytotoxic drugs have an effect on myelosuppression, and manifests as leucopenia and thrombocytopenia in particular. Bleomycin has unique side-effects in that it can cause pneumonitis, leading ultimately to pulmonary fibrosis. Some of the anthracycline antibiotics such as daunorubicin and doxorubicin may cause a dose-related cardiotoxicity.

Mitotic inhibitors

Mitotic inhibitors can be further categorized into Vinca alkaloids and taxanes. The Vinca or plant alkaloids are derived from natural plant sources, originally the pink periwinkle plant (*Vinca roseus*).[9] This group are able to stop mitosis by binding themselves to microtubular proteins, which are essential for formation of the mitotic spindle. All of these drugs are vesicants, and therefore the method of their administration needs to be considered. Patients receiving these drugs may experience neurotoxicity, and peripheral neuropathy is also common.[9] The taxanes are a newer category of cytotoxic drug within this classification. Taxanes are also plant derivatives, and come from the yew tree family. They bind to microtubules and inhibit cell proliferation.[9] Neutropenia is the most profound side-effect seen with this group of drugs.

Topoisomerase inhibitors

Topoisomerase inhibitors interact with Top2, an enzyme required for replication of DNA.[9] These drugs are also associated with a dose-dependent myelosuppression, which occurs in virtually all patients treated with them.[12]

Tumours that are actively growing are going through rapid cell division; consequently, they will be more receptive to the effects of cytotoxic drugs. The rate of growth of a tumour can be roughly calculated by considering the tumour doubling time; this is the amount of time a tumour takes to double its size.[12] Some cancers are known to be very fast growing, such as those that are testicular in origin: such tumours are thought to have a doubling time of 21 days.[12] Due to the rapid cell replication that occurs in such tumours, chemotherapy is able to have a greater effect, and therefore cell kill, which leads to a more favourable prognosis and probable cure for such patients.

ASSESSING RISK PRIOR TO CHEMOTHERAPY

Before commencing treatment with chemotherapy, it is important to consider the impact that the proposed treatment may have on an individual's physiological and emotional status. Consideration should also be given to the patient's lifestyle, support network, ability to cope with equipment and potential compliance. For example, it might be inappropriate to place a semipermanent central venous catheter in a patient who lives alone and is visually impaired. If the prescribed treatment may lead to side-effects, then the patient's ability to cope and report these side-effects would need to be assessed to ensure the patient's safety in relation to receiving a specific treatment.

Assessment of physiological status prior to chemotherapy, especially in patients from vulnerable groups such as the elderly or those with advanced cancer, is important in identifying the potential hazards of chemotherapy. The higher incidence of cancer in older people means that many patients undergoing chemotherapy are older and have physiological changes or co-morbid disease that may influence morbidity.[13] Ageing is an individualized process but, over time, the function of many organ systems declines, resulting in changes in the way the body reacts to chemotherapy. Elderly patients may have a slower gastrointestinal mobility, influencing oral drug absorption, mucosal integrity and muscle strength. These can have consequences on side-effect profiles as well as on fatigue levels. In addition, the elderly tend to have lower glomerular filtration rates, which result in reduced ability to remove cytotoxic drugs, resulting in greater nephrotoxicity. Age alone is not predictive of the effects of chemotherapy treatment – more the frailty of individuals and their respective body systems.[14,15] Ascertaining whether a person is fit for chemotherapy treatment often involves a wide range of investigations, including full blood count, renal function via ethylene diamine tetra-acetic acid (EDTA) test and other tests dependent on possible adverse effects caused by the potential drugs, such as lung function or cardiac function.

Departments should be responsible for developing policies to ensure suitability and safety of clients receiving treatments through rigorous assessment processes undertaken by experienced personnel (for further information see Ch. 10 on decision-making).

ROUTES OF CHEMOTHERAPY ADMINISTRATION

Cytotoxic chemotherapy can be administered by a variety of routes: intravenous, intramuscular, subcutaneous, topical, intrathecal, intravesical, intraperitoneal and intrapleural as well as by the oral route (Table 14.2). Like all drugs, the effective and safe administration of chemotherapy is dependent on a partnership between the various healthcare professionals concerned, i.e. doctor, pharmacist and nurse. The manner in which chemotherapy is delivered influences the extent to which it reaches its intended site of action and this can affect patient benefits and the nature and pattern of side-effects. For example, chemotherapy may also be instilled into one area of the body so as to have a direct effect on cancer cells rather than a systemic one. One of the responsibilities of those administering chemotherapy is to ensure that the patient receives appropriate chemotherapy, in the right formulation and route, with correct dose, time and duration. Those caring for patients also need to make sure that patients receiving chemotherapy have the appropriate monitoring, safety and side-effect support to enhance efficacy of therapy. To achieve this, nurses must have a sound knowledge of the drugs being administered and the various clinical issues associated with the different routes of administration.

Table 14.2: Routes of administration of chemotherapy: clinical considerations

Route of administration	Risk assessment	Practical implications
Intravenous: peripheral venous access or central venous access device (CVAD)	Assess patient immune and blood picture prior to chemotherapy. Check patency of access: flush with 10 ml of 0.9% sodium chloride prior to administration. Observe for: resistance, swelling or pain, signs of infiltration or leakage. Check the site or injection cap also at the end of the procedure	The site should be observed for the administration of vesicants drugs. Check administration via bolus or infusion; some vesicants must not be administered as infusions into peripheral veins. Make sure that safety guidelines re administration are adhered too. Protect patient from contact with the drugs. Administer antiemetics prior to chemotherapy. Flush with 0.9% sodium chloride between and after administering drugs
Intramuscular and subcutaneous	Assess patient immune and blood picture prior to chemotherapy. Observe skin for bruising and rotate sites to avoid patient discomfort. If administered by community nurses, information should be provided for those staff	Precautions for handling chemotherapy still apply to intramuscular and subcutaneous drugs. For deep intramuscular injection, use a Z-track technique to prevent leakage from site of injection
Intrathecal	Preparation of the drug must be via an aseptic technique. Formal checks are required of intrathecal medication in line with local guidelines. Intrathecal drugs should be given after intravenous medication	Administration should be in a designated clinical area and be within normal working hours in case of complications. A formal induction process in the procedures for administration of intrathecal medication reduces risk of drug error. Post-administration observations for signs of infection, headache or increased intracranial pressure should be undertaken
Intrapleural	Give premedication prior to procedure. Assess mobility and knowledge of the procedure. Local pleural pain and signs of inflammation are common 24–48 hours post treatment and appropriate symptom control is essential	Use flexible cannula or catheters if possible to improve patient comfort. Following administration, patients should turn every 15 minutes for between 4 and 6 hours to allow drug to cover all surfaces. Observe respirations and colour during and after procedure

Intravesical	Check patency of urinary catheter and make sure bladder is empty of urine. Assess patient's immune and blood picture prior to chemotherapy	Use an aseptic technique when infusing and protect from chemotherapy spills. Allow gravity to instil chemotherapy into the urinary catheter. Rapid instillation is uncomfortable for the patient. The drug needs to be allowed to stay in the bladder 1 hour. Advise patient on fluid intake to reduce the likelihood of tissue debris in the urine
Intraperitoneal	Assess patient's condition and immune system prior to administration. Weigh patient prior to and after therapy. Observe for leakage around the drain site; precautions need to be taken for both patient and staff as for other chemotherapy drugs	Prior to installation, pre-warm infusion to body temperature to prevent cramping and discomfort for the patient. Instillation is usually 1–2 L over 10–60 minutes, dependent on regimen and is kept within the peritoneum for 1–3 hours before drainage. Assess for fever, which is a common side-effect
Intra-arterial	The tumour site determines which artery is used to deliver chemotherapy. Insertion is an operative procedure. Mobility is usually restricted post treatment, dependent on site of catheter	Dressings following surgery should not be removed but observed for signs of bleeding. Careful technique and safety is required in removing or changing equipment to avoid air embolism, infection or bleeding. The catheter should be removed by a doctor
Oral	Evaluate patient's knowledge of medications and self-medication ability prior to discharge. Appropriate information and assessment advice in relation to toxicity needs to be provided to community staff	Dose–response is very dependent on compliance of the patient in taking the medication correctly. Self-assessment of toxicities: fever, hand-foot syndrome and diarrhoea are important indicators of toxicity and should be reported

Intravenous route

By far the most common route of cytotoxic drug administration is the intravenous one. this can be performed by a central venous access device (CVAD) or a peripheral cannula.[2] Cannulas are commonly used for both bolus and short-term infusions.[2] The disadvantage of this form of administration is that it is often associated with phlebitis and needs frequent resiting.[2] Patients requiring long-term treatments or drugs that are vesicants should be considered for CVAD placement.

There are many peripheral venous access devices available. The type of cytotoxic drug, dose and stability, degree of irritation or vesicant nature and dilution should all be considered when selecting the appropriate device. With the peripheral administration route, the most commonly used sites are the large veins of the forearm (cephalic or basillic), as these give easy access but also result in fewer problems if extravasation occurs.[16] When using peripheral routes for administing cytotoxic drugs, it is important to check patency prior to administration, and observe the site for signs of phlebitis, infiltration or extravasation (see Table 14.2). When administering cytotoxic drugs, it is good practice to give all vesicants first[2,17] and to use at least 5–10 ml sodium chloride 0.9% in between each drug to ensure adequate flushing of the vein and discourage the mixing of drugs. When using any intravenous device to administer a vesicant, one should check patency by encouraging backflow of blood every 2–5 ml that is injected.[2,17]

Bolus or continuous infusion

Intravenous cytotoxic drugs may be given as bolus injections. This means quick delivery of the drug and constant supervision during its administration. If administering bolus chemotherapy via a cannula, it is possible to continuously assess the device site for signs of infiltration or extravasation, which would require immediate intervention. Administering drugs as a bolus injection has been noted[2] to cause an increased incidence of venous spasm and irritation, which may make administration traumatic for the patient. To reduce this occurring, it is more appropriate to administer bolus injections via the side arm of a fast-running drip of sodium chloride 0.9% to prevent venous spasm and irritation. This method ensures safe delivery of the drug, while diluting it and aiding rapid blood flow to carry the cytotoxic solution away from the intravenous device site.

Continuous intravenous infusions of cytotoxic drugs are more restrictive for patients, but allow drugs to be administered in very dilute states to assist in maintaining venous integrity. It should be noted that continuous infusion of vesicant drugs via the peripheral route is extremely hazardous and should be avoided. This is predominantly because it is not feasible to observe the intravenous device for the duration of an infusion, and therefore extravasation may occur unnoticed for a time. It is therefore safer that patients who require vesicant infusions should be offered a CVAD to reduce their risk of tissue damage.[2]

Intramuscular and subcutaneous injection

Intramuscular and subcutaneous infusions are useful routes of administration for certain chemotherapy drugs. It is a good route if venous access is limited but can only be used with small volumes (less than 3 ml).[18] Only a small number of cytotoxic drugs can be administered in this way (see Table 14.2). Some of the problems that arise from this route are incomplete absorption and bleeding and discomfort from regular injections.[17] Recommendations for administration are explored in Table 14.2. Although the volume and administration route are different, the preparation, assessment of risk and safety are the same as for other routes.

Intrathecal administration

Intrathecal administration is the administration of cytotoxic drugs into the central nervous system (CNS) via the cerebrospinal fluid. This route is used only for a small number of chemotherapy drugs and is used most widely in the treatment of leukaemia and lymphoma.[19] The advantage of this route is that it allows the drugs to have direct contact with the CNS, when normally they are unable to pass the blood–brain barrier. However, this route also has huge potential for harm, and has been associated with several deaths through drug error or maladministration.[18,20] The main route of delivery for intrathecal chemotherapy is through a lumbar puncture, and this may need to be performed on a weekly or monthly basis.[21] The key requirements for safe administration are indicated in Table 14.2.

Intrapleural administration

Intrapleural instillation is where chemotherapy is administered into the pleural cavity. Pleural effusion is a common secondary site of many cancers and instillation following drainage of pleural effusion can prevent or delay effusion recurrence.[19] Principles for safe intrapleural administration are explored in Table 14.2. Some patients complain of local pleural pain and inflammation post administration and this can last for 24–48 hours. The provision of adequate analgesia and patent education are essential.

Intravesical administration

Intravesical chemotherapy is instilled directly into the bladder via a urinary catheter. Drugs then have an effect on the bladder mucosa, which allows a cytotoxic effect on any superficial tumour cells that may be present without causing systemic adverse effects. Patients report few side-effects from these cytotoxic instillations; usually, the main trauma is associated with the initial access (see Table 14.2).

Intraperitoneal administration

Intraperitoneal administration is the administration of the chemotherapy into the peritoneal cavity. This is used most widely in the palliation of ascites and tumours which result from local regional disease spread within the peritoneal cavity. The peritoneal cavity is semipermeable, allowing high concentrations of the drug to affect disease with low blood levels.[18] Principles for administration are given in Table 14.2.

Intra-arterial administration

Very occasionally, and usually within specialist settings, chemotherapy may be administered directly into an artery supplying an organ. For example, the hepatic artery may be catheterized to administer cytotoxic drugs for the treatment of hepatic tumours. This method causes very few systemic side-effects but there are obvious risks associated with intra-arterial access.

Oral chemotherapy

Oral chemotherapy is a relatively new route for cytotoxic administration, as previously many cytotoxic drugs were unable to be successfully absorbed through the gastrointestinal tract. The development of new agents and oral formulations may see 20–25% of all chemotherapy drugs being given through oral administration in the future.[22] The oral route provides many advantages for patients, including shorter treatment time, improved tolerability and the independence of self-administration, which have much less impact on patient's quality of life. Oral chemotherapy also presents many challenges for health care, including variability of absorption, patient compliance and the need for self-assessment (see Table 14.2).[23]

Changes constantly occur in the routes for administration, and patients are increasingly receiving chemotherapy in their own homes. The move towards ambulatory chemotherapy has increased within the last decade. New developments in ambulatory infusion devices have revolutionized chemotherapy administration and devices are now so small as to enable patients to continue their normal lives.[24] These devices are used for small volumes and for a variety of drugs and are designed for patients to move around. Patients may choose to have a CVAD inserted and care for this themselves at home, so that intermittent treatment can be administered in a familiar setting. The advent of oral cytotoxics has also led to more home chemotherapy. Patient education, safety and assessment of potential side-effects are of the utmost importance and careful preparation for home care is very much the role of the cancer nurse.

ASSESSMENT OF PATIENTS RECEIVING CHEMOTHERAPY

Nurses, even if not administering chemotherapy drugs, require a level of skill and knowledge to enable them to adequately assess patients.[4] It may be difficult to ensure continuity of assessment for each patient, as the nurse treating them may change over time. This needs to be taken into consideration, and adequate records maintained to provide a clear clinical picture for each patient. Patient reports of symptom incidence are higher than those recorded by medical staff,[25] and with the increasing use of home care, careful monitoring through self-report is increasingly becoming the norm. Literature reviews and some studies have identified that systematic assessment has allowed clinicians to successfully manage patient problems earlier with a reduction in symptom distress.[26–28] A number of checklists and self-assessment tools are available. Dennison and Shute[29] developed a short chemotherapy checklist for outpatient staff that recorded oncology patients' concerns. Although useful in practice, it may lack comprehensiveness and validity checking. Structured assessments enable a consistent documentation and decision-making process. Brown et al[30] developed and tested a chemotherapy self-assessment scale (C-SAS) for monitoring the impact of cytotoxic drugs on patients' experiences. This was developed in association with clinicians to enhance practicality of use. Other approaches to chemotherapy symptom assessment have used more novel techniques with handheld computers and systematic measurement techniques for patient problems such as oral health, fatigue, pain and nausea and vomiting.[31]

THE NURSING ROLE WITHIN CHEMOTHERAPY

Administration and safety

The role of the nurse in the administration of cytotoxic chemotherapy is continuously developing. The importance of education and training for staff administering these treatments is widely recognized, as safety for both patient and staff is essential. The risks associated with handling chemotherapy are associated with the time, dose and routes of exposure. Cytotoxic drugs can be absorbed through the skin and this may be through handling the drug or through exposure to patient waste products as a result of drug metabolism.[16] A number of experimental studies have suggested serious effects resulting from exposure to cytotoxic drugs, e.g. infertility. The hazards of handling chemotherapy drugs are well known, and it is important that safety measures are taken in order to protect staff that administer and handle chemotherapy. This includes consideration of the safety of the environment for and the need for drugs to be reconstituted in a vertical class II or III biological safety cabinet with laminar flow.[17] Safety also includes protective clothing such as gloves[32] and disposable gowns, for both reconstitution and handling. Goggles should be worn for reconstitution and masks where there is a possibility of inhalation.[33]

Healthcare institutions where cytotoxic drugs are administered have the responsibility to ensure that protocols are available to ensure safety of the patient at all times. There is also a need for policies to be available to ensure safety for all personnel that may come into contact with these drugs. Drugs must be handled and disposed of correctly to protect the people who are working with and receiving them.[34] National guidelines may also exist which determine the conditions under which drugs considered to be hazardous may be stored, reconstituted and handled.[35]

Safety of administration also includes safety for the patient through nurses' awareness and management of extravasation. This is a condition where vesicant drugs are inadvertently administered into surrounding tissues while administering chemotherapy. This can lead to necrosis at the site of injection. Early detection and treatment are essential to prevent future problems, such as pain, physical defect, delays in treatment and possibly litigation.[16] The distress caused as a result of extravasation occurring is high for both the patient and nurse; therefore, it is important to focus on safe intravenous technique. The signs and symptoms of extravasation are acute pain and feelings of burning or stinging at the injection site, induration or swelling, erythema and blanching of the skin. The management of extravasation is controversial and there is little consensus across Europe as to the best management approach. The management of extravasation varies between centres, but the principles are to stop the delivery of the drug and to withdraw as much of the drug as possible. Follow-up is to apply a cold pack to the site and local treatment with topical dimethyl sulfoxide (DMSO) and application of topical hydrocortisone cream to reduce limb inflammation.[17] It is important to report and fully document any extravasation incident, as the patient may require follow-up care.

The nurse administering these treatments is responsible for ensuring that all drugs that need to be given alongside the cytotoxic drugs are also administered. Nurses need to be aware of the content of chemotherapy regimens, which should be standardized within their work environment through the use of protocols to ensure safety and therapeutic outcomes.[2] Protocols should also provide the necessary information to inform the nurse of acceptable clinical data to proceed with the prescribed treatment, such as full blood count parameters and other measures of client well-being.

Processes surrounding chemotherapy administration need to be closely monitored to ensure quality. Strict policies must be followed to ensure patient safety and also to allow staff to be aware of the safe parameters in which these treatments can be given.[36] By using policies and protocols, nurses can ensure that their practice is safe and also clients receive the same standard of care within the oncology setting, no matter who is delivering their treatments.

Patient education and information

Information and patient education are fundamental to the patient's experience of cancer treatment (see Ch. 11). Studies have shown that information and communication are vital to the management of a chemotherapy patient's anxiety and distress.[37] Well-informed patients find it easier to cope with their disease, to feel in control and to maintain a positive outlook.[38] Provision of information also means that patients are more likely to participate in clinical decision-making, enhancing their ability to make informed choices about chemotherapy.[39] However, it is also important not to overburden patients with non-essential information, as this can lead to emotional distress and reduced cooperation.[40] Much of the literature on information provision in chemotherapy looks at the giving of information from the healthcare providers' view rather than the viewpoint of patients relating to their concerns and needs.

Coates et al,[41] in a study asking Australian patients to rate chemotherapy-related problems, detected 73 problems associated with chemotherapy. Problems such as 'length of time treatment takes' and 'having a needle' were ranked above psychological problems such as feeling anxious or tense. Practical problems such as parking and travel to the treatment centre can lead to frustration and increased anxiety. Therefore, information about the treatment facility and consideration of the practical aspects of care are as important as information on side-effects (Table 14.3).

Side-effect management

Adverse effects of chemotherapy treatments are dependent upon the drug given, the dose and route prescribed, previous cytotoxic exposure and, finally, the patient's age and general health prior to starting therapy. Public perceptions of cytotoxic drug toxicities are often negative through media misinterpretation and patient stories. Common misconceptions are that all drugs cause complete alopecia and cause excessive vomiting and diarrhoea. The provision of information and checking patients' understanding when first meeting, then after referral for chemotherapy, is important to dispel misconceptions and check recall. In addition, fears about side-effects can influence a patient's decision-making and play a part in treatment refusal.[42]

Side-effects and toxicities caused by cytotoxic chemotherapy can be categorized into acute and medium-term side-effects (Table 14.4): acute side-effects are those that occur within hours of the drug being administered, whereas medium-term side effects are defined as those which manifest days to weeks after treatment.[36,43] Toxicities can also be categorized to look at their effect on systemic regions of the client.[43]

Haematological toxicity

The normal haemopoietic functions of patients' bone marrow will become disrupted following delivery of the majority of cytotoxic drugs. The degree to which the disruption is manifested is

Table 14.3: Important things a patient should know about chemotherapy treatment

Delivery	Side-effects and concerns
How many cycles and frequency of chemotherapy?	Evaluate information they have received on all possible side-effects of chemotherapy
Where, when and how will they receive the drugs?	Have they received written information prior to the chemotherapy visit?
How is progress in relation to chemotherapy monitored?	Has travel arrangements and funding for hospital visits been discussed?
Are there any procedures that need to be completed prior to chemotherapy, such as blood tests?	Have they taken any prior medications before receiving chemotherapy, i.e. antiemetics?
How often are blood tests required?	Have they been assessed for a wig if they need or want one?
How will the patient know if they should stop or modify their treatment?	Do they have information on key contact telephone numbers, i.e. who to contact, when and for what?
If they are unable to attend for chemotherapy for some reason, who should they let know?	Are there any precautions they need to take at home in relation to infection?
Are they able to undertake usual physical activities with the CVAD, such as swimming or exercise?	What happens if they are suddenly unwell with side-effects? What should they do?
What happens if the infusion device stops working? What do they do?	How will they know when side-effects are worse than they should be?
	How will the community nurse know I am home?

Table 14.4: Potential side-effects of chemotherapy over time: dependent on action, duration and dose of chemotherapy

Acute: within hours of receiving chemotherapy	Medium term: days to weeks after chemotherapy	Late: months to years after chemotherapy
Nausea and vomiting	Fatigue	Cardiac toxicity
Neutropenia	Pulmonary inflammation	Pulmonary fibrosis
Alopecia	Early menopause	Skin pigmentation
Fever	Tinnitus	Photosensitivity
Vascular pain	Hand-foot syndrome	Infertility
Anaphylaxis syndrome	Mucositis	Menopause
Tumour lysis syndrome	Diarrhoea	Hearing loss
Haemorrhagic cystitis	Constipation	Secondary cancer
	Thrombocytopenia	
	Anaemia	
	Neurotoxicity	

dependent upon the individual drug, the dose and the patient's existing clinical state. Some of the effects on bone marrow will not be displayed immediately, such as anaemia. The average life span of an erythrocyte is 100–120 days;[44] therefore, the demand for this cell type is minimal in comparison to that of a neutrophil, which may only live for up to a few days.[44] Nurses administering chemotherapy need to have an awareness of potential haematological toxicities associated with the drugs that they are administering in order to educate their clients on important clinical signs that should be reported. For example, clients at risk of thrombocytopenia should be asked to report any signs of bruising or bleeding immediately, as they may require platelet transfusions to prevent haemorrhage. Anaemia can be a very distressing side-effect to patients receiving chemotherapy. As previously explained, it is likely to occur towards the end of a course of chemotherapy, when the patient may also have developed cumulative fatigue from the treatment. Anaemia may therefore be overlooked, unless blood results are carefully monitored.

Neurological toxicity

Many of the side-effects within this category can be very distressing for the chemotherapy patients and their significant others. Some of these toxicities are also likely to have long-term consequences. For example, patients treated with platinum-based therapies should be monitored for loss of hearing. If ignored, this can lead to irreversible ototoxicity.[11,43] Other common indicators are muscle weakness and loss of sensation; these signs should be assessed prior to chemotherapy treatment. Peripheral nerve toxicity is a distressing side-effect that manifests as a neuropathy. If untreated, by either dose reduction and/or pharmacological intervention, this can have long-lasting and disabling effects such as loss of balance, strength and sensation.[45] Severe neurotoxicity may be seen in patients receiving drugs such as high-dose vincristine and cytosine arabinoside (cytarabine); these effects will be further exacerbated if the client also receives radiotherapy to the CNS.[9]

Renal and bladder toxicity

Many cytotoxic drugs or their metabolites are excreted by the kidneys. To ensure patient safety, it is necessary to assess renal function prior to commencing treatment. Drugs which are known to cause toxicity to the kidneys, e.g. cisplatin, should be given with caution and diuresis monitored. Often, forced diuresis may be used to help reduce the impact of these drugs.[9] Some other drugs are known to have a direct effect on the bladder mucosa and it may be necessary to administer prophylactic medication as an adjuvant therapy. An example of this would be when administering high-dose cyclophosphamide; the patient should be encouraged to have a high fluid input and their urine should be monitored for the presence of blood.

Dermatological toxicity

Alopecia is commonly seen when clients receive anthracycline antibiotics, Vinka alkaloids and taxane treatments. Patients who desire a wig should be encouraged to obtain one prior to treatment commencing. Certain groups of patients may be able to access measures to prevent or reduce alopecia induced by cytotoxic drugs, such as scalp hypothermia. There are a variety of methods available to achieve this and results in patients with normal liver function are beneficial.[8] Certain groups of patients are not eligible to receive scalp cooling, where blood supply to the head is essential to ensure that the drugs have a cytotoxic action, such as in the case of leukaemia. Local policies should state which clients are suitable to be offered scalp hypothermia as a method to prevent alopecia. Patients should also understand that hair loss due to chemotherapy is not permanent and that their hair will grow back following completion of the treatment course.

Organ toxicity

Cardiotoxicity causing arrhythmias and heart failure is seen in patients who have received anthracycline antibiotic therapy. The effect of these drugs on cardiac tissue is cumulative and may also be exacerbated by other treatments and any underlying conditions. Patients receiving anthracycline treatment should have a cardiac assessment prior to commencing treatment and be regularly assessed for any deterioration.[2,10,36] All major organs are at risk of toxicity. Pulmonary toxicity is commonly associated with the use of many cytotoxic drugs.[10,43] Alkylating agents are associated with inducing pulmonary fibrosis and, in particular, busulfan is more likely to cause this[10] than many of the other drugs in this group. Hepatotoxicity can be caused by a number of cytotoxic drugs, which display a rise in plasma enzymes. Permanent hepatic failure is rare, but is occasionally seen with the use of antimetabolites.[10,43]

Hepatotoxicity is an uncommon side-effect of chemotherapy.[9] However, the liver plays a large part in drug metabolism and there is a therefore a risk. The reason that this risk is minimal is due to the slow cell replication that occurs in the hepatocytes,[44] cells of the liver, which makes them less vulnerable than rapidly dividing cells. Liver function should be assessed prior to commencing chemotherapy and, if drugs are known to be hepatotoxic, more vigilant monitoring should become routine.

Gastrointestinal toxicity

The mucosal cells of the oral cavity are extremely susceptible to the effects of chemotherapy. It is estimated that about 40% of adults receiving chemotherapy will develop some form of oral complication.[9] The mouth is commonly affected, either directly by the cytotoxic drugs or the myelosuppressive effects that the drugs have on the bone marrow. Complications of the mouth can be very varied and their management is dependent on isolating an accurate cause and diagnosis through vigilant assessment.

Nausea and vomiting are often the most feared side-effects by clients. Prescribing appropriate antiemetic regimes in accordance with the emetogenic potential of specific cytotoxic drugs is essential in preventing these side effects.[2] Antiemetic drugs should be reviewed for their suitability, as they may indeed bring with them other undesirable side-effects. Antiemetics should commence prior to treatment and then continue for at least 3 days after completion of the regimen.[43] Antiemetics should be selected for their ability to combat emesis induced by chemotherapy, depending on their emetogenic potential. It is also important to ensure that any antiemetics prescribed are given at the correct dose and type specified for the chemotherapy being given.[8] Other non-pharmacological methods of preventing this distressing and disruptive side-effect may also be employed by the client. Nurses should have an awareness of other interventions, such as bland diet, eating little and often and distraction therapies.[2,3,11,43] (See Ch. 20 for more in-depth consideration of the management of nausea and vomiting.)

Fatigue

Fatigue is the most frequently cited side-effect of chemotherapy and can occur during and after administration.[46] This has been found to have a greater impact than other chemotherapy side-effect on the patient's self-care ability.[40] The aetiology of chemotherapy-related fatigue is unknown; however, neutropenia and anaemia can contribute to fatigue. Fatigue is usually reported 3–4 days following administration of chemotherapy. It is frequently related to the treatment cycle, with fatigue decreasing prior to the next cycle of chemotherapy.[47] Fatigue patterns vary with chemotherapy regimen, disease and treatment duration, but tend to become more pronounced about 10 days following chemotherapy.[48] Despite its frequent occurrence, the pattern of fatigue is unclear, and interventions such as exercise and education have been used with good effect in some patient groups. (For more in-depth information on fatigue management, see Ch. 30.)

Hand-foot syndrome

Hand-foot syndrome (HFS), which is also know as palmar-plantar erythrodysaesthesia, is seen more commonly with drugs such as 5-fluorouracil (5-FU) and doxorubicin. This condition is rarely life-threatening, but can cause patient distress and be indicative of enhanced toxicity. Symptoms of HFS are erythema, numbness, tingling and paraesthesia on the palms or soles of the feet. Patients often describe difficulty in holding objects, painful rashes and swelling. The hands tend to be more commonly affected than the feet. The aetiology of HFS is unclear, but is linked to the dose and duration of drug. With dose reduction, HFS disappears and the skin can heal over in several days to weeks, depending on severity. There is little evidence as to the best approaches for managing this adverse effect, but several studies suggest the use of topical emollients or corticosteroids can reduce inflammation.[49]

Flu-like symptoms

Flu-like symptoms and fever are reactions that are seen in some patients receiving drugs such as bleomycin, mitomycin C and aspariginase. These clients should be warned of the potential side-effects and treated with paracetamol and steroids in order to prevent what can be very distressing consequences of their treatment.[2,11,43]

There are a number of long-term effects of chemotherapy which may arise years after treatment (see Table 14.4). Amongst these iare infertility, onset of early menopause and the potential of a second malignancy. Cytotoxic drugs interfere with DNA, and therefore may cause mutations.[9] It should be noted, however, that the benefits of chemotherapy outweigh the risk of a second malignancy developing.

Ongoing support for chemotherapy patients

The ongoing support of patients both during and after chemotherapy is reliant not only on the sound assessment skills of the nurse but also the effective management of side-effects. Poor management can lead to further complications: uncontrolled nausea, for example, can lead to metabolite imbalance, anorexia and general deterioration of the patient's physical condition. Over recent years, there have been many drug developments that can enhance support and recovery for patients undergoing chemotherapy, including new generations of antiemetics and antibiotics and the growth factors. Erythropoietin, a glycoprotein hormone produced by the kidney in response to tissue hypoxia, increases red blood cell activity, and with this hormone it is possible to increase patients' red blood cell recovery as a result of chemotherapy. Although well-tolerated by patients, it is expensive and also is not effective in all patients.[50]

Chemotherapy treatment is associated with a high level of psychological distress not only as a result of side-effects of the drugs but also as a result of the continuous nature of the cycles of chemotherapy and their impact on daily life. Psychological difficulties commonly experienced by chemotherapy patients include anxiety, depression, distress and mood swings. Studies indicate that women undergoing chemotherapy experience more severe anxiety than women receiving radiotherapy or surgery.[51] Ekman et al,[52] in a qualitative study of women's perceptions of receiving chemotherapy for ovarian cancer, found that the psychosocial issues were focused on trying to maintain normality and accepting the chemotherapy (Box 14.1).

Interventions for psychological problems as a result of cancer treatment focus on information provision, communication and limited counselling, as well as enhancing an individual's coping skills. Newell et al,[53] in a systematic review of psychological interventions, found that despite the poor quality of the evidence base, interventions such as group therapy, education, counselling and cognitive behavioural therapy offered the most benefit for patients. An example of the use of such techniques within chemotherapy is that of relaxation techniques and distraction interventions. Studies have shown that these interventions can have a significant effect on chemotherapy-related symptom distress and in improving patients' quality of life.[54]

INNOVATIONS IN CHEMOTHERAPY TREATMENT

In order for current treatments to advance and therefore improve both quality of life and survival rates for clients with cancer, there is a need for ongoing developments and innovations in the way treatments are delivered as well as new therapeutic agents. Testing these new developments and evaluating healthcare change are important in enhancing chemotherapy services. Clinical trials are therefore essential in leading the way in developing new chemotherapy regimens. Without comparison of new treatments against traditional ones, little change would occur that would be of benefit to the patient.

A number of studies have tried to identify key issues in the support of patients undergoing clinical trials.[55,56] Decisions to participate in clinical trials are complex, involving a balance between individual decision-making and beliefs about the possible benefits of participation.[57] The main focus is around the processes of ensuring that informed consent to enter a clinical trial is obtained. To ensure understanding and comprehension, the clinical trials nurse must be an astute assessor who has an in-depth knowledge of the clinical trial and all of its processes.[58] A clear expectation needs to be provided to the patient as to what the goals of the trial are. Despite the importance of clinical trials in the development of cancer treatment, participation is reported to be as low as 2–3% in the USA for adults[59] and, depending on cancer site, less than 5% in the UK.[60]

New and forthcoming treatments

Over the last two decades or more, a wealth of knowledge has emerged that has helped us to understand at the molecular level the biological events that lead to the development of human cancer. It has been crucial to identify the biological features of cancerous cells that make them different from normal, healthy cells so that new, more effective therapies that tar-

---

Box 14.1

Perceptions of receiving chemotherapy

Ekman and colleagues[52] report that women during chemotherapy for ovarian cancer found that the chemotherapy and alopecia reinforced their cancer diagnosis. There was fear that the cancer could return but also hope that the chemotherapy would provide a cure.

One women described the chemotherapy as: 'It must be something very strong in the medicines in that you feel so sick, but it will surely take away the cancer cells'. The perception that the women needs to suffer and that side-effects were to be expected is often expressed by patients. Other patients in the above study tried to remain positive, with the perception that positive thinking would reduce side-effects: 'I am not sick anymore'; 'this therapy will make me healthy'; and 'I will live as usual because the treatment will take the cancer away' (p179). Despite these thoughts, there was an underlying threat that the treatment may not work: 'What will happen if the treatment does not work?'. The acceptance of having to have chemotherapy as a necessary part of treatment was expressed by many of the women in the study. One woman said: 'I feel alright, and I understand the treatment had to be done. The chemotherapy is a good poison that I believe in. You know that you will feel ill after the treatment, but after a few days you are normal again' (p180).

get those same abnormalities can be developed. The overwhelming problems associated with the current portfolio of cytotoxic agents is their inherent toxicities, which can be life-threatening. It can be said that the vast majority of anticancer drugs target DNA (by inhibiting its synthesis or by direct damage to its structure), whether it be in the tumour or in normal tissue. Consequently, there is a lack of specificity for tumour cells, and this is the underlying cause of the toxicity associated with cancer chemotherapy. The idea of using therapies that target specific features of the cancer cell has come about in an effort to circumvent unwanted side-effects of cancer treatment. New targets on which to base new anticancer therapies include signalling pathways that regulate cellular growth and differentiation, agents that target abnormal cancer-associated genes (oncogenes), components of the cell cycle machinery and the growth and spread of cancer via metastases. The current ethos is to consider many of the new, targeted cancer therapies for use in combination with standard chemotherapy, with a dose reduction of the latter to minimize toxicity. A selection of new anticancer agents at various stages of development will be considered below.

Glivec

A common feature of chronic myeloid leukaemia (CML) is the presence of an abnormal chromosome, sometimes referred to as the Philadelphia chromosome. This comes about when part of chromosome 9 becomes attached (translocated) to part of chromosome 22. The presence of the abnormal chromosome results in the production of a protein referred to as Bcr-Abl. It was subsequently discovered that Bcr-Abl possessed an abnormally high level of an enzyme, tyrosine kinase, crucial to cell signalling processes, ultimately dictating the rate of cell proliferation. The drug Glivec (imatinib), developed as an orally active agent, was designed to inhibit the abnormal tyrosine kinase enzyme activity (by blocking its function) associated with Bcr-Abl and the Philadelphia chromosome. The clinical trials of Glivec were first carried out in 1998 and were watched with great interest, with response rates achieved over and above what might have been

expected for an antitumour agent. Indeed, the rapid success of Glivec has meant that it has now replaced the majority of treatments used for chronic-phase CML. Interestingly, Glivec is capable of inhibiting other biological mechanisms associated with cancer, in addition to Bcr-Abl tyrosine kinase. The most notable of these is the c-kit tyrosine kinase in the case of gastrointestinal stromal tumours (GISTs). Due to the presence of a mutation, c-kit in GIST behaves abnormally and is resistant to normal control mechanisms, in much the same way as Bcr-Abl. Glivec has now been licensed for use as a single agent in GIST, following a very rapid clinical development phase.[12,61]

Herceptin

The human epidermal growth factor receptor-2 (HER2) is located on the surface of the cell and is involved in signal transduction pathways essential for cell growth and differentiation. In human breast cancers, HER2 is overexpressed in 15–25% of cases, a feature correlated with poor clinical outcome in women with node-positive or node-negative disease.[62] The antibody Herceptin (trastuzumab) was specifically designed to target HER2 positive breast cancers. The clinical development of Herceptin included its assessment either as monotherapy or in combination with cytotoxic agents such as anthracyclines or paclitaxel. Based on favourable efficacy and safety, Herceptin was approved for use in the USA for monotherapy or first line in combination with paclitaxel for the treatment of HER2-positive metastatic breast cancer.[63] It subsequently received regulatory approval in 72 countries worldwide. There are other agents under various stages of clinical development designed to inhibit the activity of growth factor receptors such as Iressa and C225, a monoclonal antibody which targets epidermal growth factor receptor (EGFR).[64]

Antiangiogenic agents

Angiogenesis is the process of generating new capillary blood vessels. Tumour growth and metastasis are dependent on efficient angiogenesis. Many regulators of angiogenesis are growth factors and receptor tyrosine kinases involved in the migration and proliferation of endothelial cells. A number of drugs are currently being developed to inhibit vascular endothelial growth factor (VEGF) and agents that target its associated receptors Flt-1 and Flk-1. Arastin, a monoclonal antibody that targets VEGF has been licensed for use in metastatic colon cancer in the USA.

One of the important elements leading to successful angiogenesis is the breakdown of the extracellular matrix, which is carried out by enzymes with a specialist function called matrix metalloproteinases (MMPs). These enzyme complexes actually digest components in tissue, allowing the budding of new blood vessels and also contributing to the process of metastasis. Agents in the category of MMP inhibitors include marimistat, Bay12-9566 and BMS-275291, which are in various stages of clinical development.[65]

Cancer gene therapy

Gene therapy has been considered as an approach in oncology, but the field is still relatively new.[66,67] As with all gene therapies, the gene of interest has to be delivered into the body via a carrier system, typically an inactivated virus. The use of so-called viral vectors in other branches of medicine employing gene therapy has highlighted many problems and hazards associated with this procedure. However, cancer clinical trials employing gene therapy are continuing and the results are eagerly awaited (for more information see Ch. 15 on biological therapies).

CONCLUSION

Chemotherapy is a major treatment modality for cancer and can have a substantial impact on patients' physical function and quality of life. Many common cancers are treated with cytotoxic chemotherapy on an inpatient as well as an outpatient basis; therefore, nurses have a pivotal role in the care of the patient undergoing chemotherapy. There is a considerable amount of research on the physical effects and management of chemotherapy but less on the psychological impact of this treatment. Short-term complications have been well-defined and interventions such as those for nausea and vomiting

have had considerable investment from pharmaceutical companies in trying to ameliorate chemotherapy's adverse effects. Despite this, many patients still experience symptoms and distress as a result of chemotherapy, and more complex and intractable problems such as fatigue and early menopause as a result of chemotherapy are harder to resolve. Accessibility of chemotherapy, such as physical access to hospital, waiting lists, waiting times and scheduling of treatment continue to be issues for many patients across Europe. The treatment environment is critical to the successful and safe administration of chemotherapy in reducing patient anxiety and distress. Cancer nurses can influence this environment in many ways not only by understanding patients' experiences but also by considering the patient pathway from treatment decision to chemotherapy administration.

REFERENCES

1. Jack CM. Innovations in cancer therapeutics. In: Clarke D, Flanagan J, Kendrick K, eds. Advancing nursing practice in cancer and palliative care. Palgrave: Macmillan; 2002:93–116.

2. Dougherty L. Safe handling and administration of intravenous cytotoxic drugs. In: Dougherty L, Lamb J, eds. Intravenous therapy in nursing practice. London: Churchill Livingstone; 1999: 447–480.

3. Wilkes GM, Ingwersen K, Barton-Burke M. Introduction to chemotherapy drugs. In: Wilkes et al. Oncology nursing drug handbook. London: Jones and Bartlett; 2001:2–31.

4. Department of Health. The NHS Cancer Plan. London: HMSO; 2000.

5. Sitzia J, Wood N. Patient satisfaction with cancer chemotherapy nursing: a review of the literature. Int J Nurs Stud 1998; 35:1–2.

6. Moliterni A, Bonadonna G, Valagussa O, Ferrari L, Zambetti M. Cyclophosphamide, methotrexate and fluorouracil with and without doxorubicin in the adjuvant treatment of resectable breast cancer with one to three positive axillary nodes. J Clin Oncol 1991; 9:1124–1130.

7. Deery P, Faithfull S. Developing a patient pathway to deliver a new oral chemotherapy. Prof Nurse 2003; 19(2):102–106.

8. Moran P. Cellular effects of cancer chemotherapy. administration. J IV Nurs 2000; 23(1):44.

9. Holmes S. Cancer chemotherapy: a guide for practice. Dorking: Asset Books; 1997. http://www.continuingeducation.com/pharmtech/trainingsafety/ 24 July 2001.

10. Souhami R, Tobias J. Cancer and its management. 3rd edn. Oxford: Blackwell Science; 1998.

11. Otto S. Oncology nursing. 3rd edn. St Louis: Mosby Year Book; 1997

12. Cadeville R.,Buchdunger E, Zimmermann J, Matter A. Glivec (STI571; imatinib) a rationally developed, targeted anticancer drug. Nat Rev Drug Discov 2002; 1:493-502.

13. Hood LE. Chemotherapy in the elderly: supportive measures for chemotherapy-induced myelotoxicity. Clin J Oncol Nurs 2003; 7(2):185–190.

14. Balducci L, Yates J. General guidelines for the management of older patients with cancer. Oncology 2000; 19:1583–1584.

15. Bailey C, Corner J. Older people, care, and cancer: a critical perspective FACET. Eur J Cancer Care, March 2003: www.blackwellpublishing.com/journals/ecc

16. Weinstein S. Antineoplastic therapy. In: Plumer's principles and practice of intravenous therapy. 7th edn. Philadelphia: JB Lippincott; 2000:474–548.

17. Dougherty L, Lister S. Drug administration: cytotoxic drugs – Royal Marsden Hospital manual of clinical nursing procedures. Oxford: Blackwell Science; 2002.

18. Sewell G, Summerhayes M, Stanley A. Administration of chemotherapy. In: Allwood M, Stanley A, Wright P, eds. The cytotoxic handbook. 4th edn. Oxford: Radcliffe Medical Press; 2002.

19. Goodman M. Chemotherapy: principles of administration. In: Yarbro CH, Frogge MH, Goodman M, eds. Cancer nursing – principles and practice. Boston: Jones and Bartlett; 2000.

20. Schulmeister L. A complication of vascular access device insertion. J Intrav Nurs 1998; 21(4):197–202.

21. Stanley A. Managing complications of chemotherapy administration. In: Allwood M, Stanley A, Wright P, eds. The cytotoxic handbook. 4th edn. Oxford: Radcliffe Medical Press; 2002.

22. Bedell CH. A changing paradigm for cancer treatment: the advent of new oral chemotherapy agents. Clin J Oncol Nurs Suppl 2003; 7(6):5–9.

23. Faithfull S, Deery P. Implementation of capecitabine (Xeloda) into a UK cancer centre: UK experience. Eur J Oncol Nurs 2004; 8:S54–62.

24. Perucca R. Types of infusion therapy equipment. In: Hankins J, Walldman Lonsway RA, Hedrick C, Perdue M, eds. Infusion therapy in clinical practice. 2nd edn. Philadelphia: WB Saunders; 2001.

25. Williams PD, Ducey KA, Sears AM, et al. Treatment type symptom severity among oncology patients by self report. Int J Nurs Stud 2001; 38:359–367.

26. Dodd M. Managing side effects of chemotherapy. In: Fitzpatrick J, Stevenson J, eds. Annual review of nursing research. New York: Springer; 1993:77–104.

27. Larson P, Kohlman V Dodd M, et al. A model for symptom management. Image: J Nurs Scholarship 1994; 26:272–276.

28. Sarna L. Effectiveness of structured nursing assessment of symptom distress in advanced lung cancer. Oncol Nurs Forum 1998; 25(6):1041–1048.

29. Dennison S, Shute T. Identifying patient concerns: improving the quality of patient visits to the oncology out-patient department – a pilot audit. Eur J Oncol Nurs 2000; 4:91–98.

30. Brown V, Sitzia J, Richardson A, et al. The development of the chemotherapy symptom assessment scale (C-SAS): a scale for the routine clinical assessment of the symptom experiences of patients receiving cytotoxic chemotherapy. Int J Nurs Stud 2001; 38:497–510.

31. Kearney N. Classifying nursing care to improve patient outcomes: the example of WISECARE. NT Res 2001; 6(4):747–756.

32. Worthington K. Hazardous drugs: handling medications can pose dangers to nurses. Am J Nurs 2002; 102(5):120.

33. Labuhn K, Valanis B, Schoeny R, Loveday K, Vollmer W. Nurses' and pharmacists' exposure to antineoplastic drugs: findings from industrial hygiene scans and urine mutagenicity tests. Cancer Nurs 1998; 21(2):79–89.

34. Allwood M, Stanley A, Wright P. The cytotoxic handbook. 4th edn. Oxford: Radcliffe Medical Press; 1997.

35. Training, safety and quality when preparing chemotherapy agents. Continuing Education online. Available: http://www.continuingeducation.com/pharmtech/trainingsafety/ 24 July 2001.

36. Tanghe A, Paidaens R, Evans G, et al. Case study of quality assurance in the administration of chemotherapy. Cancer Nurs 1996; 19(6):447–454.

37. Meyerowitz B, Watkins I, Sparks F. Quality of life for breast cancer patients receiving adjuvant chemotherapy. Am J Nurs 1983; 83:232–235.

38. Thomas R, Dalya M, Perryman C, Stockfond D. Forewarned is forearmed – benefits of preparatory information on video cassette for patients receiving chemotherapy or radiotherapy – a randomised controlled trial. Eur J Cancer 2000; 36: 1536-1543.

39. Van De Molen B. Relating information needs to the cancer experience: 1 Information as a key coping strategy. Eur J Cancer Care 1999; 8:238–244.

40. Ream E, Richardson A. The role of information in patients' adaption to chemotherapy and radiotherapy: a review of the literature. Eur J Cancer Care 1996; 5:132–138.

41. Coates A, Abraham S, Kaye SB, et al. On the receiving end – patient perception of the side effects of cancer chemotherapy. Eur J Cancer Clin Oncol 1983; 19:203–208.

42. Tierney AJ, Taylor J, Closs SJ. Knowledge, expectations and experiences of patients receiving chemotherapy for breast cancer. Scand J Caring Sci 1992; 6:75–80.

43. Lilly Oncology. Cytotoxic chemotherapy. 5th edn. Hants: Eli Lilly Company Limited; 1997.

44. Marieb EN. Human anatomy and physiology. 5th edn. Menlo Park, CA: Benjamin Cummings; 2001.

45. Visovsky C, Daly BJ. Clinical evaluation and patterns of chemotherapy-induced peripheral neuropathy. J Am Acad Nurse Pract 2004; 16(8)353–359.

46. Winningham ML, Nail LM, Barton Burke M, et al. Fatigue and the cancer experience: the state of the knowledge. Oncol Nurs Forum 1994; 21:23–36.

47. Berger AM. Patterns of fatigue and activity and rest during adjuvant breast cancer chemotherapy. Oncol Nurs Forum 1998; 25:51–62.

48. Richardson A, Ream E. Self care behaviours initiated by chemotherapy patients in response to fatigue. Int J Nurs Stud 1997; 34(1): 35–43.

49. Lassere Y, Hoff P. Management of hand-foot syndrome in patients treated with capecitabine (Xeloda). Eur J Oncol Nurs 2004; 8:s31–40.

50. Crawford J, Cella D, Cleeland CS, et al. Relationship between changes in haemoglobin level and quality of life during chemotherapy in anaemic cancer patients receiving epoietin alfa therapy. Cancer 2002; 95:888–895.

51. Schreier AM, Williams SA. Anxiety and quality of life of women who receive radiation or chemotherapy for breast cancer. Oncol Nurs Forum 2004; 31(1):127–130.

52. Ekman I, Bergbom I, Ekman T, Berhold H, Mahsneh SM. Maintaining normality and support are central issues when receiving chemotherapy for ovarian cancer. Cancer Nurs 2004; 27(3):177–182.

53. Newell SA, Sanson-Fisher RW, Savolainen NJ. Systematic review of psychological therapies for cancer patients: overview and recommendations for future research. J Natl Cancer Inst 2002; 94(8):558–584.

54. Schneider SM, Prince-Paul M, Allen MJ, Silverman P, Talaba D. Virtual reality as a distraction intervention for women receiving chemotherapy. Oncol Nurs Forum 2004; 31(1):81–88.

55. Verheggen FWSM, Nieman F, Jonkers R. Determinants of patient participation in clinical studies requiring informed consent: Why patients enter a clinical trail. Patient Educ Couns 1998; 35:111–125.

56. Cox K. Assessing the quality of life of patients in phase I and II anti-cancer drug trials: interviews versus questionnaires. Soc Sci Med 2003; 56(5):921–934.

57. Cox K, McGarry J. Why patients don't take part in cancer clinical trials: an overview of the literature. Eur J Cancer Care 2003; 12:114–122.

58. Ocker B, Pawlik Plank D. The research nurse role in a clinic-based oncology research setting. Cancer Nurs 2000; 23(4):286–292.

59. Collyar D. The value of clinical trials from a patient perspective. Breast J 2000; 6:310–314.

60. Jenkins V, Fallowfield L. Reasons for accepting or declining to participate in randomized clinical trials for cancer therapy. Br J Cancer 2000; 82:1783–1788.

61. Mauro MJ, O'Dwyer M, Heinrich MC, Druker BJ. STI571: a paradigm of new agents for cancer therapeutics. J Clin Oncol 2002; 20:325–334.

62. Hynes NE, Stern DF. The biology of erbB-2/neu/HER-2 and its role in cancer. Biochim Biophys Acta 1994; 1198:165–184.drug. Nature Reviews 2002; 1:493–502.

63. Bell R. What can we learn from Herceptin trials in metastatic breast cancer? Oncology 2002; 63:39–46.

64. Ciardiello F, Tortora G. A novel approach in the treatment of cancer: targeting the epidermal growth factor receptor. Clin Cancer Res 2001; 7:2958–2970.

65. Hidalgo M, Eckhardt SG. Development of matrix metalloproteinase inhibitors in cancer therapy. J Natl Cancer Inst 2001; 93: 178–193.

66. Curiel DT, Gerritsen WR, Krul MRL. Progress in cancer gene therapy. Cancer Gene Ther 2000; 7:1197–1199.

67. Nielsen LL, Maneval DC. P53 tumor suppressor gene therapy for cancer. Cancer Gene Ther 1998; 5:52–63.

CHAPTER 15

Biological Therapy

DIANE BATCHELOR

CHAPTER CONTENTS

Introduction	303		Angiogenesis inhibitors	312
Definition of biotherapy	303		Gene therapy	312
Historical perspectives in biological			Strategies for gene therapy and diagnoses	313
therapy	304		Important aspects of gene therapy	314
Rationale for biological therapy	305		Nursing care	314
Biotechnological advancement and the			Side-effects	316
development of biological therapies	306		Coordination of care	326
New drug development and biological			The future	326
therapies	307		Novel delivery of cytokines	326
Immunotherapy	307		Radioimmunotherapy	327
Cytokines	307			
Monoclonal antibodies	310		Conclusion	327
Vaccines	311		References	327

INTRODUCTION

This chapter will provide an insight into biological therapies and the nursing care of patients who receive them. Biological therapy is the fourth modality for treating cancer and has received considerable interest in the last 20 years. The identification of genes and genetic engineering has spawned a booming biotechnology industry that is producing agents of the future. Harnessing the bodies' own defences and manipulating them has increased treatment options for patients with cancer.

This chapter will give an overview of the various forms of biotherapy and their mode of action. This is placed against an historical backdrop. The rationale for biological therapies and present applications within cancer care will be described. The nature of the side-effects experienced as well as the interventions commonly used for their relief are discussed. Important aspects of nursing care are explored. Finally, the potential for biological therapy to change the face of cancer care in the future is presented.

DEFINITION OF BIOTHERAPY

Biological therapy (biotherapy) can be defined as the use of naturally occurring proteins (derived from biological sources) that modify or augment the body's natural response to disease processes or agents that affect biological processes.[1] Biological therapies are being used to treat viral and bacterial infections, AIDS, autoimmune illnesses and cancer among many other conditions. Biological therapy in oncology (including both solid tumours and haematological malignancies) is used to modify biological processes and tumour environments in order to prevent and treat or arrest the growth of cancer.

Although the biological processes of cancer are extremely complex, in the last 30 years further insight has been gained into the mechanisms of tumour microbiology, the host–tumour relationship and their components. This has resulted in the development of agents that can alter these processes and result in antitumour activity. Biological processes that can presently be modified by biological agents are the immune response, immunity, angiogenesis, oncogenesis and tumour suppression. These processes have all been described in Chapter 7.

For the purposes of this chapter, biological therapy is considered to fall into four categories: immunotherapy, vaccination therapy, angiogenesis inhibition and gene therapy. Immunotherapy comprises the use of products derived from the immune system to stimulate or modify the immune response. Vaccination therapy encompasses the use of tumour cells or cell products to produce tumour immunity. Gene therapy is the transfer of genes to cells to alter their processes and protein production. Finally, angiogenesis inhibition is the inhibition of tumour blood vessel development.

HISTORICAL PERSPECTIVES IN BIOLOGICAL THERAPY

Biological therapy using immunological principles began during the Middle Ages. Naive attempts were made at immunizing humans against infectious disease using vaccines. The word *vaccine* was derived from the Latin word *vaccus*, which means cow. This word was probably chosen as the first vaccines developed were used to treat cowpox. It had been observed that individuals who were exposed to or once recovered from cowpox did not become infected again. The underlying principle of vaccination/immunisation is that injecting a weakened strain of bacteria/virus

could develop immunity to those bacteria. Edward Jenner, who developed the cowpox vaccine in 1798, was one of the first to apply this principle and to succeed. Louis Pasteur, who is the godfather of bacteriology, carried this principle of developing immunity to infection forward.

The first application of immunotherapy in oncology was Coley's toxins (in the early 1890s). Dr Coley observed that patients who had developed spontaneous regression of their tumour had recently undergone an infection.[2] He derived his toxins by purifying bacterial byproducts and injecting them. These toxins acted as non-specific immunostimulatory agents and induced an immune response that attempted to reduce the tumour.[3] The response rate achieved around the turn of the last century was ±18–20%. Although these remissions were quite remarkable for that time, Coley's toxins fell out of favour when interest in radiotherapy began.

Only in the 1960s did immunotherapy once again reach the clinic setting for the treatment of cancer. Bacille Calmette-Guérin (BCG), developed from the virus *Mycobacterium bovis*, had been used for many years as a vaccination for tuberculosis.[2] Some objective responses were seen in patients with in-transit melanoma following intralesional administration of BCG. BCG has also been used in patients with haematological malignancies as well as various other solid tumours. Using the scarification method, metastatic disease was treated, but response rates were not promising. BCG was also tested as an intravesicular treatment in patients with superficial bladder carcinoma with success. It has since been registered as a treatment for this disease.

In the 1970s, with the discovery of the interferons – interferon alpha (IFNα), beta (IFNβ) and gamma (IFNγ) – the era of the cytokines was born. Cytokines are protein cell regulators developed by the immune system.[2] IFNα was originally derived by manual extraction from human white blood cells,[4] but since the development of genetic engineering, the interferons and other cytokines have been produced by the DNA recombinant technique. The interferons are antiviral agents that prevent the infection of cells by viruses. Interferons have been used for viral illnesses such as condyloma acuminata (IFNα), multiple sclerosis (IFNβ) and certain types of hepatitis (IFNα), as well as for cancer. The first registered indication for IFNα in oncology was hairy cell leukaemia.[5]

The interleukins IL-1 to IL-12 and other interleukins were developed and researched but never achieved registration for use in oncology. The cytokine IL-2 has been registered for the treatment of renal cell cancer. The growth factors granulocyte colony-stimulating factor (GCSF) and granulocyte–macrophage colony-stimulating factor (GM–CSF) have been registered primarily for use in patients with leucocytopenia following treatment with myelosuppressive chemotherapy.

The cytokines, IFNα, IL-2 and the growth factors GCSF and GM-CSF were given in the past as an intravenous solution in high doses. The administration of high-dose cytokines is associated with severe multi-organ toxicity, which has contributed to re-examining their use within the context of therapeutic response in relation to toxicity. This research revealed that activity could be achieved with lower doses and longer treatment schedules, making the subcutaneous route an attractive option.[6] Cytokines are now primarily administered through the subcutaneous route.

Cellular therapy began around the mid 1980s. The most well-known cellular therapies were the lymphokine-activated killer (LAK) cells and tumour-infiltrating lymphocytes (TILs). These approaches were developed by Dr Rosenberg from the National Cancer Institute in Bethesda, Maryland. After patients had received an IL-2 infusion for approximately 5 days, their lymphocytes multiplied and became more active. Lymphocytes (which continued to multiply) were then harvested from the patient and cultured for several days with IL-2. The LAK cells were then reinfused to the patient in daily portions for 3 days, while the patient also received continuous administration of IL-2. Although successes were seen, subsequent studies did not prove any benefit above IL-2 alone,[2] and the toxicity profile was severe.

The principle of TILs was similar to LAK, except that the activated lymphocytes were harvested from the patient's tumour. It was found that these lymphocytes not only had the ability to penetrate tumours but also to lyse tumour cells. It was felt that these lymphocytes were tumour-specific and therefore would be more potent. Although they were more potent than LAK cells, the addition of TILs did not increase response and was highly toxic and expensive.[2]

In the 1980s, with the development of the hybridoma technique, monoclonal antibodies began to enter the clinical setting in the form of a targeted therapy against cancer. One of the first monoclonal antibodies to be developed was Oncoscint, which was registered for use as a diagnostic tool to identify ovarian carcinoma cells. Panorex was discovered to target colon carcinoma cells and was developed for therapeutic indications. Recently, Herceptin (trastuzumab) and rituximab have been registered as treatments for breast cancer and B-cell non-Hodgkin's lymphoma, respectively.

Tumour vaccines mark the development of a new era in tumour-specific therapy. Numerous studies have been carried out such as injecting autologous tumour cell preparations to induce active specific immunity (ASI). This strategy was applied in colon cancer patients. The same principles exist as with other vaccinations. The injection of tumour antigens stimulates the immune system to induce tumour immunity.

With the identification of DNA by Watson and Crick in the 1950s and the Human Genome Project, subsequently, the opportunity has been created to manipulate DNA to the benefit of the host and prevent disease. Dr French Anderson started the first gene laboratory in 1968[7] and the first gene therapy trial took place in 1990, in the National Institutes of Health in Bethesda, Maryland, USA.

This section has provided a brief overview of the history of biological therapy. The next section will discuss the rationale for this mode of cancer treatment.

RATIONALE FOR BIOLOGICAL THERAPY

Tumour development is a multi-stage process that encompasses numerous genetic changes, as described in Chapter 5. Changes in genes (tumour genes, such as proto-oncogenes,

oncogenes and tumour suppressor genes) alter the gene products they produce and the expression of protein on the cell surface. Recognition of proteins (tumour antigens) on the cell surface can stimulate an immune response. The immune response is our protective mechanism that uses white blood cells and proteins (such as cytokines, growth factors and antibodies) to fight off bacterial and viral infections as well as tumour cells.

Once tumours and their metastases develop, they need to survive. Vascular endothelial growth factors contribute to the formation of blood vessels (angiogenesis). All these biological mechanisms can be manipulated with the use of immunotherapy, gene therapy and angiogenesis inhibitors with varying measures of success and will be described in the following section.

But first it is probably worth addressing the questions of why we need a new type of therapy to treat cancer and why we should devote more resources when we are still learning about the potential and applications of existing therapies? Possible answers include the following:

- New therapies are always needed to fight cancer, as a significant number of cancers remain without cure. In addition, the best treatment results are often achieved through multi-modality treatments that create more choices.

- New developments in microbiology and biotechnology have allowed scientists to discover new pathways for treating cancer. This knowledge has provided the possibility of more tumour-specific therapies that can prevent the destruction of normal cells.

- A direct relationship has been found between the biological (immune) system and cancer: i.e. carcinogenesis, angiogenesis, TILs, an increased risk of cancer in individuals who are immunosuppressed and spontaneous regression of tumours.

- A more tumor-specific class of agents needs to be developed to spare patients the multi-organ toxicity that has been seen in the past.

Biotechnological advancement and the development of biological therapies

With the discovery of DNA, genes and proteins that govern the functions of our bodies, scientists looked ahead to finding new ways to develop drugs that could mimic substances and processes in our own bodies. The DNA recombinant technique is a form of genetic engineering whereby DNA is made by recombining fragments of DNA from different organisms. This allows cytokines to be produced in large quantities for clinical applications. The gene that is responsible for producing a cytokine is isolated and inserted into a gene sequence, which is then introduced into a rapidly growing bacteria, usually *Escherichia coli*. The bacteria then acts as a production factory, producing large amounts of the cytokine. Following the purification of the bacteria, a large quantity of cytokine is available for use. This process is used to produce the interferons, interleukins and growth factors.

Subsequently, hybridoma technology was discovered which introduced the monoclonal antibodies (MoAbs) into our biological repertoire. Simplified, this process consists of the introduction of a tumour antigen/receptor into a mouse. Subsequently, the mouse develops antibodies specific to that antigen/receptor. In order to produce the MoAbs in large quantities, the plasma cells that produce the antibody are harvested and united with rapidly growing cells. This combination produces cell fusion factories that produce the MoAbs on a large scale. Due to MoAbs originating from mouse protein, allergic reactions can occur during their infusion, as antibodies develop to the mouse protein: i.e. HAMA (human anti-mouse antibody). Scientists have continued to perfect the production of MoAbs by constructing chimeric antibodies. Chimeric antibodies are molecules that are part mouse (at the binding site) and part human. This prevents HAMA formations and possibly an infusion reaction.

These two techniques marked the beginning of immunotherapy drug development. Immunotherapy using vaccines derived from a variety of antigens does not have one consistent development process. Gene therapy uses viral vectors for transferring the gene to the cell, in order to carry out its function. Gene transfer is so variable that it has not yet been completely standardized. This falls outside the scope of this chapter.

NEW DRUG DEVELOPMENT AND BIOLOGICAL THERAPIES

It is essential to look at drug development with biological agents differently to that with chemotherapy agents. In chemotherapy trials, one looks at the distribution and availability of the agents (pharmacokinetics) and what the chemotherapy does in the body (pharmacodynamics).[8] Other determining factors are maximum tolerated dose (MTD) and the dose-limiting toxicity (DLT), terms often associated with traditional phase 1 studies with chemotherapy. This principle implies that more is better, specifically in terms of tumour cell death. In terms of toxicity, it means that the patient is encountering doses at the limits of what the body can accept.

With biological studies, the principles of dosing and evaluation of distribution are different. There will be an MTD, but an optimal biological response modifier dose (OBRMD) is the aim. Studies have shown that more is not necessarily better when stimulating the immune system. In addition, cell therapies require certain numbers of cells to achieve the desired immune cell/tumour cell response. In terms of monoclonal antibodies, the receptors on tumour cells need to be bound to the MoAb, which might require that the first dose be actually greater than subsequent doses. With vaccines, a small amount of tumour antigen might stimulate the required immune response, or dose increases might be based on biological responses. Inability to measure the level of tumour immunity, the decision to repeat the vaccine and at what moment might be difficult to ascertain.

Thus, dosing and scheduling are complex issues with biological therapies and are dependent on the type of therapy, the dose, the route and the response that is aimed for. Drug development is challenging.

Agents that have been developed and are registered for use can be found in Table 15.1.

IMMUNOTHERAPY

Immunotherapy is a treatment modality that modifies, stimulates or controls processes of the immune system to the benefit of the host[9] (see Ch. 7). Most of the agents used today are proteins, and several have been registered for the treatment of cancer. Immunotherapy consists of the use of cytokines/haemopoietic growth factors (HGFs), monoclonal antibodies and vaccines.

Immunotherapy has three applications:

- Diagnostic: monoclonal antibodies that target for a particular antigen can be labelled and injected. These will migrate to the tumour and be picked up by radiographic equipment and demonstrate the location of tumour. In addition, MoAbs can be used to identify cell types in pathology – immunohistochemistry.

- Supportive: with the help of the HGFs, the length and severity of chemotherapy-induced leucopenia can be decreased.[9]

- Therapeutic: cytokines and MoAbs can be used to treat cancer.

Cytokines

Cytokines are glycoprotein messengers that mobilize white blood cells to perform many different functions. Cytokines can be categorized as either monokines (derived from monocytes) or lymphokines (derived from lymphocytes), although these names are rarely used in clinical practice. When secreted from blood cells or administered, they are taken up through receptors on the membranes of white cells and trigger them to multiply and carry out their respective functions.

Interferon is a cytokine that is produced by cells when they come in to contact with a virus. Interferon is the general name given to a family of cytokines best known for their immunomodulatory function and, in particular, their unique ability to interfere with viral replication. The interferon protects the other cells

307

Table 15.1: Summary of biological agents, rationale for use and applications in oncology

Immunotherapy	Class of biological therapy	Trade name	Generic name	Rationale for use	Application in oncology	Side-effects
Cytokines *Definition* Glycoproteins derived from the immune system that play a major role in an immune response	Interferon	Interferon alpha	Roferon Pegasus	Enhance tumour cell differentiation, inhibit oncogenes Stimulate an immune response	Melanoma, renal cell carcinoma, AIDS-related Kaposi's sarcoma (KS), follicular lymphoma, hairy cell leukaemia, and chronic myelogenous leukaemia	1–6, 10–20, 22,23,27
		Pegylated Interferon alpha long-acting	IntronA Peg Intron	Antiproliferative Anti-angiogenic Antiviral Cytotoxic Impede blood cell differentiation		see above
	Interleukins	Interleukin 2	Proleukin	Activation of T and B lymphocytes, NK cells and macrophages Stimulate development of secondary cytokines that activate an immune response	Renal cell carcinoma Melanoma (US only)	1–6, 8–27, 30
	Haemopoietic growth factors	Granulocyte colony-stimulating factor	Granocyte Neupogen Neulasta (long-acting)	Promotes the proliferation and differentiation of hematopoeitic cells	Non-myeloid malignancies receiving myelosuppressive anticancer drugs associated with a significant incidence of febrile neutropenia	1–5 mild in nature
		Granulocyte-macrophage colony-stimulating factor (GM-CSF)	Leucomax	Granulocytes, macrophages. The antigen-presenting cells: dendrites	Non-myeloid malignancies receiving myelosuppressive anticancer drugs associated with a significant incidence of febrile neutropenia	1–7

Monoclonal antibodies						
Definition Antibodies developed via the hybridoma technique and specific to a receptor or antigen. They can be used to diagnose and treat cancer and manage side-effects	Signal transduction inhibitor	Herceptin	Traztuzumab	Binds HER-2, a receptor for epidermal growth factor (EGF) that is found on some tumor cells	HER2 protein overexpressing metastatic breast cancer; first line with paclitaxel	1–5, 7
	Antigen specific	Mab Thera	Rituximab	Binds to the CD20 molecule (antigen) found on most B cells	Relapsed or refractory low-grade or follicular, CD20+, B-cell non-Hodgkin's lymphoma (NHL)	1–5, 7 All infusion-related side effects from start of therapy to ± 6 hours following therapy
	Antigen-specific	Mab Campath	Alemtuzumab	Binds to CD52, a molecule found on white blood cells.	B-cell chronic lymphocytic leukaemia failed on fludarabine	1–5, 7 Anti-infective regimen essential with Campath
	Antigen-specific (diagnostic)	Oncoscint	Satumomab Pendetide	Delivery of a radioactive agent to the cell	Radiographic visualization of tumours for imaging	

The numbers in the far right column refer to the side effects associated with the agent in Table 15.4.

from being infected: hence the name. The most frequently used interferon is IFNα. The antiproliferative, antiviral and immunomodulatory activities of the interferons have stimulated interest in the application of these agents for the treatment of a number of disorders, including neoplastic as well as viral and microbial diseases.

Interleukins are cytokines that are produced by white blood cells during an immune response. Interleukins regulate the production, development and interaction of diverse white blood cells. There are more than 18 known interleukins and interleukin-2 (IL-2) is the most frequently used. IL-2, a protein produced naturally in the body in very small amounts, is an immune modulator. It is produced by T lymphocytes during an immune response and is responsible for increases in CD4+ counts and T-helper cells.

Haematopoietic growth factors are also cytokines with a specific function. They are responsible for proliferation and differentiation of various types of blood cells. GCSF stimulates the neutrophil granulocytes to multiply. Neutrophils are white blood cells involved in fighting bacterial infections. GM-CSF is not only responsible for the development of granulocytes but also macrophages, which are responsible for tumour antigen presentation.

Monoclonal antibodies

Monoclonal antibodies are antibodies that can recognize, bind and categorize tumour antigens or tumour receptors. Therefore, they can be used for many functions. There are two parts to an antibody: the variable region and the constant region. The variable region locks onto the antigen/receptor, and the constant region sends signals out to the immune system to assist in destroying the cell. We have millions of antibodies in our bodies, and each has a different sequence within the binding region – hence the name 'variable region.' This occurs because the variable region must fit the unique receptor or antigen correctly, just like a key in a lock. Each antibody binds to a particular antigenic determinant on a receptor of a specific tumour cell.

Originally, MoAbs were completely made in the mouse. However, mouse MoAbs may cause problems in patients, because they are foreign proteins. When administered to humans, they can induce allergic reactions and/or the generation of HAMA upon retreatment. HAMA can reduce efficacy of MoAbs by increasing their sequestration and degradation. As production techniques have become more sophisticated, MoAbs are being constructed to make most of the molecule human in sequence (humanized MoAbs), whereby only the binding areas (the variable region) remain of mouse origin. In that way, the body does not recognize them as mouse proteins, thus significantly reducing the risk of allergic reactions and the generation of HAMA.[10] A vast array of MoAbs has been developed and are being used as diagnostic tools to classify tumours in pathological immunohistochemistry. Oncoscint is an MoAb that is presently being used to characterize cancer cells at diagnosis. Certain MoAbs are not only capable of recognizing tumour cells but also of destroying cancer cells with assistance of cells from the immune system (Mabthera, MabCampath). Other MoAbs inhibit signal transduction (Herceptin) necessary for tumour cell division. MoAbs can target and carry other therapies to tumour cells such as radiotherapy, chemotherapy and toxins. These are referred to as conjugated antibodies. A MoAb conjugated with yttrium is called a radio-labelled MoAb. A summary of the applications of the less frequently used MoAbs and radiolabelled MoAbs can be found in Box 15.1.

MoAbs have a different effect on tumours than chemotherapy. Many MoAbs halt tumour cell growth (cytostatic), as opposed to the cells being destroyed by chemotherapy (cytotoxic). Tumour cell death as a result of a MoAb's action is slower to achieve and occurs via other mechanisms. The tumour may not become larger, and it might take a while before it shrinks and becomes smaller. This is especially true in the treatment of solid tumours. Overall, it is important to make patients aware of how MoAbs can affect tumours, so that the hope that patients have for these promising targeted therapies remains realistic.

Although MoAbs show great therapeutic promise, they are not applicable in all patients with a specific cancer. Not all tumours over express the target receptor/antigen (e.g. only

Box 15.1

Applications of less-frequently used monoclonal antibodies (MoABs) and radiolabelled MoAbs

Therapeutic: targeted to tumour cells:

- Gemtuzumab ozogamicin (Mylotarg). Mylotarg is an agent approved for the treatment of CD33-positive acute myeloid leukaemia (AML) in first relapse
- Cetuximab (Erbitux) is a monoclonal antibody that targets and inhibits epidermal growth factor receptor (EGFR). EGFR is overexpressed in more than 35% of all solid malignant tumours
- Tositumomab (Bexxar) is a monoclonal antibody that has a radioactive substance (iodine-131) attached to it. It binds to the CD20 receptor located on B-lymphocyte cells
- Ibritumomab tiuxetan (Zevalin) is a monoclonal antibody linked to the radioactive isotope yttrium-90. The monoclonal antibody targets the CD20 antigen on mature B cells and B-cell tumors. Radiation is delivered directly to tumour cells

Therapeutic: targeted to vascular endothelial growth receptors (angiogenesis inhibitors):

- Vitaxin binds to a vascular integrin (alpha-v/beta-3) found on the blood vessels of tumours but not on the blood vessels supplying normal tissues. In phase 2 clinical trials
- Bevacizumab (Avastin) is an anti-vascular endothelial growth factor receptor (VEGF) monoclonal antibody for the treatment of solid tumours

20–50% of breast cancers overexpress the Her2 receptor). Depending on tumour type, only some tumours, at a defined maturation stage, express the specific receptor/antigen (e.g. CD20 is expressed by only a subset of B-cell lymphomas).

When MoAbs are administered in the appropriate patient population, they will not be 100% effective for all patients for one or more of the following reasons. Tumour cells are very savvy at surviving and they can change their receptor/antigen status (through down-regulation or shedding of the receptor/antigen) when attacked. Tumour antigens, usually bound to the cell surface, can be spontaneously shed into the circulation. If this occurs, then the MoAb binds to the soluble antigen in the bloodstream, thus being prevented from reaching the tumour. Solid tumours can be quite dense and the circulatory network quite narrow. MoAbs are fairly large molecules and may have difficulty in entering deep into solid tumour masses with low-vessel density.

Patients who are treated with MoAbs may be on long-term treatment, with some receiving this therapy for up to 1 year depending on response, and they be treated more frequently than with other therapies to keep their tumours under control. This has effects on daily life and possibly quality of life.

Vaccines

Vaccines, which have been used since the Middle Ages to prevent infection, can now be used as antitumour therapy. By injecting a weak strain of an antigen, e.g. tumour antigen, memory cells (B lymphocytes) can be stimulated to develop antibodies and subsequently immunity to a specific antigen. There are different types of tumour vaccines. Autologous and allogeneic tumour vaccines may be injected as tumour cell suspensions or are combined with an adjuvant, a substance which by itself is capable of inducing an immune response. BCG is one substance that has been used as an adjuvant. A specific immunization ASI is one type of vaccine showing promise. Vaccination using tumour antigens may incur antitumour immunity. These approaches remain under study and, as yet, there have been no tumour vaccines registered for treating cancer.

Another type of antitumour vaccine approach is to deliver antigens packed in dendrites. Dendrites, the gatekeepers of the immune system, are potent cells that play a principal role in directing immune responses and are antigen-presenting cells capable of stimulating a T-cell-mediated immune response. A dendrite vaccine is a subject of current research, whereby it is loaded with cancer proteins.[11]

The results of this study and many others will offer insights into the ability of vaccine-mediated immune responses to achieve therapeutic benefit as well as providing increased knowledge on effective ways to confer tumour immunity.

ANGIOGENESIS INHIBITORS

Angiogenesis is fundamental to the reproduction, development and repair of blood vessels.[12] Blood vessels are formed from endothelial cells that are stimulated by numerous proangiogenic and antiangiogenic factors. The development of blood vessels for tumour nourishment occurs through the release of several proteins/growth factors directly from the receptors on tumour cell membranes. Blocking tumour cell receptors indirectly or directly may play a role in preventing the process of angiogenesis. MoAbs that block the receptors are one approach. Not all growth factors, receptors and their functions are understood. Therefore, these agents remain under study and have not been registered. Indirect angiogenesis inhibition takes place with thalidomide, an agent that has undergone a rebirth and is showing promise, but it is an agent that is not derived from biological processes and affects angiogenesis very differently than the MoABs. The cytokine IFNα also has indirect angiogenesis inhibition and is used as a treatment for this goal.

Nursing care for patients receiving angiogenesis inhibitors is in its infancy. Nobody currently knows what type of nursing care will be required to manage patients on antiangiogenic treatment.[12]

GENE THERAPY

Gene therapy is one of the most important developments to occur in medicine because it will change modern medicine and the diagnosis and treatment of many diseases. Feasibly, in patients with an hereditary disposition to cancer, gene vaccines could be developed that prevent cancer from occurring. Expanding knowledge in the field of genetics and cancer is also influencing the future of cancer diagnosis and treatment. Cancer is one of approximately 5000 diseases that can be caused by changes in the gene. It is generally believed that tumour growth, in many cases, results from faults in the genes (accumulation of mutations), alteration of cell multiplication (proliferation) and cell specialization (differentiation); e.g. oncogenes and tumour suppressor genes.[13] Gene therapy is the introduction of genetic material into a patients' tissues with the aim of a therapeutic benefit.[14] Transferring genes, which alter cell processes and change the function of the cell or repair genetic alterations, can directly affect the production or the growth of tumour cells. This form of therapy is currently under intensive investigation. Since the gene changes with cancer are complex, it will probably not be effective to correct only one gene and, through this correction, achieve a cure for cancer.

Genes may be marked for recognition and tracking of their behaviour. Gene therapy can reduce multi-drug resistance, induce tumour cell death, improve immunogenicity of tumour cells for destruction or sensitize tumour cells for destruction by other agents. There are several gene therapy approaches but, to this day, none have been registered for the treatment of cancer.

To realize the effects of this therapy, certain developments were needed, such as gene delivery systems. These systems, which use viruses to transport genes into tumour cells, are essential to the success of gene transfer,[14] but are not yet without challenges. Their safety and efficacy are not yet completely assured.

Viral vectors are used as a transfer vehicle for genes because they have the ability to transfect cells with DNA. The vector enters the nucleus of the cell and delivers the gene to the appropriate place in the DNA, in such a way that the gene can be expressed for a period of time. Two broad approaches have been used to deliver genes to cells, namely viral vectors and non-viral vectors, which have different advantages as regards efficiency, ease of production, quality and safety.

Although a number of viruses have been developed, interest has centred on four types: recombinant retroviruses (including lentiviruses), adenoviruses, adeno-associated viruses (AAV) and herpes simplex virus type 1.[15]

Retroviruses are a class of enveloped viruses that, following infection, is reverse transcribed into double-stranded DNA, which then integrates into the host genome and is expressed as a protein. Some retroviruses contain proto-oncogenes, which, when mutated, may cause cancers. Retroviruses can also transform cells by integrating near to a cellular proto-oncogene, or by disrupting a tumour suppresser gene. This event is termed insertional mutagenesis, and, although extremely rare, could still occur when retroviruses are used as vectors. Lentiviruses are a subclass of retroviruses that are able to infect both proliferating and non-proliferating cells.

Adenoviruses are viruses, most of which cause respiratory tract infections. Adenovirus-based vectors are promising vehicles for gene replacement therapy due to their ability to efficiently transduce a wide variety of proliferating and non-proliferating cells for gene replacement therapy.[16] Instead of integrating in the host genome, they replicate, reducing the risk of insertional mutagenesis. Immune responses to the vector might occur, although scientists are continually altering the virus to prevent that from occurring. This means that adenoviruses can, besides gene replacement therapy, become the basis of vaccine delivery vehicles. They are attractive vaccine vectors, as they induce both innate and adaptive immune responses in humans.[17]

Adeno-associated viruses are non-pathogenic human viruses that are dependent on a helper virus, usually an adenovirus, to proliferate. AAV are capable of infecting both dividing and non-dividing cells and integrate into a specific point of the host genome; they are less immunogenic than adenoviruses.[18]

The herpes simplex virus is used as a vector for gene transfer to the nervous system. A particular advantage of the herpes simplex system is that the virus is neurotropic and is therefore suited for gene therapy to the nervous system.[19]

Viral vectors can induce an immunological response to some degree and may have safety risks such as insertional mutagenesis and toxicity problems. Furthermore, their capacity is limited and large-scale production is expensive and fraught with quality control issues and may be difficult to achieve.

Circumventing the immune response to the vector is a major challenge with all vector types. Viral vectors are the most likely to induce an immune response, especially those, like adenovirus and AAV, which are immunogenic. The first immune response occurring after vector transfer emerges from the innate immune system, mainly consisting of a rapid (few hours) inflammatory cytokines and chemokines secretion around the administration site. This reaction is high with adenoviral vectors and almost null with AAV.[20]

DNA can be directly injected into muscle cells or attached to gold particles that are bombarded into the tissue using a gene gun. They are unaffected by the immune response and can be expressed for longer periods of time; this technique is relatively inexpensive.

Strategies for gene therapy and diagnoses

Gene marking

Marker genes are used in haematology to identify abnormal white cells that are present following autologous bone marrow transplantation. By doing this, if the disease exacerbates the leukaemic cells can be examined for their origin.[21]

Multi-drug resistance gene therapy

The multi-drug resistance (MDR) gene is responsible for chemotherapy failing by making tumour cells resistant to chemotherapy. If the tumour cell has the MDR gene, the chemotherapy will be pumped out and the treatment will be ineffective. By inserting the MDR gene into blood and bone marrow cells, they will become resistant to chemotherapy, so that higher doses can be given and life-threatening toxicity can be diminished.

Suicide gene implantation in tumours

This elegant strategy is used to infect tumour cells with the herpes simplex virus and, subsequently, to treat them with ganciclovir, causing tumour cell death. Some limitations of this technique exist, the main one being delivery and extent of transfection.[19] Some success has been seen with gliomas.[22]

Allogeneic bone marrow transplantation as a cure for leukaemia and lymphoma is limited by the development of graft versus host disease (GvHD), an immunological reaction of the donor's T lymphocytes against the host's normal tissues. One option to treat GvHD is the transfer of 'suicide' genes into the donor's T lymphocytes to render them susceptible to prodrug administration. This procedure should permit the elimination of unwanted T lymphocytes in GvHD.[23]

Gene immunotherapy

One way to fight cancer with gene therapy is to increase immunity to cancer cells. Tumour cells could be changed to increase their immunogenicity, whereby immune cells can recognize and destroy them better. This can be done by vaccinating with genetically manipulated tumour cells that produce a cytokine that assists in antigen presentation.[24]

Important aspects of gene therapy

Due to the complexity of gene therapy, it takes place in very few institutes around the world. The introduction of a gene therapy clinical trial has a long route to follow before it can actually be implemented. The government, environmental safety organizations and health departments are usually the first step. This is to establish safety, followed by quality control of the viral vectors. Subsequently, ethical committees, biological safety departments in the institutes and nursing departments evaluate the study.

Toxicity

With gene therapy, a new toxicity profile will be seen for each approach. The toxicity is dependent on the gene, the vector, the target organ and the length of time it is expressed. Specifically, in the adenovirusses, the immune system can be activated and develops an immune response against the therapy, possibly interfering with its activity. An allergic reaction is also feasible.

Long-term effects or effects in the genome are not known and will not be apparent for a long time. Possible long-term effects that could occur are increased incidence of second tumours, effects to germ cells and reactivation of the injected viruses (recombination).

There have been no registered indications for gene therapy as yet. It is still too soon to say what the promise of this therapy is. Nurses have the responsibility of sharing their experiences of preparing and caring for patients with other colleagues, e.g. through publications.

Gene therapy should only be performed in carefully monitored research centres, by trained staff skilled in research and able to evaluate the findings that are emanating from these studies. These groups of healthcare workers carry a great responsibility for enabling the potential of gene therapy. Its administration must be deemed safe for the patient and the environment, and potential side-effects should be identified.[25] As new approaches and gene agents become available, hospitals and other agencies should review these agents diligently to determine whether they should be classified as hazardous.[26] Table 15.2 describes aspects that might need to be considered by a clinical area preparing to integrate gene therapy into practice.

NURSING CARE

The principles of biotherapy nursing need to be integrated into all aspects of oncology nursing. The nursing care of patients who receive biotherapy, which differs greatly from other therapies in terms of its side-effect profile and presentation, has emerged to become a subspecialty of oncology nursing. For example, the three most frequently occurring side-effects of immunotherapy are a flu-like syndrome, mild nausea and vomiting and fatigue. Whereas the three most frequently occurring side-effects of chemotherapy are bone marrow depression, nausea and vomiting and alopecia. To minimize treatment-associated anxiety, patients and their families need a fundamental understanding of the side-effects and their management.

Table 15.2: Actions needed to prepare to integrate gene therapy into a clinical department

Action	Components
Develop a multidisciplinary team to discuss integration on the department	Physicians Scientist Head nurse Staff nurses Specialist nurses Research nurses Infection prevention team Environmental/biological safety officer Laboratory personnel Pharmacy personnel
Integration issues that should be discussed	National guidelines for gene therapy implementation National approval of the gene therapy protocol Educating key personnel How logistics will be coordinated New delivery measures, compatibility issues Safety of formulation and delivery Conditions for safe handling Isolation procedures if using infectious viral vectors What observations and documentation will be done Spill and risk management How healthcare professionals will be registered How to determine the educational need of patients and families about the therapy
Information needed about the gene therapy product	Name of the gene product Vector or carrier of the gene Packaging form Dose or cell dose Stability/storage Reconstitution and dilution Route Precautions Contraindications Expected side-effects Spillage measures Extravasation measures Handling of excreta Disposal of used materials: bed sheets, etc. Onset of action, peak action, duration of action

(continues)

Table 15.2: Actions needed to prepare to integrate gene therapy into a clinical department—cont'd

Action	Components
Management issues	Assess acuity; How many nursing personnel will be needed? Assess new nursing delivery models Contract for boundaries of nursing care delivery Provide a framework for integrating genetics into practice Teach personnel Where will gene therapy be delivered on the department? Who will deliver gene therapy? How will multidisciplinary collaboration be developed? Planning issues
Educational preparation for staff	Basis of genetics Basics of genes and their functions Genetic terminology How are genes isolated and identified: The Genome Project Genetic technologies and their applications Types of gene therapy Vectors and gene transfer techniques Gene therapy administration Gene therapy precautions and safe handling Side-effect assessment and management Isolation techniques

Side-effects

General information

Biological therapy is responsible for a number of side-effects. It is important to look at the type of agent, how it is produced and which biological mechanism is altered or modulated in order to understand which toxicities may occur. Table 15.3 provides a description of common side-effects and possible management strategies, both pharmacological and non-pharmacological.

Mechanism of toxicity

As with many other therapies, the side-effects of biotherapeutic agents are drug-, dose-, schedule- and route-dependent. There are also agent-specific side-effect profiles. It is thought that the side-effects of biotherapeutic agents are the result of the release of secondary cytokines such as tumour necrosis factor (TNF) and IFNγ and/or reactions to the administration of protein. As secondary cytokine release can occur throughout the body, toxicity can be expected in any or all of the organ systems. Side-effects are usually reversible within 24–72 hours following completion of therapy, except for fatigue and skin changes. Nurses should become familiar with the side-effect profiles of individual therapies. No long-term side-effects have been observed.

Patterns of side-effects

Each agent has its own toxicity pattern . It is extremely important to be aware of the patterns of toxicity, which will guide the patient information and nursing care process.

Side effect patterns can be characterized temporally as:

- Cumulative side effects: seen with IL-2. The longer it is administered, the more severe the side-effects are.

- Diminishing numbers and severity of side effects (tachyphylaxis): seen with IFNα.

Table 15.3: Nature and characteristics of common side-effects associated with biological therapy and associated management strategies

Common side-effects	Characteristics as related to biotherapy	Possible pharmacological symptom management strategies	Common non-pharmacological management strategies
1. Chills and rigors	A feeling of being cold followed by goose bumps and uncontrolled shaking until core body temperature has risen. Begins approx. 30 minutes following administration and can last up to 90 minutes. It is often accompanied by increased blood pressure and occasional nausea and vomiting	Pethidine (Demerol) Diazepam	Warmth: hot water bottles, extra blankets, warm drinks Severe chills: warming blankets Provide reassurance
2. Fever	A rise in core body temperature above normal and occurs following chills and rigors. Temperature increases vary per individual. Usually accompanied by headache, tachycardia and hypotension. Often 1–3 hours following injection	Paracetamol Non-steroidal anti-inflammatory drugs (NSAIDs)	Pre- or postmedicate with paracetamol Sponge baths with tepid water Keep the patient as cool as possible Encourage increased food and fluid intake to restore the metabolic and fluid demands of fever such as water, juice and bouillon and light high caloric snacks
3. Sweating	Loss of fluid via the dermis as a cooling mechanism. Following sweating, temperature will decrease	None	Keep patient dry to prevent further cooling and rebound temperature elevations Encourage increased fluid intake to replace insensible fluid loss
4. Body pains	Headache, muscle pain, joint pain. Bone pain usually occurs concurrently with fever	Paracetamol	Provide encouragement, warmth and comfort measures
5. Malaise	Feeling unwell, a diminished desire to undertake activities, including self-care activities. Occurs concurrently with fever	None	Provide encouragement, comfort and reassurance. Encourage a good diet and mobility, not to stay the whole day in bed

(continues)

Table 15.3: Nature and characteristics of common side-effects associated with biological therapy and associated management strategies—cont'd

Common side-effects	Characteristics as related to biotherapy	Possible pharmacological symptom management strategies	Common non-pharmacological management strategies
6. Fatigue	Different than malaise. Diminished energy level (some patients complain about heavy legs). Affects cognition: can cause difficulty concentrating or forgetfulness. Can be accompanied by emotional lability and mood changes. Can be cumulative and dose-limiting. Can occur anytime following administration. Life-disrupting severity, altered sleep patterns[31]	Sedatives, if related to altered sleeping patterns and frequent dreaming. Antidepressants. Stimulants	Interventions for fatigue: see Ch. 30. Rule out thyroid dysfunction. Rule out anaemia. Monitor: psychosocial status, mood, depression, sleeping patterns, neurological status. Encourage adequate sleep hygiene
7. Allergic reactions	An immune reaction to foreign proteins usually occurring 1–120 minutes following administration: generalized flush, urticaria, tickle in throat, desire to urinate or defecate, feeling of impending doom, followed by pallor or cyanosis may precede the reaction[36]	As directed: varies per institution	Provide encouragement, comfort and reassurance. Slowing the infusion rate if applicable
8. Dyspnoea	Increased respiratory rate due to the metabolic needs of fever or due to extreme fatigue. Usually occurs after a couple of days of therapy	None	Provide encouragement, comfort and reassurance. Provide fans, positioning breathing techniques, relaxation and O$_2$ p.r.n.
9. Cough	Can be related to leucocyte invasion in the lung in the presence of lung metastases. Usually occurs after a couple of days of therapy	Codeine. Bronchodilators	Provide encouragement, comfort and reassurance. Keep room air humidified

10. Altered appetite	A feeling of not wanting to eat, eating less, eating differently, full bloated feeling in the stomach. Can be accompanied by weight loss. Can begin anytime	Metoclopramide as prokinetic could improve bloating	See Ch. 29. Weight loss >3 kg, refer to dietitian Consider supplemental foods and vitamins
11. Altered taste	Food tastes different, altered perception salt and sweet sensations. Can begin anytime	None	Try foods that taste different or have little taste (cool, crisp foods such as cold fruit, drinks, yoghurt, instant breakfast)
12. Odour intolerance	Intolerance of scents that were acceptable prior to therapy	None	Avoid cooking garlic, meat or other strong smelling foods in the patient's presence Provide scent-free environment
13. Nausea	An unpleasant feeling; may be accompanied by sweating, pallor and followed by vomiting. Can begin anytime	Metoclopramide Stemetil (prochlorperazine) Motilium (domperidone) Note: dexamethasone should not be used as it can diminish the effect of immunotherapy	Encourage the patient to relax, take deep breaths, drink plenty of fluids See Ch. 20
14. Vomiting	Expelling stomach contents under pressure. Can begin anytime.	See nausea. If severe: 5HT$_3$ antagonists	Same as nausea
15. Diarrhoea	Increased frequency and /or loss of firmness of stool. Usually begins several days following start therapy.	Immodium (loperamide)	Encourage increased fluid intake, if necessary supplemental fluids IV Encourage a bland diet

(continues)

Table 15.3: Nature and characteristics of common side-effects associated with biological therapy and associated management strategies—cont'd

Common side-effects	Characteristics as related to biotherapy	Possible pharmacological symptom management strategies	Common non-pharmacological management strategies
16. Altered mucous membranes	Reddened, inflamed, oedematous mucous membranes, open areas in the corners of the mouth. Usually begins a few days following start of therapy	None	Rinse the mouth regularly with saline, keep the teeth clean, and prevent infection Have patients see the dentist prior to treatment if pre-existing problems are present
17. Local skin change injection site reactions	Erythematous, raised lesions at the site of injection Hardened tissue under erythematous areas. Can begin anytime	Non-steroidal anti-inflammatory creams (not always available)	Avoid injecting in red, hardened areas which may detriment absorption of agents Use smaller-gauge needle Applying cool or warm compresses to injection site
18. Generalized skin changes	Redness, dryness, rash, itch, dry and/or wet desquamation. Usually begins a few days following start of therapy. Psoriatic flares (IFNα)[39] Note: be alert that rash on the chest might be related to an allergic reaction	Consider antihistamines Largactil (chlorpromazine) for severe itch	Shower or bath in lukewarm water Avoid hot baths or showers, soap products, alcohol-based skin lotions and non-perfumed bath products and encourage adequate oral hygiene When bathing, completely moisten skin, pat dry, immediately apply an oil-based crème Oatmeal baths for pruritus Encourage patients to wear sun-protective clothing
19. Hair changes	Hair thinning <50% and/or unmanageable hair beginning usually 3 months after start date 1st treatment. Vitiligo[37]	None	Have hair cut shorter if necessary or desired

		Adjust medication with antihypertensives p.r.n.	Consult cardiologist prior to therapy and p.r.n.. Possible termination of antihypertensives. Fluid replacement therapy p.r.n. Follow blood pressure over time Teach interventions for dizziness
20.	Cardiovascular changes	Increased heart rate and deceased blood pressure and dizziness during fever Increased blood pressure during chills Long-term therapy with IFNα can decrease blood pressure and cause dizziness	
21.	Fluid imbalances	Sweating, increased fluid needs due to fever, oedema due to increased capillary mobility, changes in urine; diminished amount, darker colour and increased odour. Can occur at anytime.	Lasix (furosemide) for oedema p.r.n.	Fluid replacement therapy p.r.n.
22.	Leucopenia	Decreased numbers of certain leucocyte populations. Can occur anytime following the first injection.	None	Dose reductions of causal agent, or temporarily stop therapy p.r.n.
23.	Thrombocytopenia	Decreased numbers of thrombocytes. Can occur anytime following the first injection.	None	Dose reduction of causal agent , or stop therapy
24.	Renal dysfunction	Increased creatinine, blood urea nitrogen (BUN). Can occur anytime following the first injection	None, avoid NSAIDs	Same as above; encourage fluid intake
25.	Liver dysfunction	Increased alkaline phosphatase (ALP), aspartate transaminase (ASAT), alanine aminotransferase (ALAT), lactate dehydrogenase (LDH). Can occur anytime following the first injection	None	Same as above
26.	Autoimmune dysfunction	Primarily thyroiditis. Can occur anytime but usually not in the first weeks of therapy	Corticosteroids Thyroxine	Be aware of signs of hypo- and hyperthyroidism

(continues)

Table 15.3: Nature and characteristics of common side-effects associated with biological therapy and associated management strategies—cont'd

Common side-effects	Characteristics as related to biotherapy	Possible pharmacological symptom management strategies	Common non-pharmacological management strategies
27. Depression	Mood changes, suicidal ideation, rapidly arising mood disorders[38]	Antidepressants	Primarily with long-term IFNα therapy. Monitor psychosocial status monthly. Encourage patient to express feelings of anger and anxiety about therapy
28. Neurological changes	Mental slowing, problems with concentration, lethargy, vivid dreams, confusion	None	Awareness of the temporary nature. Associated with cytokine therapy primarily. Encourage ambulation and changes of scenery, relaxation exercises, and report any changes of neurological status
29. Changed sexual activity	Altered desire Erectile dysfunction Can start following the first treatment	None	Awareness of the temporary nature of this side-effect
30. Vascular leak	Increased vascular permeability, extravasation of fluid and protein into capillary and tissue beds	Discontinue antihypertensive prior to initiating therapy Vasopressor p.r.n.	Weigh daily and assess for fluid retention Monitor urinary volume Encourage fluid intake Instruct patient when to notify Resolves quickly after ending therapy

There is a biphasic pattern with IFN. Severe acute toxicity is seen on initiating therapy, followed by a tolerance for certain toxicities developing over time.

- Unchanging side-effects: seen with HGFs. If there are side-effects, they are the same each day it is administered.

- First-dose toxicity (FDT): infusion-related side-effects are seen with MoAbs and vary with the agent given. Generally, most of the expected toxicity occurs during the infusion. The infusion-related side-effects are more severe with the first infusion, as often a loading dose is given. FDT is seen in ±40% of all patients who receive MoAbs. Long-term side-effects have not yet been characterized as most patients who have been treated with these agents have had little long-term follow-up.

Note: Patterns of toxicity have not been established for vaccines, gene therapy and many angiogenesis inhibitors as yet.

The most frequently occurring side-effect of immunotherapy is the flu-like syndrome that consists of chills and rigors, fever, sweating, diffuse body pains and malaise. This is a distinguishing side-effect of immunotherapy. Please refer back to Table 15.1 for possible side-effects of immunotherapy

Specific information about treatment with IFNα and its nursing care

One of the most frequently administered immunological agents is IFNα. It is most often prescribed as long-term subcutaneous therapy. Scheduling is characterized by an initiation and maintenance phase. The initiation phase is 4 weeks and is characterized by daily intensive subcutaneous/intravenous dosing (daily × 5 or daily × 7). The maintenance phase begins in week 5 and can extend from 1 to 5 years, depending on the type of cancer. Maintenance is characterized by a less-intensive dose, either 3 times/week, daily × 5 or daily. Patients who receive this treatment must be provided with ongoing education to assist them to cope with the therapy and its side-effects: i.e. the side-effect pattern with IFNα is more intensive during the first weeks, tapering off during maintenance. A graduated teaching programme is

advised. Educational programmes using the principles of self-management and self-efficacy, such as those used to initiate and maintain insulin for diabetics, should be considered.

Patients are overwhelmed at the beginning of therapy and need vigilant observation to assist them to cope with side-effect management. An example is given in Case Study 15.1.

During the toxicity assessment, Mrs J was asked about the timing, length and severity of the chills and fever, as well as the time of paracetamol ingestion, sleeping and general well-being. Pharmacological and non-pharmacological interventions should be adapted as needed, and teaching reinforced. She was encouraged to call back during the week if necessary, and was advised to return to clinic on a weekly basis for the first month, which is consistent with current practice.

After the first month, when the maintenance phase begins, patients should have all teaching

CASE STUDY 15.1

Mrs J was to receive adjuvant therapy with IFNα for 2 years. Prior to treatment initiation, she was taught about IFN, self-injection and the side-effects. She returned home with written materials to read in preparation for the next visit. Subsequently, during the next session, she was taught how to self-inject herself. She felt so confident in her ability to self-inject that she chose to do so at home before going to bed that evening. (Night-time dosing has been suggested in the literature as patients might sleep through most of the side-effects. Note: be aware that not all patients sleep well as a result. Ongoing evaluation of the time of administration is essential.) The day following the first injection, Mrs J called the nurse to relate her experience with the first dose. The nurse assessed the toxicity. Mrs J stated that at the time of injection, she took a premedication of 1000 mg of paracetamol. Ninety minutes following injection, she began to feel cold, followed by chills and rigors that lasted over 1 hour. She couldn't believe how the bed was shaking. Three hours after injecting, she had a fever of 39.4°C and vomited twice. She took 2 more paracetamol suppositories and tried to sleep. After sweating profusely, 2 hours later the fever had broken and she began to feel a bit better. In the morning when she woke, she felt sluggish and not completely rested.

reinforced and be prepared for a shift to chronic side-effects. The chronic symptoms experienced by patients on IFN include fatigue (70–100% of patients), anorexia (40–70%) and neuropsychiatric symptoms (up to 30%) which appear to be dose-related, and cumulative, worsening over time.[27] In general, patients with cancer have a higher risk of developing clinical depression.[28] A minority of patients on IFNα therapy become depressed, in some cases leading to suicide. A variety of educational materials, videotapes and publications are available to assist in teaching patients.[29] Monthly appointments should be made to support patients in integrating the therapy into their daily lives. Monthly or more frequent assessments of fatigue and psychosocial concerns are imperative. Discussing roles in the family, return-to-work issues and dealing with side-effects are essential to assist patients in coping with treatment and in maintaining quality of life. Adjustment to both side-effects and treatment regimen has been characterized by apprehension and impatience.[30] Patients and their families must be made aware of all adverse reactions and be taught when they should contact healthcare professionals with their concerns. Individualized exercise programmes can be developed for those at risk for deconditioning due to fatigue. A thorough psychosocial assessment should be done at each visit and referrals to the social worker/psychologist made as necessary. Boredom is often associated with cognitive fatigue and inability to accomplish work and other tasks. Finding ways to manage and intervene with the compounding effect of boredom on the perception of fatigue is an important implication for practice.[31]

Specific issues to be addressed in the nursing assessment

Before patients receive treatment with biological agents, a thorough assessment should take place, just as with any other therapy. Each biological agent has its own mechanism of action and side-effects. Modules that address the unique issues with each agent, such as the setting, dose and schedule as well as nature of the therapy, should be used as an adjunct to the basic nursing assessment. It is essential to do baseline screening for all disease-related symptoms. A comprehensive toxicity assessment tool, such as the National Cancer Institute of Canada (NCIC) toxicity grading scale, could be used for this purpose. Subsequently, an in-depth assessment of existing symptoms as well as those symptoms that patients would be expected to develop as a result of the agent should be taken. This will eventually assist in evaluating treatment-related toxicity: i.e. with IFN, ask about the patient's history of fevers and what their normal fever temperature is. Patients who will receive IL-2 are at risk for vascular leak syndrome; therefore, is there a history of fluid retention or pre-existing conditions that place the patient at greater risk for oedema?

A history of autoimmune illnesses, infections and allergies gives insight into the present functioning of the immune system. Underlying cardiac problems, psychiatric problems or nutritional or weight loss problems can contribute to or place patients at risk for some treatment toxicities, and may be indicators of a poor prognosis. The presence of tumour sweats can compound fever from therapies and patients may have pre-existing dehydration.

Although previous experiences with cancer therapies, specifically immunotherapies, are not contraindicated, they can give you information about earlier side-effect profiles which may be a predictor of future side-effects.

Assessing the patients' ability to cope and ability to perform self-care, especially in relation to outpatient subcutaneous therapy is extremely important. Many patients are unable to cope with these therapies if they live alone, especially the elderly. What or who are the patient's support systems? Does the patient live far from the healthcare facility? Who can the patient contact on short notice when in need. Is the family physician up to date on the treatment and its plan as well as community nurses? Do patients have the appropriate support and resources in the home for dealing with the side-effects?

A history of current medications – specifically, antihypertensives, corticosteroids and NSAIDs (non-steroidal anti-inflammatory drugs) – should be taken. The following drugs could affect either the biological response modifier's mechanism of action or the side-effects:

- corticosteroids, by their inhibitory effect on immune function
- NSAIDs such as naproxen, ibuprofen or diclofenac, by their effect on white blood cells and anti-inflammatory effects
- antihypertensives, by increasing the risk of hypotension
- antidepressants, by their possible effect on antiemetic pathways.

Assessing the level of knowledge about the treatment and the treatment plan as well as personal capabilities will assist in developing strategies for patient education. Ongoing assessment of patients is to be determined by the therapy and its pattern of toxicity. Close monitoring and constant evaluation of patients are key to the management of toxicities.[32]

Administration

As new biological treatments are continually entering the workplace, nurses should familiarize themselves with the issues and concerns specific to their use, especially because many of these issues differ from those of conventional chemotherapy. Nurses should be aware of the proper method of administering the agent. In addition, nurses should educate patients and their families about the course of treatment, possible side-effects, planned interventions for those side-effects and potential disease response.[33]

Routes

There are many ways biological agents can be given, although the oral route is the least likely. Almost all of the agents are proteins and the molecules are too unstable for oral formulation.

BCG is given intravesically for superficial bladder cancer. BCG is also used as an adjuvant (co-stimulatory agent) for some vaccines, whereby the subcutaneous route is chosen. The cytokines/HGFs are presently most frequently given via the subcutaneous route and on an outpatient basis. The monoclonal antibodies are all given intravenously. Vaccines can be given either subcutaneously or intradermally. Gene therapy is now given intravenously, but

has also been given as inhalations, subcutaneous injections and when it reaches its potential will have some very unique delivery systems. The angiogenetic inhibitors are given intravenously but thalidomide is a tablet and differs in its composition and mechanism of action (it is also not a biological agent)

Preparation and safety of biological agents

The Oncology Nursing Society (ONS) of America has published chemotherapy and biotherapy safe handling guidelines. Herein, one finds instructions for preparing biological agents in general. There are no specific guidelines for the administration of each biological agent.

Usually only the direct subcutaneous injectables are prepared by nurses or patients, such as the HGFs, IL-2 and IFNα. These agents are made available in ampoules or prefilled syringes of solution or lyophilized powder, a dissolvable protein with diluent. Other agents for direct infusion are prepared by the pharmacy or are available as a solution with the cytokines.

The ONS chemotherapy and biotherapy guidelines refer to the *IARC Monographs Overall Evaluations of Carcinogenicity to Humans*, Volumes 1–88[34] for toxicology of biological agents. This list contains all hazards evaluated to date, according to the type of hazard posed and to the type of exposure. INF and thalidomide are considered to be hazardous agents and, as such, should be handled according to strict precautions for healthcare professionals, as designated by current policy within their institutes. All other agents receive no mention and may have been on the market too briefly and have limited toxicology data. Most biological agents, as stated earlier, are proteins and are therefore easily biodegradable. The majority of biological agents do not affect the DNA, and therefore are not considered genotoxic. It is best to avoid direct contact with skin and avoid generating aerosols. It is important to teach patients who self-inject at home to dispose of their materials in accordance with local policies. More research is needed to establish safety profiles with each agent.

The issue of safe handling of gene therapy and their viral transfer methods remains obscure, and nurses need to consult with local biological safety advisors as well as pharmacy to provide the safest conditions under which the staff and the environment are exposed to these agents.

Premedication

Almost all agents, except for BCG, vaccines and gene therapy, require a premedication to prepare patients for either initial toxicity or infusion-related events.

For the cytokines, IL-2, IFNα and GM-CSF, premedication with paracetamol will help reduce and delay the chills and fever that begin 45–90 minutes following administration. With GCSF, premedication is not needed unless the patient has developed a flu-like syndrome with prior injections.

MoAbs have an infusion-related event approximately 40% of the time and the characteristics of the event differ with each agent. Therefore the premedication varies according to agent. Patients should be monitored carefully throughout treatment. Vital signs (i.e. temperature, pulse, respiration and blood pressure) should be taken at baseline, before infusion, as needed during infusion and immediately at the end of infusion. These measurements should be repeated, as needed, for as long as 4 hours after treatment. Infusion-related symptoms generally occur shortly after the start of the infusion and are resolved by halting the infusion and providing supportive therapy. When controlled, the infusion may be restarted, if deemed safe, at a slower rate. Excellent teaching materials are available from each of the pharmaceutical industries that have developed MoAbs.

Vaccine therapy has few side-effects associated with administration. Premedications are not required.

Coordination of care

The most notable issues in ambulatory oncology nursing are time, setting, staffing and continuity of care. The chronic multisystem nature of cancer makes it difficult to manage, especially during periods of intense therapy.[34a] The preparation, education and delivery of these agents challenge nurses to provide quality care. Assessing the home situation and the ability to self-monitor at home for administration and side-effects is essential. Assuring that all the prerequisites are in place for patients to self-inject takes time and coordination as well as teaching patients to manage side-effects of therapy administered on an inpatient or ambulatory setting. Prerequisites such as equipment needed to treat at home, education about the treatment and its side-effects, self-assessment, follow-up by community nursing, contact with family physician, prescriptions for necessary comedication, blood slips and appointments at laboratories close to home, telephone numbers for emergencies and report to on-call physicians are just a few of the tasks to be performed to achieve coordination of care for patients receiving biological therapies.

THE FUTURE

What will the future bring with biological therapies? Knowledge of microbiology will increase and influence the development of more unique compounds with unique mechanisms of action. With the discovery of DNA microarrays, the pathologists of the future may be able to detect cancer using gene chips before tumours have formed. Possibly, by altering genes with prophylactic gene therapy, tumours may be prevented. Pharmacogenetics will be able to determine individual responses to therapy. This might lead to making many current forms of therapy for some obsolete. Tumour immunization in childhood; is that the future if we can detect cancer predisposition and vaccinate against it? People who are at high risk for developing cancer may be identified and could receive prophylactic vaccines.[35] The sky is the limit if you just imagine the limitless possibilities of gene therapy, but they will all have consequences for oncology nurses.

Novel delivery of cytokines

Immunotherapy with cytokines is being given in new forms. Pegylating cytokines increases their half-life and diminishes the need for frequent administration. This has already been introduced to the clinical arena in the form of pegylated IFNα and GCSF. Other forms will follow.

Radioimmunotherapy

Agents called radioimmunoconjugates have already entered the clinical arena. These are MoAbs that are linked with a radioactive isotope such as iodine-131 or yttrium-90. By infusing the MoAb that is tumour cell specific and combining it with small amounts of radioactivity, tumour-targeted therapy takes place via two mechanisms: the action of the MoAb and the action of the radioisotope. Two agents are nearing registration: tositumomab and ibritumomab for use in lymphoma. These agents will have safe handling issues for nurses. Please refer to local guidelines.

CONCLUSION

It is difficult to envisage all the possible implications that new developments in biological therapy will have on oncology nursing. Although there is hope that genetics and gene therapy will offer promise for a future diagnosis and treatment of cancer, one must keep in mind that cancer is the result of many complex changes within the cell, making this goal a challenging one. There are so many new approaches developing that will continually challenge the delivery of quality nursing care.

Biotherapy will remain innovative, reflecting scientific discoveries and requiring the nurse to be flexible but to offer structure to patients. The nursing process will remain the best framework to assist nurses in providing this structure while serving the needs of professional enhancement in oncology nursing.[25] Nurses who work in clinical trials, as well as nurse practitioners and clinical nurse specialists, are at the cutting edge of these new developments and of developing the nursing care of the future.

REFERENCES

1. Oldham R. Cancer biotherapy: general principles. In: Oldham R, ed. Principles of cancer biotherapy. 3rd edn. Dordrecht, Netherlands: Kluwer Academic Press; 1998:1–15.
2. Reiger PT, ed. Biotherapy and overview in biotherapy. In: A comprehensive overview. Boston: Jones and Bartlett; 2001:3–23.
3. Hall S. A commotion in the blood: life, death and the immune system. New York, NY: Henry Holt and Company; 1997.
4. Cantell K, Hervonen S, Cavalletto L, et al. Human leukocyte interferon production, purification and animal experiments. In: Waymouth C, ed. In vitro. Baltimore: Baltimore Tissue Culture Association; 1975:35–38.
5. Cuaron L, Thompson J. The interferons. In: Trahan Reiger P, ed. Biotherapy: a comprehensive overview. Maine: Jones and Bartlett, 2001:125–194.
6. Atzpodien J, Poliwoda H, Kirtchner H. Alpha interferon and interleukin-2 in renal cell carcinoma: studies in non-hospitalised patients. Semin Oncol 1991; 18(5 Suppl 7):108–112.
7. Jenkins J, Wheeler V. Gene therapy for cancer. Cancer Nurs 1994; 17(6):447–456.
8. Van Wijk A. Pharmacokinetics. Early clinical studies group research nurses. Manual for research nurses. In: Van Wijk A, Batchelor DM, Dubbelman AC, eds. The Netherlands: Koopmans; 2001:79–85.
9. Batchelor D, de Gast GC, Mallo HA. Biotherapie: In Van Den Berg J, van Rees, eds. de Kankerpatient. 5th edn. The Netherlands: Bohn Stafleu; 2001:155–179.
10. Batchelor D. How do monoclonal antibodies work? Medscape Nurs 2004; April 14, www.medscape.com
11. DeMeyer E, Barr J. Dendritic cells: the sentry cells of the immune system. Educational Monograph. Oncol Educ Serv 2003:18–20.
12. Camp-Sorrel D. Angiogenesis: the fifth cancer treatment modality. Oncol Nurs Forum 2003; 30(6):934–942.
13. Blankenstein T. 1994 Increasing tumor immunogenicity by genetic modification. Eur J Cancer 1994; 30(A8):1182–1187.
14. Young A, Kerr DJ. Genetic and immunological therapy for cancer. J R Soc Med 2000; 93:10–14.
15. Robbins PD, Tahara H, Ghivizzani SC. Viral vectors for gene therapy. Trends Biotechnol 1998;16(1):35–40.
16. Cao H, Koehler DR, Hu J. Adenoviral vectors. Viral Immunol 2004;17(3):327–333.
17. Tatsis N, Ertl HC. Adenoviruses as vaccine vectors. Mol Ther 2004; 10(4):616–629.
18. Buning H, Braun-Falco M, Hallek M. Progress in the use of adeno-associated viral vectors for gene therapy. Cells Tissues Organs 2004; 177(3):139–150.
19. Yenari MA, Sapolsky RM. Gene therapy in neurological disease. Methods Mol Med 2004; 104:75–88.
20. Bessis N, GarciaCozar FJ, Boissier MC. Immune responses to gene therapy vectors: influence on vector function and effector mechanisms. Gene Ther 2004; 11(Suppl 1):S10–17.
21. Larochelle A, Dunbar CE. Genetic manipulation of hematopoietic stem cells. Semin Hematol 2004; 41(4):257–271.

22. Immonen A, Vapalahti M, Tyynela K, et al. AdvHSV-tk gene therapy with intravenous ganciclovir improves survival in human malignant glioma: a randomised, controlled study. Mol Ther 2004; 10(5):967–972.

23. Introna M, Rambaldi A. Suicide gene therapy and the control of graft-vs-host disease. Best Pract Res Clin Haematol. 2004; 17(3):453–463.

24. Alves A, Vibert E, Trajcevski S, et al. Adjuvant interleukin-12 gene therapy for the management of colorectal liver metastases. Cancer Gene Ther 2004; 11(12):782–789.

25. Batchelor D. Genetics and cancer: the future impact on oncology nursing. Oncol Nurs Today 1997; 2(1):

26. Blecher CS, Glynn-Tucker E, McDiarmid, Newton S. Safe handling of hazardous drugs. In: Polovich, ed. Chemotherapy and biotherapy guidelines and recommendations. Pittsburg, PA: Oncology Nursing Society; 2002.

27. Weiss K. Safety profile of interferon-alpha therapy. Semin Oncol 1998;25(Suppl 1):9–13.

28. Valentine AD, Meyers CA, Kling MA, et al. Mood and cognitive side effects of interferon alfa therapy. Semin Oncol 1998; 25(Suppl 1):39–47.

29. Moldawer N. High dose interleukin-2 therapy for metastatic renal cell carcinoma: administration in a non-intensive care unit setting in the oncology ward. Biother Consid Oncol Nurs 2004; 7(1):5–8.

30. Garvey E, Matutat R, Bolten D. 1983 Care of the patient undergoing interferon therapy. Cancer Nurs 1983; 8:303–306.

31. Porock D, Junger JA. Just go with the flow: a qualitative study of fatigue in biotherapy. Eur J Cancer Care 2004; 13(4):356–361.

32. Brophy L, Sharp E. Physical symptoms of combination biotherapy: a quality of life issue. Oncol Nurs Forum Suppl 1991; 18(1):25–30.

33. Shannon-Dorcy K. Nursing implications of Mylotarg®: a novel antibody-targeted chemotherapy for CD33+ acute myeloid leukemia in first relapse. Oncol Nurs Forum 2002; 29(4):E52–59.

34. Brown KH, Esper P, Keeleher LO, et al, eds Chemotherapy and biotherapy guidelines for practice. Pittsburg PA: Oncology Nursing Society Publication; 2001.

34a. Seeley K, DeMeyer E. Nursing care of patients receiving Campath. Clin J Oncol Nurs 2002; 6(3): 138–143.

35. Timmerman J. Levy R. The history of the development of vaccines for the treatment of lymphoma. Clin Lymphoma 1(2):129–139.

36. Kosits C, Callaghan M. Rituximab: a new monoclonal antibody therapy for non-Hodgkin's lymphoma. Oncol Nurs Forum 2000; 27(1):51–59.

37. Fox V, Guindon K. Cutaneous reactions associated with alpha interferon therapy. Clin J Oncol Nurs 2000; 4(4):164–168.

38. Gool A, Kruit WHJ, Cornelissen JJ, et al. Management of psychiatric Adverse events with immunotherapy with interferon alpha. Acta Neuropsychiatrica 1999; 11:120–124.

39. Stafford-Fox V, Guindon K. Cutaneous reactions associated with alpha interferon therapy. Clin J Oncol Nurs 2000; 4(4):164–168.

CHAPTER 16

Bone Marrow Transplantation

BARRY QUINN AND MOIRA STEPHENS

CHAPTER CONTENTS

Introduction	329	Anaemia	343
		Graft versus host disease	343
History of bone marrow transplants	330	Electrolyte imbalance/renal failure	344
		Hepatic toxicity/veno-occlusive	
Principles of bone marrow		disease	345
transplantation	330	Mucositis/gastrointestinal toxicity	345
		Psychological and spiritual issues	345
Types of transplant	331		
Haematopoetic stem cell transplant	331	Multi-professional team work	346
Tissue typing	332		
Donor issues	333	Long-term side effects	346
Harvesting and cryopreservation of		Physical symptoms and restrictions	347
stem cells	334	Fertility	347
High-dose treatment in preparation		Cataracts	347
for HSCT	335	Secondary malignancies	347
Allogeneic transplants with reduced			
conditioning regimen	337	Follow-up care	347
The transplant process	337	Immunity and vaccination post	
Pre transplant	337	transplant	348
Engraftment period	339		
		Survivorship issues	348
Supportive care	339		
		Conclusion	349
Short-term side effects and their			
management	340	References	349
Immunosuppression	340		
Thrombocytopenia and bleeding			
disorders	343		

INTRODUCTION

Blood and marrow (stem cell) transplantation (BMT) is now used to treat a wide variety of malignant and non-malignant conditions, including haematological and non-haematological disorders. The overall aim of transplantation is to ablate (clear) the existing marrow and to replace it with healthy stem cells.[1]

Since the introduction of transplantation, much progress has been made in attempting to reduce the toxicities associated with the treatment while ensuring the removal of residual disease. The transplant team are required to balance the desire to cure or induce long-term remission and improve the quality of a person's life without the risk of increased treatment-related morbidity and mortality.

Many nurses choose to commit most of their careers to working in this constantly challenging and developing field of cancer care. Nurses specializing in transplant care can work in a variety of roles, including ward-based nurse, clinical nurse specialist, research nurse, transplant coordinator, donor coordinator, nurse manager or nurse consultant. Nurses who are not working directly in the transplant setting will still care for patients who are preparing for their transplant or who are experiencing transplant-related morbidity. Whatever their role, all cancer nurses encountering patients undergoing bone marrow transplants require a high level of clinical and psychological skill so as to support patients and their families through treatments that are associated with a substantial risk of long-term morbidity and mortality.

This chapter will outline the history of bone marrow transplantation, principles of treatment, types of transplant, procedures, supportive care, side effects and follow-up issues related to this complex area of cancer care.

HISTORY OF BONE MARROW TRANSPLANTS

The use of bone marrow transplantation was first documented as early as the 19th century when medical practitioners attempted to use this poorly understood treatment option as a last attempt to treat disease.[2] At that time, bone marrow rich in stem cells was injected and sometimes fed to patients in an attempt to treat disease.[2] By the early 1960s, bone marrow transplantation was beginning to be used to treat haematological diseases and, through the work of clinicians such as George Mathe[3] and Donall Thomas,[4] many advances were made. Further developments, including a better understanding of chemotherapy agents, tissue typing and supportive therapies such as antibacterial, antifungals, antiviral and growth factors, have enabled what was once an experimental procedure to become a widely established treatment for a variety of serious disorders.[1]

Up until the 1980s, stem cells were harvested from bone marrow cavities, but new developments have enabled circulating peripheral stem cells (found in the bloodstream) to be collected and harvested for use in the transplant process.[5]

During the 1990s, transplantation developed further to include the use of stem cells collected from the umbilical cords of newborn babies,[6] although the collection and storage of umbilical cord blood remains controversial. Due to the insufficient number of stem cells found in umbilical cord blood, such transplants are generally restricted to the paediatric field.[7]

The number of transplants being performed throughout Europe has increased dramatically and, in 2001, the European Group for Blood and Marrow Transplantation recorded nearly 20,000 transplants.[8] Blood and marrow transplantation is an increasingly important curative treatment in the management of a wide range of diseases, including haematological malignancies, breast, lung and testis cancer and autoimmune and non-malignant haematological disorders.[8]

Bone marrow transplantation may be necessary when the bone marrow does not function correctly (as in aplastic anaemia or sickle cell disease), when it is diseased (as in leukaemia) or when it is suppressed following intensive treatment.[9] Bone marrow can be replaced by the patient's own cells (autologous transplant) or by donor cells (allogeneic transplant). Specific conditions for which blood or marrow stem cell transplantation may be indicated are listed in Box 16.1.

PRINCIPLES OF BONE MARROW TRANSPLANTATION

The underlying rationale for stem cell transplantation is based on two key principles:

1 The dose intensity of most chemotherapeutic agents is limited by dose-related marrow toxicity.

2 Transplanted stem cells reconstitute (replenish) the patient's haemopoietic and immunological system after high-dose chemotherapy and/or total body irradiation.

Before high-dose treatment is given, stem cells are removed from the patient or selected donor and harvested. Following high-dose chemotherapy ± radiotherapy, harvested stem

Transplantation indications

Autologous
Accepted indications:
Relapsed non-Hodgkin's lymphoma (intermediate and high grade)
Relapsed Hodgkin's lymphoma
Acute myeloid leukaemia (poor risk factor first or second complete remission with no allogenic option)
Multiple myeloma

Possible indications:
Relapsed germ cell tumours
Ewing's sarcoma
Neuroblastoma
Soft tissue sarcoma
Auto-immune disease (multiple sclerosis, rheumatoid arthritis, systemic lupus erythematosus)

Allogenic
Acute myeloid leukaemia (poor risk first or second complete remission)
Acute lymphoblastic leukaemia (poor risk first or second complete remission)
Severe aplastic anaemia
Chronic myeloid leukaemia
Myelodysplasia
Multiple myeloma (stage II/III)
Primary immunodeficiency syndromes
Thalassaemia
Sickle-cell disease
Inborn errors of metabolism
Relapsed aggressive non-Hodgkin's lymphoma
Relapsed Hodgkin's lymphoma

Source: Provan et al.[10]

cells are transplanted back into the patient. These infused stem cells find their way to the marrow and repopulate. The mechanism by which this occurs is unknown.[1]

TYPES OF TRANSPLANT

Haemopoietic stem cell transplantation

Haemopoietic stem cell transplantion (HSCT) refers to any procedure that involves trans-

planting the stem cell population into a recipient (the patient), with the intent to repopulate or replace the haemopoietic system, either totally or partially, for transient or permanent periods of time.[10] HSCT may be autologous or allogeneic. Key aspects of both types of HSCT are compared in Table 16.1.

Autografts

Autologous stem cell transplantation involves rescuing the patient from high-dose chemotherapy with or without radiotherapy using the patient's own stem cells collected from the bone marrow or peripheral blood. Autografting is usually used, and seems to work more effectively, after chemotherapy has induced a state of remission, i.e. where there is no detectable disease.[1] Because patients are being 'rescued' with their own stem cells, the procedure is generally uncomplicated and is associated with low transplant-related mortality.[7] There is, however, a risk that the transplanted cells may contain malignant cells. For this reason the harvested cells may be purged of any residual disease by treating them with immunomagnetic approaches, monocolonal antibodies or chemotherapy (known as negative selection) or by purposefully reinfusing only cells carrying the cluster differentiation 34 (CD34+) receptor, which act as the precursors to haemopoietic cells (known as positive selection).[9,11]

Allografts

Allogeneic stem cell transplantation involves the administration of bone marrow or peripheral blood stem cells from a source other than the patient himself. The source may be a close family member (a matched sibling donor or a partially matched family donor known as a mismatched donor). In the case of a related donor, transplants may be carried out using a twin (sygenic), a sibling, a member of the extended family or indeed a parent (haploidentical). The ideal donor is a matched family member but, in the absence of a family donor, national and international registries can be searched so as to find an unrelated donor (matched unrelated donor, MUD). Most countries in Europe have national registries and the IBMTR (International Bone Marrow Transplant Registry) provides a global registry

Table 16.1: Comparison of autologous and allogeneic haemopoietic stem cell transplantion (HSCT)

Parameter	Allogeneic	Autologous
Indications	Haematological malignancies, aplastic anaemia, congenital bone marrow disorders, immune deficiency states, some inborn errors of metabolism	Haematological malignancies and solid tumours. Possible role in autoimmune disorders. Future role in combination with gene therapy to treat genetic disorders, HIV, etc.
Stem cell source	Marrow, peripheral blood, cord blood, family donors, unrelated donors, HLA matched or partially matched	Autologous marrow or peripheral stem cells
Preparative regimen	Required to provide immunosuppression to allow engraftment. Intensive therapy for malignant disease	Primarily designed to provide intensive myeloablative or myelosuppressive treatment to eradicate malignant disease
Post-transplant treatment	Supportive care, transfusions, growth factors, immune manipulation, prophylaxis of graft versus host disease (GvHD)	Supportive care, transfusions, growth factors, immune manipulation
Infectious complication risk	High – sustained risk of infection for months or years	Low – mainly in the early transplant period
Major complications	Conditioning regimen toxicity. Disease recurrence/progression. GvHD. Immune deficiency. Treatment-related mortality 5–35%, depending on many patient, donor and disease-related factors	Preparative regimen toxicity. Disease recurrence/progression. Treatment-related mortality usually <5%

of unrelated donors. Addresses of donor registries are available at www.bmdw.org.

Tissue typing

Patients are 'matched' with their donors by a process called tissue typing using blood tests from both the donor and recipient. Tissue typing refers to the detection of antigens on the lymphocyte. These antigens are collectively known as human leucocyte antigens (HLAs) and are determined by an individual's inherited major histocompatibility complex (MHC). MHC genes are located on chromosome 6, and one chromosome is inherited from each parent. Three of these antigens (HLA-A, HLA-B and HLA-DR) are thought to be the most important in determining donor compatibility.[10] Matching is achieved by comparing the HLA of the possible donor and recipient.

In each case, the more closely matched the donor and the recipient, the fewer complications are thought to occur. While mismatched transplants (where one or more of the above antigens is not a true match) may be carried out, they carry greater risk.[1] Amongst siblings there is 1:4 chance of having an HLA matched donor (Fig. 16.1). Currently, there are more than five million voluntary donors registered worldwide. Unfortunately, donors are not always available. Whereas 80–90% of Caucasians will find a possible donor match, only 20–30% of non-Caucasians will have a possible unrelated donor.[12] The chance of matching someone in the general population is thought to be 1 in 20,000.

Even though allogeneic transplantation is based on accurate matching, differences between donors and patients are inevitable. Many of the major complications of allogeneic transplantation arise from these areas of mismatch: see Case Study 16.1 for discussion of some of these issues.

Donor issues

Once a suitable donor has been found, the donor needs to be supported and prepared for harvesting. Unfortunately, the psychological implications of donating bone marrow are often overlooked. Little attention has been paid to the experience of the donor, but research suggests that bone marrow donation can be stressful, and that donors are often ill prepared.[13]

The opportunity to help another person, through donating one's bone marrow, can be seen as a wonderful experience. It is not uncommon to hear donors say that it is one of the most important things they have ever done. However, if things go wrong, donors may blame themselves for transplant complications, graft failure or graft versus host disease (GvHD).[14,15] The care of donors has been guided and directed by such organizations as the World Marrow Donor Organization (WMDA) and national groups such as the Anthony Nolan Trust (UK), Eurodonor (NL) and The National Marrow Donor Program (US). The WMDA have set out very clear

CASE STUDY 16.1

Jim is a 23-year-old man with a diagnosis of acute myeloid leukaemia (AML) M1. At presentation he had a white blood cell count of 103 and abnormal cytogenetics (he had a deletion of chromosome 7). He is in remission and has completed 3 courses of anthracycline/cytosine-based chemotherapy. He is now fit and well. He has 4 siblings, 2 of whom are matched to his tissue type. He asks you what treatment options are available to him.

What key factors would be important in determining his options for future treatment such as transplant?
Jim, having considered his position of being at high risk of relapse, his young age and good performance status and the availability of 2 potential sibling matched donors, decides to go ahead with allogeneic transplant. Of his 2 donors, one is his 45-year-old sister who is CMV* negative and a mother of 4, and the other is his 26-year-old brother who is CMV positive.

Which donor would you consider to be Jim's best option and why?
Jim is CMV positive and therefore potentially at risk of reactivating his CMV during immunosupression anyway. If the recipient is CMV negative, then a CMV negative donor may be preferred. As his sister is multiparous, she will be allosensitized, have antibodies and therefore her donated cells may have a greater probability for graft versus host disease (GvHD). Both donors are young and healthy; therefore, donor health is not an issue on this occasion. Older donors may be associated with an increased incidence of GvHD. If the donors were equal choices, ABO blood group compatibility may then be taken into consideration.

*CMV, cytomegalovirus, is a virus belonging to the herpes simplex group. The virus may lie dormant but may become life threatening in a person who is severely immunocompromised, leading to conditions such as interstitial pneumonitis and hepatitis.

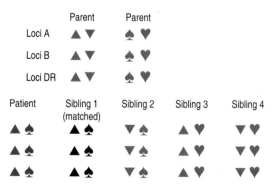

Figure 16.1: Inheritance of MHC, demonstrating 1:4 chance of a match.

guidelines that protect the rights of the donor while recognizing the needs of patients.[12]

Organizations such as WMDA strongly advocate that the donor needs to be cared for by a team not directly involved in the recipient's transplant;[12] however, this is not always feasible with related donors. Related donors who are cared for by members of the transplant team may not always get the support they require. Nurses need to be aware that, at times, related donors may feel somewhat coerced by the transplant team or by family members into donating bone marrow or stem cells. It must be remembered that some of the investigations performed (including human immunodeficiency virus (HIV) and hepatitis screening) and side effects from treatments may have a long-lasting effect on the donor. Other ethical issues include informed consent for minors who may be approached to be donors.[11] While many larger cancer centres have appointed a donor coordinator to support donors, other centres may not have similar resources. The transplant team thus has a duty to care for donors not only during the harvesting phase but also following the transplant procedure. Nurses need to be able to listen and to respond to the concerns of all donors and to be aware of their fears, hopes and at times unrealistic dreams. It may help a transplant team to explore with donors what they find helpful or unhelpful. A related donor who has previously experienced the donating procedure may be willing to talk to other concerned potential donors.

Harvesting and cryopreservation of stem cells

Whether for allogeneic or autologous transplant, the method of collection for both bone marrow and peripheral stem cells is principally the same. The greatest percentage of stem cells live in the bone marrow and so may be collected directly from the marrow,[10] but, as previously stated, stem cells may also be mobilized and collected from the peripheral blood, or, in relatively small amounts, from umbilical cord blood.

Bone marrow

In most centres, the donor (or patient) is admitted to the hospital either the day before or on the day of donation, and this time can be used to ensure the donor is fully aware of what is about to take place. Due to the requirement of a general anaesthesia, most centres will require the donor to stay in hospital for at least one night after the procedure; however, some centres allow the donor home on the same day.[7]

Bone marrow may be removed from the iliac crests or the sternum. A number of small incisions are made in the pelvic or sternum region; a large needle is then inserted to draw marrow from the bones. This procedure generally lasts for 1–2 hours and normally 500–1000 ml of the donor's marrow is taken.[1] Because this represents only a small percentage of the body's bone marrow, levels normally return to normal within a few weeks. Discomfort around the incision sites may last for a few days, and mild analgesia may be required. Tiredness is also a common side effect.

Although donor complications are rare, nurses need to be aware of potential problems. Possible complications may include infection or uncontrolled pain at the incision sites and blood loss. Some centres store one to two units of the donor's own blood before the procedure and return this to them during or after bone marrow harvesting.

After the bone marrow is harvested, it is then processed to remove blood and bone fragments. Marrow that is to be stored for later use is preserved using dimethyl sulfoxide (DMSO) and stored in liquid nitrogen at -130–$160°C$.[1] Autologous bone marrow harvests are treated in a similar way, although up to 2 litres may be required if there is a need to purge the marrow to remove any potential cancerous cells. If this is the case, a greater number of incisions and a longer period for the body's marrow to return to a normal level are required. Possible complications are listed in Box 16.2.

Peripheral stem cells

In most centres, the use of peripheral stem cells has now overtaken the use of bone marrow.[16] Because the vast percentage of stem cells live in the bone marrow rather than the peripheral blood, the number of circulating stem cells in the peripheral blood needs to be increased before harvesting occurs. This is achieved, through a process of mobilization, in one of two ways:

1 Granulocyte colony-stimulating factor (GCSF), a naturally occurring haemopoietic growth factor, is

Possible side effects of granulocyte colony-stimulating factor (GCSF)

Flu-like symptoms
Fever
Muscle pain
Bone pain
Headache
Raised alkaline phosphatase levels
Rarely, lung infiltrates, breathlessness, cough
Splenic pain and infarction (rare)

administered once daily for 3–5 days at a dose of 5–16 µg/kg, given as a subcutaneous injection. The patient or community/clinic nurse usually administers the injections. Although the risks associated with GCSF are few, patients and donors need to be aware of all the possible side effects (see Box 16.2). Bone pain is the commonest reported symptom.

2 The level of stem cells circulating in the peripheral blood is known to rise following a course of chemotherapy.[17] Cytotoxic drugs such as ifosfamide, cyclophosphamide or etoposide, with or without GCSF, may be administered to mobilize and increase the number of stem cells in the peripheral blood so that they can be collected (harvested). The addition of GCSF is thought to increase the circulating stem cell population by 500- to 1000-fold.

Following mobilization, peripheral stem cells are removed through a process known as apheresis. In the apheresis procedure, blood is taken from an intravenous catheter or a large vein in the arm and is passed through a cell separator machine, which removes stem cells before the blood is returned to the patient. This procedure normally lasts for 2–4 hours and it is not unusual for the patient to go through the apheresis process several times in order for a sufficient number of cells to be collected. The stem cells collected in this manner are then processed and cryopreserved in a similar way to bone marrow cells.

Cord blood collection

Stem cells can be collected at the birth of a newborn infant by venepuncture from the umbilical cord and placental blood. The stem cells are only present in small numbers and so this source is more useful for paediatric recipients, as the number of stem cells required for successful engraftment is determined by the recipient's weight.[16,18] The few cord blood transplants undertaken in Europe for adult recipients have required stem cells from up to 9 cords. Some parents have been encouraged and have chosen to bank their child's cord blood in specifically appointed blood banks in Europe and the United States,[1] although the usefulness of such banks is the subject of much debate.

Donor lymphocyte infusions

Donor lymphocyte infusions (DLI) refers to any situation where lymphocytes from a previous donor of stem cells are given to the same recipient with the intention of shifting the balance between donor and recipient haemopoiesis towards donor type. DLI may be used in situations such as relapse following a sibling allograft or MUD transplant. The newly infused lymphocytes mount an immune response causing a graft-versus-tumour effect, thereby attacking the reoccurring cancer cells.[19]

The advantages and disadvantages of using peripheral blood, bone marrow and umbilical cord stem cells are detailed in Table 16.2.

High-dose treatment in preparation for HSCT

Following a successful bone marrow or stem cell harvest, patients who have been selected for HSCT will undergo high-dose treatment with the aim of destroying any remaining cancer cells. Such treatment is often referred to as the conditioning regimen.

The conditioning regimen will vary according to the patient's disease and medical condition, as well as according to local protocol. All regimens use single agent or combination chemotherapy with or without radiotherapy. The conditioning regimen serves two key functions (see Table 16.3):

Table 16.2: Stem cell sources – indications, advantages and disadvantages

Source	Indications	Advantages	Disadvantages
Peripheral blood	Autologous transplant Allogeneic transplant Syngeneic transplant Donor lymphocyte infusion	Can be undertaken as an outpatient More rapid engraftment of neutrophils and platelets	Growth factors ± chemotherapy required to mobilize stem cells. There may be an increased incidence of chronic graft versus host disease (GvHD). Possible risks to donor include bone pain
Cord blood	Allogeneic transplant Syngeneic transplant Haplo-identical or partially mismatched transplant	Relatively low levels of GvHD despite use of mismatched grafts Unrelated donor cells increasingly available from cord blood banks Additional source for small or low weight children without siblings	Only small numbers of cells in collections (recipient cell dose is weight related, therefore not suitable for adults)
Bone marrow	Autologous transplant Allogeneic transplant Syngeneic transplant	Can be harvested on day of transplant (for an allograft)	Risks associated with general anaesthetic, infection at harvest sites, bacteraemia, fractured iliac crest or sternum, haematomas, pain at harvest sites Usually involves an inpatient stay

- to destroy malignant cells throughout the body more effectively than through conventional treatment
- to destroy the cells of the immune system (immunosuppression) in patients undergoing allogeneic transplantation, therefore reducing the risk that the recipient will reject the graft.

The conditioning regimen sets the stage for potential cure but is also responsible for many transplant-related complications. The ideal conditioning regimen therefore eradicates malignant disease while causing tolerable side effects.[20]

High-dose chemotherapy may be given over a course of 1–6 days. If total body irradiation (TBI) is used, it may be given in one dose or in multiple doses over the course of several days (fractionated radiotherapy). There is evidence that the complications associated with radiother-apy are less intense if a fractionated dose is used.[7] Researchers are currently exploring methods of targeting radiotherapy more specifically, so as to reduce the complications seen with TBI.

Side effects of TBI and/or chemotherapy include:

- bone marrow depression
- multiple infections
- gastrointestinal disturbance
- bladder damage
- alopecia
- disruption to skin integrity
- fatigue
- veno-occlusive disease (VOD)
- interstitial pneumonitis
- cataracts
- infertility

Table 16.3: Examples of conditioning regimens

Primary purpose – elimination of remaining disease	Primary purpose – immunosuppression	Both purposes
Busulfan	Antithymocyte globulin	Cyclophosphamide
Carboplatin	Corticosteroids	Melphalan
Carmustine	Fludarabine	Thiotepa
Cytarabine	Total lymphocyte irradiation	Total body irradiation
Diaziquone	Various monoclonal antibody	
Etoposide	preparations	
Mitoxantrone		
Paclitaxel		

Allogeneic transplants with reduced conditioning regimen

The late 1990s saw the introduction of lower-dose conditioning regimes, also referred to as 'mini transplants' or 'transplant-light'. These mini transplants utilize reduced-intensity conditioning regimens to maximize the immunological benefits of the graft-versus-tumour effect, while reducing the risk of transplant-related mortality without increasing the risk of relapse.[21,22] Long-term results are as yet unknown. Allo-HSCT with reduced conditioning may provide a potentially curative option for those whom a full allograft is considered to be very high risk (e.g. older patients with co-morbidities). However, current procedures are ill defined, and further research is needed to establish the role and efficacy of mini transplants. Complications evident in early studies appear to be GvHD and infections, notable cytomegalovirus (CMV) reactivation.[23]

THE TRANSPLANT PROCESS

The transplant process can be simply divided into three phases:

1 pre transplant
2 transplant and engraftment
3 post transplant.

Nurses have a key role to play in the supportive care of patients throughout the transplant process.

Pre transplant

An essential element of the transplant process is the assessment of the risks and benefits related to the individual patient.[7] Although there have been many developments in the reduction of treatment-related mortality and long-term morbidity, the risks are still considerable. An important and sometimes overlooked aspect of nursing in the transplant setting is the role of advocacy, whereby the nurse can work with team members to carefully explain each step of the transplant process and enable the patient to make an informed choice. A comprehensive assessment should include a careful evaluation of the patient, his disease and donor availability. Factors that need to be addressed are covered below:

* The appropriateness of transplant for the individual – this needs to be assessed using the guidelines for transplant according to disease type and status. Despite efforts to coordinate guidelines across Europe, most transplant centres have slightly different practices. It is possible that one centre might regard a transplant as inappropriate, where another centre would consider it a viable option for an individual.

337

- Age – advancing age is usually associated with higher transplant-related toxicity and poorer long-term survival.[1]

- Performance status – low performance status at the beginning of the transplant process increases the risk of mortality. Poor performance status can be related to earlier complications such as the person's disease, previous treatment or co-morbidity factors. Organ impairment, such as renal failure secondary to multiple myeloma or other illness is a particular concern.

- Psychological assessment – this is often overlooked in the early transplant process. Psychological assessment needs to include the level and source of support available to the patient. The transplant process and its long-term effects can be extremely demanding for patients and their families.[11] Numerous studies have identified adjustment problems amongst survivors of bone marrow transplant,[24] and it is important that psychological assessment and intervention become a more central part of transplant care.[25]

- Nutritional assessment – optimizing a patient's nutritional status before transplant is extremely important. Patients can be advised of ways in which they can supplement their nutritional intake through snacks, supplementary food and drinks before and during the transplant process.[35] If the patient is already malnourished, the placing of a percutaneous endoscopic gastrostomy (PEG) or nasogastric tube early in the transplant process may need to be considered.[26] Providing nutritional support to a transplant patient often calls for creativity on the part of the team. Encouraging snacks, nourishing drinks and small amounts 'little and often' can greatly help in the transplant preparation and later in the healing process.

- Potential sources of infection – any possible sources should be assessed, including a full dental examination,[27] so as to identify and deal with any potential complications.

- Physical assessment – this should include an accurate diagnosis of disease, with kidney, lung and heart function tests as well as a full screening as indicated:[1]
  - chest X-ray
  - echocardiogram
  - pulmonary functioning
  - creatinine clearance
  - full blood count
  - biochemistry, liver functioning & clotting screen
  - virology screen
  - genetics
  - disease status.

- Fertility and sexual issues – these should be addressed sensitively and accurately.[28,29] Conditioning regimens, including chemotherapy and TBI, are known to affect fertility. The physical and psychological effects of the transplant itself can often affect the patients' perceptions of themselves and how they express and see themselves sexually.

Preparing the family is also an integral part of the assessment process. If they wish, family members can be helped to feel part of the caring. A patient may benefit from the support of the presence of a family member on the actual day of transplantation. Children can be encouraged to make gifts, such as drawings, for the parent undergoing the transplant, which may help to bring some sense of normality to this 'abnormal situation'. In turn, the parent has reminders in his room of those close to him. One father who had set aside his interest in art took it up again during the transplant process and used his spare time to make drawings for his children. When the children were asked at school, 'Where is your daddy?', they replied, 'Daddy is in hospital making drawings for us'. Where family support is lacking, or where there are already family problems, it is important that other sources of psychosocial support are considered and appropriate referrals made to members of the multidisciplinary team. Because of the toxicity associated with transplantation and the extensive period of time patients often spend in hospital, financial and practical concerns should also be addressed.

The transplant process is complex and the side effects are often far reaching; hence, it is vital that patients and family members are adequately informed and can be active members in their care.

Unfortunately, patients often talk of their frustration at their lack of knowledge during the treatment process.[30] Knowledge needs to be shared at a level that the patient and family understands. Written and verbal information should be provided throughout the transplant process, covering the following key areas:

- the type of transplant to be carried out
- the potential short- and long-term complications of the procedure
- the risks of undergoing or not undergoing the transplant procedure
- alternative treatment options
- guidance on local practice, such as isolation and diet policy
- the roles of team members.

Numerous written resources exist, including comprehensive patient information booklets such as those produced by cancer charities and research foundations. These can be a useful resource when explaining complex aspects of the transplant process.

Engraftment period

The actual infusion of bone marrow or peripheral stem cells (often referred to as the 'rescue process') is usually uncomplicated, and in many ways resembles the infusion of other blood products. Donated or autologous stem cells are administered intravenously, and a nurse should stay with the patient throughout the procedure to monitor vital signs and observe for any reaction. Patients may be premedicated with diphenhydramine and/or hydrocortisone to minimize any reaction to the cells being infused or to the preservative that may have been used to protect the cells during the freezing process.[7]

Although the rescue process is usually straightforward, it may be a time of anticipation and anxiety for the patient. It is also the beginning of an unknown period of waiting for engraftment to take place. During this time, daily blood tests are performed so as to assess bone marrow function. As already mentioned, engraftment involves the stem cells migrating to the recipient's bone marrow space and beginning to regenerate.[10] The period leading up to engraftment is a stressful time for all concerned, but especially for the patient and family members. Patients will often monitor the results of their daily blood tests, firstly for signs of the relevant counts dropping following their conditioning treatment and then for the hopeful signs of engraftment. Many patients will go through a period of asking themselves questions such as, 'Will the treatment work for me?',[31] and taking time each day to discuss the implications of blood results may be very important. Unfortunately, some patients will not recover their blood counts, and graft failure is seen in 5–15% of transplants.[32]

The engraftment period lasts from 2 to 4 weeks and will very much depend on the type of transplant used and the individuality of the patient's response to treatment.[1] During the pre-engraftment period, the patient will experience severe pancytopenia (reduction in number of all types of blood cells), leading to severe immunosuppression. The complete recovery of the patient's immune system will take anything from months to years, depending on the nature of the transplant carried out.[1] During pre-engraftment and the early engraftment period, the emphasis of nursing care is on the prevention, recognition and timely management of complications. These are listed in Box 16.3.

SUPPORTIVE CARE

Cancer nurses play a key role in the supportive care of patients during the pre-engraftment and early engraftment period. Preventing and managing complications is a priority, but providing psychological support is also crucial at this vulnerable time. Complications can occur as a result of:

- dose-intensive conditioning regimens, e.g. infection, bleeding, organ toxicity
- GvHD
- supportive medications being used to treat transplant complications (e.g. amphotericin B)
- treatment failure, e.g. relapse.

Supportive care techniques can sustain the recipient until stabilized engraftment.[11]

Box 16.3

Possible complications of bone marrow or stem cell transplant

Early complications:

Infection – bacterial, fungal, viral, protozoa

Gastrointestinal disturbance

Haemorrhage

Acute graft versus host disease (GvHD)

Graft failure

Renal toxicity

Haemorrhagic cystitis

Interstitial pneunomitis

Veno-occlusive disease

Cardiac failure

Psychological issues, including the isolation experience

Late complications:

Infections – cytomegalovirus, *Pneumocystis carinii* pneumonia

Chronic GvHD

Chronic pulmonary complications

Infertility

Secondary malignancies

Relapse

Cataract

Autoimmune disorders

Hypothyrodism

Psychological disturbance

Source: Provan et al[10] and Hoffbrand et al.[7]

Both high-dose chemotherapy and radiotherapy can cause temporary and sometimes permanent damage to any organ, but may particularly affect the gastrointestinal tract, lungs, liver and kidneys.[16] The prolonged period of pancytopenia following transplant allows for infections to take hold of the patient with a severely deficient immune system. Further complications such as GvHD, VOD and disseminated intravascular disease (DIC) need to be considered and addressed.

It is only through an experienced and multi-skilled team working closely together that transplant-related complications can be addressed and dealt with swiftly. For this reason, transplant procedures should be carried out in accredited transplant units, where sufficient facilities, including highly skilled personnel, are present to deal with transplant-related issues.

Since 2002 all transplant units are encouraged to gain accreditation through Joint Accreditation Committee (JACIE) of the International Society for Cellular Therapy (ISCT) and the European Group for Blood and Marrow Transplantation (EBMT). The aim of this group is to set out and publish standards to which all centres performing transplant must conform. These standards apply to the processing and transplantation of all sources of haemopoietic progenitor cells and all phases of collection, processing and administration of these cells.[33] Because of the level of expertise required for transplantation, all accredited centres must be able to show that the necessary resources are in place. These include a high level of specialist medical and nursing expertise. Centres must also have access to other specialized areas of care to which referral can be made, such as renal, pulmonary, cardiology, dermatology, infectious disease, gastroenterological and intensive care facilities. Essential laboratory facilities include cytogenetics, molecular studies, specialist virology, tissue typing, pathology and transfusion services.[33] Centres are required to work closely with fertility clinics to support patients facing the prospect of infertility. It is through continuing collaboration and the utilization of these resources that improved patient care can be achieved.

Box 16.4 lists some of the core aspects of nursing care required during the transplantation process. Partnership with the patient and a multidisciplinary approach are fundamental to all aspects of supportive care.

SHORT TERM SIDE-EFFECTS AND THEIR MANAGEMENT

Immunosuppression

Profound neutropenia (a white blood cell count of less than $0.5 \times 10^9/L$) is an inevitable consequence of bone marrow transplantation. Supportive care to address immunosuppression will demand a degree of protective isolation. However, isolation procedures vary considerably from centre to centre and the

Box 16.4

Core aspects of nursing care during transplantation

- Fluid balance monitoring and maintenance of hydration
- Nutritional assessment and care, including supplements as appropriate
- Oral assessment and oral care to promote comfort and reduce infection
- Assessment and management of other symptoms of gastrointestinal disturbance, e.g. diarrhoea, nausea and vomiting
- Monitoring for signs and possible sources of infection
- Assessment and minimization of sleep disturbance and promotion of comfort
- Advice and encouragement of gentle exercise and breathing
- Assessment of psychological/spiritual well-being, listening to worries and addressing concerns
- Personal hygiene
- Assessment of any drug reactions
- Monitoring daily blood counts

Source: EBMT.[16]

debate continues as to the extent to which isolation is necessary.[34] The physical and psychological impact of a transplant centre's isolation practice should be carefully considered. Some patients are cared for in a single room, with or without Hepa air filtration and positive air pressure, whereas others may be cared for in open bays or increasingly in patients' own homes.[11] There is, as yet, no clear evidence to support the use of one environment over another and nurses have an important role to play in questioning some of the isolation procedures that patients are asked to endure. Ambulatory transplants are gaining in popularity, and there may be considerable benefits to patients and families (both psychological and physical) from being cared for at home.[8]

Patients receiving an autologous or allogeneic transplant will be at risk of infection due to the conditioning regimen causing extensive pancytopenia. The length of pancytopenia will depend on a multitude of factors, including the conditioning treatment, the origin of stem cells and whether growth factors are administered. Patients receiving an allograft will require some form of immunosuppressive therapy, such as ciclosporin, to prevent or reduce GvHD, thereby depressing T-cell functioning. B-cell and T-cell dysfunction may continue for months and sometimes years, especially in cases where patients develop chronic GvHD.[1]

The careful hand washing of patients, staff and visitors remains one of the most important practices in preventing the spread of infection.[35] Again, local practice will determine the protective clothing required by staff and visitors, ranging from hand washing to masks, gown, gloves and other types of protective clothing. One of the ironies of isolation is that many of the infections, which place patients at risk, are, in fact, endogenous. Patients may, therefore, need particular support in meeting their hygiene needs so as to reduce infection and provide comfort.

Because of the treatment administered, patients will often not be able to mount a normal immune response and at times the only indication of a growing infection may be a raised temperature.[35] Other considerations such as drug reactions and GvHD need to be considered when pyrexia occurs (see Case Study 16.2). Because of underlying neutropenia and possible skin or mucosal breakdown, Gram-positive and Gram-negative bacterial infections are common. Prompt treatment with broad-spectrum antibiotics is required to prevent sepsis-related endotoxin release and septic shock[10] (see Ch. 35). If pyrexia occurs, close monitoring of the patient and a full screening is required (Box 16.5). Fungal infections are difficult to confirm and antifungal treatment is often started when pyrexia does not resolve. Viral infections such as respiratory syncytial virus, *Candida*, herpes simplex and CMV may occur anytime post transplant.

The risks and benefits of prophylactic treatments such as antibiotics, antiviral and antifungal agents continue to be debated. While many centres are reluctant to use antibiotics due to concerns surrounding developing resistance, some centres advocate the use of one of the quinolenes such as ciprofloxacin to reduce the risk of Gram-negative infections.[1]

341

CASE STUDY 16.2

Louie is a 35-year-old man with a diagnosis of acute myeloid leukaemia (AML) M1 admitted for a sibling transplant from his sister. His conditioning regimen includes etoposide and total body irradiation (TBI). Previously, Louie has attended the pre-transplant clinic, where his treatment plan has been explained and pre-transplant screening has been completed. Louie is welcomed to the Unit and shown to a single room with washing facilities. The admitting nurse explains the plan of care and introduces him to members of the team. The bone marrow transplant coordinator will visit or make contact with the ward team regularly. **What issues may be concerning Louie at this time?**

Having completed his conditioning treatment, Louie receives an infusion of his sister's stem cells. Five days following the transplant, Louie's neutrophils fall, as expected, to 0.2×10^9/L, his platelets are 34 and haemoglobin 10. Later that evening Louie develops a raised temperature 38.4°C. Blood pressure is 130/85, pulse 95 and respiratory rate 16. **What are the priorities for Louie's nursing care?**

Working together, the team take blood cultures from Louie via his peripheral and central lines. Further screening for infection is carried out, including samples of mid stream urine, sputum and faeces. Swabs are sent for microbiology, culturing and sensitivity and investigations are ordered. You note that Louie is haemodynamically stable and has passed urine within the last hour. Having been reviewed by the medical team he is commenced on broad-spectrum intravenous antibiotics. **You are asked to monitor Louie closely. What would you monitor?**

Forty-eight hours later, and despite antibiotic therapy, Louie remains pyrexial. Further blood cultures are taken and antibiotics are reviewed and he is commenced on second-line antibiotics. A further 24 hours later Louie remains pyrexial and is commenced on intravenous antifungal therapy and a high-resolution CT scan is arranged to rule out *Aspergillus*. Nurses closely monitor Louie for signs of shock, dehydration and changes in breathing patterns. Louie has severe oral mucositis and ulceration and is given analgesics. Louie is commenced on high-dose aciclovir and intravenous fluids to supplement his fluid intake. Louie is encouraged to sip fluids. On day 10, his temperature appears to be settling. On day 17, his neutrophils show signs of beginning to rise. Louie feels tired but is pleased to see his counts rising.

Box 16.5

Screening required in the event of pyrexia

- Peripheral and central line blood cultures
- Mid stream urine
- Possible sputum sample for productive cough
- Mouth/throat swab
- Faecal sample
- Wound swab

Invasive fungal infections carry a high degree of mortality if not treated swiftly. The findings of studies have led to recommendations of a range of antifungal prophylaxis agents, such as fluconazole.[36] All patients undergoing allografts will receive prophylactic treatment against *Pneumocystis carinii* with trimethoprim–sulfamethoxazole (co-trimoxazole) or pentamidine nebulizers.[32] Patients who are known to have been exposed to fungal infections in the past also tend to be given antifungal prophylaxis.

Antiviral prophylaxis is generally advocated throughout the transplant procedure,[7] usually beginning with an oral version of an antiviral such as aciclovir and converting to an intravenous dose when required. Interstitial pneumonitis is the most common cause of death immediately post transplant and over 50% are caused by CMV.[1] The prompt recognition and treatment of a suspected infection are central to a successful outcome.

Many centres advocate the use of haemopoietic growth factors such as GCSF or granulocyte–macrophage colony-stimulating factor (GM-CSF). This naturally occurring growth factor helps increase the number of neutrophils, thereby reducing the length of immunosuppression and decreasing the time span during which infections can occur.

Patients undergoing a transplant continue to be at risk of infection for many months following engraftment. *Cytomegaloviruses*, *Aspergillus* and *P. carinii* can be fatal if left untreated.[7] Patients can experience the reactivation of herpes simplex virus in the form of oral or genital herpes, and may need to be readmitted with painful conditions such as herpes zoster (shingles).

Thrombocytopenia and bleeding disorders

Thrombocytopenia (a platelet count less than $150 \times 10^9/L$) is frequently directly related to the treatment being used to tackle the underlying malignancy (i.e. chemotherapy or radiotherapy). Thrombocytopenia may be the result of bone marrow involvement, coagulation disorders such as DIC or platelet abnormalities secondary to immune-mediated reactions such as thrombotic thrombocytopenic purpura (TPP).[37]

Bleeding is often seen in the mucous membranes of the nose and mouth, as well as under the skin, in the gastrointestinal tract, nervous system or lungs. Platelet transfusions are given if there is any evidence of bleeding and/or to maintain the platelet count so as to prevent bleeding. Although the definition of a minimum platelet count may vary between centres, it is widely recognized that spontaneous bleeding may occur when the platelet count is lower than $100 \times 10^9/L$, and major haemorrhage is more likely to occur when the platelet counts falls below $20 \times 10^9/L$.[37] Patients should be monitored for refractory thrombocytopenia, which is caused by the patient's ability to develop antibodies that attack the donated platelets, preventing adequate platelet increments occurring after transfusion. In this case, single donor HLA-matched platelets may be required.

In addition to working closely with the patient to observe for any signs of bruising or bleeding, a full blood count to monitor platelet numbers is generally carried out daily. A coagulation screen should be performed to monitor for any abnormalities, especially if the patient is bleeding or septic. Fresh frozen plasma and/or cryoprecipitate may be given to correct clotting abnormalities. DIC may be seen in septic patients, particularly if a Gram-negative sepsis is present (see Ch. 35). Other rarer complications include TTP and haemolytic uraemic syndrome (HUS). Both conditions consist of platelet microthrombi partly occluding the vascular lumen of arterioles, capillaries and overlying proliferating endothelial cells. Neurological disturbances and renal failure may be present. In both these conditions, platelet transfusion is strongly contraindicated, and may contribute to death. It is believed that the transfused platelets compound the already-existing occlusion.[37]

All female patients undergoing a transplant will require a cessation of menstruation; this may need to be induced, so as to cover the period of thrombocytopenia. This usually continues until the platelets are higher than $100 \times 10^9/L$. Norethisterone tablets 5–10 mg three times a day can be taken orally or Cyclogest (progesterone) 400 mg pessaries can be given to patients who can no longer take medications. In some cases the team may need to consider oestrogen patches to control bleeding.

Anaemia

Both chemotherapy and radiotherapy treatments can damage the bone marrow's ability to produce red blood cells (RBCs), and so patients undergoing transplantation will require blood product transfusions to treat anaemia. To reduce the risk of transfusion-related GvHD, all donated blood products given to transplant patients are irradiated, thereby destroying lymphocytes that might otherwise attack the patient's cells.[37] All patients should receive CMV-negative blood products until the patient's CMV status is known. While some centres consider it safe to provide leucocyte-depleted products, due to the small risk of transmitting CMV through blood products, many centres advocate the use of only CMV-negative blood products to CMV-negative allograft patients. The decision to transfuse blood should always be taken having considered the patient's haemoglobin level and symptoms. The administration of multiple blood transfusions over a period of time can result in complications associated with iron overload in the long term.

Graft versus host disease

GvHD continues to be one of the most serious complications of an allogeneic transplant.[7] GvHD is responsible for about 25% of the mortality seen after allogeneic transplants, and is thought to affect as many as 80% of allogeneic recipients.[32] GvHD occurs because the T cells in the donated marrow identify the recipient's body as foreign and mount an attack. GvHD can be acute, occurring in the first 100 days following transplant, or chronic, appearing more than a 100 days after transplant.[7] The organs most likely to be affected are the skin, the gastrointestinal tract and the liver. Skin symptoms can range from a mild rash appearing on the hands and feet to a more generalized erythroderma leading to severe skin break down, increasing the possibility of infection. Patients may report severe cramps and distinctive green-coloured diarrhoea, suggesting gut involvement. Signs of liver involvement include elevated serum bilirubin, jaundice colour and swollen girth. All or any of these symptoms can leave the patient feeling very distressed and exhausted. The symptoms of GvHD are graded from 1 (mild), which may require little or no treatment, to 4 (severe), which may be life threatening[11] (see Case Study 16.3).

While the main aim of care is to prevent GvHD or to reduce its toxic effects, it has been recognized that the presence of GvHD has a degree of graft-versus-disease effect. Some studies suggest that patients who have a degree of GvHD are less likely to relapse than those patients with no evidence of GvHD.[38,39]

Donor cells can be treated to achieve T-cell depletion before they are infused, thereby reducing the risk of GvHD.[1] One popular treatment choice, however, is the immunosuppressant drug ciclosporin, which interferes with the functioning of T lymphocytes in the donated cells.[7] Ciclosporin may be used alone or in conjunction with the chemotherapy agent methotrexate. It is normally administered intravenously at 3 mg/kg, but close monitoring of blood levels is required and the dose should be adjusted accordingly. Ciclosporin is normally commenced immediately before the transplant and continued for 3–6 months after the transplant unless toxicities dictate otherwise. The toxicities associated with the drug include renal and liver damage, hypertension and central nervous system disturbance.

Treatment of GvHD normally includes increasing the dose of ciclosporin, administering high-dose steroids or antithymocyte glob-

---

CASE STUDY 16.3

A 34-year-old woman, Marie, 22 days after a related allogeneic bone marrow transplant, is mildly febrile and complains of a burning sensation on the palms of her hands and soles of her feet. **How will you assess her and what do you expect to find?**

Marie has a skin rash, which is painful, maculopapular and predominately involves her hands and the soles of her feet. Her vital signs are temperature 37.8°C, pulse 84, respirations 20, blood pressure 120/76. **What biochemistry blood results would you be alerted to check?**

Marie's ciclosporin level is 60 ng/ml, her liver enzymes and renal function tests are within normal limits. Marie's rash is diagnosed as acute graft versus host disease (GvHD) grade 1 and a decision is made to observe her closely. However, her ciclosporin level is slightly low and may be subtherapeutic, so her dose is increased. **What skin care would you advise for Marie?**

The following day, Marie develops diarrhoea. By mid-day, she has passed 3 litres of watery diarrhoea with a 'mincemeat' appearance. It has no odour but is increasing in quantity during the day. **What biochemistry blood results would you now check, and what would you expect to be prescribed?**

Marie's ciclosporin level is now therapeutic at 280 ng/l. Her urea is raised at 11.2, as is her serum creatinine at 119. Her potassium is low at 2.9. You suspect that she is dehydrated and has GvHD of her gut grade 3. Marie is commenced on 8 hourly litres of sodium chloride with added potassium to correct her dehydration, and methyl prednisolone 1 g intraveneously to treat her GvHD according to local guidelines.

You administer loperamide, and plan to consider codeine phosphate and octreotide if loperamide is ineffective. Marie is placed on a stool chart to assess the frequency and consistency of stools and the presence of blood or tissue.

---

ulin. Topical creams containing steroids may be applied to the skin. Monoclonal antibodies and thalidomide may be also be used.[1]

Electrolyte imbalance/renal failure

The nurse, in partnership with other members of the team, needs to monitor daily any signs of renal disturbance or electrolyte imbalance.

This will involve working with patients to monitor fluid intake and output and support their daily nutritional requirements. Secondary complications can arise as a result of the patient's inability to drink fluids and maintain nutrition due to a number of factors, including severe mucositis, poorly controlled nausea and/or vomiting, diarrhoea and lack of appetite. Many of the drugs used in the transplant setting are associated with renal toxicity and electrolyte imbalance, thus adding to the risk of problems.[20] Renal deterioration can be gradual or very rapid in its onset, quickly leading to renal failure, particularly when secondary to severe sepsis. Nurses need to be extremely vigilant in assessing signs of renal deterioration. Monitoring fluid and electrolyte balance, encouraging the patient to sip fluids and working closely with medical and dietetic staff are vitally important.

Hepatic toxicity/veno-occlusive disease

Veno-occlusive disease is one of the consequences of toxic injury to the liver. VOD tends to occur during the first 3 weeks after transplant and is characterized by a raised bilirubin, right upper quadrant pain, weight gain and ascites in the absence of other liver disease.[1] Diagnosis is made on the basis of two of the former symptoms/signs, an ultrasound and, where feasible, liver biopsy. Symptoms of VOD may indicate infection, acute GvHD or drug toxicity, so these need to be carefully assessed. The reported incidence of VOD is up to 20% in patients undergoing allogeneic transplant and 10% of patients undergoing autologous transplant.[37] Known risk factors include elevated liver enzymes pre transplant, intensity of pre-transplant chemotherapy, presence of active liver disease, type and intensity of conditioning regimen, TBI dose and rate, mismatched or unrelated donor allografts and second transplant.[1] VOD can be mild or severe, with complete recovery or with rapidly progressive hepatic failure leading to death, usually from multi-organ failure. The mortality rate is 50%.[37]

Management of VOD aims to maintain intravascular volume and renal perfusion without increasing extravascular fluid accumulation, but the best treatment remains unclear. Trials using recombinant human tissue plasminogen activator (rh-tPA) together with low-dose heparin, defibrotide (antithrombotic agents), high-dose steroids and prostaglandin E_1 have all shown some benefit with varying degrees of associated toxicity.[16]

Mucositis/gastrointestinal toxicity

Gastrointestinal (GI) symptoms such as diarrhoea, stomatitis and mucositis are commonly seen in the transplant setting and can be very distressing to patients and their families.[26] Patients should be encouraged to use prophylactic mouthwashes, which may not be able to prevent mucositis, but may help to prevent further infection secondary to mucosal breakdown.[40] It is not uncommon for patients to be unable to use mouthwashes due to nausea or pain and, if this is the case, the nurse can suggest a simple mouth gargle or rinse of normal saline to clean debris and relieve discomfort. Analgesia such as cocaine mouthwashes, opiate suspensions and subcutaneous or intravenous opiates may need to be considered.[1] Such options should be initiated early to prevent undue patient discomfort.

Severe mucositis can significantly interfere with the patient's ability to eat and drink. Because of this problem, some centres advocate the placement of a nasogastric or percutaneous tube to administer feeds, but the nutritional benefits must be considered alongside the potential intrusion for the patient of yet another tube and device. The use of total parenteral nutrition (TPN) should be considered following the advice of the team dietician. Where diarrhoea is particularly severe, TPN may be indicated.

Psychological and spiritual issues

Often patients undergoing transplants have travelled a considerable distance from their home to find themselves in a highly technical environment far from their support network. The busy clinical environment can be frightening, and if the patient is in isolation, it can feel extremely lonely. It may be in this environment that the patient begins to question what the disease and treatment has meant to them and their families.[41] Because the clinical team is often so focused on physical parameters and risks, it may be that the psychological impact of the experience is overlooked. A psychodynamic model as applied to the bone marrow transplant process suggests that it is important to identify the individual's level of psychological adjustment at the beginning of treatment.[42] Patients who display high levels of agitation and anxiety, and who have experienced unresolved loss in the past or who have previous psychiatric problems, may be particularly at risk. Those showing responses such as anger, sadness or fear, but who have a realistic balance of hope and concern for the future and a good network of support are likely to be adjusting normally to this life-changing situation. Research suggests that common psychological responses to bone marrow transplantation include depression, anxiety, body image changes and reactions indicative of post-traumatic stress disorder (PTSD).[25,43,44] Patients with high levels of psychological distress after bone marrow transplantation may have more difficulty finding meaning and purpose in their lives[24] and may experience a sense of isolation.[45]

The aggressive nature of the treatment and symptoms experienced during the transplant process can be extremely challenging, and the relationship that develops between the patient and cancer nurse can be a major source of support. Techniques such as relaxation can also be particularly helpful,[24,25] and follow-up programmes need to address psychological concerns and issues of reintegration into life.[46] Alby[47] points out that leaving hospital at the end of a bone marrow transplant can be difficult for patients, due to the fear of leaving a protected environment with skilled, supportive staff, combined with the fear of facing life with a different body and the constraints imposed by the treatment or medication.

Among the concerns that patients and family may have to face is the reality of graft failure or the fear of relapse. Not all patients will identify with a formalized religious faith, and patients and family members may turn to the nurse or a team member as they face many difficult decisions and choices.[31,48] A reprioritization of life values and beliefs may occur, and the transplant patient may describe a lasting change in outlook.[45]

MULTI-PROFESSIONAL TEAM WORK

Because of the complex nature of BMT, a high level of teamwork is required: the active involvement of the patient and family is essential.[49] Other team members include doctors, nurses, physiotherapists, dietitians, complementary therapy practitioners, laboratory staff, radiographers and the chaplaincy team. Over a period of weeks and months the patient will be introduced to a wide variety of health and social care professionals and the nurse has an important role to play in helping to coordinate care and at times to act as the patient's advocate. It may also be necessary to refer patients to the palliative care team and/or the critical care unit (CCU). If a patient needs to be transferred to a CCU setting, this can be extremely frightening. An occasional visit from the nursing transplant team can serve to act as support for the family and a resource for the critical care team, who may be less familiar with the underlying disease and transplant treatments.[50]

LONG-TERM SIDE EFFECTS

The long-term effects of BMT are multidimensional and may occur as a result of a number of factors, including:

- the delayed effects of chemoradiation therapy, including physical symptoms, fertility problems, cataracts and secondary malignancies
- the experience of facing one's own mortality
- loss of control
- fear of relapse
- adaptation to the post-transplant self, both physically and psychologically

The loss of control, fear of relapse or recurrence and sense of having to face one's own mortality are common psychological responses to a cancer diagnosis and treatment, and are explored further in Chapter 33. Specific problems in relation to BMT are discussed below.

Physical symptoms and restrictions

A study of 84 individuals in the year after BMT showed that more than half experienced fatigue and loss of strength in the first 6 months, and that problems with stamina persisted at 1 year for around 40%.[46] Concerns about changes in appearance and body image were expressed by about a third of patients, and many felt restricted in their daily lives as a result of having to avoid situations in which they might be at risk of infection or skin damage. Approximately one-third of patients were still troubled by continued health problems, including infections, difficulty concentrating, eating difficulties and gastrointestinal problems.

Fertility

Most patients who receive TBI as part of their conditioning treatment become sterile. Although some studies describe long-term problems with intimacy and sexuality, sexual desire and function usually return to normal after transplantation.[51] However, the experience of living with infertility can be extremely painful, and Schover[52] graphically describes this loss as living with 'empty arms'.

Chemotherapy drugs, especially the alkylating agents, may cause temporary or permanent reproductive difficulties.[52] The extent of these problems depends on the patient's age and gender and on the dosage and duration of treatment. Because infertility is common among those treated with chemotherapy and/or radiation therapy, nurses and the team need to be aware of the fertility preservation options and support available. Men are usually encouraged to consider sperm banking before treatment begins if they wish to father children after transplantation. Menstrual irregularities often develop in women who have received high-dose chemotherapy, and menstruation may return up to 2 years after transplantation in younger women. Women over the age of 25 are likely to go through early menopause, and hormone replacement therapy can help relieve the symptoms of menopause and may be recommended for other medical reasons such as control of osteoporosis. Today, the cryopreservation of fertilized or unfertilized eggs or ovarian tissue before transplant is possible for some women provided their induction treatment has not already caused infertility. Sterility and early menopause can be a psychologically distressing side effect and therefore should be addressed by the patient, partner, family and healthcare team before and after transplantation.

Cataracts

Roughly three-quarters of patients who receive single-dose TBI develop cataracts. The number is reduced to about 20% in patients who receive fractionated radiation doses or in those who do not receive TBI. Cataracts may occur 3–6 years after TBI and those who develop cataracts generally need corrective surgery, which often restores normal vision.[9]

Secondary malignancies

There is evidence that high-dose chemotherapy, radiotherapy, immunosuppression, stem cell mobilization, viral infection or other unknown factors related to the procedure may increase the risk for secondary cancers. Studies have shown that the risk varies considerably (between 4% and 6%), depending on the patient's age, general health, menopausal status (for women) and previous history of radiation.[53] The dosage and type of chemotherapy drug or radiation given also affect the likelihood of a second cancer developing. It is thought that transplant recipients have a six times greater likelihood of developing a tumour than non-transplanted persons,[39] although it is hoped that this risk will be reduced as targeted treatments become more widely used.

FOLLOW-UP CARE

As transplant care and practice varies throughout Europe, so discharge criteria and follow-up care may vary also according to local practice and the patient's condition. However, most centres throughout Europe follow broadly similar guidelines, advocating that patients are monitored for endocrine abnormalities, cardiac function, pulmonary function, bone density, chronic GvHD, relapse and the incidence of secondary neoplasms. Follow-up care should also provide psychological support for patients with ongoing problems and residual effects post transplant, including advice in areas such as reimmunization and fertility. The first year after transplant can be a difficult time, and patients commonly express fears about the future, a sense of loss of control, anxiety and depression and a sense of being more cautious.[46] Some also feel a sense of isolation, partly because of an inability to socialize in the way they used to, and partly because the experience of surviving a near-death experience makes them feel 'different'.

The assessment of quality of life throughout the BMT process can illuminate aspects of life in which patients need particular support. Numerous quality of life instruments exist, but there has been increasing interest in the potential for specific tools such as the Functional Assessment of Cancer Therapy-Bone Marrow Transplant (FACT-BMT) scale to identify important dimensions of quality of life in this patient group.[54] The routine clinical assessment of quality of life before transplant, at the time of discharge and several months after transplant would provide a meaningful starting point for the development of supportive follow-up care.

Some patients will need to return to the hospital's outpatient department daily for the first 2 weeks after transplant, whereas others are seen less frequently. Follow-up visits to the transplant clinic continue every 1–2 weeks for the first few months, to ensure that blood counts are returning to normal. Patients are then seen every month for about 6 months. The schedule of checkups should be based on the needs of each individual patient. Generally, checkups are performed every 2–6 months: most include bone marrow aspiration to determine the condition of the marrow.

Allograft recipients receiving immunosuppressive therapy need to be monitored carefully for toxicity. Ciclosporin is normally discontinued by 6 months post transplantation. Prophylaxis against specific infections is required, usually involving the administration of penicillin to prevent pneumococcal sepsis secondary to hyposplenism, aciclovir to prevent reactivation of the herpes simplex virus and the herpes zoster virus, and co-trimoxazole or pentamidine to prevent infection with *P. carinii*.[10]

IMMUNITY AND VACCINATION POST TRANSPLANT

Immune reactivity during the first month post transplant is extremely low. Some white cells such as cytotoxic and phagocytic cells resume function by day 100, but the more specialized functions of T and B lymphocytes may remain impaired for a year or more. The immune system remains suppressed for longer in patients with chronic GvHD due to the mechanism of GvHD and the immunosuppressive drugs used to treat it.[1] There are limited data on the effect of donor age, recepient age, disease and conditioning regimen on immune reactivity. More evidence is required around the need for immunization and its efficacy and outcome in transplanted patients. However, certain groups should not be given live vaccination after transplant (Box 16.6).

SURVIVORSHIP ISSUES

Many patients need a full year to recover physically and psychologically from a bone marrow transplant, although most return to an active,

---

Box 16.6

Patients who should not be considered eligible for live vaccination after blood or bone marrow transplant

- All autograft recipients for 2 years
- All allograft recipients for 2 years
- Patients on immunosuppressive therapy for any reason
- Patients suffering from chronic graft versus host disease (GvHD)
- Patients suffering from recurrent malignancy after transplantation

working life. However, the extent to which patients successfully readapt to life after transplant depends on a number of factors.[45,55] These include the clinical status of the disease, prior treatment, physical and psychological characteristics of the patient and available social support. Relatively little attention has been paid to the rehabilitation of patients following BMT, although interest in this area is now increasing.[31,55] Survivorship encompasses the individual's ability to function physically, as well as feelings about self, wholeness and normality. Baker et al's study[46] demonstrated that a significant number of BMT survivors have difficulty returning to former roles and resuming social relationships. Financial and work problems were also prominent. Many patients find it extremely difficult to re-establish 'normal' life, particularly as they may need to continue medication indefinitely, or may have to adapt their lifestyle considerably so as to prevent fatigue, avoid infectious diseases and cope with the long-term effects of treatment. Changes in liver and gastrointestinal function may also require alterations in diet. In addition, it can be difficult to adapt to bodily changes such as dry eyes, skin changes and sensitivity. Altered body image, sexuality and fertility can continue to challenge an individual's sense of self. Some patients experience changes in their self-image because they have received part of their body from someone else; on the other hand, some people think of their transplantation date as a new 'birthday'. Chapter 36 discusses rehabilitation and survivorship issues in more depth.

CONCLUSION

Despite the risk of morbidity and mortality, the option of bone marrow transplantation holds out real hope to many people living with cancer. More effective conditioning regimens with less toxicity are being developed, including more targeted therapies based on the identification of leukaemia and tumour-specific antigens.[1] As scientists continue to increase their understanding of the benefits of the graft-versus-disease effect, conditioning regimens continue to advance in the transplant setting.

The debate persists over the feasibility of ambulatory transplants, and it is vital that such debate should not merely focus on saving money, but more importantly on the physical and psychological benefits to patients. The ongoing work of gene therapy and the ability to manipulate stem cells in the laboratory promises even greater advances in this field of cancer care.[10] There is a real need for nurses to be actively involved in these developments while continuing to focus on improving the whole experience of patients undergoing transplantation.[45] Nurses in the transplant setting or beyond have a vital role to play in the supportive care they offer to patients and their families throughout the transplant journey.

REFERENCES

1. Childs RW. Allogeneic stem cell transplantation. In: De Vito, VT, Hellman S, Rosenberg SA, eds. Cancer principles and practice. 6th Edn. Philadelphia Lippincott, Williams & Wilkins, 2001:2779–2798.

2. Benjamin, S. Introduction. In: Treleaven J, Wiernik P, eds. Colour atlas and text of bone marrow transplantation. London: Mosby-Wolfe, 1995:9–17.

3. Mathe G, Amiel JL, Schwarzenberg L, et al. (1963) Haematopoietic chimera in man after allogenic bone marrow transplantation. BMJ 1963: 2:1633–1635.

4. Thomas ED, Storb R, Clift RA. Bone marrow transplantation. N Engl J Med 1975; 292:832.

5. Russell NH. Peripheral blood stem cells for allogenic transplantation. Bone Marrow Transplant 1994; 13:353–355.

6. Gluckman E, Rocha V, Boyer-Chammard A, et al. Outcome of cord blood transplantation from related and unrelated donors. N Engl J Med 1997; 337(6): 373–381.

7. Hoffbrand AV, Pettit JE, Moss PAH. Essential haematology. 4th edn. Oxford Blackwell Science; 2001.

8. European Group for Blood and Marrow Transplantation.2002; www.ebmt.org

9. Areman H, Deeg J, Sacher RA. Bone marrow and stem cell processing: a manual of current techniques. Philadelphia: FA Davis; 1992.

10. Provan D, Baglin T, Lilleyman J, Singer C, Oxford handbook of clinical haematology. 2nd edn. Oxford: Oxford University Press; 2004.

11. Buchsel P. Bone marrow transplantation. In: Miaskowski C, Buchsel P, eds. Oncology nursing:

assessment and clinical care. St Louis: Mosby; 1999:143–186.

12. Cleaver SA, Warren P, Kern M, et al. Special report: donor work-up and transport of bone marrow. World Marrow Donor Association; 1997.

13. Molassiotis A, Holroyd E. Assessment of psychosocial adjustment in Chinese unrelated bone marrow donors. Bone Marrow Transplant 1999; 24:903–910.

14. Switzer GE, Dew MA, Magistro CA, et al. The effects of bereavement on adult sibling bone marrow donors' psychological well-being and reactions to donation. Bone Marrow Transplant 1998; 21:181–188.

15. Smith ME. Facing death: donor and recipient responses to the gift of life. Holistic Nurs Pract 1998; 13(1):32–40.

16. European Group for Blood and Marrow Transplantation. The EBMT handbook: blood and marrow transplantation. Paris: European School of Haematology; 1998.

17. Buchsel P, Kapustay P. Peripheral stem cell transplantation. In: Miaskowski C, Buchsel P, Eds. Oncology nursing: assessment and clinical care. St Louis: Mosby; 1999:187–208.

18. Gluckman E, Rocha V, Garnier F, et al. Analysis of factors associated with engraftment after umbilical cord blood transplantation. European Group for Blood and Marrow Transplantation. Nature 2001; 27(1).

19. Weiden PL, Sullivan KM, Flournoy N, Storb R, Thomas ED. Anti-leukaemic effect of chronic graft versus leukaemic disease: contribution to improved survival after allogeneic marrow transplantation. N Engl J Med 1981; 304(25):1529–1533.

20. Souhami R, Tobias J. Cancer and its management. 3rd edn. Oxford: Blackwell Science; 2003.

21. Valcarcel D, Canals C, Martino R, et al. Allogeneic haemopoietic transplantation from HLA-identical siblings: independent prognostic effect of age, diagnosis, and reduced-intensity conditioning. Bone Marrow Transplant Suppl 2003; 31(1):58.

22. Crawley C, Szydio R, Lalancette G, et al. Sibling and unrelated reduced-intensity conditioned allogenic transplantation for multiple myeloma. Bone Marrow Transplant Suppl 2003; 31(1):56.

23. Michallet M, Le Q, Bilger F, et al. Long-term follow-up of 92 haemopoietic stem cell transplantation patients after non-myeloablative conditioning regimens. Bone Marrow Transplant Suppl 2003; 31(1):58.

24. Johnson Vickberg SM, Duhamel KN, Smith MY, et al. Global meaning and psychological adjustment among survivors of bone marrow transplant. Psycho Oncology 2001; 10:29–39.

25. Molassiotis A. A conceptual model of adaptation to illness and quality of life for cancer patients treated with bone marrow transplants. J Adv Nurs 1997; 26:572–579.

26. Stiff P. Mucositis associated with stem cell transplantation: current status and innovative approaches to management. Bone Marrow Transplant 2001; 27:S3–S11.

27. Graber J, de Almeida JC, Javaheri D, et al. Dental health and viridans streptococcal bacteremia in allogenic haematopoietic stem cell transplant recipients. Bone Marrow Transplant 2001; 27:537–542.

28. Nishimoto PW. Sex and sexuality in the cancer patient. Nurse Pract Forum 1995; 6(4):221–227.

29. Quinn B, Kelly D. Sperm-banking in cancer care. Eur J Oncol Nurs 2000; 4(1):55–58.

30. Stacey J. Teratologies: a cultural study of cancer. London: Routledge; 1997.

31. Steeves R. Patients who have undergone bone marrow transplantation: their quest in meaning. Oncol Nurs Forum 1992; 19:899–905.

32. Barrett J, Treleaven J. Bone marrow transplantation in practice. Edinburgh: Churchill Livingstone; 1998.

33. JACIE Joint Accreditation Committee of (i) International Society for Haemopoetic and Graft Engineering – ISHAGE and (ii) European Group for Bone and Marrow Transplantation – EBMT.1998 www.jacie.org

34. Poe SS, Larson E, McGuire D, Krumm S. A national survey of infection prevention practices on bone marrow transplant units. Oncol Nurs Forum 1994; 21(10):1687–1694.

35. Hart S. Prevention of infection. In: Grundy M, ed. Nursing in haematological oncology. Edinburgh: Baillière Tindall; 2000.

36. Goodman JL, Winston DJ, Greenfield RA, et al. A controlled trial of fluconazole to prevent fungal infections in patients undergoing bone marrow transplants. N Engl J Med 1992; 326:845.

37. O'Connell N, McCann SR. Haematologic emergencies. In: Johnston PG, Spence RAJ, eds. Oncologic emergencies. Oxford: Oxford University Press; 2002:289–308.

38. Kolb HJ, Mittermuller J, Clemm CH, et al. Donor leukocyte transfusions for treatment of recurrent chronic myeloid leukaemia in marrow transplanted patients. Blood 1990; 76(12):2462–2465.

39. Deeg HJ, Klingemann H, Philips GL. A guide to bone marrow transplantation. New York: Springer-Verlag; 1992.

40. Miller M, Kearney N. Oral care for patients with cancer: a review of the literature. Cancer Nurs 2001; 24(4):241–253.

41. Quinn B. Making sense of cancer. Bone Marrow Transplant Suppl 2004; 32(1).

42. Futterman AD, Wellisch DK. Psychodynamic themes of bone marrow transplantation: when I becomes thou. Haematol Clin N Am 1990; 4;699–709.

43. Jacobsen PB, Widows MR, Hann DM, Andrykowski MA, Kronish LE. Posttraumatic stress disorder symptoms after bone marrow transplant in cancer. Psychosom Med 1998; 60:366–371.

44. McQuellon RP, Craven BL, Russell GB, et al. Quality of life in breast cancer patients before and after autologous bone marrow transplantation. Bone Marrow Transplant 1996; 18(3):579–584.

45. Stephens M. The lived experience post autologous transplant for a haematological malignancy: a phenomenological study. Eur J Oncol Nurs 2005: in press.

46. Baker F, Zabora J, Polland A, Wingard J. Reintegration after bone marrow transplantation. Cancer Pract 1999; 7(4):190–197.

47. Alby N. Leukaemia bone marrow transplantation. In: Watson M, ed. Cancer patient care. Cambridge: British Psychological Society/Cambridge University Press; 1991.

48. Quinn B. Exploring nurses' experience of supporting a cancer patient in their search for meaning. Eur J Oncol Nur 2002; 7(3):164–171.

49. Department of Health. NHS Cancer Plan. London: Department of Health; 2000.

50. Vos H, Trout G. Issues concerning the transfer of haematology patients to intensive care. Bone Marrow Transplant Suppl 2002; 29(2):252.

51. Quinn B. Sexual health in cancer care. Nurs Times 2003; 99(4):32–34.

52. Schover LP. Sexuality and fertility after cancer. New York: Wiley & Sons; 1997.

53. Trealeven J. In: Treleaven J, Wiernik P, eds. Colour atlas and text of bone marrow transplantation. London: Mosby-Wolfe; 1995:193–200.

54. McQuellon RP, Russell GB, Cella DF, et al. Quality of life measurement in bone marrow transplantation; development of the Functional Assessment of Cancer Therapy-Bone Marrow Transplant (FACT-BMT) scale. Bone Marrow Transplant 1997; 19(4):357–368.

55. Hjermstad MJ, Kaasa S. Quality of life in adult cancer patients treated with bone marrow transplantation – a review of the literature. Eur J Cancer 1995; 31(2):163–173.

CHAPTER 17

Hormone Therapy

DEBORAH FENLON

CHAPTER CONTENTS

Introduction	353	Side effects of hormone therapy	361
Understanding the principles of hormone therapy	354	Side effects of hormone therapy in breast cancer	361
		Maintenance of general health	370
Breast cancer	354	Other side effects of hormone therapy in women	371
Uses in breast cancer	354		
Principles of treatment of breast cancer	356	Side effects of hormone therapy in prostate cancer	373
Prostate cancer	358		
Uses in prostate cancer	358	Conclusion and forward directions	375
Principles of treatment	360	References	375
Other cancers	361		
Endometrium	361		
Thyroid	361		

INTRODUCTION

Hormone, or endocrine, therapies are rarely used as first-line treatment for any cancer. However, they may provide useful treatment options for tumours in sites that are normally under hormonal control. They are generally associated with a low rate of side effects and in carefully selected patients there is a good response rate. For this reason, they can be an extremely useful treatment option in people with cancer. The two major cancers for which hormone therapies are useful are breast and prostate cancer. Hormone therapies have been used in other cancers, but with limited success, and other cancer therapies are more useful in these cases. The focus in this chapter is therefore largely on breast and prostate cancer.

Cancer nurses need to have an understanding of the way in which hormone therapies work, to be familiar with the side effects and to have an appreciation of the options available to help minimize the impact of side effects. This is often a neglected area for cancer nurses as they are more familiar with the acute problems experienced by people with cancer who are experiencing inpatient hospital care. However, hormone therapies are likely to be taken over a long period of time by a large number of people with cancer and their need to be adequately informed should not be underestimated. The rationale for the use of hormone therapies is complex and many of the issues do not have clear-cut answers. Furthermore, there is frequent reference to new research about hormones and cancer within the public media; therefore, users have an increased need for accurate and up-to-date information about the risks and benefits of treatments available.

Breast and prostate cancers account for a large proportion of cancer in the European Union. In the UK a woman has a 1 in 9 chance of developing breast cancer in her lifetime.[1] This is the highest incidence of breast cancer in the world, closely followed by other European countries such as Denmark, Ireland and the Netherlands.[2] A high percentage of these will have adjuvant hormone therapies and many will subsequently require hormone therapy for metastatic disease.

Prostate cancer is the second most common cancer in men within the European Union, with an estimated 134,000 cases and 55,700 deaths in 1996.[1] Endocrine therapy in prostate cancer is generally reserved for use in metastatic disease. However, as 50–60% present with metastatic disease and prostate cancer accounts for 6% of all cancer, a substantial number of people will therefore be treated with hormone therapy.[3]

Whereas hormone therapies are usually associated with a low incidence of side effects, these are often underreported by physicians.[4] As they are not used with curative intent, the balance of side effects in relation to the benefit gained needs to be weighed carefully with full involvement of the patient. This chapter will consider the rationale for use of hormone therapies, the various drugs used and their side effects and offer some possibilities for the management of these side effects.

UNDERSTANDING THE PRINCIPLES OF HORMONE THERAPY

In order for a tumour to be responsive to hormone therapies, the cells present in the tumour need to have hormone receptors. These are proteins found on the surface of the cell which bind specific hormones and enable the passage of the hormone into the nucleus of the cell where it is able to exert its effect. Tumours that contain these hormone receptors arise from tissue which would also normally contain many hormone receptors. However, it is not always possible to predict which tumours will contain

hormone receptors, as tumours may be very mixed, with some cells which resemble the original tissue from which they arose and some being very different. In general, those tumours which are more similar to the original tissue are more likely to contain hormone receptors, to be more responsive to hormone treatments and to behave in a less aggressive fashion.[5]

Predictions can be made about the effect that any hormone therapy might have in the body, but these cannot be made with certainty as there are complex interactions between hormones which influence each other's behaviour by switching on and off hormone receptors in different parts of the body. This means that any theory about the safety or efficacy of a drug or other preparations always needs to be fully tested before it can be promoted for widespread use.

The normal role of some hormones, such as oestrogen, is to promote the growth of tissues including breast and endometrium and that of others, such as progesterone, is to promote maturation of tissue.[6] It can be postulated that those hormones which promote normal tissue growth might also stimulate tumour growth, and this has been demonstrated for oestrogen and breast cancer. Depriving these tumours of oestrogen will cause regression. The underlying principle, therefore, of hormone therapies is to deprive a tumour of the hormone on which it is dependent for growth.[7]

There are a variety of ways in which a tumour can be deprived of hormone: these usually entail removing or reducing the hormone in the body by surgery, radiotherapy or hormonal manipulation. Introducing hormones which interfere with the action of the target hormone can also be effective. These methods will be dealt with for each tumour site individually.

BREAST CANCER

Uses in breast cancer

In breast cancer there are a wide variety of uses of hormone therapies, which can be used in conjunction with other treatments or on their own. Clinical use of different hormones has led to better understanding of the role of hormones in cancer development and the most exciting area currently being investigated is the possibility that hormone manipulation might lead to the prevention of breast cancer.

Metastatic disease

Hormone therapies were initially used in the treatment of metastatic breast cancer, because as a single treatment they are not enough to bring about a cure. Once breast cancer has returned it is not possible to eliminate cancer completely, but the use of hormone therapies has been shown to keep the disease under control. It is possible to see tumours in regression for many years solely on hormone treatment, but the average response rate is around 18 months. Overall, only about 30% of women with metastatic disease will respond to hormone therapy,[8] but if treatment is targeted at selected groups that have been demonstrated to have oestrogen receptor positive (ER+ve) tumours, then the response rate goes up to about 45%.[9] There is no increased benefit by giving combined hormonal therapies as there would be with chemotherapy, but it is possible to see response to a succession of different hormone treatments.[10] Women who are premenopausal should undergo oophorectomy, either surgically or with luteinizing hormone releasing hormone (LHRH) analogues.[10] For postmenopausal women, tamoxifen has been used for many years as the first-line treatment, although some studies have now demonstrated anastrozole to be equally as effective as tamoxifen.[11] Hormones can be given sequentially and should be continued until progression of disease. Once tamoxifen and the aromatase inhibitors have been used, progestogens may also be useful, with the use of androgens, high-dose oestrogen and aminoglutethimide now becoming rare.[10]

Adjuvant therapy

Once it had been established that hormone therapy was useful in metastatic disease, it was then pursued as an adjuvant treatment in the hope of preventing cancer recurrence. It has now been clearly established that adjuvant tamoxifen reduces the chance of recurrence and mortality from breast cancer by 47% in those women who have ER+ve tumours.[12] More recently, it has also been shown that anastrozole can also prevent breast cancer recurrence without the risks of endometrial cancer.[13] However, some women experience joint aches and pains, and there is a concern that anastrozole may increase the risk of osteoporosis. Women who have oestrogen receptor negative (ER−ve) tumours do not benefit from tamoxifen.[14] Current guidelines recommend that only women with ER+ve tumours be given tamoxifen as an adjuvant treatment. It has been shown that there is no additional benefit in continuing tamoxifen for more than 5 years in those women who have had no axillary lymph nodes involved at primary surgery.[15] There is still some debate as to whether to recommend continued tamoxifen after 5 years for women who had disease in the axillary nodes at primary surgery. However, the risks from continued treatment might outweigh benefits if given indefinitely, and so current recommendations are to discontinue treatment at 5 years. If tamoxifen is given in combination with chemotherapy, there may be an increased risk of thromboembolic events,[16] and so it is probably better to reserve tamoxifen use until after chemotherapy has been completed. Ovarian ablation, either by surgery or use of LHRH analogues, may also be recommended as an adjuvant treatment for premenopausal women.[13] The benefit of this has been disputed, as it could be argued that chemotherapy that suppresses ovarian function has a hormonal effect as well as a direct cytotoxic effect.

Prevention of disease

Women who were using tamoxifen to prevent recurrence were noted to have a reduced incidence of new primary breast cancers in the unaffected breast.[17] It was therefore postulated that tamoxifen might even prevent the development of breast cancer. Work in the United States has supported this hypothesis,[18] although there are still many questions to be asked about the role of tamoxifen as a preventative agent. Other major studies in the UK[19] and Italy[20] have not been able to demonstrate a reduction in breast cancer. This may be due to the nature of the cohort of women studied. For example, the British study drew largely from women at a very high risk of breast cancer and may have had a large percentage of women with an altered gene which predisposed them to cancer. This might suggest that tamoxifen is not helpful in this particular group. If tamoxifen is to be used as a preventative agent, then it needs to be established for whom it will be effective, how long it should be used for and how should the risk of side effects be reduced.

Male breast cancer

There are no controlled studies to determine the most appropriate adjuvant treatment for male breast cancer. However, 85% of male breast cancers are ER+ve and 70% are progesterone receptor-positive.[21] As response to hormone therapy correlates to the presence of receptors, it is presumed that there is a survival benefit to giving adjuvant tamoxifen to men. It is associated with a high rate of symptoms, such as hot flushes and impotence.[22] In metastatic disease, orchidectomy or the use of LHRH analogues may be useful. Tamoxifen, progesterones and aromatase inhibitors may also be used in the same way as for female breast cancer.

Principles of treatment of breast cancer

The rationale for depriving breast tumours of oestrogen has been supported by clinical observation as long ago as 1899, when Beatson demonstrated that women with metastatic breast cancers could achieve remission of disease when their ovaries were removed.[23] In the 1970s, the mechanism for this was discovered when oestrogen receptors were demonstrated.[24] Oestrogen receptors are found in cells throughout the body in nearly all the major organs, including the brain, skin, bones and periurethral tract.[24] Not all breast cancers contain oestrogen receptors, and those that are ER–ve are much less likely to respond to hormonal manipulation. Oestrogen has remained the most important hormone when considering treatment for breast cancer. All the hormonal treatments available are based on reducing the amount of oestrogen or opposing its action in some way.

Oestrogen is mainly produced in the ovaries, although about 10% of oestrogen is produced in subcutaneous tissue under the control of the adrenal gland. This peripheral oestrogen continues to be produced after menopause and so hormonal treatments of breast cancer are effective both before and after the menopause. Both the ovaries and the adrenal gland are under the influence of the pituitary. When there are low levels of sex hormones such as oestrogen in the body, the pituitary is stimulated to release the gonadotrophic hormones – luteinizing hormone (LH) and follicle-stimulating hormone (FSH). Once these reach the gonads (ovaries in women and testes in men), they stimulate the gonads to produce sex hormones. In the female, the ovaries will produce oestrogen and progesterone; in the male, the testes will produce testosterone. The adrenal gland is under the influence of adrenocorticotrophic hormone (ACTH). In turn, the pituitary is governed by the hypothalamus. The hormone that induces the pituitary to release LH and FSH is called luteinizing hormone releasing hormone (LHRH) or gonadotrophic hormone releasing hormone (GHRH). If there are high levels of end hormone, such as oestrogen, in the body, then the pituitary will stop producing LHRH. This is known as the negative feedback effect (Fig. 17.1).

The primary way to prevent oestrogen production is to remove the ovaries. A further reduction in oestrogen production could then be to remove the adrenal gland and, subsequently, a hypophysectomy could reduce oestrogen levels further. Historically, all these operations have been performed with some success, causing regression of breast cancer tumours. However, adrenalectomy and hypophysectomy are associated with high levels of morbidity (and even mortality) and have now been replaced by more subtle methods. Oophorectomy is rarely performed, as production of oestrogen by the ovaries can be halted in other ways. Irradiation of the ovaries will bring about permanent menopause, but is associated with significant side effects. The use of adjuvant chemotherapy will usually interfere with ovarian function and this can sometimes be permanent. The nearer that a woman is to her natural menopause, then the more likely it is that her periods will cease altogether.[25] See Table 17.1 for a summary of all the breast cancer treatments.

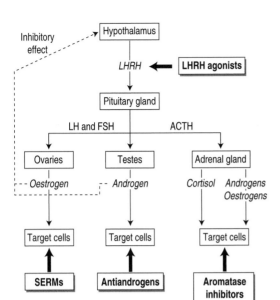

Figure 17.1: Sites of action of endocrine therapies. ACTH, adrenocorticotrophic hormone; LH, luteinizing hormone; FSH, follicle-stimulating hormone; LHRH, luteinizing hormone releasing hormone; SERMS, selective oestrogen receptor modulators.

Gonadotrophins

Gonadotrophins are hormones which have an effect on the gonads. The main one is LHRH. A reversible menopause can be brought about by the use of LHRH analogues, such as leuprorelin or goserelin (Zoladex). These work by mimicking the action of natural LHRH and bind to receptor sites on the pituitary. Initially, they will stimulate the pituitary and cause a release of gonadotrophins. However, they are a great deal more potent than natural LHRH and so permanently occupy the receptor sites in the pituitary. Once the sites are blocked, they are no longer receptive to new waves of LHRH and so are unable to fulfil their function and cause the release of gonadotrophins. Without stimulation from the pituitary, the ovary ceases hormone production. Once gonadotrophins are present in the system again, the ovary recovers. It has been proposed that while the ovaries are quiescent in this way they may be protected from the detrimental effects of chemotherapy. Therefore, it has been proposed that young women undergoing chemotherapy who wish to retain their fertility

may choose to have LHRH treatment in order to preserve ovarian function.

Aromatase inhibitors

In postmenopausal women there is still some circulating oestrogen made in subcutaneous fatty tissue. Women who are obese have higher levels of oestrogen, and obesity has been shown to be a risk factor for the onset of breast cancer.[26] Oestrogen produced in this way can be reduced by interfering with the chain of chemical reactions which produce oestrogen.[27] One of the major enzymes that is involved with facilitating these chemical processes is the aromatase enzyme. Molecules that bind with this enzyme are known as aromatase inhibitors: they hinder the action of the enzyme, which results in a lower production of the end hormone.[28] A number of these molecules have been developed and are now widely used in the treatment of postmenopausal breast cancer. The earliest known was aminoglutethimide;[27] however, this also interfered with other pathways and so had a significant amount of unacceptable side effects.[29] It was also necessary to give hydrocortisone with aminoglutethimide, as this interferes with cortisol production. The newer molecules are highly specific and associated with very low levels of side effects. The side effects that are found are more related to the resulting low levels of oestrogen than to inadvertent effects of the drug. The drugs that are now in use are formestane, Aromasin (exemestane), letrozole and anastrozole. Reduction of oestrogen may result in oestrogen withdrawal symptoms, such as hot flushes and dry vagina.[30] Long-term use may also be associated with musculoskeletal changes, causing aching joints and possibly a loss of bone density. Although joint pains and fractures are increased, there is a lower side-effect profile with anastrozole over tamoxifen, and anastrozole increases disease-free survival, so may now be recommended as first-line adjuvant therapy for postmenopausal women with hormone receptor positive breast cancer.[30a]

There are a number of other methods of hormone therapy that rely on interfering with the action of oestrogen at the target cell site. The mechanism of action of these drugs is only

357

partially understood and usually results in a mixture of blocking and enabling of hormone responses. Progesterones and testosterone both have actions that oppose that of oestrogen and have been shown to be effective in treating breast cancer. However, they have hormonal effects of their own, which may be significant and unacceptable. Synthetic progestogens can be useful in the treatment of breast cancer. The main ones used are medroxyprogesterone acetate (Farlutal or Provera)[31] and megestrol acetate (Megace).[32] The incidence of side effects is low and some people experience a feeling of well-being when taking progestogens, which makes them particularly useful in palliative care. The main side effect noted is increased appetite and consequent weight gain.[31] Long-term use may also result in cushingoid changes, such as a redistribution of body fat, which results in a classic moon face and thoracic hump. Earlier changes noted may be increase in sebum production and thinning of hair. Glucose intolerance can be induced, so diabetes should be monitored for. The synthetic drug tamoxifen (Nolvadex, Soltamox) has been found to have mixed oestrogenic and antioestrogenic activity and has been a mainstay of breast cancer treatment for many years.[33]

Selective oestrogen receptor modulators

There is normally a small amount of circulating oestrogen in the body after the menopause; this is known to have a beneficial effect in a variety of ways, including prevention of bone loss, improved cardiovascular features[34] and protection of the brain from the onset of Alzheimer's disease.[35] An ideal molecule would be one which retained these positive oestrogenic effects but did not cause breast cancer cells to grow. A number of molecules have now been identified which have a mixture of oestrogenic and non-oestrogenic effects. These are known as selective oestrogen receptor modulators (SERMs).[36] The perfect SERM has not yet been identified. Tamoxifen, the best known of this group, prevents breast cancer growth and also appears to have a weak beneficial effect on bone[37] and possibly the cardiovascular system.[38] However, it can stimulate endometrial growth, causing thickening of the lining of the womb, which leads to polyps and rarely cancer.[39] Other SERMs have been developed to obtain the ideal profile: toremifene and raloxifene are available. Raloxifene has been licensed for use in osteoporosis, and is currently being investigated for its potential role in the prevention of breast cancer.[40] Many plants contain molecules which are similar to animal oestrogens; these are called phytoestrogens. Phytoestrogens are the active component in soy food products. They appear to have mild oestrogenic effects in the body and there is currently much research to evaluate their uses. Claims have been made that they may be able to reduce menopausal symptoms or even to prevent breast cancer, but there is little direct evidence as yet to support these claims.

PROSTATE CANCER

Uses in prostate cancer

Hormone treatment in the form of androgen deprivation has been the mainstay of treatment of metastatic prostate cancer since the 1940s and produces effective and reliable responses in around 80% of patients.[3]

It is now increasingly common to give hormone therapies as an adjuvant to primary surgery or radiotherapy, with the aim of facilitating local control and improving survival. Hormones given before surgery (neoadjuvant therapy) can reduce the size of the initial tumour, but it is uncertain whether this will translate into improved quality of life or survival. In the radiotherapy setting, neoadjuvant hormonal therapy improves local control, although survival data is not available. Adjuvant LHRH agonists improve both local control and survival after radiotherapy.[44] Currently, the LHRH agonists are the drugs of choice for adjuvant therapy, whereas combined androgen blockade has generally been used as neoadjuvant therapy. Monotherapy with a non-steroidal antiandrogen has considerable potential in both settings. Areas for future studies include appropriate end points for clinical studies, comparative drug efficacy and the effect of treatment on quality of life.[44]

Table 17.1: Summary of hormone therapies used to treat breast cancer

Treatment modality	Generic drug name	Trade names	Side effects	Notes
Surgery	Oophorectomy		Early menopause	May be used for treatment in premenopausal women or for prevention
	Adrenalectomy			No longer used
	Hypophysectomy			No longer used
Radiotherapy	Ovarian ablation		Menopause	Occasionally used
Drugs	LHRH analogues	Goserelin Leuprorelin	Zoladex Prostap	Temporary menopause	Subcutaneous injection once per month
	Aromatase inhibitors	Aminoglutethimide	Orimeten	Drowsiness, lethargy, rash	Rarely used – corticosteroid replacement necessary
		Anastrozole Letrozole	Arimidex Femara	Hot flushes Joint pains	
	Progesterones	Medroxyprogesterone acetate	Farlutal Provera Depo-Provera	Weight gain, tremors, sweating, Cushing-like features, muscular cramps, nausea/vomiting[31]	
		Megestrol acetate	Megace	Weight gain, vaginal bleeding, nausea, hot flushes and hypertension[32]	
	Testosterone		Durabolin	Masculinization	Rarely used
	SERMs	Tamoxifen	Nolvadex Soltamox	Hot flushes[41] Vaginal dryness[41] Endometrial cancer[39] Venous thrombosis[42] Hepatotoxicity[43]	
		Raloxifene Toremifene	Evista Fareston	Hot flushes, vaginal bleeding, endometrial cancer	

Principles of treatment

In the same way that the treatment of breast cancer depends on manipulation of the oestrogenic environment, so in prostate cancer a reduction in the levels of testosterone can bring about regression of disease. Huggins and Bergenstal[45] first observed that the prostate gland is dependent on androgens, mainly testosterone, and demonstrated a response in patients with advanced prostatic cancer by removal of the testes (orchidectomy). Androgen receptors are found in target cells that will respond to changes in levels of androgens. Androgen deprivation can produce symptomatic relief in 80–85% of patients, with a mean duration of response of about 18 months. This high response rate makes it the treatment of choice for metastatic prostate cancer. However, as with breast cancer, this does not represent a cure, and most patients will subsequently relapse after treatment with endocrine therapy (see Table 17.2 for an overview of treatments).

Orchidectomy

The removal of the testes reduces testosterone by around 90%.[46] This takes place very quickly and, where rapid relief of symptoms is required, such as spinal cord compression, makes surgery the treatment of choice. Bone metastases respond well to this treatment option, with up to 90% relief from bony pain.[47] However, some men find surgery unacceptable due to the negative image associated with castration and the side effects of impotence and loss of libido, present in up to 60% of men. A further disadvantage is that the active androgen, dihydrotestosterone (DHT) is only reduced by 60–70%.[46] These androgens are produced in the adrenal gland. Although the response rate is high, it is not universal and so some men may have unnecessary surgery that is irreversible.

Gonadotrophins

LHRH analogues, such as goserelin, work in the same way in men as they do in women by suppressing the function of the gonads. In men, they prevent the testes from producing testosterone. This is known as a medical castration and reduces androgen to the same levels as surgical castration within 2–4 weeks.[46] Where surgery is not an option, then this is a useful alternative to orchidectomy. It is also reversible, so that if there is no benefit then treatment can be stopped. Both orchidectomy and the use of LHRH analogues interfere with sexual function. A preference for medical castration over surgery has been shown by 80% of patients.[48] In some countries, the ongoing cost associated with medication may make surgery the preferred choice.

Antiandrogens

Following treatment with either LHRH analogues or orchidectomy, testosterone is still produced by the adrenal glands, which is normally about 5% of circulating testosterone.[3] Antiandrogens may be used to oppose the action of this testosterone. These compete with androgens for binding sites at the androgen receptor in the nucleus of prostate cancer cells. There are two classes of antiandrogens:

- steroidal, such as cyproterone acetate (Cyprostat) or megestrol acetate (Megace)

- non-steroidal, such as flutamide (Drogenil), nilutamide or bicalutamide (Casodex).

The steroidal antiandrogens not only block androgen receptors, but also inhibit the release of LH, thus causing a reduction in testosterone production. They may be used as a first-line treatment instead of orchidectomy or LHRH analogues. Cyproterone acetate has been shown to be as effective as oestrogen, with a response rate of 40–55%.[44] It is unclear whether the non-steroidal antiandrogens are as effective as castration when they are used as single agents, but they are becoming more widely used because of the chance of retaining sexual function.

To reduce androgens to a minimum, both orchidectomy and antiandrogens may be used. This is known as combined androgen blockade (CAB) or maximum androgen blockade (MAB). This may result in an increased response, with longer to progression than castration alone, although it is still debated.[49]

A further benefit of using LHRH analogues rather than orchidectomy is the ability to give androgen blockade intermittently. This is done by monitoring disease levels by the presence of prostate-specific antigen (PSA) and administering androgen blockade with evidence of tumour progression. By giving a break from treatment, it is suggested that tumour cells do not develop resistance to androgen treatment and so patients with limited disease could stay on intermittent therapy indefinitely.

Other drugs

The administration of oestrogen, such as diethylstilbestrol, will achieve the same levels of testosterone as orchidectomy. This is due to negative feedback on the pituitary gland. There may also be a direct effect, as there are oestrogen receptors in the prostate. However, this approach is not often used due to complications from myocardial infarction, cerebrovascular accident and pulmonary embolism. Other side effects include loss of libido, impotence and gynaecomastia. Oestrogens used to be the treatment of choice, but are now usually replaced by medical or surgical castration due to cardiovascular toxicity.

Aromatase inhibitors, such as aminoglutethimide given with hydrocortisone, may have a role in second-line hormone treatment, but they are accompanied by a high rate of side effects. Where a rapid response is required but surgery is not an option, ketoconazole may be used. This produces castrate levels of testosterone within 24–48 hours.[46] However, it causes liver damage and adrenal suppression and so is not suitable for long-term use. Corticosteroids used alone may have a use in patients who have relapsed after first-line hormonal treatment, as they reduce concentrations of ACTH and so interfere with the production of adrenal androgens. Second-line treatments have a much lower response rate of 30% at best.[3]

OTHER CANCERS

Endometrium

The primary treatment for cancer of the endometrium (uterus) is surgery and radiotherapy. Hormone therapy may be given as an adjuvant treatment, but the evidence to support this is poor and hormone therapy is usually reserved for treatment of metastatic disease. However, endometrial cancer is hormone-dependent and responds to progestogens such as medroxyprogesterone acetate (100–500 mg daily) or megestrol acetate (40–320 mg daily). Tamoxifen, LHRH analogues and danazol may also be useful. Overall, a 20–30% response rate is seen with hormone therapy.

Thyroid

The treatment of thyroid cancer is thyroid ablation, usually by surgery or radiotherapy, followed by physiological hormone replacement therapy (HRT). This prevents hypothyroidism and maintains thyroid-stimulating hormone (TSH) at low levels to minimize the chance of recurrence of a TSH-dependent tumour. Elderly patients who are unfit for surgery and have small, well-differentiated tumours which are dependent on TSH for growth, may be treated by levothyroxine alone. This inhibits the secretion of TSH by negative feedback control.

SIDE EFFECTS OF HORMONE THERAPY

For breast and prostate cancer, the hormone manipulations that are available are largely effective through influencing the sex hormones of oestrogen and testosterone. Many of the side effects are therefore related to sexual characteristics. This makes it necessary to address the side effects separately for men and women. The first part of this section will therefore concentrate on the side effects of hormonal treatment for breast cancer and the second part will consider side effects of hormonal treatments for prostate cancer.

Side effects of hormone therapy in breast cancer

Many of the problems caused by hormonal treatments for women with breast cancer are similar to the normal changes that would be seen in the body with varying hormone levels. One of the most dramatic of these is when the

Table 17.2: Summary of hormone therapies used to treat prostate cancer

Treatment modality	Generic drug name	Trade names	Side effects	Notes
Surgery	Orchidectomy		Loss of libido Impotence May be unacceptable to some	Quick acting, but irreversible
Drugs	LHRH analogues Goserelin Leuprorelin Triptorelin Buserilin	Zoladex Prostap Decapeptyl Suprefact	Loss of libido Impotence Tumour flare	Subcutaneous injection once per month s.c. 3× daily and then intranasally 6× daily
	Progesterones Medroxyprogesterone acetate (also has antiandrogen properties)	Farlutal Provera Depo-Provera	Weight gain, tremors, sweating, Cushing-like features, muscular cramps, nausea/vomiting[31]	
	Megestrol acetate	Megace	Weight gain, vaginal bleeding, nausea, hot flushes and hypertension[32]	
	Oestrogen Diethylstilbestrol Ethinyloestradiol	Ethinyloestradiol	Cardiovascular problems, nausea Loss of libido Gynaecomastia	Rarely used
	Antiandrogens Steroidal – Cyproterone acetate	Cyprostat	Loss of libido, impotence, disturbances in liver function, thromboembolism Steroidal effects (e.g. weight gain & fluid retention)[44]	Avoids surgery, as effective as oestrogen[46]
	Non-steroidal – Flutamide – Nilutamide – Bicalutamide	Drogenil Casodex	Gynaecomastia, diarrhoea	
	Aromatase inhibitors Aminoglutethimide Ketoconazole	Orimeten	Drowsiness, lethargy, rash Liver damage	

ovaries cease to produce oestrogen and the menopause comes about. Without any hormonal manipulation, the ovaries decrease oestrogen production over a period of many years, which finally results in cessation of menstruation around the age of 51 years old. Women who have treatment for breast cancer may have menopause induced early, either by direct hormonal manipulation or as a consequence of chemotherapy. Menopause will be considered here in the context of breast cancer and then other side effects of hormone therapy in breast cancer will be examined.

Menopause – causes

Menopausal difficulties are frequently seen after breast cancer. It has been demonstrated that 60% of all women treated for breast cancer will suffer menopausal difficulties.[50] This is for a number of reasons. It should not be forgotten that many women will be naturally menopausal at the time that breast cancer occurs. Breast cancer starts to become common after the age of 50 years old, and this is also the average time of menopause. It is current practice to recommend that women do not take HRT once they have had breast cancer. This means that there is a group of women who are suffering problems with the natural menopause but who are limited in their options of controlling their symptoms.

Women who are required to cease use of HRT when they are diagnosed with breast cancer will experience a recurrence of the symptoms from which they sought relief at the time of menopause. Symptoms that occur at this time can be as severe as those that initially stimulated the women to take HRT. A further difficulty at this time is the belief that many women have that the HRT actually caused their breast cancer.

A further group of women will experience menopause as a consequence of their treatment for breast cancer. The LHRH analogues such as Zoladex are used to induce menopause, and the consequences of menopausal symptoms will occur as would be expected. Chemotherapy suppresses ovarian function and many women will have a temporary or permanent cessation of their menstruation. Thirty per cent of all premenopausal women will be amenorrhoeic one

year after chemotherapy and many more will suffer disruptions to the menstrual cycle.[51] This depends to some extent on the agent used, as some chemotherapy agents are more likely to affect the ovaries than others. As a general rule, women who are under 40 years old are more likely to recover ovarian function; for those over the age of 40 years old, periods are less likely to return.[52] Menopausal difficulties, in particular hot flushes and night sweats, may occur with suppression of ovarian function, whether this is temporary or permanent. There is some evidence to suggest that these symptoms are worse with an induced menopause than if it had occurred naturally.[53]

Although the exact mechanism of hot flushes is not known, there is a link with declining oestrogen levels. Hormone therapies which have an effect on oestrogen levels in the body may also cause symptoms associated with changes in oestrogen levels, such as hot flushes. The aromatase inhibitors and tamoxifen have also been shown to aggravate hot flushes;[32] in a postmenopausal woman, these are not usually severe, as the adjustment to low oestrogen levels has already been made.

Menopause – experience

For a woman to experience menopause as a consequence of treatment for breast cancer adds an additional burden to the cancer and its treatment. For many, this is seen as secondary to the cancer, but often comes back as an issue once treatment has been completed. At this time, the permanence of the changes may bring the realization of losses, such as the ability to bear children. A normal menopause may be for many woman a positive time, free from menstruation and contraception. However, for a woman who has undergone an early menopause, her feelings may be dominated by concerns over ageing and changing self-image. Work by Singer and Hunter[54] shows that women who have premature menopause suffer negative repercussions to their self-esteem and body image and feelings of bereavement surrounding their lost 'life plan' and lost fertility. They also suggest that the extent to which early menopause was perceived as a problem depended on what else was happening in the woman's life. In the context of ill health it was less of a problem.

Work by Knobf[55] showed that those women with breast cancer who undergo menopause due to chemotherapy have similar experiences to those women who undergo a natural menopause. She found that while women were undergoing active treatment, menopausal symptoms were minimized and women responded by ignoring them. As time went by, menopausal symptoms became more of a dominant concern, especially for those women who suffered moderate or severe distress or significant disruption to their roles and daily life. Further work by Knobf[56] showed that healthcare professionals tended to focus in on treatment and related side effects. Although they informed women that their periods would stop, they did not look at menopause as a whole and what the implications might be for the women:

> Saying that your periods may stop doesn't sound like you are going to have menopause ... they are not giving the full message.[56]

Women found that they had to rely on themselves to find a way to cope. They became more wary about their health, being careful about medication and adopting healthy lifestyle choices. Cancer and menopause were two major life events for these women which they experienced simultaneously and, subsequently, had to integrate into a coherent strategy for carrying on with life.

Davis et al[57] found similar issues and identified that taking and keeping control were an important concern for women with breast cancer. They identified that this could be done through information and support. Other significant issues they found for women with breast cancer were:

> Maintaining a coherent sense of self and the desire to return to 'normal'.

Women often begin the cancer experience with the belief that once they have completed their treatment they will be able to return to normal. However, they begin to realize that some of these changes are more permanent, which challenge their sense of identity. The fact that several changes are occurring simultaneously makes this process more difficult.

At the time of menopause, women are often met by a 'cloak of silence',[58] where it becomes hard to find understanding and information about their concerns. This is legitimized in cancer care when a physician's focus is orientated around more immediately life-threatening concerns. Women are receiving the message that menopause is 'secondary' and, consequently, they make it so, independent of their actual experience.

Women with breast cancer have been found to have a high number of menopausal difficulties.[59] Harris et al[53] found that after breast cancer women were five times more likely to be experiencing symptoms than women who had not had breast cancer. This may be partly due to the fact that after breast cancer women are much less likely to take HRT to help symptoms. Carpenter and Andrykowski[59] outlined the incidence of a range of symptoms (Table 17.3), but acknowledged that for women with breast cancer there may be multiple causes of some of these symptoms and so they may not be entirely due to the menopause. Women who have had chemotherapy and radiotherapy without undergoing menopause may also suffer joint pains, difficulty sleeping and feeling tired. Nevertheless, hot flushes and night sweats appear to be more prevalent and more severe amongst this population than the normal population.

For women with breast cancer there are difficulties in separating out the experience of breast cancer and that of menopause. For example, some women during menopause experience a sensation known as formication and described by some as 'skin crawls'. This is a sensation of irritation or prickling under the skin often felt in the chest wall. Women with breast cancer may interpret this as cancer in their chest wall or lymph glands. Some women have been heard to describe this as evidence that their chemotherapy is working because 'they can feel it'. Experiences that are identified as hormonal will automatically be ascribed to hormonal treatments, such as tamoxifen, whether this is the case or not. Women who have been treated with chemotherapy may be going through menopause due to ovarian suppression due to the cytotoxic effect on the ovaries. While tamoxifen can cause hot flushes, ovarian suppression causes a dramatic change in hormonal levels, with particularly low

Table 17.3: Incidence of menopausal symptoms in women after breast cancer

Symptom	Percentage
Joint pain	77%
Feeling tired	75%
Difficulty sleeping	68%
Hot flushes	66%
Headaches	55%
Irritable and nervous	54%
Depressed	51%
Numbness and tingling	40%
Vaginal dryness	36%
Dizzy spells	25%
Pounding heart	25%
Painful intercourse	21%
Skin crawls	18%

Source: Carpenter and Andrykowski.[59]

oestrogen levels, which may result in severe hot flushes and night sweats. Side effects from chemotherapy, such as tiredness, are almost impossible to tease out from menopausal experiences. It may be that tiredness following chemotherapy is extended due to the menopause, but this cannot be identified for certain.

When under stress, one is more likely to interpret normal body sensations as indicative of important and worrying symptoms.[60] Kleinman also discusses how after serious or chronic illness confidence is lost in the body and the expectation of health. After breast cancer, it is common to interpret body sensations as cancer returning. Where there are new sensations as a consequence of menopause, then it is unsurprising that these can be alarming and that more attention

would be paid to them than if they had not occurred in the context of life-threatening illness.

Hot flushes

Hot flushes are a commonly reported sign of menopause, but vary widely in their manifestation. They can be frequent and severe and have been reported with up to 240 occurring in a 24-hour period.[61] Descriptions vary from being a mild feeling of warmth in the upper body and face with mild perspiration through to severe flushes that feel like 'a raging furnace' or 'burning up'.[62] Several studies have now shown that around 65% women who have been treated for breast cancer will experience hot flushes,[59,63,64] with one study showing up to 70%.[50] The severity of the flushes was reported as 29% mild, 37% moderate and 34% severe by Couzi[63] with similar ratings shown by Carpenter and Andrykowski.[59] Further studies by Carpenter et al[64] and McPhail[65] in the UK, comparing women who had been treated for breast cancer with women who were naturally menopausal, reported that the breast cancer survivors experienced hot flushes that were significantly more frequent, severe, bothersome and of greater duration. When the menopause is induced by chemotherapy or surgically, the resultant levels of circulating oestrogen are much less than with natural menopause. There is also a lower level of other hormones, such as testosterone,[66] which may also have an impact on the severity of menopausal symptoms. Tamoxifen also causes hot flushes, although the exact mechanism behind this is not clear.[67]

Menopause – treatment

Menopause within the context of breast cancer is a complex occurrence. The symptoms experienced, the possibilities for management and the meaning that it has for the individual are all complicated by the presence of breast cancer. It is important therefore for healthcare professionals to hear the patients' experiences and work with them to help them understand the changes that are occurring in their bodies, so that they can implement strategies that are appropriate to their own lives and circumstances, in order to deal with the difficulties they have to face.

An approach advocated by Kleinman[60] for women suffering chronic conditions is to construct a mini-ethnography of the woman's life and then work with her to address those areas which have significance or cause disruption to daily living. Once individuals have been able to discuss what their own personal issues are with this transition, then they can begin to construct a way to deal with them. The role of the professional is to facilitate an understanding of the processes that are occurring and thus to help the individual to construct personal meaning and significance in the process. Specific interventions may be useful to help women to adjust to these changes. Ganz et al[68] adopted an approach of this nature for women with menopausal difficulties after breast cancer by using in-depth assessment and an intervention programme based on mutually identified goals. They showed significant improvement in menopausal difficulties and sexual activity. An approach of this nature is suggested in Box 17.1. The assessment focuses on the problems as defined by the woman herself and the role of the nurse is to help the woman understand what is happening to her and explore the options available to help her manage her difficulties. Together they will put together a package of strategies, including pharmacological and non-pharmacological methods, to help the woman deal with her physical symptoms and cope with the changes that are occurring to her. Although it is generally contraindicated, some women will be experiencing sufficiently severe difficulties to want to consider the possibility of using hormone replacement therapy. There is currently much controversy on the advisability of using HRT in this situation, and each woman will need to consider carefully the risks and benefits that apply to her individual circumstances.

Hormone replacement therapy

Because oestrogen may be implicated in the development of breast cancer it is generally considered that HRT is unsafe to use after breast cancer.[6,7] The main hormone in HRT is oestrogen; however, this is known to

---

Box 17.1

A nursing approach to the management of menopausal difficulties in breast cancer

- In-depth assessment of menopausal difficulties experienced
- Exploration of the meaning of menopause, including heralding of old age, change in social status, etc.
- Exploration of the impact of menopause as a consequence of treatment for breast cancer
- Information and education around difficulties encountered
- Behavioural techniques to cope with hot flushes, e.g. distraction, paced respiration
- Advice on stress management
- Specific strategies for managing vaginal dryness and painful intercourse
- Discussion regarding appropriateness of pharmacological intervention
- Advice regarding complementary and herbal therapies and diet
- Advice on maintaining health

---

increase the risk of uterine cancer, and so progesterone is added as a protection for the uterus. Those women who have had a hysterectomy require oestrogen alone. It is known that oestrogen causes growth of breast tumours,[6] and there is a small but significant increase in the incidence of breast cancer in women taking HRT.[69] It is now known that HRT delivered in a combined form of both oestrogen and progesterone is associated with a much higher risk of developing breast cancer than oestrogen-only preparations[70] (Table 17.4). However, there is no direct evidence that the use of HRT in women who have had breast cancer will increase recurrence, and this is the subject of current debate. Cancers that occur while women are taking HRT appear to be less aggressive and carry a good prognosis.[71] There has been no increase in mortality from breast cancer associated with HRT use.[71] One study has shown that women with breast cancer who take HRT actually have a lower incidence of cancer recurrence than those who do not.[72] This may be due to selection bias, but is an early indication that HRT may be safe if given for short periods of time. A large-scale trial is currently underway to investigate this question.[73] It will remain difficult to tease out the relative differences between different kinds of HRT. Questions that will remain for some time will be about dose, length of treatment and combination or oestrogen-only preparations. Still other forms of HRT are becoming available, such as tibolone (Livial). This is a synthetic hormone that has some oestrogenic activity, but also has progestogenic and androgenic activity. Further laboratory and clinical trials will be needed to evaluate the safety of these drugs.

While some women will say that the problem of menopause is small in relation to cancer, others will say that it is a continuing reminder that they have had cancer and that it is the last thing preventing them from return to normal. For some, the problem is so great that quality of life is intolerable and they feel that they would be prepared to sacrifice long-term survival in order to improve their current life. This group of women is prepared to consider the use of HRT even when the medical recommendation is that it is regarded to be unsafe. Some would prefer to take other medication and still others will say that they would rather not have any more medicine but allow menopause to take its natural course.

Pharmacological measures for the control of hot flushes

For those women that prefer not to take HRT, there are a number of other pharmacological measures that have some effect in relieving hot flushes, although these are not as effective as HRT and all have side effects. Clonidine 0.1 mg/day is effective in reducing hot flushes in tamoxifen-induced hot flushes by 20%,[74] although some women have dry mouth or constipation.

Some studies have shown that selective serotonin re-uptake inhibitors (SSRIs) may be effective in reducing hot flushes. Blood levels of serotonin appear to be diminished in menopausal women[75] and oestrogen replacement therapy appears to augment serotonin activity.[76] Pilot studies have been conducted using venlafaxine (12.5 mg twice daily)[77] and paroxetine (20 mg daily).[78] These have shown that 55–67% women show at least a 50% reduction in the incidence of hot flushes and 58–73% reduction in the severity of hot flushes. Unwanted effects of these drugs include dry mouth, nausea, somnolence, nightmares, disorientation and a stimulation of anxiety. Although these early studies appear promising, personal experience has shown a high level of side effects that women find totally unacceptable.

Progesterone therapy, such as Megace (20 mg twice daily) has been found to be effective

Table 17.4: Incidence of breast and endometrial cancer with and without hormone replacement therapy (HRT)

HRT use	Length of use	Number of cancers per 1000 in women aged 50–65 years old	
		Breast	Endometrium
No HRT		32	5
Oestrogen only	5 years	33.5	9
	10 years	37	15
Oestrogen and progesterone	5 years	38	Not known
	10 years	51	6–7

Source: based on information in Million Women Study Collaborators.[70]

in reducing hot flushes in women with breast cancer.[79] However, there are little data on the long-term safety of the use of progesterone after breast cancer.

Many women take herbal remedies for hot flushes.[80,81] Ernst[82] suggests that there is a growing body of data to support the efficacy of some of these popular herbal medicinal products, and the potential for doing good seems greater than that for doing harm. However, he stresses that no herbal medicines are free of adverse effects. Because the evidence is incomplete, risk–benefit assessments are not completely reliable, and much knowledge is still lacking. The most interesting group of herbal remedies is the phytoestrogens.

Phytoestrogens

There is growing interest in the role of phytoestrogens both in breast cancer and menopause: these molecules are found in plants and have a similar molecular structure to oestrogen. They can be part of the diet or found in herbal remedies, and include many substances classified as lignans, isoflavones and coumestans. Intestinal flora convert inactive plant precursors into compounds active in the human.[83] They are found in plant sources such as soya beans and soya foods, linseed, sunflower and flax seeds, bean sprouts, whole grains, fruit and vegetables. They are also provided in herbal remedies such as red clover (*Trifolium pratense*), black cohosh (*Cimicifuga racemosa*), chaste berry (*Vitex agnus castus*), dong quai (*Angelica sinensis*), hops (*Humulus lupulus*) and liquorice (*Glycyrrhiza glabra*).[84] In oriental countries where the intake of phytoestrogens is high, both breast cancer and menopausal difficulties are lower in incidence than in the West.[85] It is thought that they may be able to influence the development of breast cancer[85,86] and to reduce hot flushes after menopause.

The evidence for the reduction in hot flushes due to phytoestrogens is conflicting. It has been shown that soya, red clover, hops and chaste berry have oestrogenic effects and liquorice and dong quai have a mild oestrogenic activity.[84] Therefore, this might result in oestrogenic benefits such as the reduction of flushes. The majority of work has been conducted on soya, with several studies showing a

reduction in flushing[87,88] and others showing no change.[89,90] There are mild gastrointestinal disturbances. The difficulties with achieving standardization of results may be due to types and amount of product used. Many of the soya products available in the West are alcohol-washed and this may reduce the isoflavone content.[91] If soya products are effective, it is not clear whether supplements should be used or whether the effect will be greater by incorporating soya into the diet.

Black cohosh (*Cimicifuga racemosa*), does not appear to have oestrogenic effects in the body.[84,92] Again, evidence is conflicting, with Jacobson et al[93] showing no reduction in flushing, but Lieberman[94] and Liske et al[92] showing a benefit. There is growing use of black cohosh (sold as RemiFemin) for alleviation of hot flushes;[95] as it does not appear to have oestrogenic effects, it might be presumed to be safe after breast cancer,[91] although this raises a question about its mechanism of action.

There is also a trend towards the use of red clover, which has a clear oestrogenic effect. Van der Weijer and Berentsen[96] showed a benefit, but Fugh-Berman and Kronenberg[97] showed no reduction of flushing. Red clover may have benefits to the heart and bone,[98] but has been shown to cause infertility in animals[99] and contains coumarins, which may affect clotting.[97]

There are still many questions and difficulties surrounding the use of phytoestrogens. Supplements that are available are expensive, and the long-term safety of phytoestrogens is unknown. Oestrogenic effects may include the reduction of hot flushes, benefits to heart, bone and vagina.[100] Where it is claimed that a substance has an oestrogenic effect in the body, it must therefore follow that there is a potential risk of stimulating breast cancer growth. Until more evidence is available, it cannot be assumed that the use of herbal preparations for the relief of hot flushes is safe.

Natural progesterone or wild yam (Dioscorea villosa)

Wild yam cream is usually promoted for its progesterone content. However, it also contains oestrogen-like substances. If wild yam is introduced into the body, then it will be metabolized into a number of different compounds, including oestrogens, androgens and even steroids. However, it is unlikely that enough is absorbed through application to the skin to have any significant effect. It is difficult to control the dose when used as a cream, as people will use different amounts. Work done by Komesaroff et al[101] showed that wild yam cream (Biogest) did not help hot flushes, nor did it have any effect on other hormones. Blood progesterone levels were not measurably raised. There are no long-term data to suggest that the use of progesterones, natural or otherwise, for the control of hot flushes is safe after breast cancer.

Non-pharmacological approaches to managing hot flushes

As menopause is seen as a natural event, many women take the approach that they would rather manage their problems themselves using a variety of self-help measures. They use behavioural strategies, cognitive techniques, changes to diet and complementary therapies such as homeopathy and acupuncture to help hot flushes. Harris et al[53] have shown that women are 5 times more likely to suffer severe menopausal symptoms after breast cancer than after normal menopause and to use soya products to try to reduce flushing. Research on these approaches is notoriously difficult, and there is very little evidence available to support their use. There is a growing body of anecdotal evidence that supports benefits from these approaches, and they may increase a sense of control and well-being in women that use them. Evening primrose oil is often recommended for hot flushes, but there is little evidence to support this.[102] Vitamin E supplements have been shown to decrease the number of flushes experienced, although this is a small effect.[103] Smoking increases the number of hot flushes that women have,[104] so smoking cessation should be encouraged. There is some evidence that women who exercise regularly have less hot flushes than those who are more sedentary.[105]

Women, themselves, manage hot flushes with a variety of coping mechanisms. These

---

Box 17.2

Behavioural strategies employed by women to reduce discomfort due to hot flushes

- Keeping a note of when hot flushes occur to identify patterns to be more prepared.
- Wearing cotton (or silk) clothing (more absorbent materials which provide warmth after a flush is over).
- Wearing layers of clothing that can be taken off or put on as body temperature changes.
- Avoiding close-fitting clothes and choosing open necks.
- Using several layers of bedclothes (natural fabrics are better) that can be removed as required.
- Using sprays or moist wipes to help lower skin temperature (some add pleasant smelling oils to the spray, such as peppermint, which has cooling properties, or lavender, which has a relaxing effect).
- Using an electric fan to help lower skin temperature.
- If not sleeping well because of flushes, trying to find time to have a rest during the day.
- Trying to avoid warm, stuffy rooms as they can make flushes worse.
- Drinking plenty of cold water.
- Identifying foods that trigger flushing and avoid. These include hot or spicy foods, alcohol and caffeine.
- Use of refrigerated cool gel packs. Using at night under pillows or any time in the day.
- Learning not to fight against the flushes.

---

can be largely divided into behavioural and cognitive strategies. Behavioural strategies include adopting means to increase body cooling, such as choice of appropriate clothing; cotton is more absorbent than synthetic fibres, layers of thin clothing are easier to adjust, and loose fitting clothing may be more comfortable than tailored clothes (Box 17.2). However, some women may feel disadvantaged by the necessity to wear less feminine clothing and may not wish to alter their clothing, but rather maintain their normal social image.

For the healthcare professional, Reynolds[106] provides a guide which suggests 5 areas of cognitive strategies for helping women deal with hot flushes (Box 17.3). As discussed

Box 17.3

Guide to cognitive strategies to help women deal with hot flushes

- Need for empowering through information and support
- Helping to think about physical sensations in a different way
- Challenging fears and planning coping strategies
- Relaxation techniques
- Maintaining/increasing self-esteem and self-acceptance

Source: Reynolds.[106]

above, when symptoms and experiences are better understood, then they are less likely to cause anxiety and are more easily dealt with simply by obtaining accurate information.

Some hot flush sensations may be accompanied by feelings of panic and loss of control. These feelings can spiral into increased anxiety, so that women undergo real fears of the consequences. Where they are able to recognize and identify these fears and then reinterpret the experience in less catastrophic terms, they may be able to reduce the intensity of the distress caused. This extreme anxiety may also be reduced where women are able to learn specific relaxation techniques to focus on and which help the woman's sense of control. Once women have learnt not to fight the wave of heat that comes over them, but accept it, then it often peaks at a lower level and passes more quickly. Some women describe how they reinterpret the heat as a positive experience, e.g. reminding themselves of enjoyable summer holidays.

Fears of being unable to cope in social situations are common and often accompanied by embarrassment and inability to concentrate on tasks at hand. Some women are able to challenge these fears by asking for honest feedback from those they trust about socially embarrassing occurrences such as body odour. Coping strategies such as going back over work done during a flush, or taking a few minutes out for deep breathing, can also help minimize distress.

Relaxation therapy using paced breathing techniques has been shown to be effective in reducing flushing in women who have not had breast cancer.[107] Pilot work by Fenlon[108] has shown a 30% reduction in hot flushes in women who use relaxation techniques after breast cancer. Fenlon[108] also showed that daily relaxation therapy reduced anxiety in this group, which it could be suggested might help women experience a sense of increased control over their life as a whole and therefore make them better able to cope with difficulties that they may face. The increased sense of control may reduce intolerable menopausal difficulties to a level that is tolerable. Finally, one of the most distressing problems caused by hot flushes is sleep disturbance and resulting chronic tiredness. Daily relaxation may help to improve sleep and increase feelings of being rested and, again, increase tolerance for difficult symptoms (Case Study 17.1).

Maintenance of general health

After menopause, there is a marked increase in both heart disease and osteoporosis. Women need to consider their long-term health at this time and appropriate diet, exercise and the cessation of smoking can all do much to help reduce the risks of heart disease and osteoporosis. Some women may have particular concerns about the possibility of developing osteoporosis in later life, especially if they have undergone premature menopause due to cancer treatment or where there is osteoporosis in the family. Tamoxifen may protect against bone loss in postmenopausal women but other hormone treatments may exacerbate it.[109] It is clear that HRT can reduce bone loss and therefore reduce the risk of fracture. However, this protection is only given while hormones are still being taken and the incidence of fractures after the age of 75, when most fractures occur, is the same.[110] Weight-bearing exercise will prevent bone loss, although it will not increase bone density.[111] It can also help to improve fitness and muscle strength, which will contribute to the prevention of falls and a lower risk of fracture.[112] In conjunction with advice to increase dietary calcium, exercise plays a significant part in a lifestyle prescrip-

Other side effects of hormone therapy in women

Weight gain

An increase in appetite and subsequent gain in weight are clearly associated with the use of progesterone. However, other weight gain is not clearly related to hormone use. It is the norm for women to increase their weight with age, and after menopause the distribution of body fat will change so that it is more concentrated around the abdomen.[113] Davies et al.[114] showed that weight gain is an age-related effect and is not influenced either by cessation of ovarian function or by the use of HRT. A number of studies have shown that it is common to gain weight during the year following a diagnosis of breast cancer, whether or not adjuvant treatment is given,[25,115,116] although the use of chemotherapy is closely correlated with weight gain.[117] Goodwin et al[25] showed that weight gain is greatest for those who have chemotherapy (1.6 kg) and least for those who have no adjuvant therapy (0.6 kg). Women on tamoxifen gained an average of 1.3 kg. Premenopausal women gain more weight than postmenopausal women do. The most important controlling factor in weight gain is physical exercise.[118] De George et al[119] showed that exercise and dietary measures could be effective in controlling weight gain, even after breast cancer treatment.

Body image changes

Although the relative contributions of hormone therapy, chemotherapy and menopause are unclear, it is the case that weight gain does occur in women undergoing adjuvant therapy for breast cancer. Western societies put undue pressure on women to conform to the ideal of young, beautiful and slim,[120] and so to increase weight is to emphasize change and loss in women who are already undergoing significant change and losses due to facing a life-threatening illness. It may be possible for women to reduce weight by a programme of exercise and dieting, but this may also be very difficult in the face of a regimen of aggressive treatments with debilitating effects.

CASE STUDY 17.1

Management of menopause after breast cancer

Mrs Y is a 48-year-old PE teacher who finds hot flushes intolerable. She returns to work after 6 months sick leave following surgery, radiotherapy and chemotherapy. She finds her hot flushes particularly bothersome during lessons, particularly as they are aggravated by physical exercise. Mrs Y is feeling very stressed at work due to high levels of bureaucracy. She is also struggling with her relationship with her husband due to the major changes occurring in her life, which are making her review her priorities. She also has problems with painful sexual intercourse, due to having a dry vagina. The nursing intervention is to spend some time in discussion with Mrs Y, evaluating her problems by listening to her story. During the course of the interview advice is given about:

- management of flushes with a variety of strategies, including HRT, other prescription medicines, stress management, complementary medicines and behavioural techniques
- diet and exercise to maintain long-term health of cardiovascular and skeletal systems
- control of vaginal dryness and pelvic floor exercises
- marriage guidance counselling.

Mrs Y decides to re-evaluate what is important in her life by finding ways to reduce her stress. She has 3 months of HRT to help her through a difficult time. She reduces her working hours and takes up yoga for relaxation. As a PE teacher she already has a healthy lifestyle and eats well, but she starts to play tennis again to increase her weight-bearing exercise. At the end of 3 months HRT, she cuts it down gradually. Although the flushes increase again, she feels more in control. She is feeling less stressed and sleeping better and the flushes bother her less and are less frequent. At work she has a handheld electric fan and wears open neck cotton shirts with extra layers for warmth. She has chosen to manage her vaginal dryness with a vaginal moisturizer and she and her husband have started to attend marriage guidance counselling.

tion for reducing fractures in later life. Women who have had breast cancer may be at increased risk for osteoporosis and may choose to have increased monitoring for bone density to facilitate early detection and treatment.

371

Some women also suffer other body image changes such as thinning hair with tamoxifen, and an increase in oily skin with progesterones. If androgens are used in women, then virilization will occur. This takes the form of increase in body and facial hair, male pattern hair loss, increase in oily skin and a lowering of the voice. It may also be accompanied by an increase in libido.

The process of undergoing menopause may also contribute to significant body image change in some women. Most cancer treatments are for a defined period, something to be endured and which ultimately comes to an end, but menopause is an irreversible change to the body. The woman may feel that she is no longer the person that she used to be. She must now think of herself as an old woman instead of a young woman. Menopause is a constant reminder of all the losses due to the cancer experience.[57]

Sexual health

It may appear self-evident that altering the hormonal balance in women might interfere with their sexuality. However, work by Berglund et al[121] has shown that chemotherapy has a much greater impact on sexual health in women with breast cancer than hormone therapy and that this effect lasts for up to 3 years after treatment. Changes in sexuality can occur with hormone treatments, but are more likely to be part of the overall changes that occur at this time. Cancer treatment can have an impact on the quality of sexual relationships due to the discomfort of breast surgery, the fatigue of chemotherapy and the disruption to sleep caused by hot flushes. Alterations in circulating sex hormones are only one of the contributing factors to changing sexual relations.[122] The use of androgens can increase libido in women.

Treatments that induce early menopause can cause sexual difficulties due to a dry and painful vagina. Goserelin increases sexual dysfunction during treatment among patients without chemotherapy, but the disturbances of sexual functioning are reversible. The use of adjuvant chemotherapy is associated with continued sexual problems, even after 3 years.[121]

It is clear that vaginal dryness may lead to dyspareunia and thus interfere with sexual rela-tionships, but again this cannot be taken in isolation from the other changes that are occurring in a woman's life at this time. Work done by Cawood and Bancroft[123] showed that the most important predictors of sexuality in menopausal women were not physiological but social: these were other aspects of the sexual relationship, sexual attitudes and measures of well-being. The best predictor of both well-being and depression was tiredness.[123] Therefore, while advising on vaginal dryness this should not be taken in isolation from general assessment and discussion regarding general health and well-being.

Vaginal dryness

Couzi et al[63] has shown that 48% of post-menopausal women experience vaginal dryness after breast cancer. This may be a mild irritation or can be severe, causing pain and inhibiting intercourse, and 26% complain of pain on intercourse.[63] The use of simple moisturizers may be of benefit. These include gels such as Astroglide, GyneMoistrin and Moist Again. A polycarbophil moisturizing gel such as Replens can improve vaginal moisture and elasticity and is found to be of benefit in up to 80% of women.[124] Several studies found this to be an effective alternative to local oestrogen therapy.[125,126] This works by adhering to the wall of the vagina and allowing moisture to be absorbed over a period of time. It has the advantage of only needing to be applied 3 times per week.

For some women it may be appropriate to consider the use of local oestrogen. This is very poorly absorbed and, indeed, when the vagina is particularly dry, will not be absorbed at all. Oestrogen preparations should be chosen with care as some are larger doses which may be absorbed and raise serum oestrogen levels, e.g. oestrogen creams such as Ovestine (estriol 0.1%). The oestrogen tablet Vagifem has been shown not to influence serum oestrogen levels, and some centres therefore consider it safe to use after breast cancer (Table 17.5).

Tumour flare

Tumour flare is a rare phenomenon that may happen in patients with metastatic disease. The use of oestrogen, LHRH analogues or, rarely,

Table 17.5: Products to use with vaginal dryness

Generic (proprietary name)	Formulation	Regimen	Notes
Vaginal lubricants (Astroglide, GyneMoistrin, Moist Again)	Gels	As required	
Vaginal moisturizing gel (Replens)	Polycarbophil gel	Use applicator: insert gel 3 nights per week	
Oestrogen tablet (Vagifem)	25 µg oestradiol	Insert 1 tablet daily for 2 weeks; then reduce to 1 tablet twice weekly	Discontinue after 3 months to assess need for further treatment

tamoxifen may cause an initial worsening of the disease due to a temporary surge of circulating oestrogen. In women with bone disease, this may cause an increase in pain and a release of calcium into the bloodstream. This can result in hypercalcaemia, which is a potentially life-threatening condition. Women should be taught to be aware of the effects of hypercalcaemia and report them immediately.

Thromboembolism

Oestrogens increase the risk of embolism and cause a rise in deep vein thrombosis and pulmonary embolism. A small rise in thromboembolic events has also been observed with tamoxifen.[18]

Vaginal bleeding

Vaginal bleeding can occur as a response to withdrawing treatment with some hormones, such as the progesterones. It is also an indicator of endometrial hyperplasia or even cancer. Tamoxifen increases the risk of endometrial cancer, so any unexplained bleeding should be followed up.[127]

Side effects of hormone therapy in prostate cancer

Many of the problems that occur with hormone therapy in breast cancer are similar to those that occur with prostate cancer in men. Body image changes are closely linked to gen-

der, and alterations in sexuality may be a problem for both men and women. However, there is little literature available in this area and in clinical practice the side effects of hormone therapy in men are often underreported and underrated, with the consequence that they are largely ignored. Although prostate cancer can occur in men younger than 50 years old, it is largely a disease of older men and 50% of all new cases occur above the age of 75.[128] This means that many of these men will already be living with significant losses, such as retirement, death of family members and the onset of other chronic diseases. For some, these may lead to a sudden sense of feeling old. In this context, the changes brought about by hormonal therapies may have a significant impact on an individual's self-image and self-esteem.

Body image changes

The symbolic nature of the loss of the testicles has the potential to cause men to have concerns about their masculinity and body image.[129] Weight gain can be a problem in men during androgen suppression.[130] A reduction in testosterone can result in breast swelling: this is generally low, with one study reporting an incidence of 4.8%[131] with the use of LHRH analogues. With oestrogen use, this can be greater. Where gynaecomastia is likely to be a problem, this can be prevented by the use of radiation. Penile atrophy and a reduction in facial and body hair may also occur with androgen suppression.

373

Sexuality

A reduction of androgen causes a loss of libido and difficulty with obtaining erections. Coupled with the body image changes and general fatigue that men may experience when being treated for prostate cancer, sexual activity can be greatly decreased.[129] The use of LHRH analogues will suppress the function of the testes in the same way as ovarian function is suppressed in women. This will result in a medical orchidectomy and deprive the tumour of androgens. After either a medical or surgical orchidectomy, men will usually lose their sex drive and ability to develop erections, with only 20% retaining sexual function,[132] although Schover[133] has reported one case study of a man who was capable of full sexual function after 6 months of LHRH treatment. The effects on sexuality were limited to a reduced desire and a longer time to achieve erection and orgasm. However, even where sexual function is maintained, many men experience an inability to maintain an erection, loss of libido, dry orgasm, less intense orgasm and pain during orgasm. Although this effect is well known by the medical profession, there is little literature on the subject and it is rarely raised as an issue with patients.

Knowing that one has the ability to perform sexually is an important part of sexual self-image of a person and adjusting to the loss of sexual capability is rarely a 'non-event', even in celibate individuals. A change in a man's sexuality will also affect his self-image of himself as a man. Where a man's sexual ability is affected, then this may also have an effect on his relationship with a partner. Partners will not initiate sexual relations for fear of embarrassing their partner and men stay away from sexual behaviour for fear of not being able to satisfy their partner.

Prostate cancer is more common in older men, with a peak incidence in the 70- to 80-year-old age group, but it should not be assumed that problems with sexuality are therefore not relevant. Several major studies have shown that older men are still interested in sexual activity even where frequency is diminished: 79% of men in the 70- to 91-year-old age group are still sexually active on a regular basis.[129]

Although most nurses accept that changes in sexuality can be a problem for men with prostate cancer, it is still rare for them to be adequately dealt with. During active treatment, sexuality is often seen as less important and after treatment is completed sexual relationships may need to be recreated. However, physicians often do not raise the issue, as they believe nothing can be done about it and men themselves may not feel that this is an appropriate problem to discuss with their oncologist. Batchelor and van Ravensberg[128] discuss how men in a sexual dysfunction clinic often find it extremely difficult to ask for help and are afraid of being laughed at, many using humour to deal with the effects of their treatment. Kelly[134] suggests that men are more likely to discuss normally private issues if they have had the opportunity to build up a rapport with the healthcare professional and direct questioning about sexual dysfunction by the professional is most likely to discover any problems. Evaluation of a clinic for sexual dysfunction in Amsterdam showed that partners often felt the need for more information than the patient, so that addressing the patient and partner at the same time was considered vital:[128] 80% also thought that it was important to have both a doctor and a nurse present in their consultations.

There are a variety of approaches that can be used to help male sexuality after cancer treatment, such as Viagra (sildenafil) and suction devices. Viagra improves erectile function by increasing the blood flow to the vasculature of the penis and vacuum cylinders can be used to mimic the natural process of creating and maintaining an erection.[135] Injections of prostaglandins, phentolamine or papaverine into the base of the penis can also be used to stimulate erection.[136] Kelly[134] warns that only an appropriate health professional trained in the psychosexual care of cancer patients should explore the use of such interventions.

Hot flushes

Hot flushes are a common problem after orchidectomy or treatment with LHRH analogues, occurring in 50–66% of these men.[130] They appear to have a similar manifestation to those that occur in women at menopause and cause similar distress. Men may be reluctant to talk about flushing, perceiving it to be a woman's problem and so not a problem they wish to be identified with. Flushing may be accompanied by drenching sweats, can occur many times a day and be disruptive of sleep. Similar treatment options to those used for women have been used with variable success. Clonidine, megestrol acetate and the SSRIs (such as sertraline) have all been used with some success.[137] Soya products and phyto-estrogens may also be of use in this group, although the same concerns about long-term safety and the effect of these drugs on prostate cancer should be properly assessed. Low-dose oestrogen may be of benefit, as it may simultaneously reduce hot flushes and the risk of osteoporosis in men receiving long-term androgen suppression therapy. However, the potential for cardiovascular complications must be considered. The long-term efficacy and safety of these treatments is still unclear and the range of alternative therapies available to women for hot flushes may also be of interest to men.

Tumour flare

Due to the initial stimulation of the pituitary, in the same way as is seen in women, LHRH analogues may cause an increase in symptoms or 'flare' in the first 1–2 weeks of treatment. As bone metastases are common in prostate cancer, this can be a problem with increased pain or raised calcium levels. This may be seen in up to 5% of patients.[131] The effect can be blocked by giving an antiandrogen for several days before and for 2 weeks after commencing treatment with LHRH.[3]

Other side effects of hormone therapy in prostate cancer

Side effects of antiandrogens include nausea and vomiting and gynaecomastia. Breast tenderness occurs[138] and liver dysfunction and fatigue have also been reported.[3] Nilutamide is associated with 20% visual abnormalities and alcohol intolerance.[139] Flutamide may cause diarrhoea in up to 29% of people. Bicalutamide has been reported to cause diarrhoea, but in a lesser incidence (2.5%).[44] Liver damage is reported with ketoconazole and flutamide.

CONCLUSION AND FORWARD DIRECTIONS

The use of hormone therapies in selected tumours can give impressive results and often with minimal side effects. The impact of side effects needs to be carefully considered when the treatment is given either for metastatic disease, and cure is not an option, or for the purposes of prevention, where the recipient may never experience cancer. The search for new and better agents to improve quality of life for people with breast and prostate cancer will continue. Information gained in this field is likely to give clues about the development of new primary disease, and the potential for prevention of cancer will become a priority. The links between diet, lifestyle and endogenous hormones may point to alterations in diet being most promising for the prevention of disease. Current areas being investigated are the use of soya isoflavones to protect against both breast[140] and prostate cancer.[86] As Western populations continue to age, breast and prostate cancer will continue to increase in incidence, but there will also be an increasing population of people who survive these diseases. Long-term health and protection from cardiovascular disease and osteoporosis will then become more important. Although hormone manipulation may rarely be the treatment of choice for many cancers, it will become ever more important in long-term survivorship.

REFERENCES

1. Cancer Research UK. 2003. Incidence. http://cancerresearchuk.org/aboutcancer/statistics/statsmisc/pdfs/cancerstats_incidence.pdf 2003.

2. Tominga S, Kuroishi T, Aoki K. Cancer mortality statistics in 33 countries. Vol. 2003: UICC – International Union Against Cancer; 1998.

3. Dearnaley DP. Cancer of the prostate. BMJ 1994; 308:780–784.

4. Fellowes D, Fallowfield LJ, Saunders CM, Houghton J. Tolerability of hormone therapies for breast cancer: how informative are documented symptom profiles in medical notes for 'well-tolerated' treatments? Breast Cancer Res Treat 2001; 66:73–81.

5. Garnick MB. The dilemmas of prostate cancer. Sci Am 1994; 270:72–81.

6. Mokbel K, ed. Hormones and mammary carcinogenesis. In: Endocrine and biological therapy of breast cancer into the twenty-first century. Newbury: Petroc Press; 2001.

7. Mokbel K, ed. The physiological basis. In: Endocrine and biological therapy of breast cancer into the twenty-first century. Newbury: Petroc Press; 2001.

8. Kaufmann M. A review of endocrine options for the treatment of advanced breast cancer. Oncology 1997; 54:2–5.

9. Mokbel K, Benson J. Tamoxifen. In: Mokbel K, ed. Endocrine and biological therapy of breast cancer into the twenty-first century. Newbury: Petroc Press; 2001.

10. Buzdar A. Hortobagyi G. Update on endocrine therapy for breast cancer. Clin Cancer Res 1998; 4:527–534.

11. Bonneterre J, Thurlimann, Robertson JF. et al. Anastrozole versus tamoxifen as first-line therapy for advanced breast cancer in 668 postmenopausal women: results of the Tamoxifen or Arimidex Randomized Group Efficacy and Tolerability study. J Clin Oncol 2000; 18:3748–3757.

12. Harvey JM, Clark GM, Osborne CK, Allred DC. Estrogen receptor status by immunohistochemistry is superior to the ligand-binding assay for predicting response to adjuvant endocrine therapy in breast cancer. J Clin Oncol 1999; 17:1474–1481.

13. Baum M. A vision for the future? Br J Cancer 2001; 85(Suppl 2):15–18.

14. Fisher B, Jeong JH, Dignam J, et al. Findings from recent national surgical adjuvant breast and bowel project adjuvant studies in stage I breast cancer. J Natl Cancer Inst Monogr 2001; 30:62–66.

15. Fisher B, Dignam J, Bryant J, Wolmark N. Five versus more than five years of tamoxifen for lymph node-negative breast cancer: updated findings from the National Surgical Adjuvant Breast and Bowel Project B-14 randomized trial. J Natl Cancer Inst 2001; 93:684–690.

16. Pritchard KI, Paterson AH, Paul NA, et al. Increased thromboembolic complications with concurrent tamoxifen and chemotherapy in a randomized trial of adjuvant therapy for women with breast cancer. National Cancer Institute of Canada Clinical Trials Group Breast Cancer Site Group. J Clin Oncol 1996; 14:2731–2737.

17. Nayfield SG, Karp JE, Ford LG, Dorr FA, Kramer BS. Potential role of tamoxifen in prevention of breast cancer. J Natl Cancer Inst 1991; 83:1450–1459.

18. Fisher B, Costantino JP, Wickerham DL, et al. Tamoxifen for prevention of breast cancer: report of the National Surgical Adjuvant Breast and Bowel Project P-1 Study. J Natl Cancer Inst 1998; 90:1371–1388.

19. Powles T, Eeles R, Ashley S, et al. Interim analysis of the incidence of breast cancer in the Royal Marsden Hospital tamoxifen randomised chemoprevention trial. Lancet 1998; 352:98–101.

20. Veronesi U, Maisonneuve P, Costa A, et al. Prevention of breast cancer with tamoxifen: preliminary findings from the Italian randomised trial among hysterectomised women. Italian Tamoxifen Prevention Study. Lancet 1998; 352:93–97.

21. Jaiyesimi IA, Buzdar AU, Sahin AA, Ross MA. Carcinoma of the male breast. Ann Intern Med 1992; 117:771–777.

22. Anelli TF, Anelli A, Tran KN, Lebwohl DE, Borgen PI. Tamoxifen administration is associated with a high rate of treatment-limiting symptoms in male breast cancer patients. Cancer 1994; 74:74–77.

23. Forrest AP. Beatson: hormones and the management of breast cancer. J R Coll Surg Edinb 1982; 27:253–263.

24. Barnes DM, Hanby AM. Oestrogen and progesterone receptors in breast cancer: past, present and future. Histopathology 2001; 38:271–274.

25. Goodwin PJ, Ennis M, Pritchard KI, et al. Adjuvant treatment and onset of menopause predict weight gain after breast cancer diagnosis. J Clin Oncol 1999; 17:120–129.

26. Mezzetti M, La-Vecchia C, Decarli A, et al. Population attributable risk for breast cancer: diet, nutrition, and physical exercise. J Natl Cancer Inst 1998; 90:389–394.

27. Santen RJ. Aromatase inhibitors: 1. In: Powles TJ, Smith IE, eds. The medical management of breast cancer. London: Martin Dunitz; 1991.

28. Brodie AM, Njar VC. Aromatase inhibitors and their application in breast cancer treatment. Steroids 2000; 65:171–179.

29. Coombes RC, Evans TRJ. Aromatase inhibitors. In: Powles TJ, Smith IE, eds. The medical management of breast cancer. London: Martin Dunitz; 1991.

30. Clemett D, Lamb HM. Exemestane: a review of its use in postmenopausal women with advanced breast cancer. Drugs 2000; 59:1279–1296.

30a. Howell A, Cuzick J, Baum M, et al and ATAC Trialists' Group. Results of the ATAC (Arimidex, Tamoxifen, Alone or in Combination) trial after completion of 5 years' adjuvant treatment for breast cancer. Lancet 2005; 365:60–62.

31. Pannuti F, Martoni A, Zamagni C, Melotti B. Progestins I: medroxyprogesterone acetate. In: Powles T, Smith I, eds. The medical management of breast cancer. Cambridge: Martin Dunitz; 1993.

32. Powles T. Progestins II: megestrol acetate. In: Powles T, Smith I, eds. The medical management of breast cancer. Cambridge: Martin Dunitz; 1993.

33. Jordan VC. Tamoxifen: a personal retrospective. Lancet Oncol 2000; 1:43–49.

34. Rees M. The benefits and risks of hormone replacement therapy. In: Hope S, Rees M, Brockie J, eds. Hormone replacement therapy: a guide for primary care. Oxford: Oxford University Press; 1999.

35. Silva I, Mor G, Naftolin F. Estrogen and the aging brain. Maturitas 2001; 38:95–100; discussion 100–101.

36. Jordan VC, Gapstur S, Morrow M. Selective estrogen receptor modulation and reduction in risk of breast cancer, osteoporosis, and coronary heart disease. J Natl Cancer Inst 2001; 93:1449–1457.

37. Love RR., Cameron L, Connell BL, Leventhal H. Symptoms associated with tamoxifen treatment in postmenopausal women. Arch Intern Med 1991; 151:1842–1847.

38. Costantino JP, Kuller LH, Ives DG, Fisher B, Dignam J. Coronary heart disease mortality and adjuvant tamoxifen therapy. J Natl Cancer Inst 1997; 89:776–782.

39. Stearns V, Gelmann E. Does tamoxifen cause cancer in humans? J Clin Oncol 1998; 16:779–792.

40. Cummings SR, Eckert S, Krueger KA, et al. The effect of raloxifene on risk of breast cancer in postmenopausal women: results from the MORE randomized trial. Multiple Outcomes of Raloxifene Evaluation. JAMA 1999; 281:2189–2197.

41. Love RR, Barden HS, Mazess RB, Epstein S, Chappell RJ. Effect of tamoxifen on lumbar spine bone mineral density in postmenopausal women after 5 years. Arch Intern Med 1994; 154:2585–2588.

42. Fisher B, Dignam J, Bryant J. Five versus more than five years of tamoxifen therapy for breast cancer patients with negative lymph nodes and estrogen receptor-positive tumors. J Natl Cancer Inst 1996; 88:1526–1542.

43. Blackburn A, Amiel S, Millis R. Tamoxifen and liver damage. Br Med J 1984; 289:288.

44. Tyrrell CJ. Adjuvant and neoadjuvant hormonal therapy for prostate cancer. Eur Urol 1999; 36:549–558.

45. Huggins C, Bergenstal D. Inhibition of human mammary and prostatic cancer by adrenalectomy. Cancer Res 1952; 12:134–141.

46. Tyrrell CJ. Controversies in the management of advanced prostate cancer. Br J Cancer 1999; 79:146–155.

47. Kaisary AV, Tyrrell CJ, Peeling WB, Griffiths K. Comparison of LHRH analogue (Zoladex) with orchiectomy in patients with metastatic prostatic carcinoma. Br J Urol 1991; 67:502–508.

48. Fossa SD, Opjordsmoen S, Haug E. Androgen replacement and quality of life in patients treated for bilateral testicular cancer. Eur J Cancer 1999; 35:1220–1225.

49. Schellhammer P, Sharifi R, Block N, et al. Clinical benefits of bicalutamide compared with flutamide in combined androgen blockade for patients with advanced prostatic carcinoma: final report of a double-blind, randomized, multicenter trial. Urology 1997; 50:330–336.

50. Canney PA, Hatton MQ. The prevalence of menopausal symptoms in patients treated for breast cancer. Clin Oncol 1994; 6:297–299.

51. Lower EE, Blau R, Gazder P, Tummala R. The risk of premature menopause induced by chemotherapy for early breast cancer. J Womens Health Gend Based Med 1999; 8:949–954.

52. Goodwin PJ, Ennis M, Pritchard KI, Trudeau M, Hood N. Risk of menopause during the first year after breast cancer diagnosis. J Clin Oncol 1999; 17:2365–2370.

53. Harris PF, Remington PL, Trentham-Dietz A, Allen CI, Newcomb PA. Prevalence and treatment of menopausal symptoms among breast cancer survivors. J Pain Symptom Manage 2002; 23:501–509.

54. Singer D, Hunter M. The experience of premature menopause: a thematic discourse analysis. J Reprod Infant Psychol 1999; 17:63–81.

55. Knobf MT. The menopausal symptom experience in young mid-life women with breast cancer. Cancer Nurs 2001; 24:201–210; quiz 210–211.

56. Knobf MT. Carrying on: the experience of premature menopause in women with early stage breast cancer. Nurs Res 2002; 51:9–17.

57. Davis CS, Zinkand JE, Fitch MI. Cancer treatment-induced menopause: meaning for breast and gynecological cancer survivors. Can Oncol Nurs J 2000; 10:14–21.

58. Dickson GL. A feminist poststructuralist analysis of the knowledge of menopause. Adv Nurs Sci 1990; 12:15–31.

59. Carpenter JS, Andrykowski MA. Menopausal symptoms in breast cancer survivors. Oncol Nurs Forum 1999; 26:1311–1317.

60. Kleinman A. The illness narratives: suffering, healing and the human condition. New York: Basic Books; 1988.

61. Levine-Silverman S. The menopausal hot flash: a procrustean bed of research. J Adv Nurs 1989; 14:939–949.

62. Finck G, Barton DL, Loprinzi CL, Quella SK, Sloan JA. Definitions of hot flashes in breast cancer survivors. J Pain Symptom Manage 1998; 16:327–333.

63. Couzi RJ, Helzlsouer KJ, Fetting JH. Prevalence of menopausal symptoms among women with a history of breast cancer and attitudes toward estrogen replacement therapy. J Clin Oncol 1995; 13:2737–2744.

64. Carpenter JS, Johnson D, Wagner L, Andrykowski M. Hot flashes and related outcomes in breast cancer survivors and matched comparison women. Oncol Nurs Forum 2002; 29:E16–25.

65. McPhail G, Smith LN. Acute menopause symptoms during adjuvant systemic treatment for breast cancer: a case-control study. Cancer Nurs 2000; 23:430–443.

377

66. Kaplan HS. A neglected issue: the sexual side effects of current treatments for breast cancer. J Sex Marital Ther 1992; 18:3–19.

67. Mourits MJ, Bockermann I, de Vries EG, et al. Tamoxifen effects on subjective and psychosexual well-being, in a randomised breast cancer study comparing high-dose and standard-dose chemotherapy. Br J Cancer 2002; 86:1546–1550.

68. Ganz PA, Greendale GA, Petersen L, et al. Managing menopausal symptoms in breast cancer survivors: results of a randomized controlled trial [see comments]. J Natl Cancer Inst 2000; 92:1054–1064.

69. Schairer C, Lubin J, Troisi R, et al. Menopausal estrogen and estrogen-progestin replacement therapy and breast cancer risk. JAMA 2000; 283:485–491.

70. Million Women Study Collaborators. Breast cancer and hormone-replacement therapy in the Million Women Study. Lancet 2003; 362:19–427.

71. Holli K, Isola J, Cuzick J. Low biologic aggressiveness in breast cancer in women using hormone replacement therapy. J Clin Oncol 1998; 16:3115–3120.

72. O'Meara ES, Rossing MA, Daling JR, et al. 2001. Hormone replacement therapy after a diagnosis of breast cancer in relation to recurrence and mortality. J Natl Cancer Inst 2001; 93:754–762.

73. Marsden J. Hormone replacement therapy and breast cancer. Maturitas 2000; 34(Suppl 2):S11–S24.

74. Goldberg RM, Loprinzi CL, O'Fallon JR, et al. Transdermal clonidine for ameliorating tamoxifen-induced hot flashes [published erratum appears in J Clin Oncol 1996; 14(8):2411]. J Clin Oncol 1994; 12:155–158.

75. Gonzales GF, Carrillo C. Blood serotonin levels in postmenopausal women: effects of age and serum oestradiol levels. Maturitas 1993; 17:23–29.

76. Stearns V, Ullmer L, Lopez JF, et al. Hot flushes. Lancet 2002; 360:1851–1861.

77. Loprinzi CL, Pisansky TM, Fonseca R, et al. Pilot evaluation of venlafaxine hydrochloride for the therapy of hot flashes in cancer survivors. J Clin Oncol 1998; 16:2377–2381.

78. Stearns V, Beebe K, Iyengar M, Smith Y. 2003. Randomized, double-blind study of controlled release paroxetine in treatment of menopausal hot flash. Obstetr Gynecol 2003; 101:97S.

79. Loprinzi CL, Michalak JC, Quella SK, et al. Megestrol acetate for the prevention of hot flashes. N Engl J Med 1994; 331:347–352.

80. Pick M. Herbal treatments for menopause. Black cohosh, soy and micronized progesterone. Adv Nurse Pract 2000; 8:29–30.

81. Gardner C. Ease through menopause with homeopathic and herbal medicine. J Perianesth Nurs 1999; 14:139–143.

82. Ernst E. The risk-benefit profile of commonly used herbal therapies: Ginkgo, St. John's Wort, Ginseng, Echinacea, Saw Palmetto, and Kava. Ann Intern Med 2002; 136:42–53.

83. Adlercreutz H, Mazur W. Phyto-oestrogens and Western diseases. Ann Med 1997; 29:95–120.

84. Liu J, Burdette JE, Xu H, et al. Evaluation of estrogenic activity of plant extracts for the potential treatment of menopausal symptoms. J Agric Food Chem 2001; 49:2472–2479.

85. Stephens FO. 1997. Breast cancer: aetiological factors and associations (a possible protective role of phytoestrogens). Aust NZ J Surg 1997; 67:755–760.

86. Adlercreutz H. Phyto-oestrogens and cancer. Lancet Oncol 2002; 3:364–373.

87. Albertazzi P, Pansini F, Bonaccorsi G, et al. The effect of dietary soy supplementation on hot flushes. Obstet Gynecol 1998; 91:6–11.

88. Murkies AL, Lombard C, Strauss BJ, et al. Dietary flour supplementation decreases post-menopausal hot flushes: effect of soy and wheat. Maturitas 1995; 21:189–195.

89. Quella SK, Loprinzi CL, Barton DL, et al. Evaluation of soy phytoestrogens for the treatment of hot flashes in breast cancer survivors: A North Central Cancer Treatment Group Trial. J Clin Oncol 2000; 18: 1068–1074.

90. Van Patten CL, Olivotto IA, Chambers GK, et al. 2002. Effect of soy phytoestrogens on hot flashes in postmenopausal women with breast cancer: a randomized, controlled clinical trial. J Clin Oncol 2002; 20:1449–1455.

91. Gass ML, Taylor MB. Alternatives for women through menopause. Am J Obstet Gynecol 2001; 185:S47–56.

92. Liske E, Hanggi W, Henneicke-von Zepelin HH, et al. 2002. Physiological investigation of a unique extract of black cohosh (Cimicifugae racemosae rhizoma): a 6-month clinical study demonstrates no systemic estrogenic effect. J Womens Health Gend Based Med 2002; 11:163–174.

93. Jacobson JS, Troxel AB, Evans J, et al. Randomized trial of black cohosh for the treatment of hot flashes among women with a history of breast cancer. J Clin Oncol 2001; 19:2739–2745.

94. Lieberman S. A review of the effectiveness of Cimicifuga racemosa (black cohosh) for the symptoms of menopause. J Womens Health 1998; 7:525–529.

95. McKenna DJ, Jones K, Humphrey S, Hughes K. Black cohosh: efficacy, safety, and use in clinical and preclinical applications. Altern Ther Health Med 2001; 7:93–100.

96. van de Weijer P, Barentsen R. Isoflavones from red clover (Promensil) significantly reduce menopausal hot flush symptoms compared with placebo. Maturitas 2002; 42:187.

97. Fugh-Berman A, Kronenberg F. Red clover (*Trifolium pratense*) for menopausal women: current state of knowledge. Menopause 2001; 8:333–337.

98. Clifton-Bligh PB, Baber RJ, Fulcher GR, Nery ML, Moreton T. The effect of isoflavones extracted from red clover (Rimostil) on lipid and bone metabolism. Menopause 2001; 8:259–265.

99. Vincent A, Fitzpatrick LA. Soy isoflavones: are they useful in menopause? Mayo Clin Proc 2000; 75:1174–1184.

100. Eden J. Phytoestrogens and the menopause. Baillière's Clin Endocrinol Metab 1998; 12:581–587.

101. Komesaroff PA., Black CV, Cable V, Sudhir K. Effects of wild yam extract on menopausal symptoms, lipids and sex hormones in healthy menopausal women. Climacteric 2001; 4:144–150.

102. Chenoy R, Hussain S, Tayob Y, et al. The effect of oral gamolenic acid from evening primrose oil on menopausal flushing. Br Med J 1994; 308:501–503.

103. Barton D, Loprinzi CL, Quella SK, et al. Prospective evaluation of vitamin E for hot flashes in breast cancer survivors. J Clin Oncol 1998;16:495–500.

104. Obermeyer CM, Ghorayeb F, Reynolds R. 1999. Symptom reporting around the menopause in Beirut, Lebanon. Maturitas 1999; 33:249–258.

105. Hammar M, Berg G, Lindgren R. Does physical exercise influence the frequency of postmenopausal hot flushes? Acta Obstet Gynecol Scand 1990; 69:409–412.

106. Reynolds F. Psychological responses to menopausal hot flushes: implications of a qualitative study for counselling interventions. Counselling Psychol Q 1997; 10:309–321.

107. Freedman RR, Woodward S. Behavioral treatment of menopausal hot flushes: evaluation by ambulatory monitoring. Am J Obstet Gynecol 1992; 167:436–439.

108. Fenlon D. Relaxation therapy as an intervention for hot flushes in women with breast cancer. Eur J Oncol Nurs 1999; 3:223–231.

109. Baum M. Tamoxifen – the treatment of choice. "Why look for alternatives?" Br J Cancer 1998; 78:1–4.

110. te Velde E, van Leusden H. 1994. Hormonal treatment for the climacteric: alleviation of symptoms and prevention of postmenopausal disease. Lancet 1994; 343:654–658.

111. Sharkey NA, Williams NI, Guerin JB. The role of exercise in the prevention and treatment of osteoporosis and osteoarthritis. Nurs Clin North Am 2000; 35:209–221.

112. Forwood MR, Larsen JA. Exercise recommendations for osteoporosis. A position statement of the Australian and New Zealand Bone and Mineral Society. Aust Fam Physician 2000; 29:761–764.

113. Astrup A. Physical activity and weight gain and fat distribution changes with menopause: current evidence and research issues. Med Sci Sports Exerc 1999; 31:S564–567.

114. Davies KM, Heaney RP, Recker RR, Barger-Lux MJ, Lappe JM. Hormones, weight change and menopause. Int J Obes Relat Metab Disord 2001; 25:874–879.

115. Hoskin PJ, Ashley S, Yarnold JR. Weight gain after primary surgery for breast cancer – effect of tamoxifen. Breast Cancer Res Treat 1992; 22:129–132.

116. Kumar NB, Allen K, Cantor A, et al. Weight gain associated with adjuvant tamoxifen therapy in stage I and II breast cancer: fact or artifact?" Breast Cancer Res Treat 1997; 44:135–143.

117. McInnes JA, Knobf MT. Weight gain and quality of life in women treated with adjuvant chemotherapy for early-stage breast cancer. Oncol Nurs Forum 2001; 28:675–684.

118. Simkin-Silverman LR, Wing RR. Weight gain during menopause. Is it inevitable or can it be prevented? Postgrad Med 2000; 108:47–50, 53–56.

119. DeGeorge D, Gray JJ, Fetting JH, Rolls BJ. Weight gain in patients with breast cancer receiving adjuvant treatment as a function of restraint, disinhibition, and hunger. Oncol Nurs Forum 1990; 17:23–28; discussion 28–30.

120. Greer G. The change: women, ageing and the menopause. London: Penguin; 1991.

121. Berglund G, Nystedt M, Bolund C, Sjoden PO, Rutquist LE. Effect of endocrine treatment on sexuality in premenopausal breast cancer patients: a prospective randomized study. J Clin Oncol 2001; 19:2788–2796.

122. Greendale GA, Petersen L, Zibecchi L, Ganz PA. Factors related to sexual function in postmenopausal women with a history of breast cancer. Menopause 2001; 8:111–119.

123. Cawood EH, Bancroft J. Steroid hormones, the menopause, sexuality and well-being of women. Psychol Med 1996; 26:925–936.

124. Gelfand MM, Wendman E. Treating vaginal dryness in breast cancer patients: results of applying a polycarbophil moisturizing gel. J Women's Health 1994; 3:427–434.

125. Nachtigall LE. 1994. Comparative study: Replens versus local estrogen in menopausal women. Fertil Steril 1994; 61:178–180.

126. Bygdeman M, Swahn ML. Replens versus dienoestrol cream in the symptomatic treatment of vaginal atrophy in postmenopausal women. Maturitas 1996; 23:259–263.

127. Mourits MJ, De Vries EG, Willemse PH, et al. Tamoxifen treatment and gynecologic side effects: a review. Obstet Gynecol 2001; 97:855–866.

128. Batchelor D, Van Ravensberg S. Altered patterns of male sexuality in prostate cancer. Oncol Nurses Today 2001; 6:14–18.

129. Ofman U. Sexual quality of life in men with prostate cancer. Cancer 1995; 75:1949–1953.

130. Moyad MA. Complementary/alternative therapies for reducing hot flashes in prostate cancer patients: reevaluating the existing indirect data from studies of breast cancer and postmenopausal women. Urology 2002; 59:20–33.

131. Denis L, Murphy GP. Overview of phase III trials on combined androgen treatment in patients with metastatic prostate cancer. Cancer 1993; 72:3888–3895.

132. Rousseau L, Dupont A, Labrie F, Couture M. 1988. Sexuality changes in prostate cancer patients receiving antihormonal therapy combining the antiandrogen flutamide with medical (LHRH agonist) or surgical castration. Arch Sex Behav 1988; 17:87–98.

133. Schover LR. Sexuality and fertility in urologic cancer patients. Cancer 1987; 60:553–558.

134. Kelly D. Altered patterns of male sexuality in prostate cancer. Oncol Nurs Today 2001; 6:19–20.

135. Nadig PW. Vacuum erection devices: a review. World J Urol 1990; 8:114–117.

136. Floth A, Schramek P. Intracavernous injection of prostaglandin E, in combination with papaverine enhanced effectiveness in comparison with papaverine plus phentolamine and prostaglandin E alone. J Urol 1991; 145:56–59.

137. Roth AJ, Scher HI. Sertraline relieves hot flashes secondary to medical castration as treatment of advanced prostate cancer. Psychooncology 1998; 7:129–132.

138. McLeod DG, Benson RC Jr, Eisenberger MA, et al. The use of flutamide in hormone-refractory metastatic prostate cancer. Cancer 1993; 72:3870–3873.

139. Decensi AU, Boccardo F, Guarneri D, et al. 1991. Monotherapy with nilutamide, a pure nonsteroidal antiandrogen, in untreated patients with metastatic carcinoma of the prostate. The Italian Prostatic Cancer Project. J Urol 1991; 146:377–381.

140. Ingram D, Sanders K, Kolybaba M, Lopez D. 1997. Case-control study of phyto-oestrogens and breast cancer. Lancet 1997; 350:990–994.

CHAPTER 18

Complementary and Alternative Therapies

ALEXANDER MOLASSIOTIS, ANNE CAWTHORN AND PETER A MACKERETH

CHAPTER CONTENTS

Introduction	381
Definitions of complementary and alternative medicine	381
Popularity of complementary and alternative medicine	382
Access to complementary and alternative medicine	383
Reasons for using complementary and alternative medicine	383
The integrative model of cancer care	384
Effectiveness of complementary and alternative medicine	384
Body–mind interventions	385
Touch and bodywork modalities	386
Herbs	391
Homeopathy	391
Acupuncture	391
Energy therapies	391
Caring for informal and professional carers	392
Regulation issues	392
Legal, professional and managerial issues	392
Supervision and support for CAM therapists	393
Integrating complementary and alternative medicine into conventional practice	395
Conclusion	395
References	396

INTRODUCTION

The potential for complementary and alternative medicine (CAM) to manage stress and alleviate other health problems is an area of growing interest amongst the general population. People with cancer are increasingly using CAM to treat the cancer or improve physical and psychological well-being. Patients often ask advice about CAM from healthcare professionals, and hence nurses need to be knowledgeable enough to provide information regarding access to and appropriateness of CAM therapies. Furthermore, many nurses are developing skills in CAM and are using these in their day-to-day work, as well as taking responsibility for coordinating services

and undertaking research in this area. This chapter is not a prescriptive or definitive guide to CAM therapies but aims to discuss some of the key issues around the use of CAM, including definitions available, reasons for using CAM, the current legal situation and the clinical and service integration issues relevant to practice.

DEFINITIONS OF COMPLEMENTARY AND ALTERNATIVE MEDICINE

Discussions surrounding the use and definitions of complementary and alternative therapies have been ongoing during the past 20 years with a number of reports adding to the debate.[1-4] Most recently, the National Guidelines for the Use of Complementary Therapies in Supportive and Palliative Care used the term 'complementary' to describe therapies used alongside conventional health care.[5] Stone[6(p55)] suggests that both in the UK and USA there has been a significant shift towards 'integrated (or integrative) health care' and greater tolerance towards the inclusion of complementary therapies by governments and the medical fraternity. The Foundation for Integrated Medicine discussion document on Integrated Healthcare in the UK[2] (a body established by HRH the Prince of Wales) examined practical ways in which conventional and complementary therapists could develop a working partnership. It was suggested that the way forward is to combine the best of conventional and complementary medicine. However, despite more consensus being achieved in relation to integration of therapies into health care, and more specifically into cancer care, there still seems to be some conceptual confusion as to how therapies are defined and why they are chosen. Part of this confusion arises as a result of the number of different terms used to describe CAM, including unorthodox medicine, unconventional medicine and unproven medicine.

Broad definitions exist, such as that used by the National Center for Complementary and Alternative Medicine (NCCAM) in the USA, which defines CAM as a group of diverse medical and healthcare systems, practices, and products that are not currently considered to be part of conventional medicine. A more holistic definition was introduced in the mid 1990s, defining CAM as:

> Any diagnosis, treatment or prevention that complements mainstream medicine by contributing to a common whole, by satisfying a demand not met by orthodoxy or by diversifying the conceptual framework of medicine.[7(p506)]

A number of models have been developed in an attempt to clarify and categorize the many therapies that fall under the umbrella definition of CAM. The British House of Lords Report on complementary and alternative medicine[3] divided therapies into three areas:

1 Professionally organized alternative therapies such as acupuncture, chiropractic, herbal medicine, homeopathy and osteopathy.

2 Complementary therapies such as aromatherapy, reflexology, body work therapies and mind–body therapies.

3 Alternative disciplines:
   • long-established and traditional systems of health care such as Ayurvedic medicine, Chinese herbal medicine and Eastern medicine
   • other alternative disciplines such as crystal healing, iridology and kinesiology.

A more comprehensive categorization of CAM therapies has been also proposed by the NCCAM and divides CAM into five broad types (http://nccam.nih.gov/health/whatis-cam/), including:

1 Alternative medical systems, which are traditional systems of medicine with a long history, such as traditional Chinese medicine, Ayurveda, homeopathy or naturopathy.

2 Mind–body interventions, such as meditation, art therapy, spiritual healing, psychological interventions, music therapy or prayer as a therapy.

3 Biologically based therapies, such as herbs, dietary supplements, medicinal teas or animal extracts (i.e. shark cartilage).

4 Manipulative and body-based methods, such as chiropractic, osteopathy or massage.

5 Energy therapies, such as electromagnetic therapy, Qi Gong or Reiki.

POPULARITY OF COMPLEMENTARY AND ALTERNATIVE MEDICINE

Surveys conducted in the UK and in Australia indicate that between 25% and 50% of the general population use CAM on a regular basis, often at their own expense.[8,9] The huge growth of CAM has been particularly evident in the field of cancer and palliative care,[10] and Tavares[5] suggests that a significant number of people use complementary therapies after a cancer diagnosis. Risberg et al[11] state that surveys of CAM amongst cancer patients in Scandinavia and across the world during the last 5–10 years report a prevalence rate of use ranging from 10% to over 50%. Surveys by Rees et al[12] and Lewith et al[13] in the UK have found that over 30% of people with cancer use complementary therapies. However, Lewith et al's suggestion that another 49% would have liked the opportunity to receive a therapy had it been available, supports the view that 'the majority of cancer patients at some stage in their illness will explore the use of complementary therapies'.[14(p4)]

More recent work across Europe showed that 35.9% of cancer patients ($n = 956$) used some form of CAM after the diagnosis of cancer, and that patients with pancreatic, liver, bone and brain cancer showed the highest rates of use.[15] Furthermore, use of CAM is equally high in the paediatric cancer population, with rates of use as high as 42%[16] in Canada or 32.7% in the UK.[17]

ACCESS TO COMPLEMENTARY AND ALTERNATIVE MEDICINE

Access to CAM varies considerably within healthcare settings. The greatest increase in the provision of CAM over the past decade is in the field of cancer and palliative care. Kohn[14] evaluated the provision of CAM within cancer and palliative care in the UK, finding that hospices are the greatest providers (36%), with hospitals providing 31% and the voluntary sector providing a further 20%. The Macmillan Directory of Complementary Therapy Services lists the range of services available for patients and their carers.[14] Within general practice, Thomas et al[18] identified that 39.5% of GP partnerships in England provide some form of complementary therapy. The Royal College of Nursing[4] found that nurses were most likely to offer massage, aromatherapy and reflexology in their practice.

REASONS FOR USING COMPLEMENTARY AND ALTERNATIVE MEDICINE

Corner and Harewood[8] categorized motivation for the use of CAM by patients with cancer under two distinct headings: first, as a means of either curing the cancer or reducing the tumour burden, with 'alternative treatments' used as adjuncts to conventional cancer treatment with the aim of preventing recurrence or managing symptoms; the second motivation for patients choosing therapies is to maximise their quality of life during cancer treatment, and to assist return to a normal life once medical intervention has ceased.

A number of studies have investigated the reasons behind and benefits of using CAM. Coss et al[19] undertook a telephone survey of cancer patients ($n = 503$) in California, finding that people turned to alternative therapy for the following reasons:

- a desire to be treated as a whole person
- to participate in their own care
- because of a sense that conventional medicine has failed to meet their spiritual or psychological needs.

In addition, it was found that patients were looking for improved quality of life to help with the side effects of cancer such as fear, anxiety, hopelessness, changes in body image and stress.

Montbriand[20] conducted interviews ($n = 400$) to explore the reasons why American patients with cancer used alternative therapies. A strong reason for choosing to use CAM was to gain control. A study by Swisher et al[21] evaluated the effects of using CAM on women with gynaecological cancer ($n = 113$). Prior to commencement of therapy, the women identified that they hoped to achieve a wide range of potential benefits, from improved well-being to anticancer effects. The study found that actual benefits included improvements in psychosocial well-being, specifically an increased sense of hope or optimism. Other more recent studies have shown that cancer patients use CAM for a variety of reasons, including to directly treat the disease, to increase the body's ability to fight the cancer, to improve physical and emotional well-being and increase hope and optimism, to counteract ill effects from the tumour or cancer treatment and to do everything possible to overcome the disease.[15,20] These results suggest that using CAM may fulfil certain needs that are not met by conventional treatment and care.

THE INTEGRATIVE MODEL OF CANCER CARE

A means of conceptualizing the use of CAM within cancer care is through the development of a model of delivery. The integrative model of cancer care (IMCC) is suggested here as bridging (Fig. 18.1) conventional and complementary approaches. The IMCC was in part influenced by the inspirational work of Michael Kearney, a palliative care consultant who has used dreamwork and guided imagery to help reduce existential anxiety. Working in the field of cancer often involves supporting patients who are coming to terms with threats to their own mortality; Kearney[22] refers to this profoundly felt struggle as 'soul pain'. He uses 'soul' in the more classical sense, referring to the 'psyche'. Working with the soul involves offering support at a deeper level, through creating an environment that best facilitates the process of inner healing.[23] Cawthorn[24] has adopted this approach with a cancer patient whose dreams were linked to her impending death. Through being given the opportunity to work through the dreams, the patient's existential anxiety was significantly reduced.

The IMCC aims to work with the whole person – mind, body and soul – in supporting them through the unique response to their illness using the three key bridging approaches shown in Figure 18.1. The model involves offering mind–body therapies alongside medical care, to *work with the person*, within their own healing journey. Daniel[25] suggests that the therapist and patient can 'work in partnership to achieve the best levels of health, energy, emotional and spiritual well-being' even in the presence of illness and adversity.[25(p19)] The main benefits of fostering an integrative approach are that healthcare staff and practitioners providing

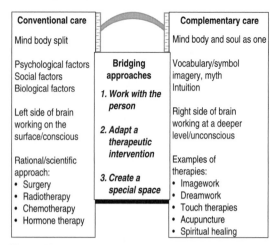

Figure 18.1: Integrative model.

therapies can work more closely together and can develop a closer relationship with the patient. Within this environment, CAM therapists can *adapt a therapeutic intervention*, such as massage, with a greater understanding of conventional treatment regimens. Similarly, medical and nursing staff are more aware of the contribution of CAM to overall care. There is now an increasing body of evidence which demonstrates that CAM used in this way can also play an important role in helping to reduce the side effects of treatments.[5,26]

The third aspect at the core of IMCC is to *create a special space*. This can be anywhere, even in a busy ward, and is about creating a holding environment where one person can attune to the other person's needs. It is akin to Bion's[27] definition of containment, which involves 'being with' another person in their suffering. Healthcare professionals often feel frustrated when they are unable to relieve suffering. By introducing techniques such as massage, relaxation techniques or visualization, nurses can help create special spaces within clinical environments.

EFFECTIVENESS OF COMPLEMENTARY AND ALTERNATIVE MEDICINE

Evidence of the effectiveness of most CAM therapies is lacking. However, a number of studies of CAM therapies have shown promising results, suggesting that CAM may be able to alleviate psychological and/or physical symptoms and improve quality of life in patients with cancer. Nonetheless, much of the research has been criticized for major methodological limitations, including small sample sizes, non-comparative designs and lack of control of confounding variables. There is an urgent need for positive results to be verified in larger studies using methodologies appropriate and sensitive to CAM concepts. A brief review of some of the studies of selected CAM therapies follows.

Body–mind interventions

A study of 181 women with breast cancer receiving either group support or CAM support (including meditation, affirmation, imagery and ritual) found that, although both groups had improved quality of life, the CAM support group showed additional improvements in spiritual integration and decreased avoidance.[28] The importance of integrating mind, body and spirit in order to have physical and emotional health has been discussed extensively.[29]

Autogenic training

Autogenic training is a type of meditation or self-hypnosis. Recent data from a pilot randomized study in 31 breast cancer patients suggest that this technique significantly decreased anxiety and depression levels and improved immune system parameters (CD8 count)[30]. Women also reported improvements in their sleep quality, although this outcome was not directly measured. Those women who were observed to be in a meditative state were more likely to experience positive effects on their psychological health.[30]

Imagery and psychoneuroimmunology

The use of imagery to treat cancer patients with advanced disease was pioneered by Simonton et al.[31] The connection between imagery and the immune system is part of the growing field of psychoneuroimmunology (PNI). Watkins[32] asserts that PNI research has generated hard scientific data that provide irrefutable evidence that virtually all the body's

defence systems are under the control of the central nervous system. There is now a substantial amount of evidence into the mind (psychology), the brain (neurology) and the body's natural defences (immunology) to suggest that the mind and body communicate with each other.[33]

Anderson and Walker[34] summarise the findings of studies evaluating survival following PNI interventions. They report that 5 randomized trials demonstrate prolonged survival and 6 trials do not. They, like others, suggest the need for more research into the psychological aspects of cancer, pointing out that many studies evaluate a combination of relaxation therapy, guided imagery, hypnotherapy or cognitive therapy and that there is a need to clarify the effects of individual interventions.

The therapeutic use of imagery is an extension of the idea that images affect body function. Under the guidance of a therapist, patients are encouraged to imagine beneficial changes such as healing.[22,23,35,36] This approach can be divided into active/aggressive imagery, and non-aggressive imagery. Using the aggressive approach, patients are encouraged to imagine the cancer cells being eaten or destroyed by whatever medium is acceptable to them, e.g. by laser guns, sharks or conventional chemotherapy. Non-aggressive imagery uses a 'balancing' approach, encouraging patients to visualize a golden light filling each of the organs, or to imagine the chemotherapy aiding the healing process. The authors' recent experience of using this type of imagery in a cancer centre suggests that it helps patients to cope with investigations and treatments by allowing them to switch their thoughts from the unpleasant situation they are in. Patients can be taught to access memories of a pleasant experience (a beach, or a time when they have achieved something) while they are undergoing chemotherapy or having an MRI (magnetic resonance imaging) scan.

Giedt[37] suggests how the use of guided imagery as a nursing intervention using PNI principles can also assist in the management of distressing symptoms such as pain. Giedt[37] works on the principle that pain causes both a physical sensation and a mental image, and suggests that therapists work by paying attention

385

to the metaphors used by the patient to describe both the pain sensation and the image it creates. A burning sensation, for example, can be relieved by encouraging the patient to imagine a contrasting sensation, such as cool water.

Touch and bodywork modalities

The use of touch in human relationships is complex. Nursing scholars have examined the phenomenon of touch, acknowledging that is used to signal caring, achieve nursing goals and provide comfort in a variety of healthcare settings.[38-40] Nurses and complementary therapists often use touch as part of a physical and emotional assessment. Chang[41] gave an example of touch as a vehicle for assessment, reporting a nurse in his study who said: 'frequently I would hold a patient's hand and at the same time I would try to observe temperature, pulse and emotional state'.[41(p823)] In a massage session the therapist might palpate soft tissue and provide effleurage (stroking) at the same time as noticing the patient's breathing as a possible indicator of enjoyment or discomfort with treatment.

Touch therapies

The manipulation of soft tissue, in the form of massage, aromatherapy or reflexology, carries with it other many possible benefits, some as yet not fully understood or evaluated within cancer care. Concerns continue to be raised by health professionals as to whether soft tissue work might promote metastasis. The work of the Touch Research Institute and others has helped to clarify the benefits of massage for people with cancer and diminish these concerns. Additionally, Stringer[42] has reported on the benefits of aromatherapy and massage for people with leukaemia, showing that treatments can be adapted safely even where there are concerns about an individual's haematological status.

Using a number of validated physiological and psychological measures, massage has been demonstrated to reduce cortisol levels, anxiety and pain.[43] A recent systematic review shows that massage and aromatherapy are associated with short-term improvements in psychologi-

cal well-being, with the most consistent effects demonstrated on levels of anxiety.[44] An uncontrolled evaluation of healing by gentle touch in patients with cancer ($n = 35$) showed improvements in ratings of relaxation and stress, severe pain/discomfort and depression/anxiety, with those experiencing more severe symptoms on entry to the study showing higher improvements.[45] Another recent trial did not demonstrate any long-term effects of massage in a sample of 42 palliative care patients, with the exception of sleep scores.[46] Evidence is mixed as to whether aromatherapy adds any benefit over and above the effects of massage alone. However, a trial of massage with or without aromatherapy showed improvements in quality of life in the aromatherapy group.[92] See Table 18.1 for a summary of studies using touch therapy.

Touch therapies in practice

The nursing literature suggests that complementary therapies such as reflexology and foot massage could be introduced into healthcare settings as an ideal non-pharmacological method of reducing stress and anxiety and managing difficult symptoms such as pain and nausea.[47,48] Relatives may also benefit from sitting in on treatments and seeing the effects for themselves. Cromwell et al[49] have reported that relatives valued the provision of reflexology, judging its availability to be a special treat. Brief reviews of recent studies are given in Table 18.1.

There is evidence to suggest that an increasing number of UK hospitals are employing therapists or allowing volunteer practitioners to provide therapies such as massage, aromatherapy and reflexology.[50,51] Many nurses are also attempting to include CAM therapies within their roles. Typically, these healthcare professionals have self-funded their training and are very enthusiastic about integrating therapies within their practice settings, despite existing workloads and some resistance from colleagues. A UK survey by Graham et al[51] identified that some hospitals were reluctant to fund treatments, because of concerns about research evidence, insurance and the quality of practitioner training. Achieving continued funding for complementary therapies, so as to

Table 18.1: Summary of studies using touch therapies (massage and reflexology) with cancer patients

Recent research	Title	Design	Method/ treatment	Measures	Findings	Limitations/issues
Penson[80]	An evaluation of a complementary therapy service in palliative care	Qualitative study $n = 38$	9 complementary therapies including reflexology 4 focus groups	Discussion of the experience facilitated by an independent researcher	The personal qualities of the therapists were deemed as crucial. Massage most popular. Peak effects reported at the 4th week	Focus groups reported to be therapeutic. Included 6 carers, which might have inhibited critical comments from patients. Author acknowledges that patients with cancer can be overly grateful and 'nice'
Dryden et al[85]	Evaluation of a pilot complementary therapy service	Non-randomized & no control group $n = 18$	Foot/hand massage incorporating reflexology techniques	Heart rate & blood pressure. Practitioner diaries & treatment records. Follow-up semi-structured questionnaire	Significant reduction in systolic blood pressure and heart rate. Self-reporting of relaxation post treatment that was cumulative	Possible bias as all authors participated in the study as practitioners. No control or randomization
Wilkinson et al[90]	An evaluation of aromatherapy massage in palliative care	Randomized controlled study $n = 103$	Massage with or without aromatherapy (Roman Camomile)	State Trait Anxiety Inventory. Rotterdam Symptom Checklist. Semi-structured interview	Massage with or without aromatherapy reduced levels of anxiety. Significant improvement in quality of life with the addition of aromatherapy	Attrition rate was high –16 left the study due to deterioration in condition or death. Patients condition variable across the group. No double-blind features so they were therapist knew they were administering aromatherapy

(continues)

Table 18.1: Summary of studies using touch therapies (massage and reflexology) with cancer patients—cont'd

Recent research	Title	Design	Method/treatment	Measures	Findings	Limitations/issues
Field[43]	Effects of massage on women with breast cancer	Randomized control study n = 20	30 minutes body massage twice a week for 5 weeks (n = 10) Control Group (n = 10)	State Trait Anxiety Inventory (STAI). Profile of Mood States Depression Scale (POMS). Short-form McGill Pain Questionnaire (SF-MPQ). Visual Analogue Scale (VAS) Symptom Checklist. Functional Assessment of Cancer Therapy (FACT) Scale. Immune & biochemical measures.	Significant by group reduction in anxiety and depression. Significant increase in immune function	Short duration of the study – unable to assess effects on cancer remission
Grealish et al[47]	To assess the effects of foot massage on nausea, pain and relaxation in hospitalized patients with cancer	Quasi-experimental. Random assignment to 3 different protocols of massage and relaxation. n = 87	2 sessions of foot massage and one relaxation activity	Heart rate. Pain (VAS). Nausea (VAS). Self-report of relaxation (VAS)	Significant difference in all measures. Improving relaxation and reducing nausea and pain	No control for medication. Anecdotal comments about massage as satisfactory nursing intervention. No exploration of lasting effects

Stephenson et al[48]	To assess the effects of reflexology on pain and anxiety in patients with lung and breast cancer	Quasi-experimental Cross-over trial. n = 23	Reflexology. No intervention period	Pain (SF-MPQ). Anxiety (VAS)	Significant decrease in anxiety following reflexology for both groups. Significant decrease in pain for breast cancer group	Only 2 out of the 10 lung cancer patients reported pain compared to 11 out of 13 in the breast cancer group Gender difference in the group and effects of pain relief makes it difficult to interpret results
Lively et al[91]	An economic evaluation of the cost savings of massage therapy in alleviating high-dose chemotherapy-induced nausea and vomiting	n = 31. 14 controls received antiemetics. 17 received massage as an adjunct to antiemetics	Thrice weekly massage sessions with 50% of patients receiving a maximum of 5 treatments	Record of days with: 1. nausea & vomiting 2. total parenteral nutrition 3. control with antiemetics in treatment programme	The use of massage therapy in the 17 patients resulted in a significant cost saving of $2853 10 per patient	Small sample size. Only one masseuse used. Nursing costs not included. One chemotherapy regimen assessed. Did not quantify effects on anxiety or stress
Lawvere[92]	The effects of massage therapy in ovarian cancer patients	Cross-over trial pilot study. n = 7	30-minute massage compared with 30-minute rest	Speilberger State Anxiety Inventory. Visual Analogue Mood Scale. Memorial Pain Assessment	Significant reduction in anxiety. Reported reductions in depressed mood and pain but not significant	Small sample. Not generalizable (all white females). Not blinded to treatment sequence. Short washout period

(continues)

Table 18.1: Summary of studies using touch therapies (massage and reflexology) with cancer patients—cont'd

Recent research	Title	Design	Method/ treatment	Measures	Findings	Limitations/issues
Wright et al[93]	Clients' perception of the benefits of reflexology on their quality of life	Retrospective analysis of client's view of benefit (n = 47)	Random selection of treatment records for between 1 and 16 treatments	Quality of life indicators and domains	34% increase in relaxation. 29.8% improved sense of self. 29.8% improved sleep. 27.6% improved energy. 23% improved pain relief	Anecdotal. Non-validated measure. Details of random selection not given. Unclear as to whether the views were sought by the herapists – halo effect may have influenced responses
Stephenson et al[94]	The effect of foot reflexology on pain in patients with metastatic cancer	A pilot study (n = 36). Randomized sample. Control group (n = 17)	Foot massage. No treatment (Control group was offered reflexology at the end of the project	10 point Pain Scale	Immediate positive effect for treatment group (p) <0.01) Self-reported Not significant at 3 or 24 hours)	Small numbers. One measure only

ensure an integrative service, remains a considerable challenge.

Herbs

Given the popularity of herbal medicines among cancer patients,[15, 52] it is surprising that little clinical research has been undertaken in this field. In-vitro experimental studies have shown that some individual herbs have biological activity, such as antioxidant, antitumour, antioestrogenic and immunostimulant actions. Examples include:

- Red ginseng, which has been shown, in vitro, to have potent tumour therapeutic activity and improve the cell immune system.[53]

- *Ganoderma lucidum*, in spore or powder form, which has also demonstrated strong antitumour activity against breast and prostate cancer cells.[54]

- Greek Labiatae herbs (including *Mentha pulegium* and *Thymus parnassicus* Halácsy)[55] and extract of *Herba scutellaria*,[56] all of which have shown cytotoxic activity

- Chinese motherwort herb,[57] which has shown antiproliferation activity (apoptosis)

- *Astragalus* and *Ligusticum*, which appear to have immunopotentiating effects and may be useful adjuncts to conventional cancer treatments.[58]

Anecdotal reports also advocate the popular herb essiac, for its alleged anticancer activity.[59] A review of a number of herbs with potential anticancer effects is presented by Montbriand.[60]

Much discussion has also been directed at PC-SPES, a commercially available product that includes 8 different types of herbs (i.e. *Ganoderma*) and which is used as a non-oestrogenic treatment for prostate cancer, significantly decreasing prostate-specific antigen (PSA) levels.[61] Controversy about this product exists and the US Food and Drug Administration (FDA) have recalled it from the market. However, it may, in future, become a therapeutic option for prostate cancer patients.[62]

Controversy exists over the use of black cohosh for hot flushes, a common problem in breast and prostate cancer patients. Positive[63] and negative[64] results have been published and studies have shown that black cohosh is associated with a number of side effects, including gastrointestinal upsets and rashes. Other products advocated for hot flushes include vitamin E, soya or red clover, antidepressant supplements (St John's wort) and acupuncture.[65] Further research to support these claims is still required.

Homeopathy

Homeopathy is also commonly used by cancer patients,[15] and it may well have a role in the supportive care of patients with cancer.[66] Studies suggest that homeopathic preparations may be useful in alleviating radiotherapy skin reactions[67] and hot flushes (especially in breast cancer patients receiving tamoxifen).[68,69] Homeopathy may also have effects on fatigue and mood disturbance.[67] However, the range of possibilities for homeopathy in the symptom management of cancer patients has not been fully explored and methodologically rigorous studies are needed.

Acupuncture

Acupuncture is gaining in popularity as a treatment for chronic illness and cancer symptoms. It has shown to be effective in the management of nausea and vomiting (see Ch. 20), and there are suggestions that it is also helpful in the management of pain, especially in palliative care settings. Acupuncture has also been associated with significant improvements in breathlessness, with patients showing a marked change in visual analogue scores, relaxation and anxiety and reductions in respiratory rate. These changes were sustained for 90 minutes post acupuncture.[70]

Energy therapies

There is some evidence that Reiki is useful in conjunction with opioid therapy, one study showing an association with significantly lower pain scores following therapy.[71] In another phase II trial, participants who received Reiki experienced improved pain control and quality of life, although opioid use was similar in the two groups.[72]

CARING FOR INFORMAL AND PROFESSIONAL CARERS

The potential for burnout and work-related stress is well acknowledged in the medical and nursing literature.[73,74] Field et al[75] conducted a study in which hospital workers were given a 10-minute chair massage, after which decreases in anxiety, depression and fatigue were reported alongside increases in vigour. Katz et al[76] conducted a small pilot study evaluating 8 sessions of on-site chair massage, also given to hospital staff. Relaxation and mood states received higher scores after the treatment, along with reduced tension and pain intensity. In another larger study involving 100 health-care workers, subjects were randomized into 2 groups, one group ($n = 50$) receiving 20 minutes of chair massage and the other, the control group ($n = 50$), resting for an equal time period.[77] Subjects who received chair massage exhibited decreases in blood pressure recordings, anxiety and sleep disturbances, and improvements in well-being and emotional control. Positive comments and high satisfaction were also reported by staff in a cancer hospital who were offered chair massage as part of a clinical initiative to improve working lives.[78]

The emotional and physical impact of caring for someone with cancer is well acknowledged and the potential for carers to benefit from CAM is also attracting attention. A service project providing massage to carers has been the subject of a published evaluation in the USA.[79] Thirteen caregivers were provided with an average of 6 massage sessions, after which 85% reported reductions in their emotional and physical stress levels, 77% reported reductions in physical pain and 54% reported improved sleep patterns. In the UK, a massage service for family members of patients receiving palliative care has been well evaluated in a focus group study.[80] A service providing chair massage for carers in an acute cancer setting has reported improvements in well-being,

sleep and stress following 15-minute massage sessions provided on the ward.[81]

REGULATION ISSUES

The training and regulation of therapists is a key concern for patients, practitioners and health-care professionals.[1–3] Lead professional bodies are keen to advance the reputation of CAM so as to reassure and protect both the public and the practitioners. Given that such a wide range of therapies exist, Budd and Mills[82] believe that statutory control of CAM is unrealistic. They suggest that the way forward is self-regulation, in which individual therapy groups comply with a number of activities (Box 18.1). In the UK, the government is supporting the exploration of statutory regulation for acupuncture and herbalism, because these therapies may be associated with greater risk of harm to patients.

Legal, professional and managerial issues

Although CAM therapies are not usually seen as a core component of conventional care, nonetheless, they represent interventions that

---

Box 18.1

Voluntary self-regulation activities

- Maintains a register of individual members or member organizations
- Sets educational standards and an independent accreditation system for training establishments
- Maintains professional competence amongst its members with an adequate programme of continuing development
- Provides codes of conduct, ethics and practice
- Has in place a complaints procedure that is accessible to the public
- Requires members to have adequate professional indemnity insurance
- Has the capacity to represent the whole profession
- Includes external representation on executive councils to represent patients or clients and the wider public interest

Source: Budd and Mills.[82]

require management and delivery by skilled and accountable therapists. Stone[83] asserts that the ethical duty to provide benefit to patients is enshrined in the legal concept of duty of care, which requires therapists to treat their patients with all due skill and care. Because many CAM therapies involve touch, the civil action of 'battery' (or trespass to the person), which upholds respect for the patient's bodily autonomy, is of particular importance. A battery is said to occur when touch is used, e.g. in the course of the treatment, without first having obtained consent.[83]

Although surveys have been conducted on the popularity of complementary therapies, little quantifiable data exist on the delivery of CAM within healthcare services and/or the patients who are receiving them. Some healthcare organisations have established Complementary Therapy Committees, so as to share this type of information and agree policies and protocols. Ideally, the membership of such a committee should include representation from practitioners, management and, if possible, service users. Alternatively, this work can be subsumed under a general Policy and Practice Committee, which can delegate activities such as auditing and drafting of protocols and policies to specific working groups. A number of UK hospitals have been proactive in this work and can be approached for advice and copies of protocols and policies.[84] Important first steps in the planning of services include:

- Conducting surveys of interest in CAM by patients and clinical staff.
- Gathering information about existing CAM-related skills and training amongst staff.
- Preparing and revising treatment records so that data can be collected for audit purposes. Documentation should include details of reasons for the referral, evaluation comments from the patient and a record of treatment times and observed responses to treatment.

Reports from the Foundation for Integrated Medicine and the House of Lords in the UK have both made many important recommendations for the regulation and training of CAM practitioners providing services in healthcare settings. The use of volunteers in the provision of CAM treatments to patients is an area of considerable debate. Although all therapists should, ideally, be part of the core workforce, the reality is that volunteers currently provide many existing CAM services. This situation does enable volunteers to feel a sense of reciprocity from their contribution,[5] as they can be part of a team, gaining from the experience and giving freely to others without financial gain. Additionally, some volunteers may use their experience as a step to paid employment, either within the organization or elsewhere. However, the use of volunteers can be problematic. Adequate support and supervisory review are not always in place, yet it is suggested that in order to safeguard patients and CAM professional practice, respectful use of volunteers requires that they be given the same consideration as paid therapists.[5] For example, volunteers need careful recruitment, orientation, induction, support for continuing professional development and planned review of their activities and professional aspirations.

Supervision and support for CAM therapists

Reflective practice and supervision have been identified as effective ways of exploring the therapeutic role, safeguarding an individual practitioner's scope of professional practice and supporting quality care.[86] Typically, supervision involves meeting with a facilitator, individually or as part of a group. The establishment of a supervision contract forms an important part of the process and the development of a supervisory relationship. It has been suggested that supervision can help nurses using CAM to become more 'potent' in their therapeutic work,[87] but supervision can also operate as a risk management tool, possibly reducing complaints and even cases of litigation.[88]

Table 18.2 illustrates the key managerial issues that may arise in relation to two different types of provision: by voluntary therapists or existing healthcare professionals. Practical issues for CAM therapists are discussed in Box 18.2.

393

Table 18.2: Different types of CAM provision in healthcare organizations: managerial issues and strategies to resolve these

Type of practitioners	Management issues	Possible strategies
Volunteer CAM practitioners (non-healthcare professionals)	Need to identify means of monitoring and supervising No formal contract to manage their services Variable knowledge of health and illness Provision can cease if volunteers remove their services	Employment of a Complementary Therapy Coordinator to manage volunteers Provision of inservice education and support for further training Audit of service to develop a case for funded session work
Role expansion for healthcare staff (qualified therapists)	Competition with existing role and duties	Allocated set hours for the activity Different uniform and role title Consider providing CAM interventions in a different, but linked clinical area

Box 18.2

Practice points for healthcare settings

Preparation
- Ensure you have consent from the patient, their consultant and the departmental head nurse.
- Encourage the patient to inform their family/and or partner that they are considering receiving a CAM intervention.
- Ensure you have made a workable contract with the patient. For example, identify how they might like to feel at the end of the session: e.g. energized, relaxed or more comfortable (NB: CAM is not a substitute for prescribed pain medication).
- Adhere to hospital infection control policies – strict hand washing, use of a clean towel with each patient and correct disposal of paper towels.
- Consider factors, which might interfere with treatment: e.g. time, dress and place. For example, Dryden et al[85] found that nursing staff providing reflexology were less likely to get interrupted during the afternoons when visitors were at a mimimum, and when they wore a different uniform. Make sure that the environment and the position you are working in are comfortable at all times.

During and post treatment
- Check with the patient intermittently that they are comfortable and happy to continue (ongoing consent).
- If a patient's visitor wishes to be present (and the patient agrees) make sure that they are briefed beforehand. For example, relatives often feel that they have to talk, so being told that they will need to sit quietly can be useful.
- Acknowledge background noise and distractions in busy clinical settings by noticing them but coming back to the work (you can ask the patient to do likewise).
- Make sure that you can monitor the patient's post-treatment responses. For example, avoid treating a patient just before finishing your shift.
- Record the treatment(s) within the patient's existing records and maintain your own confidential records.

Source: adapted from Mackereth et al.[81]

Box 18.3

Recommendations for developing and integrating model CAM services

- Evaluate existing and developing CAM services to examine best integrative practice
- Share best practice in integrative CAM in oncology journals, conference and seminar events
- Establish and/or participate in CAM research, practice networks and specialist interest groups to obtain support and share best practice.
- Establish and/or participate in the local Complementary Therapy Committee or equivalent
- Establish transparent recruitment practices, management support and appropriate supervision for therapists, whether voluntary or funded
- Develop criteria for CAM posts, detailing preferred prior experience, acceptable qualifications and means of maintaining professional development
- Consider establishing lead roles or coordinator posts to manage, conduct evaluation activities and supervise CAM practitioners

Coordinator/practitioner roles for complementary therapies are beginning to develop, and these will be pivotal to the management of volunteers and paid session therapists. As well as providing a resource for healthcare staff and patients, these coordinators can facilitate and organize inservice training courses and income generation through consultative and educational work. Another important aspect of these roles will be the auditing of existing services, so as to contribute to evidence that will help to secure permanent funding for CAM therapies.

INTEGRATING COMPLEMENTARY AND ALTERNATIVE MEDICINE INTO CONVENTIONAL PRACTICE

Despite evidence that selective CAM therapies can benefit cancer patients and increase overall satisfaction with health care, many conventional healthcare settings have been unable to integrate CAM into their services. Although patients can access CAM outside the conventional healthcare setting, the benefits of integrating services are clear. In an integrated service, both conventional and CAM-related care are supervised and monitored by knowledgeable healthcare professionals, thus improving communication, increasing trust, improving safety, empowering patients and potentially contributing to improved symptom management and supportive care.

Successful integration is more likely to occur when there is a demand for CAM services within a context of secure funding, commitment and realism from senior staff in the conventional setting. An integrated service includes protected time for education, ongoing evaluation of services, development of jointly agreed protocols or guidelines (between conventional and CAM practitioners) and adherence to careful selection and supervision of CAM practitioners (Box 18.3). Two other important issues for successful integration are the establishment of links with other conventional settings using CAM services and political or managerial support.[2,89] It is imperative that services are planned to meet demand, and that referral criteria are understood and adhered to, so as to avoid conflict between practitioners due to unresolved differences in perspective.[2,89]

Integration may, however, fail to materialize for a number of practical reasons, including financial insecurity, staff time constraints, lack of appropriate premises, unrealistic expectations (of both staff and patients), real or perceived lack of evidence of effectiveness, and lack of resources or time for reflection and evaluation.

CONCLUSION

The benefits of using CAM therapies for patients with cancer can be numerous, especially in relation to supportive care. However, the lack of evidence for CAM and the safety issues continue to fuel debate about the appropriateness of integrating CAM into conventional care settings.[95] There is an urgent need to expand the evidence base for CAM and to evaluate the safety and efficacy of CAM in cancer care. The reality is that patients are increasingly attracted to CAM, and healthcare professionals need to become much more knowledgeable in the field. Pre- and post-registration courses for doctors, nurses and allied health professionals must address knowledge and attitudes towards CAM, so as to develop understanding and encourage critical awareness. We also need to be in a position to educate patients and provide them with high-quality information about the risks and benefits of CAM in relation to cancer, so that we can assist patients to make informed and appropriate decisions in their care. In the clinical sector, we need to evaluate models of integrated service provision and examine the skills and support required to ensure that therapists working in cancer care are 'fit for practice'. Consensus guidelines and agreement on training and regulation amongst stakeholders in Europe will help to ensure that CAM therapies provided to patients with cancer are safe, effective and adequately evaluated.

REFERENCES

1. British Medical Association. Complementary medicine new approaches to good practice. London: British Medical Association; 1993.
2. Foundation for Integrated Medicine. Integrated healthcare: a way forward for the next five years. London: FIM; 1997.
3. House of Lords: Select Committee on Science and Technology. Complementary and alternative medicine. HL Paper 123.London: House of Lords; 2000.
4. Royal College of Nursing. Complementary therapies in nursing, midwifery and health visiting practice. RCN guidance on integrating complementary therapies into clinical care. London: Royal College of Nursing; 2003.
5. Tavares M. National guidelines for the use of complementary therapies in supportive and palliative care. The Prince of Wales's Foundation for Integrated Health & the National Council for Hospice and Specialist Palliative Services. London: The Prince of Wales's Foundation for Integrated Health; 2003.
6. Stone J. How might traditional remedies be incorporated into discussions of integrated medicine? Complement Therap Nurs Midwifery 2001; 7(2):55–58.
7. Ernst E, Resch KL, Mills S, et al. Complementary medicine – a definition. Br J Gen Pract 1995; 45:506.
8. Corner J, Harewood J. Exploring the use of complementary and alternative medicine by people with cancer. Nurs Times Res 2004; 9(2):101–109.
9. Ernst E The current position of complementary/alternative medicine in cancer. Eur J Cancer 2003; 39(16):2273–2277.
10. Ernst E, White A. The BBC survey of complementary therapy medicine used in the UK. Complement Therap Med 2000; 8:32–36.
11. Risberg T, Vickers A, Bremmes RM, et al. Does use of alternative medicine predict survival from cancer? Eur J Cancer 2003; 39:372–377.
12. Rees RW, Feigal I, Vickers A, et al. Prevalence of complementary therapy use by women with breast cancer: a population-based survey. Eur J Cancer 2000; 36:1359–1364
13. Lewith GT, Broomfield J, Prescott P. 2002 Complementary therapies in Southampton: a survey of staff and patients. Complement Therap Med 2002; 10:100–106.
14. Kohn M. Directory of complementary therapy services in UK cancer care. London: Macmillan Cancer Relief; 2002.
15. Molassiotis A, Fernadez-Ortega P, Pud D, et al. Use of complementary and alternative medicine in cancer patients: a European survey. Ann Oncol 2005; 16–655–663.
16. Fernadez CV, Stutzer CA, MacWilliam L, Fryer C. Alternative and complementary therapy use in paediatric oncology patients in British Columbia: prevalence and reasons for use and nonuse. J Clin Oncol 1998; 16:1279–1286.
17. Molassiotis A, Cubbin D. 'Thinking outside the box': complementary and alternative therapies use in paediatric oncology patients. Eur J Oncol Nurs 2004; 8:50–60.
18. Thomas KJ, Nicholl JP, Fall M. Access to complementary medicine via general practice. Br J Gen Pract 2001; 51(462):25–30.
19. Coss RA, McGrath P, Caggiano V. Alternative care: patient choices for adjunct therapies within a cancer centre. Cancer Pract 1998; 3:176–181.
20. Montbriand MJ. Decision tree model describing alternate health care choices made by oncology patients. Cancer Nurs 1995; 18:104–117.
21. Swisher EM, Cohn DE, Goff BA, et al. Use of complementary and alternative medicine among women with gynaecological cancers. Gynecolog Oncol 2002; 84:363–367.
22. Kearney M. Mortally wounded stories of soul pain, death and healing. New York: Touchstone; 1997.
23. Kearney M. A place of healing: working with suffering in living and dying. Oxford: Oxford University Press; 2000.
24. Cawthorn A. Using imagework for adjustment anxiety in a patient diagnosed with advanced cancer. Unpublished MSc thesis. University of Wales; 2002.

25. Daniel R. Holistic approaches to cancer: general principles and the assessment of the patient. In: Barraclough J, ed. Integrated cancer care. Oxford: Oxford University Press; 2001.

26. Russo H 2000 Integrated healthcare: a guide to good practice. London: The Foundation for Integrated Medicine; 2000.

27. Bion WR. The psycho-analytic study of thinking. A theory of thinking. Int J Psychoanal 1962; 43:306–310.

28. Targ EF, Levine EG. The efficacy of a mind-body-spirit group for women with breast cancer: a randomized controlled trial. Gen Hosp Psychiatry 2002; 24:238–248.

29. Mytko JJ, Knight SJ. Body, mind and spirit: towards the integration of religiosity and spirituality in cancer quality of life research. Psycho-Oncol 1999; 8:439–450.

30. Hidderley M, Holt M. A pilot randomized trial assessing the effects of autogenic training in early stage cancer patients in relation to psychological status and immune system responses. Eur J Oncol Nursing 2004; 8:61–65.

31. Simonton OC, Matthews-Simonton S, Sparks TF. Psychological interventions in the treatment of cancer. Psychosomatics 1980; 21:226–233.

32. Watkins A. Mind-body medicine. New York: Churchill Livingstone; 1997.

33. Ader R. Historical perspectives on psychoneuroimmunology. In: Friedman H, Klien TW, Friedman AL, eds. Psychoneuroimmunology, stress and infection. Boca Raton, Fl: CRC Press; 1996.

34. Anderson J, Walker LG. Psychological factors and cancer progression: involvement of behavioural pathways. In: Lewis CE, O'Brian RM, Barraclough J, eds. The Psycho-Immunonology of Cancer. 2nd edn. Oxford: University Press Oxford; 2003.

35. Cunningham AJ. The healing journey: overcoming the crisis of cancer. Toronto; Key Porter Books; 2000.

36. Kearney M. Imagework in a case of intractable pain. Palliat Med 1992; 6:152–157.

37. Giedt MS. Guided imagery. A psychoneuroimmunological intervention in holistic nursing practice. J Holist Nurs Assoc 1997; 15:112–127.

38. Butts JB. Outcomes of comfort touch in institutionalized elderly female residents. Geriatr Nurs 2001; 22:180–184.

39. Harrison LL, Williams AK, Berbaum ML, Stem JT, Leeper J. Physiologic & behavioural effects of gentle human touch on preterm infants. Res Nurs Health 2000; 23:435–446.

40. Verity S. Communicating with sedated ventilated patients in intensive care: focusing on the use of touch. Intens Crit Care Nurs 1996; 12:354–358.

41. Chang SO. The conceptual structure of physical touch in caring. J Adv Nurs 2001; 33:820–827.

42. Stringer J. Massage and aromatherapy on a Leukaemia Unit. Complement Ther Nurs Midwifery 2000; 6:72–76.

43. Field T. Touch therapy. London: Harcourt Press; 2000.

44. Fellowes D, Barnes K, Wilkinson S. Aromatherapy and massage for symptom relief in patients with cancer. Cochrane Pain, Palliative Care and Supportive Care Group. Cochrane Database of Syst Rev 2004 (2) CD063751.

45. Weze C, Leathard HL, Grange J, Tiplady P, Stevens G. Evaluation of healing by gentle touch in 35 clients with cancer. Eur J Oncol Nurs 2004; 8:40–49.

46. Soden K, Vincent K, Craske S, Lucas C, Ashley S. A randomised controlled trial of aromatherapy massage in a hospice setting. Palliat Med 2004; 18:87–92.

47. Grealish L, Lomasney A, Whiteman B. Foot massage: a nursing intervention to modify the distressing symptoms of pain and nausea in patients hospitalised with cancer. Cancer Nurs 2000; 23:237–243.

48. Stephenson NLN, Weinrich SP. The effects of foot reflexology on anxiety and pain in patients with breast and lung cancer. Oncol Nurs Forum 2000; 27:67–72.

49. Cromwell C, Dryden S, Jones D, Mackereth P. 'Just the ticket'; case studies, reflections and clinical supervision (Part 111). Complement Ther Nurs Midwifery 1999; 5:42–45.

50. Rankin-Box D. Therapies in practice: a survey assessing nurses' use of complementary therapies. Complement Ther Nurs Midwifery 1997; 3:92–99.

51. Graham L, Goldstone L, Ejindu A, Baker J, Asiedu-Addo E. Penetration of complementary therapies into NHS trust and private hospital practice. Complement Ther Nurs Midwifery 1998; 4:160–165.

52. Richardson MA, Sanders T, Palmer JL, Greisinger A, Singletary SE. Complementary/alternative medicine use in a comprehensive cancer center and the implications for oncology. J Clin Oncol 2000; 18:2505–2514.

53. Xiaoguang C, Hongyan L, Xiaohong L, et al. Cancer chemopreventive and therapeutic activities of red ginseng. J Ethnopharmacol 1998; 60:71–78.

54. Sliva D, Sedlak M, Slivova V, et al. Biologic activity of spores and dried powder from *Ganoderma lucidum* for the inhibition of highly invasive human breast and prostate cancer cells. J Altern Complement Med 2003; 9:491–497.

55. Badisa RB, Tzakou O, Couladis M, Pilarinou E. Cytotoxic activities of some Greek Labiatae herbs. Phytother Res 2003; 17:472–476.

56. Powell CB, Fung P, Jackson J, et al. Aqueous extract of *Herba Scutellaria barbatae*, a Chinese herb used for ovarian cancer, induces apoptosis of ovarian cancer cell lines. Gynecolog Oncol 2003; 91:332–340.

57. Chinwala MG, Gao M, Dai J, Shao J. In vitro anticancer activities of *Leonurus heterophyllus* sweet (Chinese motherwort herb). J Altern Complement Med 2003; 9:511–518.

58. Sinclair S. Chinese herbs: a clinical review of *Astragalus, Ligusticum* and *Schizandrae*. Altern Med Rev 1998; 3:338–344.

59. Tamayo C, Richardson MA, Diamond S, Skoda I. The chemistry and biological activity of herbs used in Flor-Essence herbal tonic and Essiac. Phytother Res 2000; 14:1–14.

60. Montbriand MJ. Past and present herbs used to treat cancer: medicine, magic, or poison? Oncol Nurs Forum 1999; 26:49–60.

61. Cordell GA. PC-SPES: a brief overview. Integr Cancer Ther 2002; 1:271–286.

62. Pirani JF. The effects of phytotherapeutic agents on prostate cancer: an overview of recent clinical trials of PC SPES. Urology 2001; 58(2 Suppl 1):36–38.

63. Kronenberg F, Fugh-Berman A. Complementary and alternative medicine for menopausal symptoms: a review of randomized, controlled trials. Ann Intern Med 2002; 137:805–813.

64. Jacobson JS, Troxel AB, Evans J, et al. Randomized trial of black cohosh for the treatment of hot flashes among women with a history of breast cancer. J Clin Oncol 2001; 19:2739–2745.

65. Moyad MA. Complementary/alternative therapies for reducing hot flashes in prostate cancer patients: reevaluating the existing indirect data from studies of breast cancer and postmenopausal women. Urology 2002; 59(Suppl 1):20–33.

66. Thompson EA. Using homeopathy to offer supportive cancer care, in a National Health Service outpatient setting. Complement Ther Nurs Midwifery 1999; 5:37–41.

67. Balzarini A, Felisi E, Martini A, De Conno F. Efficacy of homeopathic treatment of skin reactions during radiotherapy for breast cancer: a randomized, double-blind clinical trial. Br Homeopath J 2000; 89:8–12.

68. Clover A, Ratsey D. Homeopathic treatment of hot flashes: a pilot study. Homeopathy 2002; 91:75–79.

69. Thompson EA, Reilly D. The homeopathic approach to the treatment of symptoms of oestrogen withdrawal in breast cancer patients. A prospective observational study. Homeopathy 2003; 92:131–134.

70. Filshie J, Penn K, Ashley S, Davis CL. Acupuncture for the relief of cancer-related breathlessness. Palliat Med 1996; 10:145–150.

71. Olson K, Hanson J. Using Reiki to manage pain: a preliminary report. Cancer Prev Control 1997; 1:108–113.

72. Olson K, Hanson J, Michaud M. 2003. A phase II trial of Reiki for the management of pain in advanced cancer patients. J Pain Symptom Manage 2003; 26: 990–997.

73. Kash KM, Holland JC, Breitbart W, et al. Stress and burnout in oncology. Oncology (Huntingt) 2000; 14:1621–1633.

74. Fitch MI, Bakker D, Conlon M. Important issues in clinical practice: perspectives of oncology nurses. Can Oncol Nurse J 1999; 9:151–164.

75. Field T, Quintino O, Henteleff T, Wells-Keife L, Delvecchio-Feinberg G. Job stress reduction therapies. Altern Ther Health Med 1997; 3(4):54–56.

76. Katz J, Wowk A, Culp D, Wakeling H. Pain and tension are reduced among hospital nurses after on-site massage treatments: a pilot study. J Perianesth Nurs 1999; 14:128–133.

77. Hodge M, Robinson C, Boehmer J, Klein S. Employee outcomes following work-site acupressure and massage. Massage Ther J 2000; 39:48–64.

78. Mackereth PA, White K, Cawthorn A, Lynch B. Improving stressful working lives: complementary therapies, counselling and clinical supervision for staff. Eur J Oncol Nurs 2005.

79. Oregon Hospice Association and East-West College of Healing Arts. Massage as a respite intervention for primary caregivers. Am J Hospice Palliat Med 1998; Jan/Feb:43–47.

80. Penson J. Complementary therapies: making a difference in palliative care. Complement Ther Nurs Midwifery 1998; 4:77–81.

81. Mackereth P, Stringer J, Lynch B, Campbell G. How CAM helps at acute cancer hospital. J Holistic Healthcare 2004; 1:33–38.

82. Budd S, Mills S. Regulatory prospects for complementary and alternative medicine: information pack. Centre for Complementary Health Studies University of Exeter on behalf of the Department of Health, UK; 2000.

83. Stone J. An ethical framework for complementary and alternative therapies. London: Routledge; 2002.

84. Rankin Box D, McVey M. Policy development. In: Rankin-Box, D, ed. The nurse's handbook of complementary therapies. 2nd edn. London: Harcourt; 2001.

85. Dryden S, Holden S, Mackereth P. 'Just the ticket'; the findings of a pilot complementary therapy service (Part II). Complement Ther Nurs Midwifery 1999; 5(1):15–18.

86. Mackereth P. Clinical supervision and complementary therapies. In: Rankin-Box, D, ed. The nurse's handbook of complementary therapies. London: Churchill Livingstone; 2000.

87. Mackereth P. Clinical supervision for 'potent' practice. Complement Ther Nurs Midwifery 1997; 3:38–41.

88. Tingle J. Clinical supervision is an effective risk management tool. Br J Nurs 1995; 4(14):794–795.

89. Shapiro DA, Safer M. 2002. Integrating complementary therapies into a traditional oncology practice. M.D. Oncol Issues 2002; 17:35–40.

90. Wilkinson S. An evaluation of aromatherapy massage in palliative care. Palliat Med 1999; 13(5):409–417.

91. Lively BT, Holiday-Goodman M, Black C, Arondekar B. Massage therapy for chemotherapy-induced emesis. In: Rich GJ, ed. Massage therapy: the evidence for practice. London: Harcourt Brace; 2002.

92. Lawvere S. 2002 The effect of massage therapy in ovarian cancer patients. In: Rich GJ, ed.

Massage therapy: the evidence for practice. London: Harcourt Brace; 2002.

93. Wright S, Courtney C, Donnelly C, Kenny T, Lavin C. Client's perceptions of the benefits of reflexology on their quality of life. Complement Ther Nurs Midwifery 2002; 8:69–76.

94. Stephenson N, Dalton JA, Carlson J. The effect of foot reflexology on pain in patients with metastatic cancer. Appl Nurs Res 2003; 16(4):284–286.

95. Molassiotis A. The evil complementary and alternative medicine! ... the debate continues! Eur J Oncol Nurs 2005; 9:112-114.

SECTION 5

Symptom management

19. Haematological Support 403

20. Nausea and Vomiting 415

21. Pain 439

22. Constipation and Diarrhoea 481

23. Breathlessness 507

24. Skin and Wound Care 527

25. Lymphoedema 559

26. Oral Complications in Patients
    with Cancer 575

27. Alopecia 601

28. Malignant Effusions 619

29. Anorexia, Cachexia and Malnutrition . . . 633

30. Cancer-Related Fatigue 657

31. The Impact of Cancer and Cancer
    Therapy on Sexual and Reproductive
    Health. 675

32. Altered Body Image 701

33. Psychological Care for Patients
    with Cancer 717

CHAPTER 19

Haematological Support

JACQUI STRINGER, JANE COLLINS AND ANGELA LEATHER

CHAPTER CONTENTS

Introduction to the increasing needs to support bone marrow suppression in oncology nursing	403	
Haematological implications of cancer		
Low red blood cells (erythrocytopenia/ anaemia)	404	
Low white blood cells (leucopenia)	404	
Low platelets (thrombocytopenia)	405	
Pancytopenia	405	
Venous thromboembolism	405	
Blood product support	405	
Red cells	405	
Platelets	406	
Fresh frozen plasma	406	
Albumin	407	
Immunoglobulins	407	
Haematopoietic stem cells	407	
Special requirements	408	
Administration	408	

Transfusion reactions	408
Management of acute transfusion reactions	408
Transfusion-transmitted infection	409
Safety	409
Patient information	409
Safe administration of treatment	410
Planning nursing care	410
Ethical issues	411
New approaches to haematological support	412
Erythropoietin	412
Haematopoietic growth factors	412
Donor granulocytes	413
Coagulation factors	413
Community care	413
Conclusion	413
References	414

INTRODUCTION TO THE INCREASING NEEDS TO SUPPORT BONE MARROW SUPPRESSION IN ONCOLOGY NURSING

This chapter will provide an overview of the impact that cancer treatments can have on the bone marrow and the basic supportive care required by the patient. Blood product support required and issues relating to patients and staff safety will be highlighted. Issues around patients declining haematological support will also be discussed.

Patients undergoing treatment for cancer require haematological support for three main reasons. It may be that their bone marrow is not functioning effectively as a direct consequence of their disease, as it would be in the case of patients suffering with haematological malignancies. Excessive blood loss through surgery or damage to the marrow due to radiation therapy can also lead to the need for haematological support. However, the most common reason for haematological support in the field of cancer care is because of the effects of chemotherapy (see also Ch. 14)

Chemotherapy involves drugs being given to destroy cells while they are dividing. The majority of drugs are only active to cells at a certain phase in mitosis or cell division; consequently, above a certain optimal dosage, the drug's effectiveness will plateau. However, some drugs, such as alkylating agents, are not phase-specific and they kill more cells with increasing dosage.

Clinicians are constantly learning more about the development of tumours. The number of chemotherapy agents available is also expanding, as is the variety and strength of the combinations in which they are used. This knowledge culminates in extremely potent chemotherapy regimens being used earlier and earlier in the patient's cancer journey.

Unfortunately, so far, there are no drugs in clinical use with action specific to malignant cells. Cancer cells are a result of cell mutation; malignant cells often proliferate faster than normal cells. However, normal cells do proliferate and, until relatively recently, the main dose-limiting factor for chemotherapy dosage was specifically myelosuppression. Bone marrow is very sensitive to chemotherapy, as the haematopoietic stem cells (HSC) are some of the fastest replicating cells in the body and, as such, are easily damaged by many chemotherapy agents. Historically, the only support therapies available were transfusion of blood products, dose reduction and delay in chemotherapy administration and the use of antibiotics.[1] Although these approaches are still used, in recent years a much wider range of products have been developed to support the patient's bone marrow, including HSC rescue, which allows clinicians to use higher doses of chemotherapy as curative treatments for a number of solid tumours, e.g. breast cancer and teratoma. Consequently, bone marrow suppression is no longer seen as the major limiting factor to the intensity of the chemotherapy prescribed.

HAEMATOLOGICAL IMPLICATIONS OF CANCER

To understand the impact of myelosuppression on the body, it is necessary to be aware of the normal blood count for a healthy individual. The most important elements are presented below, along with examples of potential problems encountered by patients undergoing treatment for malignant conditions because of either the disease process or the treatment:[2]

- haemoglobin – male 13.5–17.5 g/dl; female 11.5–15.5 g/dl
- leucocytes (white cells) – male and female $4.0–11.0 \times 10^9/L$
- neutrophils – male and female $2.5–7.5 \times 10^9/L$
- lymphocytes – male and female $1.5–3.5 \times 10^9/L$
- platelets – male and female $150–400 \times 10^9/L$

Low red blood cells (erythrocytopenia/ anaemia)

Haemoglobin is carried on the red blood cells and is responsible for carrying oxygen to the cells of the body. When myelosuppression occurs, a patient's haemoglobin can reach critical levels of as low as 4 g/dl; however, the patient becomes symptomatic of anaemia before reaching such low levels of haemaglobin, showing signs such as excessive fatigue and breathlessness.

Anaemia in patients with cancer may be due to the following causes:[3]

- chemotherapy and/or radiotherapy
- surgical intervention
- bone marrow tumour infiltration
- anaemia of chronic disease
- haematinic (iron, vitamin B_{12}, folate) deficiency
- bleeding and coagulopathy
- haemolysis
- decreased erythropoietin (EPO) production
- decreased responsiveness to EPO

Low white blood cells (leucopenia)

The leucocyte or total white cell count shows the level of immune system functioning. The most important component of the white cell count is the number of neutrophils or polymorphonuclear neutrophils (PMNs) present, as these cells protect the body from opportunistic infections (e.g. the common cold) becoming potentially life-threatening in nature. These innate or 'non-adaptive cells' are one of the body's first line of defence when under attack and account for 60–70% of leucocytes in adults.[4] When a patient becomes neutropenic (with a neutrophil count below $1.0 \times 10^9/L$, and often as low as $0.0 \times 10^9/L$, with or without other leucocyte values) it is very important to protect them from infection. It becomes the role of the medical and nursing staff to take over the protection offered by the immune system. This is done through measures such as isolation nursing, administration of prophylactic antimicrobial drugs and strict hygiene procedures for all involved in the care of the patient. If, despite these measures, the patient contracts an infection – seen through symptoms such as high temperatures, sweats, feeling cold, shivering (rigors) and sometimes a dramatic drop in blood pressure – at this point intravenous antibiotics are required.

Low platelets (thrombocytopenia)

Platelets are responsible for minimizing bleeding following vascular injury. The clotting cascade assists in permanently sealing the area by forming a 'plug' over the damaged area. Thrombocytopenia is the reduction in the number of circulating platelets and can occur as a result of bone marrow failure caused by disease, myelotoxic treatment or inherited platelet disorders.[5]

Following chemotherapy, a patient's platelet count reaches a nadir (lowest point), 10–14 days post-chemotherapy,[6] and can fall to values of less than $10 \times 10^9/L$. At this time, the patient is vulnerable to active bleeding from internal organs (e.g. haematemesis or haemoptysis), following minimal trauma, but much more commonly, through seepage of blood from small blood vessels. Signs of a low platelet count include nosebleeds, excessive bruising or tiny pinprick bruises that have a rash-like appearance, known as petechiae. A low platelet count also puts a patient at risk of major bleeds such as a brain haemorrhage, which can be fatal. It is therefore imperative that medical/nursing staff monitor the patient's platelet count and observe for signs of active bleeding. Patient education is vital in ensuring that bleeding risks are minimized: e.g. performing oral hygiene using a soft toothbrush. When patients are seen to be at higher risk of bleeding (platelet count below 10 $\times 10^9/L$), they are supported by platelet trans-

fusions, although this varies from place to place depending on local policy.

Pancytopenia

When all elements within bone marrow are lower than the normal range, i.e. red cells, white cells and platelets, this is known as pancytopenia, and the patient requires care related to all these factors.

Venous thromboembolism

Patients with cancer are also at high risk of venous thromboembolism (VTE), a condition that is relatively uncommon in healthy adults. This is diagnosed clinically as between 11 and 15% of patient's ante mortem and up to 50% show evidence of VTE post mortem.[7] There are many reasons for this increased risk, including the fact that all tumour cells activate the clotting cascade,[8] surgery and some cytotoxic agents (e.g. thalidomide) trigger similar mechanisms.[9] These factors, combined with immobility and blood vessel wall injury, interact to put the patient at high risk of VTE. As many patients receive treatment as outpatients, oncology nurses play a crucial role in the coordination of at-risk patients.[10]

BLOOD PRODUCT SUPPORT

The most frequently used blood products to support patients with cancer are red cells, platelets and plasma. Immunoglobulins, single-factor clotting concentrates and donor granulocytes are also used in supporting some patients with cancer through the intensive periods of their treatment. Overall, a third of all patients with cancer require at least one blood transfusion: for example, 1 in 5 patients with breast cancer and half of all patients with malignant lung disease. The likelihood of receiving a transfusion is unrelated to the patient's age, but varies with tumour type and stage.[11]

Red cells

Red cell transfusions are indicated to improve the delivery of oxygen to the tissues within a short period of time. There is no agreed haemo-globin threshold from which red cells should be transfused – this can range between 7 and 10 g/dl.[12] Patients with a pre-treatment haemaglo-bin of less than 11 g/dl are more likely to require a transfusion than those not anaemic prior to commencing chemotherapy.[11] It is important not to rely solely on haemoglobin levels as a trig-ger for transfusion, as individual patients with cancer will experience differing degrees of symp-toms relating to anaemia, including malaise, pal-lor and dyspnoea on exertion, or even at rest. Equally, other factors need to be taken into con-sideration. These include the patient's age, gen-eral health, co-morbidity (such as respiratory or cardiac disease) as well as the rate of fall of the haemoglobin concentration. Consideration of the patient's clinical condition is a vital part of the decision whether or not to transfuse red cells; this requires individual patient assessment. Involvement in such decisions is an integral part of the role of the oncology nurse. An important consideration when assessing the patient is that the side-effects of the patient's treatment and the malignancy itself can result in patients experienc-ing the same symptoms as that of anaemia.

The majority of red cells are supplied resus-pended in an additive solution (e.g. SAGM – saline, adenine, glucose and mannitol) in order to maintain the red cells in good condition dur-ing storage. The packed cell volume (PCV) is between 55 and 65%. One unit of red cells would expect to raise the haemoglobin by approximately 1 g/dl.[13] Once removed from an approved blood refrigerator, red cells should be transfused over a specified time period (varied by local policy) to prevent bacterial proliferation and potential transfusion-transmitted infection. All blood products transfused must be ABO and RhD compatible with the patient's own blood group, to minimize the risk of acute haemolytic reaction. The development of red cell antibodies in some patients following multiple blood trans-fusions requires the selection of blood units from donations that do not have the corresponding antigen present on the surface of the red cells.

Platelets

Platelet transfusions may be used prophylacti-cally to prevent bleeding in thrombocytopenic patients or therapeutically to arrest haemor-rhage.[5] In myelosuppressed patients, platelet transfusions may be required daily, and patients with infections or who are actively bleeding will also have a high demand for platelets. Platelets are stored at room temperature; they have a lim-ited life span following donation, due to the risk of bacterial proliferation during storage. A sin-gle unit of platelets would normally increase the platelet count by at least a value of $20 \times 10^9/L$. However, some patients will fail to gain benefit from platelet transfusions. This situation can be due to either immune (human leucocyte anti-gen (HLA) or human platelet antigen (HPA) antibodies, immune complexes) and/or non-immune causes (infection, splenomegaly, dis-seminated intravascular coagulation (DIC), bleeding) and occurs in more than 50% of patients receiving multiple platelet transfu-sions.[14] Refractory patients require platelets specifically selected to their HLA type if anti-bodies to HLA Class 1 antigens have been iden-tified. To effectively monitor the response from the transfusion of HLA-selected platelet units, the patient's platelet count should ideally be remeasured 1 hour following comple-tion of the transfusion. Platelet units must be stored on a platelet agitator, transfused over 20–30 minutes and should be ABO compatible with the patient's own blood group. ABO com-patibility is essential to minimize the risk of haemolysis caused by transfusion of levels of anti-A and/or anti-B antibody in the donor plasma, which may react with the patient's red cells.

Fresh frozen plasma

Fresh frozen plasma (FFP) transfusion is indi-cated to correct abnormal coagulation by replacing the patient's clotting factors in the presence of bleeding in situations such as:

- liver disease
- acute DIC
- following 'massive transfusion' (the replacement of a patient's total blood volume within 24 hours)
- plasma exchange for treatment of thrombotic thrombocytopenic purpura (TTP).

FFP is also used prophylactically prior to invasive procedures when there is significant risk of bleeding and laboratory investigations have indicated that the product is likely to correct the coagulopathy, although there is little evidence for the effectiveness of prophylactic use.[15] FFP is thawed in the laboratory and transfused over 30 minutes, at a dosage of 10–15 ml of plasma per kg of patient's body weight.[16] Cryoprecipitate is prepared from FFP and contains higher concentrations of the clotting factors factor VIII, fibrinogen and von Willebrand factor. This product is indicated when a patient has a low fibrinogen level (less than 1 g/L), or has congenital or acquired deficiencies in fibrinogen, factor VIII and factor XIII when single-factor concentrates are unavailable. As with platelet transfusions, FFP should be ABO compatible with the patient's own blood group.

Albumin

Human albumin solution (HAS) is derived from pooled human plasma and the main indications for transfusion include hypoproteinaemia, paracentesis of ascites and therapeutic plasma exchange for haematological conditions which result in hyperviscosity or require large-volume leucodepletion using a cell separator machine. Human albumin is suitable for all blood groups – cross-matching the product with the patient's own red cells is not required.

Immunoglobulins

Either 'normal' or 'specific' human immunoglobulin products can be used to protect susceptible immunosuppressed patients against infection, e.g. patients post bone marrow transplant. Normal human immunoglobulin, used in most cases, is prepared from blood donations and reflects the immune status of the general population. Specific human immunoglobulin is selected from donors who are known to have high antibody levels against a particular antigen (e.g. anti-D or anti-hepatitis B) and is used to treat at-risk patients who have been exposed to a particular antigen. Immunoglobulin can be transfused regardless of the patient's blood group.

Haematopoietic stem cells

As well as using blood products to support patients undergoing treatment for solid tumours, it is also possible (and indeed it is becoming increasingly more common) to offer the patient intensive regimens of chemotherapy and/or radiotherapy followed by 'rescue' with haematopoietic stem cells (HSC). However, for many patients suffering from haematological malignancies the use of HSC from self, sibling or unrelated donor is the treatment of choice but can lead to challenges relating to the provision of blood products. A clear example is the case of ABO-incompatible allogeneic haematopoietic stem cell transplantation (HSCT), which can increase transplant-associated complications.[17] Around 15–25% of HLA identical sibling donor/recipient pairs differ in ABO groups. This figure is higher in unrelated donor transplants. The incompatibility can be major or minor.

Major ABO incompatibility

The patient has antibodies to the donor cells. The presence of anti-A and/or anti-B in the patient's plasma can react with the donor's red cells, e.g. donor Group A, patient group O. Following transplant, the patient's ABO type red cells should be given until the patient's original ABO antibodies are no longer detected and donor ABO cells are present. From this time, donor type ABO red cells must be given. Donor ABO type platelets and plasma should be given from the day of transplantation.

Minor ABO incompatibility

The donor product has antibodies to the patient's cells. The presence of anti-A and/or anti-B in the donor's plasma can react with the patient's red cells, e.g. donor Group O, patient Group A. Following transplant, donor ABO type red cells should be given. Platelets and plasma of the patient's original ABO type should be given until the patient's original ABO antibodies are no longer detected. Thereafter, donor ABO type platelets and plasma should be given.

Major and minor ABO incompatibility

The presence of both patient and donor antibodies. Following transplant, Group O red cells should be used, until the patient's original

ABO antibodies are no longer detected. From this point on, donor ABO type red cells must be transfused. Group AB plasma and platelets must be given until the patient's ABO type cells are no longer detected; then donor platelets and plasma are given (for full review of nursing care see Ch. 16).

Special requirements

In certain cases, patients with cancer may require specially selected blood products, such as the following.

CMV-negative blood products

Cytomegalovirus (CMV) seronegative allogeneic transplant patients will require CMV-negative blood products to minimize the risk of a clinical CMV infection or reactivation of dormant disease when the patient becomes immunocompromised.

Gamma irradiation

Some patients with cancer – e.g. Hodgkin's disease patients, stem cell transplant patients or patients who have received purine analogue chemotherapy agents – are at risk of transfusion-associated graft versus host disease (TA GvHD) if blood products transfused to them are not irradiated.

HLA-selected platelets

Patients who have known HLA antibodies require HLA-selected platelets. Refer to local policy for specific indications.

ADMINISTRATION

The whole transfusion process of sampling, storage, collection, prescription administration, observation, management of adverse events, documentation and disposal should follow strict local policy, protocols and guidelines based upon evidence from national guidelines in order to minimize risk to the transfused patients. All staff involved in this process should have induction training and annual updates in order to make blood transfusion safer. Training and education form a major part of the emerging role of transfusion practitioners in clinical practice, disseminating evidence based on best practice across the multidisciplinary team.

Transfusion reactions

Although serious acute transfusion complications are rare, it is very important to be vigilant for signs and symptoms of a transfusion reaction. These usually present during the first 15 minutes of the transfusion. A patient with a severe reaction can deteriorate rapidly.

Acute complications of transfusion include:

- acute haemolytic reaction (incompatible red cells reacting with patients' anti-A and/or anti-B antibodies)
- bacterial contamination from blood product unit
- transfusion-related acute lung injury (TRALI) (antibodies in donor plasma reacting with patients' white cells)
- fluid overload
- severe allergic/anaphylactic reaction.

Clinical signs include:

- fever
- hypotension
- oozing from any wounds or puncture sites
- haemoglobinaemia (haemoglobin detected in the blood)
- haemoglobinuria (haemoglobin detected in the urine)
- fever is often due to a cause other than acute haemolysis.

Symptoms include:

- feeling of apprehension or 'something wrong'
- agitation
- flushing
- pain at venepuncture site
- pain experienced in chest, abdomen or flank/loin (lower back).

Management of acute transfusion reactions

Local protocols should be followed, but management should include the following actions:

1 If the only feature is a rise in temperature of less than 1.5°C from baseline or an urticarial (itchy) rash:

- Recheck that the correct blood is being transfused.
- Give prescribed antipyretics for fever.
- Give prescribed antihistamine for urticaria.
- Recommence the transfusion at a slower rate, following confirmation from medical staff.
- Observe more frequently than routine practice.

2 If severe acute reaction is suspected:

- Stop the transfusion – disconnect the transfusion line, including any connecting/extension lines, and maintain intravenous access with normal saline.
- Call a doctor urgently and record patient's temperature, blood pressure, pulse and respiratory rate.
- Check for respiratory signs – dyspnoea, tachypnoea, wheeze and cyanosis.
- Recheck the identity of patient against the blood unit and documentation.
- Notify blood bank
- Check blood gases or oxygen saturation, as indicated.
- Ensure further care and management is provided according to the patient's developing clinical features.

All suspected transfusion reactions should be reported as soon as possible to the transfusion laboratory as well as the medical team caring for the patient and events clearly recorded in the patient's nursing and medical records.

Transfusion-transmitted infection

The risk of transmission of viral infections such as hepatitis B, C, HIV, HTLV and CMV and bacterial infections such as syphilis via blood components is minimal. This is mainly due to developments in product testing and more stringent donor health screening. However, there are still risks associated with each blood product transfused. Precautionary measures to reduce the incidence of transmission of infection via blood components are in place in all countries. An example of such measures are those that have been taken in the UK to reduce the risk of transmission of variant Creutzfeldt–Jakob disease (vCJD). This involves the removal of white cells from all blood products, plus the extension of the exclusion criteria of blood donors and sources of plasma products from outside of the UK.[13] The educational role of the oncology nurse is vital in ensuring patients with cancer are aware of the risks and benefits associated with blood product supportive therapy.

Safety

Haemovigilance schemes such as the Serious Hazards of Transfusion 'SHOT' scheme in the UK operate to provide an analysis of serious transfusion complications. The scheme acts as an evidence base for blood safety initiatives, policies and guidelines by collecting confidential and anonymized data on adverse events, and publishing results in an annual report.[18] The most frequently reported incident category is 'incorrect blood component transfused', where a patient is transfused with a blood component or plasma product which did not meet the appropriate requirements or which was intended for another patient. Categories of reporting include non-infectious adverse events and transfusion-transmitted infections. Similar schemes operate in other countries. It is important that nursing staff report any adverse events to the medical team and assist the blood transfusion laboratory staff in investigating such events by effective interpersonal communication as well as by maintaining accurate and comprehensive documentation.

Patient information

Although written consent to receive a blood product transfusion (in the UK) is not currently a mandatory requirement, it is important that prior to commencing any transfusion every patient has access to information relating to the benefits, known risks and procedural aspects of the process. Equally, they are entitled to the opportunity to discuss appropriate alternatives to allogeneic transfusion with either nursing or medical staff. Patients who have special blood product requirements such as CMV-negative or irradiated cellular blood products need to be aware of these requirements, particularly when shared care is being delivered but also in case of an emergency situation. Systems and protocols must be present in all clinical departments, facilitating access to relevant patient and product information. These would avoid delays and prevent errors that may otherwise lead to patients receiving incorrect blood products.

SAFE ADMINISTRATION OF TREATMENT

The safe administration of treatment for the various aspects of bone marrow failure is essential to avoid unnecessary complications – all wards/units participating in such care should have up-to-date policies and guidelines based on current evidence.

Planning nursing care

There are two levels of nursing care required that relate to the administration of haematological support products:

- dealing with the patient at risk as a consequence of bone marrow suppression/failure
- caring for the patient receiving blood products and related treatments.

Caring for the patient at risk due to bone marrow suppression

Caring for the patient at risk due to bone marrow suppression and their family requires the nurse to demonstrate understanding of the patient's physical, psychological, social and spiritual needs. Primarily, these needs will be met through effective communication and adequate education of the family members, enabling them to understand the implications of symptoms such as breathlessness, coughing, pyrexia and bruising. Without such education, these symptoms may frighten both the patient and

their family, as they may misinterpret the symptoms as signs of the cancer returning/progressing. The reassurance of regular hospital/doctor appointments during 'at-risk' periods of treatment are an essential aspect of the patient's care. Patients also require guidance as to what action to take if signs and symptoms are present, such as a high fever, that give them a cause for concern. Patients should be advised by the nurse regarding infection risks (e.g. being in crowded spaces such as trains or cinemas during any period of risk) and should be educated to be vigilant to any problems arising. If they feel unwell or have a high temperature, patients should be advised to contact their centre straightaway, as early treatment can prevent further complications, which may become life-threatening. Any information given to patients must include contact details for a member of staff whom they know (usually the oncology nurse specialist), giving them direct access to the team in charge of the their clinical care. This enables the patient and family to feel secure in the knowledge that even at home they have access to those who are caring for them. Patients can then maintain a large element of control, enabling them to be actively involved in the decision-making process through open communication with the multidisciplinary team.

The nursing care of a patient receiving blood products

The nursing care of a patient receiving blood products requires the nurse to communicate effectively with both the patient and family, thus ensuring their peace of mind and that of the rest of the multidisciplinary team. An important issue relating to the care of the patient in need of haematological support is to ensure safe administration of any blood products (see Administration section). However, there are associated issues to be reflected upon, which are now considered.

Infection control

Patients requiring support with blood products will often have a generalized reduction in cell counts (pancytopaenia) and, as such, be at risk of infection. If they are neutropenic (neutrophil count less than 1×10^9/L), supportive strategies include minimizing the length of neutropenia through the use of growth factors and protective isolation nursing. There is a growing body of evidence to suggest that optimal hygiene on the part of the patient, their relatives and the multidisciplinary team in conjunction with the use of alcohol hand rub has made such practices outmoded.[19] Regardless of the presence or absence of neutropenia, any nurse using an intravenous access device to administer blood products is putting a patient at potential risk of septicaemia. Therefore, it is essential that all nurses are trained in aseptic intravenous access technique, and that a local policy is in place to maintain good practice. Equally, it is essential for nurses to be able to recognize the signs and symptoms of acute neutropenic septicaemia (pyrexia, rigors, hypotension, tachycardia) in case, despite appropriate precautions, infection does occur.

Fluid balance

It is important to be aware that a patient requiring large amounts of blood products is at risk of fluid overload. This risk can be minimized by the use of, for example, packed cells rather than whole blood, and administering prescribed diuretics. However, it is still vital for the nurse to monitor and record a patient's fluid input and output and be aware of any concurrent risk factors such as renal dysfunction, cardiac complications and breathlessness due to pericardial effusion or ascites.

Psychological support

As with all physical symptoms relating to care of the patient with cancer, there is a large element of psychological care required. The oncology nurse has a duty to make certain that each patient has an understanding of the symptoms associated with bone marrow suppression and appropriate actions to take. Reassurance may be required to reinforce patient understanding that symptoms such as breathlessness or fatigue may be a result of anaemia – especially if anaemia was also a presenting symptom at diagnosis. The consequences of bone marrow suppression may result in a change of role for the patient, possibly causing disruption to the family unit. Assisting the family to adjust to such changes is the responsibility of the oncology nurse. A patient with cancer may require support in coming to terms with changes in body image, for example due to pallor, presence of a central line or excessive bruising.

ETHICAL ISSUES

Ethical dilemmas present themselves in all aspects of nursing, and provide thought-provoking issues for consideration; the delivery of haematological support is no exception. Ethical challenges can arise for a wide variety of reasons. If, for example, a patient is taken unconscious to an emergency department and a blood transfusion is urgently required to save the patient's life, doctors have the right to provide such treatment without the patient's consent unless the patient has a card (or other identifying item) stating the patient's wishes or beliefs. In the case of an infant requiring a blood transfusion, the medical profession usually accepts that a parent is entitled, on behalf of the infant, to consent or reject treatment in the infant's best interests. However, where doctors and parents disagree, it can be left up to the court to decide.

For some patients, religious and personal beliefs lead them to be reluctant to receive blood transfusions that would otherwise be given to support the effects of their cancer treatment. This stance may be held despite the possible negative impact on survival and/or recovery. All patients have a right to be treated with respect to their wishes, and staff must be sensitive to their individual values, beliefs and cultural needs.

Examples where conflicting beliefs should be considered include:

- Jehovah's Witnesses, who seek alternatives to certain blood transfusions as they strongly believe that a human must not sustain his or her life with another person's blood, knowingly accepting a blood transfusion damages their relationship with God.
- Animal-rights campaigners may refuse a treatment if it has been tested on animals. Many drug and treatment research

411

primarily involves animals before proceeding to human trials. Some products themselves are animal-derived, e.g. antilymphocyte and antithymocyte globulins, which are often used as a treatment to induce immunosuppression prior to bone marrow transplantation.

As discussed above, the effects of chemotherapy and radiotherapy cause severe disruption to the bone marrow and immunity of a patient with cancer. If a patient declines haematological support, then their physician is obliged to tailor the treatment prescribed significantly to reduce any myelosuppressive side-effects despite this being a potentially less-effective means of treating their disease. It is important as an oncology nurse to be aware of a patient's views and encourage them to make these beliefs known. It is also essential that patients thinking of declining blood product support be given the opportunity to discuss their feelings with their doctor in order to reach an autonomous and informed decision. A conflict of opinion concerning the nature of treatment may pose ethical problems, as discussed above. Consequently oncology nurses may experience a conflict of interest between their obligation to act as advocates for the patient and family when these interests differ from that of the oncology team.[20]

NEW APPROACHES TO HAEMATOLOGICAL SUPPORT

As discussed in the Blood Product Support section, for a small proportion of patients, difficulties may be faced in providing optimal blood product support due to the development of red cell, HLA and/or platelet antibodies directed against cell-specific antigens. Antibodies can occur following multiple transfusions and/or pregnancy in females that can cause immunological reactions in patients unless specifically selected products are transfused.

In some circumstances, other treatments are available for use instead of blood product transfusions. These are now considered.

Erythropoietin

Treatment-induced anaemia is widespread. It is an under-recognized and undertreated problem in patients with cancer, especially those receiving platinum-based chemotherapy, which appears to increase the incidence of anaemia.[21] Erythropoietin (EPO) is a type of protein that occurs naturally in the body and stimulates the bone marrow to produce erythrocytes. Anaemia can be a poor prognostic factor in several cancer settings, such as in head and neck and cervical cancers; it can affect a patient's quality of life significantly as well as impacting on the patient's compliance and ability to tolerate treatment. Erythropoietic agents have been shown to be well tolerated and highly effective in correcting the anaemia associated with cancer.[22] Such agents are usually given as a subcutaneous injection. Although they can be administered intravenously, subcutaneous is the preferred route through injections two to three times weekly. Iron stores within the body are critical in maintaining the EPO uptake, and parenteral iron can be given to increase this response. The UK's National Institute for Clinical Excellence (NICE) is currently reviewing the evidence surrounding the use of EPO in patients with cancer.[23]

Haematopoietic growth factors

Due to immunosuppression from cancer treatments, infections can be a significant life-threatening risk; therefore, neutropenic support and monitoring of patients' vital signs and clinical assessment is essential. Prolonged neutropenia can delay further treatments and may significantly change a treatment plan. Febrile neutropenia is a frequent event for patients with cancer undergoing chemotherapy and can lead to potentially life-threatening situations. Haematopoietic growth factors, such as granulocyte colony-stimulating factor (GCSF), are available to increase the speed of neutrophil recovery, thus reducing the length of neutropenia and its associated risks of sepsis. Colony-stimulating factors (CSFs) are cytokines that stimulate and accelerate the production of one or more cellular lines in bone marrow;[24] they are given by a daily subcutaneous injection. A number of patients may experience side-effects from these injections such as flu-like symptoms or bony pain, some of which can be relieved with simple analgesia. A meta-analytical study revealed that CSFs in patients with febrile neutropenia due to cancer chemotherapy do not affect the overall mortality but reduce the length of hospital admissions and neutrophil recovery period.

Donor granulocytes

Infusing granulocytes is an effective way of treating and speeding the recovery from severe bacterial or fungal infections, which are often caused through prolonged neutropenia.[25] Granulocytes are white cells that have been collected from volunteer donors. These are prepared by pooling white cells from units of donated whole blood. However, due to the small amount of circulating granulocytes in a healthy individual, several units (10–20) of whole blood would need to be centrifuged to collect sufficient levels of granulocytes for optimal results. Using multiple products from different donors, however, has the potential to cause problems with the development of antibodies. The most effective method of collecting granulocytes is to stimulate and harvest from a single, healthy volunteer donor. However, this has risks to the donor, as it requires an injection of GCSF and a small dose of steroid (dexamethasone) 12 hours prior to collection. The premedication is necessary to boost the granulocyte population into the peripheral circulation, where they are then collected by apheresis (cell separation). As with whole blood donation, it is essential to select ABO-compatible donors and ensure serological tests are negative. Cross-matching of donor and recipient blood compatibility is required and all granulocytes require gamma irradiation prior to transfusion to prevent TA GvHD. Some reactions commonly occur with granulocyte transfusions. These include mild to moderate fever with minor arterial oxygen desaturation, which may require slowing of the transfusion, antipyretics, antihistamines and steroids.[26] More severe reactions are less common but include hypotension, pulmonary infiltration and respiratory distress.

Coagulation factors

Other haematological complications, such as clotting abnormalities, can occur as a result of cancer treatments and sometimes the disease itself. Clotting abnormalities can often be corrected by agents such as FFP or medications such as vitamin K. In recent clinical trials, researchers have looked at the effectiveness of recombinant factor VIIa, and reported that it can be administered to manage bleeding and correct clotting abnormalities in patients with thrombocytopenia caused by impaired platelet production or bone marrow suppression.[27]

Community care

Recently, there has been a vast increase in the number of patients being treated, where possible, in their own homes. Training nurses to administer and monitor blood transfusions and other specialist treatments such as chemotherapy and intravenous antibiotics in the community has led to an improvement in resources and improved quality of life for patients.[28,29]

CONCLUSION

Patients with cancer require haematological support as a result of the malignant disease process and associated treatment options, particularly if chemotherapy is the treatment of choice. The oncology nurse plays a vital role in ensuring that patients receive safe and competent care throughout their cancer journey. The provision of appropriate haematological support through the safe use of blood products and alternative strategies is an integral part of that role. It is imperative that all nurses working and patients undergoing treatment for cancer are aware of local policies and guidelines relating to the provision of haematological support. Nurses should be aware of patients' beliefs in relation to blood product support, be vigilant in the monitoring of patients receiving blood product transfusion and conscientious in educating the patients and families with regard to the side-effects of cancer treatment.

REFERENCES

1. Howell S, Demetri GD, Crawford J. Haematopoietic growth factors. In: Pazdur R, Coia LR, Hoskins WJ, Wagman LD, eds. Cancer management: a multidisciplinary approach. Newyork: CMP; 2004, pp. 883-898.

2. Hoffbrand AV, Pettit JE, Moss PAH. Essential haematology. 4th edn. London: Mosby. 2001.

3. Taylor C. Transfusion triggers in medical patients with chronic anaemia. In: Thomas D, Thompson J, Ridler B, eds. A manual for blood conservation. Harley: TFM; 2005:181.

4. Roitt I, Brostoff J, Male D. Immunology. 6th edn. Edinburgh: Mosby; 2001.

5. British Committee for Standards in Haematology, Blood Transfusion Task Force. Guidelines for the use of platelet transfusions. Br J Haematol 2003; 122:10-23.

6. Dunleavy R. Bone marrow suppression: infection and bleeding. In: Corner J, Bailey C, eds. Cancer nursing, care in context. Oxford: Blackwell; 2001.

7. Kirkova J, Fainsinger RL. Thrombosis and anticoagulation in palliative care: an evolving challenge. J Palliat Care 2004; 20(2):101-104.

8. De Cicco M. The prothrombic state of cancer: pathogenic mechanisms. Crit Rev Oncol Haematol 2004; 50:187-196.

9. Viale PH, Schwartz RN. Venous thromboembolism in patients with cancer, part I: survey of oncology nurses' attitudes and treatment practices for ambulatory settings. Clin J Oncol Nurs 2004; 8(5):455-461.

10. Van-Gerpen R, Mast ME. Thromboembolic disorders in cancer. Clin J Oncol Nurs 2004; 8(3):289-299.

11. Barrett-Lee PJ, Bailey NP, O'Brien MER, Wager E. Large-scale UK audit of blood transfusion requirements and anaemia in patients receiving cytotoxic chemotherapy. Br J Cancer 2000; 82(1):93-97.

12. British Committee for Standards in Haematology, Blood Transfusion Task Force. Guidelines for the clinical use of red cell transfusions. Br J Haematol 2001; 113:24-31.

13. McClelland DBL, ed. Handbook of transfusion medicine. Blood transfusion services of the United Kingdom. 3rd edn. Norwich: HMSO; 2001.

14. Murphy M, Pamphilon DH, eds. Practical transfusion medicine. Oxford: Blackwell Science; 2001.

15. Stanworth SJ, Brunskill SJ, Hyde CJ, McLelland DBL, Murphy MF. Is fresh frozen plasma clinically effective? A systematic review of randomised controlled trials. Br J Haematol 2004; 126:139-152.

16. British Committee for Standards in Haematology, Blood Transfusion Task Force. Guidelines for the use of fresh-frozen plasma, cryoprecipitate and cryosupernatant. Br J Haematol 2004; 126:11-28.

17. Worel N, Kalhs P, Keil F, et al. ABO mismatch increases transplant-related morbidity and mortality in patients given nonmyeloablative allogeneic HPC transplantation. Transfusion 2003; 43:1153-1161.

18. Stainsby D, Cohen H, Jones H, et al. Serious Hazards of Transfusion (SHOT). Annual report 2003. Manchester: Serious Hazards of Transfusion Steering Group; 2004.

19. Mank A, Van der Lelie H. Is there still an indication for nursing patients with prolonged neutropenia in protective isolation? An evidence-based nursing and medical study of 4 years experience for nursing patients without isolation. Eu J Oncol Nurs 2003; 7:17-23.

20. Gates B. Advocacy; a nurses' guide. London: Scutari Press; 1994.

21. Atterbury C, Howell C. Haematology & Bone Marrow Transplantation News. Royal College of Nursing Haematology and Bone Marrow Transplant Forum. Newsletter Winter 2004/2005.

22. Smith RE. Erythropoietin agents in the management of cancer patients. Anaemia, quality of life and possible effects on survival. J Support Oncol 2003; 1(4):249-256.

23. NICE guidelines for anaemia (cancer treatment induced), erythropoietin and darbepoetin. Pending, for issue: Dec. 2005. Website: www.nice.org.uk

24. Clark OAC, Lyman G, Castro AA, Clark LGO, Djulbegovic B. Colony stimulating factor for chemotherapy induced febrile neutropenia. Chichester: Wiley; The Cochrane Library; 2005. issue 2.

25. Hubel K, Carter RA, Conrad Liles W, et al. Granulocyte transfusion therapy for infections in candidates and recipients of HPC transplantation: a comparative analysis of feasibility and outcome for community donors versus related donors. Transfusion 2002; 42:1414-1421.

26. Price TH, Bowden RA, Boeckh M, et al. Phase I/II trial of neutrophil transfusions from donors stimulated with G-CSF and dexamethasone for treatment of patients with infections in haematopoietic stem cell transplantation. Blood 2000; 95:3302-3309.

27. Kristensen J, Killander A, Hippe E. Clinical experience with recombinant factor VIIa in patients with thrombocytopenia. Haemostasis 1996; 26(Suppl 1):159-164.

28. Craig JIO, Milligan P, Cairns J, McClelland DBL, Parker AC. (1999) Nurse practitioner support for transfusion in patients with haematological disorders in hospital and at home. Transfusion Med 1999; 9:31-36.

29. Green J, Pirie L. Framework for the safe delivery of a blood transfusion service in the community setting (draft 7). English National Blood Transfusion Committee.

CHAPTER 20

Nausea and Vomiting

ALEXANDER MOLASSIOTIS AND SUSSANNE BÖRJESON

CHAPTER CONTENTS

Introduction	415	Anticipatory nausea and vomiting	423
Significance of nausea and vomiting	415	Nausea and vomiting in advanced cancer	424
Definitions	416	Assessment of nausea and vomiting	424
Mechanisms of nausea and vomiting	417	Management of nausea and vomiting	425
Chemotherapy-related nausea and vomiting	419	Pharmacological treatment	425
Factors associated with chemotherapy-related nausea and vomiting	421	Psychoeducational and behavioural techniques	428
		Diet	430
Nausea and vomiting after radiation therapy	422	Complementary and alternative therapies	431
Nausea and vomiting after surgery	423	Effects of nausea and vomiting on quality of life	431
Nausea and vomiting after biological therapies	423	Conclusion	432
		References	432

INTRODUCTION

Treatment or disease-induced nausea and vomiting remain a major problem in patients with cancer. This chapter will discuss how nausea and vomiting develop, associated factors, different types of nausea and vomiting (i.e. acute, delayed or anticipatory nausea and vomiting) and issues related to assessment and measurement. Pharmacological and non-pharmacological management will be presented in detail, with special focus on the management of treatment failures, as well as development and use of evidence-based antiemetic guidelines. Finally, the effects of nausea and vomiting on patients' quality of life will be summarized.

SIGNIFICANCE OF NAUSEA AND VOMITING

As early as 1983 it was shown that the possibility of experiencing treatment-related nausea and vomiting was considered to be one of the most important and dreaded side effects for patients.[1] The most important and severe side effect reported was 'being sick' (vomiting) followed by 'feeling sick' (nausea).[1] This perception has persisted over the last 20 years,[2-5] even though new antiemetics have been introduced in the management of nausea and vomiting. The more recent studies looking at the effects of nausea and vomiting on quality of life of patients with cancer clearly demonstrate that a range of social, work-related and daily activity-related domains of health-related quality of life are significantly affected.[6-8] Also, uncontrolled nausea and vomiting can have major physiological effects, including:

- fluid and electrolyte imbalance
- dehydration
- anorexia, weight loss or aversion to foods (see Ch. 29)
- decreased absorption or renal elimination of medication.[9-11]

Because of the severity of these two symptoms, lower doses of chemotherapy may be used or some patients may decide not to complete their chemotherapy course, decreasing their chances of survival.[6,12] Ten years after the early study by Coates et al,[1] nausea remained one of the most distressing symptoms for patients with cancer. Vomiting, which in 1983 was the most important side effect, ranked fifth in 1993.[5] The latter study shows that, although improvements in antiemetic medications and treatment protocols may have decreased the severity of vomiting, it may have increased the severity of nausea. This is further confirmed in a recent study, where it was shown that, although the duration of vomiting was reduced in a sample of 1413 patients treated in the community, the duration of nausea was increased.[13]

DEFINITIONS

Nausea, vomiting and retching are discrete symptoms that must be clearly defined and understood in order to accurately assess and measure these separate concepts.[14] Misunderstanding over terms may lead to confusion and, subsequently, poor management. The term 'emesis' has been used for collectively describing both vomiting and retching[15] or all three symptoms (nausea, vomiting, retching):[16]

- *Nausea* is a subjective, unobservable phenomenon of an unpleasant sensation often associated with a feeling that vomiting is imminent.[17] It is often associated with unpleasant sensations experienced in the back of the throat and the epigastrium and can be described as 'feeling sick at stomach'.[14] Nausea can be accompanied by autonomic nervous system activity such as pupil dilatation, cutaneous vasoconstriction, sweating and salivation, as well as tachycardia and gastric relaxation.[18]

- *Vomiting* is the forceful expulsion of the contents of the stomach through the oral or nasal cavity and can, in contrast to nausea, be objectively measured and can be described as 'throwing up'.[14,19]

- *Retching* is the attempt to vomit without bringing anything up and can be measured both subjectively and objectively.[19] According to Rhodes et al, it may be described by terms such as 'dry heaves', 'gagging' or 'attempting to vomit without results'.[14]

Chemotherapy-induced nausea and vomiting (CINV) is further classified into three phases of time related to chemotherapy administration: acute, delayed and anticipatory nausea and vomiting. Further, two types of nausea and vomiting related to the treatment of the symptoms are described – breakthrough and refractory nausea and vomiting.

- *Acute CINV* occurs within the first 24 hours following chemotherapy administration. The symptoms generally begin 1–2 hours following most chemotherapy administration but exceptions exist, e.g. cyclophosphamide and carboplatin.[20,21]

- *Delayed CINV* is defined as symptoms beginning after the day of chemotherapy treatment. The timing of the actual start of delayed CINV is poorly documented and may differ depending on the chemotherapy. Recent studies indicate that it may begin 16–24 hours after drug administration.[22] For most patients, delayed symptoms disappear within the first week after chemotherapy.

- *Anticipatory CINV* is also referred to as conditioned, learned or psychological nausea and vomiting and these symptoms only occur if the patient previously has experienced acute and/or delayed

CINV.[23] Anticipatory CINV is characterized by the patient experiencing nausea and/or vomiting prior to administration of chemotherapy or at any time when the patient thinks of aspects related to the experience of nausea and vomiting.[24] Anticipatory CINV tends to increase with the number of cycles received [25] and the symptoms may persist for a long time after the completion of chemotherapy.[26]

- *Breakthrough CINV* is nausea and vomiting that occurs despite optimal preventative therapy, in either the acute or the delayed phase.[27]

- *Refractory CINV* is defined as failure to respond to prevention and/or intervention in the previous cycle of treatment.[27]

MECHANISMS OF NAUSEA AND VOMITING

Patients with cancer can experience nausea, vomiting and retching for a wide variety of reasons,[28,29] the most common being chemotherapy. The feature that the different reasons have in common is that they are all able to activate the emetic reflex, one of the body's mechanisms, which protects against accidental ingestion of toxins in rather the same way that the cough reflex protects the airways.[28] The emetic reflex in humans provides a mechanism for the removal of poisons from the body. Nausea gives an early indication of the presence of a toxin, and, along with vomiting, provides a conditioning stimulus for the development of an aversion to future exposure to the same stimulus. In essence, the food already ingested is ejected and the learned aversion limits further consumption of the toxic agent.[28] In the context of ingestion of contaminated food, these responses are 'appropriate' and lead to expulsion of the toxin. However, when activated by a therapeutic agent such as chemotherapy, the response is clearly 'inappropriate', since the toxin is in the circulation and vomiting thus has little effect on removing it from the body. In addition, the aversion

induced may give rise to anticipatory nausea and vomiting and fear or avoidance of further treatment.[17]

To trigger nausea and vomiting, all that is required is that the causative factor, such as a cytotoxic drug or radiation (which can be regarded as 'cellular poisons'), access and activate one or more of the systems that are presumed to have evolved for the detection of toxins in the food. By considering the parallels between nausea and vomiting induced in the 'natural' as opposed to the 'clinical' environment, it becomes apparent that the best way of preventing the symptoms is to prevent the initial activation of the emetic inputs. In addition, optimal antiemetic therapy should be given at the first course of treatment and not be reserved for 'failures' because of the increased probability of inducing anticipatory nausea and vomiting and possible avoidance of further therapy.[17]

The mechanism by which chemotherapy induces nausea and vomiting is complex and still not completely understood. Mechanisms for acute CINV are different than the mechanisms for delayed or anticipatory CINV. Further, the mechanism associated with one chemotherapy agent may be different to that of another. Additionally, the dose or schedule of one drug may be affected by another drug. The impact of combining anticancer strategies such as chemotherapy and radiotherapy or biotherapy may also influence the profile of the patient's nausea and vomiting. This complexity helps us to understand why there is no one antiemetic regimen that is effective all of the time or in all settings.

Our understanding of the emetic mechanisms has mainly derived from animal experiments, pioneered by Borison and Wang over 50 years ago.[30,31] They made a distinction between the 'vomiting centre' in the reticular formation of the medulla in the hindbrain, which coordinates the forces required for emesis to occur, and the emetic detection sites, which give input to the vomiting centre to trigger the emetic reflex. The current view is that there is unlikely to be a single anatomical site that could be called the vomiting centre. Instead, it has been suggested that the vomiting centre is a neural network receiving information from various sites and coordinating the emetic response.[17] Sources of emetic inputs to the vomiting centre include the abdominal viscera, heart, vestibular system, area postrema and higher brain centres.[32]

All of the afferent inputs received by the vomiting centre are controlled by neurotransmitters and their receptors, e.g. dopamine, acetylcholine, histamine and serotonin.[33] The inputs most likely involved in triggering the emetic response to cytotoxic drugs and radiotherapy come primarily from the area postrema (popularly referred to as the chemoreceptor trigger zone for emesis) and abdominal vagal afferents.[34] The mechanism by which chemotherapy stimulates nausea and vomiting was only partially understood until it was identified that the antiemetic effect of metoclopramide was not through blockade of dopamine receptor but instead due to blockade of serotonin type 3 ($5\text{-}HT_3$) receptors.[35] Serotonin is found in high concentrations within the enterochromaffin cells in the gut as well as in the CNS and platelets. $5\text{-}HT_3$ receptors are widely distributed both in peripheral tissue and in the region of area postrema where vagal afferents enter the brain. It is hypothesized that chemotherapy and radiation cause release of serotonin from enterochromaffin cells in the gut, which then activates the abdominal vagal afferents.[33] Furthermore, the vomiting centre coordinates autonomic and somatic reactions, leading to nausea and vomiting.

Comprehensive reviews of the area of mechanisms for nausea and vomiting are available.[17,34] The above is a simplified summary of a very complicated system, parts of which are unknown. Even if the release of $5\text{-}HT_3$ seems to be the major cause of acute nausea and vomiting in patients receiving chemotherapy, a number of other sources, acting through different mechanisms may also result in the symptoms in patients with cancer.

The above model refers to acute nausea and vomiting. Less is known about the mechanisms underlying the delayed symptoms.[36,37] In a recent review article, Roila et al[38] describe some of the postulated underlying mechanisms:

1 Disruption of the blood–brain barrier: antineoplastic agents, especially cisplatin, can disrupt the blood–brain barrier, determining a mild and reversible cerebral oedema. The increased intracranial pressure may potentiate other emetic inputs. The documented activity of corticosteroids in the treatment of cerebral oedema and delayed nausea and vomiting give some support to this hypothesis.

2 Disruption of gastrointestinal motility and/or permeability: chemotherapy agents, in particular cisplatin, can cause temporary disturbances in the gastrointestinal tract function, such as hypomotility and gastroparesis that are capable of inducing protracted nausea and vomiting. The cytotoxic effect of drugs such as cisplatin can stimulate the release of hormones, many of which can induce emesis.[39,40]

3 Role of endogenous or exogenous adrenal hormones: corticosteroids and noradrenaline (norepinephrine) may play a role in delayed nausea and vomiting. Urinary cortisol and noradrenaline excretion have been shown to be related to the intensity of delayed nausea. The anti-inflammatory properties of cortisol may act as an antiemetic by preventing the release of serotonin in the gut or preventing the activation of $5\text{-}HT_3$ receptors in the gastrointestinal system. Noradrenaline may promote the release of serotonin in the gut or affect the sensitivity of $5\text{-}HT_3$ receptors.[41,42] Abrupt discontinuation of corticosteroid treatment can bring about adrenal failure, leading to delayed nausea and vomiting.[43]

4 Accumulation of emetogenic metabolites from chemotherapy agents: such as those of cisplatin, which have been identified in the body fluid and tissues over 24 hours after its administration.

The authors concluded that delayed nausea and vomiting is a multifactorial phenomenon with relative contributions from each of the above factors or others not yet determined. Delayed nausea and vomiting have been studied mainly in patients treated with cisplatin. Since the incidence and characteristics of the symptoms differ between patients receiving cisplatin-based chemotherapy and those receiving moderately emetogenic chemotherapy, different mechanisms may be involved.[38] This has been highlighted in a study investigating methotrexate-induced emesis in dogs, where the authors found a probable involvement of serotonin as an agonist for a $5\text{-}HT_4$ receptor in the induction of delayed nausea and vomiting.[44]

Recently, basic and clinical research has focused on a new type of antiemetic, the neurokinin type 1 (or NK_1) receptor antagonists. These new agents block substance P, a neuropeptide that affects this receptor.[37] Substance P is found within the central and peripheral nervous system and is known to be involved in a number of inflammatory and pain settings. Studies indicate that substance P induces vomiting in ferrets, and that agents which block NK_1 receptors are potent antiemetics for a wide variety of emetic stimuli in animal models.[34] A limited number of studies have been performed showing effect mainly for delayed nausea and vomiting[45–48] but the NK_1 receptors may also provide additional benefit in the prevention of acute symptoms when combined with a $5\text{-}HT_3$ receptor antagonist and a corticosteroid.[48] This would imply that the NK_1 receptors represent a valuable new approach and novel mechanism of action for the prevention of nausea and vomiting.

Therapeutic irradiation to any part of the body has the potential to cause nausea and vomiting. However, symptoms occur most commonly when radiation fields include the gastrointestinal (GI) tract (especially the upper abdomen) or brain or when total body irradiation is administered.[49,50] Like chemotherapy-induced nausea and vomiting, the exact mechanism by which irradiation induces nausea and vomiting is not known. Since drugs that block the actions of dopamine and serotonin can attenuate nausea and vomiting following radiotherapy, it has been suggested that irradiation leads to the release of neurotransmitters including dopamine and serotonin somewhere in the body, which in turn initiates the emetic reflex.[51] Hypothetically, two different mechanisms have been postulated: either a passive cell damage mechanism which could release transmitters that induce nausea and vomiting or an active functional defence mechanism through release of mediators by functioning cells. These two possible mechanisms may work together in the induction of nausea and vomiting. The passive cell damage mechanism has been supported by the fact that it seems to be a release of free radicals immediately after irradiation, which may release histamines and other transmitters. Further, damage of the enterochromaffin cells of the GI mucosa by irradiation seems to release serotonin, which initiates the emetogenic response in the same way as for chemotherapy-induced nausea and vomiting.[49]

Anticipatory nausea and vomiting usually develops as a result of psychological processes. Although a physiological involvement may exist (i.e. GI cancer involvement), the most prominent explanations around the development of anticipatory nausea and vomiting are psychological in nature. These may range from a psychodynamic conceptualization, coping model, the influence of anxiety, to a learning paradigm involving classical conditioning.[52–54]. The latter seems to be the most widely accepted explanation based on circumstantial evidence, although such conclusions derive from studies with low methodological quality. The fact that anticipatory nausea and vomiting respond well to behavioural treatments is another indication of the psychological processes behind their development.

CHEMOTHERAPY-RELATED NAUSEA AND VOMITING

Most chemotherapy agents will produce nausea and vomiting, although their emetogenic profile may vary, depending on a combination of factors as explained later in the chapter. As many as 76–88% or more of patients receiving chemotherapy may develop acute nausea.[55,56] Further, in a group of 522 patients receiving ondansetron and 4 different doses of dexamethasone as antiemetic prophylaxis, it was reported that despite best prophylaxis 57.1% of patients experienced delayed nausea and 37.4% delayed vomiting.[36] Patients also feel that nausea and vomiting are not well-managed or controlled, as shown in a large multicentre UK study, where only 13.2% of the patients (n = 281) felt these symptoms were well-managed.[57] Nausea and vomiting, especially the delayed phase, is less prevalent in children than in adults.[58]

Commonly, the emetogenic potential of different chemotherapeutic agents is categorized into:

- highly emetogenic agents, carrying the risk of acute and delayed vomiting (>90%)
- moderately emetogenic agents, carrying significant acute vomiting risk (30–90%) but a lower risk for delayed vomiting
- low emetogenicity, carrying low risk for acute vomiting (10–30%)
- minimal or no risk for delayed vomiting, and minimal emetogenicity, which includes chemotherapy that carries minimal (<10%) risk for acute and delayed vomiting or none at all[59] (Box 20.1).

Box 20.1

Emetogenic potential of chemotherapy

High (>90%)
Cisplatin
Carmustine (>250 mg/m^2)
Cyclophosphamide (>1500 mg/m^2)
Dacarbazine (>500 mg/m^2)
Dactinomycin
Lomustine (>60 mg/m^2)
Mechlorethamine
Pentostatin
Streptozocin

Moderate (30–90%)
Carboplatin
Carmustine (<250 mg/m^2)
Cisplatin (<50 mg/m^2)
Cyclophosphamide (<1500 mg/m^2)
Cyclophosphamide (oral)[a]
Cytarabine (>1 g/m^2)
Daunorubicin
Doxorubicin
Epirubicin[a]
Hexamethylamine (oral)[ab]
Idarubicin[a]
Ifosfamide[a]
Imitinib (oral)
Irinotecan[a]
Melphalan
Mitoxantrone (>12 mg/m^2)

Box 20.1

Oxaliplatin
Procarbazine (oral)[b]
Temozolomide (oral)
Vinorelbine (oral)

Low (10–30%)
Aldesleukin (IL-2)
Asparaginase
Bortezomib
Cetuximab
Cytarabine (<1 g/m^2)
Docetaxel
Doxorubicin (<20 mg/m^2)
Etoposide (oral)
Fluorouracil (<1000 mg/m^2)
Gemcitabine
Methotrexate (>100 mg/m^2)
Mitomycin
Mitoxantrone (<12 mg/m^2)
Paclitaxel
Temozolomide
Thiotepa
Topotecan
Emetogenic potential of chemotherapy

Minimal (<10%)
Bevacizumab
Bleomycin
Busulfan
Capecitabine[c]
Chlorambucil
2-Chlorodeoxyadenosine
Etoposide/teniposide (i.v.)
Methotrexate (<100 mg/m^2)
Fludarabine
Gefitinib (oral)
Hydroxyurea
L-phenylalanine mustard
Rituximab
Trastuzumab[c]
Vincristine
Vinblastine
Vinorelbine (i.v.)

Source: Drug names used are generic: reproduced from Koeller et al[59] and Antiemetic guidelines.[62]
[a]30–60% risk of emesis in Hesketh et al.[63]
[b]High emetic potential in Koeller et al.[59]
[c]Low emetic potential in Koeller et al.[59]

A number of other classifications of the emetic potential of chemotherapy agents do exist,[16,60–64] but they are all opinion-based rather than evidence-based classifications. Better differentiation of risk of acute emesis is necessary, as some aspects are debatable and they may add to the existing confusion clinicians are already in, as discussed in an editorial by Roila.[65]

In relation to classification systems of emetic risk, it is important to consider that these are dose-related and higher-than-standard doses of most chemotherapy agents should be classified in the next higher level.[11] As expected, classification systems differ, as they are based mostly on opinions;[65] e.g. nurses tend to rate most chemotherapeutic agents as more emetogenic than the doctors.[11] Furthermore, as it is more common to use combination chemotherapy nowadays, two or more agents given together will have much higher emetic risk than that classified as single agents, making the utilization of such guidelines in practice difficult.[65]

Factors associated with chemotherapy-related nausea and vomiting

It is important to be able to assess individual factors contributing to nausea and vomiting development, as patients at risk can be identified and treated with more aggressive or tailor-made interventions. A large number of factors contribute to the development of nausea and vomiting – some physiological, some psychological, some personality and some individual in nature. Researchers/clinicians interested in the management of nausea and vomiting have typically followed a single-model approach. However, in order to produce better outcomes, a multidimensional approach to nausea and vomiting may be more appropriate. For example, using a behavioural technique (acting on psychological level and partially on physical arousal) in combination with antiemetics (acting on a physiological level/neurotransmitter pathways), nausea and vomiting may be decreased by as much as half or more.[66] Indeed, Morrow et al[18] discuss such a need to merge views, and they present a biobehavioural model of explanation for nausea and vomiting, reviewing some of the key findings in the area from the past 20 or so years. In this model, patient expectation, individual characteristics and the emetogenicity of chemotherapy affect the hypothalamic–pituitary–adrenal axis and the autonomic nervous system, producing the different types of nausea and vomiting (anticipatory, acute, delayed emesis).

Patient expectations of developing nausea after treatment are consistently shown to be associated with post-treatment nausea in a number of studies,[13,67–69] although studies that report no such relationship do exist.[70,71] Results about expectations of vomiting are, however, less consistent. Other psychological constructs such as anxiety[67,71–74] and 'conditioning effects'[53] are well-known causative factors for nausea and vomiting, and expectations may be influencing the development of anxiety rather than directly linked with nausea and vomiting, but the correlational data presented in the literature leave little room for clear causative explanations. A number of other factors have been identified as potentially or partly responsible for nausea and vomiting development, including:

- younger age[67,75] (<50 years old or <40 years old in some studies)
- female gender[6,76]
- susceptibility to nausea when eating certain foods[72]
- taste of drugs during the infusion of chemotherapy[73]
- desire for control and choice of antiemetics[77]
- low alcohol use[6]
- psychological status and stress[78]
- labyrinthitis/vestibular dysfunction[67]
- susceptibility to motion sickness.[75,79,80]

In a study of 306 patients receiving cisplatin, it was shown that stressed patients were twice as likely to develop nausea or retching compared to those without stress indicators, whereas patients less than 40 years old were almost 3 times more likely to experience retching compared to older patients.[78] Furthermore, one of the strongest predictors of delayed nausea and vomiting is acute nausea and vomiting.[50,67] All these characteristics, in different combinations, which vary from individual to individual, explain part of the variance in the development of nausea and vomiting, together with the emetogenicity of the chemotherapy used, stage of disease[67] and other treatment or disease-related characteristics.

Patients developing anticipatory nausea and/or vomiting may be more depressed or anxious than those who do not develop anticipatory symptoms, with a personality profile characterized by future despair, social alienation and inhibited style.[81] Morrow et al[75] assessed the predictive value of eight clinical characteristics in the development of anticipatory nausea. Characteristics included experiencing nausea and vomiting after the first chemotherapy, nausea after treatment described as 'moderate, severe or intolerable', age under 50 years old, susceptibility to motion sickness, feelings of generalized weakness, feeling warm or hot after treatment, and sweating after chemotherapy. They reported that patients who had 4 or more of these characteristics developed significantly more nausea and vomiting by the fourth chemotherapy cycle than those who had fewer than 4. Such findings confirm the biobehavioural nature of the symptoms and lead us to the idea that nausea and vomiting are multifactorial experiences and their management may need multiple interventions. However, more work is necessary in this area, as many inconsistencies exist across studies and in some cases the emetogenicity of the chemotherapy given or the type of antiemetics used are more associated with nausea and vomiting than by patient or environmental factors.[82]

NAUSEA AND VOMITING AFTER RADIATION THERAPY

Radiation therapy does produce similar toxicity to chemotherapy, but the patterns are different and mostly dose- and site-related. In a study of 914 patients receiving radiation therapy in 51 Italian centres, nausea or vomiting occurred in 37.3% and 17.1%, respectively, and 38.7% of the patients experienced both nausea and vomiting.[50] Acute vomiting is usually the norm in patients receiving radiation therapy, especially after single-fraction radiation, with prolonged (or delayed) nausea and vomiting lasting 2–3 days seen in about 40% of patients, and anticipatory nausea and vomiting is extremely low.[51] Vomiting may develop from 30 minutes to 4 hours post-irradiation[51] and within minutes when total body irradiation as preparation for a bone marrow transplant is given.[11] Although the intensity of these two symptoms may be relatively low, it may become a major and distressing problem for patients and affect their daily life, especially when patients experience these feelings over a prolonged period of time as in the case of patients receiving fractionated irradiation.[83] Treatment interruptions have been reported in 20% of patients undergoing fractionated irradiation,[84] and this may decrease the chances of complete control of the tumour and affect survival.

The most common factors behind radiation-induced nausea and vomiting include the radiation site (especially the abdominal area) and radiation fields >400 m² (including total body and hemibody irradiation).[50] As enterochromaffin cells (involved in the mechanisms of nausea and vomiting development) are located in the upper epigastric area, this may explain why irradiation of the abdominal area is a high-risk factor for nausea and vomiting. Other factors can be seen in Box 20.2. Higher rates of nausea and vomiting may also be seen in patients receiving radiation to the thorax or head and neck.[50]

It is interesting that, although the evidence clearly demonstrates that patients receiving radiation therapy do experience nausea and vomiting, they are not routinely offered antiemetic support, unless they are receiving single high-dose radiation to the abdomen.[84] In a large multicentre study it was shown that only 14% of patients receiving radiation therapy received antiemetics, and these were prescribed mostly for symptomatic management rather than preventatively.[50] Thus, clinicians in radiation therapy centres need to be more aware of the presence and effects of the distressing

---

Box 20.2

Factors associated with radiation-induced nausea and vomiting

- Single and total dose, dose rate
- Fractionation
- Field size (irradiation volume)
- Site of irradiation, organs included in the radiation field
- Patient positioning
- Radiation technique (energy, beam quality)
- Previous or simultaneous influencing therapy
- General health status of the patient

Source: adapted from Feyer et al.[49]

symptoms of nausea and vomiting in their patients and manage them more effectively. Also, a need for evidence-based approaches to the management of radiation-induced nausea and vomiting is pressing.

NAUSEA AND VOMITING AFTER SURGERY

Postoperative nausea and vomiting, although less common with the use of newer anaesthetic drugs, is still a problem for some patients. Different anaesthetic agents produce different levels of nausea and vomiting. For example, in a study involving patients undergoing surgery for breast cancer it was shown that desflurane produced nausea and vomiting in 67% of the women, sevoflurane in 36% and isoflurane in 22% during a 24-hour period, even though the emergence from anaesthesia was not different in the three groups.[85] The authors suggest an anaesthetic agent based on its low nausea and vomiting profile should be considered. Also, co-induction with other drugs may help the situation, as in the case of clonidine in a recent study of 68 women undergoing breast surgery, where it was shown to almost halve the experience of postoperative nausea and vomiting compared to a control group.[86]

Postoperative nausea and vomiting is considerably more common in women (about twice or three times) compared to males,[87] and gynaecological surgical procedures are known to be associated with a high incidence of nausea and vomiting.[88] Further, patients with breast cancer undergoing surgery with general anaesthesia develop very high rates of postoperative nausea and vomiting (60–81.5%).[89,90] These high-risk groups of patients may benefit from antiemetic prophylaxis, but more research is necessary in this area to establish best management protocols.

NAUSEA AND VOMITING AFTER BIOLOGICAL THERAPIES

The use of biotherapies as single or combined treatment modality is becoming more common. Although little research has been directed to the symptom experience of patients with cancer receiving biotherapies, the evidence suggests that about a third of patients develop a number of toxicities, including grade 3 or 4 nausea and vomiting, depending on the rate of infusion and the specific biological therapy used. In a recent study of 49 patients with metastatic melanoma treated with Bryostatin either over 24 or 72 hours, the former regimen was associated with a 35% incidence of grade 3/4 nausea and vomiting, whereas the latter regimen was associated with only a 5% incidence.[91] Other studies have combined chemotherapy and biotherapies, in which case it is not clear which contributes to the incidence of nausea and vomiting. Nevertheless, such studies show generally higher rates of nausea and vomiting than those expected with chemotherapy only. For example, in a study of 28 patients with melanoma treated with a chemotherapy combination protocol of highly emetogenic agents, interleukin-2 and interferon-alpha, it was shown that significant toxicity developed, including nausea and vomiting in 96% of the patients.[92]

Furthermore, Foelber[93] (in a review) suggests that toxicities that can be ascribed to low-dose interleukin-2 after autologous stem cell transplant include nausea and vomiting, together with diarrhoea and skin rashes. Similar considerable toxicity (grade 3/4 nausea and vomiting) was further observed in a study of 13 patients with colorectal cancer using 5-fluorouracil (5-FU), leucovorin (calcium folinate) and interferon-alpha.[94] The limited evidence and information about side effects and biotherapies should be increased with good-quality studies, especially as treatment with biotherapies is becoming more commonplace for a range of cancers.

ANTICIPATORY NAUSEA AND VOMITING

Depending on the definition of anticipatory nausea and vomiting, which is not always consistent, studies have shown that the median prevalence of anticipatory nausea is 33% (range 14–63%) and that of anticipatory vomiting is 12% (range 9–27%).[52] A number of factors can contribute to the development of anticipatory nausea and vomiting, which Morrow and Dobkin[52] have categorized into three groups in their detailed review article:

- demographic factors (i.e. age)
- clinical variables (i.e. susceptibility to motion sickness)
- psychological variables (i.e. anxiety or depression).

Many of these, however, are not consistent across studies. Expectations for developing anticipatory nausea and vomiting seem to be a more consistent predictor of anticipatory nausea and vomiting.[54,95,96] Previous experience of nausea and vomiting in earlier courses of chemotherapy is also a common predictor of anticipatory nausea and vomiting,[96] which further supports the conditioned response in their development. The conditioned response seen in adults is also evident in paediatrics.[97]

NAUSEA AND VOMITING IN ADVANCED CANCER

Nausea and vomiting in advanced cancer is very common, with typical rates ranging from 50 to 60%; it is more common in patients under 65 years old, females and those with cancer of the stomach and breast.[98] In advanced cancer, nausea and vomiting can be even more complicated than that experienced due to chemoradiotherapy or other treatments. Besides the reasons described earlier, nausea and vomiting in advanced cancer can develop as a result of gastric stasis or intestinal obstruction, pharyngeal irritation, opioid use, morphine-related constipation, paraneoplastic syndrome, pain, hypercalcaemia, brain metastasis, renal failure, raised intracranial pressure and tumour burden.[14,98,99] Opioid-induced nausea and vomiting is common, with 30% of patients receiving morphine, feeling nausea during the first week of treatment.[98] In palliative care, before resorting to antiemetics, it is important to treat the reversible causes of nausea and vomiting (i.e. pain or intracranial pressure). For example, a laxative may be effective in relieving nausea and vomiting if constipation is the

causative factor or stopping non-steroidal anti-inflammatory drugs (NSAIDS) if gastric irritation is the cause. The cause of nausea and vomiting may be evident by the pattern of vomiting, associated symptoms, review of the medications taken and physical examination.[100] In addition, nausea and vomiting in advanced disease may mask other conditions. Thus, a careful assessment and 'attention to detail', as suggested by Twycross,[101] is important as well as better utilization of what is already available, including non-pharmacological therapies. Intractable nausea and vomiting, especially in patients with GI and brain metastasis may be a condition that is serious and difficult to manage, but it has received little attention in the literature.

ASSESSMENT OF NAUSEA AND VOMITING

Assessment and documentation of symptoms, such as nausea and emesis, and evaluation of the effect of treatment given are crucial components for optimal symptom control[102] and therefore important tasks for nurses caring for patients with cancer. Assessment is an ongoing process that begins with the initial patient contact and continues through the patient's entire treatment period. Skillful observation and effective, efficient techniques for gathering data are required. Assessment tools that can be completed and reviewed quickly utilize less patient energy and nursing time. Nausea may occur without vomiting and or/retching, and vice versa. Therefore, when evaluating the symptoms, it is important to separate the three phenomena rather than taking a global approach to all symptoms.[14] Patients may not use the same descriptor for the symptoms as the clinician.[103] It is therefore crucial that questionnaires, self-report instruments or interviews use words that have the same meaning for all participants.

To have an accurate and complete picture of the patient's symptoms it is important to assess not only the frequency of nausea and vomiting but also to include the dimensions of intensity, duration and perceived symptom distress.[102,104] Nausea and vomiting can be evaluated as part of a comprehensive assessment of treatment-related symptoms or with instruments specifically developed to measure nausea and vomiting. Several comprehensive instruments that include assessment of one or more of the components are available.[105–109] Clinicians may see some of them as too extensive, limiting their usefulness in daily clinical practice. Visual analogue scales (VAS) and simple categorical scales are often chosen by clinicians due to their simplicity both for the patient and for the caregiver. A study investigating the concordance between a four-point verbal category scale and a VAS in assessing nausea intensity showed a good agreement between the two methods,[110] indicating that either method could be used. However, the VAS may have advantages if the focus is on detecting small but possibly clinically significant changes on individual patients.

The introduction of 5-HT$_3$ receptor antagonists greatly improved the possibilities of preventing acute nausea and vomiting associated with chemotherapy. This has made it possible for most patients with cancer to receive chemotherapy on an outpatient basis. One drawback of this otherwise positive development is the impaired communication between patients and hospital staff post chemotherapy, when delayed symptoms occur. In clinical studies, patient outcomes are carefully documented, often using patient diaries. This is unfortunately rarely the case in clinical practice, increasing the risk of underestimating the extent of patients' symptoms. The use of patient logs or daily diaries provides useful assessment information. They can also help family caregivers and patients develop experience in problem-solving, a greater sense of control and improved self-care.[14]

Recently, a quality assurance system using patient diaries to evaluate patient outcomes both for individual patients and groups of patients was reported.[111] This quality assurance system consists of evidence-based antiemetic practice guidelines, a nausea and emesis diary, a computer database and regular clinical audit procedures 2–3 times a year. In this system the diary is not only used for the evaluation of outcomes for the individual patient at the next cycle but also to evaluate the effectiveness of the guidelines for whole groups of patients.

This makes it possible to review and, if necessary, change the antiemetic guidelines accordingly, based on systematically collected clinical data.

MANAGEMENT OF NAUSEA AND VOMITING

Pharmacological treatment

The symptoms of nausea and vomiting are most frequently managed with antiemetic drug therapy where the goal is to prevent nausea and vomiting completely. However, patients with cancer can experience nausea and vomiting from a variety of different causes and no single antiemetic drug is capable of dealing with all of them. Therefore, the goal of complete protection in all patients during the course of their disease is not realistic. Even so, if nausea and vomiting occur despite prophylactic antiemetic treatment, relief can be offered if the underlying cause is identified or if changes in the antiemetic treatment can be made. A thorough investigation of possible underlying causes and type of nausea is needed in order to choose the most appropriate antiemetic. Also, to achieve optimal symptom control, it may be necessary to combine drugs with different modes of action or alter the time schedule for antiemetic dosing. Table 20.1 provides an overview of the most common classes of drugs used for prevention and treatment of nausea and vomiting.

Many antiemetic drugs are, to a greater or lesser extent, dopamine receptor antagonists that act either by increasing the GI motility or by blocking dopamine receptors. Since patients with cancer may experience nausea and vomiting from different causes at the same time, it is important to investigate the underlying cause and choose the antiemetic drug or combination of drugs that are relevant. It should be emphasized that many drugs have a similar antiemetic action and combining them may increase the risk of side effects.

Despite advances in the area, treatment-related nausea and vomiting still represents one of the great challenges for nurses working with patients with cancer. The introduction of

Table 20.1: Drugs used for prevention and treatment of nausea and vomiting due to different causes

Class	Example	Mode of action
5-HT$_3$ receptor antagonists	Dolasetron Granisetron Ondansetron Tropisetron	Inhibition of selective 5-HT$_3$ receptor sites both centrally and in the GI tract
NK$_1$ receptor antagonist	Aprepitant	Acts centrally
Benzamides	Metoclopramide	Dopamine receptor and 5-HT$_3$ receptor (low-affinity) inhibition, increase in gastric emptying
Corticosteroids	Dexamethasone Betamethasone	Uncertain
Benzodiazepines	Lorazepam Diazepam	Anxiolytic, sedative
Phenothiazines	Prochlorperazine Dixyrazine	Mainly dopamine receptor blockade
Butyrophenones	Haloperidol Droperidol	Mainly dopamine receptor blockade
Anticholinergics	Scopolamine	Reduces GI secretion and motility, central antiemetic action
Antihistamines	Cyclizine Thiethylperazine	Histamine (H$_1$) and dopamine receptor blockade, block labyrinth impulses
Cannabinoids	Nabilone Dronabinol	Cannabinoid receptor blockade

5-HT$_3$ receptor antagonists was a major breakthrough for chemotherapy-induced nausea and vomiting, at least during the acute phase. In patients receiving highly emetogenic therapy (such as cisplatin), complete control of acute symptoms have risen from less than 1% in 1981[112] to about 60% in 1998.[113] Aprepitant, the new neurokinin antagonist, has shown promising early results, with improvements in control of emesis by 20% or more in patients receiving highly emetogenic chemotherpy, especially in delayed emesis.[114] For more moderately emetogenic drugs (such as anthracyclines, carboplatin or cyclophosphamide), current control is now in the 70–80% range.[37] However, during the delayed phase, up to 60% of patients still suffer from nausea and vomiting.[38]

Adequate pharmacological treatment is crucial to achieve optimal control of chemotherapy-induced nausea and vomiting. During the last 20 years, a large number of clinical trials have been carried out to establish the most effective pharmacological treatment. For clinicians, it may be difficult to synthesize the information available in the studies to make it applicable to the patient. Therefore, several groups and organizations have recently reviewed and synthesized the information, elaborating guidelines to aid clinical practice.[16,60,61,62,64,115] The guidelines are extensive, including a large number of references summarizing the evidence presented in the literature. For clinicians, the documents may be too extensive and technical in nature and thereby difficult to use in daily practice. Therefore, experts representing different disciplines and organizations have recently held consensus meetings that aim to produce and publish condensed summaries of the available antiemetic guidelines.[59,116] Some general statements, listed in Box 20.3 were agreed upon. Tables 20.2A and 20.2B shows suggested treatment options based on emetogenic risk of the chemotherapy given and the suggested doses for common antiemetics.

Studies with combination treatments based on the best available treatment and the new NK_1 receptor antagonist have recently started. In a randomized study by Campos et al[48] the additive effect of an NK_1 receptor antagonist was evaluated compared to a combination of granisetron and dexamethasone: 80% of the patients receiving the three drug combination were without vomiting during the acute phase compared to 57% of the patients receiving granisetron and dexamethasone. During the delayed phase the patients received either the NK_1 receptor antagonist or placebo, indicating a suboptimal control arm since a corticosteroid was not given.[60] This also affected the control rate. A maximum of 50% of the patients were free from nausea during the study period (days 1–5), irrespective of treatment arm. A maxi-

mum of 63% of the patients were free of vomiting during the delayed phase (day 2–5). This highlights the importance of proper study design based on the best treatment available when evaluating new drugs or drug combinations. The patients in the Campos study all received chemotherapy comprising high-dose (>70 mg/m^2) cisplatin. Further studies are needed to confirm these results in other chemotherapy regimens.

Box 20.3

Basic antiemetic standards

- Antiemetics should always be given prophylactically
- If patients receive a combination of chemotherapy, treat according to the agent with the maximum emetogenic risk
- When given at appropriate doses, the available 5-HT$_3$ receptor antagonists are equivalent both in terms of efficacy and side effects
- The lowest fully effective dose of each agent should be given
- Oral antiemetics (in proper doses) are as effective as similar intravenous formulations
- Single-dose administration of antiemetics is as effective as multiple doses
- Use dexamethasone together with 5-HT$_3$ receptor antagonists before chemotherapy
- Acute and delayed chemotherapy-induced nausea and vomiting should be separately assessed and treated

Table 20.2A: Suggested treatment of chemotherapy-induced nausea and vomiting (based on consensus statements)

Risk category	Acute phase (day 1 of chemotherapy)	Delayed phase (day 2+)
High	5-HT$_3$ receptor antagonist + aprepitant + steroid	Steroid + aprepitant (more superior results) or seroid + 5-HT$_3$ receptor antagonist
Moderate	5-HT$_3$ receptor antagonist + steroid	Steroid alone or 5-HT$_3$ receptor antagonist
Low	Single agents: (steroid or other[a] agents)	No preventative measures
Minimal	No preventative measures	No preventative measures

[a]Other agents may be: dopamine receptor antagonists, phenothiazines, butyrophenones.

Table 20.2B: Suggested treatment of chemotherapy-induced nausea and vomiting (based on consensus statements)

Drug (dosage)	Acute phase (day 1)	Delayed phase (day 2+)
Dolasetron	iv: 100 mg or 1.8 mg/kg po: 100 mg	po: 100 mg daily
Granisetron	iv: 1 mg or 10 μg/kg po: 2 mg	po: 1 mg bid
Ondansetron	iv: 8 mg or 0.15 mg/kg po: 16 mg	po: 8 mg bid
Tropisetron	iv: 5 mg po: 5 mg	po: 5 mg daily
Metoclopramide	Not recommended	20-40 mg bid – qid
Aprepitant	125 mg orally, once	80 mg orally once, for 2 days
Dexamethasone: In high-risk situations In moderate-risk situations In low-risk situations	iv: 20 mg po: 20 mg 8 mg once 4–8 mg once	po: 8 mg b.i.d. 8 mg daily for 2–3 days or po: 4 bid No preventative measure

Treatment failures

In a recent review article, Aapro [27] suggests that breakthrough or refractory nausea and vomiting following chemotherapy may be related to inadequate therapy. This is an important point, stressing the need to use and implement the evidence-based antiemetic guidelines that have been published.[16,60,62,115] Of the patients that actually do receive the best treatment available and still experience nausea and vomiting, suggestions for treatment are available, although few adequate studies in the area have been performed. The suggestions are summarized in Box 20.4.

Psychoeducational and behavioural techniques

A large amount of research has been conducted on the effects of behavioural and psychological interventions in the management of chemotherapy-related nausea and vomiting, especially in the 1980s. Almost consistently, research supports the positive effects of these techniques, with relaxation training and guided imagery the most well-researched and most effective techniques.

Progressive muscle relaxation training (PMRT) is the most common technique used and it involves active relaxation and tensing-releasing of groups of muscles, often combined with guided imagery (thinking in pictures through the voice of the therapist). In their excellent review, Burish and Tope[53] summarize the work they (and others) have done over the preceding decade. In relation to the use of PMRT, the conclusion is that it can be effective in reducing the distress from chemotherapy, including conditioned nausea and vomiting, negative affect and physiological arousal and, if taught before the chemotherapy, it can prevent or at least significantly delay the onset of conditioned symptoms.[53] Later studies using improved methodology and larger sample sizes confirmed the results. For example, Arakawa[117] showed that total scores of nausea, vomiting and retching after chemotherapy were decreased as well as feel-

Box 20.4

Suggestions for treatment failures

1. If optimal treatment has been given as prophylaxis, repeat dosing of the same agent is unlikely to be successful. Attempt to give a rescue drug of a different pharmacological class.
2. If nausea and vomiting occur despite optimal prophylaxis, other causes of the symptoms should be considered, such as concomitant medications, bowel obstruction, migraine or brain metastases.
3. In patients who experience nausea and vomiting despite optimal prophylactic treatment with a 5-HT$_3$ receptor antagonists plus a corticosteroid, the addition of metopimazine or another D2 receptor antagonist may increase the protection during the following cycle. Also propofol has shown activity but is difficult to use because of its narrow therapeutic window.
4. If treatment based on one of the 5-HT$_3$ receptor antagonists has failed, a switch to another may be worthwhile.
5. In case of breakthrough nausea and vomiting and when nothing else seems to help, sedating the patients may be of value.

Source: adapted from Aapro.[27]

ings of anxiety in a group of 60 patients. In a recent study of PMRT use, Molassiotis et al[66] have also demonstrated that frequency and duration of both nausea and vomiting were significantly lower in the PMRT group as compared to a control group during the first 4 days of the chemotherapy. The results were less clear with respect to psychological status and anxiety, as no significant differences were found, but it was evident that anxiety and mood improved in the experimental group and worsened in the control group. In terms of delivery techniques, Carey and Burish[118] suggest that PMRT delivery by a professional therapist is more effective than audiotapes or use of trained volunteers, but this is an area needing further exploration. In a more recent work, use of audiotapes was well-received and led to significant changes in quality of life domains of patients with colorectal cancer,[119] and such findings indicate that the role of audiotapes or other cost-effective methods

may have a place in the delivery of relaxation techniques.

Guided imagery has also demonstrated significant effects in reducing nausea and vomiting, either combined with PMRT[120] or on its own.[121] Guided imagery may also act indirectly in lowering nausea and vomiting, as studies have shown that guided imagery can decrease anxiety,[122] which is known to produce conditioning symptoms. Another potentially useful method for selective patients, although logistically difficult to use in everyday practice, is *biofeedback*. This is a technique where people learn to control various physiological processes when they are given moment-to-moment information in select physiological responses.[53] Early positive findings in the 1980s have not been replicated successfully.[123] Positive findings with biofeedback, however, may have been influenced by the fact that these patients also received PMRT.[53,123] Also, *systematic desensitization* has been shown to decrease anticipatory and post-treatment nausea and vomiting.[124] Furthermore, *hypnosis and mental preparation* through an audiotape were used in a study of 50 women undergoing breast surgery and it was reported that patients in the experimental group had considerably less postoperative vomiting than the control group (39% vs 68%) and less postoperative nausea.[125] However, the strong element of relaxation or imagery in this study should be considered in interpreting the results. Nevertheless, hypnosis or cognitive-behavioural training in a study of bone marrow transplant patients did not show any effect in reducing nausea and vomiting.[126]

Diverting attention may be a more easy and cost-effective way to manage nausea and vomiting more effectively. All the relaxation techniques described earlier have a common element, i.e. diverting the patient's attention.[53] When PMRT was compared with cognitive distraction, it was shown that both reduced the experience of nausea and both had equal effect.[127] This is further confirmed in the paediatric oncology setting, where nausea and vomiting were reduced in children receiving chemotherapy who were given computer games to play with.[128] Music therapy may also be an appropriate distraction method that is useful in

429

decreasing nausea and vomiting,[129–131] but limited evidence on this topic exists.

Coping preparation or other psychoeducational techniques have also been effective not only in reducing nausea and vomiting but also other negative affects.[53,132] Burish et al[133] assessed the effectiveness of a coping preparation programme (PREP) and PMRT, both individually and combined. The coping preparation included a tour of the oncology clinic, a videotaped presentation about chemotherapy, a discussion session with both patients and family members and a booklet for patients/families to take home (single session of 90 minutes in all). Results indicated that the PREP not only significantly reduced nausea and vomiting but also increased patients' knowledge, improved general coping ability and decreased negative affect.[133] The combination group of PREP and PMRT did not offer any significant advantage from only the PREP. Moreover, another coping strategy programme was developed and tested in patients with breast cancer undergoing autologous bone marrow transplantation.[134] The programme consisted of preparatory information, cognitive restructuring and relaxation with guided imagery. In this large randomized trial ($n = 110$), nausea was significantly lower in patients assigned the coping strategy programme as compared to patients in the control group, even after controlling for relevant variables.[134] Further, a 'blunting' or distraction-oriented coping style may be associated with less anticipatory and post-treatment nausea.[132] In children with cancer, a range of coping strategies are employed to deal with nausea and vomiting (most frequently distraction, emotional regulation and wishful thinking), with most helpful strategies (reported by 40–60% of children) being sleeping, social support and emotional regulation.[135]

Although the evidence in some of these psychobehavioural techniques is overwhelming, they are not often incorporated in the care of patients with cancer. The unfamiliarity of nursing and medical staff with these techniques, the time needed to deliver the interventions, the lack of preparation and costs involved may be some of the reasons behind this phenomenon.[66] Less time-consuming and more cost-effective methods of delivering these interventions is necessary and this should be a major focus of symptom management research. Furthermore, it is argued that providing these interventions in a simplistic way without careful assessment and preparation may result in suboptimal care and deleterious responses.[136]

Diet

Malnutrition is a common problem in 40–80% of patients with cancer[137] (see Ch. 29). If the patient experiences nausea and vomiting, the risk of insufficient nutritional intake increases, resulting in further weight loss, which may interfere with the possibility of giving adequate antitumour treatment. There is also a risk of developing conditioned symptoms related to the smell or sight of food.[26] Therefore, potentially nauseating stimuli in the patient's environment should be reduced or eliminated. The patient should be encouraged to eat at times when the risk of nausea and vomiting is less. This is especially important for patients having multiple days of treatment such as chemotherapy or radiation therapy. Cool, carbonated beverages and bland food served at room temperature is often well tolerated. During the time period when there is risk of nausea and vomiting, large meals should be avoided. Attractively prepared food presented as small but frequent meals served during nausea-free periods might be a better choice. During chemotherapy, foods may taste differently, indicating the need to avoid certain dishes or flavours.[138] Sweet, fatty and spicy food should be avoided. Lightly salted food such as sour pickles or snacks, as well as lemons and dry crackers/toast, may also be helpful, especially if the patient is already nauseated. Other recommended food includes yoghurt, oatmeal, baked or grilled chicken (without skin), fruits and vegetables that are soft or bland, such as canned peaches, chilled drinks sipped slowly between meals, ice lollies, flat ginger ale, flat cola and fruit juice. Foods to avoid include fatty, greasy or fried foods, sweets, biscuits or cake, and foods with strong smells; in addition, patients should avoid drinking too much fluid together with a meal.

Complementary and alternative therapies

One of the very few complementary and alternative medicine (CAM) therapies showing an overwhelming positive effect on health is that of acupuncture in the management of nausea and vomiting. This method is based on traditional Chinese medicine philosophies and involves stimulation of a specific point by fine needles. The point (Pericardium 6 or P6 point) is located in the ventral surface of the wrist. In a systematic review of the literature, Vickers[139] reports that from the 12 randomized, placebo-controlled, double-blind studies of nausea and vomiting related to chemotherapy, pregnancy and anaesthesia, 11 favour acupuncture. More studies have been carried out since the systematic review by Vickers,[139] and most present data in favour of the technique. One of the most well-conducted studies in the field is the one by Shen et al[140] who compared electroacupuncture, sham acupuncture and antiemetics only in women undergoing myeloablative chemotherapy ($n = 104$). Vomiting during days 1–5 occurred on average 6.3 times in the electroacupuncture group, 10.7 in the sham acupuncture group and 13.4 times in the pharmacotherapy-only group.

A less-invasive form of acupuncture is acupressure, which is based on the same principles as acupuncture but uses pressure on the P6 point instead of needling. Finger acupressure to P6 and another point (Stomach 36 in the knee) was effective in managing both the experience and intensity of nausea in a group of 17 women.[141] Use of P6 acustimulation wristbands (incorporating a battery-operated device that provides transcutaneous electrical nerve stimulation) in another study led to trends towards improvements in delayed nausea ($p < 0.06$) and significantly fewer antiemetic tablets.[142] Improved severity of nausea, especially in days 2–4 post treatment have also been reported in a study of 18 patients receiving cisplatin.[143] Nevertheless, results are not conclusive, as a number of acupressure studies have failed to demonstrate a significant effect, perhaps as a result of methodological inadequacies and small sample sizes.

A 10-minute food massage may also have significant effects on patients' nausea, as demonstrated in one study.[144] Aromatherapy and reflexology may also have an effect on nausea and vomiting, and systematic reviews on their effects are currently underway. Ginger is thought to help with nausea and vomiting (in teas or biscuits). Other herbal medications that are advocated to assist in the management of nausea and vomiting include:

- peppermint
- a combination of herbs such as alfalfa leaf, catnip, peppermint leaf, cinnamon bark, ginger root, and lobelia
- kelp (bladderack)
- the homeopathic remedy ipecac.

Little, if any, scientific evidence exists about their effectiveness. Smoking cannabis can also be effective in reducing nausea and vomiting, for patients receiving chemotherapy, decreasing nausea and vomiting by as much as 70–100% [145]. However, the latter review incorporates a number of studies with low methodological rigour, which were conducted before the $5\text{-}HT_3$ antiemetic introduction.

EFFECTS OF NAUSEA AND VOMITING ON QUALITY OF LIFE

As nausea and vomiting can impact on the patient's daily activities due to their distressing nature, it is inevitable they will affect a patient's quality of life. Indeed, Osoba et al[6] have shown in a large study of 832 patients experiencing both nausea and vomiting that they had statistically worse fatigue, anorexia, insomnia, physical, social, cognitive and global quality of life than patients who experienced no nausea and vomiting or those experiencing only nausea. Increased severity of vomiting (>2 episodes) was not associated with worse functioning compared to those experiencing only 1–2 episodes of vomiting except in terms of anorexia and overall quality of life.[6]

Furthermore, in a hypothetical scenario of presence or absence of nausea and vomiting, patients ($n = 30$) reported a mean quality of life score of 79 out of 100 in the absence of nausea and vomiting and 27 out of 100 with nausea and vomiting, indicating that a relief of

431

nausea and vomiting can have a significant impact on a patient's quality of life.[8] In another study of 119 patients it was also shown that post-chemotherapy nausea and vomiting had a significant impact on quality of life, as patients experiencing either nausea or vomiting lowered their quality of life score from pretreatment on 6 functioning and 5 symptom scales (EORTC-QOL-C30 scale) at day 2 and on 4 functioning and 4 symptom scales on day 6.[146] A substantial correlation ($r = 0.58$) between 'nausea and vomiting burden' and 'overall treatment burden' has also been reported,[147] indicating the significant burden nausea and vomiting place on a patient's treatment journey. Others, however, have disagreed that nausea and vomiting contribute substantially to any of the quality of life areas.[148]

An often-forgotten concept behind patient perception of symptom bother that affects the perception of quality of life is culture. There may be a degree of cultural variability in nausea and vomiting, as there are different levels of nausea and vomiting across studies from place to place, even when the same chemotherapy and antiemetics have been used. This is further supported by an economic study conducted in four different countries about the value patients were willing to pay in order to improve acute and delayed vomiting by 20 and 30%, respectively.[149] Results indicated that different cultural groups value benefit and improved quality of life in a different way, which may have implications in the evaluation of the relationship between nausea/vomiting and quality of life.

CONCLUSION

Irrespective of the tremendous amount of work that has been directed to the symptoms of nausea and vomiting over the past 20 or so years, which no other symptom (with the exception of pain) has seen so far, they remain major problems for patients and we need to learn more about them before we manage them well. Confidently applying the best knowledge available in practice will enhance desired outcomes. But new knowledge and new directions in the management of nausea and vomiting are neces-

sary. The role of nursing is paramount in the management of patients experiencing nausea and vomiting, acting as patient educators and supporting them with a number of interventions to manage these distressing symptoms. The focus needs to be on imaginative, multidimensional and multidisciplinary management of these symptoms. The areas where we have limited knowledge require greater exploration – i.e. nausea and vomiting in patients receiving radiotherapy and after biological therapies – and interventions need to be developed, incorporating the breadth of information we have available.

REFERENCES

1. Coates A, Abraham S, Kaye SB. On the receiving end – patient perception of the side-effects of cancer chemotherapy. Eur J Cancer Clin Oncol 1983; 19(2):203–208.
2. Laszlo J, ed. Antiemetics and cancer chemotherapy. Baltimore: Williams & Wilkins; 1983.
3. Richardson JL, Marks G, Levine A. The influence of symptoms of disease and side effects of treatment on compliance with cancer therapy. J Clin Oncol 1988; 6:1746–1752.
4. Lindley CM, Bernard S, Fields SM. Incidence and duration of chemotherapy-induced nausea and vomiting in the outpatient oncology population. J Clin Oncol 1989; 7:1142–1149.
5. Griffin AM, Butow PN, Coates AS, et al. On the receiving end. V: Patient perceptions of the side effects of cancer chemotherapy in 1993. Ann Oncol 1996; 7:189–195.
6. Osoba D, Zee B, Warr D, et al. Effect of postchemotherapy nausea and vomiting on health-related quality of life. Support Care Cancer 1997; 5:307–313.
7. Osoba D, Zee B, Warr D, et al J. Quality of life studies in chemotherapy-induced emesis. Oncology 1996; 53(Suppl 1):92–95.
8. Grunberg S, Boutin N, Ireland A, et al. Impact of nausea/vomiting on quality of life as a visual analogue scale-derived utility score. Support Care Cancer 1996; 4:435–439.
9. Hawthorn J. Understanding and management of nausea and vomiting. Oxford: Blackwell Science; 1995.
10. Joss RA., Brand BC, Buser KS, Cerny T. The symptomatic control of cytostatic drug-induced emesis. A recent history and review. Eur J Cancer 1990; 26(Suppl 1):S2–8.
11. Wickham R. Nausea and vomiting: are they still a problem? In: Gates RA, Fink RM, eds. Oncology nursing secrets. Philadelphia: Hanley & Belfus; 1997:250–261.

12. Gilbar O. The quality of life of cancer patients who refuse chemotherapy. Soc Sci Med 1991; 32:1337–1340.

13. Roscoe JA, Morrow GR, Hickok JT, Stern RM. Nausea and vomiting remain a significant clinical problem: trends over time in controlling chemotherapy-induced nausea and vomiting in 1413 patients treated in community clinical practices. J Pain Symptom Manage 2000; 20:113–121.

14. Rhodes VA, McDaniel RW. Nausea, vomiting, and retching: complex problems in palliative care. CA Cancer J Clinic 2001; 51:232–248.

15. Hesketh PJ, Gralla RJ, du Bois A, Tonato M. Methodology of antiemetic trials: response assessment, evaluation of new agents and definition of chemotherapy emetogenicity. Support Care Cancer 1998; 6:221–227.

16. Anonymous. Prevention of chemotherapy- and radiotherapy-induced emesis: results of Perugia Consensus Conference. Antiemetic Subcommittee of the Multinational Association of Supportive Care in Cancer (MASCC). Ann Oncol 1998; 9:811–819.

17. Andrews PLR. The mechanism of emesis induced by chemotherapy and radiotherapy. In: Tonato M, ed. Antiemetics in the supportive care of cancer patients. Berlin: Springer-Verlag; 1996:3–24.

18. Morrow GR, Roscoe JA, Hickok JT, Andrews PLR, Matteson S. Nausea and emesis: evidence for a biobehavioral perspective. Support Care Cancer 2002; 10:96–105.

19. Rhodes VA, Watson PM, Johnson MH, Madsen RW, Beck NC. Patterns of nausea, vomiting, and distress in patients receiving antineoplastic drug protocols. Oncol Nurs Forum 1987; 14:35–44.

20. Fetting JH, Grochow LB, Folstein MF, Ettinger DS, Colvin M. The course of nausea and vomiting after high-dose cyclophosphamide. Cancer Treat Rep 1982; 66:1487–1493.

21. Martin M, Diaz-Rubio E, Sanchez A, Almenarez J, Lopez-Vega JM. The natural course of emesis after carboplatin treatment. Acta Oncol 1990; 29:593–595.

22. Kris MG, Pisters KM, Hinkley L. Delayed emesis following anticancer chemotherapy. Support Care Cancer 1994; 2:297–300.

23. Morrow GR, Roscoe JA, Kirshner JJ, Hynes HE, Rosenbluth RJ. Anticipatory nausea and vomiting in the era of 5-HT3 antiemetics. Support Care Cancer 1998; 6:244–247.

24. Carey MP, Burish TG. Etiology and treatment of the psychological side effects associated with cancer chemotherapy: a critical review and discussion. Psychol Bull 1988; 104(3):307–325.

25. Matteson S, Roscoe J, Hickok J, Morrow GR. The role of behavioral conditioning in the development of nausea. Am J Obstet Gynecol 2002; 185(5 Suppl):S239–S243.

26. Hursti T, Fredrikson M, Börjeson S, et al. Association between personality characteristics and the prevalence and extinction of conditioned nausea after chemotherapy. J Psychosoc Oncol 1992; 10:59–77.

27. Aapro MS. How do we manage patients with refractory or breakthrough emesis? Support Care Cancer 2002; 10:106–109.

28. Andrews PLR. , Sanger GJ, eds. The problem of emesis in anti-cancer therapy: an introduction. In: Emesis in anti-cancer therapy. Mechanisms and treatment. London: Chapman & Hall Medical; 1993:1–7.

29. Grant M, Ropka ME. Management of major clinical nursing problems. Alterations in nutrition. In: McCorkle R, Grant M, Frank-Stromborg M, Baird SB, eds. Cancer nursing. A comprehensive textbook. Philadelphia: WB Saunders; 1996:919–943.

30. Borison HL, Wang SC. Functional localisation of the central coordinating mechansim for emesis in cat. J Neurophysiol 1949; 12:304–313.

31. Borison HL, Wang SC. Physiology and pharmacology of vomiting. Pharmac Rev 1953; 5:193–230.

32. Miller AD. Central mechanisms of vomiting. Dig Dis Sci 1999; 44(8 Suppl):39S–43S.

33. Gregory RE. Ettinger DS. 5-HT3 receptor antagonists for the prevention of chemotherapy-induced nausea and vomiting. A comparison of their pharmacology and clinical efficacy. Drugs 1998; 55:173–189.

34. Andrews PL, Naylor RJ, Joss RA. Neuropharmacology of emesis and its relevance to anti-emetic therapy. Consensus and controversies. Support Care Cancer 1998; 6:197–203.

35. Miner WD, Sanger GJ. Inhibition of cisplatin-induced vomiting by selective 5-hydroxytryptamine M-receptor antagonism. Br J Pharmacol 1986; 88(3):497–499.

36. The Italian Group for Antiemetic Research. Prevention of cisplatin-induced delayed emesis: still unsatisfactory. Italian Group for Antiemetic Research. Support Care Cancer 2000; 8:229–232.

37. Gralla RJ. New agents, new treatment, and antiemetic therapy. Semin Oncol 2002; 29(1 Suppl 4):119–124.

38. Roila F, Donati D, Tamberi S, Margutti G. Delayed emesis: incidence, pattern, prognostic factors and optimal treatment. Support Care Cancer 2002; 10:88–95.

39. Cunningham D, Morgan RJ, Mills PR. Functional and structural changes of the human proximal small intestine after cytotoxic therapy. J Clin Pathol 1985; 38:265–270.

40. Allan SG, Smyth JF. Small intestinal mucosal toxicity of cis-platinum – comparison of toxicity with platinum analogues and dexamethasone. Br J Cancer 1986; 53:355–360.

41. Fredrikson M, Hursti T, Furst CJ et al. Nausea in cancer chemotherapy is inversely related to urinary cortisol excretion. Br J Cancer 1992; 65:779–780.

42. Fredrikson M, Hursti TJ, Steineck G, et al. Delayed chemotherapy-induced nausea is augmented by high levels of endogenous noradrenaline. Br J Cancer 1994; 70:642–645.

43. Alberola V, Garcia J, Lluch A, et al. Relation between adrenal failure and delayed emesis in patients receiving dexamethasone to prevent gastrointestinal toxicity of high-dose cisplatin. Cancer Chemother Pharmacol 1986; 18(Suppl 1):A2.

44. Yamakuni H, Sawai H, Maeda V, et al. Probable involvement of the 5-hydroxytryptamine(4) receptor in methotrexate-induced delayed emesis in dogs. J Pharmacol Exp Ther 2000; 292:1002–1007.

45. Hesketh PJ, Gralla RJ, Webb RT, et al. Randomized phase II study of the neurokinin 1 receptor antagonist CJ-11,974 in the control of cisplatin-induced emesis. J Clin Oncol 1999; 17:338–343.

46. de Wit R, Herrstedt J, Rapoport B, et al. The oral NK(1) antagonist, aprepitant, given with standard antiemetics provides protection against nausea and vomiting over multiple cycles of cisplatin-based chemotherapy: a combined analysis of two randomised, placebo-controlled phase III clinical studies. Eur J Cancer 2004; 40:403–410.

47. Hesketh PJ, Grunberg SM, Gralla RJ, et al. The oral neurokinin-1 antagonist aprepitant for the prevention of chemotherapy-induced nausea and vomiting: a multinational, randomised, double-blind, placebo-controlled trial in patients receiving high-dose cisplatin – the Aprepitant Protocol 052 Study Group. J Clin Oncol 2003; 21:4112–4119.

48. Campos D, Pereira JR, Reinhardt RR, et al. Prevention of cisplatin-induced emesis by the oral neurokinin-1 antagonist, MK-869, in combination with granisetron and dexamethasone or with dexamethasone alone. J Clin Oncol 2001; 19:1759–1767.

49. Feyer PC, Stewart AL, Titlbach O. Aetiology and prevention of emesis induced by radiotherapy. Support Care Cancer 1998; 6:253–260.

50. Anonymous. Radiation-induced emesis: a prospective observational multicentre Italian trial. The Italian Group for Antiemetic Research in Radiotherapy. Int J Radiat Oncol Biol Phys 1999; 44:619–625.

51. Pisters KM, Kris MG. Treatment-related nausea and vomiting. In: Berger A, Portenoy RK, Weissman DE, eds. Principles and practice of supportive oncology. Philadelphia: Lippincott-Raven; 1998:165–177.

52. Morrow GR, Dobkin PL. Anticipatory nausea and vomiting in cancer patients undergoing chemotheraphy treatment: prevalence, etiology, and behavioural interventions. Clin Psychol Rev 1988; 8:517–556.

53. Burish TG, Tope DM. Psychological techniques for controlling the adverse side effects of cancer chemotherapy: findings from a decade of research. J Pain Symptom Manage 1992; 7:287–301.

54. Montgomery GH, Bovbjerg DH. The development of anticipatory nausea in patients receiving adjuvant chemotherapy for breast cancer. Physiol Behav 1997; 61: 737–741.

55. Hickok JT, Roscoe JA, Morrow GR, et al. Nausea and emesis remain significant problems of chemotherapy despite prophylaxis with 5-hydroxytryptamine-3 antiemetics: a University of Rochester James P. Wilmot Cancer Center Community Clinical Oncology Program Study of 360 cancer patients treated in the community. Cancer 2003; 97:2880–2886.

56. Molassiotis A, Mok Ts, Yam BM, et al. An analysis of the antiemetic protection of metoclopramide plus dexamethasone in Chinese patients receiving moderately high emetogenic chemotherapy. Eur J Cancer Care 2002; 11:108–113.

57. Stone P, Richardson A, Ream E, et al. Cancer-related fatigue: inevitable, unimportant and untreatable? Results of a multi-centre patient surgery. Ann Oncol 2000; 11:971–975.

58. Lee Dupuis L, Lau R, Greenberg ML. Delayed nausea and vomiting in children receiving antineoplastics. Med Pediatr Oncol 2001; 37:115–121.

59. Koeller JM, Aapro MS, Gralla RJ, et al. Antiemetic guidelines: creating a more practical treatment approach. Support Care Cancer 2002; 10:519–522.

60. Gralla RJ, Osoba D, Kris MG, et al. Recommendations for the use of antiemetics: evidence-based, clinical practice guidelines. American Society of Clinical Oncology. J Clin Oncol 1999; 17:2971–2994.

61. American Society of Health-System Pharmacists (ASHSP). ASHSP therapeutic guidelines on the pharmacological management of nausea and vomiting in adult and pediatric patients receiving chemotherapy or radiation therapy or undergoing surgery. Am J Health Syst Pharm 1999; 56:729–764.

62. Antiemetic Guidelines, Multidational Association for Supportive Care in Cancer, 2004; can be viewed at: www.mascc.org

63. Hesketh PJ, Kris MG, Grunberg SM, et al. Proposal for classifying the acute emetogenicity of cancer chemotherapy. J Clin Oncol 1997; 15:103–109.

64. National Comprehensive Cancer Network (NCCN). NCCN antiemesis practice guidelines. Oncology 1997; 11:57–89.

65. Roila F. Do we need new antiemetic guidelines? Support Care Cancer 2002; 10:517–518.

66. Molassiotis A, Yung HP, Yam BM, et al. The effectiveness of progressive muscle relaxation training in managing chemotherapy-induced nausea and vomiting in Chinese breast cancer

patients: a randomised controlled trial. Support Care Cancer 2002; 10:237–246.

67. Molassiotis A, Yam BM, Yung H, et al. Pretreatment factors predicting the development of postchemotherapy nausea and vomiting in Chinese breast cancer patients. Support Care Cancer 2002; 10:139–145.

68. Haut MW, Beckwith B, Laurie JA, Klatt N. Postchemotherapy nausea and vomiting in cancer patients receiving outpatient chemotherapy. J Psychosoc Oncol 1991; 9:117–130.

69. Rhodes VA, Johnson MH, McDaniel RW. Nausea, vomiting, and retching: the management of the symptom experience. Semin Oncol Nurs 1995; 11:256–265.

70. Cassileth BR, Lusk EJ, Bodenheimer BJ, et al. Chemotherapeutic toxicity – the relationship between patients' pretreatment expectations and posttreatment results. Am J Clin Oncol 1985; 8:419–425.

71. Andrykowski MA, Gregg ME. The role of psychological variables in post-chemotherapy nausea: anxiety and expectation. Psychosom Med 1992; 54:48–58.

72. Jacobsen PB, Andrykowski MA, Redd WH, et al. Nonpharmacologic factors in the development of posttreatment nausea with adjuvant chemotherapy for breast cancer. Cancer 1988; 61:379–385.

73. Nerenz DR, Leventhal H, Douglas VE, Love RR. Anxiety and drug taste as predictors of anticipatory nausea in cancer chemotherapy. J Clin Oncol 1986; 4:224–233.

74. Carey MP, Burish TG. Anxiety as a predictor of behavioural therapy outcome for cancer chemotherapy patients. J Consult Clin Psychol 1985; 53:860–865.

75. Morrow GR, Lindke J, Black PM. Predicting development of anticipatory nausea in cancer patients: prospective examination of eight clinical characteristics. J Pain Symptom Manage 1991; 6:215–223.

76. du Bois A, Meerpohl HG, Vach W, et al. Course, patterns, and risk-factors for chemotherapy-induced emesis in cisplatin-pretreated patients: a study with ondansetron. Eur J Cancer 1992; 28(2–3):450–457.

77. Wallston KA, Pointer Smith RA, King JE, et al. Desire for control and choice of antiemetic treatment for cancer chemotherapy. West J Nurs Res 1991; 13:12–29.

78. Tsavaris N, Kosmas C, Mylonakis N, et al. Parameters that influence the outcome of nausea and emesis in cisplatin based chemotherapy. Anticancer Res 2000; 20(6C):4777–4783.

79. Leventhal H, Easterling DV, Nerenz DR, Love RR. The role of motion sickness in predicting anticipatory nausea. J Behav Med 1988; 11:117–129.

80. Morrow GR. The effect of a susceptibility to motion sickness on the side effects of cancer chemotherapy. Cancer 1985; 55:2766–2770.

81. Van Komen RW, Redd WJ. Personality factors associated with anticipatory nausea/vomiting in patients receiving cancer chemotherapy. Health Psychol 1985; 4:189–202.

82. Pater J, Slamet L, Zee B, et al. Inconsistency of prognostic factors for post-chemotherapy nausea and vomiting. Supp Care Cancer 1994; 2: 161–166.

83. Roberts JT, Priestman TJ. A review of ondansetron in the management of radiotherapy-induced emesis. Oncology 1993; 50:173–179.

84. Feyer PC, Zimmermann JS, Titlbach OJ, et al. Radiotherapy-induced emesis. An overview. Strahlentherapie und Onkologie 1998; 174(Suppl 3):56–61.

85. Karlsen KL, Persson E, Wennberg E, Stenqvist O. Anaesthesia, recovery and postoperative nausea and vomiting after breast surgery. A comparison between desflurane, sevoflurane and isoflurane anaesthesia. Acta Anaesthesiol Scand 2000; 44:489–493.

86. Oddby-Muhrbeck E, Eskborg S, Bergendahl HTD, Muhrbeck O, Lönnqvist PA. Effects of clonidine on postoperative nausea and vomiting in breast cancer surgery. Anesthesiology 2002; 96:1109–1114.

87. Watcha MF, White PF. Postoperative nausea and vomiting: its etiology, treatment and prevention. Anesthesiology 1992; 77:162–184.

88. Tang Tang J, Watcha MF, White MF. A comparison of costs and efficacy of ondansetron and droperidol as prophylactic antiemetic therapy for elective outpatient gynaecologic procedures. Anesth Analg 1996; 83:304–313.

89. Oddby-Muhrbeck E, Jakobsson J, Andersson L, Askergren J. Postoperative nausea and vomiting: a comparison between intravenous and inhalation anaesthesia in breast surgery. Acta Anaesthesiol Scand 1994; 38:52–56.

90. Sadhasivam S, Saxena A, Kathirvel S, et al. The safety and efficacy of prophylactic ondansetron in patients undergoing modified radical mastectomy. Anesth Analg 1999; 89:1340–1345.

91. Bedikian AY, Plager C, Stewart JR, et al. Phase II evaluation of bryostatin-1 in metastatic melanoma. Melanoma Res 2001; 11:183–188.

92. Dillman RO, Soori G, Wiemann MC, et al. Phase II trial of subcutaneous interleukin-2, subcutaneous interferon-alpha, intravenous combination chemotherapy, and oral tamoxifen in the treatment of metastatic melanoma: final results of cancer biotherapy research group 94-11. Cancer Biother Radiopharm 2000; 15:487–494.

93. Foelber R. Autologous stem cell transplant plus interleukin-2 for breast cancer: review and nursing management. Oncol Nurs Forum 1998; 25:563–568.

94. Soori GS, Oldham RK, Dobbs TW, et al. Chemo-biotherapy with 5-fluorouracil, leucovorin, and alpha interferon in metastatic carcinoma of the colon – a Cancer Biotherapy

Research Group (CBRG) phase II study. Cancer Biother Radiopharm 2000; 15:175–183.

95. Hickok JT, Roscoe JA, Morrow GR, et al. The role of patients' expectations in the development of anticipatory nausea related to chemotherapy for cancer. J Pain Symptom Manage 2001; 22:843–850.

96. Watson M, Meyer L, Thomson A, Osofsky S. Psychological factors predicting nausea and vomiting in breast cancer patients on chemotherapy. Eur J Cancer 1998; 34:831–837.

97. Stockhorst U, Spennes-Saleh S, Körholz D, et al. Anticipatory symptoms and anticipatory immune responses in pediatric cancer patients receiving chemotherapy: features of a classically conditioned response? Brain, Behaviour, and Immunity 2000; 14:198–218

98. Baines MJ. ABC of palliative care: nausea, vomiting and intestinal obstruction. BMJ 1997; 315:1148–1150.

99. Twycross R, Back I. Nausea and vomiting in advanced cancer. Eur J Palliat Care 1998; 5:39–45.

100. Davis MP, Walsh D. Treatment of nausea and vomiting in advanced cancer. Support Care Cancer 2000; 8:444–452.

101. Twycross RG. Attention to detail. Progr Palliat Care 1994; 2:222–227.

102. Rhodes VA. Criteria for assessment of nausea, vomiting, and retching. Oncol Nurs Forum 1997; 24(7 Suppl):13–19.

103. Rhodes VA, Watson PM, Johnson MH. Development of reliable and valid measures of nausea and vomiting. Cancer Nurs 1984; 7:33–41.

104. Rhodes VA, McDaniel RW, Homan SS, Johnson M, Madsen R. An instrument to measure symptom experience. Symptom occurrence and symptom distress. Cancer Nurs 2000; 23:49–54.

105. Morrow GR. The assessment of nausea and vomiting. Past problems, current issues and suggestions for future research. Cancer 1984; 53:2267–2278.

106. Lindley CM, Hirsch JD, O'Neill CV, et al. Quality of life consequences of chemotherapy-induced emesis. Qual Life Res 1992; 1:331–340.

107. Portenoy RK, Thaler HT, Kornblith AB, et al. The Memorial Symptom Assessment Scale: an instrument for the evaluation of symptom prevalence, characteristics and distress. Eur J Cancer 1994; 9:1326–1336.

108. McDaniel RW, Rhodes VA. Symptom experience. Semin Oncol Nurs 1995; 11:232–234.

109. Rhodes VA, McDaniel RW. The Index of Nausea, Vomiting, and Retching: a new format of the Index of Nausea and Vomiting. Oncol Nurs Forum 1999; 26:889–894.

110. Börjeson S , Hursti TJ, Peterson C, et al. Similarities and differences in assessing nausea on a verbal category scale and a visual analogue scale. Cancer Nurs 1997; 20:260–266.

111. Jederud C, Börjeson S, Andersson B, et al. Development of LINES – a quality assurance system for evaluation of nausea and emesis following chemotherapy. 3rd European Oncology Nursing Society, Venice, Italy, 2002.

112. Gralla RJ, Itri LM, Pisko SE, et al. Antiemetic efficacy of high-dose metoclopramide: randomized trials with placebo and prochlorperazine in patients with chemotherapy-induced nausea and vomiting. N Engl J Med 1981; 305:905–909.

113. Gralla RJ, Navari RM, Hesketh PJ, et al. Single-dose oral granisetron has equivalent antiemetic efficacy to intravenous ondansetron for highly emetogenic cisplatin-based chemotherapy. J Clin Oncol 1998; 16:1568–1573.

114. Olver IN. Aprepitant in antiemetic combinations to prevent chemotherapy-induced nausea and vomiting. Int J Clin Pract 2004; 58:201–206.

115. ESMO Guidelines Task Force. ESMO Recommendations for prophylaxis of chemotherapy-induced nausea and vomiting (NV). Ann Oncol 2001; 12:1059–1060.

116. Börjeson, S. Creating practical antiemetic guidelines. EONS Newsletter 2002; September:4–5.

117. Arakawa S. (1997). Relaxation to reduce nausea, vomiting, and anxiety induced by chemotherapy in Japanese patients. Cancer Nurs 1997; 20:342–349.

118. Carey MP, Burish TG. Providing relaxation training to cancer chemotherapy patients: a comparison of three delivery techniques. J Consult Clin Psychol 1987; 55:732–737.

119. Cheung YL, Molassiotis A, Chang AM. The effect of progressive muscle relaxation training on anxiety and quality of life after stoma surgery in colorectal cancer patients. Psycho-Oncology 2003; 12:254–266.

120. Burish TG, Carey MP, Krozely MG, Greco FA. Conditioned side effects induced by cancer chemotherapy: prevention through behavioural treatment. J Consult Clin Psychol 1987; 55:42–48.

121. Troesch LM, Rodehaver CB, Delaney EA, Yanes B. The influence of guided imagery on chemotherapy-related nausea and vomiting. Oncol Nurs Forum 1993; 20:1179–1185.

122. King JV. A holistic technique to lower anxiety: relaxation with guided imagery. J Holist Nurs 1988; 6:16–20.

123. Burish TG, Jenkins RA. Effectiveness of biofeedback and relaxation training in reducing the side effects of cancer chemotherapy. Health Psychol 1992; 11:17–23.

124. Morrow GR, Asbury R, Hammon S, et al. Comparing the effectiveness of behavioural treatment for chemotherapy-induced nausea and vomiting when administered by oncologists, oncology nurses, and clinical psychologists. Health Psychol 1992; 11:250–256.

125. Enqvist B, Bjorkland C, Engman M, Jakobsson J. Preoperative hypnosis reduced postoperative vomiting after surgery of the breasts. A prospective, randomized and blinded study. Acta Anaesthesiol Scand 1997; 41:1028–1032.

126. Syrjala KL, Cummings C, Donaldson GW. Hypnosis or cognitive behavioural training for the reduction of pain and nausea during cancer treatment: a controlled clinical trial. Pain 1992; 48:137–146.

127. Vasterling J, Jenkins R, Matt Tope D, Burish TG. Cognitive distraction and relaxation training for the control of side effects due to cancer chemotherapy. J Behav Med 1993; 16:65–80.

128. Redd WH, Jacobsen PB, Die-Trill M, et al. Cognitive/attentional distraction in the control of conditioned nausea in pediatric cancer patients receiving chemotherapy. J Consult Clin Psychol 1987; 55:391–395.

129. Frank JM. The effects of music therapy and guided visual imagery on chemotherapy induced nausea and vomiting. Oncol Nurs Forum 1985; 12:47–52.

130. Burns SJI, Harbuz MS, Hucklebridge F, Bunt L. A pilot study into the therapeutic effects of music therapy at a cancer help center. Altern Ther Health Med 2001; 7:48–56.

131. Ezzone S, Baker C, Rosselet R, Terepka E. Music as an adjunct to antiemetic therapy. Oncol Nurs Forum 1998; 25:1551–1556.

132. Lerman C, Rimer B, Blumberg B, et al. Effects of coping style and relaxation on cancer chemotherapy side effects and emotional responses. Cancer Nurs 1990; 13:308–315.

133. Burish TG, Snyder SL, Jenkins RA. Preparing patients for cancer chemotherapy: effect of coping preparation and relaxation interventions. J Consult Clin Psychol 1991; 59:518–525.

134. Gaston-Johansson F, Fall-Dickson J, Nanda J, et al. The effectiveness of the comprehensive coping strategy program on clinical outcomes in breast cancer autologous bone marrow transplantation. Cancer Nurs 2000; 23:277–285.

135. Tyc VL, Mulhern RK, Jayawardene D, Fairclough D. Chemotherapy-induced nausea and emesis in pediatric cancer patients: an analysis of coping strategies. J Pain Symptom Manage 1995; 10:338–347.

136. Van Fleet S. Relaxation and imagery for symptom management: improving patient assessment and individualizing treatment. Oncol Nurs Forum 2000; 27:501–510.

137. Foltz AT. Nutritional disturbances. In:. Yarbro H, Frogge MH, Goodman M, Groenwald SL, eds. Cancer nursing: principles and practice. Boston: Jones and Bartlett; 2000:754–775.

138. Wickham RS, Rehwaldt M, Kefer C, et al. Taste changes experienced by patients receiving chemotherapy. Oncol Nurs Forum 1999; 26:697–706.

139. Vickers AJ. Can acupuncture have specific effects on health? A systematic review of acupuncture antiemesis trials. J R Soc Med 1996; 89:303–311.

140. Shen J, Wegner N, Glaspy J, et al. Electroacupuncture for control of myeloablative chemotherapy-induced emesis: a randomized controlled trial. JAMA 2000; 284:2755–2761.

141. Dibble SL, Chapman J, Mack KA, Shih A. Acupressure for nausea: results of a pilot study. Oncol Nurs Forum 2000; 27:41–47.

142. Roscoe JA, Morrow GR, Bushunow P, Tian L, Matteson S. Acustimulation wristbands for the relief of chemotherapy-induced nausea. Altern Ther Health Med 2002; 8:56–63.

143. Pearl ML, Fischer M, McCauley DL, Valea FA, Chalas E. Transcutaneous electrical nerve stimulation as an adjunct for controlling chemotherapy-induced nausea and vomiting in gynecologic oncology patients. Cancer Nurs 1999; 22:307–311.

144. Grealish L, Lomansney A, Whiteman B. Foot massage: a nursing intervention to modify the distressing symptoms of pain and nausea in patients hospitalized with cancer. Cancer Nurs 2000; 23:237–243.

145. Musty RE, Rossi R. Effects of smoked cannabis and oral tetrahydocannabinol on nausea and emesis after cancer chemotherapy: a review of state clinical trials. J Cannabis Therapeutics 2000; 1:29–42.

146. Rusthoven JJ, Osoba D, Butts CA, et al. The impact of postchemotherapy nausea and vomiting on quality of life after moderately emetogenic chemotherapy. Support Care Cancer 1998; 6:389–395.

147. Bernhard J, Maibach R, Thülimann B, Sessa C, Aapro MS. Patients' estimation of overall treatment burden: Why not ask the obvious? J Clin Oncol 2002; 20:65–72.

148. Bliss JM, Robertson B, Selby PJ. The impact of nausea and vomiting upon quality of life measures. Br J Cancer 1992; 66(Suppl. XIX):S14–S23.

149. Dranitsaris G, Leung P, Ciotti R, et al. Implementing evidence based antiemetic guidelines in the oncology setting: results of a 4-month prospective intervention study. Support Care Cancer 2001; 9:611–618.

CHAPTER 21

Pain

Emile Maassen and Elisabeth Patiraki

CHAPTER CONTENTS

Introduction	439	Treatment options on the basis of pain assessment	452
The importance of controlling cancer pain	440	Improving the quality of care of patients with cancer pain	465
Definition(s) of pain	440	Quality assurance in the treatment of cancer pain	465
Epidemiology of cancer pain	440	Standards, guidelines and critical pathways	466
Theories and mechanisms of pain	441	Improving pain management	467
Types and causes of pain in cancer patients	444	Pain in specific patient populations	467
Total pain: the multiple dimensions of cancer pain	447	Educational interventions for improving knowledge of nurses, patients and caregivers	469
Consequences of unrelieved cancer pain	448	Conclusion	471
Effective cancer pain management	449	References	472
The assessment and documentation of pain	449		

INTRODUCTION

Despite advances in knowledge and technology, pain management continues to challenge oncology nurses and other healthcare professionals. In an effort to improve pain management, the focus of nurses has shifted in recent years from managing the individual patient's pain to a broader institutional perspective. As members of interdisciplinary teams involved in practice, administration, education and research, nurses are pivotal to improving pain outcomes. This requires nurses to become more knowledgeable, be up to date with the many advances in pain management and be capable of working in interdisciplinary teams to change institutional practices. As cancer pain poses such a significant burden worldwide, this chapter will explore what constitutes the significance of this problem: the available pharmacological and non-pharmacological therapeutic options on the basis of individualized pain assessment and their limitations as well as innovative ways that enhance the quality of care in patients with cancer.

A large part of the chapter will be devoted to the pathophysiology of pain, because understanding the mechanisms and causes of cancer pain provides nurses with the rationale for decision-making, dispels common misconceptions and helps nurses to overcome the barriers they often face. A section of the chapter will discuss the Pain Arch Model, which provides an example of a framework that enables healthcare providers to define the 'path' that the pain follows, identify the appropriate therapies and interventions and select the most appropriate methods or tools to evaluate their effectiveness. The need for quality improvement processes to monitor and ultimately ameliorate the quality of the care provided and educational interventions for improving the knowledge of nurses, patients and caregivers will also be discussed. Throughout the chapter cancer pain is viewed as an emergency and cancer pain relief as a professional mandate and challenge for every individual nurse.

THE IMPORTANCE OF CONTROLLING CANCER PAIN

Definition(s) of pain

Many different definitions of pain are used in everyday life; definitions used by healthcare professionals, general (linguistic) definitions and individual definitions. Every one of these tries to describe the essence of pain. In 1986, the World Health Organization (WHO) adopted the definition of pain from the International Association for the Study of Pain (IASP), which was formulated by Merskey et al in 1979.[1] It states 'pain is an unpleasant sensory and emotional experience associated with actual or potential tissue damage, or described in terms of such damage'. In order to determine if someone has pain, the person has to describe his sensory and emotional experience as unpleasant and in terms of (actual or potential) tissue damage. Within the nursing profession, a well-recognized definition by McCaffery[2] has been widely used for many years. McCaffery states that 'pain is whatever the experiencing person says it is, existing whenever the experiencing person says it does'. Therefore the diagnosis of 'pain' relies on the information provided by 'the experiencing person'.

Every definition of pain has its limitations. The limitation of the WHO definition lies primarily in the addition of the word 'unpleasant'. The word 'unpleasant refers only to the negative-affective aspects of pain, omitting its effect on behavioural responses. That same 'unpleasant experience' makes people cry, scream, curse, seek or demand help, seclude themselves from their significant others or even commit suicide. Also the addition '. . . or described in terms of such damage' can rule out the most frequent pain in Western society: *headache*. It is seldom associated with actual or potential tissue damage, but more often with stress. The use of adjectives and their meanings differ greatly among persons, countries, generations or cultures.[3] The awareness of these differences contributes to the understanding of its underlying message.

Melzack and Wall said that the diversity of pain experiences explains why it has been impossible, so far, to achieve a satisfactory definition of pain. At present, we must be content with guidelines *towards* a definition rather than a definition itself.[4] With regard to this last sentence, the 'guideline' from McCaffery is very useful. Only the patient can lead us to the definition of his experience of pain, so a precondition is that we need to ask the patient in order to learn what pain is to him. The way a patient defines or describes his pain can be regarded as a message that is definitive or not. Nevertheless, the members of a multidisciplinary team may well interpret that message differently. This can result in a delay in treatment, and therefore suboptimal care. An initiative to eliminate this risk of miscommunication amongst healthcare workers is to reach an understanding within the professional team on one common definition and vision of pain. Together with a multidisciplinary assessment tool, it facilitates optimal pain management. Also, as important as the definition of pain, is the definition of *pain management*. In 1994, nurses in the Netherlands reached a consensus,[5] defining 'pain management as the prevention, and if this is not possible, the termination, or at least the alleviation of pain'. This definition prioritizes specifically the order of goals in pain management (Box 21.1).

Epidemiology of cancer pain

Pain is one of the most common symptoms experienced by patients with cancer through the course of their disease.[6] Cancer pain is a widely recognized serious worldwide problem.[7,8] The magnitude of this problem reflects our failure to recognize and treat it effectively, since pain remains persistently among

Prioritization of goals in pain management[5]

1. Prevention
People instantly assess risks and decide what would be the best way to prevent tissue damage. Prevention is omnipresent in the acting/activities of persons, both patients and healthcare workers.

2. Termination
If at any time prevention fails or was not possible, the next treatment goal would be to terminate the pain. This can be achieved through cure of the underlying cause and/or by symptom management, so that the patient is pain-free.

3. Alleviation
If the first two steps are not achievable, the only treatment option left is to reduce pain as much as possible.

the major problems reported by hospitalized individuals.[9–11] Although large-scale epidemiological studies of the incidence and severity of cancer pain are lacking, reviews of numerous studies in specialized cancer care settings have demonstrated that the prevalence of pain increases with the progression of disease.[12,13] Existing studies suggest that as many as 30–40% of patients with cancer at the time of diagnosis and 65–85% undergoing treatment or in the terminal phase of disease have unrelieved pain.[14–16] Other studies have demonstrated that up to 77% of patients with advanced disease report pain of severe intensity, and 70–80% experience more than one pain syndrome and have numerous causes of pain.[17,18] Results from a recent study in the Netherlands documented that the majority of patients with cancer reported their average pain intensity to be at least moderate.[19] It is estimated that 50% of patients of Western societies and 90% of those living in undeveloped countries continue to experience unacceptable levels of pain.[20] Nowadays, it is frustrating to find that patients with cancer continue to experience some degree of pain even during the last period of their life. Several studies examining family members of patients with cancer include increased number of reports that their loved ones suffered severe pain in the last weeks of their life.[21,22]

Theories and mechanisms of pain

Pain is a fundamental protective mechanism or warning system that is activated in response to potential or actual tissue damage.[23] Its primary function is to draw attention, or demand care for a wound, or force people to take some rest. These reactions are aimed at preventing the injury becoming worse and/or stimulating the process of healing.

Pain models

In the history of mankind, there has always been a need to explain pain, as it is connected with suffering.[3] With limited knowledge of physiology, the need to give meaning to suffering could only be provided by a higher power such as religion. The word 'pain' is derived from the Latin word 'Puna', which means punishment. In religious scriptures like The Bible, many examples of the guilty and not guilty suffering can be found. One of the oldest known explanations of pain comes from Hippocrates (460–370BC), who argued that any disturbance at the four elements of the body (light, air, earth and water) caused pain.[24,25] Later, Aristotle (384–322 BC) explained pain as an emotion like joy.[26] Almost two millennia later, Descartes[27] explained pain by a model that still is referred to as 'the rope–bell model'. Scientists like Müller[28] and Frey[29] in the 19th century discovered more about the working of the nervous system. Their contribution to our knowledge of pain was that there is no specific nerve type or system for pain. Receptors of all nerve types play a role in the detection of (noxious) stimuli through transduction, which is one of the five phases in the process of awareness to a sensible sensation. Noordenbos[30] proposed a model based on the presence of parallel fibre systems – also called the 'evolution model'. In the process of transmission of information to the brain, 'fast' A fibres at any level within the nervous system (NS) can most often inhibit information passed through by 'slow' C fibres. This means that fast fibre activity runs ahead of slow fibre activity. It can alarm the central nervous system (CNS) of the arrival of nociceptive information from slow fibres.

The gate control theory by Melzack and Wall[31] takes it one step further. The alarming of the CNS by fast A fibres can also result in 'feedback' from the so-called decision stations that in return regulate the transmission of information to the brain (gate control theory). Information passes through several of these stations, where it is selected and filtered on the basis of other information like sensory and motor activity and memory.

Mechanisms of pain

There is some overlap in definitions of pain, nociception and suffering. However, the neural mechanisms of nociception and pain have been examined extensively, whereas the neural mechanisms of suffering are virtually unknown. Although pain is associated with emotional, cognitive and learned behaviours, two anatomical sites are essential for pain processing: the primary sensory neurons and the dorsal horn of the spinal cord, where sensory neurons make synaptic connections.[32] The pain process comprises five major phases: transduction, transmission, modulation, perception and projection (Fig. 21.1).

The first step in the pain process is transduction. Noxious stimuli provoking tissue damage are either mechanical (pressure), chemical (both endogenous and/or exogenous) or thermal (cold or heat). All pain due to tissue damage is reducible to one of these factors. The severity of tissue damage is responsible for the release of substances from the bloodstream or from within the tissue cell. These substances are primarily potassium, prostaglandin and bradykinin, which sensitize (activate) free nerve endings[35] (Fig. 21.2). A secondary risk factor for pain is the damage of nerve tissue. This tissue damage can result in different types of neuropathic pain.

Nociceptors are a heterogeneous group of neurons that differ on a variety of factors ranging from the neurotransmitters and receptors they contain to their response to noxious stimuli and conduction of action potentials following activation. They are classified to A fibre nociceptors (Aβ, A delta), mediating fast prickly pain, and C fibre nociceptors, mediating slow burning pain.[36] The dualism of pain between the different nerve fibres can be experienced in everyday life. For example, at a venepuncture site A fibres transmit information quickly and carry so-called 'first pain'.[37] Sensitized by the noxious stimulus of the puncture, this results in a sharp, well-localized pain for a relatively short period of time.[34] C fibres transmit information slowly. Sensitized by that same stimulus, this results in diffuse dull pain that can last for hours to days. Once the noxious stimuli have been transduced and the primary afferent nociceptor (PAN) action potential has been generated, the action potential must be transmitted to and through the CNS before pain is perceived. Nociceptive sig-

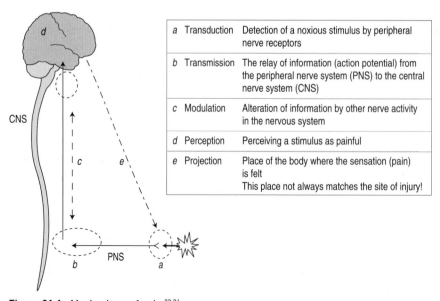

a	Transduction	Detection of a noxious stimulus by peripheral nerve receptors
b	Transmission	The relay of information (action potential) from the peripheral nerve system (PNS) to the central nerve system (CNS)
c	Modulation	Alteration of information by other nerve activity in the nervous system
d	Perception	Perceiving a stimulus as painful
e	Projection	Place of the body where the sensation (pain) is felt. This place not always matches the site of injury!

Figure 21.1: Mechanisms of pain.[33,34]

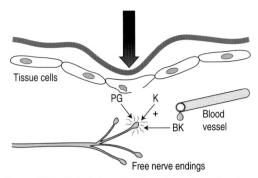

Figure 21.2: Principles of nociceptive pain: potassium (K), prostaglandin (P) and bradykinin (BK).[35]

nal transmission is accomplished in three steps: (1) projector to the CNS, (2) processing within the dorsal horn of the spinal cord and (3) transmission to the brain. The precise location at which pain is perceived is unclear. Some authors indicate that perception is at the thalamus but others suggest that pain perception is at cerebral levels.[38]

A growing body of evidence suggests that pain is not a static or passive consequence of defined peripheral input, but rather an active process that is generated partially in the peripheral nervous system (PNS) and partially in the CNS, and then subsequently transferred to a pain centre within the brain.[39] Pain results from diverse mechanisms that occur either solely in one condition or are expressed in multiple syndromes at different times.[40]

Neurobiology of pain

Recent breakthroughs in our understanding of pain mechanisms can be traced to the introduction of molecular biology techniques into pain research. New ion channel proteins involved in generating, modulating and propagating action potential along nociceptor axons have been cloned and characterized using molecular biology techniques. These techniques continue to reveal nociceptive mechanisms involving molecules, receptors and neural networks that underlie neural reorganization (plasticity) in the spinal cord and brainstem after peripheral tissue damage or nerve injury.[41]

Under acute pain conditions, nociceptor response is stable and the pain sensation is reflective of the intensity, localization and duration of the stimulus. Conversely, with chronic pain, repeated stimulation or modification in the chemical milieu surrounding the nociceptors leads to hypersensitivity at the site of damage and in the surrounding area.[42] Inflammatory and neuropathic pain are characterized by this hypersensitivity, which may be irreversible depending on nociceptor sensitivity and responsiveness, alterations in ion channel conduction and the degree of disinhibition. Neurotransmitters, nerve factors, molecular processes, receptors and phenotypic neuron expression contribute to the sensation known as pain and its reversible or intractable nature.[23]

Pain that occurs during inflammation is related to an increase in noxious inputs peripherally and to central sensitization.[43] Not only do inflammatory cells trigger sensitization of primary afferent neurons in the periphery, but they also produce chemical signals that penetrate the CNS and generate cyclooxygenase (COX),[43] which is involved in the synthesis of prostaglandins. Two COX enzymes, COX-1 and COX-2, compromise the COX pathway and contribute to inflammation and the synthesis of prostaglandins. A second important pathway involved in peripheral nociceptor sensitization is the lypoxygenase (LOX), which plays a critical role in inducing the synthesis of proinflammatory mediators such as interleukin-8 and platelet activating factor.[44] Some inflammatory mediators directly activate nociceptor terminals and others sensitize them by reducing their transduction thresholds. One of the many molecules expressed by nociceptors that has been implicated recently in this action is the tetrodoxin (TTX) resistant sodium channel, which is medicated by activation of intracellular kinases and increases in intracellular calcium.[45] Vanilloid receptors, temperature-sensitive ion channels, participate in the sensation of inflammatory pain and play an important role in peripheral sensitization.[43] Central sensitization is a process driven by activation of intracellular signal transduction cascades, an increase in neuronal membrane synaptic excitability and a loss of pain inhibition.[23] A key receptor involved in central sensitization is the N-methyl-D-aspartate (NMDA) receptor critical for the development of hyperalgesia and the maintenance of pathological pain following inflammation or nerve injury.[43]

443

Peripheral nerve injury leads to complex changes in sensory neurons. Nerve injury also causes synaptic reorganization, whereby the low threshold Aβ fibre neurons, whose axons normally terminate in the deep dorsal horn, begin to grow into lamina II, which normally receives only nociceptive information from C fibres that terminate there. This change results in mechanical allodynia (touch is interpreted as pain). The changed synaptic connectivity may play an important role in the intractable nature of many neuropathic pain syndromes.[39]

Types and causes of pain in cancer patients

Types of pain

General classification of pain by neurophysiological (Table 21.1) and temporal characteristics (Table 21.2) provides clinicians with invaluable information about the possible origin of a pain, its possible treatment sensitiveness and therefore goal. However, cancer pain is viewed as a multidimensional phenomenon; therefore, these classifications are rather crude as they only

Table 21.1: Neurophysiological classification[35,46–50]	
Nociceptive pain	**Pain due to activation of nociceptors (A delta and C fibres) by noxious stimuli**
a Somatic pain	Tissue damage to skin, muscles, tendons or bones can result in somatic pain that is mostly well localized or 'projected'
b Visceral pain (Unreferred pain)	Tissue damage to organs within the abdominal or thoracic cavity can result in visceral pain that is often described as 'deep, diffuse pain' around the effected organ
Referred pain[a]	Visceral pain is felt in a place other than the affected organ, mostly in a dermatome or myotome (part of the skin or a muscle that is innervated by one nerve branch). Their nerves connect at the same level with the central nervous system as the affected organ. Due to this misinterpretation pain is projected to a different but related site that does not match with the site of injury
Neuropathic pain	**Pain as the result of neural injury or irritation in either the PNS or CNS**
a Peripheral neuropathic pain	Nerve compression (carpal tunnel syndrome, Pan Coast syndrome); root compression (hernia nucleous pulposa); neuralgia, neuromata (stump pain); phantom pain; polyneuropathies (diabetes) and plexus avulsion
b Central neuropathic pain	Cerebral or spinal lesions by CVA, SAH, trauma, complications of (diagnostic) procedures/neurosurgery, tumour/metastases, infection/abscess, thalamus syndrome or spinal ischaemic conditions
c Deafferentation pain	Deafferentation pain caused by the interruption of normal nerve input can be seen as an advanced form of neuropathic pain. In reaction to this sensory loss, the nervous system tries to establish a new balance within the CNS. If this balance cannot be restored it will result in almost incurable pain despite the absence of noxious stimuli (phantom limb, brachial plexus avulsion).
Psychogenic pain	**Pain presumed to exist when no nociceptive or neuropathic mechanism can be identified next to psychological symptoms like depression. This classification is controversial.**

[a]This phenomenon is also seen in deep somatic pain.

Table 21.2: Temporal classification of pain[51-53]

Pain	Description
Acute pain	Sudden onset Sharp Often direct relation with tissue damage Relation with the progress of the healing process Well projected to the site of injury Well reacting to non- and pharmacological peripheral acting therapies
Chronic pain	Slow onset Often no direct relation with tissue damage Existing longer than the duration of the expected healing process (> 6 months) Not well projected to site of injury/deep diffuse pain Poorly reacting to non- and pharmacological peripherally acting therapies
Constant	A frequently unpredictable (periodic) recurrence of pain on a background of absence of pain, or periodic absence of normally stable chronic pain
Intermittent	A frequently (periodic) recurrence of pain on a background of absence of pain, or periodic absence of normally stable chronic pain
Breakthrough	A transitory exacerbation of pain that occurs on a background of otherwise stable persistent pain
Incidental	Due to specific activity such as eating, defecation, walking, socializing
Spontaneous or idiopathic pain exacerbation	Not linked to scheduled analgesic dose and occurs at the end of dosing interval of around the clock opioid therapy

apply to mechanisms and components of the physiological and sensory dimension.

Nociceptive pain (predominately acute pain) is initiated when intense or damaging noxious stimuli activate nociceptors of primary sensory neurons. The pain continues as long as the noxious stimulus persists or until healing occurs. The pain is typically localized and initially is sharp but then becomes dull and aching. Visceral pain is usually purely localized and is perceived as a deep crampy, squeezing pain. The patient with acute pain could have autonomic symptoms such as diaphoresis, nausea and vomiting.[54]

Neuropathic pain is pain that arises from the nervous system. It can be the result of an increase in afferent information (towards the brain) by either excitation or disinhibition. It can also be caused by compression of a nerve or nerve structure[55] by a tumour, oedema, haematoma, abscess, blood vessel, hernia, scar tissue or foreign body. The pain continues after the noxious stimulus is thought to have dissipated. It is perceived as burning, numbing, stabbing, shooting or electric-like. It can be very distressing to patients not only because of its seemingly neverending, sickening quality, but because, managing this type of pain is difficult and frustrating.[54] Diagnosis depends upon (1) the neuroanatomical distribution of pain and (2) by evidence of sensory dysfunction involving peripheral nerves, plexus, nerve root or central pathway. If the affected nerve or pathway is mixed motor and sensory, then

445

weakness muscle atrophy or reflex abnormalities may provide additional clues to neural involvement. Impaired sensation is often evident during a central examination. Sensory dysfunction may be manifested as hypo- and/or hyperaesthesia for one or more modalities, increasing pain to normally painful stimuli (hyperalgesia) or pain due to normally non-painful stimuli (allodynia). Temporal and spatial sensory dysfunctions are also common. However, there are few carefully designed treatment trials for neurogenic pain.[56]

Breakthrough pain may be caused by somatic, visceral or neuropathic pathophysiology, and it is most often related to the same mechanism that causes persistent pain.[57] The main characteristics of breakthrough pain are rapid onset, often paroxysmal (peaking in intensity within 3 minutes), short duration (1–240 minutes), moderate to severe intensity and with relatively low daily frequency.[53] Breakthrough pain may be classified according to precipitating events. When flares of pain are associated with movement or activity, this is described as incident pain, with most common triggers being walking, sitting up, coughing and defecating.[58] When breakthrough pain is not linked to scheduled analgesic doses and not related to movement or function, it is called spontaneous or idiopathic breakthrough pain. Finally, end-of-dose failures are termed pain exacerbations and typically occur at the end of the dosing interval of an around the clock opioid therapy.

Causes and classification of cancer pain

The pain seen in patients with cancer is pathophysiologically and biochemically similar to, but aetiologically and clinically different from, the pain seen in other individuals.[59] Cancer pain is either nociceptive or neuropathic; it can be acute, chronic or intermittent and is rarely accompanied by signs of sympathetic nervous system arousal.[60] A well-recognized phenomenon in patients with cancer is the concept of breakthrough pain. The prevalence among patients with cancer ranges from approximately 51% to 90%.[53] In the only prospective study found, breakthrough pain was reported by 80% of patients with cancer.[61] Most patients will feel pain of varying duration and degree at

some point during their cancer experience. Furthermore, patients often have more than one pain at a time. Foley's[62] classification of individuals suffering from cancer pain is helpful to healthcare workers in managing the multidimensional issues occurring in these patients. She groups patients with cancer into one of the following five groups:

1. Patients with acute cancer-related pain associated with diagnosis or cancer therapy (surgery, chemotherapy, radiotherapy)

2. Patients with chronic cancer-related pain associated with cancer progression or cancer therapy

3. Patients with pre-existing chronic pain and cancer-related pain

4. Patients with a history of drug administration and cancer-related pain, including patients actively involved in illicit drug use, in a methadone maintenance programme or with a past history of drug abuse

5. Dying patients with cancer-related pain.

A common useful classification of cancer pain is by its organic aetiology.[63] Tumours cause pain by invading, destroying or compressing the affected area. The most common cause of cancer-related pain is bone metastasis from cancer of the breast, lung or prostate.[64] The three major causes are cancer itself, anticancer treatment and causes unrelated to either tumour or treatment (Box 21.2). In addition, various physical (immobility, insomnia, constipation, diarrhoea, wounds, dysphagia, urinary retention), psychosocial (social isolation, anxiety, depression, fear, hopelessness, economic problems, unwanted role changes) and environmental factors (noise, restraints, too hot or too cold temperature, dislike of facility, lack of privacy) can negatively influence the pain experience.[54]

The uniqueness of cancer pain results from the likelihood that a person will be experiencing pain from more than one aetiology, at more than one site, causing more than one pain syndrome manifested in varied patterns, intensities and duration.[59]

Box 21.2

Causes of pain in patients with cancer[13,54,63,65]

The disease
Pain due to direct tumour involvement
Primary or metastatic bone disease
Tumour invading viscera or fungating through mucous membranes
Nerve compression or infiltration (tumour invasion of the brachial or lumbo-sacral plexus, post-herpetic neuralgia)

Anticancer therapy
Diagnostic interventions: biopsy, injection, dressings change, positioning on hard table
Nursing procedures: injection, venepuncture, dressing change, movement of painful body parts
Delivery of treatment:
- post-surgical pain: acute postoperative pain, chronic pain syndromes (post-mastectomy pain, post-radical neck dissection pain, stump and phantom limb pain)
- chemotherapy syndromes: headache, oral mucositis, musculoskeletal pain and corticosteroid pain
- post-radiation pain syndromes oropharyngeal mucositis, radiation enteritis and proctocolitis, fibrosis of nerve plexus and painful peripheral neuropathy, osteoradionecrosis
- post-biotherapy pain: myalgia/arthralgia, neuropathy
- pain associated with inflammation, pain related to reflex activity, nerve compression and deafferentation pain

Unrelated to disease or treatment
Pain indirectly associated with cancer: pain due to bedsores, muscle spasm, constipation, deep vein thrombosis, candidiasis and herpetic and post-herpetic neuralgia
Pre-existing, painful conditions: degenerative arthritis, diabetic peripheral neuropathy, migraines or other non-malignant pain conditions

Total pain: the multiple dimensions of cancer pain

Cancer pain originates in noxious physical pathology, but is modified by a number of factors. The complexities of the pain experience are reflected in the multiplicity of theories that have arisen to describe it. Starting from LeShan's work[66] examining 'the universe of the patient in chronic pain', a growing body of research data and clinical observations have further clarified many of the factors that influence the experience of pain in the patient with cancer. It has become increasingly evident that pain may be most helpfully viewed not as solely a 'physical' or 'emotional' pain but as a total experience. Saunders coined the term 'total pain'[67] to describe the all-encompassing nature of intractable cancer pain and the need to assess and treat all of its components; physical–psychological–interpersonal–financial–spiritual (Fig. 21.3).

It has long been appreciated that the perceived meaning of pain modifies the pain experience. Cancer pain may simultaneously have a cognitive meaning, an affective meaning, a bodily meaning and a transcendent or spiritual meaning for the patient.[68] Moreover, Saunders dictum that the patient and family, rather than the patient alone, must be seen as the unit of care[67] is well founded on research data demonstrating significant marital difficulties between patients with chronic pain and their spouses.[69] Failure to assess what pain means to the patient and family and what the family dynamics are, before a therapeutic plan is developed, would be negligent. Nowadays, provision of palliative care to relieve pain and suffering is based on the conceptual model of the whole person experiencing total pain. The various components must be addressed simultaneously. Physical aspects of pain cannot be treated in isolation from other aspects, nor can patients' anxieties be effectively addressed when patients are suffering physically. Relief from pain should therefore be seen as part of a comprehensive pattern of care encompassing the physical, psychological, social and spiritual aspects of suffering.[67]

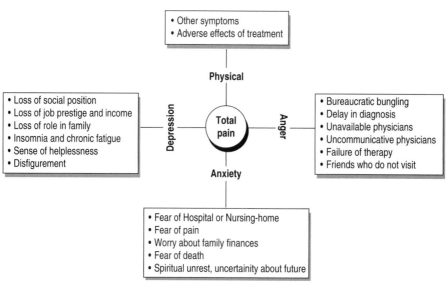

Figure 21.3: Total pain concept. (Reproduced with permission from Twycross R. Pain relief in advanced cancer. Edinbugh: Churchill Livingstone; 1994:28.)

The conceptualization of pain as a multidimensional phenomenon is based on the work of several researchers over the last three decades.[70-73] Ahles et al[71] were the first to examine cancer-related pain from a multidisciplinary point of view. Expanding the conceptual model proposed by Melzack and Casey,[70] they hypothesized five separate components of the cancer pain experience:

- physiological (organic causes of pain)
- sensory (intensity, location, quality)
- affective (anxiety, depression, modus states, locus of control)
- cognitive (thought processes, views of self, meaning of pain)
- behavioural (communication of pain, activity level, use of medications).

Additionally, a sixth dimension, 'socio-cultural' (ethnic background, demographic variables) was added by McGuire[72] and a seventh dimension, 'spiritual', is proposed by Spross and Burke to present a more complete picture of factors affecting the perception and interpretation of pain.[74]

This multifactorial perspective provides the foundation for assessing and ultimately managing pain. Each of the dimensions of cancer pain

requires different approaches, actions and the input from various healthcare providers. This multidisciplinary approach to pain control is recommended by the WHO,[8,75] referring to a team that includes doctors, nurses and other health professionals, each bringing their own expertise. Nurses are key workers in this process as they spend more time than any other member of the team with the person in pain. They are in the most prominent position to support, inform and empower the patient with cancer and their families to alleviate their pain and suffering,[76] as the assessment of the patient is centred on understanding and responding to the needs of the whole person as a unique individual.[77]

Consequences of unrelieved cancer pain

The effect of cancer pain in terms of suffering, disability and declining quality of life is high.[78] It is estimated that one-third of adults with metastatic cancer report pain that reduces their activity level, and requires the use of analgesics.[63] Unrelieved pain can further weaken the already debilitated patients. Uncontrolled pain merits a high priority not only for those with advanced disease but also for the patients whose condition is stable, or their life expectancy is long, because it prevents them from working productively, enjoying recreation or taking pleasure in their usual role in the family and society.[79]

The costs of uncontrolled pain are classified as physiological, psychological and economic.[80–82] The physiological costs include delays in recovery, impairment of immune function, impairment in movement, loss of appetite and sleep and possibly partial or complete disability. The various psychological costs incorporate anxiety, depression, frustration, hostility, loss of enjoyment in life, interference with relations and intimacy and even suicidal ideation. Economic costs consist of repeated hospital admissions and extended lengths of stay, unplanned visits and loss of income and insurance coverage. Pain reduces the patient's option to exercise control; it is a constant threat to self-image and life, and a lack of a basis for hope.[79] From the patient perspective, pain is a constant reminder of the disease and of death.[83] It worsens patients' helplessness, anxiety and depression. It can consume every aspect of their life and, consequently, exert a major influence on all dimensions of quality of life (physical well-being, psychological well-being and social and spiritual well-being).[84,85] The quality of life of patients with cancer with pain, and their family caregivers, is significantly worse than that of patients with cancer without pain.[86] Moreover, families of patients with cancer share the loss of control and suffering of their loved ones in pain. They also experience psychological and social stresses and impaired quality of life, while they have inadequate knowledge about pain management.[87]

EFFECTIVE CANCER PAIN MANAGEMENT

A multidisciplinary, multimodal approach to managing pain is the appropriate way to achieve optimal patient, family, caregiver and institutional outcomes.[72] Additionally, patients and their families or significant others should be active contributors in the process. In the Oncology Nursing Society's position paper on cancer pain, the key leadership and coordinating role of the nurse in the multidisciplinary

process of managing cancer pain is highlighted.[88] However, there are a number of common errors that can occur in the management of pain.[89] These can be divided into four categories (Box 21.3). Hence, preconditions for effective management of cancer pain are to work with the correct diagnosis; assess pain with the right tools; choose the proper combination of interventions; and evaluate pain regularly. Sound documentation contributes to the quality and continuity of care provided.[87]

The assessment and documentation of pain

Pain assessment is the cornerstone of pain management.[76] Collection of pain assessment data should be systematic, organized and ongoing. Incorporating a framework into the assessment process assists in obtaining data and identifying missing elements.[90] All the basic elements of assessment are included in the 1994 Agency for Health Care Policy and Research (AHCPR) guideline on the management of cancer pain.[15] Every patient with cancer experiencing pain has the right to expect an accurate, timely assessment of that pain experience and a concerted effort on the part of the involved caregivers to help patients find a way to adequately control the pain experienced.[91]

Box 21.3	
Common errors in pain management	
1st	Pain complaints remain unnoticed; therefore, the (nursing) diagnosis is not established
2nd	The individual pain is insufficiently analysed in relation to cause, appearance, meaning and consequences; the use of a (multidimensional) assessment tool is not common
3rd	Lack of knowledge about different pain interventions and their mechanism of action entails the risk of over- or undertreatment of pain
4th	Ignorance towards the mechanism of an action intervention will result in difficulty evaluating its effect

An initial comprehensive pain evaluation should include a detailed history, including an assessment of pain intensity and characteristics, a physical examination, a psychological and social assessment and a diagnostic evaluation of signs and symptoms associated with the common cancer pain syndromes.[92] A multidimensional assessment is usually interdisciplinary. If the setting does not provide for the team approach, nurses or doctors trained in pain assessment should be considered. Comprehensive assessment of certain dimensions of pain syndromes is often performed by various members of the team but nurses observe or collect data in all dimensions of pain.[83] According to Donovan, the eight dimensions considered to be essential for a thorough nursing assessment of pain are location, intensity, factors influencing the occurrence of pain, observed behaviours including vital signs, psychological and social modifiers, effects of pain, effects of therapy and established patterns of coping.[91] If nurses lack the time to complete long assessment tools, they should obtain at the very least information about the location and severity for each pain.

Assessment should primarily focus on the patient's perspective, but use of the significant other's input may be useful. The characteristics of each pain should be evaluated and the patient's perspective on the pain that is most distressing disruptive or disabling elicited. The nurse should note whether medications are being administered and taken as prescribed.[54] Privacy in a comfortable area is fundamental to the assessment process. Through minimizing distractions, interruptions and extraneous information, the process will take less time and be more productive. Other requirements include simple and easy assessment tools, reliable not time-consuming, and clearly understood tools that separately assess sensory-intensive and affective dimensions of pain.[93] Moreover, pain assessments should be documented clearly, completely and regularly.

Assessment instruments

The use of subjective self-reports of pain is recommended with the exception of individuals with cognitive impairment or problems with verbal ability precluding self-report.[83] There are many available unidimensional and multidimensional tools for pain assessment.[91,94] Unidimensional tools measure only one dimension of pain such as intensity, location, relief or observable indications, in contrast to multidimensional tools, which combine two or more dimensions of pain allowing assessment of sensory, affective and behavioural pain aspects. It should be remembered that not all dimensions are necessarily present or important in every patient with pain. The widely used and the simplest pain intensity scales in clinical practice are the numerical analogue scale (NAS), numerical graphic rating scale (NRS), verbal graphic rating scale (VGRS),[95] visual analogue scale (VAS)[96] and faces or Oucher scale.[97] It is reported that the most widely used and the simplest measures of pain are VAS and V(G)RS.[98] The 0–10 scale is more practical than 0–5 and 0–100 numerical scales.[54] Kremer et al compared the different types of scales and found that patients preferred the verbal pain rating scale.[99]

Different multidimensional questionnaires are designed to assess pain. Four instruments have been considered short enough for routine clinical use for patients with cancer: the Brief Pain Inventory, the Memorial Pain Assessment Card, the Short Form McGill Pain Questionnaire and the Edmonton Symptom Assessment Scale.[100–106]

The McGill Pain Questionnaire[101] (MPQ) was developed from a list of words describing the different qualities of pain. Three major classes (sensory, affective and evaluative) are subdivided into 20 subclasses. These classes are used to indicate perceptual attributes, emotional component and magnitude, respectively. A body drawing is provided to indicate the location of pain. The MPQ is sensitive for qualitative and quantitative measurements as well as for distinguishing acute from chronic pain. It has been extensively translated and evaluated in various countries. Acute pain scores higher in the sensory category, whereas chronic pain scores higher in the affective category. Controversy exists as to whether three categories are sufficient to establish stable validity; however, most evidence indicates that it is a valid test.[93] In 1987 Melzack developed the *MPQ-short form*, which includes 15 words, sensory, affective and total descriptors, to describe pain.[102]

The *Wisconsin Brief Pain Questionnaire* (BPQ) was designed to assess pain in cancer and other diseases. It has been evaluated with regard to both reliability and validity and proved to be sufficiently reliable and valid for research purposes.[103] The BPQ is shorter than the MPQ and devised specifically to assess patients with cancer pain.[55] From this questionnaire, a validated 'short form' was also developed, the Brief Pain Inventory or BPI-SF, which can be completed in 5–15 minutes. It is self-administered and has been translated into several languages.

The *Memorial Pain Assessment Card* (MPAC) is a brief validated measure that uses VAS scales to characterize pain intensity, pain relief and mood and an 8-point verbal rating score to further characterize pain intensity.[104]

The *Edmonton Symptom Assessment Scale* (ESAS) is a 9-item patient-rated symptom VAS developed for use in assessing the symptoms of patients receiving palliative care.[105] Some research[106] suggests that this is a simple and useful method for the regular assessment of symptom distress, including pain, in the palliative care setting.

Furthermore, *pain assessment charts* and *pain diaries* are useful tools in clinical practice to document the dynamic nature of cancer pain over a period of time. They have been shown to encourage communication between the patients, their family and health professionals.[54] Pain diaries can be of particular use in the community setting, if patients are well educated in reporting prompt changes in their pain.[76] Another useful way in which we can record patients' pain over a period of time is to use an integrated care pathway for pain.[211]

It is important to carefully select the appropriate tool for a given clinical environment and patient population. The instrument(s) of choice in pain assessment is determined by several factors:[94]

- the duration of pain (acute/chronic)
- the goal of measurement – adjustment of therapy/clinical research
- the patient himself – age/capacity to respond
- the psychometric properties of the instruments – reliability/validity
- realities of the clinical setting – time and staff availability/ability to score and use results.

Consistent use of a valid pain measurement scale by all disciplines can guide clinical decisions concerning additional assessment and therapy.

The pain-arch model

The pain-arch model is not an assessment instrument as such, but can be used as a pain management tool. The pain-arch model[89] was developed after merging the Van Cranenburg pain model[107] and the Dutch consensus conference 'Nursing on Pain'.[5] It is made up of 3 elements. On the two pillars Therapy and Evaluation rests the arch that consists of 5 levels (Fig. 21.4). In this model pain is regarded as a process where one or more steps can be identified as 'applicable' to the patient. In sequence these are risk, cause, awareness, experience and reaction. Each step corresponds with one of the five levels of the arch (Table 21.3).

The model enables healthcare workers to:

1. Define the steps applicable to their patient, also called 'the pain path'.
2. Identify therapies and interventions which are appropriate.
3. Select the proper methods of tools to evaluate the effect.

This 'path' is formed by a straight line from the dot in the centre of the arch to one of the numbers I up to IX inclusive. By reasoning out which subsequent levels apply to the patient in pain, the line should cross just these levels. This is done in opposite order, from the top level of 'pain behaviour' downwards. The assessment could take as little as 60 seconds. The levels involved correspond with forms of therapy that can be considered (Therapy – left pillar). Each intervention correlates with a specific assessment/evaluation method (Evaluation – right pillar). The effect of an intervention can be measured on the corresponding and higher levels.

This 'path' can be defined by reasoning out if a level applies to the patient in pain. This is done in opposite order, from the top level of 'pain behaviour' downwards. In the sector PAIN! the numbers IV, V and VI have in common that the

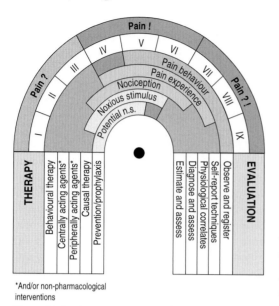

*And/or non-pharmacological interventions

Figure 21.4: The pain-arch model.[89]

levels 'pain experience', 'nociception' and 'noxious stimulus' are *always* involved. Sometimes the alarm sounds, although no actual damage to the body can be determined. If *no* potential and noxious stimulus can be indicated, the pain path ends in the sector PAIN?! (numbers VII, VIII or IX). This does not mean that the pain experienced is not real or has no function. Absence of pain is not always a question of a failing alarm system. A non-painful bruise on a patient, of which it is unclear how long it exists and how it

got there, would show a 'pain path' that ends in number II or III. In the sector PAIN? there is *never* a pain experience, and therefore no pain behaviour. One can wonder if pain one does not feel (minimal tissue damage) or cannot feel (failing alarm system) is really pain and therefore should be managed. Nevertheless, a potential or noxious stimulus can be treated with the corresponding interventions (prevention/prophylaxis and/or causal therapy) to prevent the exceeding of the pain threshold at a later stage.

Treatment options on the basis of pain assessment

The multidimensional framework of cancer-related pain provides an excellent conceptual approach to managing pain.[83] The IASP[108] has emphasized the need for multidisciplinary management of patients with chronic pain and for attention to the physical, psychological, social, vocational, recreational and other functional aspects of persons with pain-related disabilities. Next to prevention, the management of cancer-related pain may be divided into two distinct approaches: causal therapy (primary control of the disease process itself) and symptomatic management (pharmacological, invasive (reversible–irreversible) and non-pharmacological approaches).[109] The choice for any combination of therapies depends on the (contra-) indications, the availability of

Table 21.3: Pain-arch model[89]

Step	Level	Description
Risk	Potential noxious stimulus	Every stimulus that has the potential of damaging tissue but has not yet reached the body or has not yet arisen from the body
Cause	Noxious stimulus	Any stimulus that reaches the body or arises from the body and damages tissue
Awareness	Nociception	Signal that reaches the brain and is evoked by exposure to a noxious stimulus or, in absence, is perceived as such
Experience	Pain experience	Subjective experience of a painful sensation: intensity, time aspects (like duration), character, course and hindrance
Reaction	Pain behaviour	The numerous reactions & changes in behaviour evoked by pain that can be observed

therapy, the expertise by the caregivers and the acceptability by the patient.

Prevention/prophylactic therapy

Prevention is the best form of 'therapy' aimed to withhold a potential noxious stimulus from the body or to keep the body away from the stimulus. *Prophylactic* therapy is used preceding causal therapy when there is a strong suspicion that prevention will fail or cannot be achieved at all. For example, a prophylactic measure is the use of EMLA, a topical anaesthetic that can be applied on the skin previous to a painful procedure (biopsy, insertion of an intravenous cannula). It temporarily prevents the transduction of noxious stimuli by numbing the peripheral nerve receptors.

Causal therapy

Pain management begins with an attempt to reverse the underlying cause of pain.[90] In relation to cancer pain, causal therapy means removal or reduction of the tumour mass through an operation and/or the use of chemotherapy or radiotherapy. This may reduce the pressure on, or stretching of tissue in the surrounding organs, blood vessels and nerves by the tumour/metastasis. Radiotherapy provides an effective symptomatic treatment for local bone pain and can be another method for treating breakthrough pain that may be the cause of poor opioid responsiveness.[110] Over 40% of patients with painful bone metastases can expect at least 50% pain relief and just under 30% can expect complete relief at 1 month.[111] In patients with advanced cancer with a limited life expectancy and poor performance status, radiotherapy with single fractions may be more convenient than protracted courses.[110] There is little discernible difference in efficacy between the fractionation schedules and indeed between different doses at the same schedule.[111] In the presence of multiple areas of pain hemibody radiation has been suggested, although toxicity is a concern. Radioisotopes are more easily administered, less toxic and effective in subclinical sites of metastasis. The most clinically used bone-seeking radioisotopes in patients with bone metastasis from breast or prostate cancer are

strontium-89, rhenium-186 and samarium-153. Three trials (192 patients) with radioisotopes alone produced similar extent of relief with similar onset and duration to that provided by radiotherapy.[112–114]

Chemotherapy used to treat particular painful conditions (pancreatic or prostate cancer) may also lessen pain. For this reason, agents such as gemcitabine[115] and mitoxantrone[116] have been approved for palliative care. Surgical means of pain relief (denervation or joint replacement) are generally reserved for highly specific situations or severe intractable pain.[57] Sometimes a primary antineoplastic treatment may not be curative, but may substantially alleviate pain. Indeed, active antineoplastic treatment and pain therapy should be used together, although the need to increase pain management strategies typically arises during the later stages of the disease.[8] Primary therapies sometimes do not treat the pain directly. For example, stool softeners may lessen pain associated with defecation, and breakthrough pain due to coughing may be controlled by an antitussive agent.[57]

Effective pharmacological approaches

Pain cannot always be managed by removing the direct cause. Drug therapy is the mainstay of treatment of cancer pain in all age groups because it is effective, inexpensive, with relatively low risk, and usually rapid onset. The goal of analgesic pharmacotherapy is optimizing pain relief while minimizing side effects and inconvenience to the patient. Specifically, the goals of cancer pain pharmacological therapy are to find the right dose of around-the-clock medications to control persistent pain and the right dose of supplemental medication to relieve breakthrough pain. The unpredictable individual response in terms of analgesia and toxicity depends on patient-related factors, drug-selective effects and pain-related factors. An essential principle in using medications to manage cancer pain is to individualize the regimen to the patient.[15] A simple well-validated and effective method for assuring the rational titration of therapy for cancer pain has been devised by the WHO.[75] The WHO analgesic ladder (Fig. 21.5) offers an important framework for pharmacological interventions at the level of nociception and pain experience.

The ultimate goal of the analgesic ladder is freedom from cancer pain. Pain intensity is the main evaluation criterion in the choice to move up or down the ladder. The first step in this approach is the use of acetaminophen (paracetamol), aspirin or another non-steroidal anti-inflammatory drug (NSAID) for mild to moderate pain. When pain persists or increases, an opioid such as codeine or hydrocodeine should be added (not substituted by the NSAID). Pain that is persistent or moderate to severe at the onset should be treated by increasing opioid potency using higher doses. The five essential concepts of the WHO approach to drug therapy of cancer pain are by the mouth, by the clock, by the ladder, for the individual and with attention to detail. Optimal use of the WHO ladder has been shown to be effective in relieving pain for approximately 90% of patients with cancer and over 75% of patients with cancer who are terminally ill.[58]

Non-opioid analgesics

Non-opioid analgesics are merely peripherally acting agents that intervene in the nociception, specifically in the phases of transduction and transmission. Their effect on the modulation of noxious stimuli is considered to be a central action. Peripherally acting agents intervene in nociception by inhibiting peripheral nerve activity in such way that the pain threshold is not exceeded at all, or limited to a minimum. The best-known peripherally acting agents are paracetamol and the group of NSAIDs, including salicylates (aspirin).[15] This last group intervenes specifically in the transduction of noxious stimuli. The well-known peripheral actions of NSAIDs are achieved through the previously mentioned inhibiting effect on the release of prostaglandin and the reduction of oedema as a result of their anti-inflammatory effect at the site of injury. However, a sound body of evidence also supports a central action, although the underlying mechanisms have not been well established. NSAIDs may interact centrally with the opioid system, the serotonergic system or with central nitric oxide mechanisms. Even administered peripherally, NSAIDs can deliver effective levels of drug to the CNS.[110]

NSAIDs are used as initial therapy in mild pain because they are effective, are often available over the counter and can be used effectively in combination with opioids and adjuvant analgesics if pain intensity increases.[75] No single-dose trial has shown any efficacy advantage of one NSAID over another. Used as single agents, NSAIDs have a ceiling effect on their analgesic potential, so the use of doses higher than those specified in the package insert is not recommended. Adverse effects of NSAIDs that may appear at any time include renal failure, hepatic dysfunction, bleeding and gastric ulceration. The efficacy dose–response curve for NSAIDs is said to be flat compared with the dose–response curve for adverse effects such as gastrointestinal symptoms, dizziness and drowsiness.[117] Increasing the dose is therefore more likely to increase adverse effects than to improve analgesia. The risk of NSAID-induced gastric bleeding (lowest with ibuprofen) increases with age.[118] Therefore, when age is greater than 75 years old, cardiovascular diseases or history of peptic ulcer, prophylactic misoprostol should be considered for preventing NSAID gastrointestinal complications.[119] There is no evidence that NSAIDs given rectally or by injection perform better (or faster) than the same dose given by mouth.[111]

These other routes become appropriate when patients cannot swallow. NSAIDs may benefit diverse types of pain, particularly bone pain. Intermittent use may be beneficial in breakthrough pain (headache, incident pain due to bone metastases) and neuropathic pain unre-

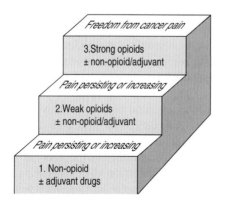

Figure 21.5: WHO analgesic ladder.

sponsive to conventional treatment. Spinal administration of several NSAIDs reduces the behavioural hyperalgesia evoked by the spinal action of substance P and NMDA at doses that are 100–800 times lower than those required for other systemic administration.[110] Also, local anaesthetics belong to the category of peripheral-acting agents. They either block the transduction of noxious stimuli by numbing the nerve endings or block the transmission of noxious stimuli. Both mechanisms are reversible. Arner et al showed that the duration of pain relief could far outlast the duration of local anaesthetic action, and that prolonged relief could result from a series of blocks.[120]

Opioids

'Opioid' is a general term for morphine derived from the opium poppy and semisynthetic or synthetic drugs with morphine-like activity. Their mechanism of action in pain management is the binding to opioid receptors, the μ (mu) and δ (delta) and/or κ (kappa) receptors, on the surfaces of nerve cells throughout the CNS.[4] Agents that bind to specific receptors are termed ligands. This binding to the different receptors can be complete (agonist), incomplete (antagonist), partial (partial agonist) or mixed (mixed agonist – antagonist)[33] (Fig. 21.6).

Commonly used full agonists include morphine, hydromorphone, codeine, oxycodon, hydrocodone, methadone, levorphanol and fentanyl. These opioids do not have a ceiling to their analgesic efficacy and will not reverse or antagonize the effects of other opioids within this class given simultaneously. Buprenorphine is a partial agonist, which, in comparison to full agonists, displays a ceiling effect to analgesia. In clinical use, mixed agonists include pentazocine, butorphanol tartate, dezocine and nalbuphine hydrochloride, which also have a ceiling effect. In contrast to full agonists, they block opioid analgesia at one type or receptor (μ) or at neutral at the receptor while simultaneously activating a different opioid receptor (κ).[15] Therefore, patients receiving full agonists should not be given a mixed agonist antagonist because this may precipitate a withdrawal syndrome and increase pain. Because opioids alter the perception of pain, patients

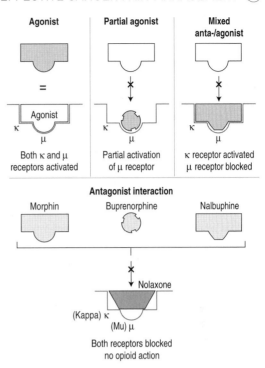

Figure 21.6: Antagonist/agonist mechanism of action.

report frequently that they still feel the pain but that it is less discomforting.[121]

There is no compelling evidence that one opioid is better than another but there is good evidence that pethidine has a specific disadvantage[122] and no specific advantage. Given in multiple doses, the metabolite norpethidine can accumulate and act as a CNS irritant, ultimately causing convulsions, especially in renal dysfunction. Morphine and relatives diamorphine and codeine have an active rather than a toxic metabolite, morphine-6-glucoronide. In renal dysfunction this metabolite can accumulate and result in greater effect from a given dose, because it is more active than morphine.[111] Morphine remains the first choice for reasons of familiarity, bioavailability and cost rather than proven superiority. Initial problems with nausea and dizziness commonly settle. Prophylactic use of laxatives is indicated for all patients.[15] The systemic availability of morphine by the oral route is poor (20–30%) and this contributes to a sometimes unpredictable onset of action and great interindividual variability in dose requirements and response. Some types of pain, and notably neuropathic pain, do not always respond well or completely to morphine. However, none of the alternatives to morphine has so far demonstrated advantage, which could make it preferable as the first-line oral opioid for cancer pain.[111]

In pain management, many routes are available for the administration of opioids: oral, transdermal, rectal, subcutaneous, intravenous and spinal (epidural or intrathecal).[15,20] Recommendations and guidelines by the WHO,[8,75] European Association of Palliative Care (EAPS),[123] American Pain Society (APS)[124] and US Department of Health and Human Services[15] give guidance on the use of morphine and the alternative strong opioid analgesics. The oral route is the simplest and most acceptable to patients. Ideally, two types of formulation are required: normal release (for dose titration) and modified release (for maintenance treatment). For patients who cannot swallow, alternative routes are transdermal, rectal or subcutaneous administration. Intramuscular administration should be avoided because this route can be painful and absorption is not reliable. A continuous intravenous infusion provides the most consistent level of analgesia and is easily accomplished for patients who have permanent intravenous access for other purposes. If intravenous access is not available or desirable, continuous subcutaneous opioid infusion offers a practical alternative in the hospital and home. Patient-controlled analgesia (PCA) can be accomplished by mouth or by the use of a special pump set to prescribed parameters to administer the drug intravenously or epidurally. Many studies support that PCA is safe both at home and with hospitalized patients, but it is contraindicated for sedated and confused patients.[125]

Breakthrough pain is a clinical challenge due to its severity and rapid onset. A balance between relieving pain and producing analgesic side effects must be achieved to manage it appropriately. Supplemental analgesia and sometimes a re-evaluation of the around-the-clock dosage is necessary. The supplemental analgesic should be a pure μ-opioid agonist, rapidly absorbed, highly efficacious with relatively short duration effect and, when possible, a route that is convenient for the patient.

Newer routes of administration such as oral transmucosal, because of their rapid onset of analgesia and convenience, provide more patient-friendly means of relieving breakthrough pain than the oral or intravenous route.[57] Dose escalation of opioids should be done by titration. The individual, gradual increment of the opioid dose aims to provide effective pain control, with a minimum of side effects. The intervals between escalations in titration depends on the type, form and route of opioids used. The size of steps in dose escalation also depends on patient conditions such as renal impairment, previous opioid use and/or alcohol abuse.[33]

When opioid-related side effects occur before satisfactory analgesia is achieved, a change to an alternative opioid or a change in the route of administration should be considered. Hydrocodone or oxycodone, if available in both normal release and modified release formulation for oral administration, are effective alternatives to oral morphine.[111] Transdermal fentanyl may be a useful non-invasive alternative in patients with stable doses. An informal accepted conversion ratio for substituting methadone is currently not available. Published equivalent doses for opioid analgesics vary in the suggested doses that are equianalgesic to morphine. Clinical response is the criterion that must be applied for each patient, and titration to clinical response is necessary.[15]

The most common traditional side effects of opioid agonists (sedation, nausea, constipation, pruritus, sweating, anaphylaxis and urinary retention) are rarely a cause for halting analgesic treatment.[126] Although there is no clear evidence that one particular opioid agonist has a significant lower prevalence or intensity of sedation, nausea or constipation compared to other agonists, there is a general consensus that a patient may experience fewer side effects with a given opioid agonist. However, there is good evidence that the risk of adverse effects is increased when high-tech approaches are used for drug administration.[127] The most recently recognized side effects with the exception of pulmonary edema[126] (cognitive failure, delirium, myoclonus/grand mal seizures, hyperalgesia, severe sedation–coma) are of a neuropsychiatric nature. Enthusiastic opioid titration may be associated with severe neurotoxicity. Nurses' efforts must be concentrated to rapidly identify and manage these complex syndromes. Strategies that have been proposed for the management of opioid neurotoxicity are opioid rotation, dose reduction, circadian modulation, hydration, psychostimulants and sedatives. Aggressive management of side effects is an appropriate strategy to address poor opioid responsiveness. Interventions that may reduce opioid side effects include antiemetics for nausea and vomiting, hydration or psychotropic drugs (benzodiazepines or neuroleptics) for confusion, benzodiazepines for myoclonus and, psychostimulants for severe drowsiness.[110]

Myths and misconceptions in opioid use

Common myths and misconceptions which may underpin dubious and sometimes unethical practices include fears of respiratory depression, addiction and the beliefs that opioids should be withheld until pain is intolerable and that patients are lying about their pain if they respond to the administration of a placebo.[128] Morphine does not cause clinically important respiratory depression in patients with cancer in pain.[129] Pain acts as an antagonist to respiratory depression. Appropriate use indicates regular evaluation and monitoring for signs of overdose. If respiratory depression does occur, administration of opioids should be temporarily ceased, while naloxone is titrated to respiratory rate and consciousness until the side effect is reversed.[15] However, close monitoring should be continued as naloxone often has a shorter half-life than opioids. Opiophobia is one of the most frequently cited reasons for poor pain management.[130] Adequate doses of opioids are often not available or not given, primarily because of fear of addiction. Opioids used for people who are not in pain can induce physical and psychological dependency (addiction) but psychological dependency or addiction is rarely seen in patients with cancer-related pain (less than 1:10,000).[131,132] Unfortunately, some governments restrict medical availability on the grounds that if drugs are available medically this will worsen the street addiction problem. However, there is no evidence for this view.[111]

In clinical practice, terms frequently used incorrectly and interchangeably are tolerance, physical dependence and addiction.[133] The presence of opioid tolerance and physical dependence does not equate with addiction. The need to increase the opioid dose could potentially be related to the development of analgesic tolerance. Tolerance in opioid therapy is the need for a higher dose to control pain because of a diminishing analgesic effect over time.[134] Dose escalation can restore adequate pain relief.[135] However, the main reason for increasing the dose is not pharmacological tolerance but progression of the disease. Although pharmacological tolerance exists, it is argued among clinicians that an increased need for opioids in pain management is driven by disease rather than by pharmacological tolerance.[136,137] Most patients requiring a dose escalation to manage increasing pain demonstrate progression of disease.[132,138]

Physical dependence on opioids is revealed when the opioid is abruptly discontinued or when naloxone is administered and is typically manifested as anxiety, irritability, joint pains, chills and hot flushes, nausea, vomiting, abdominal cramps and diarrhoea. Cessation of opioid therapy without withdrawal symptoms can be achieved by halving or quartering the dose of opioid every 1–2 days until the daily equivalent of about 15 mg of oral morphine is reached.[139] Endorphins may explain the placebo effect, and the analgesic effect of some forms of alternative non-pharmacological approaches such as acupuncture or transcutaneous electrical nerve stimulation (TENS). Endorphins or endogenous opiates are substances produced by the body itself that have a similar effect to morphine.[4] Endorphins play an important role in the endogenous analgesic system. The spinal fluid transports the ligands to receptors on neurons throughout the CNS. Due to their relatively large molecules compared to morphine, endorphins cannot pass the brain–blood barrier; therefore, they cannot bind to opioid receptors outside the CNS.

Adjuvant analgesics

Adjuvant analgesics, also known as co-analgesics, are useful in controlling pain, primarily by enhancing the activity of pain medication,

457

treating concurrent symptoms that exacerbate pain and providing independent analgesia.[15,55,139] Commonly used agents, described in Table 21.4, can be used separately or in combination with conventional analgesics such as opioids and/or NSAIDs. The dose is usually lower than that for its primary indication and should be carefully given. When given in combination with opioids, close monitoring of side effects is required. These co-analgesics should be considered for the treatment of all types of cancer pain but are particularly important for pain syndromes relatively unresponsive to morphine alone.[109]

Some adjuvant analgesics may produce independent analgesic effects: antidepressants, sodium channel blocking agents, glucocorticoids, bisphosphonates, nitrous oxide and other drugs for neuropathic pain (e.g. anticonvulsant agents, benzodiazepines or endogeuous adenosine). Examples of drugs that enhance analgesia produced by opioids are NMDA antagonists, calcium channel antagonists, clonidine, cholinergic agonists and neostigmine.[110] There is a clinical impression that these pharmacological classes of drugs are useful in cancer pain management. For example, antidepressants and anticonvulsants have been used for pain control in neuropathic pain for more than 30 years. However, we still need to determine the relative risk and benefit of the best and most appropriate anticonvulsant and the best and most appropriate antidepressant and then compare them directly in neuropathic pain.[111]

Invasive analgesic interventions

Between 70% and 90% of all cancer pain can be controlled with oral medication.[140] Appropriate use of invasive measures in the remaining 10–30% of patients – most often those with advanced disease – who fail oral therapy can relieve nearly all cancer pain. Invasive analgesic procedures include epidural and intrathecal analgesia, nerve blocks, neurolytic blocks, cordotomy and surgical stabilization of bony disease.[141]

The rationale for the spinal route's ability to provide increased opioid effectiveness while decreasing toxicity is related to the opioid placement near the CNS which is in close proximity to the opioid receptors. The perceived benefit of invasive analgesia is supported by a prospective randomized study with matched groups: patients receiving intrathecal analgesics achieved statistically more significant improvement in their pain and symptom relief score than those receiving comprehensive medical management.[142] Contraindications for intraspinal therapy include allergic reactions to implanted materials, tumour encroachment of the thecal sac, occult or systemic infections or lack of support systems to manage the catheter and the pump effectively.[143]

Nerve blocks work to disrupt nerve signals. These blocks may be temporary or permanent, based on the solution injected. The benefit of these procedures is to decrease well-localized pain following a nerve root distribution (e.g pain with herpes zoster).[151] Three studies compared intravenous lidocaine 5 mg/kg with saline in cancer-related pain.[111] Most patients in the sample were on regular analgesics. Despite that, each study examined a different pain state (pain due to bony metastases,[145] tumour invasion of the nerve plexus[146] and chemotherapy-induced polyneuropathy or radiotherapy-induced plexopath[147]); lidocaine had no significant effect. Neurolytic blocks are permanent blocks that interrupt the NS by essentially destroying the appropriate nerve pathway.[144] Neurolyitic substances like ethanol or phenol are often employed, but also electricity, cold/heat or surgery are all used to interrupt the transmission of sensory information. Besides the neurological deficits that may occur, there is one other major disadvantage: pain can return even more vigorously than before, and this deafferentation pain is more difficult to treat. However, these neurolytic block procedures do have a place in cancer pain management, when life expectancy is less than 3 months or where other simpler techniques have failed, or are not possible.[148] For example, pain associated with pancreatic cancer responds well to coeliac plexus block,[149] which may also help those with abdominal or perineal pain from tumour in the pelvis. Research demonstrates significant improvement in quality of life and survival, and improvements in pain levels with the possibility of being pain-free for the remainder of the individual's life.[150]

Table 21.4: Adjuvant analgesics[8,15,110,111]

Adjuvants	Indication	Examples	Mechanism of action
Antidepressants	Neuropathic pain (burning and shooting)	Amitriptyline, clomipramine	Unknown, possible inhibiting noradrenaline re-uptake
Anticonvulsants	Neuralgia (lancinating pain) complicating nerve injury	Carbamazepine, phenytoin	Unclear, possible acting as antagonists on the N-methyl D-aspartate (NMDA) mechanism
Muscle relaxants	Muscle tension due to pain	Diazepam, cyclopenzaprine	Purely analgesic action unknown
Neuroleptics	Neuropathic pain (central)	Haloperidol, levomepromazine	Reduction anxiety/restlessness
Corticosteroids	Pain with inflammatory component	Dexamethasone, methylprednisolone	Pressure relief by reduction of oedema
Bisphosphonates osteoclast- and calcitonin	Bone pain	Pamidronate, calcitonin	Potent inhibitor of induced bone resorption
Sodium channel blocking agents	Neuropathic pain	Systemic local anesthetics, carbamazepine phenytoin, open sodium channel blockers	Inhibit sodium channels of hyperactive and depolarized nerves
NMDA antagonists	Poorly responsive pain symptoms, predictable breakthrough pains	Ketamine, haloperidol,	Block the activity of NMDA-receptors
Calcium channel antagonists	May potentiate opioid nociception	Nifedipine (nimodipine)	May modify chronic opioid effects, including the expression of tolerance
Clonidine	Refractory neuropathic pain	Clonidine	Inhibits primary afferent transmission, including the inhibitor of substance P release from nociceptive nervous in the spinal cord
Nitrous oxide	Control of breakthrough pain	50% nitrous oxide and 50% oxygen	Analgesic, anxiolytic and sedative agent
Placebo	None		Possible: release of endorphins

Few patients require surgical intervention to interrupt central or peripheral nociceptive pathways. The most commonly performed surgical procedure for cancer pain relief is anterolateral cordotomy, carrying significant morbidity when done by an open technique.[151] Percutaneous cordotomy, however, has largely replaced the open method but is usually ineffective in neuropathic pain. Immediate pain relief is achieved in the majority of patients, but pain recurs in roughly half of these patients by 6–12 months when paraesthesias or dysaesthesias are developed. Placement of an Omaya reservoir under the scalp, connected to a catheter whose tip lies within the lateral cerebral ventricle, may provide satisfactory analgesia, with relatively few side effects.[152] Invasive analgesic interventions require intense patient education to understand the burden related with these therapies, including increased travel for analgesic titration or refills, potential surgery and working in partnership with pain specialists.

Non-pharmacological approaches

Non-pharmacological, non-invasive, treatments of pain are being increasingly utilized, especially in comprehensive pain centres. The purpose of development of non-pharmacological approaches is not to replace somatic interventions but to treat the affective cognitive and behavioural aspects of cancer-related pain.[153] The classification of non-invasive pain treatments led by Fernandez[154] (interpersonal/spiritual, cognitive, behavioural, physical and environmental) is used to present the various categories of interventions in pain management (Box 21.4). Muscular tension, autonomic arousal and mental distress are thought to exacerbate pain.[55] Non-pharmacological, centrally acting interventions alter the perception of pain by influencing one or more of these factors.

Interpersonal/spiritual non-pharmacological interventions

These interventions focus on establishing and enhancing therapeutic relationships between nurses and patients.[156] The therapeutic *nurse–patient relationship* enables the nurse to understand the patient as a whole person and

---

Box 21.4

Non-pharmacological measures[74,155]

Interpersonal/ spiritual non-invasive measures
- The nurse–patient relationship
- Therapeutic touch
- Spiritual interventions

Cognitive interventions
- Imagery
- Patient education
- Rhythmic cognitive activity
- Attention – diversion (audiotapes, humour, music, videos)

Behavioural interventions
- Counselling–support (individual or family)
- Hypnosis
- Biofeedback
- Pain diary
- Self-monitoring
- Expectancy
- Perceived controllability
- Attribution

Physical interventions
- Relaxation
- Breathing
- Cutaneous techniques
- Positioning
- Movement and exercise

Environmental manipulations
- Manipulation of the environment
- Attention of temperature or amount of light or noise
- Tapes of pleasant sounds
- Flexibility in usual routines of the setting

---

the suffering component of the pain experience. In a trusting therapeutic environment, numerous opportunities for holistic interventions that provide comfort to patients and their significant others can be offered.[157] The climate of the therapeutic nurse–patient relationship is the foundation for the use of other non-invasive interventions.

Therapeutic touch (TT) is difficult to categorize, but it is claimed that its mechanism of action does not interfere with the nervous system but with energy fields in the body.[155] As part of this method, TT enables patients to mobilize their own inner resources so that self-healing can take place. It is at this point that deep relaxation can occur and anxiety or physical and emotional pain can be relieved.[158] In a number of case studies, a positive effect of TT on pain has been reported, although none demonstrated a coherent cause–effect relationship. Attempts to explain the mechanism of action behind TT adequately in a scientific way have failed and the possibility of a placebo effect could not be ruled out.

Spiritual interventions that may be practiced by nurses, family members or a pastor include praying with patients, consoling, encouraging, being present, talking, smiling and touching, and providing (religious) music. Spiritual counselling may increase the patient's coping skills and provide spiritual and emotional support.[156,157]

Cognitive interventions

Cognitive interventions include patient education, imagery, rhythmic cognitive activity, attention diversion and self-statements. These interventions primarily address the cognitive dimension of the pain experience. However, modifying or changing one's thoughts can ameliorate spiritual distress and influence affective, behavioural and sociocultural aspects of the pain experience. Using strategies to revise negative and discouraging thoughts can enable patients to regain some control when they are feeling powerless.[74]

Patent education should emphasize that pain can be effectively managed. Nowadays, multiple teaching aids are available but professional time is required to teach pain management. Patient education is effective in decreasing pain by promoting self-care, improving ability to comply with the pain regimen and preventing side effects. Ferrell et al developed a comprehensive pain programme for elderly patients with cancer. The programme had a large educational component but also used audiotapes for progressive muscle relaxation and guided imagery. Compared to randomized controls, the intervention was effective in decreasing pain and anxiety and improving sleep.[159]

Focusing or distraction techniques make use of the principle of focusing attention on stimuli other than pain, such as another physiological sensation (breathing, heartbeat, touch and movement), a positive emotion through mem-

ory, visual distraction (external) as guided imagery (internal), auditory input such as music, etc. The result of 'focusing' is distraction – away from the pain – and, through this, reduction of mental distress caused by the pain. The effect can last for several minutes up to an hour.[76] *Re-framing* may influence the patient's 'coping style'. It is a form of patient education that is often incorporated into daily nursing practice. With this technique, cognitive reappraisal, patients learn to monitor and evaluate negative thoughts and replace them with positive thoughts and images. Patients are taught on a basic level to handle signals from the body, communicate adequately in relation to emotions, fears, disease and limitations, handle uncertainty, adapt to changes, accept consequences of choices, alter self-image, and acquire pain-diminishing interventions or activities.

Imagery for the purpose of pain relief may be defined as using one's imagination to develop sensory images that decrease the intensity of pain or focus on a pleasant, more acceptable or non-painful substitute of pain. Images may vary from brief ones, such as those used in ordinary conversation, to lengthy ones, such as those developed systematically by the individual (therapeutic guided imagery). A nurse may assist patients doing this by guiding them through the use of an imagery technique.[76]

Music may reduce pain perception by evoking emotions that result in releasing endogenous opiates and reducing muscle tension. Music interventions may be competing effectively for neurological pathways, thus reducing the transmission of pain messages. Moreover, they can improve mood by diminishing feelings of anxiety, powerless and helplessness.[74] Music relaxation can be used as a support and distraction during medical and nursing interventions.[160] There are few well-designed studies with music therapy and no recommendations can be made based on data thus far, although some evidence of controlling pain in patients with cancer does exist.[161]

Behavioural interventions

Behavioural interventions include those requiring some degree of external control (e.g hypnosis, operant conditioning, biofeedback) and others requiring low external control (e.g expectancy, controllability and attribution). Behaviours in the latter category are under the patient's control; therefore, they are probably learned as a result of the therapist's intervention in the cognitive domain. *Counselling and supporting individuals – family* can enhance the effectiveness of the analgesics in addition to helping instil a sense of control and self-efficacy in patients. Behavioural therapy consists of a number of different modules. Every form of behavioural therapy influences 'coping style' and focuses on patient education. It is specifically used in patients with chronic pain syndromes and/or traumatic pain experiences in the past that result in suffering.

Hypnosis can be defined as 'an artificially induced state of consciousness characterized by a heightened receptivity to suggestion'.[162] That state of consciousness is one of alertness and intense concentration through diminished peripheral awareness. To achieve this state of consciousness, a combination of different techniques is used in the process of hypnosis. It includes 'ego strengthening', 'imagery', 'attention fixation', narrowing the field of external influences and achieving a deep state of relaxation. Hypnosis has a long history of use in the treatment of cancer-related pain. Unfortunately, most of the studies reported in the literature are anecdotal case reports. However, Spiegel and Bloom found that hypnosis was effective in reducing pain in patients with metastatic breast cancer assigned to a supportive-expressive group therapy compared to a control group.[163]

Biofeedback is a technique where patients are trained to monitor individual exacerbating factors of pain as muscular tension, autonomic arousal and mental distress. Once patients have learned to identify the relation between the different physiological reactions and their pain threshold, they may recognize symptoms without the help of these measuring devises. They can then make preventative use of the different non-invasive complementary therapies to reduce exacerbating factors. This technique is scarcely used in cancer pain, as it requires a prolonged training period[55] and its effectiveness has not been examined yet. Melzack and Wall state that biofeedback does add something important to the psychological therapy of pain. It is a useful vehicle for distraction, relaxation, suggestion and for providing patients with a sense of control over their pain.[4]

Physical interventions

Physical interventions may reduce pain through direct effects on the musculoskeletal, integumentary and nervous system. Indications for these interventions are muscle tension, localized pain, anxiety or pain prevention. Common non-invasive physical interventions include relaxation, breathing techniques, cutaneous techniques, positioning, movement and exercise.

In relaxation, attention and imagination are focused on the dissipation of tension in successive muscle groups.[164] Deep relaxation through hypnosis not only reduces muscular tension and mental distress but is also most likely to be responsible for physiological changes such as reduced oxygen consumption, respiratory rate and heart rate, and a normalization of blood pressure.[165] In cancer pain, there is limited evidence to assess the role of relaxation.[166] Curtis concluded that music can benefit relaxation in pain relief.[167] Relaxation with imagery was also found to improve pain in patients with oral mucositis.[168]

Cutaneous interventions are non-pharmacological equivalents to the peripherally acting agents, providing pain relief through neuromodulation by cutaneous stimulation (the altering of nerve activity through stimulation of the skin). Forms of cutaneous stimulation are temperature (cold/heat), external pressure (massage, vibration) and peripheral stimulation such as nerve stimulation by TENS (non-invasive) or acupuncture (invasive). These non-pharmacological interventions can not only *decrease* the transmission of noxious stimuli but also *increase* the transmission of *non*-noxious stimuli (gate control theory).[31] Cutaneous interventions can be used interchangeably for various durations. As no minimum or maximum times have been established, the best guidelines are based on patient's comfort and safety.[74]

Temperature is probably one of the oldest and most used non-pharmacological intervention used by patients to reduce pain.[169] Both cold and heat are often overlooked as treatments of pain as they can relieve pain through counterirritation or hyperstimulation (the use of a pain stimulus to relieve pain, e.g ice massage to the site of chronic pain).[74] Heat improves the blood flow and cell metabolism and, with it, the elimination of pain-causing substances. It can also relax muscle spasm and decrease joint stiffness.[170] Cold decreases peripheral blood flow through vasoconstriction, which reduces or prevents swelling. Also, cell metabolism can decrease in the cooled area, which inhibits the release of pain-causing substances. A third mechanism of action is probably the inhibiting effect of cold on the conduction of impulses by nerve fibres.[171] The combination of these factors probably explains why the pain-diminishing effect of cold lasts longer than that of heat. Nevertheless, patients often prefer the use of heat.[172] Contraindications for the use of cold are diseases where vascular constriction increases symptoms, e.g. peripheral vascular diseases.

Massage includes stroking, friction and kneading of muscles and soft tissues; stroking massage decreases oedema and produces muscle relaxation, whereas friction and kneading massage break down intramuscular adhesions and prepare muscles and soft tissues for stretching.[173] External pressure in the form of massage or vibration can either be superficial or deep. Deep stimulation or pressure massage is best applied in acute pain. Pressure can relieve acute pain by applying a stronger but less painful stimulus mostly proximal to the wound or pain site (deep stimulation). The sharper pain of the injury will be overruled through the increase in both intensity and pattern of *non*-noxious stimuli. This mechanism is also known as counterirritation or stimulation.[174] Superficial massage is most commonly used at the back/shoulder area and extremities and it mainly relaxes the muscles. In superficial massage, this effect on pain relief is probably greater than the effect of counterstimulation, as opposed to vibration therapy. The use of a simple handheld 'vibrator' is an undervalued intervention, despite the fact that its effect generally lasts longer than that of superficial massage.[175–177] The main contraindication for both kinds of therapy is non-acceptance by the patient. Massage therapy may provide immediate but not prolonged pain relief in patients with cancer,[178] with men responding better than women.[179]

TENS involves the delivery of electric energy across the surface of the skin and stimulation of the peripheral nervous system. The rationale is based on the gate control theory of pain modulation. In pain management, TENS is better valued for its stimulating effect on the sensory nerves, especially the A fibres. McCaffrey and Beebe state that the success of TENS is strongly dependent upon the skill of the person administering it.[76] TENS is most effective in neuropathic pain, phantom pain and postherpetic neuralgia.[169] For TENS in chronic pain we have lack of evidence of effect (rather than evidence of lack of effect).[111] The only reported systematic review of its use in chronic pain examining acute labour and chronic pain concluded that TENS has not undergone sufficiently strict and rigorous clinical evaluation. Case series[180,181] and a small randomized control trial[182] also suggest that TENS may provide short-term pain relief in dying patients or in patients with intractable cancer pain.

Acupuncture is a technique of peripheral sensory stimulation because it targets the neural network for endogenous pain modulation. Different acupuncture modes and parameters activate different inhibitory mechanisms at various sites within the endogenous system.[183] Acupuncture may be helpful in relieving advanced or refractory cancer pain, although data stem only from uncontrolled studies.[184] Indeed, a recent randomized trial in 90 cancer patients experiencing pain randomized to receive two sessions of ear acupuncture or sham acupuncture showed that pain intensity decreased by 36% at 2 months from baseline in the group receiving acupuncture; there was little change for patients receiving placebo (2%).[281] Hence, acupuncture in managing cancer pain shows a promising role that needs to be further explored in the future.

Environmental manipulations

Finally, an important but often overlooked category of non-pharmacological interventions for cancer pain is the manipulation of patient's environment. A number of environmental factors, including light, noise, temperature and

463

ambience may alter the external background of human painful experience and are often under the nurse's control.[74]

None of the non-pharmacological approaches described are inherently incompatible with the use of analgesics. In fact, a likely advantage of non-pharmacological approaches is the reduction of analgesics needed for pain management and a reduction in the negative side effects associated with high doses of analgesics. It is obvious that little research has been conducted to evaluate the effectiveness of these strategies systematically or to develop guidelines for their use.[111] Published literature of adults with cancer pain revealed few controlled studies, weak theoretical frameworks, few complete descriptions of the nature of the pain problem and lack of control over the interventions.[185–187] However, preliminary evidence supports the view that non-drug approaches appear to hold promise for reducing pain and suffering in patients with cancer.

The success of these approaches is strongly dependent upon the skill of the person administering them. The qualifications and training necessary for the effective use of the procedures varies with each technique. Within the cancer pain literature, the majority of professionals utilizing hypnosis or biofeedback are primarily psychologists. Main services offered by physiotherapists are therapeutic touch, advice on hot/cold applications, provision of TENS machines, acupuncture, massage, relaxation techniques, advice and provision of walking aids and gait re-education. Adaptive techniques in the activities of daily living, relaxation techniques, purposeful activity and creative activity are usually services provided by occupational therapists.[153]

Oncology nurses should be aware of the range of available non-pharmacological interventions and be skilled at the application of some of them. They should always look for measures that their patients have previously found effective. Some of these treatments require time, energy and concentration on the part of the patient. Thus, the identification of patients in need of pain management is a problem that needs attention. A combination of non-invasive interventions can easily be combined and included in the nursing plan (e.g. heat can be used during relaxation or imagery).

It seems that nurses tend not to apply non-invasive measures systematically in the everyday pain management of patients with cancer. Time, expense, belief systems and a poor evidence base are factors that may all limit the way in which these therapies may be included in the patient's care plan. Despite the many difficulties encountered in conducting psychological/behavioural research with patients with cancer a great deal of research is necessary to validate the efficacy of those techniques.[111]

Evaluation

No matter what therapy is utilized for pain management, its effectiveness should be evaluated. As cancer pain is closely related to the course of the disease, pain assessment should be performed at regular intervals, and the therapeutic effect of the pain interventions can be evaluated several times a day.[188] Evaluating pain should be regarded as a process that has a number of dimensions, as detailed in Box 21.5.

In the evaluation of *pain behaviour*, changes compared to the initial pain assessment are monitored and reported. 'Behaviour' in this sense means that the patient has at least some extent of control over pain behaviour compared with autonomic physiological reactions. Table 21.5 presents a list of common pain behaviours that are observed.

Behavioural measures should never replace self-report measures, as long as the patient is capable of doing these. However, lack of behav-

---

Box 21.5

Three dimensions of evaluation in pain management[89]

1. Evaluation of an intervention for its primary effect (corresponding level in pain arch model): e.g. the effect of paracetamol on nociception, or of morphine on pain experience.

2. Evaluation of the secondary effect of this intervention (on the higher levels): e.g. the effect of paracetamol on pain experience and pain behaviour.

3. Always assess the possibility that new threatening and/or damaging stimuli arise: e.g. changes on the lower levels.

Table 21.5: Pain behaviour[49,189]

(Non)-verbal communication	Facial expressions (frowning, clenched teeth, screwed up eyes) vocalization (crying, moaning, whining, complaining)
Locomotive apparatus	Posture, impaired mobility, inactivity, protective movement, urge to move/restlessness, pinching/rubbing painful part
Psychological aspects	Social seclusion/altered relations, inconsolableness, preoccupation, irritability and other symptoms of depression-like loss of appetite or interest
Healthcare consumption	Doctor visits and the use of pain medication can also be considered as pain behaviour

ioural cues does not mean that pain is absent, whether this is caused by the disease or as a result of palliative treatment (opioids or sedatives). In relation to *pain experience*, we can only make use of self-report techniques such as pain questionnaires, pain charts, inventories or diaries. They are particularly useful in the regular assessment of pain and should register:

- the projection site(s) of pain
- the different time aspects (onset, time of day, duration)
- the intensity
- the character or quality of pain (stabbing, burning, pinching, etc.)
- influencing factors (e.g. the effect of pain on mood and vice versa).

In between these regular assessments, pain can be evaluated daily or multiple times a day by the use of VAS, especially if there is a change in pain, after analgesic administration or after any modifications in the pain management plan. A VAS is simple, fast, reliable, sensitive and accurately reflects the perceived magnitude of the stimulus.[93]

Physiological reactions that correlate with pain are observed best in neonates. Examples are increase of heart rate, elevation of blood pressure, decrease of saturation and/or CO_2 or O_2 levels in blood, hyperglycaemia, palmar sweating (as of 37 weeks), changes in colour of the skin or dilated pupils. Along with ageing, the correlation between pain and the above-mentioned reactions becomes less significant. In adults experiencing acute pain, physiological adaptation occurs relatively quickly, often within minutes after the injury.[76] Due to this phenomenon,

the effect of peripherally acting agents and their non-pharmacological equivalents can best be evaluated by their secondary effect on the higher levels: pain experience and pain behaviour.

The effect of causal treatment can be evaluated by reassessment of initial diagnosed noxious stimuli as the cause of pain, e.g. the reduction of tumour size after radiation. In the acute care setting, initial pain assessment should be undertaken on admission and reassessment daily or more frequently, depending on the severity of pain. In the community, pain should be assessed at each visit, the timing depending on each patient's individual circumstances. Assessment must be an ongoing process because of the changes in nature of pain, disease and patient response. Sudden severe pain is a medical emergency and patients should be assessed as soon as possible.[54]

IMPROVING THE QUALITY OF CARE OF PATIENTS WITH CANCER PAIN

Quality assurance in the treatment of cancer pain

Cancer pain management has surfaced worldwide as a significant quality care outcome for researchers and clinicians.[84] It is an important issue that is increasingly used to evaluate the effectiveness of nursing care. A number of obstacles to successful pain management do exist and can be attributed to healthcare professionals, patients, families and the healthcare system. Lack of pain management knowledge by healthcare professionals has emerged as one of the significant problems related to ineffective pain management worldwide.[190–193] Additional barriers, besides the nurse's knowledge and attitudes, exist and are similar across countries.[194] These include patients' hesitance to communicate their pain,[19,195–199] lack of knowledge by physicians,[200] lack of resources and organisational support,[19,190] opioid regulations,[201] and a lack of appropriate and consistent definition of addiction.[202]

Recognition of the widespread undertreatment of cancer pain has prompted recent corrective efforts from healthcare disciplines, professional and consumer organizations and governments throughout the world. As cancer pain control is a problem of international scope, the WHO has urged that every nation give high priority to establishing a cancer pain relief policy.[8] Guidelines, standards of care, position papers and principles of professional practice are increasingly available to improve effectiveness and cost-effectiveness of care. Numerous organizations (Ad Hoc Committee on Cancer Pain of the American Society of Clinical Oncology, American Pain Society, Health and Public Policy Committee, European Association of Palliative Care, European Organization for the Research & Treatment of Cancer, American College of Physicians) have produced guidelines and policy statements on the management of cancer pain.[15,20,88,203]

Standards, guidelines and critical pathways

Standards, guidelines and critical pathways are clinical tools that operationalize the implementation of evidence-based practice.[204] They are statements assisting the practitioner and patient to make decisions about appropriate health care for specific clinical conditions as recommendations on pain assessment and management guidelines. They are available in formats suitable for healthcare practitioners, the scientific community, educators and consumers.[205]

Standards

Standards are authoritative statements that provide a framework against which quality of care can be measured and constantly improved.[206] Standards tend to be stable over time and describe the responsibilities for which professionals are accountable for. The Joint Commission on Accreditation of Healthcare Organizations has mandated standards for pain assessment and management for hospitals, nursing homes and other facilities.[207] Standards incorporate basic principles of pain assessment and treatment into patterns of daily practice, including standards of practice, documentation systems, policies and procedures, orientation and continuing education programmes and quality improvement programmes.

Guidelines

Guidelines reflect the state of knowledge, current at the time of publication, on effective and appropriate care and change as knowledge advances. In every setting, the clinical guideline development process has made positive contributions to the quality of care.[208] However, decisions to adopt any particular recommendation must be made in light of available resources and circumstances presented by individual patients. According to clinical needs and constraints, practice guidelines may be adopted, modified or rejected by the care setting.[209] Schmid et al explain the complex process of implementation of clinical practice guidelines in a large setting.[210] The Oncology Nursing Society (ONS) in the United States has developed an online evidence-based practice resource centre to provide a guide for nurses in solving clinical problems and developing guidelines (http://www.ons.org/).

Critical pathways and algorithms

Critical pathways and algorithms that define patient outcomes for specific medical conditions provide useful strategies for nurses to monitor and manage the processes of patient care. They delineate the optimal sequence of timing of interventions. Their use is intended to reduce variation in practice and cost.[211] In a study evaluating 14 pain management clinical pathways, it was found that patients whose caregivers used the pathways had less pain across the hospital stay, less interference by pain in nearly all quality of life indicators and greater satisfaction with caregiver responsiveness to their pain. However, these improvements reversed after discharge.[212]

Improving pain management

Continuous quality improvement processes are organization-wide activities designed to monitor and ultimately improve the quality of the care provided. The methods and tools used provide powerful means to design and test strategies to improve pain management.[213] Patients with cancer receive care in hospitals, clinicians' offices, ambulatory care centres, homes, nursing homes and hospices. Thus, when evaluating quality of care, the multiplicity of centres where cancer care is provided should be considered. Pain management should be evaluated at points of transition in the provision of services to ensure that optimal pain management is achieved and maintained.[214]

To improve the quality of pain management, nurses need to take leadership roles in their own organizations by participating actively in interdisciplinary organizations and local or national cancer pain initiatives. The process of developing a quality improvement programme for pain management practices at the nursing unit or organizational level is described by a step-by-step guide, ranging from establishing a multidisciplinary pain management committee to the selection of pain-intensity scales and staff education activities.[215]

The common proposed steps[216] towards quality improvement in pain management are the following:

- To develop an interdisciplinary workgroup
- To examine and analyse current practice within the institution (organizational needs assessment, knowledge and attitudes surveys)
- To articulate and implement standards of practice and guidelines to improve pain management – agreement on ways of pain-intensity and pain-relief documentation; recourses/policies guiding the use of specialized technologies; clarify lines of responsibility in the setting; promise patients a quick pain response; provide readily available information about pharmacological and non-

pharmacological interventions to clinicians to facilitate order writing and interpretation of orders
- To develop and provide educational opportunities for nursing staff, patients and caregivers
- Ongoing evaluation and improving pain management quality.

The quality of pain management in the outpatient setting can be evaluated by retrospective and prospective methods. It is suggested that prospective evaluations of the quality of cancer pain management with patient diaries in the outpatient/home-care setting can help clinicians do 'real time' evaluations and modify pain management plans for individuals.[215] Morse investigated the experience of cancer pain at home from the concurrent perspectives of the patient caregiver and home-care nurse. Authors recommended a need for improved communication and collaboration among health professionals as well as further professional, patient and family education in relation to pain.[217] Structured pain education yielded enhanced knowledge and attitudes about pain, quality of life and pain management, but there are still many challenges within the current home-care environment to optimal integration of pain education.[218]

Pain in specific patient populations

Populations at particular risk of poor pain management are infants and children, elderly people, those from ethnic minorities, persons with a history of chemical dependency and persons with cognitive impairment or learning disabilities.[15] Current evidence suggests that these patients continue to be vulnerable to inadequate pain assessment, limited opportunities to offer self-reports of pain (the gold standard for pain assessment) and the resulting chronic undertreatment of pain leading to needless suffering.[219]

Children

Pain in children with cancer arises more often from the treatment than from the disease.[220] Multiple myths exist about pain in children. It is wrongly believed that children are not as sensitive as adults, that the smaller the children the less the pain experience is remembered, that children cannot be assessed reliably and that because of their immature metabolic systems, opioids are not safe to be administered to them.[221] The many factors shaping children's pain are developmental, emotional and cognitive state, physical condition, past experiences, the stage of disease, the meaning of pain, attitudes and reactions of family, personality traits, cultural background and environment.[222] Assessment of pain involves self-reports (e.g. Faces Pain Scale by Bieri et al[223]), proxy reports, observations and physiological measures. The Gustave Roussy Child Pain Scale is the only observation tool developed for children with cancer.[224] Tailoring assessment and management strategies is necessary for children with developmental delays, learning disabilities, emotional disturbances and language barriers.

Elderly

Although among the institutionalized elderly the prevalence of pain may be over 70%, pain management in elderly people with cancer has been minimally studied and is underreported in the literature.[225] Underreporting of pain in elderly patients with cancer pain is due to many reasons, such as inappropriate beliefs about pain sensitivity, pain tolerance and ability to use opioids.[15] For many of these patients, pain is seen as a metaphor for advancing illness and even proceeding death.[226] A common myth is that pain perception is altered by age.[227] Often, elderly people report pain differently than younger patients due to organic, psychological and cultural changes associated with ageing.[228] Clinicians dealing with older people who may have impaired recall of pain due to alterations in memory need to combine some kind of verbal screen for the presence of pain with the use of other clinical tools to evaluate self-report consistency.[229] The same WHO three-step ladder that applies to younger patients should apply to the elderly with the only difference that lower doses should be used. The risk for gastric and renal toxicity with NSAIDs and unusual reactions including cognitive impairment, headache and constipation are increased among elderly patients.[230]

Culturally diverse populations

Populations are rarely homogeneous due to human migration, intermarriage and genetic polymorphism. The immigrant population in most European countries is constantly increasing. In the last decade, over 200 articles explored the relationship between ethnicity and pain, but it seems that most studies address cultural influences in patients with acute pain, fewer with chronic pain and even less with cancer pain.[231] Various studies using diverse methods suggest that culture does play a crucial role in the individual experience of pain but the role of culture in shaping the experience of pain within specific ethnic groups is only just beginning to be studied.[232]

If a healthcare provider and the patient are from different cultural or socioeconomic backgrounds or speak a different language, the patient is at high risk for poor pain management.[231] For the improvement of pain management programmes, the patient and family members' cultural beliefs and approaches should be incorporated in the treatment plan.[233]

To understand pain and the cultural perception patients and staff hold about pain, it is crucial to developing a pain management programme that complies with Joint Commission requirements.[234] The challenge of ethnicity is to understand how far the human experience embodies not only measurable differences that distinguish specific groups but also deep similarities that bind people together despite their diverse cultural and ethnic backgrounds. Clinical awareness of cultural meanings and normal standards of behaviour and acceptable communication can improve patient assessment and management.[235] If the patient speaks another language, efforts should be made to find a translator to determine a convenient way to assess pain. Recognizing the special needs of minority cultural groups, a cancer pain education programme using focus group methods developed a culturally sensitive, linguistically appropriate cancer pain education booklet in 11 languages for 11 ethnic groups.[236]

People with cognitive impairment

Patients with mental or psychiatric illness require careful differential assessment before their pain is dismissed as part of the mental illness, rather than actually having pain. In persons with Alzheimer's disease or severe cognitive impairment, pain assessment by means of self-report techniques may be inconclusive.[237] Feldt critiques the existing literature on pain assessment instruments for cognitively impaired elderly and reports findings of a pilot testing of a Checklist of Nonverbal Pain Indicators.[238] Patients with cognitive impairment, in addition to being assessed for physical pain when immobile or resting, should be assessed for non-physical pain and its impact on activities of daily living.[239] More knowledge is needed about assessment and management of pain in adults with substance abuse disorders or mental illness, in persons with alterations in cognition, in persons suffering from sensory alterations and/or neuropathic pain and in critically or acutely ill adults. Although the influence of instruction in tool use is apparent in patients' self-reports of pain, instructions about use of pain scales and assessment tools have not been studied in this population.

Educational interventions for improving knowledge of nurses, patients and caregivers

Knowledge deficits of nurses

Educating and supporting nurses to undertake more effective pain management remains a worldwide high priority for nursing and health care. It is clearly reflected in the literature that pain is addressed in a limited fashion in basic nursing education.[240,241] As a result, nurses feel ill-prepared to care for patients suffering pain and make incorrect decisions about pain management.[128] Although nurses are recognized as the principal providers of patient care and the cornerstone in palliative care, many studies have shown that significant knowledge deficits regarding effective pain management continue to exist among nurses. In the majority of knowledge and attitudes surveys, using different instruments, nurses answered less than 70% of the questions correctly,[242–244] indicating that many nurses continue to lack sufficient knowledge regarding pain management. The main nursing knowledge deficits emerging from a recent literature review[245] are:

1 Poor assessment of pain.[19,191,195,196,242,246,247]

2 Lack of pharmacological information and knowledge[242,243,246,248,249]

3 Misconceptions in the use of analgesics such as:

- exaggerated fears from the appearance of psychological dependence[191,242,243,244]
- respiratory depression[195,244,250]
- sedation[195,244,250]
- inability to use equianalgesic conversion charts.[242,243,249]

Cancer nurses have been found to be more knowledgeable about pain management than other nurses.[195,196,244,246] The longer a country has a palliative care programme in place, the more likely nurses are to have correct information about cancer pain.[191]

A state-wide survey of nurses across speciality areas revealed that many nurses were unaware of the beneficial effects of non-pharmacological treatments for severe pain.[242] Although a wide variety of non-pharmacological pain control strategies were used by up to 86.5% of nurses in a British study,[251] lack of knowledge and use of these complementary methods of pain control is the norm. Few nurses identified use of relaxation, distraction and massage[252] and 90% of the charts audited in another study had no documentation of the use of these nursing interventions to decrease pain.[257]

Personal and professional pain experiences of nurses

Although numerous studies exist regarding nurses' attitudes and knowledge about pain management, only a few have been conducted to examine the relationship between nurses' personal and professional pain experiences and their pain management knowledge.[253–256] In a study, 42% of cancer nurses stated that they altered their pain management practices (i.e. more timely analgesia administration) as a result of their own feelings about pain.[255] However, two studies did not support a relationship between pain experience and pain management knowledge.[257,258] The conflicting findings cast doubt on the relationship between pain experience and pain management knowledge by nurses and suggest a need for further research. If a relationship does exist, further clarification might suggest ways to enhance pain management education by incorporating relevant approaches.

The great majority of nurses in the previous studies were American. Since pain experiences entail cognitive and cultural factors, examining nurses from other countries might further advance the understanding of pain experience and pain knowledge. The purpose of a recent exploratory study was to describe Greek nurses' personal and professional pain experiences and to examine the relationship with their pain management knowledge. Reporting a personal pain experience was associated with describing a positive professional pain experience. Nurses reporting positive professional experiences with pain scored higher in pain management knowledge than nurses reporting negative professional experiences.[259]

Education of nurses, patients and families /caregivers

Evidence exists in the literature that continuous education of nurses can improve their knowledge and attitudes to pain management.[10,195,260–263] However, few studies have examined the ability of educational interventions to demonstrate a sustained benefit. From those available, results are equivocal, possibly owing to differences in the interventions utilized, knowledge and attitude surveys used and administration support in the various institutions for practice changes. However, structured educational interventions have been successful in demonstrating significant and sustained increases in nurses' knowledge and attitudes regarding pain management in several studies.[264–266]

Education of the patient and family/caregiver should be systematic in order to provide the appropriate knowledge and ensure safe care outside the structured healthcare setting. It is essential to assure not only compliance with the prescribed medical and nursing plan but also to enable a proactive approach to cancer pain management. For ambulatory patients, pain diaries are especially helpful in facilitating pain assessment, evaluating how pain is being managed and the need for further education. Patient education is recognized by cancer nursing professional organisations[88] as an essential element of cancer pain management and a primary responsibility for nurses. Cancer nurses are challenged to design educational approaches for patients and their caregivers depending on where they are located (in the hospital, in ambulatory care settings or in the home setting). Data from a qualitative study of 85 caregivers found the various roles they had to assume, such as assessing pain, keeping records, deciding what drug and non-drug approaches to use and communicating with the physician.[267] Patients with cancer and their family caregivers share the same misconceptions and lack of knowledge about cancer pain. Furthermore, family members may experience tremendous burden being in charge of pain management due to their inadequate knowledge and attitudes about pain and its management. In any intervention to improve patients' knowledge and skills, it is essential to include family members due to different perceptions of family caregivers about patients' pain reported.[268] In a recent review of evaluation and research in cancer-related patient education during the past decade, the great need for patient education concerning medications and pain management has been highlighted.[269] Moreover, older patients were found to have significantly less knowledge about pain management than younger patients.[86,87] Coaching patients tends to result in their pain assessments being similar to nurses' assessments.[270] In the conclusions of a systematic review of educational interventions to improve cancer pain control, it is supported that further progress in cancer pain control in ambulatory settings may occur through brief nursing interventions targeting patients in combination with a daily pain diary.[271]

Patient education for cancer pain control should include five phases: assessment, goal setting, selection of educational strategies, implementation and reassessment.[272] Pain information can be provided with verbal discussion or written materials and must be followed by an evaluation of the content learned and used toward achieving appropriate pain relief. Pain education programmes based on different models, such as individualization,[273-275] in groups[276] or with media,[277] showed improvements in knowledge and decreased pain intensity. Furthermore, in an experimental study of 149 patients with cancer cared for at home, structured pain education yielded enhanced knowledge and attitudes about pain, quality of life and pain management.[218] A recent study evaluated the effect of an individualized education and coaching intervention on pain outcomes and pain-related knowledge among outpatients with cancer pain. Compared with provision of standard educational materials and counselling, a brief individualized education and coaching intervention for outpatients with cancer pain was associated with improvement in average pain levels but, as authors suggested, larger studies are needed to validate these effects and elucidate their mechanisms.[278] In another study, the impact of pain education on 50 family members providing home care to elderly patients with cancer was evaluated prior to initiation of the programme and at 1 and 3 weeks following the intervention. Pain education was found effective in improving knowledge and attitudes regarding pain management.[274] Also, the PRO-SELF pain control programme is supported as an effective approach to help patients with metastatic bone pain and their family caregivers obtain the knowledge and skills to increase analgesic intake and lower the severity of pain and number of hours per day in pain. This educational programme combined face-to-face sessions and telephone calls to provide teaching and coaching sessions.[268]

An essential element of improved pain management is pain education of the public. An article by Ferrell and Juarez reported on the implementation of a national training project, the Cancer Pain Education for Patients and the Public.[279] National cancer organizations (e.g. American Cancer Society) and cancer pain initiatives (e.g. Wisconsin Cancer Pain Initiative) have produced booklets with questions and answers about pain control for adults, children and adolescents with cancer pain, offering great help in patients' education.

Patient teaching combined with novel approaches to deliver appropriate pain content can lead to increased patient compliance with the prescribed pain regimen. The remaining challenge is to find ways to overcome significant barriers such as limited time and resources to improve cancer care of patients in pain by providing patient education.[280] As nurses, we need to continue to learn what works and does not work for patients and families in our practice settings and stay active in developing and testing quality improvement models, tools and interventions toward better patient–family care provision.

CONCLUSION

Pain relief is the essence of cancer care. As management of cancer pain is a multidisciplinary challenge, it requires close collaboration between healthcare professionals for an integrated approach combining pharmacological and non-pharmacological techniques. Optimal pain control is still prohibited by erroneous clinical decisions, poor collection and interpretation of data, patient reluctance or ability to report pain, non-compliance with pain control regimens and various factors influencing therapeutic decision-making.

Because nurses have sustained contact with patients across all care settings, they are in a position to identify underestimated and untreated pain. They should advocate for their patients' needs for pain relief and comfort by examining systematically their practice and environment. If any barriers are identified, they should speak up and demand changes. It is the responsibility of every nurse to use his/her position within the healthcare team to ensure that effective pain management occurs. More educational efforts need to focus on equipping health professionals, patients and their caregivers with the necessary knowledge, skills and attitudes to participate in undertaking comprehensive regular pain assessment and decision-making on the best-available treatment option for each individual and his family. Furthermore, significant efforts are required to secure institutional commitment in addressing the main underlying reasons for suboptimal pain management, such as ritualistic and bureaucratic practices, lack of resources and breakdown in continuity and quality of care.

REFERENCES

1. IASP Subcommittee on Taxonomy. Pain terms: a list with definitions and notes on usage. Recommended by the IASP Subcommittee on Taxonomy. Pain 1979; 6:249.

2. McCaffery M. Nursing management of the patient with pain. 1st edn. Philadelphia: Lippincott: 1972.

3. Morris DB. The culture of pain. 1st edn. Berkeley: University of California Press; 1991.

4. Melzack R, Wall PD. The challenge of pain. 2nd edn. London: Penguin Books; 1988.

5. Consensusbijeenkomst Verpleegkunde bij Pijn 1994 CBO (Report on the Consensus Meeting Nursing and Pain, The Netherlands: Quality Institute for Healthcare CBO; 1994.) [in Dutch]

6. Flatow FA, Long S. Specialized care at the terminal ill. In: De Vita VJ, Hellman S, Rosenberg SA, eds. Cancer: principles and practice of oncology. 6th edn. Philadelphia: Lippincott, Williams and Wilkins; 2001:3077–3088.

7. Brecia FJ. Pain management issues as part of the comprehensive care of the cancer patient. Semin Oncol 1993; 20(1 Suppl. A):48–52.

8. World Health Organization.Cancer pain relief and palliative care. Report of a WHO Expert Committee, Technical Report, Geneva; 1990.

9. Coyne PJ. International efforts in cancer pain relief. Semin Oncol Nurs 1997;13:57–62.

10. De Rond MEJ, De Wit R, VanDam FSAM, Muller MJ. A pain monitoring program for nurses: effect on the administration of analgesics. Pain 2000; 89:25–38.

11. Twycross A. Educating nurses about pain management: the way forward. J Clin Nurs 2002; 11:705–714.

12. Daut R, Cleeland C. The prevalence and severity of pain in cancer. Cancer 1982; 50:1913–1918.

13. Coyle N, Foley K. Prevalence and profile of pain syndromes in cancer patients. In: McGuire D, Yarbro CH, eds. Cancer pain management. Orlando, Florida: Crune and Stratton; 1987:21–46.

14. Desbiens NA, Wu AW, Broste SK, et al. Pain and satisfaction with pain control in seriously ill hospitalized adults: findings from the SUPPORT research investigations. Crit Care Med 1996; 24:1953–1961.

15. United States. Management of Cancer Pain Guideline Panel; United States. Agency for Health Care Policy and Research. Management of cancer pain/Management of Cancer Pain Guideline Panel No 9. Rockville, MD, US Dept. of Health and Human Services, Public Health Service, Agency for Health Care Policy and Research; 1994.

16. Zhukovsky DS, Corowski E, Hausdorff J, Napolitano B, Lesser M. Unmet analgesic needs in cancer patients. J Pain Symptom Manage 1995; 10:113–119.

17. Grond S, Zech D, Diefenbach C, Radbruch L, Lehmann KA. Assessment of cancer pain: a prospective evaluation in 2266 cancer patients referred to a pain service. Pain 1996; 64:107–114.

18. Twycross R, Harcourt J, Bergl S. A survey of pain in patients with advanced cancer. J Pain Symptom Manage 1996; 12:273–282.

19. De Wit R, Van Dam F, Vielvoye-Kerkmeer A, Mattern C, Abu-Saas H. The treatment of chronic cancer pain in a cancer hospital in the Netherlands. J Pain Symptom Manage 1999; 17:333–350.

20. Hanks GW, de Conno F, Hanna M, et al. Morphine in cancer pain: modes of administration. BMJ 1996; 312: 823–826.

21. Lynn J, Teno J, Phillips R, et al. Perceptions by family members of the dying experience of older and seriously ill patients. Ann Intern Med1997; 126:97–106.

22. Tolle S, Tilden V, Hickman S, Rosenfeld A. Family reports of pain in dying hospitalized patients: a structured telephone survey. West J Med 2000; 172:347–377.

23. Miaskowski C. Recent advances in understanding pain mechanisms provide future directions for pain management. Oncol Nurs Forum 2004; 31(4 Suppl):25–35.

24. Smith WD. The Hippocratic tradition. Ithaca: Cornell University Press; 1979.

25. Kordiolis N. Critical comments on pain management in Ancient Greece. Hellenic Oncol 1989; 25:46–55. [in Greek]

26. Barnes AJ. The complete works of Aristotle [the revised Oxford translation]. Princeton: Princeton University Press; 1984.

27. Descartes R, Steele HT. Treatise of man. [French text with translation and commentary by Thomas Steele Hall]. Cambridge: Harvard University Press; 1972.

28. Müller J. Elements of physiology. London: Taylor and Walton; 1842.

29. Von Frey M. Beitrage zur Sinnespsychologie der Haut. Ber. d kgl sachs Ges d Wiss, math-phys Kl 47 (1895) 166-184.

30. Noordenbos W. Pain; problems pertaining to the transmission of nerve impulses which give rise to pain. Preliminary statement. Amsterdam: Elsevier Press; 1959.

31. Melzack R, Wall PD. Pain mechanisms: a new theory. Science 1965; 3669(150): 971–979.

32. Basbaum AI, Woolf CJ. Pain. Curr Biol 1999; 9(12):R429–431.

33. Hawthorn J, Redmond K. Pain: causes and management. Oxford, Malden, MA: Blackwell Science; 1998:173

34. van Cranenburgh B. Inleiding in de toegepaste neurowetenschappen. 2de herziene druk. Lochem: Tijdstroom; 1987 [in Dutch].

35. Fields HL. Pain. New York: McGraw-Hill; 1987.

36. Stucky CL, Gold MS, Zhang X. Mechanisms of pain. Proc Natl Acad Sci USA 2001; 98(21):11845–11846.

37. Hamill RJ, Rowlingson JC. Handbook of critical care pain management. New York: McGraw-Hill; 1994.

38. Wilkie DJ. Neural mechanisms of pain: a foundation for cancer pain assessment and management. In: McGuire D, Yarbro C, Ferrell BR, eds. Cancer pain management. London: Jones and Bartlett; 1995:61–87.

39. Woolf CJ, Salter MW. Neuronal plasticity: increasing the gain in pain. Science 2000; 288:1765–1768.

40. Scholz J, Woolf CJ. Can we conquer pain? Nature Neurosci 2002; 5(Suppl.): 1062–1067.

41. Noguchi K, Tohyama M. Molecular biology of pain: should clinicians care? Pain Clinical Updates, IASP 2000; VIII(2):1–4.

42. Woolf CJ, Decosterd I. Implications of recent advances in the understanding of pain pathophysiology for the assessment of pain in patients. Pain 1999; 82(Suppl. 6): S141–S147.

43. Bolay H, Moskowitz MA. Mechanisms of pain modulation in chronic syndromes. Neurology 2002; 59(5 Suppl. 2):S2–S7.

44. Miaskowski C. Biology of mucosal pain. J Natl Cancer Instit Monogr 2001; 29:37–40.

45. Woolf CJ, Mannion RJ. Neuropathic pain: etiology, symptoms, mechanisms, and management. Lancet 1999; 353:1959–1964.

46. Procacci P, Zoppi M. Pathophysiology and clinical aspects of visceral and referred pain. In: Bonica JJ, Lindblom U, Iggo A, eds. Proc Third World Congress on Pain. New York: Raven Press; 1983:21–28.

47. Woolf CJ. The pathophysiology of peripheral neuropathic pain – abnormal peripheral input and abnormal central processing. Acta Neurochirurg Suppl (Wien) 1993; 58:125–130.

48. Bowsher D. Central pain: clinical and physiological characteristics. J Neurol Neurosurg Psychiatry 1996; 61:62–69.

49. Szasz TS. Pain and pleasure: a study of bodily feelings. 2nd edn. New York: Basic Books; 1975.

50. Menges JL. Chronic pain patients: some psychological aspects. In: Persistent pain, Vol III. London: Academic Press; 1981.

51. Bonica JJ. Definitions and taxonomy of pain. In: Bonica JJ, ed. The management of pain. 2nd edn. Philadelphia: Lee and Febiger; 1990.

52. Duarte RA. Classification of pain. In: Kanner R, ed. Pain management secrets. Philadelphia: Hanley and Belfus; 1997:5–7.

53. Portenoy RK, Hagen NA. Breakthrough pain: definition, prevalence and characteristics. Pain 1990; 41:273–281.

54. Collins PM. Pain. In: Johnson BL, Gross J, eds. Handbook of oncology nurses. 3rd edn. Boston: Jones and Bartlett Publishers; 1998:305–336.

55. Patt RB. Cancer pain. Philadelphia: JB Lippincott; 1993.

56. Hansson P. Neurogenic pain: diagnosis and treatment. Pain Clinical Updates, IASP 1994; II(3):1–4.

57. Simmons M. Management of breakthrough pain due to cancer. Oncology 1999; 13:1103–1108.

58. Sykes J, Johnson R, Hanks GW. Difficult pain problems. In: Fallon MT, O'Neil B, eds. ABC of palliative care. London: BMJ Books; 1998:5–7.

59. McGuire DB. Cancer pain: pathophysiology of pain in cancer. Cancer Nurs 1989; 12:310–315.

60. Payne R. Cancer pain, anatomy, physiology, and pharmacology. Cancer 1989; 63:2266–2274.

61. Farrar JT, Cleary J, Rauck R, Busch M, Nordbrock E. Oral transmucosal fentanyl citrate: randomized, double-blinded, placebo-controlled trial for treatment of breakthrough pain in cancer patients. J Natl Cancer Inst 1998; 90:611–616.

62. Foley KM. The treatment of pain in the patient with cancer. CA Cancer J Clin 1986; 36:104–214.

63. Foley KM. Acute and chronic cancer pain syndromes. In: Doyle D, Hanks G, Cherny N, Calman K, eds. Oxford textbook of palliative medicine. Oxford: Oxford University Press: 2004:298–316.

64. Gonzales GR. Cancer pain syndromes. In: Kanner R, ed. Pain management secrets. Philadelphia: Hanley and Belfus; 1997:107–112.

65. Chapman CR, Kornell J, Syrjala KL. Pain complications of cancer diagnosis and therapy. In: McGuire D, Yarbro CH, eds. Cancer pain management. Orlando, Florida: Crune and Stratton; 1987:47–67.

66. LeShan L. The world of the patient in severe pain of long duration. J Chron Dis 1964; 17:119–126.

67. Saunders C. The management of terminal illness. London: Hospital Medication Publication; 1967.

68. Melzack R. The puzzle of pain. Harmondsworth: Penguin Books; 1973.

69. Waring EM. The relationship of chronic pain to depression, marital adjustment and family dynamics. Pain 1978; 5(3):285–292.

70. Melzack R, Casey KL. Sensory, motivational and central control determinants of pain: a new conceptual model. In: Kenshalo D, ed. The skin senses. Proceedings of the First International Symposium on the Skin Senses. Springfield, IL: Thomas; 1968: 423–439.

473

71. Ahles TA, Blanchard EB, Ruckdeschel JC. The multidimensional nature of cancer-related pain. Pain 1983; 17:277–288.

72. McGuire DB. The multidimensional phenomenon of cancer pain. In: McGuire D, Yarbro CH, eds. Cancer pain management. Orlando, Florida: Crune and Stratton; 1987:1–20.

73. Bates MS. Ethnicity and pain: a biocultural model. Soc Sci Med 1987; 24:47–50.

74. Spross JA, Burke MW. Nonpharmachological management of cancer pain. In: McGuire D, Yarbro C, Ferrell BR, eds. Cancer pain management. London: Jones and Bartlett; 1995:159–205.

75. World Health Organisation. Cancer pain relief. Geneva: WHO; 1986.

76. McCaffery M, Beebe A, eds. Clinical manual for nursing practice. St Louis: CV Mosby; 1989.

77. Krishnasamy M. Pain. In: Corner J, Bailey C, eds. Cancer nursing care in context. Oxford: Blackwell Science; 2001:339–349.

78. Kuuppelomaki M, Lauri S. Cancer patients' reported experiences of suffering. Cancer Nurs 1998; 21(5):364–369.

79. Moinpour CM, Chapman CR. Pain management and quality of life in cancer patients. In: Lehmann RKA, Zech D, eds. Transdermal fentanyl: a new approach to prolonged pain control. Berlin: Springer-Verlag; 1991:42–63.

80. Dodd MJ, Miaskowski C, Paul SM. Symptom clusters and their effect on the functional status of patients with cancer. Oncol Nurs Forum 2001; 28:465–470.

81. Glover J, Miaskowski C, Dibble S, Dodd MJ. Mood states of oncology outpatients: Does pain make a difference? J Pain Symptom Manage 1995; 10(2):120–128.

82. Miaskowski C, Lee KA. Pain, fatigue and sleep disturbances in oncology outpatients receiving radiation therapy for bone metastasis: a pilot study. J Pain Symptom Manage 1999; 17:320–332.

83. McGuire DB. The multiple dimensions of cancer pain: a framework for assessment and management. In: McGuire D, Yarbro C, Ferrell BR, eds. Cancer pain management. London: Jones and Bartlett; 1995:1–17.

84. Ferrell BR, Rhiner M, Cohen MZ. Pain as a metaphor illness. Part I: Impact of cancer pain on family caregivers. Oncol Nurs Forum 1991; 18:1303–1309.

85. Padilla GV. Validity of health related quality of life subscales. Progr Cardiovasc Nurs 1992; 7(7):13–20.

86. Miaskowski C, Kragness L Dibble SL, Wallhagen M. Differences in mood states, health status, and perceived strain between caregivers of oncology outpatients with and without cancer-related pain. J Pain Symptom Manage 1997; 13:138–147.

87. Yeager KA, Miaskowski C, Dibble S, Wallhagen M. Advances in pain knowledge in cancer patients with and without pain. Cancer Pract 1997; 5:39–45.

88. Spross JA, McGuire DB, Schmitt RM. Oncology Nursing Society Position Paper on Cancer Pain. Oncol Nurs Forum 1990; 17:595–614, 751–760, 825, 943–955.

89. Maassen E. Het pijnboogmodel; de brug tussen therapie en evaluatie. Verslagboek 14ᶜ VvOV Congres, Dutch Oncology Nursing Society, 1995: 71–74 [in Dutch].

90. Abrahm JL, Snyder L. Pain assessment and management. Primary Care 2001; 28(2):269–297.

91. Donovan MI. Clinical assessment of cancer pain. In: McGuire D, Yarbro CH, eds. Cancer pain management. Orlando, Florida: Crune and Stratton; 1987:105–131.

92. Vallerand AH. Measurement issues in the comphrehensive assessment or cancer pain. Semin Oncol Nurs 1997; 13:16–24.

93. Olsen S, Nolan MF, Kori S. Pain measurement. An overview of two commonly used methods. Anesth Rev 1992; 19(6):11–15

94. Syrjala KL. The measurement of pain. In: McGuire D, Yarbro CH, eds. Cancer pain management. Orlando, Florida: Crune and Stratton; 1987:133–150.

95. McGuire DB. Comprehensive and multidimensional assessment and measurement of pain. J Pain Symptom Manage 1992; 7:312–319.

96. Giff AG. Visual analogue scales: measurement of subjective phenomena. Nurs Res 1989; 38:286–288.

97. McGrath PJ, Umruh AM, Finley GA. Pain management in childern. Pain Clinical Updates, IASP 1995; III(2):1–4.

98. Hovi SL, Lauri S. Patients and nurses assessment of cancer pain. Eur J Cancer Care 1999; 8:213–219.

99. Kremer E, Atkinson JH, Ignelzi RJ. Measurement of pain: patient preference does not confound pain mesurement. Pain 1981; 10:241–248.

100. Fink R, Gates R. Pain assessment. In: Ferrell BR, Coyle N, eds. Palliative nursing., Oxford: Oxford University Press; 2001:53–71.

101. Melzack R. The McGill Pain Questionnaire: major properties and scoring methods. Pain 1975; 1:277–299.

102. Melzack R. The short form McGill Pain Questionnaire. Pain 1987; 30:191–197.

103. Daut RL, Cleeland CS, Flanery RC. Development of the Wisconsin Brief Pain Questionnaire to assess pain in cancer and other diseases. Pain 1983; 17:197–210.

104. Fishman B, Pasternak S, Wallenstein SL, et al. The Memorial Pain Assessment Card. A valid instrument for the evaluation of cancer pain. Cancer 1987; 60:1151–1158.

105. Chang VT, Hwang SS, Feuerman M. Validation of the Edmonton Symptom Assessment Scale. Cancer 2000; 88:2164–2171.

106. Bruera E, Kuehn N, Miller MJ, Selmser P, Macmillan K. The Edmonton Symptom Assessment System (ESAS): a simple method for the assessment of palliative care patients. J Palliat Care 1991; 7(2):6–9.

107. van Cranenburgh B, Kobus M. Pijn en pijnbestrijding. In: Jaarboek Fysiotherapie. Utrecht: Bohn, Scheltema en Holkema; 1989:5–15 [in Dutch].

108. International Association for the Study of Pain, Task Force on Guidelines for Desirable Characteristics for Pain Treatment Facilities. Desirable characteristics for pain treatment facilities. Standards for physician fellowship in pain management. Seattle, WA: International Association for the Study of Pain; 1990.

109. Catalano RB. Pharmacologic management in the treatment of cancer pain. In: McGuire D, Yarbro CH, eds. Cancer pain management. Orlando, Florida: Crune and Stratton; 1987:115–201.

110. Mercadante S, Portenoy RK. Opioid poorly-respnonsive cancer pain. Part 3. Clinical strategies to improve opioid responsiveness. J Pain Symptom Manage 2001; 21:338–353

111. McQuay H, Moore A. An evidence-based resource for pain relief. Oxford: Oxford University Press; 2000.

112. Porter AT, McEwan AJ, Rowe JE, et al. Results of a randomized phase-III trial to evaluate the efficacy of strontium-89 adjuvant to local field external beam irradiation in the management of endocrine resistant metastatic prostate cancer. Int J Radiat Oncol Biol Phys 1993; 25:805–813.

113. Quilty PM, Kirk D, Bolger JJ, et al. A comparison of the palliative effects of strontium-89 and external beam radiotherapy in metastatic prostate cancer. Radiother Oncol 1994; 31:33–40.

114. Poulter CA, Cosmatos D, Rubin P, et al. A report of RTOG 8206: a phase III study of whether the addition of single dose hemibody irradiation to standard fractionated local field irradiation is more effective than local field irradiation alone in the treatment of symptomatic osseous metastases. Int J Radiat Oncol Biol Phys 1992; 23(1):207–214.

115. Burris HA 3rd, Moore MJ, Andersen J, et al. Improvements in survival and clinical benefit with gemcitabine as first line therapy in patients with advanced pancreas cancer: a randomized trial. J Clin Oncol 1997; 15:2403–2413.

116. Tannock IF, Osoba D, Stockler MR, et al. Chemotherapy with mitoxantrone plus prednisone or prednisone alone for symptomatic hormone resistant prostate cancer: a Canadian randomized trial with palliative endpoints. J Clin Oncol 1996; 14:1756–1764.

117. Eisenberg E, Berkey CS, Carr DB, Mosteller F, Chalmers TC. Efficacy and safety on nonsteroidal antiflammatory drugs for cancer pain: a meta-analysis. J Clin Oncol 1994; 12:2756–2765.

118. Henry D, Lim L, Garcia Rodrigues LA, et al. Variability in risk of gastrointestinal complications with individual non-steroidal anti-inflammatory drugs: results of a collaborative meta-analysis. BMJ 1996; 312:1563–1566.

119. Shield MJ, Morant SV. Misoprostol in patients taking non-steroidal anti-inflammatory drugs. BMJ 1996; 312: 846.

120. Arner A, Lindblom U, Meyerson BA, Molander C. Prolonged relief of neuralgia after regional anesthetic blocks. A call for further experimental and systematic clinical studies. Pain 1990; 43:287–297.

121. Reisine T, Pasternak G. Opioid analgesics and antagonists. In: Hardman JG, Limbird LE, Molinoff PB, Ruddon RW, Goodman Gilman A, eds. The pharmacological basis of therapeutics. New York: McGraw-Hill; 1996:Chapter 9.

122. Szeto HH, Inturrisi CE, Houde R, et al. Accumulation of norperidine, an active metabolite of meperidine, in patients with renal failure or cancer. Ann Intern Med 1977; 86:738–741.

123. Hanks GW, de Conno F, Cherny N, et al. Morphine and alternative opioids in cancer pain: the EAPC Recommendations. Br J Cancer 2001; 84:587–593.

124. American Pain Society. Principles of analgesic use in the treatment of acute pain and cancer pain. 4th edn. Glenview IL: American Pain Society;, 1999.

125. Swanson G, Smith J, Bulich R, New P, Shiffman R. Patients-controlled analgesics for chronic cancer pain in the ambulatory setting: a report of 117 patients. J Clin Oncol 1989; 5:1903–1908.

126. Bruera E, Pereira J. Recent developments in palliative cancer care. Acta Oncologica 1998; 37:749–757.

127. Bates DW, Cullen DJ, Laird N, et al. Incidence of adverse drug events and potential adverse drugs events. JAMA 1995; 274:29–34.

128. Redmond K. Barriers to the effective management of pain. Int J Palliat Nurs 1998; 4(6):276–278, 280–283

129. Twycross R. Symptom management in advanced cancer. 2nd edn. Abingdon: Radcliffe Medical Press; 1997:30.

130. McCaffery M, Ferrell BR, Turner M. Ethical issues in the use of placebos in cancer pain management. Oncol Nurs Forum 1996; 23:1587–1593.

131. Porter J, Jick H. Addiction rare in patients treated with narcotics. N Engl J Med 1980; 302(2):123.

132. Kanner RM, Foley KM. Patterns of narcotic drug use in a cancer pain clinic. Ann NY Acad Sci 1981; 362:161–172.

133. McGuire L. Pain management. In: Otto SE, ed. Oncology nursing. St. Louis: Mosby Year Book; 1991:388–410.

134. Vaccarino AL. Tolerance to morphine analgesia: basic issues to consider. Pain Forum 1999; 8(1):25–28.

135. Portenoy RK, Foley KM, Inturrisi CE. The nature of opioid responsiveness and its implications for neuropathic pain: new hypotheses derived from studies of opioid infusions. Pain 1990; 43:273–286.

136. Twycross RG. Opioids In: Wall BD, Melzak R, eds. Textbook of pain. 3rd edn. Edinburgh, Churchill Livingstone; 1994:934–962.

137. McQuay HJ. Opioids in chronic pain. Br J Anaesth 1989; 63:213–226.

138. Foley KM. Clinical tolerance to opioids. In: Basbaum BIA, Dahlem JMR, eds. Towards a new pharmocotherapy of pain. Chichester: John Wiley; 181–204.

139. Foley KM, Inturrisi CE. Analgesic drug therapy in cancer pain: Principles and practice. Med Clin N Am 1987; 71:207–232.

140. Zech DF, Grond S, Lynch J, Hertel D, Lehmann KA. Validation of World Health Organization Guidelines for cancer pain relief: a 10-year prospective study. Pain 1995; 63(1):65–76.

141. Cullinane CM, Chu D, Mamelak A. Current surgical options in the control of cancer pain. Cancer Pract 2002; 10(Suppl 1):S21–26.

142. Smith T, Staats P, Deer T, et al. Randomized clinical trial of an implantable drug delivery system compared with comprehensive medical management for refractory cancer pain: impact on pain, drug-related toxicity, and survival. J Clin Oncol 2002; 20:4040–4049.

143. Ferrante M, Bedder M, Caplan R, et al. Practice guidelines for cancer pain management. Anesthesiology 1996; 84:1243–1257.

144. Coyne PJ. When the World Health Organization analgesic therapies ladder fails: the role of invasive analgesic therapies. Oncol Nurs Forum 2003; 30:777–783.

145. Sjogren P, Banning AM, Hebsgaard K, Petersen P, Gefke K. Intravenos lidokain i behandlingen af kroniske smerter forarsaget af knoglemetastser. Ugeskrift for Laeger 1989; 151:2144–2146 [in Danish].

146. Bruera E, Ripamonti C, Brenneis C, Macmillan K, Hanson J. A randomized double-blind crossover trial of intravenous lidocaine in the treatment of neuropathic cancer pain. J Pain Symptom Manage 1992; 7:138–140.

147. Ellemann K, Sjogren P, Banning A, et al. Trial of intravenous lidocaine on painful neuropathy in cancer patients. Clin J Pain 1989; 5:291–294.

148. Swarm RA, Karanikolas M, Cousins MJ. Anaesthetic techniques for pain control. In: Doyle D, Hanks G, Cherney N, Calman K, eds. Oxford textbook of palliative medicine. Oxford: Oxford University Press; 2004:378–396.

149. Eisenberg E, Carr DB, Chalmers TC. Neurolytic celiac plexus block for treatment of cancer pain: a meta-analysis. Anesth Analg 1995; 81(1):213.

150. Staats P, Hekmat H, Sauter P, Lillemoe K. The effects of alcohol celiac plexus block pain and mood on longevity in patients with unresectable pancreatic cancer: a double-blind randomized placebo controlled study. Pain Med 200; 2:28–34.

151. Lema MJ. Invasive procedures for cancer pain. Pain Clinical Updates, IASP 1998; VI(I):1–4.

152. Saberski L, Ligham D. Neuroablative techniques for cancer pain management. Techn Regional Anesth Pain Manage 1997; 1:53–58.

153. Ahles A. Psychological techniques for the management of cancer-related pain. In: McGuire D, Yarbro CH, eds. Cancer pain management. Orlando, Florida: Crune and Stratton; 1987:245–258.

154. Fernandez E. A classification system of cognitive coping strategies for pain. Pain 1986; 26:141–151.

155. Owens KM, Ehrenreich D. Literature review of nonpharmocologic methods for the treatment of chronic pain. Holist Nurs Pract 1991; 6:24–31.

156. Spross J. Pain, suffering, and spiritual well-being; assesments and interventions. Quality of Life: A Nursing Challenge 1993; 2:71–79.

157. Stiles M. The shining stranger: nurse–family spiritual relationship. Cancer Nurs 1990; 13:235–245.

158. Stevensen C. Nursing perspective. In: Barraclough J, ed. Integrated cancer care. Holistic complementary, and creative approaches. Oxford: Oxford University Press; 2001:234–243.

159. Ferrell BR, Ferrell BA, Ahn C, Tran K. Pain management for elderly patients with cancer at home. Cancer 1994; 74:2139–2146.

160. Pocket-Munro S. Music therapy. In: Doyle D, ed. Oxford textbook of palliative medicine. Oxford: Oxford University Press; 1993:555–559.

161. Zimmerman L, Pozehl B, Schmitz R. Effects of music in patients who had chronic pain. West J Nurs Res 1989; 11:298–309.

162. Salerno E, Willens JS, eds. Pain management handbook: an interdisciplinary approach. St. Louis: Mosby; 1996.

163. Spiegel D, Bloom JR. Pain in metastatic breast cancer. Cancer 1982; 52:341–345.

164. Thomas EM, Weiss SM. Non-pharmocological interventions with chronic cancer pain in adults. Cancer Control 2000; 7:157–164.

165. Benson H, Beary JF, Carol MP. The relaxation response. Psychiatry 1974; 37:37–46.

166. Carroll D, Seers K. Relaxation for the relief of chronic pain: a systematic review. J Adv Nurs 1998; 27:476–487.

167. Curtis S. The effect of music on pain relief and relaxation of the terminally ill. J Music Ther 1986; 23:10–14.

168. Syrjala KL, Donaldson GW, Davis MW, Kippes ME, Carr JE. Relaxation and imagery and cognitive-behavioral training reduce pain during cancer treatment: a controlled clinical trial. Pain 1995; 63:189–198.

169. Vasudevan SV. Physical rehabilitation in managing pain. Pain Clinical Updates, IASP 1997; V(3):1–4.

170. Mobily P, Herr K, Nicholson A. Validation of cutaneous stimulation interventions for pain management. Int J Nurs Stud 1994; 31:533–544.

171. Lehmann JF, deLatour BJ. Ultrasound short wave, micro wave, superficial heat, and cold in the treatment of pain. In: Wall PD, Melzak R, eds. Textbook of pain. Edinburgh: Churchill Livingstone; 1984:717–774.

172. McCaffery M. Nursing approaches to nonpharmacological pain control. Int J Nurs Stud 1990; 27:1–5

173. Kottke FJ, Lehnmann JF, eds. Krusen's handbook of physical medicine and rehabilitation. Philadelphia: WB Saunders; 1990.

174. Melzack R. Folk medicine and the sensory modulation of pain. In: Wall PD, Melzak R, eds. Textbook of pain. Edinburgh: Churchill Livingstone; 1984:1209–1217.

175. Bini G, Cruccu G, Hagbarth KE, Schady W, Torebjork E. Analgesic effects of vibration and cooling on pain induced by intra-neural electrical stimulation. Pain 1984; 18:239–248.

176. Lundeberg T. Long-term results of vibration stimulation as a pain relieving measure for chronic pain. Pain 1984; 20:13–23.

177. Lundeberg T, Nordemar R, Ottoson D. Pain alleviation by vibratory stimulation. Pain 1984; 20: 5–44.

178. Weinrich SP, Weinrich MC. The effects of massage on pain in cancer patients. Appl Nurs Res 1990; 3:140–145.

179. Ferrell-Torry AT, Click OJ. The use of therapeutic massage as a nursing intervention to modify anxiety and the perception of cancer pain. Cancer Nurs 1993; 16:93–101.

180. Ostrowski MJ. Pain control in advanced malignant disease using transcutaneous nerve stimulation. Br J Clin Pract 1979; 33:157–162.

181. Wen HL. Cancer pain treated with acupuncture and electrical stimulation. Mod Med Asia 1977; 13:12–16.

182. Gadsby JG, Franks A, Jarvis P, et al. Acupuncture-like transcutaneous electrical nerve stimulation within palliative care: a pilot study. Complement Ther Med 1997; 5:13–18.

183. Moolamanil T, Lundeberg T. Does acupuncture work? Pain Clinical Updates 1996; IV(3):1–4.

184. Xu S, Liu Z, Li Y. Treatment of cancerous abdominal pain by acupuncture on Zusanli (ST-36): a report of 92 cases. J Trad Chinese Med 1995; 15:189–191.

185. Wallace KG. Analysis of recent literature concerning relaxation and imagery interventions for cancer pain. Cancer Nurs 1997; 20:79–87.

186. Sindhu F. Are non pharmacological nursing interventions for the management of pain effective? – a meta-analysis. J Adv Nurs 1996; 24:1152–1159.

187. Smith MC, Stullenbarger E. An intergrative review and meta-analysis of oncology nursing research: 1981–1990. Cancer Nurs 1995; 18:167–179.

188. De Rond M. Pain from zero to ten: effects of a pain monitoring program for nurses (Thesis). Amsterdam: University of Amsterdam; 2001 [in Dutch].

189. Chapman CR, Casey KL, Dubner R, et al. Pain measurement: an overview. Pain 1985; 22:1–31.

190. Beck S. An ethnographic study of factors influencing cancer pain management in South Africa. Cancer Nurs 2000; 23:91–99.

191. McCaffery M, Ferrell B. Nurses' knowledge about cancer pain: a survey of five countries. J Pain Symptom Manage 1995; 10:356–367.

192. Patiraki-Kourbani E, Lanara V, Monos D, et al. Nursing assessment of pain in cancer patients: the Greek picture. Eur J Oncol Nurs 1998; 2:133–135.

193. Patiraki-Kourbani E. Nursing assessment of cancer patients' pain. (Dissertation). Athens: University of Athens; 1995 [in Greek].

194. Cleeland CS. Strategies for improving cancer pain management. J Pain Symptom Manage 1993; 8:361–364.

195. Howell D, Butler L, Vincent L, Watt-Watson J, Stearns N. Influencing nurses' knowledge, attitudes, and practice in cancer pain management. Cancer Nurs 2000; 23:55–63.

196. O'Brien S, Dalton JA, Konsler G, Carlson J. The knowledge and attitudes of experienced oncology nurses regarding the management of cancer related pain. Oncol Nurs Forum 1996; 23:515–521.

197. Pederson C. Nonpharmacologic interventions to manage children's pain: immediate and short-term effects of continuing education program. J Cont Educ Nurs 1996; 27:131–140.

198. Al-Hassan M, Alkhalil M, Ma'Aitah R. Jordanian nurses' roles in the management of postoperative pain in the postanesthesia unit. J Perianesth Nurs 1999; 14:384–389.

199. MacDonald DD, McNulty J, Erickson K, Weiskopf C. Communicating pain and pain management needs after surgery. Appl Nurs Res 2000; 13:70–75.

200. Von Roenn J, Cleeland C, Gonin R, Hatfeld A, Pandaya K. Physicians attitudes and practice in cancer pain management: a survey from the Eastern Cooperative Group. Ann Intern Med 1993; 119:121–126.

201. Angarola RT. National and international regulation of opioid drugs: purpose, structures,

benefits and risks. J Pain Symptom Manage 1990; 5(2 Suppl):6–11.

202. Joranson DE. Federal and state regulation of opioids. J Pain Symptom Manage 1990; 5(2 Suppl):12–23.

203. Committee on Quality Assurance Standards, American Pain Society. American Pain Society quality assurance standards for relief of acute pain and cancer pain. In: Bond MR, Charlton JE, Woolf CJ, eds. Proceedings of the VIth World Congress on Pain. Amsterdam: Elsevier Science, 1991:185–189.

204. Mead P. Clinical guidelines: promoting clinical effectiveness or a professional minefield. J Adv Nurs 2000; 31:110–116.

205. Smith T, Hillner B. Ensuring quality cancer care by the use of clinical practice guidelines and critical pathways. J Clin Oncol 2001; 19:2886–2897.

206. Yoos H, Malone K, McMullen A, et al. Standards and practice guidelines as a foundation for clinical practice. J Nurs Care Qual 1997; 11(5):48–54.

207. Gordon DB, Dahl JL, Stevenson KK. Building an institutional commitment to pain management: the Wisconsin Resource Manual, 2nd edn. Madison, WI: University of Wisconsin-Madison Board of Regents available from www.wisc.edu/trc; 2000.

208. Duff L, Kitson A, Seers K, Humphris D. Clinical guidelines: an introduction to their development and implementation. J Adv Nurs 1996; 23:887–895.

209. Practice guidelines for cancer pain management. A report by the American Society of Anesthesiologists Task Force on Pain Management, Cancer Pain Section. Anesthesiology 1996; 84:1243–1257.

210. Schmidt KL, Alpen MA, Rakel BA. Implementation of the Agency for Health Care Policy and Research Pain Guidelines. Clinical Issues Advanced Practice in Acute and Critical Care 1996; 7:425–435.

211. Gordon DB. Critical pathways: a road to institutionalizing pain management. J Pain Symptom Manage 1996; 11:252–259.

212. Dufault A, Willey-Lessne C. Using a collaborative research utilization model to develop and test the effects of clinical pathways for pain management. J Nurs Care Qual 1999; 13(4):19–33.

213. Ferrell BR, Whedon M, Rollins B. Pain and quality assessment improvement. J Nurs Care Qual 1995; 9:69–85.

214. Bookbinder M. Improving the quality of care across all settings. In: Ferrell BR, Coyle N, eds. Textbook of palliative care. New York: Oxford University Press; 2001:503–530.

215. Miaskowski C. New approaches for evaluating the quality of cancer pain management in the outpatient setting. Pain Manage Nurs 2001; 2:7–12.

216. Gordon D, Stevenson K, Berry P. Institutionalizing effective pain management practices institutional needs assessment. Am Alliance Cancer Pain Initiatives 2001.

217. Morse LK. Commentary on pain management at home: struggle, comfort, and mission. ONS Nursing Scan Oncol 1993.

218. Ferrell BR, Juarez G, Borneman T, Ter Veer A. Outcomes of pain education in community home care. J Hospice Palliat Nurs 1999 26:1655–1661.

219. Rutledge DN, Donaldson NE, Pravikoff DS. Pain assessment and documentation. Special populations of adults. Online Journal of Clinical Innovations, 2002 CINAHL Accession Number:2002045794

220. Miser AW, Dothage JA, Wesley RA, Miser JS. The prevalence of pain in a pediatric and young adult cancer population. Clin J Pain 1987; 29:73–83.

221. Hester NO. Integrating pain assessment and management into the care of children with cancer. In: McGuire D, Yarbro C, Ferrell BR, eds. Cancer pain management. London: Jones and Bartlett; 1995:231–271.

222. Hester NO, Foster RL, Beyer JE. Clinical judgment in assessing children's pain. In: Watt-Watson JH, Donovan MI, eds. Pain management: nursing perspective. St Louis: Mosby Yearbook; 1992:236–294.

223. Bieri D, Reeve RA, Champion GD, Addicoat L, Ziegler JB. The Faces Pain Scale for the self-assessment of the severity of pain experienced by children: development, initial validation, and preliminary investigation for ratio scale properties. Pain 1990; 41:139–150.

224. Gauvain-Piquard A, Rodary C, Rezvani A, Lemerle J. Pain in children aged 2–6 years: a new observational rating scale elaborated in a pediatric oncology unit – preliminary report. Pain 1987; 31:177–188.

225. Closs SJ. Pain in elderly patients: a neglected phenomenon? J Adv Nurs 1994; 19: 1072–1081.

226. Ferrell BR, Ferrell BA. Pain in elderly persons. In: McGuire D, Yarbro C, Ferrell BR, eds. Cancer pain management. London: Jones and Bartlett; 1995:273–287.

227. Kanner R. Pain in the elderly. In: Kanner R, ed. Pain management secrets. Philadelphia: Hanley and Belfus; 1997:163–166.

228. Fordyce WE. Evaluating and managing chronic pain. Geriatrics, 1978; 33:59–62.

229. Kamel HK, Phlavan M, Malekgoudarzi B, Gogel P, Morley JE. Utilizing pain assessment scales increases the frequency of diagnosing pain among the elderly nursing home residents. J Pain Symptom Manage 2000; 21:450–455.

230. Wall RT. Use of analgesic in the elderly. Clin Geriatr Med 1990; 6:345–364.

231. Morris DB. Ethnicity and pain. PAIN Clinical Updates, IASP 2001; IX(4):1–4.

232. Spivey N, ed. Enduring creation: art, pain, and fortitude. Berkeley: University of California Press; 2001.

233. Fink RS, Gates R. Cultural diversity and cancer pain. In: McGuire D, Yarbro C, Ferrell BR, eds. Cancer pain management. London: Jones and Bartlett; 1995:19–39.

234. Smith R, Curci M, Silverman A. Pain management: the global connection. Nurs Manage 2002; 33(6):26–29.

235. Juarez G, Ferrell B, Borneman T. Cultural considerations in education for cancer pain management. J Cancer Educ 1999; 14:168–173.

236. Lasch KE. Culture, pain, and culturally sensitive pain care. Pain Manage Nurs 2000; 1(3 Suppl 1):16–22.

237. Marzinski, LR. The tragedy of dementia: clinically assessing pain in the confused nonverbal elderly. J Gerontolog Nurs 1991; 17:25–28

238. Feldt KS. The Checklist of Nonverbal Pain Indicators (CNPI). Pain Manage Nurs 2000; 1:13–21.

239. Parke B. Pain in the cognitively impaired elderly. Canadian Nurse 1992; 88:17–20

240. Ferrell BR, McCaffery M, Rhiner M. Pain and addiction: an urgent need for change in nursing education. J Pain Symptom Manage 1992; 7:117–124.

241. Ferrell BR, McGuire D, Donovan M. Knowledge and beliefs regarding pain in a sample of nursing faculty. J Prof Nurs Educ 1993; 9:79–88.

242. Kuberka K, Simon J, Boettcher J. Pain management knowledge of hospital-based nurses in a rural Appalachian area. J Adv Nurs 1996; 23:861–867.

243. Brown ST, Bowman JM, Eason FR. Assessment of nurses' attitudes and knowledge regarding pain management. J Contin Educ Nurs 1999; 30:132–139.

244. Brunier G, Carson MG, Harrison DE. What do nurses know and believe about patients with pain? Results of a hospital survey. J Pain Symptom Manage 1995; 10:436–445.

245. Patiraki-Kourbani E, Lemonidou Ch. Nurses' knowledge on cancer pain relief: a review. Nosileftiki 2002; 1:28–33 [in Greek].

246. Ryan P, Vortherms R, Ward S. Cancer pain: knowledge, attitudes of pharmacologic management. J Gerontol Nurs 1994; 20:7–16.

247. Au E, Loprinzi CL, Dhodapkar M, et al. Regular use of a verbal pain scale improves the understanding of oncology inpatient pain intensity. J Clin Oncol 1994; 12:2751–2755.

248. Pederson C, Parran L. Bone marrow transplant nurses' knowledge, benefits and attitudes regarding pain management. Onocol Nurs Forum 1997; 24:1563–1571.

249. Ferrell BR, McCaffery M. Nurses' knowledge about equianalgesia and opioid dosing. Cancer Nurs 1997; 20:201–212.

250. Sjostrom B, Haljamae H, Dahlgren LO, Lindstrom B. Assessment of post-operative pain: impact of clinical experience and professional role. Acta Anaesthesiol Scand 1997; 41:339–344.

251. Closs SJ. Pain and elderly patients: a survey of nurses' knowledge and experience. J Adv Nurs 1996; 23:237–242.

252. Fothergill-Bourbonnais F, Wilson-Barnett J. A comparison study of intensive therapy and hospice nurses' knowledge on pain management. J Adv Nurs 1992; 17:362–372.

253. Wessman A, McDonald D. Nurses' personal pain experiences and their pain management knowledge. J Contin Educ Nurs 1999; 30:152–157.

254. Holm K, Cohen F, Dudas J, Medema P, Allen B. Effects of personal pain experience on pain assessment. Image 1989; 12:72–75.

255. Dalton J. Nurses' perceptions of their pain assessment skills, pain management practices, and attitudes towards pain. Oncol Nurs Forum, 1989; 16:225–231.

256. Davitz JR, Davitz LL. Inferences of patients' pain and psychological distress, studies of nursing behaviours. New York: Springer; 1981.

257. Clarke E, French B, Bilodeau M, et al. Pain management knowledge, attitudes and clinical practice: the impact of nurses' characteristics and education. Journal of Pain and Symptom Management, 1996; 11: 18-31.

258. Ketonouri H. Nurses' and patients' perception of wound pain and administration of analgesics. J Pain Symptom Manage 1987; 2:213–218.

259. Patiraki-Kourbani E, Tafas CA, McDonald DD, et al. Personal and professional pain experiences and pain management knowledge among Greek nurses. Int J Nurs Stud 2004; 41:345–354.

260. Dalton JA, Blaw W, Carlson J, et al. Changing the relationship among nurses' knowledge, self-reported behaviour, and documented behaviour in pain management: does education make a difference? J Pain Symptom Manage 1996; 12:308–319.

261. Janjan NA, Marti C, Rayn R, et al. Teaching cancer pain management: durability of educational effects on a role model program. Cancer 1996; 77:996–1001.

262. Weissman D, Dahl J. Update on the cancer pain role model education program. J Pain Symptom Manage 1995; 10:1–7.

263. Tafas CA, Patiraki E, McDonald DD, Lemonidou Ch. Testing an instrument measuring Greek nurses' knowledge and attitudes regarding pain. Cancer Nurs 2002; 25(1):8–14.

264. Barnason S, Merboth M, Pozehl B, Tietjen MJ. Utilizing an outcomes approach to improve pain management by nurses: a pilot study. Clin Nurse Spec 1998; 12:28–36.

265. Stratton L. Evaluating the effectiveness of a hospital's pain management program. J Nurs Care Qual 1999; 13(4):8–18.

266. White CL. Changing pain management practice and impacting on patient outcomes. Clin Nurse Spec 1999; 13:166–172.

267. Ferrell BR, Eberts MT, McCaffery M. Clinical decision-making and pain. Cancer Nurs 1991; 14:289–297.

268. West CM, Dodd MJ, Paul SM, et al. The PROSELF(c): Pain Control Program – an effective approach for cancer pain management. Oncol Nurs Forum 2003; 30:65–73.

269. Chelf JH, Agre P, Axelrod A, et al. Cancer-related patient education: an overview of the last decade of evaluation and research. Oncol Nurs Forum 2001; 28:1139–1147.

270. Wilkie DJ, Williams AR, Grevstad P, Mekwa J. Coaching persons with lung cancer to report sensory pain: literature review and pilot study findings. Cancer Nurs 1995; 18:7–15.

271. Allard P, Maunsell E, Labbe J, Dorval M. Educational interventions to improve cancer pain control: a systematic review. J Palliat Med 2001; 4:191–203.

272. Rimer BK, Kedziera P, Levy MH. The role of patient education in cancer pain control. Hosp J 1992; 8:171–191.

273. de Wit R, van Dam F, Zandbelt L, et al. A pain education program for chronic pain patients: follow-up results from a randomised controlled trial. Pain 1997; 73:55–69.

274. Ferrell BR, Grant M, Chan J, Ahn C, Ferrell BA. The impact of cancer pain education on family caregivers of elderly patients. Oncol Nurs Forum 1995; 22:1211–1218.

275. Ferrell BR, Grant M, Ritchey KJ, Ropchan R, Rivera LM. The pain resource nurse training program: an unique approach to pain management. J Pain Symptom Manage 1993; 8:549–556.

276. LeFort SM, Gray-Donald K, Rowat KM, Jeans ME. Randomized controlled trial of a community-based psychoeducation program for the self-management of chronic pain. Pain. 1998; 74:297–306.

277. Clotfelter CE. The effect of an educational intervention on decreasing pain intensity in elderly people with cancer. Oncol Nurs Forum 1999; 26:27–33.

278. Oliver JW, Kravitz RL, Kaplan SH, Meyers FJ. Individualized patient education and coaching to improve pain control among cancer outpatients. J Clin Oncol 2001; 19:2206–2212.

279. Ferrell BR, Juarez G. Cancer pain education for patients and the public. J Pain Symptom Manage 2002; 23:329–336.

280. Ferrell BR, Rivera LM. Cancer pain education for patients. Semin Oncol Nurs 1997; 13:42–48.

281. Alimi D, Rubino C, Pichard-Leandri E et al. Analgesic effect of auricular acupuncture for cancer pain: a randomized, blinded, controlled trial. J Clin Oncol 2003; 21: 4120-4126.

CHAPTER 22

Constipation and Diarrhoea

TANYA Y ANDREWES AND CHRISTINE NORTON

CHAPTER CONTENTS

Introduction	481	Types of diarrhoea	491
		Causes of diarrhoea	492
Normal gastrointestinal function	481	Assessment	495
		Treatment	497
Constipation	482		
Aetiology of constipation	483	Evaluation of outcomes, including	
Constipation in people with cancer	484	quality of life	502
The experience of constipation	485		
Nursing assessment	485	Conclusion	502
Planning	486		
Implementation	486	References	503
Interventions for the management of			
constipation	486		
Diarrhoea in cancer	490		

INTRODUCTION

Gastrointestinal function remains a largely taboo subject and so nursing care needs to be sensitive and appropriate. The effects of cancer itself, or of the treatments for cancer can result in a range of toxicities, including potential gastrointestinal toxicities that lead to constipation and diarrhoea. Both constipation and diarrhoea may be indicative of potentially life-limiting problems, such as bowel obstruction or systemic infection; therefore, sound assessment and astute observation are critical. Since gastrointestinal disturbances have the potential to severely impact on the quality of life[1] of the patient and the patient's family, sensitive, timely and appropriate nursing care can improve the situation.

This chapter seeks to explore the nature and experience of constipation and diarrhoea for the person with cancer. The role of the nurse, in collaboration with other healthcare professionals within the team, will be discussed and recommendations for practice proposed.

NORMAL GASTROINTESTINAL FUNCTION

The process of elimination in modern society is viewed as a highly private function. 'Normal' elimination typically takes place in allocated toilet facilities either within the home or in public places.[2] As people have grown wealthy, they have increasingly built houses with toilets reinforcing the process of elimination as a private function. Individuals are routinely socialized from early childhood to toilet independently and in private,[3] developing a neutral or positive attitude to their own excreta but a negative attitude to that of others.[4] This attitude is related to the awareness of dirt and pathogens and their influence on health.[4]

The subject of elimination is considered to be highly taboo in modern society.[2] As a result, it may be very difficult for patients to discuss their bowel function, with their families and/or with healthcare professionals. This has implications in cancer care at the stage of diagnosis and treatment, since altered bowel function may be indicative of presenting cancer[5] or progression of disease or of a toxic reaction to cancer treatments. An acknowledgement of gastrointestinal disturbance is often reluctant, tending to take place only when there are identified significant problems that the patient and/or the patient's family cannot resolve alone.[3]

The small intestines and the colon have their own characteristic patterns of motility. The small bowel undergoes forward peristalsis every 30 minutes to 1 hour, while giant contractions in the colon occur every 1–2 hours, with peaks on wakening and around midday associated with eating.[6] When individuals are healthy, food products migrate through the intestines over a period of 48–72 hours. Food products are digested in the small intestine over 1–2 hours and in the colon over a period of 24–48 hours. Throughout the migration through the intestines, the bowel contents are mixed in order to facilitate the enzymatic and bacterial breakdown of food substances and the absorption of the resulting nutrients and water.

A normal diet includes about 2 litres of fluid in food and drinks per day. The upper gastrointestinal tract secretes an additional 7–8 litres. Eight litres of this is usually reabsorbed by the small intestines, delivering about 1 litre of waste to the colon.[6] The colon absorbs 80–90% of this, leaving approximately 150 g of stool, 60–70% of which is water. When the colon is ready for the evacuation of faeces, the individual experiences a rectal sensation, commonly known as the 'call to stool' that stimulates defecation. Ignoring the 'call to stool' for any reason, intentional or not, results in increased water absorption as the faeces spends longer in the colon. The hard dry stools that develop are difficult to pass and can contribute to the experience of constipation.[7] Conversely, faster transit means that less water is reabsorbed and so may result in diarrhoea.

CONSTIPATION

There is no single clear definition for the condition of constipation. This is unsurprising since there is no clear understanding or agreement of what constitutes a 'normal' pattern of bowel evacuation. If what each individual experiences and perceives to be 'normal' is different, then it is difficult to offer a definitive statement for what is not normal. There is, however, some common agreement about the characteristics of constipation.

The management of constipation accounts for a significant annual spend of the healthcare budget. The use of laxatives accounts for at least £43 million in England alone.[8] This figure only accounts for prescription laxatives and not the range of over-the-counter laxatives that the general public can purchase. In terms of nursing time, it has been found that 10% of nursing time in the community is spent managing the condition.[9] The condition of constipation clearly accounts for a significant overall spend in the healthcare budget in terms of physical and human resources. Ideally, proactive health education interventions and nursing assessment should be combined to prevent the onset of gastrointestinal problems where possible, maximizing the patient's healthcare experience and ensuring the provision of cost-effective care.

The condition of constipation is commonly understood as difficulty in passing faeces and/or a decrease in the frequency of defecation.[6] This is often accompanied by bloating of the abdomen, abdominal pain and/or rectal pain.

It has been estimated that less than 1% of the healthy British population fail to defecate at least three times a week.[10] Although this research is very dated, the measure of three times a week has become accepted as a measure against which to assess an individual's level of defecation in Western society.[10] The norms of defecation vary not just between individuals but across cultures and countries too.[11] It may be seen as normal in some cultures or with certain diets to defecate as often as three times a day, or as little as once a week.[11]

The word constipation is thought to derive from the Latin word *constipare*, meaning 'to crowd together'. The implication is therefore of congestion. Such congestion may result in straining at stool or spending sustained periods of greater than 10 minutes in the act of defecation, two alternative objective measures for constipation.[6] It is likely that constipation will result in mild discomfort at best, but the condition has the potential to cause lethargy, bloating and general malaise,[7] worry, irritation and misery.[10] Although constipation may cause pain for the person who has cancer, it is more likely to cause distress that impacts on overall quality of life and subsequently the quality of life of the patient's relatives and carers.[9] As such, it represents a significant and challenging problem for nurses across all care settings.

Aetiology of constipation

Constipation can be split into three distinct categories, based on the causes (Table 22.1). Although not cancer-specific, these causes increase the potential for constipation in people with cancer. The co-morbidities of increasing age are a particularly significant factor and

Table 22.1: Classification of constipation

Type	Influencing factors
Primary constipation *Caused by extrinsic and/or lifestyle factors*	Inadequate privacy or time for defecation Low-fibre diet Depression Confusion Dehydration (due to factors such as poor fluid intake; vomiting; polyuria; sweating) Decreased activity and exercise Weakness and poor muscle tone Lack of energy
Secondary constipation *Caused by instrinsic and/or disease-related factors*	Primary or secondary tumour, including spinal cord compression between the thoracic 8 vertebra and lumbar 3 vertebra Metabolic effects of disease (including hypercalcaemia; hypokalaemia; uraemia; hypothyroidism) Underlying disease (including diabetes; hypothyroidism; hernia; diverticular disease; rectocele; anal fissure or stenosis; haemorrhoids and colitis)
Iatrogenic constipation *Caused by medical interventions and/or pharmacological factors*	Complications of radiation therapy Drug therapy: • Opioid analgesia (high risk) • Tricyclic antidepressants • Iron • Antispasmodics • Diuretics • Antacids • Anticonvulsants • Antihypertensives • Vincristine chemotherapy

constipation is common amongst the elderly population because they are exposed to the risk factors for primary, secondary and iatrogenic constipation.[12,13]

Norton[12] stresses the influence of posture and physical strength in the development of constipation. A good posture is essential for effective defecation. When patients are nursed in bed and have to use a bedpan, or when they are forced to use a commode, their posture may physiologically prevent or inhibit defecation. It is notable that if the patient's feet do not touch the floor when sitting on the toilet or commode, abdominal muscle function is reduced and defecation may be difficult if not impossible.[12] Immobility is similarly implicated in the development of constipation.[14] There is a reduction in colonic motility during times of immobility. This, in addition to the associated weakening of the abdominal muscles, serves to inhibit defecation.

The development of constipation is also affected by wider environmental influences. A preoccupation with avoiding creating smells[4] may lead people to repress the urge to defecate where there is a lack of toilet facilities and/or privacy.[7] Continual repression of the urge to defecate may contribute to a reduction in rectal sensitivity and a possible loss of the normal defecation reflex, increasing the potential for constipation.[8] Elimination in hospital is often considered to be particularly embarrassing because of the lack of private and comfortable facilities[2] and patients may feel compelled to ignore the call to stool because of the lack of privacy from smells that is afforded by bedside curtains.

Constipation in people with cancer

Patients with cancer are exposed to a wide range of risk factors for constipation; therefore, proactive preventative strategies and interventions are essential. Notably, the risk factors related to the diagnosis and treatment of cancer mean that constipation has the potential to affect people with any type of malignancy and not just those related to the gastrointestinal tract. Oral complications, such as the presence of *Candida* secondary to illness or treatment (chemotherapy or radiotherapy) in the person with cancer, can cause anorexia and associated nutritional problems.[7] The maintenance of oral health and the avoidance of deterioration of the oral status are therefore vital in terms of enabling dietary intake, particularly fibre, thus reducing the potential requirements for laxative use.[15,16]

Surgery

Wherever a person has surgery of the gastrointestinal tract, a potential short-term complication is paralytic ileus. Preventative measures include complete rest (nil by mouth) until bowel sounds resume and the staged reintroduction of oral fluids and then food.

Radiotherapy

Initially, radiotherapy treatment is more likely to cause diarrhoea than constipation since its action on the tissues results in inflammation and increased colonic motility (see below). A long-term complication, however, may be fibrosis of the colon walls, leading to reduced colonic motility and increasing the potential for constipation. This condition is normally associated with direct irradiation of the affected tissues and is localized. Treatment is normally with faecal softeners and stimulant laxatives.[13]

Chemotherapy

Chemotherapy treatment, except for vincristine, tends to cause diarrhoea rather than constipation, since it affects the rapidly dividing tissue in the gastrointestinal tract and increases gut motility as a result (see below). Vincristine, in particular, has the potential to cause gastrointestinal obstruction, as it causes autonomic nerve dysfunction and paralytic ileus.[15] Vigilance for potential obstruction is essential. Severe obstruction can present as 'spurious diarrhoea', typically a passive loss of foul-smelling dark brown liquid stool. This 'liquid stool' is actually faecal-stained mucus that has bypassed the impaction.

Palliative care

Constipation is most prevalent in people with advanced cancer who have been exposed to a wide range of risk factors. During the palliative care stages of the cancer journey, patients tend to be weaker and suffer from a degree of anorexia, exacerbating their overall risks.

Around 50% of people receiving hospice care in the United Kingdom suffer from constipation on admission.[6] In such cases, treatment of the underlying cause(s) may be complex and requires sound knowledge and understanding as the basis for planning, implementing and evaluating care. Thorough assessment is considered to be essential as a basis for clinical decision-making.[17,18]

Opioids are notorious for causing constipation by suppressing forward peristalsis, by increasing sphincter tone in the large intestine[8] and by reducing sensitivity to rectal distension.[19] The subcutaneous administration of morphine has been shown to slow transit and to reduce the amount of stools passed. In people with advanced cancer, anorexia and weakness, combined with the use of opioids, may result in the difficult passage of less faecal material.[17] The expenditure of undue energy on the act of defecation exacerbates the weakness and can have an adverse affect upon the patient's overall quality of life.

A confounding factor for the development of constipation in advanced cancer is the difficulty, because of generalized weakness, in assuming a sitting position on the toilet or commode long enough to defecate. Where underlying conditions are present such as spinal cord compression, rectal sensation may be absent. Consequently, there is no sensation of a 'call to stool', so the stools become very dry and hard to pass unless action is taken. The onset of constipation in a person who has had a primary diagnosis of cancer may herald the onset of spinal cord compression; therefore, vigilance is required so that a diagnosis can be made and interventions offered as appropriate.[19] Spurious diarrhoea, secondary to faecal impaction, occurs in around 10–15% of hospice patients;[20] therefore, an understanding of the physiology and treatment of both constipation and diarrhoea is vital to the provision of effective nursing care across all stages of the cancer journey.

The experience of constipation

Symptom distress has been identified as one of the main components that adversely affect the overall quality of a patient's life.[17,21,22] Carers who are witness to the pain and distress caused by constipation often experience feelings of inadequacy and frustration because they feel unable to help.[18] The associated inability of the patient to undertake fundamental activities of living such as eating and drinking while living with cancer may exacerbate stress in the carers, faced with a desire to help and preserve life at all stages of the cancer journey. For the patient, constipation and its associated problems have physical and psychosocial significance as they encounter increased pain, experience changes in body image and perhaps feel disinclined to socialize with others.

Nursing assessment

Nurses spend a significant amount of time with the patient and are therefore in an ideal position to initiate a holistic assessment of need and subsequent planned care to address the individual needs of the patient. The sensitive nature of the subject of bowel dysfunction requires the development of a therapeutic relationship so that the patient and the patient's carers feel safe to reveal sensitive and embarrassing information. The use of the nursing process offers a useful framework through which nurses are assisted to evaluate need, to plan and implement care and to monitor the outcomes of nursing interventions for constipation, through systematic evaluation. This may include maintenance of a stool chart, a patient diary, observation of the stools for blood and mucus and a symptom checklist.

Twycross and Back consider that methodical assessment is the cornerstone to effective care.[23] Initial identification of the most likely underlying cause(s) of constipation and diagnosis of the problems is considered to be essential. People with cancer are likely to have multiple pathologies and assessment must take account of this. A detailed history should be taken, considering tumour histology, local and metastatic spread (or possibility of) and any underlying pathology. Surgical intervention should be noted and drug/treatment regimens reviewed. Information regarding the pattern and speed of onset of the symptom(s) should be ascertained.[17] The former

485

and current pattern of frequency of bowel opening, change in faecal consistency and pattern of abdominal pain may provide important diagnostic information at the bedside, indicating possible intestinal obstruction.[19] It may be necessary to perform a rectal examination to rule out low faecal impaction.[24] Evaluation of biochemical status enables conditions such as hypercalcaemia to be identified or excluded from the diagnosis. Each of these factors can be incorporated into the nursing assessment on admission, or as part of the ongoing evaluation.

Physical examination is essential. The abdomen should be examined for signs of abdominal distension and presence of bowel sounds. A digital rectal assessment will confirm the presence or absence of stool, anal tone and haemorrhoids that may impact on the diagnosis and treatment plan. The presence of other factors that may impact upon, or exacerbate the symptoms of constipation, such as impaired mobility, anorexia and/or nausea and vomiting, should also be considered (see Chs 29 and 20).[23] Radiological investigation in the form of transit studies can be useful as a means to objectively identify the cause(s) of the constipation.[19]

Comprehensive assessment requires that all factors are taken into account and it is essential to assess the impact of the constipation on the patient's quality of life[17,18] There is currently no specific tool for measuring the impact of constipation on quality of life in patients with cancer; however, the Edmonton Symptom Assessment System[25] offers a useful base for assessment using a visual analogue scale system. A combined objective and subjective assessment of the impact of the symptom(s) of constipation will provide a baseline against which to measure the effectiveness of medical and nursing interventions. Self-completion of quality of life audit tools is advocated to ensure that the patient's feelings are represented accurately; however, this may be problematic for patients who are in the latter stage of their disease and/or in whom there is poor performance status.[26] In this case, objective data collection can be more difficult; however, the patient's experience can be assessed through dialogue and observation and recorded in the healthcare records, providing an additional or alternative means against which to assess the effectiveness of nursing interventions.

Planning

The provision of individualized care is a central function of nursing. Nurses working with people with cancer are responsible for planning appropriate and effective care for people with a range of complex symptoms arising from multiple pathologies.[27] Active involvement of the patient, based on shared knowledge and understanding, is fundamental to the organization of individualized treatment. On the whole, it is considered that it is a deficit in nurses' knowledge and practice that often fails to prevent constipation.[18] A key aspect of planning holistic care is education for prevention, reducing the need for reactive intervention.

Implementation

Discussion and assessment might reveal that the patient's pattern of defecation is 'normal' for the patient's condition and therefore the patient can be reassured and supported with health education as appropriate.[17] When assessment indicates that there is a potential problem of constipation, education for prevention is considered to be crucial. Compliance with treatment for constipation is directly related to the acceptability of the intervention, so active involvement, open discussion and informed choice with regard to treatment options is essential.[18]

Interventions for the management of constipation

Since the causes of constipation in people with cancer are often multifactorial (see Table 22.1) and patients often suffer the three most significant risk factors of poor food intake, impaired mobility and a requirement for opioid analgesia, successful management is complex.[6] Effective outcomes are dependent upon:

- an accurate diagnosis of cause(s)
- the choice of appropriate pharmacological intervention based on the diagnosed actual, or potential problem(s)

- an acceptable route of administration of medications for the patient that will produce the desired effect of resolving or preventing constipation
- effective treatment of reversible cause(s)
- individualized nursing care.

Non-pharmacological interventions

The management of the symptoms of constipation is complex and requires the artistic and creative application of knowledge and skills[28] to achieve sensitive care while ensuring privacy and minimizing potential disruption to the patient's daily routine. Bowel interventions should be performed in privacy in order to minimize the potential for embarrassment and to facilitate a relaxed environment for toileting functions where the patient feels supported and unhurried.[2] Alternative therapies, such as abdominal massage, may be employed as a supportive strategy for pharmacological management by the patient and/or their carer(s); however, the clinical value of such techniques remains largely unproven.[28] Massage is contraindicated over the area of a primary tumour and the associated sites of lymphatic drainage because of the belief that the resultant increase in blood circulation may encourage tumour spread;[28] although there is limited evidence to support this concept, it is suggested that massage is avoided if the patient has a primary cancer of the bowel or pelvis.

It is important for the family and carers to have the opportunity to participate in care where possible. This can be rewarding for family carers, and enables them to feel close to the patient. With appropriate education, family and carers may be able to maintain the essential health of the oral cavity. The importance of this simple role cannot be overstated, since if oral health is maintained eating and drinking are facilitated and this alone may rule out the need for pharmacological intervention.

Sykes identifies six key non-pharmacological interventions for the prophylaxis of constipation:[6]

1 Maintain good general symptom control. If the patient's nutritional and hydration status and mobility can be maintained, the potential for the development of constipation will be reduced. The symptoms of pain and nausea and vomiting in particular affect all of the above activities; therefore, control of these symptoms is crucial.

2 Encourage activity. Activity helps to maintain muscle strength and increases gut motility.

3 Maintain adequate oral fluid intake (2 litres daily). A good oral fluid intake assists the passage of food products through the gastrointestinal tract and helps to ensure that the stools have enough fluid content to be soft in preparation for defecation.

4 Maximize the fibre content of the diet. Fibre assists the passage of food products through the gastrointestinal tract. It acts as a natural stool softener; however, it can be difficult to tolerate, particularly later in the cancer journey when anorexia is present. In addition, it can cause distressing flatus. Fibre supplements should be used with great care in those who are immobile and in dehydrated people, since if transit is very slow, fibre will add to constipation.

5 Anticipate the constipating effect of medications by altering treatment or commencing prophylactic laxatives. Appropriate laxative interventions should always be prescribed when the patient is receiving opioid analgesia.

6 Create a favourable environment. If the patient is eating and drinking, one key action that aids digestion is to ensure that the patient can be seated comfortably during and after meals. The maintenance of oral hygiene assists the digestive process, so encouragement should be given to the patient or family carers to perform this care and/or assistance offered where required. The provision of a safe environment for elimination that offers privacy, warmth and comfort and that enables the patient to maintain a good posture (specifically – footstool, lean forward, padded seat if thin) is a key nursing role.

Pelvic floor exercises have been found to increase muscle tone and thus aid defecation and prevent constipation.[29] This may be a useful strategy to employ in the early stages of disease, in order to minimize the potential for constipation at later stages and to offer the patient some non-pharmacological control over their situation. It would, however, not be effective in the later stages of the cancer journey[30] when general and abdominal weakness is established, particularly in the presence of other symptoms such as pain, anorexia and nausea and vomiting.

Pharmacological interventions

There are a wide range of pharmacological preparations available for the management and prevention of constipation. They fall into four discrete categories: osmotics, stool softeners, stimulants and bulking agents (Table 22.2).[30]

Each group has a discrete action and side-effect profile. It is therefore essential that pharmacological interventions are planned according to the underlying problem and the actions of the drugs used.

The aim of pharmacological intervention for constipation is to achieve 'comfortable defecation' rather than a specific frequency of defecation.[19] Interventions should be proactive rather than reactive, preventing the onset of constipation and initiated on the basis of a risk assessment. For patients taking opioid analgesics, the regular administration of laxatives is crucial.[7] This is not only important for the comfort of the patient as a primary concern but also for encouraging the patient to continue with supportive care that is associated with the development of constipation but without which further discomfort would be inevitable.[7]

Table 22.2: Pharmacological preparations for the management of constipation

Type of preparation and action	Drug	Potential side-effects
Osmotic laxatives (onset of action is 48 hours or more) *Attract water into the bowel lumen*	Lactulose	Flatulence Abdominal discomfort Anal skin irritation
	Movicol	Abdominal distension and pain Nausea
	Milpar	Colic
Faecal softeners (onset of action is 24 hours or more) *Used to soften hard faeces, but not particularly good laxatives when used alone*	Docusate sodium	Abdominal cramps
	Liquid paraffin	Anal skin irritation Inhalational pneumonia
Stimulant laxatives (onset of action 12–24 hours) *Increase peristalsis/rectal motility* *All contraindicated in intestinal obstruction*	Senna	Abdominal cramps May colour the urine red
	Dantron (Danthron)	As above
	Bisacodyl (onset of action 10–12 hours)	Possibly carcinogenic Abdominal discomfort Should not be taken with
	Dioctyl	antacids
	Sodium picosulfate (sodium picosulphate)	Abdominal cramps Abdominal cramps

Table 22.2: Pharmacological preparations for the management of constipation—cont'd

Type of preparation and action	Drug	Side-effects
Bulk-forming laxatives (onset of action 24 hours or more) *Increase faecal mass* *High fluid intake is essential* *Not useful in faecal impaction*	Bran	Flatulence Abdominal distension Intestinal obstruction
	Isphagula husk (Fybogel/Regulan)	As above
	Methylcellulose (Celevac)	As above
	Sterculia (Normacol)	As above

Rectal preparations
 	
 Action according to type of preparation
	Micro-enema (sodium citrate)
	    Osmotic
	    Acts in 30 minutes
		Local irritation
		
		 Contraindicated in inflammatory bowel disease

	Fletchers' Phosphate Enema
	    Osmotic
	    Acts in 30 minutes
		As above

	Fletchers' Enemette (docusate sodium)
	    Faecal softener
	    Acts in 20–30 minutes
		Abdominal cramps

	Glycerin suppositories
	    Faecal softener
	    Act in 24 hours or more
		Abdominal discomfort

	Bisacodyl suppositories
	    Stimulant laxative
	    Act in 20–60 minutes
		Abdominal discomfort

A basic underpinning knowledge of the actions and side effects of each group of laxatives is required in order to ensure appropriate prescribing (see Table 22.2). Potential side-effects of chemotherapy and radiotherapy treatment, such as mucositis or nausea and vomiting, may make it difficult for the patient with cancer to take oral medications for the management or prevention of constipation. In addition, in the case of neutropenia and thrombocytopenia following chemotherapy and radiotherapy, it may be difficult or inappropriate to offer rectal medication.[27] Therefore, the importance of proactive management is clear.

Fallon and O'Neill[19] advise that rectal laxatives in the form of enemas or suppositories should not be used routinely in the patient with cancer but should be considered for incidences of faecal impaction and conditions such as spinal cord compression. Apart from having the potential to reduce rectal sensation with prolonged use, these measures are undignified and uncomfortable and they may impact negatively upon quality of life.[19] However, they can be more predictable and easier to control than oral treatments, with less likelihood of faecal incontinence. Consequently, they may be considered in the care of dependent people who do not have 24-hour carer availability at home.

The aim of care in the presence of spinal cord compression is to achieve 'controlled continence',[19] which means giving an individualized combination of oral laxatives on a daily basis, with suppositories or enemas every 2–3 days to enable rectal evacuation. The intention is to avoid faecal incontinence for those with a loss of rectal sensation.[19]

DIARRHOEA IN CANCER

Although less common than constipation, diarrhoea is not an uncommon experience for people with cancer and can be equally distressing and limiting upon quality of life. Not only is nutritional status threatened, with malnutrition and dehydration as possible consequences, but also chronic or severe diarrhoea can be exhausting and a threat to the patient's sense of control over their own body. Hogan[31] has quoted a 23-year-old man, who summarized the effect of severe diarrhoea:

> ... So many things have been taken away from me by this disease, but having diarrhoea and being afraid to leave the house is the worst .... Losing control of my bowels represents everything I have lost .... It is the ultimate in humiliating experiences.

Exact figures are not available, but it has been estimated that about 10% of patients with advanced cancer have diarrhoea.[32] Diarrhoea may be related either to the cancer, or its treatment, or incidental to both. It has often been relatively neglected as a symptom by oncology nurses, but knowledge and attention is now increasing.[33] When parents of children who had died of cancer were interviewed later, they were significantly more likely than the medical records to report that their child had a range of symptoms, including diarrhoea (40% vs <20%), and that this caused suffering (20% vs <2%), suggesting that diarrhoea may be under-recognized and undertreated, especially in the seriously ill.[34] Much assessment and treatment of diarrhoea remains empirical rather than evidence-based. If symptoms are severe during a course of radiation or chemotherapy, this can lead to interruption or even discontinuation of therapy that could otherwise be beneficial.[31] The dose of many chemotherapy drugs is limited by this unpleasant symptom. Although often the most advantageous postoperative regimen is combined chemotherapy and radiotherapy, the combination often increases the risk of diarrhoea as a side-effect, as opposed to either modality alone.[35] Nurses have a role in patient education, prevention and early symptom recognition, assessment, treatment and supportive measures.[36]

'Diarrhoea' means different things to different people, being a largely subjective symptom, and it is important to establish exactly what the patient is experiencing. There are often perceptual differences between patients, nurses and doctors.[36] Increased frequency of defecation may not be true diarrhoea if the stool is formed. Research literature often defines diarrhoea by stool volume, with more than 200 g in 24 hours as a common threshold, although again if the stool is formed this is not diarrhoea. A water content of stool greater than 70–90% is also quoted. Usual definitions combine frequency greater than 3 per day and loose stool consistency. Acute diarrhoea is usually defined as lasting for less than 14 days, persistent diarrhoea over 14 days and chronic diarrhoea as extending beyond 1 month.[37] In some patient groups (such as those with endocrine or pancreatic tumours), diarrhoea can be severe, over 3 litres/day, occasionally necessitating nursing in an intensive care unit.[38]

The American National Cancer Institute has proposed criteria for the severity of diarrhoea (Table 22.3).[36] However, this instrument does not address stool volume or characteristics. Guenter and Sweed have validated a tool to quantify stool output in tube-fed patients, which would seem to be adaptable to other causes of diarrhoea.[39] This scale identifies three choices for stool consistency (solid formed, pasty and liquid) and two volumes (large and small), giving a six-category scale. Many different criteria have been suggested in the literature, often associated with different conditions.[40]

Symptoms may include, as well as frequent loose stool, abdominal pains or cramps, urgency, blood in the stool, fever, tenesmus (constant desire to defecate),

Table 22.3: American National Cancer Institute severity of diarrhoea criteria

Severity grade	0	1	2	3	4
No. of loose stools per day	Normal	2–3	4–6	7–9	10 or more
			and/or	and/or	and/or
Symptoms		None	Nocturnal stools	Incontinence	Grossly bloody diarrhoea
			and/or	and/or	and/or
			Moderate cramping	Severe cramping	Need for parenteral support

flatulence, faecal incontinence and anal soreness.[33] It may be associated with nausea and vomiting, especially if the origin is in the upper gut. In severe or prolonged instances, dehydration, electrolyte imbalance and morbidity or even mortality can result. Rapid weight loss can lead to fatigue, even exhaustion. Diarrhoea can be socially restricting and if it persists for any length of time can be very tiring and demoralizing, significantly impairing quality of life.[33]

Types of diarrhoea

Large-volume watery diarrhoea usually indicates small bowel origin; small-volume frequent stools are more likely to be from the large bowel. Four main types of diarrhoea may be distinguished (Table 22.4) – secretory, osmotic, exudate and motility – although in some patients these may be combined. Additionally, severe constipation can present as faecal impaction with overflow 'spurious diarrhoea' (see above).

Table 22.4: Classification of diarrhoea

Type	Example conditions in cancer	Typical symptoms
Secretory	Excess fluid secretion, not balanced by reabsorption, e.g. carcinoid syndrome; thyroid; VIPoma, mucosal damage or disease, infections, endocrine tumours, GvHD, short bowel syndrome	Continues even if fasting
Osmotic	Lumenal contents have higher osmolality than gut tissue: may be carbohyrate, enteral feeds, bleeding, pancreas (inadequate digestive enzymes)	Stops if do not eat
Motility	Hyper- or hypomotility (e.g. ileus, partial obstruction), inflammation	Any
Exudate	Inflammation or ulceration (e.g. colitis), radiation colitis, colonic neoplasms	Passage of mucus, pus or blood with stool

491

Causes of diarrhoea

It is quite likely that several factors from those described below will coexist in the same individual (Table 22.5).

Type of cancer

Some cancers have a direct effect on the gut: e.g. a villous adenoma of the rectum can secrete copious amounts of mucus. Pancreatic cancer, thyroid and VIPomas of the intestine each increase the risk of secretory diarrhoea. If there is partial bowel obstruction, this may present as diarrhoea.

Surgery

There is an increasing trend to try to avoid forming a stoma in patients with a low anterior rectal cancer, instead performing a local anterior rectal resection. This can reduce rectal capacity and compliance and if the anastomosis is very low, anal sphincter function may be impaired.[41] Many patients find that, especially initially, they have an increased bowel frequency and urgency following this procedure, which may be reported as 'diarrhoea'. If treatment (chemotherapy or radiotherapy) also causes true diarrhoea, continence may be impaired.

Table 22.5: Causes of diarrhoea

Cause	Common examples
Tumour	Villous adenoma Pancreatic Colorectal Thyroid medullary carcinoma (calcitonin secretion) Oat cell lung tumours (copious secretions) Carcinoid syndrome with liver metastases (serotonin secretion) Hypersecretion of intestinal hormones (e.g. VIP, gastrin, serotonin, calcitonin) Partial bowel obstruction (mucus secretion)
Surgery	Bowel resection Gastrectomy with dumping syndrome Low anterior rectal resection Blind loop syndrome Pancreatectomy Cholecystectomy Vagotomy Graft versus host disease (GvHD) Ileocaecal bowel resection (fast transit) Palliative bypass
Radiation	Mucosal damage, inflammation, atrophy Malabsorption of bile salts
Chemotherapy	5-Fluorouracil (5-FU), methotrexate Irinotecan
Infection	Bacteria causing gastroenteritis (e.g. *Escherichia coli*, *Shigella*, *Salmonella*) *Clostridium difficile* Parasites (e.g. *Giardia*) *Candida* AIDS and its therapy

Table 22.5: Causes of diarrhoea—cont'd

Cause	Common examples
Other drugs	Laxative abuse Non-steroidal anti-inflammatory drugs Thyroxine Beta-blockers Magnesium antacids Antibiotics Diethylstilbestrol (as hormone therapy) Iron supplements Opiate withdrawal Syrups of any medication containing sorbitol as sweetener
Faecal impaction	Secondary to immobility or opiate analgesia
Nutrition	Lactose (e.g. intolerance following chemotherapy) Caffeine Sorbitol Tube feeding (especially rapid enteral feeding) Foods containing natural laxatives (e.g. prunes) Spicy or high-temperature food Excess fibre Alcohol abuse
Malabsorption	Pancreatic disease Hypoproteinaemia Malnutrition/starvation (epithelial injury) Steatorrhoea secondary to liver disease Short bowel (resection or radiation enteritis)
Other diseases/ conditions	Gastroenteritis Diabetic autonomic neuropathy Inflammatory bowel disease (e.g.ulcerative colitis, Crohn's disease) Coeliac disease Irritable bowel syndrome Scleroderma Hyperthyroidism Pancreatic disease Anxiety

Resection of a significant length of small bowel can lead to 'short bowel syndrome'. There may be insufficient mucosa to sustain nutritional status, but additionally, reabsorption of secretions may be impaired, resulting in high-volume diarrhoea. If the colon is intact, it can often compensate, but if the colon has also been removed, patients can experience troublesome stool volumes. Resection of the terminal ileum can interfere with reabsorption of bile acids. Bile acids in the colon can precipitate a secretory diarrhoea.[42]

In bone marrow transplant patients, graft versus host disease (GvHD) is recognized as causing profuse secretory diarrhoea. After gastrectomy, 'dumping syndrome' can cause high-volume urgent bowel actions after eating.

Radiation

Radiation enteritis is almost inevitable with any patient receiving radiation to the abdomen or pelvis, and is dose-dependent.[43] Troublesome symptoms probably affect 5–15% of patients, with an increasing incidence, and it is recognized as difficult to treat.[43] The small bowel is one of the most radiosensitive organs in the body because of its structure, with a huge surface area of villi, and because there is a rapid turnover of cells, with the epithelium replaced every 4–7 days.[43] Relatively low doses of radiation damage the rapidly proliferating cells of the gut mucosa, with cell loss leading to atrophy of the villi and destruction of the usual crypts in the small bowel, with damage more likely in thin patients.[43] The symptom of diarrhoea may be immediate, or may start months later, with a biphasic response, with early alteration in cell function and later abnormalities in vascular and connective tissue.[43] The protective mucus blanket is disrupted, allowing penetration of the epithelium by pathogens.[43] Some patients who had radium implants previously find that they experience a progressive diarrhoea with time. Late symptoms can include progressive diarrhoea, malabsorption, bowel wall thickening with fibrosis and possible stricture or adhesions, ischaemia, partial or complete obstruction, and even perforation and fistula formation. Radiation can reduce rectal capacity with fibrosis.[43]

Some techniques such as positioning and irradiating the pelvis when the patient has a full bladder may help minimize damage. An adequate rest period is important between doses.[43] Some chemotherapy agents such as 5-fluorouracil (5-FU) increase cellular sensitivity to radiation and interfere with recovery.[43] Surgical techniques such as insertion of mesh can prevent prolapse of the small bowel into the potential radiation field after surgical resection in the pelvis. Very old patients (over 80 years old) do not necessarily develop more symptoms than younger patients, although up to 40% undergoing pelvic radiation may have moderate-to-severe diarrhoea.[44] Taking an elemental liquid diet during radiotherapy has been found to prevent intestinal damage from radiation in an animal model,[45] and can help. However, this diet is unpalatable and poorly tolerated by many patients, particularly if they are also nauseated or anorexic, and so its use is limited in clinical practice.

Chemotherapy

Chemotherapy can result in diarrhoea in as many as 50–80% of patients on some treatment regimens.[46] Severe diarrhoea can affect 10–20% of patients on combinations such as 5-FU with leucovorin (folinic acid) or interferon.[47] It is not entirely clear why chemotherapy causes diarrhoea in some patients, and it seems likely that several different mechanisms may operate,[48] with a combination of loss of intestinal epithelium, inflammation, necrosis and secretion.[46] Antimetabolites can damage the rapidly proliferating mucosal cells of the gut, leading either to increased secretion or impaired nutrient and water absorption. Lactose malabsorption can result from chemotherapy, but is not always associated with diarrhoea. Antineoplastic drugs, particularly methotrexate, cisplatin and 5-FU, can also alter gut flora and predispose to *Clostridium difficile* infection of the gut, not necessarily associated with antibiotic use.[48,49] Relapse is common, even after the infection has been treated, and death can result if infection is not recognized or adequately treated. Irinotecan can cause early-onset diarrhoea, which may be helped by anticholinergics such as scopolamine (hyoscine) or atropine, or late onset, often accompanied by leucopenia and more likely in older patients and those who have had previous pelvic or abdominal radiation.[50] Vincristine can cause ileus.[38]

Infection

Immunocompromised patients are particularly susceptible to infections, which can lead to gastroenteritis. Repeated courses of antibiotics in turn can cause a colitis, or predispose to nosocomial infections, of which *C. difficile* is probably the most significant and can result in pseudomembranous colitis. This pathogen has been isolated from the hands of nurses attending infected patients, although environmental origin may be as important as cross-infection.[51,52] Many patients with *C. difficile* can be asymptomatic and not require treatment.[52] Person-to-person spread is implicated in pseudomembranous colitis after broad-spectrum antibiotic use, emphasizing the importance of rigorous infection control precautions with these vulnerable patients.[52–54] *Cryptosporidium* sp. has been found in stool samples of 17% of patients with neoplasia and diarrhoea in one series, with none in similar patients without diarrhoea.[55] Methicillin-resistant staphylococcal enterocolitis is reported in patients undergoing chemotherapy for leukaemia. Intestinal parasites can colonize an immunocompromised individual, particularly in countries where such parasites are prevalent.[56,57] Systemic *Candida* infection is a serious and life-threatening complication in children after bone marrow transplant and often presents with fever and severe diarrhoea, among other symptoms.[58] The American College of Gastroenterology has produced detailed guidelines on investigation and treatment of infectious diarrhoea, including in immunocompromised patients.[37]

Nutrition

Diarrhoea has been found to occur in 2–63% of patients during tube feeding, depending upon the definition of diarrhoea adopted.[42] Continuous slow infusion of nutrients into the stomach via tube feeding interferes with the normal gut secretion of digestive enzymes, which is dependent on a calorie load being delivered to the stomach and gastric distension. However, the relative contribution of feed content and altered gut secretion and motility to the diarrhoea of tube-fed patients has yet to be determined[42] and it should not be assumed that the feed is the cause in all tube-fed patients, with medications and infection as more prominent as a cause than osmotic diarrhoea in one series.[59] Addition of bulking agents such as psyllium to tube feeds can reduce diarrhoea.[60]

Malnutrition and hypoproteinaemia (with consequent oedema of tissue, including the gut wall, impairing absorption capacity) can exacerbate diarrhoea. A serum albumin of less than 2.5 mg/dl is thought to be the threshold for malabsorptive diarrhoea.

Caffeine, sorbitol and many other dietary ingredients can cause diarrhoea in selected individuals. Lactose intolerance is recognized to develop in many children after chemotherapy.[61]

Non-cancer related causes

It is important not to assume that all symptoms are inevitably cancer-related. Diarrhoea is a common symptom in the general population. Table 22.5 lists the most common causes from drugs, nutrition and other conditions. A cancer diagnosis does not preclude many of these other causes and may make them more likely.

Assessment

History and symptoms

The majority (74%) of oncology nurses have been found only to report diarrhoea as 'present' or 'absent' when describing diarrhoea, and most use a limited non-systematic evaluation.[62] Only 25% reported using a symptom diary in assessment. Patients may fear that reporting diarrhoea will result in treatment being discontinued, or they may expect diarrhoea and take it for granted as inevitable.[40] There is a need to develop and validate nursing assessment tools for this symptom.[36] Box 22.1 gives criteria suggested by an expert consensus meeting.[40]

Kelvin has given detailed suggestions for initial and weekly review assessment formats.[63] Assessment is to establish the cause of diarrhoea and to determine what effect symptoms are having on the patient and any carers involved.

Box 22.1

Criteria for optimum measurement of cancer treatment-related diarrhoea

Stool consistency graded with illustration

Liquid stool measured by volume

Assessment of tenesmus or urgency, abdominal pain and cramping

Onset and duration of diarrhoea and accompanying symptoms

Presence or absence of perianal or peristomal skin breakdown

Patient report of self-care (i.e. diaries or behaviour logs) and effect of interventions

Quality of life assessments (i.e. effect on capacity to function)

Early assessment is recommended to avoid preventable consequences of diarrhoea such as dehydration and malnutrition, and even hospitalization.[36] The unpleasantness and practical difficulties (particularly in a domestic setting) of coping with uncontrolled diarrhoea that results in faecal incontinence should not be underestimated.[64]

Pre-existing bowel habit will give an indication of how much change there has been. Irritable bowel syndrome affects 20% of the general population and many of these patients will have an existing erratic bowel habit, making it unrealistic to aim for one formed stool per day. The nature of the stool should be established. Diarrhoea may vary from pure liquid, to watery with some pieces, to mushy stool (like porridge). Patients have been found able to reliably rate their stool consistency and this correlates with water content.[65] Patients with AIDS have been found to consistently report stool consistency on a choice of pictorial stool representations and self-report of 'diarrhoea', but verbal descriptors (such as loose or semi-formed) of stool form were less useful.[66] If stool is reported as a dark foul-smelling liquid this may indicate faecal impaction with 'spurious diarrhoea'. Alternatively, stool which is foul smelling, oily, and possibly pale, may indicate fat malabsorption. It may be useful to keep a bowel diary for patients who find it difficult to remember symptoms, and to monitor the course of the diarrhoea and the success of any treatment initiated.

Associated symptoms may include tenesmus, abdominal pain or cramps. Faecal incontinence can result from urgency in someone with limited mobility, as the toilet simply cannot be reached in time. Faecal incontinence has been termed the 'unvoiced symptom' in diarrhoea,[67] and will often not be volunteered by the patient unless asked directly, and tactfully. It affects 1–2% of adults and so may pre-exist in some patients with cancer, but be exacerbated by the illness or its treatment. For women, a history of difficult childbirth or assisted vaginal delivery predisposes to difficulty controlling the bowels.[68]

History should include diet, amount and type of fluid intake, weight loss, medications, and associated nausea and vomiting. Other problems may include sleep disturbance, both for the patient and family, and effects upon social life, ability to work or travel, effect on personal relationships and added stress and anxiety. Mobility and ability to be self-caring, with availability of carers, will often determine how well diarrhoea is managed.

Examination

Blood in the stool may be bright red, suggesting anal or rectal origin, or dark and altered, suggesting bleeding higher in the bowel. Blood may not be visible, but found on occult blood testing.

If the patient has an associated fever, an infectious cause may be indicated. A history of recent exotic travel may give clues as to non-cancer causes of diarrhoea. General skin condition may indicate dehydration, as may a low urine output or dark concentrated urine or hypotension. Cardiac arrhythmias may result from electrolyte imbalance, especially in older people.

Frequent diarrhoea, especially if causing episodes of faecal incontinence, may lead to perianal excoriation, which can occasionally become extremely uncomfortable. On examination, the skin may be very inflamed and even broken and bleeding. Weight loss may indicate that diarrhoea is adversely affecting nutritional status. Guarding or rebound tenderness on abdominal palpation may indicate infection. High-pitched bowel sounds may result from partial bowel obstruction. Abdominal examination may reveal organomegaly or faecal impaction. Rectal examination will often detect impaction if present.

Further tests

If infection is suspected, a stool sample should be analysed for pathogens, including ova and parasites. Stool volume can also be measured and fat or occult blood content determined.

A hydrogen breath test is a simple non-invasive way of diagnosing lactose intolerance or bacterial overgrowth in the bowel. The patient attends, fasting overnight, and blows into a device that measures breath hydrogen. A lactose-rich meal is then given and repeat measurements taken over the next 2 hours. Normal ranges are available against which to judge the individual's test results.

Blood should be taken for a full blood count and electrolyte screen. Anaemia may indicate bleeding. A low white cell count indicates neutropenia; a high count is associated with infection. A plain abdominal X-ray will detect ileus or obstruction. Barium studies or endoscopy may be indicated to discover the cause of inflammation or bleeding and to take biopsies.

Treatment

A multidisciplinary panel has recommended practice guidelines for the management of chemotherapy-induced diarrhoea[40] (Fig. 22.1), which may also have application to other causes.

Pharmacological treatment

Antidiarrhoeal medication has been the mainstay of medical prophylaxis and treatment for diarrhoea, although, if severe, a period of bowel rest and intravenous hydration may be needed.[47] Ippoliti[69] and Cascinu[38] provide reviews of antidiarrhoeal agents in cancer, outlining drugs useful in rarer syndromes. It has been suggested that nurses should educate patients to present early and to encourage the use of over-the-counter remedies at the first sign of diarrhoea in patients undergoing chemotherapy.[46]

Constipating agents such as loperamide or codeine phosphate are usually the first option.[69] Loperamide has a small risk of precipitating paralytic ileus and, although rare, this is potentially life-threatening if massive secretion continues and ileus is unrecognized.[40] Some patients find that liquid formulation allows closer titration to symptoms. Loperamide has been found to reduce faecal incontinence, improve stool consistency and reduce stool weight compared to placebo.[70,71] There is also some evidence that loperamide increases water absorption by slowing colonic transit and, in an animal model, that it decreases internal anal sphincter relaxation in response to rectal distension[72] and increases mucosal fluid uptake.[73] Continence to rectally infused saline improved in 26 patients with chronic diarrhoea, and there was additionally a small increase in resting anal pressure.[74] Patients with diarrhoea secondary to radiation enteritis have been found to respond with slowed small gut transit and increased bile acid absorption.[75] Loperamide is best taken about 30 minutes prior

to eating, as it helps to dampen the gastrocolic response of increased gut motility upon eating.

Codeine phosphate is also effective for some patients,[76] as is diphenoxylate (Lomotil), although the dose of the latter is often limited by anticholinergic side-effects. Careful titration of dose of all antidiarrhoeals is needed to avoid constipation, as response is individual. Bulking agents such as psyllium are also used in an attempt to 'mop up' excess fluid,[77] and psyllium and gum arabic have been found to improve symptoms of faecal incontinence associated with loose stool, compared to placebo.[78]

Octreotide is a synthetic analogue of somatostatin, which is a common gut growth hormone release inhibitor. It enhances fluid and electrolyte absorption, reduces secretions, reduces small bowel motility and is an anti-inflammatory.[79] It has many different effects on the gastrointestinal tract.[80] It has been found to be more effective and faster-acting than oral loperamide in reducing chemotherapy-related diarrhoea,[81] and can be effective in patients unresponsive to loperamide.[82] It has to be given subcutaneously, and many patients can learn to self-administer, with a depot injection necessitating fewer injections. It seems to help most types of severe diarrhoea, including that associated with chemotherapy, radiation and graft versus host disease (GvHD),[83,84] where response is usually rapid.[84] It has also been found effective in preventing enterocutaneous fistulas in patients who are vulnerable after pancreatic surgery and may have a role in treating existing fistulae[79] and reducing fistula and stoma output. Octreotide is generally well tolerated, with local skin irritation as the main problem, but some tolerance may develop, necessitating increasing doses with time. Long-term high doses may promote formation of gallstones.[80] It has been reported as effective when given intravenously during chemotherapy, in combination with bowel rest (nil by mouth) and intravenous fluids for patients who could not otherwise tolerate high-dose 5-FU because of severe diarrhoea.[85]

It has been suggested that cytokines may protect the gut mucosa during chemotherapy, and this is the subject of ongoing work.[86] It is recommended that bismuth subsalicylate (Pepto-Bismol), which helps many patients with infectious diarrhoea, should not be used in

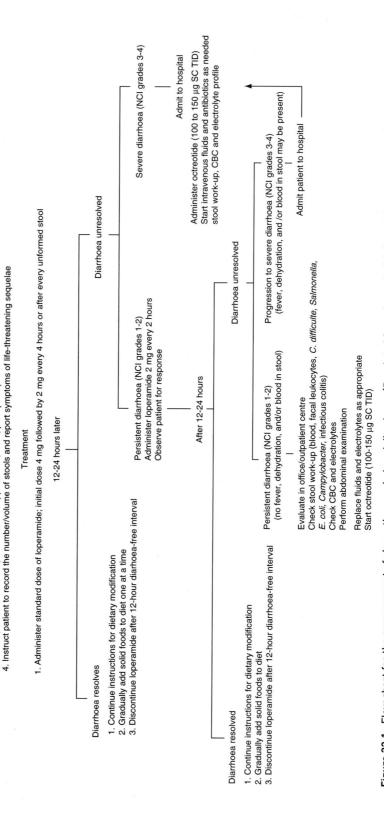

Figure 22.1: Flow chart for the management of chemotherapy-induced diarrhoea. (Reprinted from Journal of Pain and Symptom Management, Vol 19, Number 2, Kornblau SM, Benson AB, Catalano R, et al., Management of cancer treatment-related diarrhea: issues and therapeutic strategies, pp 118–129, © 2000, with permission of US Cancer Pain Relief Committee.)

498

immunocompromised patients, as encephalopathy may result.[37] Intraluminal agents such as clay and charcoal derivatives may interfere with absorption of antidiarrhoeals and other drugs and are not usually to be recommended.[69] Clonidine, which is a proabsorptive agent, has a limited role.[69] Aspirin, because of its effect of blocking prostaglandins, can also be helpful.[87]

Infectious diarrhoea should be treated with the appropriate antibiotic. *C. difficile* will often respond to metronidazole, but vancomycin may be needed if there is no response within 3 days.[38,50] However, in cases of pseudomembranous colitis following antibiotics, treatment will involve stopping the antibiotics and it is not safe to use loperamide.[38] Colestyramine (Questran) may help patients who cannot absorb bile salts after bowel resection, or after pelvic radiation.[38,88] Following pancreatic resection, pancreatic enzymes may need replacing, and are best started early after surgery, but patients need to be aware that lipase is destroyed by acid and so needs to be taken with a meal, not before or after food.[38] Additionally, antibiotics such as metronidazole can be helpful if a breath test indicates bacterial overgrowth.[88] If pain relief is needed, choice of analgesia with constipating properties (such as the opiates) may supplement the effect of antidiarrhoeal agents. Probiotics may be of value in both preventing antibiotic-associated diarrhoea and in treating infectious diarrhoea.[89] Occasionally, steroid retention enemas may be useful.[43] Other drug sensitivities should be adjusted where feasible: e.g. some patients need to change antacid, or avoid using non-steroidal anti-inflammatory drugs (NSAIDs).

Surgery

Surgery is usually best avoided if at all possible, but sometimes strictures need to be dilated (often endoscopically), and fistulae may need closing. Occasionally, a colostomy is indicated.[43]

Non-pharmacological strategies

Diet

Many people find that what they eat influences their bowel function and diet should be reviewed with each patient. The nurse supports and guides the patient in experimenting with diet and fluid modification. It is not easy to offer definitive advice on diet as the influence seems to vary from person to person, and there is very little research on which foods can make diarrhoea better or worse. What may be problematic for one person seems to have no effect at all on someone else having the same diagnosis and treatment. And, of course, eating and drinking should be a pleasure, so it would be a great pity to make life a misery by needing to constantly worry about what is eaten.

It is worth experimenting to see if each individual can find anything that exacerbates or improves diarrhoea. In clinical experience, food rich in fibre is the most common contributor to increased intestinal hurry.[90] A low-fibre diet has been recommended from the start of radiotherapy to minimize gut irritation,[63] but this can be difficult to accommodate in some diets, such as strict vegans. Martz has given detailed recommendations on low-residue and low-lactose diets.[32] A low-lactose diet can also be useful, but checks should be made that the patient does not become constipated. Softer stool is more difficult to hold during an urge to defecate, and is also more likely to passively leak.[91] Raw fruit and vegetables seem particularly aggravating for some people.[92] There are no trials on the effect of fibre reduction on diarrhoea, but clinically a lot of patients derive benefit from moderating their fibre intake. Fibre reduction must of course be taken sensibly and with awareness of the benefits of fibre to general health. Conversely, some patients find that increasing fibre helps to add bulk and substance to liquid stool. Fibre has been found to be a beneficial additive to relieve diarrhoea in tube-fed men, but not in women, for reasons which are not clear.[93] A BRATT diet (bananas, rice, applesauce or peeled cooked apples, white toast and decaffeinated tea) is often recommended in the American nursing literature,[94] although the research base for this is not available. Foods rich in pectin may help solidify stool.

Very spicy or hot food can upset some people. Other foods to consider include milk products and chocolate, which some people find make their stools looser or upsets an irritable bowel.[95] Artificial sweeteners, especially sorbitol (an ingredient in many low-calorie foods, drinks and chewing gum) have a tendency to make their stools looser. Hyperosmotic food supplements such as Ensure may exacerbate or precipitate diarrhoea. Unabsorbable sugars have a known osmotic effect, holding fluid in the gut lumen, and can provide a substrate for colonic bacteria, increasing flatus production.[96] Sports drinks are often recommended to replace lost electrolytes, but in fact do not have the best composition to do this effectively.

If patients thinks that there may be a link with what they eat, keeping a diary may reveal if there is a pattern. A course of antibiotics can upset the bowel and live natural yogurt or pro-biotics such as lactobacillus can help to restore a more regular habit. Probiotics may also be helpful to prevent or shorten the course of gas-trointestinal infections.[97] Probiotics have been shown to decrease mucosal inflammatory activity in an animal model, and also to reduce the prevalence of colon cancer secondary to chronic inflammation.[98]

Patients with lactose intolerance should omit all milk products, although the probiotic aci-dophilus is reported to convert lactose into sim-ple sugars which should be tolerated.[99] Parents of children may be tempted to encourage milk drinks, but lactose malabsorption is recognized as common after chemotherapy in children.[61] Global malabsorption may necessitate a restricted or even an elemental diet. Hot food and drink tends to stimulate peristalsis more than room temperature or cold food and so it may help to allow hot food to cool.[100] Eating small meals more frequently rather than a few large meals may also stimulate the gut less.

Some foods help to make stools firmer for some people: e.g. arrowroot as biscuits or as a flour substitute in sauces or soups, marshmal-low sweets and very ripe bananas and other foods rich in pectin may help. Bananas will also help replace lost potassium. Nutmeg has been reported as helpful.[92] Anecdotally, peppermint, fennel and ginger tea are each suggested, but with no research evidence. A high fat intake can slow down the speed with which food trav-els through the bowel, but many patients tol-erate fat poorly and a high-fat diet is obviously not healthy for other reasons and so cannot be generally recommended.

Patients requiring nutritional supplements may find some enteral feeds, particularly those with a high osmolality (500–800 mOsm/kg), promote diarrhoea, while those with a lower osmolality may be better. Rapid administration of tube or PEG (percutaneous endoscopic gas-trostomy) feeds can also induce diarrhoea.[99]

Type of fluid intake can make a difference to some people, and again this is individual and it is worth experimenting. Caffeine reduction is almost always advisable. Some people have a bowel that seems to be very sensitive to caf-feine, which is in coffee, tea, cola drinks and chocolate. Caffeine is a known gut stimu-lant,[101] and so makes the stools move through the gut faster. This means that less fluid is taken from the stools, which are then looser and more urgent. A high caffeine intake should not be stopped suddenly, as headaches can result. Alcohol seems to cause the bowels to be loose and urgent for some people. Different types of alcoholic drink can affect people in dif-ferent ways. Some find that beer is better than wine, or that white wine is better than red, or vice versa. It is impossible to be prescriptive, and so the nurse should support and guide the patient in experimenting.

Paradoxically, patients with short bowel syndrome (SBS) and diarrhoea often benefit from restricting fluid intake. This is because ingested fluid in the gut lumen has a higher osmolality than the surrounding tissue and will tend to draw fluid from the body into the gut lumen. In SBS, there is insufficient mucosa lower down the gut to reabsorb this fluid and so the more that is drunk, the more fluid will be passed. Fluid restriction is often neces-sary for patients with a high-output stoma. Ingested fluid should be as close to body fluid osmolality as possible (e.g. The World Health Organization oral rehydration fluid, see Box 22.2) and fluids such as tea and coffee should be avoided.

Nicotine is thought to slow upper gut motil-ity and increase total transit time,[102] but it seems that it can speed rectosigmoid transit,[103] and this fits with many people reporting clini-cally that smoking a cigarette facilitates initia-tion of defecation. Smoking cessation or reduction has been found useful clinically in some patients with urgency.

Box 22.2

WHO oral rehydration solution	
Sodium chloride	3.5 g
Sodium hydroxide	2.5 g
Potassium	1.5 g
Glucose	20.0 g
Distilled water	1000 ml

Biofeedback and bowel retraining

Biofeedback usually involves a combination of improving anal sphincter function by pelvic floor exercises as well as retraining rectal sensation,[104] and is usually seen as first-line therapy for patients with faecal incontinence.[105] It has been found helpful in patients with urgency and faecal incontinence after a low anterior rectal resection for rectal cancer.[106] Many people need to learn to resist the urge to defecate, thereby gradually increasing rectal capacity and decreasing urgency. Use of a rectal balloon to encourage the patient to tolerate larger volumes in the rectum before rushing to the toilet can be helpful,[104] but has only been reported occasionally as helpful in diarrhoea and not specifically in people with cancer.[107,108] It is a technique which warrants further evaluation in patients with chronic diarrhoea.

Bowel retraining is used in clinical practice, although research is not available.[104] It is not difficult to imagine how a person who has had the extremely unpleasant experience of faecal incontinence may 'learn' hypervigilance and hypersensitivity to bowel contents and experience or interpret any bowel sensation as 'urgency'. The feeling of urgency may induce an emotional reaction of anxiety, even panic, if there is no readily available toilet, because of the fear of a socially apparent bowel accident.[104] Fear of incontinence can induce a behavioural frequency in an attempt to prevent incontinent episodes. This can set up a vicious circle of hypersensitivity (monitoring the fullness of the rectum to pre-empt incontinence), urgency and anxiety.[104] It has been known that anxiety is a bowel stimulant for over 60 years,[109] increasing bowel motility and propulsive contractions.[110] Thus, anxiety makes incontinence even more likely. Anxiety leads the individual to pay more attention to somatic sensations, and possibly to misinterpret or overinterpret them.[104] The logical and natural reaction to this urgency is to find a toilet as quickly as possible and to empty the bowel, as stool in the toilet cannot cause social embarrassment. So, rather than ignoring the call to stool as most people would if the moment is not convenient, the person with previous experience of faecal incontinence responds as rapidly as possible, not even attempting to defer for fear of provoking an accident. Eventually, the individual never has the experience of an urge to defecate that diminishes, extreme urgency is felt all the time until the bowel is emptied and all urges to defecate are experienced as very urgent. A vicious circle of hypersensitivity and anxiety becomes established.

Retraining involves gradually increasing the time interval between perceived rectal fullness and defecation, slowly and incrementally. The patient is instructed to 'hold on', near the toilet initially and then progressively further away.[91] Many patients need to relearn that an urge that is resisted will wear off after a few minutes. The longer stool is retained, the more fluid is reabsorbed through the intestinal mucosa and the less liquid the stool will be. This will not help patients with acute overwhelming diarrhoea, but is found clinically useful in those who maintain an artificially high bowel frequency once acute diarrhoea has subsided because of fear of incontinence.[104]

Rectovaginal fistula may be a late complication of high-dose pelvic radiation, and is difficult to manage as the radiation will often have caused coexisting diarrhoea. If surgical repair is not possible, diversion of the faecal stream into a stoma is sometimes the best option for the patient's quality of life. An uncontrolled fistula causes great discomfort, repeated vaginal infections and soreness as well as being very difficult to manage practically, quite apart from negative impact on body image. Such patients need meticulous skin care and tremendous emotional support.

The use of frequent warm baths or bidet can be soothing to sore skin. A portable bidet is available for those without this facility (Warwick Sasco Ltd).

Products

An anal plug (Coloplast Ltd) has been found helpful in a minority of patients with faecal incontinence.[111] Use is limited by discomfort in many patients and it has not been formally evaluated in patients with diarrhoea. It is unlikely to be an option in patients with frequency, as repeated insertion and removal would cause soreness, and it may not be effective in resisting high bowel pressures often associated with severe diarrhoea. However, it may have a use in selected patients for specific occasions that provoke anxiety about faecal incontinence.

A perianal adhesive pouch is available for immobile patients with uncontrollable diarrhoea (Hollister Ltd), although many nurses seem reluctant to use this method of management.[112] Use is only suitable for a very few patients with severe debility or who are unconscious, but in a few patients with uncontrolled diarrhoea and incontinence, the pouch can protect the skin as well as making nursing management much easier. A rectal tube can also be helpful in carefully selected patients who are very ill and bed bound. Grogan and Kramer have reported that a nasopharyngeal airway was both comfortable in situ and effective for the majority of patients, and that skin integrity improved.[113]

A bedside commode may enhance access and independence. A plastic liner may minimize carer burden.[31]

EVALUATION OF OUTCOMES, INCLUDING QUALITY OF LIFE

The evaluation of outcomes of nursing interventions ensures that the patient is receiving the optimum standard of care. Objective assessment of the frequency of defecation and the characteristics of the stools provides objective data, while dialogue about the lived experience of constipation or diarrhoea captures subjective data. These data enable the nurse, together with the patient, to evaluate the patient's response to treatment. It is essential that nurses are vigilant when evaluating care, using their knowledge of potential side-effects of pharmacological treatment and the symptoms of advancing disease to inform their assessment.

Nurses commonly initiate interventions for the management of constipation and diarrhoea in collaboration with the healthcare team. Ongoing assessment and evaluation provides the basis of review of treatment regimens. Even though the decision for initiating or changing treatment may not rest with the nursing staff alone, a thorough understanding of the problems of constipation and diarrhoea ensures efficient and effective care through communication with the multidisciplinary team. Since the experience of constipation and diarrhoea is largely subjective, the only person who can really evaluate the effects of treatment is the patient. The experienced nurse will, however, be sensitive to external cues such as non-verbal signs and narrative accounts relating to the patient's comfort and can use this information to support 'objective data' about patterns of defecation. It is essential that objective and subjective observations are documented in order to inform care delivery and review, both in the context of providing effective individualized care and in the context of developing care pathways and protocols for the patient group.

CONCLUSION

Constipation and diarrhoea cause a significant problem for people with cancer, impacting on the quality of life of patients and their carers. For many patients the embarrassment that results from unresolved gastrointestinal disturbances may be as distressing as the physical discomfort. Successful management remains a unique and major challenge for nurses in cancer care. Assessment, planning, delivery and evaluation of nursing interventions, underpinned by a sound knowledge and skills base, enable nurses to deliver high-quality, individualized, effective care. Nurses ultimately need to understand the conditions of constipation and diarrhoea, be able to explain to the patient what is happening and have up-to-date knowledge about the most effective drugs available and non-pharmacological strategies in order to plan appropriate intervention.

REFERENCES

1. World Health Organisation. Cancer pain relief and palliative care. Technical Report Series 804, 1994.

2. Lawler J. Behind the screens – nursing, somology and the problem of the body. Edinburgh: Churchill Livingstone; 1991.

3. Norton C. Faecal incontinence in adults. Nurs Stand 1997; 11(46):49–54.

4. Loudon JB. On body products. In: Blacking J, ed. The anthropology of the body. London: Academic Press; 1977.

5. Campbell T. Colorectal cancer, part 1: epidemiology, aetiology, screening and diagnosis. Prof Nurse 1999; 14(12):869–872.

6. Sykes NP. Constipation and diarrhoea. In: Doyle D, Hanks GWC, Macdonald N, eds. Oxford textbook of palliative medicine. 2nd edn. Oxford: Oxford Medical Publications; 1998:513–526.

7. Winney J. Constipation. Nurs Stand 1998; 13(11):49–53.

8. Petticrew M. Treatment of constipation in older people. Nurs Times 1997; 93(48):55–56.

9. Withell B. A protocol for treating acute constipation in the community setting. Br J Community Nurs 2000; 5(3):110–117.

10. Connell AM, Hilton C, Irvine G, et al. Variation in bowel habit in two population samples. BMJ 1965; ii:1095–1099.

11. Hyde V, Jenkinson T, Koch T, Webb C. Constipation and laxative use in older community-dwelling adults. Clin Effect Nurs 1999; 3:170–180.

12. Norton C. The causes and nursing management of constipation. Br J Nurs 1996; l5(20):1252–1258.

13. Tuchmann L. Constipation. In: Gates RA, Fink RM, eds. Oncology nursing secrets. Philadelphia: Hanley and Belfus; 1997:216–225.

14. Brocklehurst J, Dickinson E, Windsor J. Laxatives and faecal incontinence in long term care. Nurs Stand 1999; 13(52):32–36.

15. Rattenbury N, Mooney G, Bowen J. Oral assessment and care for inpatients. Nurs Times 1999; 95(49):52–53.

16. Stewart E, Innes J, Mackenzie J, Downie G. A strategy to reduce laxative use among older people. Nurs Times 1997; 93(4):35–36.

17. Maestri-Banks A. An overview of constipation: causes and treatment. Int J Palliat Nurs 1998; 4(6):271–275.

18. Murray B. Preventing constipation. J Community Nurs 1997; 11(6):18–20.

19. Fallon M, O'Neill B. Constipation and diarrhoea. BMJ 1997; 315:1293–1296.

20. Levy MH, Catalano RB. Control of common physical symptoms other than pain in patients with terminal disease. Semin Oncol 1985; 12(4):411–430.

21. Clinch J, Dudgeon D, Schipper H. Quality of life assessment in palliative care. In: Doyle D, Hanks GWC, Macdonald N, eds. Oxford textbook of palliative medicine. 2nd edn. Oxford: Oxford Medical Publications; 1998:83–94.

22. Ingham J, Portenoy R. The measurement of pain and other symptoms. In: Doyle D, Hanks GWC, Macdonald N, eds. Oxford textbook of palliative medicine. 2nd edn. Oxford: Oxford Medical Publications; 1998:203–219.

23. Twycross R, Back I., Clinical management. Nausea and vomiting in advanced cancer. Eur J Palliat Care 1998; 5(2):39–45.

24. Regnard C, Hockley J. Flow diagrams in advanced cancer and other diseases. London: Edward Arnold; 1995.

25. Bruera E, Macdonald S. Audit methods: The Edmonton Symptom Assessment System. In: Higginson I, ed. Clinical audit in palliative care. Oxford: Radcliffe Medical; 1993:61–77.

26 Rees E, Hardy J, Ling J, Broadley K, A'hern R. The use of the Edmonton Symptom Assessment Scale (ESAS) within a palliative care unit in the UK. Palliat Med 1998; 12(2):75–82.

27. Camp-Sorrell D. Chemotherapy: toxicity management. In: Groenwald SL, Frogge MH, Goodman M, Yarbro CH, eds. Cancer nursing: principles and practice. 3rd edn. Boston: Jones and Bartlett; 1993.

28. Cleaveland MJ. Alternative therapies. In: Gates RA, Fink RM, eds. Oncology nursing secrets. Philadelphia: Hanley and Belfus; 1997:85–90.

29. Getliffe K, Dolman M. Promoting continence. London: Ballière Tindall; 1997.

30. Kelley A, Shepherd S. Continence. In: Mallik M, Hall C, Howard D, eds. Nursing knowledge and practice. London: Ballière Tindall; 1998:373–417.

31. Hogan CM. The nurse's role in diarrhoea management. Oncol Nurs Forum 1998; 25(5):879–886.

32. Martz CH. Diarrhea. In: Yarbro CH, ed. Cancer symptom management. Boston: Jones and Bartlett; 1999:522–536.

33. Engelking C, Rutledge DN, Ippoliti C, Neumann J, Hogan CM. Cancer-related diarrhea: a neglected cause of cancer-related symptom distress. Oncol Nurs Forum 1998; 25(5):859–860.

34. Wolfe J, Grier HE, Klar N, et al. Symptoms and suffering at the end of life in children with cancer. N Engl J Med 2000; 342:326–333.

35. Thomas PRM, Lindblad AS, Stablein DM, et al. Toxicity associated with adjuvant postoperative therapy for adenocarcinoma of the rectum. Cancer 1985; 57:1130–1134.

36. Engelking C, Wickham R, Iwamoto R. Cancer-related gastrointestinal symptoms: dilemmas in assessment and management. Develop Support Cancer Care 1996; 1(1):3–10.

37. DuPont HL. Guidelines on acute infectious diarrhea in adults. Am J Gastroenterol 1997; 92(11):1962–1975.

38. Cascinu S. Drug therapy in diarrheal diseases in oncology/hematology patients. Crit Rev Oncol Hematol 1995; 18:37–50.

39. Guenter PA, Sweed MR. A valid and reliable tool to quantify stool output in tube-fed patients. J Parenter Enteral Nutr 1998; 22(3):147–151.

40. Kornblau SM, Benson AB, Catalano R, et al. Management of cancer treatment-related diarrhea: issues and therapeutic strategies. J Pain Symptom Manage 2000; 19(2):118–129.

41. Grumann MM, Noack EM, Hoffmann IA, Schlag PM. Comparison of quality of life in patients undergoing abdominoperineal extirpation or anterior resection for rectal cancer. Ann Surg 2001; 233(2):149–156.

42. Eisenberg P. An overview of diarrhea in the patient receiving enteral nutrition. Gastroenterol Nurs 2002; 25(3):95–104.

43. Dubois A, Earnest DL. Radiation enteritis and colitis. In: Feldman M, Sleisenger MH, Scharschmidt BF, eds. Gastrointestinal and liver disease. 6th edn, Vol 2. Philadelphia: WB Saunders; 1998:1696–1707.

44. Zachariah B, Casey L, Balducci L. Radiotherapy of the oldest old cancer patients: a study of effectiveness and toxicity. J Am Geriatr Soc 1995; 43:793–795.

45. McArdle AH, Wittnich C, Freeman CR, Duguid WP. Elemental diet as prophylaxis against radiation injury. Arch Surg 1985; 120:1026–1032.

46. Cope DG. Management of chemotherapy-induced diarrhea and constipation. Nurs Clin North Am 2001; 36(4):695–707.

47. Early DS. Gastrointestinal complications of chemotherapy. In: Perry MC, ed. The chemotherapy source book. Philadelphia: Lippincott, Williams and Wilkins; 2001:477–483.

48. Anand A, Glatt AE. *Clostridium difficile* infection associated with antineoplastic chemotherapy: a review. Clin Infect Dis 1993; 17:109–113.

49. Kamthan AG, Bruckner HW, Hirschman SZ, Agus SG. *Clostridium difficile* diarrhea induced by cancer chemotherapy. Arch Intern Med 1992; 152:1715–1717.

50. Hartmann JT, Bokemeyer C. Diarrhea and constipation. Antibiot Chemother 2000; 50:184–188.

51. Schuller I, Saha V, Lin L, et al. Investigation and management of *Clostridium difficile* colonisation in a paediatric oncology unit. Arch Dis Child 1995; 72:219–222.

52. Gerard M, Defresne N, Daneau D, et al. Incidence and significance of *Clostridium difficile* in hospitalised cancer patients. Eur J Clin Microbiol Infect Dis 1988; 7(2):274–278.

53. Cudmore M, Silva J, Fekety R, Liepman MK, Kim K-H. *Clostridium difficile* colitis associated with cancer chemotherapy. Arch Intern Med 1982; 142:333–335.

54. Nolan NPM, Kelly CP, Humphreys JFH, et al. An epidemic of pseudomembranous colitis: importance of person to person spread. Gut 1987; 28:1467–1473.

55. Tanyuksel M, Doganci L. Prevalence of *Cryptosporidium* sp. in patients with neoplasia and diarrhea. Scand J Infect Dis 1995; 27:69–70.

56. Ballal M, Prabhu T, Chandran A, Shivananda PG. *Cryptosporidium* and *Isospora belli* diarrhoea in immunocompromised hosts. Indian J Cancer 1999; 36:38–42.

57. Guarner J, Matilde-Nava T, Villasenor-Flores R, Sanchez-Mejorada G. Frequency of intestinal parasites in adult cancer patients in Mexico. Arch Med Res 1997; 28(2):219–222.

58. Besnard M, Hartmann O, Valteau-Couanet D, et al. Systemic candida infection in pediatric BM autotransplantation: clinical signs, outcome and prognosis. Bone Marrow Transplant 1993; 11:465–470.

59. Edes TE, Walk BE, Austin JL. Diarrhea in tube-fed patients: feeding formula not necessarily the cause. Am J Med 1990; 88:91–93.

60. Heather DJ, Howell L, Montana M, Howell M, Hill R. Effect of a bulk-forming cathartic on diarrhea in tube-fed patients. Heart Lung 1991; 20:409–413.

61. Hyams JS, Batrus CL, Grand RJ, Sallan SE. Cancer chemotherapy-induced lactose malabsoption in children. Cancer 1982; 49:646–650.

62. Rutledge DN, Engelking C. Cancer-related diarrhea: selected findings of a national survey of oncology nurse experiences. Oncol Nurs Forum 1998; 25(5):861–872.

63. Kelvin JF. Gastrointestinal cancers. In: Dow KH, Bucholtz JD, Iwamoto RR, Fieler VK, Hilderley LJ, eds. Nursing care in radiation oncology. Philadelphia: WB Saunders; 1997:152–183.

64. Hogan CM. Cancer nursing: the art of symptom management. Oncol Nurs Forum 1997; 24(8):1335–1341.

65. Bliss DZ, Savik S, Jung H, et al. Comparison of subjective classification of stool consistency and stool water content. J Wound Ostomy Continence Nurs 1999; 26:137–141.

66. Mertz HR, Beck CK, Dixon W, et al. Validation of a new measure of diarrhea. Digest Dis Sci 1995; 40(9):1873–1882.

67. Leigh RJ, Turnberg LA. Faecal incontinence: the unvoiced symptom. Lancet 1982; 1:1349–1351.

68. Sultan AH, Kamm MA, Hudson CN, Thomas JM, Bartram CI. Anal sphincter disruption during vaginal delivery. N Engl J Med 1993; 329:1905–1911.

69. Ippoliti C. Antidiarrheal agents for the management of treatment-related diarrhea in

cancer patients. Am J Health Syst Pharm 1998; 55:1573–1580.

70. Sun WM, Read NW, Verlinden M. Effects of loperamide oxide in gastrointestinal transit time and anorectal function in patients with chronic diarrhoea and faecal incontinence. Scand J Gastroenterol 1997; 32:34–38.

71. Goke M, Ewe K, Donner K, Meyer zum Buschenfelde K-H. Influence of loperamide oxide on the anal sphincter. Dis Colon Rectum 1992; 35:857–861.

72. Rattan S, Culver PJ. Influence of loperamide on the internal anal sphincter in the opossum. Gastroenterology 1987; 93:121–128.

73. Kamm MA. Functional disorders of the colon and anorectum. Curr Opin Gastroenterol 1995; 11:9–15.

74. Read M, Read NW, Barber DC, Duthie HL. Effects of loperamide on anal sphincter function in patients complaining of chronic diarrhoea with faecal incontinence and urgency. Digest Dis Sci 1982; 27:807–814.

75. Yeoh E, Horowitz M, Russo A, et al. Gastrintestinal function in chronic radiation enteritis – effects of loperamide-N-oxide. Gut 1993; 34:476–482.

76. Palmer KR, Corbett CL, Holdsworth CD. Double-blind cross-over study comparing loperamide codeine and diphenoxylate in the treatment of chronic diarrhoea. Gastroenterology 1980; 79:1272–1275.

77. Bisanz A. Managing bowel elimination problems in patients with cancer. Oncol Nurs Forum 1997; 24(4):679–686.

78. Bliss DZ, Jung H, Savik K, et al. Supplementation with dietary fiber improves fecal incontinence. Nurs Res 2001; 50(4):203–213.

79. Gray M, Jacobsen T. Are somatostatin analogues (Octreotide and Lanreotide) effective in promoting of healing enterocutaneous fistulas? J Wound Ostomy Continence Nurs 2002; 29:228–233.

80. Lamberts SWJ, Van der Lely A-J, De Herder WW, Hofland LJ. Octreotide. N Engl J Med 1996; 334(4):246–254.

81. Gebbia V, Carreca I, Testa A, et al. Subcutaneous octreotide versus oral loperamide in the treatment of diarrhoea following chemotherapy. Anticancer Drugs 1993; 4:443–445.

82. Zidan J, Haim N, Beny A, et al. Octreotide in the treatment of severe chemotherapy-induced diarrhea. Ann Oncol 2001; 12:227–229.

83. Baillie-Johnson HR. Octreotide in the management of treatment-related diarrhoea. Anticancer Drugs 1996; 7(Suppl 1):11–15.

84. Ippoliti C, Neumann J. Octreotide in the management of diarrhea induced by graft versus host disease. Oncol Nurs Forum 1998; 25(5):873–878.

85. Petrelli NJ, Rodriguez-Bigas M, Rustum Y, Herrera L, Creaven P. Bowel rest, intravenous hydration, and continuous high-dose infusion of octreotide acetate for the treatment of chemotherapy-induced diarrhea in patients with colorectal cancer. Cancer 1993; 72:1543–1546.

86. Meropol NJ, Rustum YM, Creaven PJ, Blumenson LE, Frank C. Phase 1 and pharmacokinetic study of weekly 5-fluorouracil administered with granulocyte-macrophage colony-stimulating factor and high-dose leucovorin: a potential role for growth factor as mucosal protectant. Cancer Invest 1999; 17(1):1–9.

87. Mennie AJ, Dalley V, Dinneen LC, Collier HOJ. Treatment of radiation-induced gastrointestinal distress with acetylsalicylate. Lancet 1975; 2:942–943.

88. Danielsson A, Nyhlin H, Persson H, et al. Chronic diarrhoea after radiotherapy for gynaecological cancer: occurrence and aetiology. Gut 1991; 32:1180–1187.

89. Elmer GW, Surawicz CM, McFarland LV. Biotherapeutic agents: a neglected modality for the treatment and prevention of selected intestinal and vaginal infections. JAMA 1996; 275(11):870–876.

90. Barrett JA. Faecal incontinence and related problems in the older adult. London: Edward Arnold; 1993.

91. Norton C, Kamm MA. Bowel control – information and practical advice. Beaconsfield: Beaconsfield Publishers; 1999.

92. Anonymous. Patient pointers: what you can do about diarrhoea. Develop Support Cancer Care 1996; 1(1):27–30.

93. Mennie AJ, Dalley V. Aspirin in radiation induced diarrhea. Lancet 1973; i:1131–1133.

94. Hawkins R. Diarrhea. Clin J Oncol Nurs 2000; 4(4):183–186.

95. Ellard K. Irritable bowel syndrome. East Dereham: Neen Health Books; 1996.

96. Heaton KW. Effect of diet on intestinal function and dysfunction. In: Snape WJ, ed. Pathogenesis of functional bowel disease. New York: Plenum; 1989:79–99.

97. de Roos NM, Katan MB. Effects of probiotic bacteria on diarrhea, lipid metabolism and carcinogenesis: a review of papers between 1988 and 1998. Am J Clin Nutr 2000; 71:405–411.

98. O'Mahony L, Feeney M, O'Halloran S, et al. Probiotic impact on microbial flora, inflammation and tumour development in IL-10 knockout mice. Aliment Pharmacol Ther 2001; 15:1219–1225.

99. Basch A. Changes in elimination. Semin Oncol Nurs 1987; 3(4):287–292.

100. Charuhas PM. Dietary management during antitumor therapy of cancer patients. Topics Clin Nutr 1993; 9(1):42–53.

101. Brown SR, Cann PA, Read NW. Effect of coffee on distal colon function. Gut 1990; 31:450–453.

102. Scott AM, Kellow JE, Eckersley GM, Nolan JM, Jones MP. Cigarette smoking and nicotine delay postprandial mouth-cecum transit time. Digest Dis Sci 1992; 37(10):1544–1547.

103. Rausch T, Beglinger C, Alam N, Meier R. Effect of transdermal application of nicotine on colonic transit in healthy nonsmoking volunteers. Neurogastroenterol Mot 1998; 10:263–270.

104. Norton C, Chelvanayagam S. Methodology of biofeedback for adults with fecal incontinence – a program of care. J Wound Ostomy Continence Nurs 2001; 28:156–168.

105. Norton C, Kamm MA. Anal sphincter biofeedback and pelvic floor exercises for faecal incontinence in adults – a systematic review. Aliment Pharmacol Ther 2001; 15:1147–1154.

106. Ho YH, Chiang JM, Tan M, Low JY. Biofeedback therapy for excessive stool frequency and incontinence following anterior resection or total colectomy. Dis Colon Rectum 1996; 39(11):1289–1292.

107. Schiller LR, Santa Ana C, Davis GR, Fordtran JS. Faecal incontinence in chronic diarrhoea:

report of a case with improvement after training with rectally infused saline. Gastroenterology 1979; 77:751–753.

108. Chiarioni G, Scattolini C, Bonfante F, Vantini I. Liquid stool incontinence with severe urgency: anorectal function and effective biofeedback treatment. Gut 1993; 34:1576–1580.

109. Almy TP. Experimental studies on the irritable colon. Am J Med 1951; 10:60–67.

110. Herbst F, Kamm MA, Morris GP, et al. Gastrointestinal transit and prolonged ambulatory colonic motility in health and faecal incontinence. Gut 1997; 41:381–389.

111. Norton C, Kamm MA. Anal plug for faecal incontinence. Colorectal Dis 2001; 3: 323–327.

112. Bosley CL. Applying perianal pouches with confidence. Nursing 1995; 25(6):58–62.

113. Grogan TA, Kramer DJ. The rectal trumpet: use of a nasopharyngeal airway to contain fecal incontinence in critically ill patients. J Wound Ostomy Continence Nurs 2002; 29:193–201.

CHAPTER 23

Breathlessness

SALLY MOORE, HILARY PLANT AND MARY BREDIN

CHAPTER CONTENTS

Introduction	507	Management of breathlessness in cancer	510
		Assessment	511
The nature of breathlessness in cancer	508	Medical interventions	512
Prevalence of breathlessness in		Pharmacological strategies	513
patients with cancer	508	Non-pharmacological interventions	514
Mechanisms of breathing and			
breathlessness	508	Conclusion	523
Causes of breathlessness in cancer	509		
The experience of breathlessness	509	References	523

INTRODUCTION

Breathlessness is a common symptom for patients with advanced cancer and it causes great distress, disability, social isolation and loss of function.[1–3] This distress is partly due to the close association between being able to breathe and being able to stay alive. Yet despite its prevalence, there is evidence suggesting that breathlessness commonly goes unrecognized by health professionals,[3] who find it a difficult symptom to manage.[4,5] It is therefore not surprising that it is often poorly controlled even when specialist teams are involved.[1]

Breathlessness in advanced cancer is frequently accompanied by other debilitating symptoms such as fatigue, depression and cachexia.[2,6–8] Because these symptoms impact on the patient's experience, breathlessness cannot be treated in isolation, so optimal management must depend on a multi-professional holistic approach. Nurses, whose role includes both pharmacological and non-pharmacological approaches, are well placed to develop strategies that enable patients and their families to manage this symptom more effectively. Consequently, there is a strong argument for nurses to take a lead in the management of breathlessness.

This chapter draws on the growing literature about managing cancer-related breathlessness and our own experience of working with patients who are breathless, both in a clinic setting and on hospital wards. Over a number of years, we have sought to understand the patient's experiences of this symptom and how it impacts on all aspects of their world: physical, emotional, social and spiritual. Together with colleagues, we have learned how to respond to the problems and challenges of working with patients who are breathless, believing there is much that can be done to help patients and their families live and cope with breathlessness.

This chapter aims to provide a comprehensive and practical guide for nurses wanting to improve the experience of breathlessness for patients and their families. It is intended to give nurses the knowledge and confidence to develop their own skills, so they feel empowered to offer creative ways of managing this challenging symptom.

THE NATURE OF BREATHLESSNESS IN CANCER

Breathlessness is an unpleasant and/or uncomfortable awareness of breathing or need to breathe.[9] Dyspnoea is the common medical term used for this symptom. However, dyspnoea often has little meaning for patients, so the term 'breathlessness' is used throughout this chapter to denote a broader understanding of the patient's experience.

Prevalence of breathlessness in patients with cancer

Breathlessness is a common symptom of advanced cancer. Reported incidence varies from 15%[1] to 79%,[10] depending on the population of patients with cancer studied and the method of obtaining data. It has been reported in one study that 40% of children with cancer experience breathlessness during their illness.[11]

Patients who have lung cancer often experience breathlessness and, amongst this patient population, the incidence of breathlessness is certainly increased.[1,6,9,12,13] For example, in a study of patients with lung cancer who were receiving follow-up care after initial treatment, over 90% reported breathlessness as a problem.[14] Breathlessness is also associated with more advanced disease and correlates with shorter survival.[10,12] However, coexisting causes of breathlessness may render it a feature of less advanced disease, e.g. where a patient also suffers from a co-morbid condition such as heart failure.

Despite its prevalence, there is evidence to suggest that nurses do not always recognize when breathlessness is a problem; and some nurses have a poor understanding of the symptom and strategies that can help relieve it.[3,10] Patients report they are offered very little help and are often left to cope with the symptom in isolation.[13] Yet, apparently, patients may themselves be reluctant to report this symptom unless questioned about it directly.[3] These combined factors result in a general underassessment and undertreatment of breathlessness.

The experience of breathlessness also has a significant impact on patients' use of healthcare resources. It is not uncommon for people to attend emergency departments with acute breathlessness, or for them to be admitted to hospital.[15] Patients with breathlessness are also more likely to die in a hospital than a hospice or nursing home.[5] It seems very likely then that improved management of breathlessness would not only improve patients' experience of care but also lead to better and more appropriate use of resources.

Mechanisms of breathing and breathlessness

The underlying control of breathing entails largely involuntary processes determined by the body's oxygen levels and acid–base balance. This involuntary drive is regulated by a complex interplay of not only chemical but also neurological and musculoskeletal messages that pass between the lungs, chest wall, diaphragm and brain.[16] Coughing, talking and swallowing for instance all depend on involuntary reflexes that are linked to breathing control. In addition, however, it is also possible – in most circumstances – to exert some conscious control over breathing. It is in fact this dual control of breathing that makes it possible to work with a person who is breathless – this will be discussed later in this chapter (see Breathing retraining section).

Although the precise origin of the sensation of breathlessness is poorly understood, at least three factors are thought to contribute to this feeling:[8,17]

1 Mechanical: an obstruction or restriction within the airways or lung will provoke an increase in respiratory effort, e.g. a mass, pulmonary embolism, pleural effusion or stiffening of the lung associated with mesothelioma or fibrosis. This leads to increased exertion of the respiratory muscles in order to achieve adequate air flow.

2 Chemical: breathing patterns alter as changes in blood levels of carbon dioxide

and oxygen stimulate the respiratory centre in the brainstem.

3 Emotional: feelings – such as rage, fear, or sadness -in diverse ways, alter the rhythm and depth of breathing. These unconscious elements of breathing control are in turn affected whenever attention is focused on the breathing process and it is brought to the level of consciousness.

Causes of breathlessness in cancer

The causes of breathlessness are varied and complex. It may, for example, result from effects of the disease itself, anticancer treatment, concurrent medical conditions (either related or unrelated to having cancer) or a combination of these factors (Box 23.1). In addition, because of the likelihood of a smoking history and age, many patients with lung cancer are also likely to have chronic airways disease, which is often suboptimally treated. In one study, almost half the patients with lung cancer were found to have undiagnosed airflow obstruction, yet less than one-fifth of these patients had been prescribed a bronchodilator.[18]

It is also known that lung function decreases with age due to the normal effects of ageing on the skeleton, respiratory muscles and lung elasticity, as well as the long-term effects of chronic illness and smoking.[19,20] Therefore, since cancer is more prevalent in the elderly population, such patients are likely to have a poorer ventilatory capacity, before any effects of the disease are taken into account. Other cancer aetiology may have an affect on the mechanism of breathlessness, e.g. cachexia, muscle wasting and fatigue. Abdominal disease, ascites and even constipation may decrease lung volume and also impair breathing.

As well as pathological processes, the sensation of breathlessness can also be affected by psychological, social and spiritual factors.[21,22] This means that patients' subjective experience of breathlessness and the dysfunction it causes may not necessarily solely correlate with the underlying pathology.[8] Therefore, an understanding of the multifactorial causes of breath-

lessness will help the health professional to select the most appropriate intervention(s) for individual patients.

The experience of breathlessness

Most people have felt breathless at one time or other. Indeed, it is a normal sensation usually experienced in response to excessive physical exertion. However, in the context of illness, particularly where its reversibility is uncertain, the experience of breathlessness differs and takes on a new and more sinister meaning. In illness, e.g. chronic respiratory disease and cancer, the effects of breathlessness may impact on every aspect of a person's life and even threaten life itself.[2,23,24] In cancer, the patient's experience of

---

Box 23.1

Causes of breathlessness in patients with cancer

Cancer-related
Obstruction/compression by tumour
Lung metastases
Lung or airway collapse
Hilar or mediastinal lymphadenopathy
Lymphangitis carcinomatosa
Superior vena cava obstruction
Pleural effusion
Pericardial effusion
Consolidation
Pneumothorax
Aspiration pneumonia
Tracheo-oesophageal fistula

Treatment-related
Radiation damage to lung: e.g. fibrosis, pneumonitis
Chemotherapy damage: e.g. drug-induced pneumonitis, cardiomyopathy
Effects of surgery reducing lung capacity: e.g. pneumonectomy/lobectomy

Concurrent medical condition(s)
Ischaemic heart disease
Cardiac failure
Asthma
Chronic obstructive pulmonary disease (COPD)
Infection
Pulmonary embolis
Anaemia
Anxiety
Obesity

breathlessness (and other distressing symptoms) is inextricably linked with their experience of having a life-threatening illness.[22]

Therefore, to gain a true insight into the nature of breathlessness in people with cancer there is a need to explore the patient's own experience of the symptom. So far, much of this work has focused on patients with lung cancer.[2,3,24] These studies clearly illustrate the complex, multifaceted nature of this symptom and its impact on all aspects of the lives of patients and their families. Patients' own experiences provide powerful descriptions of the restrictive nature of breathlessness. For example, they describe the way it restricts the physical activity of breathing in terms such as '*hard to move air*' and '*it feels like it is suffocating*' or '*a tight band*'.[2,24] They also describe how it limits their physical functioning: e.g. '[it] *makes you slow right down, like a car running out of gas*'.[24] Patients find they are no longer able to perform simple daily tasks and become increasingly dependent on others, losing their social roles and become socially isolated.[2,3,24] In their own words, it leaves them feeling '*really frustrated and guilty*' and not wanting '*to live if it continued*'.[24]

From studies of patients' descriptions of breathlessness, we are able to appreciate the connection between breathlessness and feelings of fear and anxiety. Patients experience a profound loss of control, initially by the experience of having cancer and compounded by its resulting symptoms, in this case, breathlessness. Such feelings can be overwhelming, both mentally and physically, giving rise to panic, which in turn increases the sensation of breathlessness. For example, O'Driscoll et al[24] report that panic was a feature of breathlessness for 40% of the patients in their study. One woman described her breathlessness as '*a frightened feeling where you don't think you'll get another breath and because it is accompanied by fear and panic and feeling tight, you can actually feel that tightening feeling of fear in your chest and mind*'.[24]

In the context of cancer, fears and anxieties about breathlessness are often linked with a fear of death and dying.[8,24] O'Driscoll et al[24] found that 31% of patients with breathlessness described fears of impending death. Patients who are breathless often seem to fear death by

suffocation: a common belief is that breathlessness is dangerous and death might occur suddenly during an episode of breathlessness.[22,24] The following comment illustrates this fear: '*I panic a bit sometimes, because deep down I know that (this breath) could be my last one ... it's an awful feeling*'.[3]

Witnessing breathlessness can also provoke similar anxieties in others – both lay and professional carers. For those close to the patient this symptom can be extremely alarming and again may be associated with fears about death. This was reported by the wife of a man with lung cancer: '*I see him sitting there ...surviving as it were, and struggling, I just ... I think oh Lord what are you doing ... take him home now ... all this suffering*'.[25]

The fact that breathlessness may cause panic in those close to the patient can also exacerbate the symptom. This anxiety and panic can be due to the sense of helplessness friends and relatives can feel in not knowing how to support the patient. The day-to-day debilitating effects can also be difficult to live with and emotionally painful for the family, as the partner of a patient with lung cancer commented: '*and to see him ... it was just awful, to see him trying to walk up to the hospital ... it's awful, it's just a horrible feeling to see it really*'.[25] It may also cause practical problems where patients are unable to undertake their usual roles in family life.

Patterns of breathlessness may vary depending on the causes of breathlessness and extent of disease. In O'Driscoll et al's[24] study, most patients experienced intermittent breathlessness with attacks lasting between 5 and 15 minutes. Episodes of breathlessness were commonly associated with physical exertion; however, 13% were triggered by emotional factors such as crying, laughing, anger, fear, frustration, excitement and anxiety.[24] The severity of breathlessness often increases with nearness to death.[1]

MANAGEMENT OF BREATHLESSNESS IN CANCER

In the past, strategies for managing breathlessness in patients with cancer have mainly focussed on medical and pharmacological treatments, either to treat the underlying cause or to diminish the patient's perception of breathlessness. However, these strategies have largely neglected the contribution of emotional factors in exacerbating breathlessness. As a result the symptom has remained poorly controlled for many individuals.[1,6]

Corner et al[22] suggest that the emotional experience of breathlessness is inseparable from its physical experience, and that effective therapy can only be achieved once the nature and impact of breathlessness have been understood from the perspective of the individual. Therefore, Corner and colleagues have proposed an integrative model for managing breathlessness.[22,26,27] Their model combines medical and non-pharmacological approaches and is orientated towards rehabilitation: assisting individuals to manage the problem of breathlessness for themselves, rather than as passive recipients of medical care.[28] Patients are helped and supported to live with and adapt to the challenges that breathlessness imposes on them.

Within the integrative model, a range of non-pharmacological strategies have been developed which focus on both the physical and emotional aspects of breathlessness. These include:

- detailed assessment of breathlessness and factors that ameliorate or exacerbate it

- advice and support for patients and families on ways of managing breathlessness

- exploration of the meaning of breathlessness for patients, their disease and feelings about the future

- training in breathing control techniques, progressive muscle relaxation and distraction exercises

- goal setting to compliment breathing and relaxation techniques to help in the management of functional and social activities and to support the development and adoption of coping strategies

- early recognition of problems warranting pharmacological or medical intervention.[22,26.27]

The non-pharmacological intervention has been evaluated in two randomized controlled trials. Patients were randomized to receive either the non-pharmacological intervention within a nurse-led clinic or to receive 'best supportive care'. In both studies, results indicate that patients receiving the nurse-led intervention experienced significant improvements in perceived levels of breathlessness and in physical and emotional functioning.[26,27] Recently, these results have been confirmed within an outpatient specialist palliative care setting, where use of the intervention by a physiotherapist led to improvements in patients' perceived breathlessness, functioning and levels of distress.[29]

The remainder of this chapter reviews the current medical and non-pharmacological interventions, which may help patients with cancer-related breathlessness.

Assessment

The first step to managing breathlessness successfully is a detailed assessment of the problem. This will entail a medical assessment, including a thorough history, clinical examination and appropriate investigations such as chest X-ray and lung function tests to identify the possible cause(s) of breathlessness and treatments that might help to reverse it. In addition to this physical assessment, it is important to include an exploration of the patient's own perception of the problem, since we know that patients and carers often report the incidence and severity of breathlessness differently.[30] Table 23.1 offers some suggestions of areas that a nursing assessment might cover. This table is based on a breathlessness assessment tool developed by Corner and O'Driscoll.[31]

A detailed and thorough assessment can then act as a valuable guide to assist in the development of a strategic management plan, tailored to meet the needs of the individual patient. Some of the assessment may be completed quite quickly; however, discussing the emotional issues surrounding the problem of breathlessness may be difficult for both the patient and the nurse. Such issues may take time to be aired and are more likely to be spoken about when both have developed a more trusting therapeutic relationship. Time spent during the

Table 23.1: Important factors in the assessment of breathlessness

Area of focus	Factors which might influence breathlessness
Underlying pathology	For example, COPD, pneumothorax, pleural effusion, chest infection
Current medications	For example, bronchodilators, steroids, sedatives
Current respiratory symptoms	Cough, chest pain, haemoptysis
Severity of breathlessness washing, dressing (What makes the person breathless?)	For example, climbing, stairs, slopes, carrying heavy items, housework, weather, emotions
Factors that improve breathlessness	For example, slowing down, resting, gasping, relaxation, pacing activities, opening a window, fan, positive thinking, not being alone, fighting it
Impact on activity (What is the person unable to do as a result of breathlessness?)	For example, housework, answering telephone, gardening, sexual relations, social activities, work
Emotional impact of breathlessness (How does it make the person feel?)	For example, frightened, panic, lonely, choking, exhaustion, fear of dying
Impact on family/carers	For example, loss of roles (both patient and carer), financial worries, fear and anxiety
Social assessment	For example, housing and living arrangements, stairs, bathroom, shower, windows, lifts, family/social support, finances

assessment will help build the foundations of this relationship. Also during the assessment stage, listening to the patient and encouraging them to 'tell their story' will itself, be therapeutic.

No single tool has been shown to adequately assess the different components of breathlessness or be sensitive enough to change.[32] However, Corner and O'Driscoll's[31] assessment tool also incorporates three visual analogue scales, with ratings from 0 (best) to 10 (worst), for patients to self-rate their breathlessness at its best, its worst and the distress that it causes. These scales have the advantage of being simple to use and provide objective measures of the person's breathlessness, which can be repeated to assess any benefit following intervention. However, for some individuals whose disease is progressing and impacting on the severity of breathlessness, improvements on a visual analogue scale may not be demonstrated, regardless of intervention.

Medical interventions

Interventions used will depend on the underlying cause of breathlessness, the patient's general condition and sometimes the prognosis of the patient. Oncological treatments such as radiotherapy and chemotherapy can have a useful role in palliating breathlessness in between 40% and 70% of patients with lung cancer, although the effect may prove short-lived.[33–36] Radiation is usually given by external beam radiotherapy, and shorter schedules (e.g. 17 Gy in two fractions) are commonly used which reduce the burden of repeated hospital visits for patients with advanced disease and cause less side-effects.[37] In a few centres, radiotherapy can be directed straight onto the tumour by placing a radioactive source into the lung via a bronchoscopy (brachytherapy). Patients need to be fit enough to undergo a bronchoscopy for this procedure. Endobronchial laser therapy, which causes direct necrosis of the tumour, is often limited in its availability within Europe.

Chemotherapy regimens have been shown in some studies to improve symptoms, including breathlessness in patients with lung cancer, with seemingly no adverse effect on overall quality of life.[35,38] However, it is important to select patients carefully for chemotherapy and assess after each course that the benefits from treatment outweigh any adverse side-effects.

Where breathlessness occurs due to a specific event such as a new pleural effusion or pericardial effusion, active treatment should be considered. Aspiration is the definitive treatment for pleural effusion. Early pleurodesis in patients where the effusion has recurred may prevent further effusions and, consequently, limit episodes of breathlessness and improve quality of life. Pericardial aspiration may be undertaken in specialist centres and, in some instances, with repeated pericardial effusions, the creation of a 'window' to drain the fluid away into the peritoneal cavity may be considered. However, patients would need to be otherwise fit with a reasonable prognosis to make this procedure worthwhile. (For more detailed information see ch. 28.)

Breathlessness due to superior vena cava obstruction (SVCO), where there is extrinsic compression of the large central veins feeding into the heart, is usually responsive to a single dose of radiotherapy. High-dose corticosteroids may also be used to relieve the associated oedema and reduce the risk of radiotherapy-induced inflammatory reaction. Where SVCO is a feature of chemotherapy-sensitive cancers, e.g. small cell lung cancer or lymphoma, it should be considered, again depending on the patient's fitness.

Lymphangitis carcinomatosa can arise in some cancers, e.g. lung, breast, prostate or gastrointestinal tract, where there is blockage of the lymphatic drainage within the lungs. It usually causes severe and often constant breathlessness, even at rest, and can be very disabling. Radiotherapy and high-dose corticosteroids may provide some relief, but often these patients are not well enough to receive chemotherapy.

Other medical co-morbidity should be corrected where possible. Many patients with cancer will be elderly and a significant number may be smokers or ex-smokers who may also have other conditions such as asthma, chronic obstructive airways disease and heart failure. These conditions can also cause a degree of breathlessness independent of lung cancer. Optimizing the medical management of co-morbid disease is essential and a short trial of steroids, bronchodilators, diuretics and/or antibiotics may indicate a benefit in their use. Referral to other specialists within respiratory or cardiac medicine may also be appropriate.

Pharmacological strategies

Morphine is widely used in the control of breathlessness in advanced cancer and, although the precise mechanism of action is not clearly understood, it seems to modify the sensation of breathlessness for some patients by depressing respiration. A recent Cochrane review of studies exploring the benefits of opioids in relieving breathlessness suggests the use of oral or parenteral opioids may decrease the level of distress from breathlessness.[39] However, the authors admit the number of patients in the studies were small and there is no evidence to suggest any improvement in patients' functional ability with the use of opioids. There remains little evidence to guide the optimum dosage and schedule, but often starting doses of 2.5–5 mg of oral morphine are used either 4 hourly or as needed in patients who have not previously been exposed to opioids. If a patient is already taking morphine, some authors suggest a dose increment.[16,35] For patients unable to swallow, subcutaneous diamorphine can be used. Recent studies do not support the use of nebulized morphine.[39-41]

Anxiolytics such as the benzodiazepines lorazepam and diazepam are used to relieve breathlessness because of their sedative effect, which, like morphine, may depress respiration and dull the sensation of breathlessness for patients. They can also reduce some of the anxiety related to breathlessness and help breathing by their muscle relaxation effect. Although such drugs are commonly used in practice, like morphine, there are few studies confirming their benefit for patients with breathlessness or optimum dosing schedules. Commonly, lorazepam 0.5–2 mg orally or sublingually is prescribed as and when necessary. If parenteral administration is required, midazolam 2.5–5 mg (or 10–30 mg/24 hours if an infusion is necessary) is often used. From practice, we find that some patients find anxiolytic drugs particularly useful at night, when they are having trouble sleeping because of an overactive mind dwelling on the fears about what the future may hold.

Many patients with breathlessness experience intermittent breathlessness.[24] Continuous breathlessness is more commonly associated with more advanced disease. Therefore, when deciding whether to use opioids and/or anxiolytic drugs, it is important to weigh up the impact of these on the overall well-being of the individual. In the context of intermittent breathlessness, their side-effects may outweigh any potential benefit and may encourage passivity rather than enabling patients to achieve a sense of control over their symptom. The use of these drugs may be more appropriate for patients who are breathless at rest or in the last days of life.

Corticosteroids may have a useful effect on breathlessness when there is thought to be oedema around the tumour, exacerbating airways obstruction, although any beneficial effect is often temporary. They are also used if breathlessness is due to SVCO, lymphangitis carcinomatosa, radiation-induced pneumonitis, chronic airways disease or asthma. A short trial, e.g. prednisolone 30 mg for 5–10 days, will be enough to demonstrate any beneficial effect. If continued, steroids should always be used at the lowest effective dose for the shortest period of time because of the known side-effects with long-term use.

Although oxygen is widely used by patients with cancer who are breathless, there are no studies confirming its benefit in the absence of hypoxia. People without hypoxia may gain as much benefit from a cool draught of air across the face from a fan.[42] Patients may experience a placebo benefit from the use of oxygen, but for those with intermittent breathlessness, this may be associated with significant cost. We have found that for some patients, psychological dependency on oxygen decreases their physical functioning and increases social isolation. Also from observation within our own practice areas, we wonder whether some patients perceive a benefit from oxygen, because it tends to focus them on their breathing technique in the same way that learning diaphragmatic breathing might do. This may explain why in a study comparing the use of oxygen and air, patients were not able to distinguish that one was more beneficial than the other.[43]

To avoid giving oxygen inappropriately, it should be initially administered for a short trial period and only continued if the patient derives clear benefit from it. Administration using a nasal cannula, rather than a face mask, may prevent mouth dryness and reduce interference with important activities such as talking, eating and drinking.

Recently, clinicians have been investigating whether a mixture of helium and oxygen is beneficial in the context of cancer-related breathlessness.[16] Helium is a lighter gas than oxygen and is easier to breathe if there is severe airflow obstruction, e.g. in an acute asthma attack. However, research in patients with cancer is lacking.

Ahmedzai and Vora[16] advise that for some patients, particularly those troubled by dry secretions, a trial of nebulized saline may prove beneficial in helping to relieve the sensation of breathlessness. Again, there is little scientific evidence to prove its affect but anecdotally some practitioners find its use helpful.

Non-pharmacological interventions

There is a range of non-pharmacological interventions that nurses can use with patients to help them manage their breathlessness more successfully. These interventions can be used separately or together, depending on the needs of the individual, the environment and resources available. When these interventions have been offered together, within the setting of a nurse-led clinic, where environment and time are protected, they have demonstrated significant benefits for patients.[26,27] However, not all nurses will have the opportunity of working within a nurse-led clinic setting; therefore, the challenge for these practitioners will be to develop creative ways of working to incorporate these worthwhile interventions in their everyday care.

Development of a therapeutic relationship

Understanding patients' experience of their illness and what breathlessness means to them is central to being able to intervene therapeutically.[44] Therapeutic working involves nurses making themselves available to patients, allowing disclosure of difficult feelings and attempting to help find meaning in their suffering. It also involves exploring the social impact of illness and breathlessness on the patient and family in terms of lost roles, employment, relationships and sexuality. For patients with advanced cancer, some of these will never be regained, and feelings such as sadness, anger, frustration and bereavement may need to be addressed within the context of a therapeutic relationship.

Working therapeutically requires a commitment on behalf of the nurse to develop a healing relationship based on mutuality, trust and sensitivity.[45] Bailey,[46] describing the work of nurses in a breathlessness clinic, uses Bion's[47] concept of containment, to describe how the nurse may act as a container for emotions which may be intolerable for the patient. However, because of their own feelings of helplessness, nurses can often feel an overwhelming desire to be 'doing something' rather than recognizing the importance of 'being with' the patient and listening to their story. Helping patients to understand the meaning of illness is a form of healing in itself and such understanding can help patients overcome the sense of alienation, loss of self-understanding and loss of social integration that accompany life-threatening illness.[48] One nurse working in a breathlessness clinic describes how he understands this valuable therapeutic activity: '*I'm going out of my way to enter their [the patient's] world, and their world of what's going on with this breathlessness … trying to understand someone is fundamentally therapeutic in itself*'.[49]

Encouraging patients to talk about their experience of breathlessness and facilitating the exploration of feelings can allow what may have previously been 'unspoken', but nevertheless feared, to be voiced and so perhaps become less frightening. Experienced nurses can give accurate information and reassurance of fears that are irrational and those that may be grounded in realistic possibilities. For example, patients will often ask about how they are likely to die and whether it will involve pain or suffocation. Although painful for the patient to talk about such things, and uncomfortable for the nurse to hear such anguish, *not* being able to speak of these things may be more painful and increase the patient's distress. *Staying with* the patient and acknowledging such fears with openness, honesty and sensitivity is all that is necessary, since often there are no definite answers that can be given.

Breathing retraining

Patients with breathlessness often develop disordered patterns of breathing. Because of the presence of disease within the lung tissue, the elasticity of the lung may be compromised, making it harder to achieve adequate respiration. Other factors that may affect breathing include stress, fatigue, poor posture, malnutrition and emotions such as fear, depression and anxiety.[50] Frequently, patients resort to using the accessory muscles of respiration (i.e. the shoulder, neck and upper chest muscles) to breathe with, rather than using the diaphragm and lower chest muscles associated with normal breathing. Breathing, therefore, becomes shallow and rapid, leading to inadequate ventilation of the lungs, limited gaseous exchange, fatigue, increased breathlessness and anxiety.[51,52] This rapid respiratory rate also prevents the lungs from expelling air properly, leaving a greater amount of air in the lungs on expiration, resulting in less space for inspired air at the next breath.

Teaching simple diaphragmatic breathing (or breathing retraining) may be one method of helping patients to breathe more efficiently, giving them back a sense of control. Other benefits of teaching diaphragmatic breathing include:

- promote a relaxed and gentle breathing pattern
- minimize the work of breathing

515

- improve ventilation at the base of the lungs
- decrease breathlessness
- improve exercise tolerance
- promote a sense of well-being.[50]

A first step in helping the patient improve breathing technique is to explain how breathing works. This can be done with the aid of a visual diagram of the lungs. A simple explanation of how air is drawn into the lung to reach the alveoli (or air sacs), so that oxygen can then be released into the bloodstream will help patients to appreciate that it is more efficient if inhaled air has time to reach the alveoli before being expelled. It should also be explained that by taking rapid breaths in and shallow breaths out, the lungs never fully empty and a person can feel increasingly breathless.

Observing the patient's breathing pattern, its rate and rhythm at rest and during exercise, will enable the nurse to assess how the patient is breathing, before offering practical suggestions that might help. Observing the patient's posture and positioning is also important. Comfortable positions that allow the diaphragm and abdomen to move freely are preferable; shoulders and the upper chest should be relaxed so that the rib cage can move easily, allowing the lungs to expand.

Teaching diaphragmatic breathing using the lower chest and diaphragm is simple to do and may make breathing more effective, giving patients a sense of control over their breathlessness. Not all patients are able to use their diaphragm because of the location of the disease, but many are able to master the technique with encouragement and practise. We have written a simple exercise which may be helpful when teaching patients to use diaphragmatic breathing (Box 23.2).

If nurses do not feel skilled to teach breathing retraining, they should seek the support and advice of a physiotherapist who can demonstrate the necessary skills to them. Alternatively, they can refer patients to a physiotherapist for help with their breathing. Patients should be encouraged to practise diaphragmatic breathing once or twice a day. Once confident using this technique, it may be useful to patients in several ways:

- before an activity to promote an effective breathing pattern
- during an activity to decrease the level of breathlessness
- after an activity to recover from breathlessness
- as a relaxation aid, e.g. to help to get to sleep or when feeling tense
- as a tool for managing panic attacks.

We have found that even when patients are unable to use their diaphragm fully, simply talking them through the exercise and helping them to slow their breathing even slightly can give reassurance and bring back a sense of control. It can also be helpful to teach patients to slow their breathing rate by encouraging them to count as they breathe in and out. For example, 'breathe in one, two and slowly out one, two, three and four'. Encourage them to make their breath out twice as long as their breath in, as this will help stale air in the lungs to be exhaled, increasing lung capacity. Patients can breathe through either their nose or mouth, which ever they feel more comfortable with. Mouth breathing does not need to be discouraged, as it limits the length the air has to travel before it reaches the lungs. The only advantage of breathing in through the nose is that the air is moistened and filtered.

Some people find it helpful to breathe out through pursed lips. Pursed lip breathing is a pulmonary rehabilitation technique that was developed to encourage a full exhaled breath.[53] It requires the patient to purse their lips into the position to whistle or blow out.[53] This can encourage patients to exhale fully, although they should be advised not to exhale with too much force, as this can be counterproductive.

It can also be helpful to teach the patient's partner/family the breathing exercises. This can help them to encourage the patient and give them something to do in order to ease their own feelings of helplessness and panic. Sometimes asking a partner to stand behind the patient and put their hands gently on the patient's shoulders may help the patient to relax and encourage diaphragmatic breathing. However, one of the most useful things anyone can do (regardless of experience or train-

Box 23.2

Diaphragmatic breathing exercise

1. Explain what you are going to do and why:
   - *I am going to show you an exercise that will teach you how to breathe using your lower chest and abdominal muscles.*
   - *We call this type of breathing 'diaphragmatic breathing' although all I am doing is teaching you how to breathe the way you would do normally.*
   - *You might be wondering why you are not breathing with your diaphragm at the moment – this is because this strong dome-shaped muscle at the base of your lungs can be affected by such factors as stress/tension, emotions, poor posture and disease. It is possible to breathe without this muscle working very much because you have other muscles within the chest area to breathe with, although they are not quite so effective. Often the body gets into a habit of breathing inefficiently and what we have to do is to relearn this simple way of breathing once more so you get the most out of your breath.*

2. The nurse then shows the patient a diagram of the lungs and explains how breathing works – she then demonstrates what she means by diaphragmatic breathing by practising it on herself. Then she goes on to teach the patient, making sure before she begins that the patient is comfortable and the upper abdomen is in a position that aids chest expansion, i.e back fairly straight, shoulders down, arms by sides, etc.
   - *To begin with you need to be as relaxed as possible, so get really comfortable.*
   - *We need to make sure your head and back are well supported and legs are uncrossed.*
   - *Place one hand – palm down – on your upper chest, and the other hand just below your rib cage on your belly, keeping the shoulders down and relaxed.*
   - *Now picture your lungs and the dome-shaped muscle of the diaphragm underneath – as you slowly breathe in, allow the air to move all the way down to the base of your lungs and gently push the diaphragm out a little. When you do this correctly you will feel your lower hand move out a little as the lungs expand and the diaphragm is pushed out.*
   - *Now lets try that again slowly ... in your own time.*

3. The nurse needs to watch at this stage for the shoulders coming up and tensing or the person just pushing out their tummy muscles or trying to overbreathe, taking large gasps of air.
   - *It might help to close your eyes so you can concentrate on just feeling what you are doing in your body. Now again just breathe down, down into your lower hand ... staying relaxed with no effort ... and feel your hand gently being pushed out – your other hand on your upper chest should be barely moving.*
   - *Let's just breathe together for a while ... repeating what you have just learnt ... keeping yourself relaxed as you do so ....*
   - *Don't worry if you can't feel anything yet ... that's OK. I just want you to get a sense of what we are trying to do ... it sometimes takes a few sessions to feel that you are making any progress ....*

4. Towards the end of the exercise, with the patient's permission, the nurse might also put her hands on the patient's tummy to encourage the patient to breathe into her hand, so that she can feel whether or not the patient is breathing with the diaphragm. Or she could simply stand behind the patient and stroke the back using slow soft downward strokes – this is very calming, soothing and reassuring. After the exercise is finished, she should encourage patients to talk about how the exercise went, how they felt and make sure they have no further questions.

ing) is to sit with the patient, remain calm and gently encourage them, with a soft voice to relax their shoulders and slow their breathing rate down. *Staying with* someone at this frightening time will often be far more effective than disappearing off for an oxygen mask or medication.

Panic and anxiety management

It would be wrong to underestimate how difficult it is for someone to slow their breathing and gain a sense of control over their breathlessness. For some, the physical impact of breathlessness and their emotional response to the experience can be overwhelming, leading to high levels of anxiety and panic.[24] These reactions can in turn precipitate attacks of breathlessness, so that a vicious circle is established, making it difficult to disentangle the physical and emotional components of what is happening.

At such times, it can be helpful to teach patients relaxation and distraction techniques. These techniques have been used successfully with patients who are breathless due to chronic respiratory disease, resulting in decreased levels of anxiety and breathlessness.[51] Relaxation is a recognized method of helping patients cope with stress during illness, because it can help to re-establish a sense of control and well-being.[50] When a patient relaxes fully, their breathing rate slows down naturally. Once a patient feels confident in practising relaxation techniques, they can use them as part of a self-help strategy to break the cycle of anxiety and panic. Patients benefit most when taught relaxation techniques over a series of sessions in quiet, comfortable surroundings, free from distractions.[50] A simple script for relaxation is provided for nurses to use with patients who are breathless (Box 23.3).

Ideally, such an exercise can take up to 15–20 minutes. However, it is equally possible to offer a 5-minute session if time is short; patients will still find this helpful, especially if they are taught the breathing techniques as well. If facilities are available, some patients may find it useful to use a relaxation tape, which they can play when they choose, in order to relax more fully. Often, occupational therapists have access to such resources, although we have found that making our own personal tapes is more rewarding and beneficial to patients.

Distraction techniques such as visualization or guided imagery can be used together with relaxation,[50] depending on the patient's needs and the nurse's confidence in offering them. Patients can be helped to use visualization and guided imagery to distract them from unpleasant feelings and negative thoughts. For example at the end of a relaxation session, the nurse can invite them to imagine being in a beautiful and relaxing place – perhaps a place they have fond and happy memories of being in or an imaginary one. The nurse then invites them to focus on the positive feelings that place evokes. If this exercise is successful, the patient can practise imagining this scene so that it can be brought to mind at will, to control or override the vicious cycle of anxiety and panic.

In our work, we have found that visualization or guided imagery can also be useful in helping patients mentally rehearse situations or activities that they fear in advance will cause them breathlessness. For example, going on a shopping trip or attending the hospital for a scan. Rehearsing the activity or situation before carrying it out can help build the patient's confidence, making a positive outcome more likely.

There are many different relaxation and distraction methods: much will depend on which techniques the nurse is comfortable with offering and what suits the individual best. However, if nurses do not feel skilled in these techniques or their environment is not conducive to offering such therapies, referral to an occupational therapist or complementary therapist may be helpful. Bredin[50] suggests the following points may help nurses when attempting to learn and use these techniques with patients:

- create a quiet safe environment
- take time to make the patient feel comfortable
- prepare patients fully – explain what you are going to do and give the patients permission to move, cough or stop the session should they need to
- involve a family member if possible
- assess how the person is feeling before and after the session
- keep it simple
- take time at the end for the patient to recover
- be aware of the importance of keeping yourself relaxed and calm throughout the session
- be reassured it may take time for patients to learn to relax since it is a skill many people will have forgotten
- it can be helpful to practise on a friend or colleague before trying to teach a patient.

Box 23.3

Relaxation script

- Before you begin to practise this relaxation, take a little time to prepare yourself. You may want to lie down or sit in a chair, depending on where you feel most comfortable. Wherever you choose, make sure you are warm (cover yourself with a blanket if need be), your head and back should be well supported, arms and feet uncrossed.

- Try to take a relaxed attitude to this exercise; allow yourself to listen to what is going on in your body and be quite passive in your approach. If you need to stop at anytime that is fine.

- For the next few minutes you are going to practise a simple relaxation in which I am going to guide you on a journey through your body, relaxing each part in turn, beginning with your toes, working up all the way to your head ... . As sensations in your body become noticeable, observe the soft presence of relaxation where ever your awareness is focused ... .

- Now as we begin ... look up to the ceiling and then slowly, if you feel able, close your eyes.

- Don't be concerned about thoughts ... let your mind drift for a while ... allowing your thoughts to come and go ... and if you become aware of noises that's OK just let them be ... soon you won't be bothered by them at all.

- So, beginning with the tips of your toes, become aware of your toes, your feet, your ankles and notice any tension here ... then let that tension go and allow all the muscles in your feet to soften and relax ... .

- Next, become aware of your calves and your knees and just allow any tightness to disappear ... your legs beginning to feel heavy ... .

- Now notice you thighs ... letting go of any tension in your thigh muscles ... feel this part of your leg soften and become heavy too ... .

- Now, moving up the body, notice your buttocks, hips and lower back ... just allow any tension in this area to melt away, all the muscles becoming soft and loose ... .

- That sensation of softness and relaxation flowing up your spine, spreading to all the muscles in your back so it feels as if you are sinking a little deeper into the bed (or chair) behind you ... .

- Now, notice your tummy ... just imagine all the muscles here softening ... tension just flowing away with no effort ... .

- Now, turning your attention to the front of your chest, feel the movement of air as you breathe in and out ... don't try to change your breathing ... just let it come and go ... softly ... slowly ... calmly ... any tension in the chest area slowly melting away as you breathe out ... .

- Now, become aware of your shoulders and upper arms ... let your shoulders become a little heavier so it feels as if they are dropping a bit towards the floor ... all the tension you hold in this area melting easily away ... feeling a sense of relaxation in its place ... and that feeling of relaxation spreading down through your arms to the tips of your fingers ... .

- Now, notice your face and the muscles around your mouth and cheeks ... let your jaw drop slightly and lips softly part ... and feel the muscles of your face soften ... that relaxation spreading to the back of your head ... allowing your head to sink a little further into the pillow behind you ... .

- Now, as you begin to relax fully, become aware of how you are feeling and if you feel any tension returning just notice where you might be holding the tension ... and then go to that place and let go ... .

- If thoughts come into your mind just acknowledge them and let them go again ... .

- Now, just spend a few minutes quietly relaxing ... .

- Now, it's time to come back to a wakeful state ... so when you are ready slowly become aware of your surroundings once more ... notice how you feel ... then become aware of any sounds in the room ... when you are ready, slowly taking your time open your eyes ... coming back refreshed and awake ... .

Planning and pacing activities

For many patients with cancer, breathlessness is a frightening experience and they will often limit their activity to avoid the experience.[3] Over time, this may reduce their physical fitness. Teaching rehabilitative strategies may help patients achieve the highest level of functional activity that is possible within the limitations of their breathlessness.

Patients with chronic respiratory disease often develop breathlessness over a period of many years. Over this time they are able to acquire adapting and coping strategies to help them manage their breathlessness.[28] As disability increases, greater adjustments are made. However, for many patients with cancer, the onset of breathlessness is often more rapid and they will not have had time to learn coping strategies that enable them to manage their breathlessness as effectively.[28] If this is the case, it may be helpful to teach patients strategies they can use to help them remain as active as possible. Many of these will seem simple and obvious to the reader, but in our experience these strategies can offer very real and practical benefits for patients, enabling them to reach their full potential.

As described, encouraging a relaxed and slow breathing pattern before, during and following activity may reduce breathlessness. It is common for patients to actually hold their breath when undertaking an activity which they anticipate will be difficult, and it is worthwhile reminding patients to concentrate on remembering to breathe. Also giving the reassurance that being breathless itself is not actually harmful can sometimes lessen fears. Some activities such as walking and going up stairs may cause particular problems. If this is so, patients may find it helpful to match the rate of their breathing to their walking pace, by breathing in on one step and out on the next one or two steps. Patients should be also be encouraged to take frequent rests to recover their breathing before they become breathless. It is easier to recover from a slight degree of breathlessness than it is to return to normal breathing if breathlessness has become severe. This may also prevent the patient feeling that their breathing is out of control and becoming anxious.

Having something to hold on to will allow the patient to take frequent rest pauses while feeling safe that they will not fall. Using a stick or a frame allows them to stop and recover their breath safely at any time. Rails or strategically placed furniture are also useful. A chair at the top of stairs is often a good idea and will allow the patient to recover their breath before going any further. If stairs are a particular problem, it may be necessary to consider ways to limit the number of times the person has to negotiate them. If the toilet is upstairs, a commode downstairs (or a urine bottle for men) may be helpful during the day.

Many people find washing and dressing particularly exhausting, and performing these simple activities is likely to become more protracted due to breathlessness. It is worth acknowledging this with the patient. Bathrooms often get hot and steamy, making the patient feel claustrophobic and airless, increasing their feeling of breathlessness. Having a window slightly open may reduce this. Other suggestions include:

- Not having the water too hot.
- Use a stool or chair in the shower.
- Do not have water spraying directly on to the face in the shower.
- Bath towels are heavy to use – a towelling dressing gown may be better.
- Have a chair in the bathroom and sit when drying and getting dressed
- Avoid bending. Sit down when putting on socks and shoes and rest legs on the side of the bath when drying them.
- Remember to breathe when pulling clothes over the face.
- Slip arms out of a jumper first before slipping it over the head. This will limit the amount of time arms have to be held up.
- Rest frequently and recover breathing as necessary to avoid severe breathlessness.[54]

Bending or lifting items is often difficult too; and it can help to be reminded not to bend from the waist. Bending at the knees will be easier, particularly if the person has something to hold on to, e.g. a chair, which can then be used to push against on standing. Placing items such as a washing basket on a chair rather than on the ground while hanging out clothes will help reduce the amount of bending necessary. Carrying heavy objects should also be avoided when possible: a shopping bag on wheels may be more helpful.

Rushing to answer the telephone and becoming too out of breath to talk is a common difficulty. Practical suggestions such as informing family and friends that it will take longer to answer the telephone and having an answering machine to allow the person to call back at their convenience are practical suggestions to consider. Patients should also be encouraged to speak slowly, in short sentences and pause frequently to breathe.

Maintaining sexual relationships may be difficult and people frequently avoid talking about it because of embarrassment. Sometimes, just mentioning the subject can bring relief and permit the person to talk about the problem. If patients do want to talk, then sometimes suggestions such as ensuring that they find the time to relax, thinking about positions which may be comfortable, taking things slowly and, if the person uses a bronchodilator, to use this before and after lovemaking may be helpful.

Since cancer-related breathlessness often develops rapidly and patients have little time to adjust to the symptom, they may need reminding to slow down and pace their activities to enable them to be achieved. Activity pacing involves the person slowing down, planning and modifying the way in which everyday activities are carried out.[52] Nurses can help the patient identify what activities are important and what prevents them being undertaken.

We have also found that when teaching activity pacing to patients, what really makes a difference is the nurse's willingness to practise an activity with a person rather than just talk or think about it with them. For example, if a patient complains of being breathless at home when climbing up the stairs, it may be helpful for the nurse to walk with them to the nearest staircase, observe what they do and then walk with them practising slowing down, breathing and pacing. In this way the nurse will be able to observe any problems first hand, and then work together with the patient to find the most helpful solution.

It might also be helpful to prioritize activities or goals into those that the patient most wants to achieve. Sometimes, there can be discrepancies between the patient's goals and those of his family. For example, a patient may be very keen to still participate in a weekly shopping trip, whereas the partner may wish them to stay at home and rest. Together with the nurse, they can decide on what is realistic and plan what adjustments need to be made and what strategies may be helpful to enable the activity to be undertaken. Sometimes, this can mean giving up certain habits. For example, a man with lung cancer who attended the clinic des-

perately wanted to continue attending football matches with his sons. He was a proud man who did not want to give in to his breathlessness and change his habits. Nevertheless, he panicked when he could not breathe climbing up the stands in the crush of people. Acknowledging his fears about his breathlessness and then encouraging him to stop and slow his breathing and rest before becoming out of breath – pretending that he was merely stopping to look at the view – and take seats nearer the bottom of the stadium, meant that he was still able to go to football.

It may be helpful to encourage patients to plan activities ahead of time to work out tactics for coping with situations that may be difficult or may arouse panic. It is important to allow plenty of time for activities so that the patient does not feel rushed or pressured. This is particularly true with regards to going to the toilet – many patients describe how they put off going until the last moment and then become fearful that they will not get there in time. This increases their anxiety, which in turn increases their breathlessness.

Patients may need to be given permission to relinquish some former roles and tasks, and let others do more for them. The nurse can help with this process, firstly by discussing the problem, listening to concerns and then making suggestions. For example, a person may need help with domestic chores, and can be encouraged to ask friends, or involve social services. It may even be possible to claim benefits, enabling payment for such help.

The strategies in this section are aimed at the rehabilitation of the patient with breathlessness to maximize physical and social functioning. However, breathlessness is by its nature limiting, and even with activity planning and pacing, part of what is therapeutic is to acknowledge what is no longer possible and facilitate a process of grieving for those losses.[51]

Complementary therapies

There have been limited data to suggest that patients with breathlessness may benefit from acupuncture.[55,56] Other complementary therapies may also be of benefit, particularly in terms of improving patients' overall well-being and reducing anxiety. However, further rigorous evidence is required to fully understand the role of complementary therapies in the management of cancer-related breathlessness.

Managing other symptoms

It is important that breathlessness, as a symptom of cancer, is not viewed in isolation. Many patients will also experience other problems due to the effects of cancer, anticancer treatments or other co-morbidity. Common problems that patients who are breathless may also face are:[1,5]

- lack of appetite, poor diet and weight loss
- fatigue
- low mood and depression
- spiritual distress
- social isolation.

Nurses are well placed to screen for such problems and plan strategies to address them. This may involve further work with the patient by themselves or referral to other specialists such as the dietician, occupational therapist, physiotherapist, psychological support teams, social services and chaplaincy, for example.

Supporting relatives and carers

Watching a loved one struggle with breathing difficulties has a significant impact on relatives' and carers' well-being.[5,25] They often feel helpless to do anything and are frightened of the possible consequences of episodes of breathlessness. However, with support and guidance, they can play a key role in helping the patient, e.g. by learning about and encouraging breathing exercises, distraction techniques or practical changes in the running of the household. Being able to reassure the patient and having strategies to help manage breathlessness may also help alleviate their own feelings of helplessness and anxiety.

Therefore, listening to the fears and anxieties of those who are close to the patient is another important therapeutic task, since it can help to reduce and contain the distress that they too can be experiencing. If relatives feel supported, they are more likely to cope with the anxiety of witnessing the patient's breathlessness. But we acknowledge it can be challenging for the professional to support both the lay carer as well as the patient. The best solution may be to listen and work with both patient and relative together. However, sometimes partners may want to protect each other from difficult feelings, or a carer may be so anxious that it is difficult to work with the patient – and vice versa. In these cases, where there is time and if the patient is willing, it may be more appropriate to see them separately, while maintaining the confidentiality of the patient at all times.

Impact on health professionals.

Understandably, health professionals caring for patients with breathlessness may also experience feelings of anxiety and helplessness.[5,57] The helplessness they can feel when watching someone gasping for breath may lead them to develop psychological defences in order to protect themselves from such distress, and some may even withdraw from working with such patients.[57] Nurses may feel they do not have the necessary communication and counselling skills to work with patients therapeutically, fearing their lack of experience could increase the patient's distress and perhaps their own even further.

There are some important issues to consider here. The first is that nurses need to develop the self-belief and confidence that they can make a real difference in alleviating the problems associated with breathlessness. Research has shown that they can.[26,27] Secondly, developing and learning new skills to manage breathlessness successfully will take time, a valuable commodity in any healthcare system, and it is crucial that this is acknowledged and sanctioned by colleagues and managers. Thirdly, working therapeutically with very ill patients can at times be stressful, since it involves intimacy, reciprocity and risk. No matter how knowledgeable or experienced a practitioner may be, we all at times feel helpless. It is important to have the courage to stay with this feeling. Not only is it natural but also it helps us to understand more clearly the inner world of the patient and the sense of fear and helplessness they too must experience at times. This kind of work may well bring up uncomfortable emotional issues for nurses and it is therefore vital that supervision and support is available.

CONCLUSION

Breathlessness is a complex, frightening and disabling symptom for patients with advanced cancer. It can also be challenging to care for a person with breathlessness, since it is seldom relieved by medical interventions alone. In response to this, we have described how nurses can support patients and their families, to live and cope with breathlessness by adopting an integrated approach to managing the problem. This approach involves addressing both the physical and emotional aspects of the breathless experience, which can at times be demanding for practitioners, since it involves staying with the distress and fears breathlessness evokes.

Often, care and treatment environments are not conducive to the expression of distress and it is easy to overlook the genuine needs of patients and their families. Nurses must begin to think creatively about what they can offer, be prepared to develop new skills and seek ways to restructure the care and environments in which they work. It will be interesting to see whether in the next few years the recent focus on breathlessness as a symptom of advanced cancer will be translated into realistic improvements in its management for patients and their families. The challenge for us as professionals involved in cancer and supportive care is to make sure it is.

Acknowledgements

We would like to thank Dr David Peters for his help in writing the relaxation script.

REFERENCES

1. Higginson IJ, McCarthy M. Measuring symptoms in terminal cancer: are pain and dyspnea controlled? J Roy Soc Med 1989; 82:264–267.
2. Brown ML, Carrieri V, Janson-Bjerklie S, Dodd MJ. Lung cancer and dyspnea: the patients's perception. Oncol Nurs Forum 1986; 5:19–25.
3. Roberts DK, Thorne SE, Pearson C. The experience of dyspnea in late-stage cancer. Patients' and nurses' perspective. Cancer Nurs 1993; 16(4):310–320.
4. Krishnasamy M, Wilkie E. Lung cancer: patients', families' and professionals' perceptions of health care need. A national needs assessment study. London: Macmillan Practice Development Unit/Centre for Cancer and Palliative Care Studies; 1999.
5. Edmonds P, Higginson I, Altman D, et al. Is the presence of dyspnea a risk factor in morbidity in cancer patients? J Pain Symptom Manage 2000; 19(1):15–22.
6. Vainio V, Auvinen A. Prevalence of symptoms among patients with advanced cancer: an International Collaborative Study. J Pain Symptom Manage 1996; 12:3–10.
7. Hockley JM, Dunlop R, Davies RJ. Survey of distressing symptoms in dying patients and their families in hospital and the response to a symptom control team. BMJ 1988; 296:1715–1717.
8. Ripamonti C, Bruera E. Dyspnoea: pathophysiology and assessment. J Pain Symptom Manage 1997; 13:220–232.
9. Gift A. Dyspnea. Nurs Clin North Am 1990; 25(4):955–965.
10. Heyse-Moore LH, Ross V, Mullee M. How much of a problem is dyspnea in advanced cancer? Palliat Med 1991; 5:20–26.
11. Hain R, Patel N, Crabtree S, Pinkerton R. Respiratory symptoms in children dying from malignant disease. Palliat Med 1995; 9:201–206.
12. Reuben DB, Mor V. Dyspnea in terminally ill cancer patients. Chest 1986; 89:234–236.
13. Donnelly S, Walsh D, Rybicki L. The symptoms of advanced cancer: identification of clinical and research priorities by assessment of prevalence and severity. J Palliat Care 1995; 11:27–32.
14. Corner J, Moore S, Haviland J, et al. Development and evaluation of nurse led follow-up in the management of patients with lung cancer. Project No: NCP/J17/18. Final report. NHS National Cancer Research and Development Programme; 2000.
15. Escelente CP, Martin CG, Elting LS, Cantor SD. Dyspnea in cancer patients, etiology, resource utilisation and survival – implications in a managed care world. Am Cancer Soc 1996; 78:1314–1319.
16. Ahmedzai SH, Vora V. Breathlessness. In: Penson J, Fisher RA, eds. Palliative care for people with cancer. 3rd edn. London: Arnold; 2002:75–103.
17. Foote M, Sexton DL, Pawlik L. Dyspnea: a distressing sensation in lung cancer. Oncol Nurs Forum 1986; 13(5):25–31.
18. Congleton J, Muers MF. The incidence of airflow obstruction in bronchial carcinoma, its relation to breathlessness, and response to bronchodilator therapy. Respir Med 1995; 89:291–6.
19. Sykes DA, Mohanaruban K, Finucane P, Sastry BSD. Assessment of the elderly with respiratory disease. Geriatr Med 1989; 19:49–54.
20. Ahmedzai S. Palliation of respiratory symptoms. In: Doyle D, Hanks GWC, MacDonald N, eds.

Oxford textbook of palliative medicine. 2nd edn. Oxford: University Press; 1999:584–616.

21. Steele B, Shaver J. The dyspnoea experience: nociceptive properties and a model for research and practice. Adv Nurs Sci 1992; 15(1):64–76.

22. Corner J, Plant H, Warner L. Developing a nursing approach to managing dyspnoea in lung cancer. Int J Palliat Nurs 1995; 1:5–10.

23. Williams SJ. The experience of illness: chronic respiratory illness. London: Routledge; 1993.

24. O'Driscoll M, Corner J, Bailey C. The experience of breathlessness in lung cancer. Eur J Cancer Care 1999; 8:37–43.

25. Plant H. Living with cancer: understanding the experiences of close relatives of people with cancer. University of London: unpublished PhD thesis; 2000.

26. Corner J, Plant H, A'Hern R, Bailey C. Non-pharmacological intervention for breathlessness in lung cancer. Palliat Med 1996; 10:299–305.

27. Bredin M, Corner J, Krishnasamy M, et al. Multicentre randomised controlled trial of nursing intervention for breathlessness in patients with lung cancer. BMJ 1999; 318:901–904.

28. Corner J. Management of breathlessness in advanced lung cancer: new scientific evidence for developing multidisciplinary care. In: Muers MF, Macbeth F, Wells FC, Miles A, eds. The effective management of lung cancer. London: Aesculapius Medical Press; 2001:129–140.

29. Hatley J, Laurence V, Scott A, Baker R, Thomas P. Breathlessness clinics within specialist palliative care settings can improve the quality of life and functional capacity of patients with lung cancer. Palliat Med 2003: 14:410–417.

30. Maguire P, Walsh S, Jeacock J, Kingston R. Physical and psychological needs of patients dying from colo-rectal cancer. Palliat Med 1999; 13(1):45–50.

31. Corner J, O'Driscoll M. Development of a breathlessness assessment guide for use in palliative care. Palliat Med 1999; 13:375–384.

32. Van der Molen. Dyspnoea: a study of measurement instruments for the assessment of dyspnoea and their application for patients with advanced cancer. J Adv Nurs 1995; 22:948–956.

33. Numico G, Russi E, Merlan M. Best supportive care in non-small cell lung cancer: is there a role for radiotherapy and chemotherapy? Lung Cancer 2001; 32(3):213–226.

34. NHS Executive. Guidance on commissioning cancer services: improving outcomes in lung cancer. London: Department of Health; 1998.

35. Cullen MH. Trials with mitomycin, ifosfamide and cisplatin in non-small cell lung cancer. Lung Cancer 1995; 12:S95–106.

36. Ellis P, Smith IE, Hardy JR, et al. Symptom relief with MVP (mitomycin C, vinblastine and cisplatin) chemotherapy in advanced non-small cell lung cancer. Br J Cancer 1995; 71:366–370.

37. Lung Cancer Working Party. Inoperable non-small-cell lung cancer (NSCLC): a Medical Research Council randomised trial of palliative radiotherapy with two fractions or ten fractions. Br J Cancer 1991; 63:265–270.

38. Elderly Lung Cancer Vinorelbine Italian Study Group. Effects of vinorelbine on quality of life and survival of elderly patients with advanced non-small cell lung cancer. J Natl Cancer Instit 1999; 91:66–72.

39. Jennings AL, Davies AN, Higgins JPT, Broadley K. Opioids for the palliation of breathlessness in terminal illness (Cochrane Review). In: The Cochrane Library 2003; Issue 3. Oxford: Update Software.

40. Davis CL. Breathlessness, cough and other respiratory problems. BMJ 1997; 315: 931–934.

41. Davis C, Penn K, A'Hern R, et al. Single dose randomised controlled trial of nebulised morphine in patients with cancer related breathlessness. Palliat Med (Research Abstract) 1996; 10:64–65.

42. Schwartzstein RM, Lahive K, Pope A, Weinberger SE. Cold facial stimulation reduces breathlessness induced normal subjects. Am Rev Respir Dis 1987; 136:58–61.

43. Booth S, Kelly MJ, Cox MP, et al. Does oxygen help dyspnoea in patients with cancer? Am Rev Respir Crit Care Med 1996; 153:1515–18.

44. Krishnasamy M, Corner J, Bredin M, et al. Cancer nursing practice development: understanding breathlessness. J Clin Nurs 2001; 10:103–108.

45. Lanceley A. Therapeutic strategies in cancer care. In: Corner J, Bailey C, eds. Cancer nursing: care in context. Oxford: Blackwell Science; 2001:120–138.

46. Bailey C. Nursing as therapy in the management of breathlessness in lung cancer. Eur J Cancer Care 1995; 4:184–190.

47. Bion W. Learning from experience. In: Seven servants. New York: Jason Aronson; 1962.

48. Benner P, Wrubel J. The primacy of caring. Stress and coping in health and illness. Menlo Park, California: Addison-Wesley; 1989.

49. Plant H, Bredin M, Krishnasamy M, Corner J. Working with resistance, tension and objectivity: conducting a randomised controlled trial of a nursing intervention for breathlessness. NT Research 2000; 5(6):426–436.

50. Bredin M. A breath of fresh air: an interactive guide to managing breathlessness in patients with lung cancer. CD Rom. London: Macmillan Cancer Relief/Institute of Cancer Research; 2001.

51. Gift AG, Cahill CA. Psychophysiologic aspects of dyspnoea in chronic obstructive pulmonary disease: a pilot study. Heart Lung 1990; 19:252–257.

52. Epps M. Diagnostic testing for patients with lung cancer. In: Bruera E, Portnoy R. eds. Topics in

palliative care. New York: Oxford University Press; 1998:615–630.

53. Gallo-Silver L, Pollack B. Behavioural interventions for lung cancer-related breathlessness. Am Cancer Soc 2000; 8(6):268–273.

54. The Centre for Cancer and Palliative Care Studies. Living with breathlessness. London: Institute of Cancer Research; 1995.

55. Filshie J, Penn K, Ashley S, Davis CL. Acupuncture for the relief of cancer-related breathlessness. Palliat Med 1996; 10:145–150.

56. Jobst K, McPherson K, Brown V, et al. Controlled trial of acupuncture for disabling breathlessness. Lancet 1986; 20(27): 1416–1419.

57. Johnson M, Moore S. Research into practice: the reality of implementing a non-pharmacological breathlessness intervention into clinical practice. Eur J Oncol Nurs 2003; 7(1):33–38.

CHAPTER 24

Skin and Wound Care

WAYNE A NAYLOR

CHAPTER CONTENTS

Introduction	527		Wound assessment	542
Structure and function of the skin	528		Wound dressings/devices	543
Epidermal layer	528		Wounds related to cancer and cancer	
Dermal layer	529		therapies	543
Subcutaneous layer	529		Surgical wounds	544
Accessory structures of the skin	529		Extravasation wounds	544
Functions of the skin	529		Fungating malignant wounds	548
Effects of cancer therapies on the skin	529		Stoma care	550
Radiotherapy	530		Types of stoma and indications	550
Nursing care of radiotherapy skin			Appliances	552
reactions	532		Stoma siting	552
Chemotherapy	532		Stoma complications	552
Hormonal therapies	537		Fistula management	553
Biological therapies	538		Nursing care of fistulae	553
Nursing care of skin problems	538		Conclusion	554
Skin graft versus host disease	539		References	554
Wounds and wound healing	540			
The normal wound healing process	540			
Moist wound healing	541			
Impediments to healing in patients				
with cancer	542			

INTRODUCTION

Skin is not just a container for the internal organs, nor is it solely present for the purpose of providing outward physical appearance; rather, it is a complex organ composed of several layers and a number of specialized accessory structures performing many vital functions that help maintain homeostasis.

Cancer and its treatments can cause a number of changes in the skin, impairing its ability to function normally and compromising one of the body's main protective mechanisms. As well as affecting homeostasis, these changes can result in an altered appearance of the skin that results in dramatic changes in body image for the patient, causing psychological distress and social stigma. Similarly, when a wound is present, it changes the ability of the skin to fulfil its normal functions.

This chapter on skin and wound care provides an overview of the skin and its main functions, and focuses on how cancer and the therapies employed in its treatment can affect skin integrity. It also addresses the specific nursing interventions that may be employed in the management of skin changes and wounds, as well as briefly discussing the care of patients with a stoma or fistula.

STRUCTURE AND FUNCTION OF THE SKIN

The skin, also known as the integument, is one of the largest organs of the body. It completely covers the surface of the body and provides constant information about, and protects inner structures from, the external environment. The skin contains an extensive vascular and sensory network, as well as a number of specialized structures and cells.[1] There are two principal layers that combine to form the skin; these are the epidermis and dermis (Fig. 24.1). Skin sits upon fatty tissue known as the subcutaneous layer, which in turn is attached to underlying muscle and bone.[3]

Epidermal layer

The epidermis is the outer surface of the skin and has four distinct cellular layers (see Fig. 24.1). The main cells found within the epidermis are:[3–5]

- keratinocytes – the predominant cell of the epidermis (approximately 90%)
- melanocytes – pigment-producing cells
- Langerhans cells – involved in cell-mediated immune responses in the skin
- Merkel cells – closely associated with sensory nerve endings and are involved in touch sensation.

The stratum corneum is the outermost layer and comprises inactive, flat keratinocytes filled with keratin. It is impermeable to water, bacteria and a number of chemicals.[3] Below the stratum corneum lies the stratum granulosum, which contains cells that are in various stages of degeneration. The stratum spinosum is an active layer several cells' thick. Cells of this layer have numerous cellular membrane processes, called desmosomes, which bind the cells tightly together.[6]

The final and deepest layer is the stratum basale consisting of a single layer of cuboidal cells. These cells form the basis of the whole epidermis. As they multiply and differentiate, they move upwards, becoming part of the upper three layers until they are shed from the stratum corneum. The stratum basale also lines the surface of hair follicles and sweat glands.[4] In the soles and palms, an extra layer can be

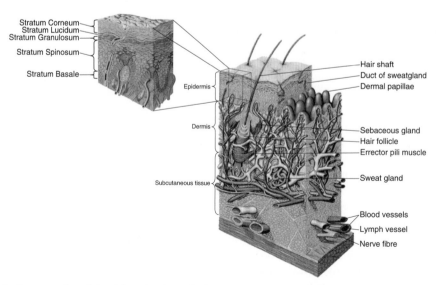

Figure 24.1: Cross-section of the skin and epidermis. (Reproduced from Global Wound Academy, Copyright © 2002 Smith & Nephew,[2] with permission of Smith & Nephew.)

found between the stratum corneum and stratum granulosum. Called the stratum lucidum, it is a specialized layer designed to provide extra cushioning against surface impact.[3] The epidermis is tightly bonded to the dermis by the basement membrane, an acellular layer composed of protein fibres.[7]

Dermal layer

Whereas the epidermis provides a tough impermeable barrier, it is the dermis that provides skin with its strength and flexibility. This is achieved by the combination of two strong elastic fibres, collagen and elastin, surrounded by a gel-like material composed of dermal proteoglycans.[3,7,8] Contained within the dermis are the blood vessels, lymphatics and sensory nerve endings of the skin (see Fig. 24.1). Cells present in the dermis include:[4]

- fibroblasts – produce collagen, elastin and ground substance
- macrophages – phagocytic cells important for fighting infection (present in the blood as monocytes)
- mast cells – part of the immune system and release histamine (responsible for allergic and hypersensitivity reactions)
- adipocytes – fat cells.

Subcutaneous layer

This fatty layer is a combination of adipose and areolar tissue, which forms a loose connective tissue. Its most important functions are the control of body temperature and an energy reservoir, in the form of fat.[4] Specialized nerve endings in this layer are sensitive to external pressure.[3]

Accessory structures of the skin

The accessory structures of the skin all arise from the dermal layer (see Fig. 24.1) and include:

- Hair – covering almost the entire body, the two main functions of hair are protection and thermal regulation. The visible part of hair is called the shaft and buried within the dermis is the hair follicle and root.

- Erector pili muscles – attached to hair follicles, these tiny muscles contract to raise hair into a more upright position ('goose pimples').
- Sebaceous glands – also associated with hair follicles, these glands secrete sebum, which has a waterproofing effect on the skin and keeps hair supple.
- Sweat glands – found over most of the skin, with the number of glands varying in different body areas, they are part of the excretion and temperature control systems of the body.
- Nails – present on the terminal end of fingers and toes, they provide a protective covering and assist in grasping small objects.

Functions of the skin

Protection

Due to its tough and durable nature, the skin is an effective barrier to external hazards, such as bacteria, chemicals and mechanical injury, as well as a containment structure to keep in substances needed by the body, e.g. water and electrolytes.[9]

Regulating body temperature is a vital part of maintaining homeostasis and the skin is one of the primary organs for heat exchange due to its extensive blood supply and large surface area. In addition, skin has a vast array of sensory nerve endings that transmit signals for pain, itch, pressure and temperature, as well as sensations of movement, vibration, stretch and touch.[1] The skin also synthesizes vitamin D, excretes water and salts as sweat and is able to absorb lipid-soluble compounds.[3,10]

The skin is often affected by cancer treatments, especially radiotherapy, in a number of ways. The mechanisms underlying skin changes after cancer treatments and their management will be detailed in the following sections.

EFFECTS OF CANCER THERAPIES ON THE SKIN

Cancer treatments are effective because they target rapidly proliferating cancer cells, impairing cell division and/or causing cell death.

Unfortunately, this effect cannot yet be confined to malignant cells alone and other tissues with a rapidly dividing cell population will also be affected. It is not uncommon therefore for patients undergoing anticancer therapy to have some form of skin involvement. This is usually due to an adverse effect on the basal cells of the epidermis and the accessory structures of the skin, as they are composed of rapidly dividing cells. Other cells within the skin may be affected, causing changes in pigmentation or sensitivity reactions.

Radiotherapy

The majority of radiotherapy is given by external beam radiation (teletherapy), which must pass through the skin to reach its target. This inevitably results in some of the radiation dose being delivered to the skin and causing damage, which results in both acute and chronic skin changes. Almost every patient will develop a degree of acute radiation-induced skin reaction due to changes in cellular proliferation within the skin.[11] Damage to cells that are dividing more slowly, e.g. in the dermis or underlying tissues such as muscle, will result in delayed and chronic skin changes.[12,13] Both acute and chronic skin changes will only occur within the radiation treatment field, including the beam exit site.[14]

Acute changes

One of the most common side-effects of radiotherapy treatment is an acute skin reaction, sometimes referred to as radiodermatitis. Up to 95% of patients treated with external beam radiotherapy will develop some form of acute skin reaction.[15] These reactions occur more frequently in areas of increased moisture and friction, e.g. the axilla, inframammary fold and perineum.[16,17] A number of factors will influence the severity of skin reactions. These comprise both extrinsic and intrinsic factors related to the method of treatment, lifestyle and health status of the patient. Factors that predispose to significant acute skin reactions include:[11,12]

- high total dose of radiation
- low-energy radiation or electrons
- treatment of the head and neck, breast or pelvic area
- large volume of normal tissue included in the area of treatment
- tangential treatment fields
- use of 'bolus' materials (e.g. a wax blanket to increase the dose of radiotherapy to the skin)
- older age
- immunosuppression
- concurrent chemotherapy or steroid therapy
- poor nutritional status
- tobacco smoking
- chronic sun exposure.

Acute skin reactions develop predominantly as a result of radiation disrupting cell division in the stratum basale, including the hair follicles and sebaceous glands.[18] Although not often subjected to radiotherapy, nails can also be affected, with a decrease in rate of growth and ridging. At high doses, the nail may be shed (onycholysis). Acute reactions usually appear within the first 2–3 weeks of treatment and may persist for up to 8 weeks post-treatment if severe.[16] They are usually classified according to the appearance of the skin and include:[14,19,20]

- Erythema – an initial transient erythema may be seen 24–48 hours after the first treatment, which is related to a local inflammatory reaction and capillary dilation. After 2–3 weeks, a more pronounced erythematous reaction will develop, accompanied by oedema and the skin may feel hot and irritable (Fig. 24.2).

- Dry desquamation – as outer layers of the epidermis are lost, the basal cells are unable to replace them and become keratinized. If the basal layer recovers it will result in the appearance of dry desquamation where the skin is dry and flaky or peeling. A decrease in the production of sweat and sebum may compound this reaction and lead to itching and irritable skin. Hair loss may occur within the treatment field (see Ch. 27 on alopecia).

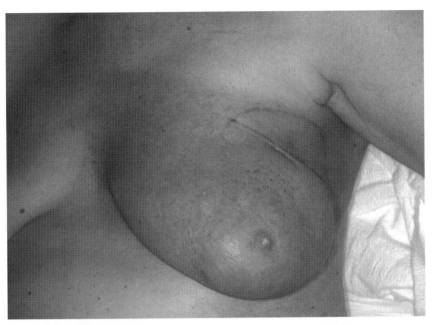

Figure 24.2: Erythema and oedema of the breast at completion of radiotherapy.

- Moist desquamation – if the basal layer does not recover, the epidermis is lost and exposure of the dermis occurs with associated exudate production, pain and the risk of infection (Fig. 24.3).
- Necrosis – although less common with modern machines and techniques used in radiotherapy, a few patients may develop skin necrosis and ulcer formation due to damage to capillaries and connective tissue.

Patients may also notice pigmentation of skin within the treatment field, which is thought to be due to radiation stimulating the production of melanin by melanocytes.[18] Pigmentation may take up to 6 months to fade, and in some cases may take longer.

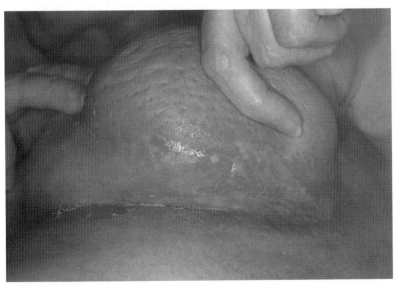

Figure 24.3: Moist desquamation in the inframammary fold at completion of radiotherapy.

Late changes

Late skin changes related to radiotherapy may begin to appear at around 3 months post-treatment or may present years after treatment. These changes are chronic in nature and occur as a result of damage to connective tissue and blood vessels of the skin. Chronic skin changes can include:[9,12,21]

- atrophy of the skin related to the loss of fibroblasts and collagen
- fibrosis and thickening of skin as a result of tissue repair following radiation exposure
- xerosis (dry skin) due to the reduction in sebaceous gland function
- pigmentation changes may include hypo- or hyperpigmentation as a result of changes in the number or function of melanocytes
- telangiectasia may develop after 1–2 years and present as multiple small, dilated red blood vessels within the skin
- necrosis and ulceration can occur following minor trauma to the area of treated skin as a result of vascular insufficiency within the irradiated skin
- radiation-induced skin cancers have been reported, although they are rare and have a long latency period.

Nursing care of radiotherapy skin reactions

The management of radiation-induced skin reactions is based upon symptom control, promoting comfort and preventing infection. The majority of strategies are aimed at maintaining the integrity and barrier functions of the epidermis through appropriate hygiene practices and the use of topical skin care and dressing products. With regard to late skin changes, there are limited treatment options available and, again, any measures are directed at maintaining skin integrity and preventing further skin damage. Surgery may be warranted for chronic radiation-induced skin ulceration.[18]

There are a number of preventative measures that may help delay onset, and reduce the severity, of skin reactions (Box 24.1).

However, it is almost inevitable that patients will develop some degree of skin reaction; hence, many skin care products have been recommended and used in the management of acute skin reactions. There are a wide variety of products and practices in use, many of which are not based on sound evidence but rather on historical practice and personal preference.[22–24] There are also a number of products that, although still used in some radiotherapy centres, are not recommended for application to the skin during radiotherapy (Box 24.2). The College of Radiographers in the United Kingdom has produced guidelines for the management of skin reactions, which are supported by a literature review.[29] Further work has supported their findings and highlighted other potential treatments for the alleviation of symptoms caused by acute skin reactions.[30] Guidelines for skin care based on this work are presented in Table 24.1.

Chemotherapy

Similar to radiotherapy, chemotherapy drugs also have a 'non-specific' effect on other cell populations within the body. Again, they act

---

Box 24.1

Preventative measures to delay onset, and reduce the severity, of acute skin reactions[29,30,171]

- Wash normally using warm water. Use non-perfumed, mild soap on the treated skin.
- Pat skin dry with a soft towel.
- Apply a recommended moisturizing cream to the skin two to three times a day to help maintain its softness.
- Avoid the use of deodorants and perfumed skin care products in the treated area.
- Avoid the use of flannels, brushes, loofah, etc., on the treated area.
- Wear loose comfortable clothing. Underwear should be the correct size and natural fibres such as cotton are recommended.
- Protect the treated skin from extreme heat, cold and sunlight during treatment.
- Continue your usual activities during treatment whenever possible (activities such as swimming should be discussed).
- Eat a balanced diet and drink plenty of fluids throughout treatment.

Products NOT recommended for skin reactions

- Petroleum jelly – difficult to remove and may build up, affecting the radiation dose to the skin.[16,25,31]
- Prophylactic topical antibiotics – may induce a sensitivity reaction and overuse could result in microbial resistance.[20,25,31]
- Topical steroids – not recommended on moist desquamation due to their adverse effect on wound healing.[14,16,20,26,31]
- Gentian violet – although shown to reduce pain from, and size of, moist desquamation,[27] it has a number of unpleasant side-effects, including drying the dermis, which may cause discomfort on movement, interfering with wound healing, masking wound changes and staining skin, clothes and work areas.[14,17,19,20,31] It has also been shown to result in permanent pigmentation of the skin if applied to granulation tissue, and is carcinogenic in animals.[28]

upon those cells with a high rate of cell division and will have a cytostatic or cytotoxic effect on the dividing cells of the skin, resulting in a number of skin changes. The most widely known effect is hair loss (see Ch. 27 on alopecia). Other common side-effects include rashes, pruritus, hyperpigmentation and photosensitivity. Nails may also be affected becoming discoloured, ridged or brittle; in rare cases, onycholysis may take place. Table 24.2 lists commonly used chemotherapy agents and their effects on the skin and its accessory structures. Pruritus or itching is perceived by cutaneous nerves and processed within the cerebral cortex in much the same way as pain. Similarly to pain, it is also a protective mechanism through the initiation of scratching as a reflex response to noxious stimuli. The sensation of pruritus occurs when sensory nerves are stimulated by histamine, proteases, prostaglandins and neuropeptides, which may be released in response to both external and internal stimuli.[44,45] Chemotherapy-induced pruritus is usually associated with the eruption of a rash or dry skin, in particular due to hypersensitivity reactions. Pruritus may be caused by a multitude of other medical conditions, such as skin disorders and diseases, hepatic or renal failure, or as

Table 24.1: Evidence-based treatments for acute radiotherapy skin reactions.[29,30]

Skin reaction type	Treatments
Erythema and dry desquamation (may be managed in the same way)	• Simple, non-perfumed hydrophilic or moisturizing cream (preferably lanolin-free) should be applied two to three times a day, as these provide symptomatic relief and may help maintain skin integrity • For itchy, irritable or burning feelings of the skin within the treatment field, apply 1% hydrocortisone cream sparingly, two to three times a day; should not be used on areas of broken or infected skin • Alternative treatments (if available) include: • hyaluronic acid 0.2% cream applied twice a day[32] • sucralfate cream applied twice a day[33]
Moist desquamation	• Hydrogel sheets may be applied to areas of moist desquamation to reduce discomfort and promote healing; their soothing and cooling properties are also beneficial for patient comfort.[34–36] • Amorphous (liquid) hydrogels may be used in skin folds or the perineum • Hydrocolloid sheet dressings may be applied to areas of moist desquamation *once radiotherapy treatment has finished*. These provide an aesthetically acceptable dressing that promotes comfort and healing[27,37] • Other modern dressing products such as semipermeable films, alginates, hydrofibre or foams may also be used and should be selected based on the presenting characteristics of the wound

Table 24.2: Effects of chemotherapeutic drugs on the skin[38–43]

Drug	Effects on skin
Amsacrine (acridinyl anisidide, m-AMSA)	Alopecia
Bleomycin	Alopecia (mild), erythema over pressure points (may progress to shallow ulcers), hand-foot syndrome, hyperkeratosis (thickening and oedema of skin), hyperpigmentation (skin or nails), peeling skin on fingertips, pruritus, radiation recall, thickening of nail beds
Busulfan	Alopecia (high dose), hyperpigmentation (hands and nail beds), rash with pruritus
Capecitabine (Xeloda)	Alopecia (uncommon), brittle and chipped nails, dermatitis, discoloration of nail beds, dry skin, hand-foot syndrome (>50%), rash/pruritus
Carboplatin (Paraplatin, JM8)	Rarely: (<3%) alopecia, rash
Carmustine (BCNU)	Generalized flushing with short infusions, marked facial flushing (lasts about 4 hours)
Chlorambucil	Rash on face, scalp and body
Cisplatin	Hand-foot syndrome, numbness or tingling in hands or feet
Cladribine (2-CdA, Leustatin)	Rash (50% of patients)
Cyclophosphamide	Alopecia, hyperpigmentation (skin and nails), hand-foot syndrome, nails may develop ridges, urticaria
Cytarabine (Ara C, cytosine arabinoside)	Alopecia, erythematous rash, hand-foot syndrome with high dose
Dacarbazine (DTIC)	Alopecia (mild), photosensitivity
Dactinomycin (actinomycin D)	Alopecia, hyperpigmentation (along vein), radiation recall, rash Severe tissue damage if extravasated
Daunorubicin	Alopecia (total), discoloration of nail beds, radiation recall, rash Severe tissue damage if extravasated
Docetaxel (Taxotere)	Alopecia (total), discoloration of nail beds, hand-foot syndrome, radiation recall, rash ± pruritus (50% of patients)
Doxorubicin	Alopecia (total), discoloration of nails, hand-foot syndrome, hyperpigmentation (skin creases), photosensitivity, radiation recall, urticaria, venous flare Severe tissue damage if extravasated
Epirubicin	Alopecia (total), discoloration of nails, hyperpigmentation, photosensitivity, radiation recall, rash ± pruritus
5-Flurouracil	Hand-foot syndrome

Table 24.2 Effects of chemotherapeutic drugs on the skin[38-43]—cont'd

Drug	Effects on skin
Estramustine (Emcyt, Estracyte)	Dry skin with pruritus, rash
Etoposide (VP16, Etopophos)	Alopecia (70% of patients), radiation recall, rash
Fludarabine	Rarely: rash
Fluorouracil (5-FU)	Alopecia (usually mild, rarely total), brittle and chipped nails, brown discoloration of skin along vein from infusion, discoloration of nail beds, hand-foot syndrome, photosensitivity, radiation recall, rash with pruritus Rarely, hyperpigmentation
Gemcitabine (Gemzar)	Alopecia (mild), radiation recall rash ± pruritus (25% of patients)
Hydroxyurea	Facial redness, radiation recall, rash Rarely: alopecia, painful leg ulcers (long-term use)
Idarubicin (Zavedos)	Alopecia (total), discoloration of nails, discoloration in skin creases, photosensitivity Rarely: radiation recall
Ifosfamide	Alopecia (total), hyperpigmentation (temporary), rash ± pruritus, ridged nails
Imatinib mesylate (Glivec)	Rash, bruising, night sweats, pruritus, petechiae
Irinotecan (Campto)	Alopecia, rash ± pruritus
Lomustine (CCNU)	Alopecia
Melphalan	Rarely: alopecia (high dose), dermatitis
Mercaptopurine (6-MP, Purinethol)	Pruritic rash Rarely: alopecia, hand-foot syndrome, hyperpigmentation on hands, feet or elbows, radiation recall
Methotrexate	Alopecia, depigmentation or hyperpigmentation, hand-foot syndrome, photosensitivity, radiation recall, rash ± pruritus
Mitomycin C	Alopecia (mild), hyperpigmentation of nails, rash ± pruritus Severe tissue damage if extravasated
Mitoxantrone	Alopecia (mild) Extravasation results in blue discoloration of skin (fades)
Mustine (chlormethine)	Alopecia, rash
Oxaliplatin	Rarely: alopecia
Paclitaxel (Taxol)	Alopecia, hand-foot syndrome, radiation recall, rash (with flu-like symptoms)

(continues)

Table 24.2: Effects of chemotherapeutic drugs on the skin[38–43]—cont'd

Drug	Effects on skin
Pentostatin	Rash + /− pruritus Rarely: alopecia
Procarbazine	Alopecia, hyperpigmentation, rash ± pruritus
Raltitrexed (Tomudex)	Alopecia (mild), rash ± pruritus
Tegafur with uracil (Uftoral)	Alopecia (mild), brittle and chipped nails, nail ridges, photosensitivity, rash ± pruritus Rarely: hyperpigmentation
Temozolomide (Temodal)	Alopecia, rash ± pruritus
Thioguanine (Lanvis, 6-TG, 6-thioguanine, Tabloid)	Rarely: rash
Thiotepa (Thioplex, Triethylenethiophosphoramide)	Alopecia (mild), flaking of skin, hyperpigmentation, pruritus, rash
Topotecan (Hycamtin)	Alopecia (60% of patients)
Vinblastine (Velban)	Alopecia (mild), photosensitivity, radiation recall, rash Severe tissue damage if extravasated
Vincristine (Oncovin)	Alopecia Severe tissue damage if extravasated
Vindesine (Eldisine)	Alopecia, rash Severe tissue damage if extravasated
Vinorelbine (Navelbine)	Alopecia (25% of patients), hyperpigmentation of vein Severe tissue damage if extravasated

a consequence of malignancy itself; in particular it is associated with leukaemia, multiple myeloma, adenocarcinoma, Hodgkin's disease and non-Hodgkin's lymphoma.[38,44] It is therefore important to accurately identify the cause, as it may not be chemotherapy-related.

Hyperpigmentation is also a consequence of some chemotherapeutic agents. The exact cause of hyperpigmentation (darkening) of the skin in patients receiving chemotherapy is not known, but may be related to an increase in melanin production as a side-effect of chemotherapy on melanocytes.[46] It is also thought that deposits of carotene, haemoglobin or the drug itself may cause changes in skin pigmentation.[47] Hyperpigmentation may be localized, diffuse or may occur where products such as dressings have been applied to the skin. In some cases, hyperpigmentation may follow the course of the vein through which the chemotherapy was administered. It is also possible for nails to become pigmented and they may develop bands of discoloration. Normal pigmentation usually returns to the skin within 4 months but may persist for longer.[38]

Patients may develop an allergic reaction to chemotherapy which may be related to the chemotherapeutic agent itself or the carrier or preservative in the drug: this is known as hypersensitivity.[46] Skin involvement may present as a generalized erythematous rash, an itchy rash (urticaria) with individual swellings (weals) caused by the release of histamine. In severe cases, the patient may experience angio-oedema (weals involving the lips, eyes and/or tongue), cutaneous vasculitis, erythema multi-forme (characterized by lesions with a 'target'-like appearance) and toxic epidermal necrolysis (formation of widespread large fluid-filled blisters followed by desquamation).[39,47] Topical chemotherapy agents may cause allergic contact dermatitis. Photosensitivity reactions occur on exposure to UV light (sunlight), with an increase in the normal skin response resembling acute sunburn. Reactions may consist of erythema, oedema, pain, tenderness or stinging and pruritus. The reaction may progress to blistering and desquamation.[38,47] This type of reaction can be identified by the fact that it only occurs on areas of the body exposed to sunlight, such as the face, arms, hands, lower legs and upper chest. There is a distinct demarcation between exposed and non-exposed skin. Nails may also be involved with tenderness of the distal one-third of the nail (photo-onycholysis). A number of chemotherapy agents can cause significant changes in the skin on the palms of the hands and soles of the feet. Commonly referred to as 'hand-foot syndrome', this reaction is also called palmar-plantar erythrodysthesia or acral erythema, and is characterized by erythema, oedema and changes in sensitivity on the palms and soles.[46,47] It may be preceded by a tingling sensation in the hands and feet and is often accompanied by pain or burning sensations. With prolonged treatment, skin changes may progress to blistering and peeling of the skin. The cause of hand-foot syndrome is not fully understood but it may be due to the accumulation and excretion of chemotherapy drugs by eccrine sweat glands, which are found in greater numbers on the palms and soles.[48] Increased blood flow, pressure and temperature associated with the palms and soles may also be a contributing factor.[49]

Radiation enhancement and recall

When chemotherapy is administered concurrently with radiation therapy, patients may suffer from an enhanced radiation skin reaction due to the combined effect on epidermal basal cells.[38] Similarly, if chemotherapy is given shortly after radiotherapy has finished, it will impair the healing of any desquamated areas. Several chemotherapy drugs can cause a recurrence of skin reactions in previously irradiated areas when given weeks to months after radiotherapy. This phenomenon is referred to as 'radiation recall', as the reaction is similar in appearance to an acute radiation-induced skin reaction and is confined to the previous radiation field. There appears to be a positive relationship between the development of radiation recall and a higher total dose of radiation.[50] A mechanism for recall reactions is unclear but hypotheses include chronic vascular damage, epithelial basal cell impairment, basal cell sensitivity to cytotoxic rechallenge and drug hypersensitivity reaction.[50]

Hormonal therapies

Hormonal therapies may be used in the control of tumours that are hormone sensitive, in particular breast, prostate and endometrial cancers. These treatments interfere with the body's naturally occurring hormones by blocking their production or their action on target tissues. Because this type of manipulation effectively 'switches off' normal hormone action within the entire body, there are a number of side-effects. Hot flushes occur with almost all hormonal drugs and manifest as a sudden heat that spreads over the body, especially the chest, face and head, often accompanied by flushing (redness) of the skin and moderate to profuse sweating. Other skin-related side-effects tend to be less severe and include:

- mild to moderate alopecia – anastrozole, Casodex (bicalutamide), letrozole
- rashes – anastrozole, flutamide, formestane, goserelin
- pruritus – flutamide, letrozole, medroxyprogesterone acetate, toremifene
- hirsutism (excessive hair on the face, chest, upper back or abdomen), which occurs in women treated with androgen therapy (male sex hormone e.g. Casodex).[40,41]

Dry skin, acne and urticaria are also possible side-effects of hormonal therapies.

Biological therapies

Biological therapy may have a direct effect on the tumour or a more general effect on bodily systems, e.g. on the haemopoietic system. Although skin side-effects are usually mild, there can be significant changes when therapies are administered at high dose or over a prolonged period. Most commonly, patients may develop a rash, which may be maculopapular in appearance and associated with pruritus, as well as dry scaly skin and hair thinning.[38,40,41] Biological agents may also induce a hypersensitivity reaction with associated skin involvement; this is a particular problem with monoclonal antibodies, such as Herceptin (trastuzumab) and Mabthera (rituximab).

NURSING CARE OF SKIN PROBLEMS

Chemotherapy, hormonal therapy and biological therapy all produce similar effects on the skin and they can therefore be managed in the same way. In general, the skin reactions induced by these therapies will subside once the drug is stopped. However, during treatment, it is essential to monitor and control symptoms to the best extent possible in order to maintain the patient's quality of life and to encourage patient compliance with treatment.

Hypersensitivity reactions should be managed symptomatically and the offending drug identified, if possible, and either removed from the patient's prescription or only given with adequate prophylaxis. Photosensitivity can be reduced if patients are aware of the possibility and given instructions on protecting their skin from sun exposure. Patients should wear protective clothing, such as a long-sleeved shirt and broad-brimmed hat, and use high protection factor sunscreen (>15+).[38] Hand-foot syndrome will only resolve once the chemotherapy is stopped and, if severe, this is the usual treatment. The chemotherapy may be restarted at a reduced dose once the symptoms have resolved. Moisturizing or emollient creams may help early in the development of hand-foot syndrome to relieve discomfort and maintain skin integrity. Cold compresses, elevation and analgesia may be useful supportive treatments.[49] Radiation enhancement and recall should be managed in the same way as acute radiotherapy skin reactions, as discussed earlier.

The management of pruritus should first include the accurate assessment and treatment of any underlying causes, including drug hypersensitivities. Good skin care is essential. Using moisturizing creams, emollient baths and encouraging an adequate fluid intake will help prevent itching associated with dry skin. Menthol (0.25–1%) in aqueous cream is a soothing alternative to calamine lotion, with the benefit of moisturizing the skin as well. Clip nails short or provide cotton gloves to prevent scratching. Drug therapies include oral antihistamines (H_1 receptor antagonists); H_2 antagonists (cimetidine, ranitidine); and non-steroidal anti-inflammatory drugs (NSAIDs) and topical or oral steroids (including dexamethasone, prednisolone and androgens, e.g. stanozolol). Pruritus associated with biliary obstruction and jaundice may respond to bile salt chelators (colestyramine); serotonin or 5-hydroxytryptamine ($5HT_3$) antagonists (e.g. granisetron, ondansetron); rifampicin; oral opioid antagonists; or an androgen (e.g. stanozolol).[44,52,53]

Sweating can present as a side-effect of chemotherapy or hormonal therapy and subsides when treatment is discontinued. However, sweating may also present as a consequence of malignant disease, especially in advanced cancer, when patients tend to suffer from excess sweating (hyperhidrosis) or night sweats (nocturnal diaphoresis).[45] With severe sweating, patients may need to change their clothing or bed linen several times during the day or night, which can be very disruptive and upsetting. Sweating may be induced by environmental temperature, emotion and fever, which may be related to infection or paraneoplastic fever related to tumour activity.[54] Lymphoma (especially Hodgkin's disease), liver metastases and carcinoid syndrome (related to carcinoid tumours that secrete serotonin) are primary causes of excessive sweating in patients with cancer, but many other malignant tumours may also cause hyperhidrosis.[55–57] Alcohol, tricyclic antidepressants and morphine can all exacerbate sweating.[44]

The treatment of excess sweating is based on correcting causes where possible and the use of drug therapies. Reducing the ambient air temperature, treating infection and using non-morphine opioids may help. Hormone replacement therapy is an option for patients who have sweating associated with hot flushes secondary to castration (common in males post orchidectomy).[44] Sweating associated with fever may be treated with antipyretics such as paracetamol or NSAIDs, along with cooling activities such as tepid sponging and using a fan. Sweating in terminal malignancy may respond to low-dose thioridazine, although side-effects of confusion and sedation may occur.[58] Alternatively, propranolol, propantheline or amitriptyline may relieve sweating.[59] Thalidomide has been used successfully in the management of sweating in patients receiving palliative care, particularly for night sweats.[60-62] Good skin hygiene is essential to prevent damage from excess moisture and to promote patient comfort. Dehydration is also a potential problem, so encouragement with oral fluids is also important.

Skin graft versus host disease

Skin is one of the main target organs for graft versus host disease (GvHD) in patients undergoing bone marrow transplantation, and skin changes can occur in either an acute (10–70 days following transplantation) or chronic (from 3 months post-transplantation) phase.[63] Skin GvHD may present in a number of forms, including pruritus, erythematous rash, blistering, cracking and/or weeping of the skin.[64] Acute GvHD of the skin may progress through stages,[65] mirroring the four clinical stages of GvHD:

- Stage 1 – maculopapular rash covering <25% of the body.
- Stage 2 – maculopapular rash covering 25–50% of the body.
- Stage 3 – extensive reddening, flaking and thickening of the skin (exfoliative dermatitis).
- Stage 4 – shedding of the outer layer of the epidermis and formation of large fluid-filled blisters (bullae) (Fig. 24.4).

Eighty to 95% of patients with chronic GvHD will have involvement of the skin, the develop-

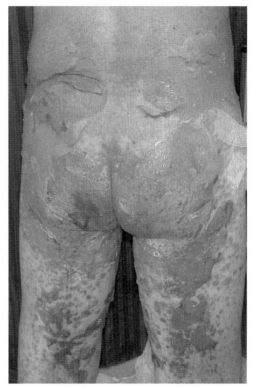

Figure 24.4: Extensive skin loss and blistering in acute graft versus host disease.

ment of which is predominantly caused by the action of T cells.[64,65] Skin changes may occur spontaneously or in areas of the body exposed to the sun, trauma or infection and can include:[65,66]

- Pruritus and erythema.
- Patchy alopecia/hair pigment loss.
- Nail changes.
- Hypo- or hyperpigmentation, particularly at sites of trauma or friction.
- Erythematous or purplish papules or plaques (similar to lichen planus).
- Sclerotic appearance with induration, thickening of the dermis and adherence to underlying fascia. May progress to tight, hyperpigmented (bronze-coloured) skin that is prone to ulceration and joint contractures.

The nursing care of cutaneous GvHD is centred on maintaining skin integrity in order to promote patient comfort and prevent superimposed infection. Skin care is the same for both acute and chronic GvHD. It is important to keep the skin clean and well moisturized through the use of warm emollient baths, gentle soaps or soap substitutes and avoiding perfumed skin care products. The use of moisturizing creams and lotions will help maintain skin suppleness and may relieve pruritus, particularly if the skin is dry and cracked. If itching is a significant problem, topical antipruretic and steroid creams may be useful.[67] Hydrogel sheet dressings may be helpful to relieve itchy, painful skin. For areas of skin breakdown or blistering, it may be necessary to use dressing products to contain exudate and also as a means of preventing infection and promoting comfort. Useful dressing products include hydrogels, alginates, hydrofibres and foams. For extensive areas of skin loss specialized burns dressings may be needed or, for extreme cases, an air-fluidized bead bed (e.g. Clinitron, FluidAir) may be appropriate.[65]

WOUNDS AND WOUND HEALING

In patients with cancer, a wound may be formed as the result of their disease or as a consequence of treatment. At its broadest definition, a wound may involve skin, soft tissues, muscle, bone or other internal structures and organs.[10] The most common cause of any wound is damage by an external agent that results in cuts, grazes, bruises, punctures and burns. However, internal factors can also cause or contribute to wound formation, e.g. an underlying disease such as venous insufficiency or diabetes. Whatever the cause of the wound, it will heal, where this is possible, by one of three methods: primary, secondary or tertiary intention healing.

- Primary intention healing – the wound edges are brought together and kept in place by the use of sutures, clips, glue or adhesive strips; there is no visible granulation tissue, e.g. surgical incision.[68]
- Secondary intention healing – the wound is open and heals from the bottom up by filling with granulation tissue. When new tissue reaches the level of the epidermis, re-epithelialization takes place, e.g.

chronic ulcer (leg, pressure), wide local excision, heavily infected wounds.[68–70]

- Tertiary (or delayed primary) intention healing – the wound is left open for several days until it is free of necrotic tissue or infection, or has enough new tissue, to allow the edges to be brought together without undue tension, e.g. large amount of tissue loss, heavily infected wound, dehisced surgical wound.[71]

The normal wound healing process

The normal process of wound healing can be divided into four separate phases, comprising haemostasis, inflammation, proliferation and maturation. While the phases must occur in sequence, they do not actually occur as distinct stages but merge together to form a seamless process.

Haemostasis occurs immediately following tissue injury and lasts for 5–10 minutes. Damaged blood vessels constrict to stem the blood flow and the coagulation cascade is initiated in response to chemical messengers released by platelets (Fig 24.5a).[72] The result is a stable clot composed of platelets, fibrin and red blood cells that seals the wound and holds the edges together. The clot eventually dries to form a scab.

The inflammatory phase also begins directly after wounding and lasts approximately 3 days, although this depends upon the extent of tissue damage, as well as microbial and foreign body contamination. This phase is characterized by local inflammation (redness, heat, oedema, discomfort and reduced function), which occurs as a result of capillary dilation and increased capillary permeability (Fig. 24.5b).[73] Neutrophils and macrophages are attracted to the wound and remove bacteria, foreign bodies and devitalized tissue. Macrophages also have an essential function in coordinating wound repair by releasing a number of growth factors that stimulate angiogenesis (growth of new blood vessels) and fibroplasia (growth and division of fibroblasts), as well as stimulating proliferation of macrophages themselves.[7,70,74]

The proliferative phase lasts around 24 days, although this depends on the extent of tissue loss. Fibroblasts are attracted to the wound and begin to produce collagen and ground sub-

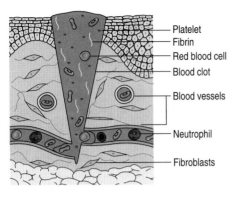

- Platelet
- Fibrin
- Red blood cell
- Blood clot
- Blood vessels
- Neutrophil
- Fibroblasts

A Haemostasis

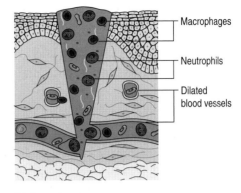

- Macrophages
- Neutrophils
- Dilated blood vessels

B Inflammatory phase

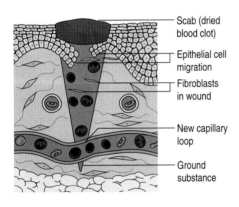

- Scab (dried blood clot)
- Epithelial cell migration
- Fibroblasts in wound
- New capillary loop
- Ground substance

C Proliferative phase

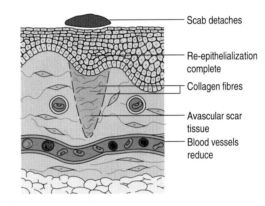

- Scab detaches
- Re-epithelialization complete
- Collagen fibres
- Avascular scar tissue
- Blood vessels reduce

D Maturation phase

Figure 24.5: Diagrammatic representations of the phases of wound healing: (A) haemostasis; (B) inflammatory phase; (C) proliferative phase; and (D) maturation phase.

stance (a mixture of fibrin, fibronectin and proteoglycans) that fills the space between collagen fibres.[69,70] Angiogenic factors stimulate endothelial cell division, resulting in new capillary loops within the collagen and ground substance. This gives rise to the development of an uneven red granular tissue in the wound bed, commonly referred to as granulation tissue (Fig. 24.5c). Wound contraction occurs during this phase and is achieved by specialized fibroblasts (myofibroblasts) that pull the wound edges inwards.[70,74] Re-epithelialization begins as basal cells from the wound margin, or hair follicles and sweat glands within the wound, begin to grow and divide to form a new epidermis.[73]

Once the wound has filled with new tissue and re-epithelialization is complete, the maturation phase begins. This phase usually begins about 21 days post injury and may last for more than a year. During maturation, the newly formed tissue is reorganized and remodelled to form the end product of healing, a scar (Fig. 25.5d). The resultant scar tissue will have around 70–80% of normal skin strength.[70,75]

Moist wound healing

In 1962, Winter[76] published a seminal work in which he proposed that epithelial cells were able to move more freely across a moist wound surface, thus producing faster rates of healing in superficial wounds dressed with an occlusive film. Further studies have confirmed this finding and established that a moist environment also encourages synthesis of collagen and ground substance, promotes angiogenesis, decreases length of inflammatory phase and promotes breakdown of necrotic tissue.[69,77–80] Moist wound healing is now a widely accepted principle of wound care and most modern wound care products provide a moist wound environment.

Impediments to healing in patients with cancer

Wound healing is reliant upon a healthy physiological state, as well as an external environment that is conducive to healing. In patients with cancer, and indeed in many other chronically ill patients, numerous factors will have an adverse effect on wound healing. These may be either internal or external and include factors such as:[10,71,81–88]

- mechanical stress, e.g. pressure, friction and shear
- wound temperature below 28°C
- desiccation and maceration
- infection
- medications, e.g. steroids, chemotherapy and immunosuppressants
- radiotherapy
- malignancy
- lifestyle, e.g. smoking
- pre-existing health problems, e.g. peripheral vascular disease and diabetes
- older age
- poor nutrition and hydration
- obesity or underweight
- stress and sleep deprivation.

WOUND ASSESSMENT

Accurate assessment of the wound environment is essential, as this provides the basis for treatment planning and allows for an evaluation of treatment efficacy. The use of a wound assessment chart will assist in this process by ensuring all relevant wound parameters are assessed and providing an ongoing record of wound progress. It is important to evaluate the effect of the wound and its treatment upon the patient in order to ensure the patient is happy with, and understands, the chosen treatment regimen. This will encourage patient compliance and promote a positive outcome, even if wound healing

is not the ultimate goal, as may be the case with a fungating wound or patient who is terminally ill. There are many aspects of a wound that can be assessed: some, such as wound volume, are not easily achieved with the resources available in most hospitals.

Measuring the size, depth and shape of the wound gives information on changes in size and therefore progress of the wound.[89,90] It also helps in selecting an appropriately sized dressing. Measurements should include the surface area of the wound if possible, and this can be achieved using grid-lined tracing material.[91] The easiest method of measuring a wound is to use a ruler to measure maximum length and width. Photography may also be a useful medium to chart wound progress.

Dressing choice is often dependent on the type of tissue present in the wound, and changes in tissue volumes are a good indicator of wound progression. A 'colour coding' system has been developed as a means of recording tissue type. The system consists of five colours that relate visually to the main types of tissue that may be present in a wound:[90,92,93]

- black (necrotic)
- yellow (sloughy)
- red (granulating)
- pink (epithelializing)
- green (infected).

In all healing wounds there is some production of exudate, which is usually serous or haemoserous in nature, but excess or purulent exudate can indicate infection. High exudate levels can lead to skin maceration and breakdown.[91] Therefore, the amount and nature of exudate should be recorded, although lack of a standard means of measuring exudate levels can be a problem. It is common to use descriptive statements such as low, medium or high, but different assessors interpret such descriptions in a different way. It may be useful to include an evaluation of whether the level and type of exudate is changing.

Wound malodour is a common complication of wound infection and may be associated with high exudate levels. Again, odour poses problems in assessment, as it is a subjective phenomenon and may be influenced by previous experiences of the assessor. The terms 'none', 'mild' and 'offensive' are commonly used to rate odour and, again, can give rise to inconsistent assessment. A descriptive scale has been proposed as an aid to odour assessment (Box 24.3) or, alternatively, patient self-assessment could be considered.[96]

Episodes of bleeding from the wound should be recorded, as this can be a significant problem in patients with cancer due to coagulation problems or malignancy in the wound. The erosion of blood vessels by a fungating tumour can result in spontaneous and heavy bleeding. Trauma during dressing changes or from adherent dressings can also cause bleeding from the wound.

Assessment of wound-related pain is essential. This includes chronic pain associated with the wound and acute pain caused by manipulation during wound care procedures. As with other forms of pain, the use of patient self-assessment is the gold standard.[96] Assessment parameters should include the type, site and frequency of pain, and effectiveness of treatments.[92,97]

As previously mentioned, excess exudate can damage peri-wound skin, as can adhesives and allergies to dressing products. Wound infection will manifest as redness, heat and oedema around the wound.[92,93] Thus, it is important to include an assessment of the surrounding skin as it may provide important information about the state of the wound.

Box 24.3

Wound odour rating scale[94,95]

- **None**: no odour evident, even when at the patient's bedside with the dressing removed
- **Slight**: wound odour is evident at close proximity to the patient when the dressing is removed
- **Moderate**: wound odour is evident upon entering the room (1.5–3 metres from the patient) with the dressing removed
- **Strong**: wound odour is evident upon entering the room (1.5–3 metres from the patient) with the dressing intact

WOUND DRESSINGS/DEVICES

There are an inordinate number of wound management products available on the market and new ones are constantly being added. This poses many problems for nurses, as it is a difficult task to remain up to date with the latest developments and know when and how to use the vast array of products they are presented with. Also, as wound care products become more sophisticated, they are increasing in price. This is often offset by the fact that many newer and more costly products are designed to be left in place for an extended period (usually up to 7 days) and to heal wounds faster. This effectively reduces the overall cost of achieving a healed wound. However, the cost-effectiveness of these products is only a reality if they are used correctly.

When deciding on which dressing or treatment to use it is vital to refer back to the wound assessment and to identify the aim of treatment. It may be inappropriate to use expensive dressings designed specifically to promote healing in a fungating wound where healing is very unlikely.[67] It is also important to consider the patient's viewpoint and their social situation. Some dressings may not be acceptable to patients even though they are the best option for their wound; there will need to be negotiation and agreement if a dressing regimen is to be successful. In some cases a single dressing may not be effective, so a combination needs to be used. It is not uncommon for fungating wounds to present a challenge in dressing fit and retention, so some experimentation may be required. Table 24.3 provides an overview of wound management products that may be useful in the care of patients with cancer along with indications and contraindications for each product and examples from each category.

WOUNDS RELATED TO CANCER AND CANCER THERAPIES

Both cancer itself and the treatments employed in its management can give rise to the formation of a wound. As previously discussed, there are many instances where the integrity of the skin is compromised by cancer therapies, but predominantly the effects are self-limiting and superficial. However, there are also occasions when the patient may experience more significant skin loss or destruction as a consequence of surgery, leakage of cytotoxic drugs into the skin (extravasation) or due to cancerous infiltration of the structures of the skin.

Surgical wounds

The treatment of many malignant tumours begins with surgery, either to remove all or part of the tumour or to take a sample of the tumour for further investigations and to clarify diagnosis. Surgery may also be performed for many other reasons, which may or may not be related to the cancer. The wound created during a surgical procedure will generally be closed and heal by primary intention. The patient may also have one or more drains placed in the wound bed to prevent the formation of a seroma (collection of serous fluid) or haematoma (collection of blood).[113] In some cases the extent of tissue removed, as in a wide local excision for melanoma, means the wound must heal by secondary intention or be repaired using a split skin graft or plastic surgical flap.[10,68,113]

Nursing care of surgical wounds

Surgical wounds healing by primary intention should require little intervention apart from regular observation of the site to assess for bleeding, infection or wound breakdown. A dressing that protects the wound from external contamination, and prevents soiling of the patient's clothing, is usually all that is necessary. The most commonly used dressings are adhesive island dressings and semipermeable films (see Table 24.3). If the wound is left open to heal by secondary intention, then it should be assessed on a regular basis (i.e. at least weekly) and an appropriate dressing selected according to the wound's appearance, e.g. necrotic, sloughy, granulating and epithelializing or infected (see Table 24.3).[67]

A closed surgical wound only needs to be covered with a dressing for 48 hours postoperatively, after which time it can be left exposed, if this is acceptable to the patient. It may be appropriate to keep the wound covered with a non-adherent dressing if the patient is distressed by the sight of the wound or if the patient experiences discomfort from clothing rubbing on the wound.[114] If the dressing becomes saturated with exudate or blood, it should be changed. The dressing should also be removed if the patient displays clinical signs of infection to allow examination of the wound site.[84]

Extravasation wounds

Extravasation of a vesicant drug can cause significant tissue damage that may result in pain, cosmetic disfigurement, nerve damage and loss of function or even amputation.[115–117] Drugs commonly associated with severe tissue damage are dactinomycin, daunorubicin, doxorubicin, mitomycin C, vinblastine and vincristine.[43] Areas with little soft tissue cover to protect underlying nerves and tendons, such as the dorsum of the hand, the forearm and the foot, are at most risk from severe extravasation injury.[118]

Following extravasation, the skin may become inflamed and oedematous with superficial skin loss. As tissue damage progresses, induration develops, followed by the formation of a necrotic ulcer, which may contain slough and/or dry black eschar.[118] Ulceration usually develops over a period of days to weeks, with maximum tissue damage evident 2–3 weeks post extravasation.[119] The ulcer may enlarge over a period of weeks or months if untreated and extend to involve underlying structures such as tendons and nerves.[117]

Nursing care of extravasation wounds

Partial- or full-thickness skin loss should be managed with a dressing that protects the wound and maintains a moist wound environment. Examples include semipermeable films, hydrocolloid sheets or hydrogel sheets.[115,120] Debridement of necrotic tissue (slough or eschar) should be performed to encourage healing and reduce the risk of infection. The removal of necrotic tissue will also allow a more accurate assessment of the extent of tissue damage.[67] Wound debridement may be achieved by several methods:

Table 24.3: Wound management products and their use[67,98–112]

Dressing category	Description	Indications	Contraindications	Examples
Activated charcoal	Attracts and binds molecules responsible for odour. May also contain other products	Malodorous wounds (e.g. fungating tumours, faecal fistulae)	Secondary dressings have no contraindications	Clinisorb, Actisorb Silver 220, CarboFlex, Kaltocarb, Lyofoam C
Adhesive island	Low-adherent, absorbent pad on an adhesive backing	Lightly exuding wounds Postoperative wounds	Heavily exuding wounds Caution on fragile or easily damaged skin	Mepore, Opsite Post-Op, Primapore, Tielle Lite
Alginates	A fibre dressing derived from an alginic acid polymer found in brown seaweed. Available as a sheet, ribbon or packing	Moderate to highly exuding wounds (sloughy, granulating) Infected/malodorous wounds Bleeding wounds/skin donor sites	Dry wounds Dry necrotic areas (eschar)	Comfeel Seasorb, Curasorb, Kaltostat, Sorbsan, Tegagen, Algisite M
Foams	Generally composed of polyurethane foam and may have one or more layers.	Light to heavily exuding superficial wounds Cavity wounds Tracheostomy and drain sites	Dry necrotic wounds Wounds with low exudate	Allevyn, Allevyn Cavity, Lyofoam, Tielle
Honey	Sterile honey for wound care is available in tubes or as impregnated dressings	Infected wounds Necrotic and sloughy wounds Fungating wounds Chronic wounds Burns	Caution in diabetes due to fructose absorption	Medihoney Antibacterial honey, Woundcare 18+, Actimel

(continues)

Table 24.3: Wound management products and their use[67,98–112]—cont'd

Dressing category	Description	Indications	Contraindications	Examples
Hydrocolloids	Usually consist of a base material containing varying amounts of gelatin, pectin and carboxymethylcellulose combined with adhesives and polymers, bonded to a semipermeable film	Light to moderately exuding wounds Clean granulating wounds Necrotic or sloughy wounds	Highly exuding wounds	Comfeel, Duoderm E, Granuflex, Hydrocoll, Tegasorb
Hydrogels	Composed of water (17.5–90% depending on the product), plus various gelling and absorptive agents. Available as sheets or gels	Light to moderately exuding wounds Rehydration of eschar Acute radiotherapy skin reactions Split skin donor sites Recipient graft sites Deep chronic wounds extending to muscle, tendon or bone Fungating and/or malodorous wounds (Novogel)	Heavily exuding wounds Caution is advised in infected wounds	Gels: Aquaform, Granugel, Intrasite Gel, Nu-Gel, Purilon, Sterigel Sheets: Geliperm, Novogel, Clearsite, Hydrosorb, Nu-Gel
Hydrofibre	Non-woven dressing composed of 100% hydrocolloid fibres (sodium carboxymethylcellulose)	Moderate to highly exuding acute and chronic wounds Cavity wounds Wounds prone to bleeding	Dry, necrotic wounds	Aquacel, Aquacel Ag (contains silver)
Semipermeable films	Thin polyurethane film with a hypoallergenic adhesive	Superficial, low-exudate wounds Surgical wounds healing by primary intention Prevention of skin breakdown As a retention dressing	Deep cavities or third-degree burns Infected wounds Moderate and highly exuding wounds	Bioclusive, Cutifilm, Epiview, Opsite Flexigrid, Opsite IV3000, Tegaderm

Skin barrier films (alcohol-free)	Liquid polymers that dry to form a protective film on the skin	Central venous catheters and long-term peripheral intravenous (IV) catheters (Opsite IV3000, Tegaderm IV) Incontinence (urine and faeces) Artificial skin openings (fistula, stoma and tracheostomy) Skin at risk of stripping by adhesive tapes Skin at risk of breakdown from moisture (e.g. exudate, urine, sweat)	Adhesive trauma may occur on removal from fragile skin Sensitivity to product or its components	Cavilon No-Sting Barrier Film, SuperSkin, No-Sting Skin-prep
Wound contact layers	Fabric net (e.g. polyamide or knitted viscose) coated with a non-adherent substance such as silicone or hydrocolloid	Acute traumatic wounds Fungating wounds Painful wounds and wounds with fragile skin Fixation of grafts Dermatological skin conditions (e.g. GvHD, blistering	Cautions: When used on bleeding wounds or wounds with very viscous exudate, cover with a moist absorbent pad dressing	Mepitel, N-A Ultra, Urgotul

Notes. In all cases dressing should not be used in patients with known sensitivity to the dressing or its components. All dressing products should be used according to manufacturer's instructions, as products within the same category may have different performance characteristics and different methods of application.

- Sharp debridement performed by a nurse (who has evidence of competency in such treatment) at the patient's bedside using scissors and scalpel.[121]

- Autolytic debridement, utilizing the body's natural debridement method by maintaining the wound in a moist environment (using hydrogels, hydrocolloids or semipermeable films).[122,123]

- Enzymatic debridement, where autolytic debridement is proving ineffective.[122,124]

- Larval therapy (sterile maggots) if patient is agreeable. The larvae produce powerful enzymes that break down necrotic tissue.[125,126]

Other treatment options include sterile honey or sugar paste, which will debride necrotic tissue, or topical negative pressure therapy (vacuum-assisted closure or VAC) on moist necrotic wounds where it will remove necrotic tissue and excess wound fluid.[102,109,127] These therapies will also encourage the formation of granulation tissue and reduce bacterial load in the wound.

Extensive tissue damage and continued pain indicate the need for surgical intervention in the form of plastic surgery.[117,118] All affected tissue needs to be excised, which usually results in a significant tissue defect that must be repaired using a delayed split skin graft or flap.[84,119]

Fungating malignant wounds

Fungating wounds are the cutaneous manifestation of malignant disease and are a devastating problem for many patients with advanced cancer. These wounds often present with a predominantly proliferative growth pattern, developing into a nodular 'fungus' or 'cauliflower'-shaped lesion (Fig. 24.6). In others cases, ulceration may predominate and produce a wound with a crater-like appearance.[96,128] It is also possible for a lesion to present with a mixed appearance of both proliferating and ulcerating areas.[129,130] In the majority of cases, healing of a fungating wound is unlikely unless there is a good response to anticancer therapy, such as radiotherapy or chemotherapy, or the wound can be surgically excised. Unfortunately, most fungating wounds will continue to deteriorate over time.

Aetiology

The aetiology of fungating wounds follows the same pattern of tumour growth and spread as elsewhere in the body. Hence, a fungating wound may develop:

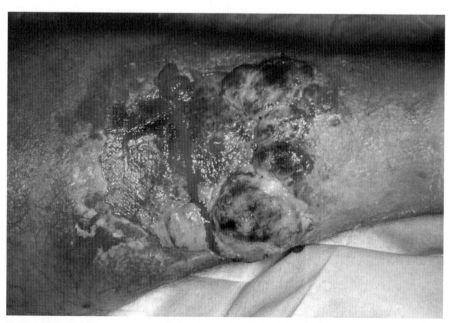

Figure 24.6: Proliferative fungating wound on the calf of a patient with malignant melanoma.

- as a result of a primary skin tumour
- by direct invasion of the skin by an underlying tumour
- by metastatic spread from a distant tumour along tissue planes, capillaries or lymph vessels
- by mechanical implantation or seeding during surgery
- by malignant change in a long-standing chronic wound (Marjolin's ulcer).

Fungating wounds tend to develop in elderly patients (>70 years old) with metastatic cancer, who are in the terminal stages of their illness.[131,132] While a fungating wound may arise anywhere on the body, the most common sites are the breast (39–62%) and the head and neck area (24–33.8%).[24,133] Tumours commonly associated with the development of malignant wounds include breast, head and neck, kidney, lung, ovary, colon, penis, bladder, lymphoma and leukaemia.[39]

The overall goals of nursing care for patients with fungating wounds are to promote comfort, confidence and a sense of well-being, prevent isolation and maintain or improve the patient's quality of life.[131,134,135] Therefore, management is focused on controlling and/or eliminating symptoms related to fungating wounds and enabling patients to manage or cope with psychological and social problems associated with their wound.[129] To achieve these goals accurate assessment of patient symptoms is vital as a means of determining patient needs and evaluating the effectiveness of symptom management interventions.[136] The most frequently reported symptoms associated with a fungating wound are exudate, malodour, bleeding and pain. These symptoms may cause or contribute to the many psychological and social problems that arise for the patient with a fungating wound.

Wound malodour is a very distressing symptom for patients and is caused by bacterial colonization or infection of the wound. This can be a particular problem where there is considerable necrotic tissue present in the wound, a state common to the majority of fungating wounds due to their poor blood supply (Fig. 24.7). Malodour may be constantly

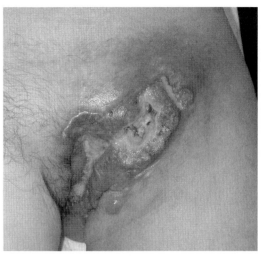

Figure 24.7: Necrotic fungating wound in the groin related to squamous cell carcinoma of the vulva.

detectable and can trigger gagging and vomiting reflexes.[39,96,137] This can be upsetting for the patient's family and caregivers, as well as healthcare professionals. The presence of a pervasive malodour can lead to embarrassment, disgust, depression and social isolation and may have a detrimental effect on sexual expression, leading to relationship problems.[135,137–139]

The copious amount of exudate produced by fungating wounds has been attributed to the increased permeability of disorganized blood vessels within the tumour and secretion of vascular permeability factor by tumour cells.[131] Wound infection can also increase exudate due to inflammation and the breakdown of tissue by bacterial proteases.[140] A common consequence of large volumes of uncontrolled exudate is leakage from the dressing, which may cause staining of the patient's clothes.[141] Poorly controlled exudate leads to similar psychosocial problems as those encountered with malodour, with embarrassment, disgust and social isolation being common.[142,143]

Pain associated with fungating wounds may be related to a number of causes. Tumour may be pressing on nerves and blood vessels or superficial ulceration may expose the dermis and its associated nerve endings.[144] This results in the characteristic superficial stinging pain often described as accompanying a fungating wound.[128] If there is nerve damage, patients may experience neuropathic pain, which may be characterized by spontaneous burning pain

549

with intermittent sharp stabbing pains. It has also been described as an 'itching', 'tingling', 'smarting' or 'stinging' pain.[145] Poor wound care practises may also cause pain, e.g. inappropriate cleansing techniques or the use of dressings that adhere to the wound bed.[139]

As well as causing pain, poor wound care practises can result in bleeding when fragile tissues are traumatized during dressing changes. The erosion of blood vessels by malignant cells may precipitate bleeding, which may be compounded by abnormal platelet function within the tumour environment. Profuse spontaneous bleeding can occur and is a very distressing event for both patients and their carers.[131]

Nursing care of fungating wounds

Chemotherapy, radiotherapy, hormone therapy or a combination of these anticancer therapies may help relieve symptoms from a fungating wound by destroying malignant cells, reducing pressure on nerves and other structures and decreasing the area of exposed tissue.[131,135,146] In particular, radiotherapy will often reduce symptoms of exudate and bleeding. However, in advanced disease these therapies may not be successful or appropriate and the patient's wound must be managed with topical products, systemic medications and other supportive therapies. Table 24.4 provides treatment options for the different symptoms associated with fungating wounds.

Cosmetic appearance

As fungating wounds tend to occur more often in the area of the breast or head and neck, the position of the wound may be a source of embarrassment and distress for the patient.[148] Appropriate wound management that attends to the patient's outward appearance can have a very positive effect on self-esteem and emotional distress.[131,135] Many patients can only continue an active social life if a socially acceptable dressing is available.[158] In most cases this may be achieved by devising a cosmetically acceptable dressing regimen that effectively manages wound symptoms and also restores body symmetry. This should be carried out in an effort to boost patient confidence and improve their ability to socialize.[158,159]

STOMA CARE

When a patient requires treatment for cancer of the bowel or urinary system they may require the formation of a stoma, which is defined as a surgically created opening of the large or small bowel, or urinary system, onto the surface of the abdomen.[160] The two main indications for stoma formation are when surgical treatment for disease requires removal of the anal sphincter or urinary bladder (e.g. abdominal perineal resection, radical cystectomy) and when distal pathology requires that bowel contents or urine be diverted, e.g. to rest or 'defunction' the lower portion of the bowel following anastomosis, or for fistula management.[161,162]

Types of stoma and indications

The type of stoma formed will depend on the organ(s) involved, location of diseased or damaged tissue and the surgical procedure. The most common type of stoma is a colostomy, followed by ileostomy and urostomy.[163] A stoma formed from small or large bowel may be fashioned as either an end stoma, where the distal portion of the bowel is removed or closed, or a loop stoma, where a loop of bowel is bought to the abdominal surface producing a proximal and distal opening (Fig. 24.8a). A colostomy is an opening into the colon and may be positioned in the sigmoid, descending, transverse or ascending colon. The stoma is usually sited in the left iliac fossa (Fig. 24.8b). If the colostomy arises from the sigmoid or descending colon, output will be formed faeces with a normal odour. A stoma arising from the transverse or ascending colon will produce copious loose stool with a strong odour.[163] An ileostomy is formed from the terminal part of the ileum, which is bought to the abdominal surface in the right iliac fossa (Fig. 24.8c).[163,164] Output from an ileostomy is usually referred to as effluent and is very soft and fluid, being similar in consistency to porridge. A urostomy or urinary diversion is most commonly fashioned using a short segment of ileum (around 10–20 cm), which forms the stoma, into which the ureters have been anastomosed (Fig. 24.8d).[161] This may also be referred to as an ileal conduit and output is urine.

Table 24.4: Symptom management strategies for fungating wounds

Symptom	Management
Malodour	Debridement of necrotic tissue to remove source of bacterial colonization/infection Metronidazole, either systemically or topically. Side-effects with systemic use and lack of an adequate blood supply to the wound may limit its usefulness.[98,147] Topical metronidazole gel applied once daily for 5–7 days is usually very effective Activated charcoal dressings Sugar paste and sterile honey Occlusive dressings may help contain wound odour Daily dressing changes and correct disposal of soiled dressings prevents build-up of stale exudate Deodorizers may mask the odour and products such as essential oils, environmental air filters or commercial deodorizers may be helpful[67]
Low exudate	Dressings that have a low absorbency so as not to dry out the wound: Examples include hydrocolloids, semipermeable films and low adherent absorbent dressings[139]
Moderate to high exudate	Dressings that will absorb the excess exudate but still maintain a moist wound environment: Alginate and hydrofibre dressings Foam dressings Non-adherent wound contact layers with a secondary absorbent pad[128,148] Stoma appliances or wound manager bags for wounds with a small opening and high exudate[139]
Pain	Assessment is the key to successful pain management, as this will identify the type of pain and therefore indicate the most appropriate treatment: Appropriate analgesia Premedication or a booster dose of usual opiate before dressing change Nitrous oxide (Entonox) gas during the procedure Morphine or diamorphine mixed with a hydrogel (0.08–0.1% mixture) and applied topically to the wound may be useful for painful ulcerating wounds[149–151] Non-adherent dressings that maintain the wound in a moist environment Dressing products that require less frequent changing Irrigation of the wound with warm saline rather than cleaning with a gauze swab[152] Complementary therapies such as relaxation, distraction or visualization may help anxious and stressed patients, who have a heightened response to pain[153,154]
Bleeding	Preventative measures are important to reduce the risk of bleeding: Non-adherent dressings that maintain a moist environment Cleansing by irrigation Oral antifibrinolytics such as tranexamic acid (Cyklokapron) may also help by reducing clot breakdown[148] Actively bleeding wounds: Sucralfate paste for light bleeding Alginate dressing for light bleeding (alginates may cause bleeding in friable wounds[155]) Haemostatic surgical sponge (e.g. Spongostan, Oxycell) Topical adrenaline or tranexamic acid (caution is advised with adrenaline as it may cause ischaemic necrosis due to local vasoconstriction)[156,157] Excessive bleeding may need referral to a vascular surgeon for cautery or ligation

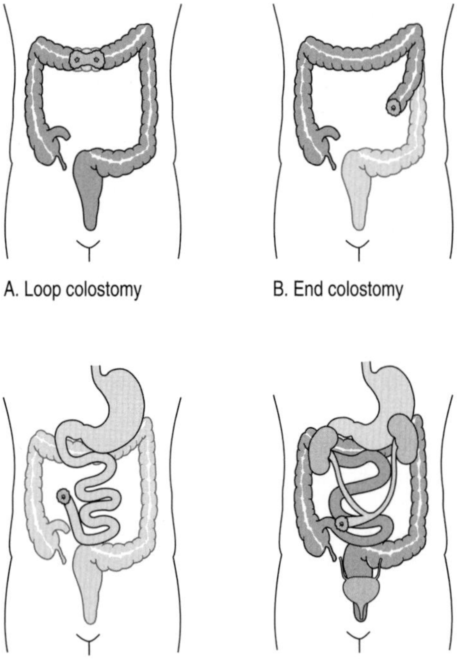

A. Loop colostomy

B. End colostomy

C. Ileostomy

D. Ileal conduit

Figure 24.8: Different types of stoma (shaded area indicates structures removed): (a) loop colostomy; (b) end colostomy; (c) ileostomy; (d) ileal conduit.

Appliances

A wide range of stoma appliances are available to suit different types of stoma and output, as well as meeting physical and lifestyle needs of patients. Modern appliances are made from clear or opaque odour-proof plastic and are either closed or drainable; most now also have an integral flatus filter. All appliances come with a hydrocolloid-type flange, possibly with an extra border of fabric tape, for fixation to the skin. The flange may be incorporated into the bag to form a one-piece appliance or it may come separately with a clip-on bag as a two-piece system. If the patient develops a retracted stoma, a convex flange may be needed. This type of flange has an outward curve that helps push the stoma out.[161]

Immediately after surgery a clear, drainable appliance will be used to allow observation of the stoma and output. As the patients move towards discharge they will generally change to an opaque appliance suitable to their type of stoma. A patient with a colostomy will generally use a closed appliance with flatus filter, whereas a patient with an ileostomy will need a

drainable appliance, as the bag will need to be emptied around six times a day.[161] For those with a urostomy, an appliance with a non-return valve and tap at the bottom is required to prevent urine backflow onto the stoma and allow drainage of urine.[163] Urostomy appliances also allow the attachment of a night drainage bag. The choice of appliance should be made by a well-informed patient with assistance from a stoma care nurse and must take into account the physical, social, cultural or religious needs of the patient.[161]

Stoma siting

The importance of correct siting of the stoma cannot be overemphasized. Inappropriate stoma placement may result in the patient being unable to see the stoma, appliance leakage, stoma retraction, prolapse and herniation.[161] Stoma siting should, ideally, take place preoperatively. The stoma site should be easily accessible to the patient and on a flat area of skin large enough to accommodate the appliance flange. It should also be located within the rectus muscle sheath to reduce peristomal herniation. If time is available, the patient should be asked to lie, sit, stand, bend, walk and wear everyday clothes to ensure that the chosen stoma site will not interfere with any normal daily activities.[162] Areas to avoid when siting a stoma include:[161,164]

- waistline, belt line
- bony prominences
- scars
- skin folds/creases, pendulous breasts, groin, umbilicus
- areas of pre-existing skin problems
- areas where weight gain or loss will alter stoma position.

Physical disabilities also need to be taken into account. This may mean that the stoma is not sited in the usual position to enable independent management of the stoma by the patient.[161]

Stoma complications

There are a number of problems that may develop with the stoma after it is fashioned;

these may occur immediately after surgery or days to months later. Most stoma complications develop within the first year post surgery.[163] Immediate complications include stoma ischaemia and necrosis, which may necessitate surgery to refashion the stoma, and bleeding.[160] Early complications occur within the first few days of stoma formation and may include:[160,162]

- high stoma output
- obstruction or non-functioning stoma
- mucocutaneous separation
- skin damage.

Late complications usually develop following discharge from hospital and can be distressing for the patient. The most common late complications are:[160,162,165]

- skin damage/contact dermatitis
- prolapse of bowel (more common in transverse loop colostomies)
- peristomal herniation
- retraction of stoma
- stenosis.

Other less common late complications include constipation, high stoma output, flatus and odour, trauma, bleeding, hypergranulation and recurrence of cancer in the stoma.[160,165] Urostomies may also present problems such as recurrent infection and oxalate crystal formation.

FISTULA MANAGEMENT

A fistula is an abnormal opening that connects two epithelial lined surfaces.[166] An enterocutaneous fistula is one that forms between the gastrointestinal tract and the skin. Fistulas tend to develop most commonly following bowel surgery and are often the result of sepsis, breakdown of an anastomosis or a distal obstruction.[67] Enterocutaneous fistula may also develop due to malignancy, radiotherapy, inflammatory bowel disease, diverticular disease or trauma.[8,167,168] The fistula may be a simple single tract or it may be complex, with multiple tracts and skin openings and possibly contain abscesses.[161]

Nursing care of fistulae

Simple fistulae generally heal with supportive care alone, whereas complex fistulae usually require surgical repair. Supportive care for an enterocutaneous fistula should always include:[67]

- protection of the surrounding skin
- collection and containment of fistula output
- control of odour
- patient support and information.

Enterocutaneous fistulae may produce extremely corrosive effluent, especially if drainage is from the upper gastrointestinal tract. This may contain proteolytic secretions that will 'digest' skin, causing excoriation, ulceration and pain. Skin protection strategies include alcohol-free skin films to prevent skin from excoriation by fistula secretions (e.g. Cavilon, SuperSkin), pastes and powders that protect mucous membranes and skin (e.g. Orabase paste, Orahesive powder) and hydrocolloid products, such as flat sheets or cohesive 'washers'. It is important that fistula drainage is contained away from the skin.[161] This is best achieved through the use of ostomy appliances or specially designed fistula and wound appliances. There are a number of products available, especially in the ostomy appliance range, and choice will depend on the volume, consistency and type of effluent. Wound management appliances (e.g. ConvaTec Wound Manager) have a wide-bore outlet for thicker effluent and may also have an access window to enable cleaning of the wound or fistula opening.[169] Fistula bags, usually smaller and narrower in design, or a urostomy pouch may be sufficient for thin watery effluent and an overnight drainage bag can be added for high-output fistulae. The majority of these appliances have a built-in charcoal filter to reduce odour or specialist ostomy products designed to control odour can also be used. Corrosive secretions will reduce the effectiveness of appliance adhesives and they may need to be replaced more often. Appliances should not be repaired if they leak, as this can result in skin damage from leaked secretions.[167,168] VAC has been used successfully in the management of enterocutaneous fistula, where it effectively contained fistula drainage and promoted healing.[170] Malnutrition and dehydration are potential problems in patients with high-output stomas and they may require dietary advice and supportive nutritional supplements.[67]

CONCLUSION

In most cases cancer is an internal entity, and to the casual observer there may be no outward signs that a person has cancer. However, this state may be changed when side-effects of treatment or the cancer itself causes changes in the skin. Patients are then faced with the prospect of others being able to see that something is wrong and of having a constant visual reminder of their disease. This can cause psychological distress, social withdrawal and possibly non-compliance with treatment. However, with knowledge, attention and good assessment of these skin problems, the nurse will be able to inform and prepare the patient for any likely adverse effects of treatment. Should skin changes occur, or if the patient develops a wound or requires stoma formation, the nurse is in a position of being able to provide support and education and find an effective solution, whether it be for symptom control or to encourage resolution of the problem.

While there is sufficient published material available on the subject of skin and wound care in patients with cancer, there is relatively little high-quality research. This is an area that nurses need to address, as they are the ones most involved in this aspect of patient care. Areas in need of further nursing research include fungating wound care, management of cutaneous GvHD and skin care in relation to cancer therapies. In particular, there is a need for further investigation of the psychosocial aspects of care in patients with skin and wound problems caused by cancer or the treatment of cancer.

REFERENCES

1. Kamel MN. Anatomy of the skin. In: Drugge R, Dunn HA, eds. The electronic textbook of dermatology. The Internet Dermatology Society; 1998. Online. Available: http://www.telemedicine.org/anatomy.htm 29 October 2002.

2. Smith & Nephew. Global Wound Academy. Smith & Nephew 2002. Online. Available: http://www.globalwoundacademy.com 7 October 2003.

3. Tortora GJ, Grabowski SR. Principles of anatomy and physiology. 10th edn. Hoboken: John Wiley; 2002.

4. Ross MH, Romrell LJ, Kaye GI. Histology a text and atlas. 3rd edn. Baltimore: Williams, and Wilkins; 1995.

5. Strete D. A color atlas of histology. New York: Harper Collins; 1995.

6. Gray H. Anatomy of the human body (revised and re-edited by WH Lewis). 20th edn. Philadelphia: Lea & Febiger; 1918. Bartleby.com; 2000. Online. Available: http://www.bartleby.com/107 7 October 2003.

7. Stocum DL. Molecular biology intelligence unit. Wound repair, regeneration and artificial tissues. Austin: RG Landes Company; 1995.

8. Bennett G, Moody M. Wound care for health professionals. London: Chapman and Hall; 1995.

9. Mortimer PS. Management of skin problems medical aspects. In: Doyle D, Hanks GWC, MacDonald N, eds. Oxford textbook of palliative medicine. 2nd edn. Oxford: Oxford University Press; 1998:617–627.

10. Collier M. The principles of optimum wound management. Nurs Stand 1996; 10(43):47–52.

11. Porock D, Kristjanson L. Skin reactions during radiotherapy for breast cancer: the use and impact of topical agents and dressings. Eur J Cancer Care 1999; 8:143–153.

12. Sitton E. Early and late radiation-induced skin alterations part 1: mechanisms of skin changes. Oncol Nurs Forum 1992; 19(5):801–807.

13. Hopewell JW. The skin: its structure and response to ionizing radiation. Int J Radiat Biol 1990; 57(4):751–773.

14. Rice AM. An introduction to radiotherapy. Nurs Stand 1997; 12(3):49–56.

15. De Conno F, Ventafridda V, Saita L. Skin problems in advanced and terminal cancer patients. J Pain Symptom Manage 1991; 6(4):247–256.

16. Blackmar A. Focus on wound care: radiation-induced skin alterations. Medsurg Nurs 1997; 6(3):172–175.

17. Rigter B, Clendon H, Kettle S. Skin reactions due to radiotherapy. New Zealand Practice Nurse 1994; Sept:17–22.

18. Sitton E. Managing side effects of skin changes and fatigue. In: Hassey Dow K, Dunn Bucholtz J, Iwamoto R, Fieler V, Hilderley L, eds. Nursing care in radiation oncology. 2nd edn. Philadelphia: WB Saunders; 1997:79–100.

19. Boots-Vickers M, Eaton K. Skin care for patients receiving radiotherapy. Prof Nurse 1999; 14(10):706–708.

20. Campbell J, Lane C. Developing a skin-care protocol in radiotherapy. Prof Nurse 1996; 12(2):105–108.

21. McDonald A. Skin ulcerations. In: Henke Yarbro C, Hansen Frogge M, Goodman M, eds. Cancer symptom management. 2nd edn. Boston: Jones and Bartlett; 1999:382–401.

22. Lavery BA. Skin care during radiotherapy: a survey of UK practice. Clin Oncol 1995; 7:184–187.

23. Barkham AM. Radiotherapy skin reactions and treatments. Prof Nurs 1993; 8:732–736.

24. Thomas S. Current practices in the management of fungating lesions and radiation damaged skin. Bridgend: The Surgical Materials Testing Laboratory; 1992.

25. Korinko A, Yurick A. Maintaining skin integrity. Am J Nurs 1997; 97(2):40–44.

26. Jones J. How to manage skin reactions to radiation therapy. Nursing98 Australasia 1998; Dec (Suppl):1–2.

27. Mak SSS, Molassiotis A, Wan W, Lee IYM, Chan ESJ. The effects of hydrocolloid dressing and gentian violet on radiation-induced moist desquamation wound healing. Cancer Nurs 2000; 23(3):220–229.

28. Hazardous Substances Data Bank TOXNET [database]. Hexamethyl-p-rosaniline chloride. Bethesda: National Library of Medicine / Specialized Information Services. Online. Available: http://toxnet.nlm.nih.gov/cgibin/sis /search/f?./temp/~2UcIdb:1 7 October 2003.

29. Glean E, Edwards S, Faithfull S, et al. Intervention for acute radiotherapy induced skin reactions in cancer patients: the development of a clinical guideline recommended for use by the College of Radiographers. J Radiother Prac 2001; 2(2):75–84.

30. Naylor W, Mallett J. Management of acute radiotherapy induced skin reactions: a literature review. Eur J Oncol Nurs 2001; 5(4):221–233.

31. Sitton E. Early and late radiation-induced skin alterations part II: nursing care of irradiated skin. Oncol Nurs Forum 1992; 19(6):907–912.

32. Liguori V, Guillemin C, Pesce GF, Mirimanoff RO, Bernier J. Double-blind, randomised clinical study comparing hyaluronic acid cream to placebo in patients treated with radiotherapy. Radiother Oncol 1997; 42:155–161.

33. Maiche A, Isokangas O, Gröhn P. Skin protection by sucralfate cream during electron beam therapy. Acta Oncol 1994; 33(2):201–203.

34. Pickering D, Warland S. The management of desquamative radiation skin reactions. The Dressing Times 1992; 5(1). Online. Available: http://www.smtl.co.uk/WMPRC/DressingsTim es/vol5.1.txt 7 October 2003.

35. Strunk B, Maher K. Collaborative nurse management of multifactorial moist desquamation in a patient undergoing radiotherapy. J ET Nurs 1993; 20(4):152–157.

36. Crane J. Extending the role of a new hydrogel. J Tissue Viability 1993; 3(3):98–99.

37. Margolin SG, Breneman JC, Denman DL, et al. Management of radiation-induced moist skin desquamation using hydrocolloid dressing. Cancer Nurs 1990; 13(2):71–80.

38. Conrad KJ. Cutaneous reactions. In: Yasko JM, ed. Nursing management of symptoms associated with chemotherapy. 5th edn. West

Conshohocken: Meniscus Health Care Communications; 2001:191–204.

39. Gallagher J. Management of cutaneous symptoms. Semin Oncol Nurs 1995; 11(4):239–247.

40. British National Formulary. BNF Number 44 (September). London: British Medical Association and the Royal Pharmaceutical Society of Great Britain; 2002.

41. CancerHelp UK. Cancer treatments; chemotherapy: side effects of specific chemotherapy drugs. Online. Available: http://www.cancerhelp.org.uk/help/default.asp ?page=177 7 October 2003.

42. Oncology Channel. Chemotherapy medications and their side effects. Online. Available: http://www.oncologychannel.com/chemotherap y/medsideeffects.shtml 7 October 2003.

43. Ramu A. Compounds and methods that reduce the risk of extravasation injury associated with the use of vesicant antineoplastic agents. Baylor College of Medicine 1996. Online.

44. Twycross R, Wilcock A. Symptom management in advanced cancer. 3rd edn. Abingdon: Radcliffe Medical Press; 2001.

45. Pittlekow MR, Loprinzi CL. Pruritus and sweating. In: Doyle D, Hanks GWC, MacDonald N, eds. Oxford textbook of palliative medicine. 2nd edn. Oxford: Oxford University Press; 1998:627–642.

46. Alley E, Green R, Schuchter L. Cutaneous toxicities of cancer therapy. Curr Opin Oncol 2002; 14(2):212–216.

47. Susser WS, Whitaker-Worth DL, Grant-Kels JM. Mucocutaneous reactions to chemotherapy. J Am Acad Dermatol 1999; 40(30):367–398.

48. Revenga Arranz F, Fernández-Durán DA, Grande C, Rodriguez Peralto JL, Vanaclocha Sebastián F. Acute and painful erythema of the hands and feet. Arch Dermatol 1997; 133(4):499–504.

49. Coyle C, Wenhold V. Picture this: painful blistered hands and feet. Clin J Oncol Nurs 2001; 5(5):230–232.

50. Camidge R, Price A. Characterizing the phenomenon of radiation recall dermatitis. Radiother Oncol 2001; 59(3):237–245.

52. MacLeod RD, Vella-Brincat J, MacLeod AD. The palliative care handbook. 2nd edn. Christchurch, New Zealand: Genesis Oncology Trust; 2002.

53. Abrahm JL. Promoting symptom control in palliative care. Semin Oncol Nurs 1998; 14(2):95–109.

54. Johnson M. Neoplastic fever. Palliat Med 1996; 10(3):217–224.

55. Lidstone V, Thorns A. Prutitus in cancer patients. Cancer Treat Rev 2001;27(5):305–312.

56. Quigley CS, Baines M. Descriptive epidemiology of sweating in a hospice population. J Palliat Care 1997; 13(1):22–26.

57. Grond S, Zech D, Diefenbach C, Bischoff A. Prevalence and pattern of symptoms in patients

with cancer: a prospective evaluation of 1635 cancer patients referred to a pain clinic. J Pain Symptom Manage 1994; 9(6):372–382.

58. Cowap J, Hardy J. Thioridazine in the management of cancer-related sweating. J Pain Symptom Manage 1998; 15(5):266.

59. Twycross R, Wilcock A, Charlesworth S, Dickman A. Palliative care formulary. 2nd edn. Abingdon: Radcliffe Medical Press; 2002.

60. Peuckmann V, Fisch M, Bruera E. Potential novel uses of thalidomide: focus on palliative care. Drugs 2000; 60(2):273–292.

61. Deaner P. Thalidomide for distressing night sweats in advanced malignant disease. Palliat Med 1998; 12(3):208.

62. Calder K, Bruera E. Thalidomide for night sweats in patients with advanced cancer. Palliat Med 2000; 14(1):77–78.

63. Outhwaite H. Blood and marrow transplantation. In: Grundy M, ed. Nursing in haematological oncology. Edinburgh: Baillière Tindall; 2000:140–155.

64. DeMeyer ES, Fletcher MA, Buschel P. Management of dermatologic complications of chronic graft versus host disease: a case study. Clin J Oncol Nurs 1997; 1(4):95–104.

65. Caudell KA. Graft-versus-host disease. In: Whedon MB, Wujcik D, eds. Blood and marrow stem cell transplantation principles, practice and nursing insights. 2nd edn. Sudbury: Jones and Bartlett; 1997:177–204.

66. Aractingi S, Chosidow O. Cutaneous graft-versus-host disease. Arch Dermatol 1998; 134:602–612.

67. Naylor W, Laverty D, Mallett J. The Royal Marsden Hospital handbook of wound management in cancer care. Oxford: Blackwell Science; 2001.

68. Miller M, Dyson M. Principles of wound care. London: Macmillan Magazines; 1996.

69. Flanagan M. The characteristics and formation of granulation tissue. J Wound Care 1998; 7(10):508–510.

70. Calvin M. Cutaneous wound repair. Wounds 1998; 10(1):12–32.

71. Sussman C. Wound healing biology and chronic wound healing. In: Sussman C, Bate-Jensen BM, eds. Wound care a collaborative practice manual for physical therapists and nurses. Maryland: Aspen Publishers; 1998:31–47.

72. Flanagan M. The physiology of wound healing. J Wound Care 2000; 9(6):299–300.

73. Flanagan M. The physiology of wound healing. In: Miller M, Glover D, eds. Wound management theory and practice. London: Nursing Times Books; 1999:14–22.

74. Flanagan M. A practical framework for wound assessment 1: physiology. Br J Nurs 1996; 5(22):1391-1397.

75. Ehrlich HP. The physiology of wound healing: a summary of normal and abnormal wound healing processes. Adv Wound Care 1999; 11(7):326–328.

76. Winter GA. Formation of the scab and rate of epithelialisation in the skin of the young domestic pig. Nature 1962; 193:293–295.

77. Eaglstein WH. The effect of occlusive dressings on collagen synthesis and re-epithelialization in superficial wounds. In: Ryan TJ, ed. An environment for healing: the role of occlusion. Royal Society of Medicine International Congress and Symposium Series No. 88. London: Royal Society of Medicine; 1985:31–34.

78. Dyson M, Young S, Pendle CL, Webster DF, Lang SM. Comparison of the effects of moist and dry conditions on dermal repair. J Invest Dermatol 1988; 91:434–439.

79. Dyson M, Young SR, Hart J, Lynch JA, Lang S. Comparison of the effects of moist and dry conditions on the process of angiogenesis during dermal repair. J Invest Dermatol 1992; 99:729–733.

80. Miller M. Moist wound healing: the evidence. Nurs Times 1998; 94(45):74–76.

81. Cutting K. Factors affecting wound healing. Nurs Stand 1994; 8(50):33–36.

82. Bowler P. The anaerobic and aerobic microbiology of wounds: a review. Wounds 1998; 10(6):170–178.

83. Thomson P. The microbiology of wounds. J Wound Care 1998; 7(9):477–478.

84. Bale S, Jones V. Wound care nursing a patient-centred approach. London: Ballière Tindall; 1997.

85. Lotti T, Rodofili C, Benci M, Menchin G. Wound-healing problems associated with cancers. J Wound Care 1998; 7(2):81–84.

86. Armstrong M. Obesity as an intrinsic factor affecting wound healing. J Wound Care 1998; 7(5):220–221.

87. Kiecolt-Glaser JK, Marucha PT, Malarkey WB, Mercado AM, Glaser R. Slowing of wound healing by psychological stress. Lancet 1995; 346(4):1194–1196.

88. Adam K, Oswald I. Protein synthesis, bodily renewal and the sleep-wake cycle. Clin Sci 1983; 65(6):561–567.

89. Miller M. Nursing assessment of Patients with non-acute wounds. Br J Nurs 1999; 8(1):10–16.

90. Flanagan M. A practical framework for wound assessment 2: methods. Br J Nurs 1997; 6(1): 6–11.

91. Moore Z. Continuing education module 2: wound care part 6: local wound assessment. World Ir Nurs 1997; 5(6):15–16.

92. Benbow M. Parameters of wound assessment. Br J Nurs 1995; 4(11):647–651.

93. Collier M. Assessing a wound. Nurs Stand 1994; 8(49 RCN Nursing Update):3–8.

94. Baker PG, Haig G. Metronidazole in the treatment of chronic pressure sores and ulcers: a comparison with standard treatments in general practice. Practitioner 1981; 225:569–573.

95. Poteete V. Case study: eliminating odours from wounds. Decubitus 1993; 6(4):43–46.

96. Collier M. The assessment of patients with malignant fungating wounds – a holistic approach: part 1. Nurs Times 1997; 93(44 Suppl):1–4.

97. Sterling C. Methods of wound assessment documentation: a study. Nurs Stand 1996; 11(10):38–41.

98. Thomas S, Fisher B, Fram P, Waring M. Odour absorbing dressings: a comparative laboratory study. World Wide Wounds 1998. Online. Available: http://www.worldwidewounds. com/1998/march/Odour-Absorbing-Dressings/odour-absorbing-dressings.html 7 October 2003.

99. Williams C. 3M cavilon no sting barrier film in the protection of vulnerable skin. Br J Nurs 1998; 7(10):613–615.

100. Young T. Reaping the benefits of foam dressings. Community Nurse 1998; 4(5):47–48.

101. Dealey C. The care of wounds. Oxford: Blackwell Science; 1999.

102. Dunford C, Cooper R, Molan P, White R. The use of honey in wound management. Nurs Stand 2000; 15(11):63–68.

103. Molan PC. The role of honey in the management of wounds. J Wound Care 1999; 8(8):415–418.

104. Williams C. Product focus: an investigation of the benefits of aquacel hydrofibre wound dressing. Br J Nurs 1999; 8(10):676–680.

105. Williams C. Product focus: the benefits and application of the lyofoam product range. Br J Nurs 1999; 8(11):745–749.

106. Jones V, Milton T. When and how to use adhesive film dressings. Nurs Times 2000; 96(14 NTPlus):3–4.

107. Jones V, Milton T. When and how to use hydrocolloid dressings. Nurs Times 2000; 96(4 NTPlus):5–7.

108. Jones V, Milton T. When and how to use hydrogels. Nurs Times 2000; 96(23 NTPlus):3–4.

109. Morgan DA. Formulary of wound management products: a guide for healthcare staff. 8th edn. Surrey: Euromed Communications; 2000.

110. Thomas S. Alginate dressings in surgery and wound management – part 1. J Wound Care 2000; 9(2):56–60.

111. Pudner R. Low/non-adherent dressings in wound management. Br J Community Nurs 2001; 15(8):12, 15–17.

112. Ballard K, Baxter H. Promoting healing in static wounds. Nurs Times 2001; 97(14):52.

113. Moore P, Foster L. Acute surgical wound care 1: an overview of treatment. Br J Nurs 1998; 7(18):1101–1106.

114. Galvani J. Not yet cut and dried. Nurs Times 1997; 93(16):88–89.

115. Stoios N. Prevention of extravasation in intravenous therapy: a review of the research evidence Nuritinga: an electronic journal of nursing 1999, 2. Online. Available: http://www.healthsci.utas.edu.au/tson/nuritinga/issue2/prevention_of_extravasation.pdf 7 October 2003.

116. Thomas S, Rowe HN, Keats J, Morgan RJH. The management of extravasation injury in neonates. World Wide Wounds 1997. Online. Available: http://www.worldwidewounds.com/1997/october/Neonates/NeonatePaper.html 7 October 2003.

117. Montrose PA. Extravasation management. Semin Oncol Nurs 1987; 3(2):128–132.

118. Murhammer JM. Management of intravenous extravasations. Virtual Hospital: P & T News: University of Iowa Health Care 1996. Online. Available: http://www.vh.org/adult/provider/pharmacy services/PTNews/1996/12.96.PTN.html 7 October 2003.

119. McCaffrey Boyle D, Engelking C. Vesicant extravasation: myths and realities. Oncol Nurs Forum 1995; 22(1):57–67.

120. Mulder GD, Haberer PA, Jeter KF. Clinicians pocket guide to chronic wound repair. Pennsylvania: Wound Care Communications Network Springhouse Corporation; 1999.

121. Vowden KR, Vowden P. Wound debridement, part 2: sharp techniques. J Wound Care 1999; 8(6):291–294.

122. Freedline A. Types of wound debridement. The Wound Care Information Network 1999. Online. Available: http://www.medicaledu.com/debridhp.htm 7 October 2003.

123. Bale S. A guide to wound debridement. J Wound Care 1997; 6(4):179–182.

124. Werner KG. Guideline for the outpatient treatment of pressure ulcer. Compliance Network Physicians/Health Force Initiative, Inc. 1999. Online. Available: http://www.cnhfi.org/pressure_ulcer/inhalt.htm#1 7 October 2003.

125. Thomas S, Jones M, Shutler S, Jones S. Maggots in wound debridement – an introduction. Surgical Materials Testing Laboratory, Bridgend. 1999. Online. Available: http://www.smtl.co.uk/WMPRC/Maggots/maggots.html 7 October 2003.

126. Thomas S, Andrews A, Jones M. The use of larval therapy in wound management. J Wound Care 1998; 7(10):521–524.

127. Morykwas MJ, Argenta LC, Shelton-Brown EI, McGuirt W. Vacuum-assisted closure: a new method for wound control and treatment: animal studies and basic foundation. Ann Plast Surg 1997; 38(6):553–562.

128. Grocott P. The management of fungating wounds. J Wound Care 1999: 8(5):232–234.

129. Young T. Wound care: the challenge of managing fungating wounds. Community Nurse 1997; 3(9 Nurse Prescriber):41–44.

130. Carville K. Caring for cancerous wounds in the community. J Wound Care 1995; 4(2):66–68.

131. Haisfield-Wolfe ME, Rund C. Malignant cutaneous wounds: a management protocol. Ostomy Wound Manage 1997; 43(1):56–66.

132. Ivetic O, Lyne PA. Fungating and ulcerating malignant lesions: a review of the literature. J Adv Nurs 1990; 15:83–88.

133. Wilks L, White K, Smeal T, Beale B. Malignant wound management: what dressings do nurses use? J Wound Care 2001; 10(3):65–70.

134. Laverty D, Cooper J, Soady S. Wound management. In: Mallett J, Dougherty L, eds. The Royal Marsden Hospital manual of clinical nursing procedures. 5th edn. Oxford: Blackwell Science; 2000:681–710.

135. Hallett A. Fungating wounds. Nurs Times 1995; 91(39):81–85.

136. Naylor W. Part 2: Symptom self-assessment in the management of fungating wounds. World Wide Wounds 2002. Online. Available: http://www.worldwidewounds.com/2002/july /Naylor-Part2/Wound-Assessment-Tool.html 7 October 2003.

137. Van Toller S. Invisible wounds: the effects of skin ulcer malodours. J Wound Care 1994; 3(2):103–105.

138. Haughton W, Young T. Common problems in wound care: malodorous wounds. Br J Nurs 1995; 4(16):959–963.

139. Jones M, Davey J, Champion A. Dressing wounds. Nurs Stand 1998; 12(39):47–52.

140. Collier M. Management of patients with fungating wounds. Nurs Stand 2000; 15(11):46–52.

141. Grocott P. The palliative management of fungating malignant wounds. J Wound Care 1995; 4(5):240–242.

142. Davis V. Goal-setting aids care. Nurs Times 1995; 91(39):72–75.

143. Boardman M, Mellor K, Neville B. Treating a patient with a heavily exuding malodorous fungating ulcer. J Wound Care 1993; 2(2):74–76.

144. Manning MP. Metastasis to skin. Semin Oncol Nurs 1998; 14(3):240–243.

145. Emflorgo CA. The assessment and treatment of wound pain. J Wound Care 1999; 8(8):384–385

146. Miller C. Management of skin problems: nursing aspects. In: Doyle D, Hanks GWC, MacDonald N, eds. Oxford textbook of palliative medicine. 2nd edn. Oxford: Oxford University Press; 1998:642–656.

147. Hampton JP. The use of metronidazole in the treatment of malodorous wounds. J Wound Care 1996; 5(9):421–426.

148. Pudner R. The management of patients with a fungating or malignant wound. Br J Community Nurs 1998; 12(9) 30, 32, 34.

149. Back IN, Finlay I. Analgesic effect of topical opioids on painful skin ulcers. J Pain Symptom Manage 1995; 10(7):493.

150. Twillman RK, Long TD, Cathers TA, Mueller DW. Treatment of painful skin ulcers with topical opioids. J Pain Symptom Manage 1999; 17(4):288–292.

151. Krajnik M, Zylicz Z. Topical morphine for cuta-neous cancer pain. Palliat Med 1997; 11(4):326 (Letter).

152. Hollinworth H. Less pain, more gain. Nurs Times 1997; 93(46):89–91

153. Ryman L, Rankin-Box D. Relaxation and visualization. In: Rankin-Box D, ed. The nurse's handbook of complementary therapies. 2nd edn. London: Baillière Tindall; 2001:251–258.

154. Downing J. Pain in the patient with cancer. Nursing Times Clinical Monographs No 5. London: NT Books; 1999.

155. Grocott P. Controlling bleeding in fragile fungating tumours. J Wound Care 1998; 7(7):342 (Letter).

156. Grocott P. Palliative management of fungating malignant wounds. J Community Nurs 2000; 14(3):31–2, 35–6, 38.

157. Dean A, Tuffin P. Fibrinolytic inhibitors for cancer-associated bleeding problems. J Pain Symptom Manage 1997; 13(1):20–24

158. Grocott P. Practical changes. Nurs Times 1993; 89(7):64–70.

159. Saunders S. Mutual support. Nurs Times 1997; 93(32):76–82.

160. Collett K. Practical aspects of stoma management. Nurs Stand 2002; 17(8): 45–52.

161. Black PK. Holistic stoma care. Edinburgh: Baillière Tindall: 2000.

162. Nicholls RJ. Surgical procedures. In Myers C, ed. Stoma care nursing a patient centred approach. London: Arnold; 1996:90–122.

163. Black P. Practical stoma care. Nurs Stand 2000; 14(41): 47–53.

164. Baxter A, Salter M. Stoma care. In: Mallett J, Dougherty L, eds. The Royal Marsden Hospital manual of clinical nursing procedures. 5th edn. Oxford: Blackwell Science; 2000:554–565.

165. Taylor P. Care of patients with complications following formation of a stoma. Prof Nurs 2001; 17(4):252–254.

166. Martin EA, ed. Concise colour medical diction-ary. Oxford: Oxford University Press; 1996.

167. Meadows C. Stoma and fistula care. In: Bruce L, Finlay TMD, eds. Nursing in gastroenterology. Edinburgh: Churchill Livingstone; 1997:85–118.

168. Forbes A, Myers C. Enterocutaneous fistula and their management. In: Myers C, ed. Stoma care nursing a patient-centred approach. London: Arnold; 1996:63–77.

169. Benbow M. The use of wound drainage bags for complex wounds. Br J Nurs 2001; 10(19):1298–1301.

170. Cro C, George KJ, Donnelly J, Irwin ST, Gardiner KR. Vacuum assisted closure system in the management of enterocutaneous fistulae. Postgrad Med J 2002; 78(920):364–365.

171. Kitchen A, Ireland J. London Standing Conference standard framework/guide: skin care for patients having radiotherapy 2002. Online. Available: http://www.london.nhs.uk/lscn/documents/LS Cradio.doc 2 September 2004.

CHAPTER 25

Lymphoedema

Julie-Ann MacLaren

CHAPTER CONTENTS

Introduction   559

Incidence and prevalence   560

Pathophysiology of cancer-related
lymphoedema   560

Differential diagnosis   561

Assessing the extent of lymphoedema   562

The patient's experience of lymphoedema   562
  Pain and altered sensation   562
  Orthopaedic problems and functional
  ability   563
  The emotional cost of lymphoedema   563
  Assessing quality of life with
  lymphoedema   564

Treatment options   565
  Complex decongestive therapy   565
  Application of compression   566
  Multi-layer lymphoedema bandaging   566
  Compression garments   566
  Promoting skin hygiene   567
  Infection   567
  Exercise and movement   568
  Strenuous exercise   568
  Lymphatic drainage   568
  Simple lymphatic drainage   569

Conclusion and implications for
practice   569

References   570

INTRODUCTION

Many patients undergoing surgery or radiotherapy for cancer are at risk of developing lymphoedema. As an incurable and progressive condition characterized by chronic swelling of the limb, trunk or head and neck,[1] it can cause significant physical, emotional and psychological morbidity.[2] Lymphoedema may also occur as a result of disease progression.[3]

Taking its lead from the practices of the lymphology clinics of Germany and Austria, conservative treatment of lymphoedema has become the remit of cancer nurses and other members of the multidisciplinary team in cancer care. Treatment facilities throughout Europe vary, leading to increasing concern about the provision of lymphoedema research,

treatment and educational preparation of nurses and therapists.[4] Despite this, innovative approaches such as statutory guarantees of treatment provision (Sweden),[5] treatment and research workgroups (the Netherlands)[6] and the possibility of yearly complex decongestive therapy (CDT) treatment through social insurance systems (Germany and Austria) have developed to meet local needs.

However, provision of services for the treatment and ongoing management of lymphoedema are only part of the story. As a relatively new area of treatment focus, lymphoedema management has yet to have the evidence base for all treatment modalities fully explored. This has led to a lack of standardization in the assessment, implementation and evaluation of treatment. This chapter will therefore consider the pathophysiology of cancer-related lymphoedema and explore the treatment options currently in use throughout Europe, identifying the evidence base and best practice within this area of cancer management.

INCIDENCE AND PREVALENCE

The incidence of lymphoedema within a cancer population is disputed within the literature, and is related to the cancer treatment received by patients, and their disease status. The key studies in this area have been British,[7,8] with little data available from other European countries. Figures of between 6% and 62% have been recorded for women receiving treatment for breast cancer.[8–13]. A combination of radiotherapy and surgery accounts for the higher incidence figures expressed.

A commonly quoted study by Kissin et al[8] reports the incidence of lymphoedema following treatment for breast cancer as 25% in women who have received either axillary surgery or radiotherapy for their disease, and a significantly greater incidence of 38.3% for those patients who have both treatment modalities. More recent research indicates that clinical advances in minimally invasive axillary surgery and radiotherapy treatment have been effective in reducing the incidence of breast cancer-related lymphoedema.[14]

The broader picture is highlighted by Stanton et al,[15] suggesting that as 1 in 12 women has a lifetime risk of developing breast cancer, almost three-quarters of a million patients with breast cancer have a lifetime risk of developing lymphoedema. Reviews of prevalence suggest that between 12.5% and 28%[8,16] of the population, having received treatment for breast cancer, will experience lymphoedema. An estimated crude prevalence of 1.33 cases per 1000 population has recently been suggested, with increased prevalence noted with age and female gender.[17]

Few data are available on the incidence and prevalence of other types of cancer-related lymphoedema. It is possible that the incidence of lower limb lymphoedema caused by cancer and its treatment mirrors that of breast cancer-related lymphoedema.[18] Incidence figures of around 16% feature in the literature,[19] but appear to have been gained through smaller-scale studies with limited scope in patient follow-up, and may, therefore be unrepresentative of the population at large.

Compression of lymphatic channels within the peritoneum due to tumour bulk has been suggested as a potential mechanism for the development of lower limb lymphoedema,[20] whereas inguinal lymph node dissection[21] and/or radiotherapy for pelvic malignancies[22] are also identified as risk factors.

Head and neck lymphoedema following neck dissection and radiotherapy are poorly represented within the literature, despite causing deformity and functional impairment.[23] Although neck and facial swelling are a feature of both post-surgical and post-irradiation recovery,[24] these tend to be transient in nature, and chronic lymphoedema a relative rarity. However, patients undergoing bilateral neck dissection and radical radiotherapy are at the greatest risk of developing chronic facial or neck oedema.[25]

PATHOPHYSIOLOGY OF CANCER-RELATED LYMPHOEDEMA

Cancer-related lymphoedema arises due to a failure of the lymphatic drainage system where an imbalance between microvascular filtration rate and lymphatic drainage rate develops due to cancer treatment damaged or obliterated lymph nodes and vessels.[26] Further to this, lymph vessels may become obstructed through infection or some inflammatory processes. Although lymph vessels are generally capable of regeneration, and can develop new collateral vessels, vessel regrowth is greatly impaired in the presence of extensive scar tissue formation or fibrosis.[27] As a result, lymphatic fluid stagnates within the interstitial spaces, leading to expansion and, consequently, swelling occurs.

Lymphatic fluid (lymph) consists of plasma protein, waste products, other macromolecules and water.[28] In initial stages, the swelling is soft and pits easily. However, the stagnation of plasma proteins causes an inflammatory response where fibrin and later collagen are deposited within the skin, increasing production of connective tissue and initiating skin thickening and loss of elasticity.[29] This also precipitates the development of skin folds, which can add to the shape and size distortion of a swollen limb,[30] as the skin stretches to accommodate the bulk of the oedema.

These changes affect the mechanical removal of lymph from the interstitium (the lymphatic pump) as the skin normally provides counterpressure to muscular movement, which propels lymph from superficial vessels to its drainage pathways in the deeper lymphatic trunks: in its swollen state, the skin is unable to provide counterpressure. Concomitant paralysis, neuropathy and limb dependency further diminish the efficiency of the lymphatic pump.[31]

DIFFERENTIAL DIAGNOSIS

A differential diagnosis of lymphoedema within the cancer setting must take into consideration many physical and psychological aspects of treatment and patient care. Many medical conditions and prescribed drugs may precipitate limb or truncal oedema, and therefore it is essential that assessment takes into consideration the aetiology of an individual's oedema. The presence of active disease must always be a consideration where lymphoedema occurs, and appropriate oncological support sought where this is suspected.

The time and nature of onset of the swelling will give an indication of the nature of the swelling. Swelling which develops immediately following surgery or radiotherapy may be due to acute inflammation and subside after a few weeks.[32] Similarly, oedema that occurs through infection, acute inflammatory episode or venous thrombosis may be acute in nature and resolve spontaneously after appropriate medical treatment. Persistent swelling may indicate lymphoedema, which is more chronic in its presentation.

Identifying trends and patterns in onset and fluctuation of swelling can give insights into the aetiology and diagnosis of swelling. Lymphoedema of sudden onset may be precipitated by trigger incidents (Box 25.1) relating to

Box 25.1

> **Potential trigger events in the development of lymphoedema**
>
> - Infection
> - Inflammatory processes
> - Metastatic or locally progressive disease
> - Limb dependence
> - Invasive or constrictive clinical procedures: e.g. sphygmomanometry, venepuncture or phlebotomy

increased physical effort, limb dependence, infection or inflammatory processes (including clinical procedures).[33] Where onset of oedema is more gradual, no trigger factors may be obvious.

The advice given to patients to avoid venepuncture, phlebotomy or blood pressure recording to the swollen area is precautionary rather than evidence-based advice,[34, 35] as the association of lymphoedema development with these clinical interventions is documented in the literature.[36] The physiological principle is that trauma to the oedematous area will increase capillary filtration rate, leading to an increase in swelling where drainage is already compromised.

Where the swelling predates cancer diagnosis and treatment, other causes of oedema must be considered. Other causes of oedema (Table 25.1) must be ruled out prior to a diagnosis of lymphoedema and subsequent treatment. Where these conditions coincide with cancer treatment-related lymphoedema, liaison with dermatology or tissue viability teams may need to be considered.

In a palliative care setting, the extent of anticancer treatment remains a factor in the aetiology of lymphoedema. However, several additional factors unique to the patient with advanced disease must be considered. Fungating tumours and skin nodules may develop where there is tumour infiltration of the skin from either local tumours or metastatic spread. These further disrupt blood and lymphatic circulation in the affected area, causing tissue necrosis.[38] Also to be considered are issues of decreased mobility and blood dyscrasias such as hypoproteinaemia, anaemia, cardiac insufficiency or failure, or the effects of medications such as steroids, which may also cause swelling.

Table 25.1: Non-lymphoedematous causes of swelling

Arm oedema	Lower limb oedema
Axillary vein thrombosis	Chronic venous or arterial insufficiency
Superior vena cava obstruction (also causing arm, hand or facial swelling)	Deep vein thrombosis
	Lipoedema (related to fat distribution)
Obesity	
Vascular obstruction: the presence of dilated or collateral veins or extremity cyanosis[37]	

ASSESSING THE EXTENT OF LYMPHOEDEMA

Assessment of lymphoedema invariably involves an estimation of the extent of swelling present. Common definitions of lymphoedema relate to the degree of swelling present within a limb, with an excess volume of greater than 200 ml or 10% in the swollen limb used as a definitive measure of lymphoedema.[39,40] The degree of fibrotic skin change within the swollen area may also be used as a measure of the extent or grade of lymphoedema present.[3]

Accuracy and precision in measuring and monitoring lymphoedema requires the adoption of standardized and reproducible assessment tools.[41,42] Measurement tools vary amongst practitioners, although the measurement of total limb volume and comparison with an unaffected side appears to be a standardized measure, and measurement techniques utilizing water immersion, tape measurement and optoelectronic scanning have been validated for use with patients.[43–45] Where bilateral limb, facial or truncal swelling occurs, comparison of limb volume measurements becomes less useful, and comparison of longitudinal differences, where achievable, in volume may provide a useful indication of volume reduction and treatment progress. Any measurement schedule implemented must be flexible to take into consideration the needs of patients at their point of the cancer trajectory and therefore adapted to suit the needs of individual patients.

THE PATIENT'S EXPERIENCE OF LYMPHOEDEMA

Physical measurement of lymphoedema is only a small part of the assessment of lymphoedema. As important as determining the extent of lymphoedema is ascertaining its effect on the daily life of the patient. The impact of lymphoedema is complex and may encompass physical, psychological and social aspects and is a source of major morbidity.[2] Symptoms such as burning sensations, irritation, dull or severe pain, exhaustion and intolerance to temperature are described alongside reports of functional diminishment, skin changes and altered body image.[46–48]

Pain and altered sensation

Pain for the patient with cancer-related lymphoedema may not be solely confined to the immediate postoperative or radiotherapy recovery period. Discomfort may be experienced due to stretching of the skin and tissues.[49–51] Where the weight of a swollen limb is considerable, the patient may complain of a deep ache due to the heaviness of the limb and associated musculoskeletal strain.[52] Patients undergoing mastectomy for breast cancer may experience postmastectomy, intercostobrachial neuralgia as a result of their treatment.[51]

However, lymphoedema should *not* cause acute or severe pain and, if this is experienced, the underlying cause must be identified and treated. The four main causes of pain occurring in a swollen limb are infection, inflammation, thrombosis and disease progression.[52] Urgent referral to an oncologist is necessary where disease progression is suspected, for further investigation and treatment.

Pain and altered sensation may occur as the result of oedema, fibrosis, nerve damage caused by treatment or advancing disease or ischaemic damage caused by microvascular injury.[53,54] Nerve damage such as carpal tunnel syndrome, brachial plexus neuropathy and cervical root entrapment have been identified in patients undergoing breast cancer treatment,[53] with an estimated 30% of patients experiencing symptoms such as partial or complete loss of function and altered sensations such as tingling, numbness and loss of grip following axillary dissection for breast cancer.[55]

Neurological deficits in a swollen limb pose two main difficulties. First, function may be compromised, leading to problems of dependency oedema due to unsupported lymphatic and venous pumps, and the associated loss of role and/or mobility. Secondly, with loss of sensation the risk of injury increases and this makes the patient particularly vulnerable to infections. Where swelling affects the head and neck region, neurological deficiency may hinder more basic functions such as respiration, eating and drinking, eyesight and effective communication.[24,25] Although rarely described in the literature, neuropathies affecting the lower limb following pelvic cancer treatment may be manifest in problems such disturbed gait, sciatic pain and foot drop.[56] Assessment by both physiotherapist and occupational therapist can be invaluable in suggesting methods of reducing discomfort, ways of supporting the limb and suitable active or passive exercises to restore function and mobility to the limbs.

Orthopaedic problems and functional ability

In the months following surgery for breast cancer, a series of physiological changes takes place. Decrease in shoulder range of movement can begin to develop as soon as 1 month after breast cancer surgery. After 6 months, there is a characteristic decrease in muscle

strength in the affected limb. At 2 months, shoulder abduction, flexion and external rotation is reduced in patients who have also undergone postoperative radiotherapy, also corresponding with increased limb volume. At the 6-month point, decrease in muscle strength has been noted for this group.[57]

The literature surrounding functional deficit within lymphoedema management focuses on the experiences of the patient with upper limb lymphoedema following breast cancer intervention. Reduction in mobility as a result of lower limb oedema is common alongside issues of early fatigue, exhaustion, lowered stamina, decreased muscle strength and inability to stand for long periods.[31,52]

Difficulty moving the limb due to its increased size, or the presence of neuropathy may mean the patient will use it less, leading to joint stiffness and associated discomfort. Incidence of shoulder stiffness and reduced movement following breast cancer treatment has been estimated at 57–75%,[16,39,49] with an estimated 31% of patients still experiencing some degree of orthopaedic-related pain 5 years after cancer treatment has ended.[39] Shoulder impairment following breast cancer treatment has been defined as an impairment of 15 degrees or more in relation to the preoperative value. The impact of shoulder stiffness is evident in difficulties in hair-brushing, and reaching overhead, while fine movements such as doing-up zippers may also be affected by neuropathy.[16] Careful pretreatment assessment of joint mobility and ongoing monitoring and treatment of impairment is therefore needed alongside interventions to reduce the volume of swelling present, to minimize the effect of neuropathic and orthopaedic discomfort on activities of daily living.

The emotional cost of lymphoedema

Patients who develop lymphoedema face a harder task in coming to terms with their cancer diagnosis than those patients who do not develop lymphoedema. This is demonstrated in the incidence of psychological morbidity, including depression, high levels of sexual, functional and social dysfunction, and poorer adjustment to disease.[58–60] The psychological responses to lymphoedema as a chronic condition may be conceptualized in terms of the stress response coping theories.

A stressful stimulus such as lymphoedema diagnosis is seen as a crisis as it forces extreme emotional and practical demands and changes upon the individual, changing radically, everyday life and expectations of the future.[61] The unpredictable nature of lymphoedema and the lack of information and prior knowledge available about it exacerbate this crisis, and compound the common assumption held by patients that lymphoedema heralds a recurrence of their cancer.[58] Stressors such as the fear of cancer recurrence or progression, the presence of new symptoms and the disparity between premorbid and illness states have been identified in the literature.[62,63]

Body image is a vulnerable part of our make-up and formed in a personal and social context.[64] Deviation from 'normal' representations of the body can cause emotional and psychological trauma to a person with lymphoedema.[61] In a study of patients with breast cancer, Woods[65] found patients with breast cancer-related lymphoedema lacked confidence in their appearance and body image, with many patients changing their style of clothing in an attempt to hide their swollen limb. Withdrawal from social interaction, hobbies and changes to occupational circumstance has also been influenced by the presence of lymphoedema.[65] The distress experienced by patients may be unrelated to the volume of lymphoedema present, with patients with minimal swelling experiencing similar problems.[66]

Experience of physical symptoms provides major psychological stressors for the patient with lymphoedema. Symptoms such as pain, discomfort, limb heaviness, reduced mobility and impaired functions have been identified in both lymphoedema and broader cancer populations as potential stressors.[52,67] However, it is those patients who experience pain alongside their lymphoedema who are most likely to suffer the highest levels of psychological distress.[59]

An individual's experience of lymphoedema is unique. Personal responses to lymphoedema stem from societal and individual expectations of what is normal and desirable. Social and cultural factors will also influence an individual's response to the swelling experienced.[68] Personal reactions to the stereotypes posed by cancer-related lymphoedema depend upon the person's usual coping mechanisms, the significance of the altered body image for the future and the level of support received from others.

The lived experience of lymphoedema is, therefore, important to comprehend. Individual differences are likely to be apparent, however. Hare[69] discusses elements of loss, anxiety and lifestyle changes caused by the presence of lymphoedema. Issues of poor information availability and the perceived lack of knowledge base of health professionals pertaining to lymphoedema have been identified as contributing to patients' psychological distress.[69]

Assessing quality of life with lymphoedema

Quality of life for patients with lymphoedema has been measured using a variety of tools, although consensus on the best approach has not been determined. The Psychological Adjustment to Illness Scale (PAIS)[70] has been used to demonstrate adjustment to illness of all domains of health care, and has been successfully validated for use with patients with cancer-related lymphoedema.[58,65,66] In comparison, the Nottingham Health Questionnaire (NHQ) has been used with good effect in assessing patients' experiences of lymphoedema.[71] Wide-scale validation of the FACT-B+4 quality of life scale assessing postoperative arm morbidity in patients with breast cancer demonstrates internal consistency and test–retest reliability, and suitability for use in longitudinal clinical trials with patients with lymphoedema.

Quality of life assessment tools are often only used within the context of research studies, and not as part of day-to-day patient assessment. This potentially leads to clinicians failing to assess and address patient-reported symptoms, and thus the true proportion of patients presenting with issues affecting quality of life may not be elucidated.[72] However, implementation of quality of life scales relevant to patients with lymphoedema should be devised with caution, as methodological weaknesses and failure to test unvalidated checklists may skew data collected in this field.[72]

TREATMENT OPTIONS

Treatment for lymphoedema at present is not curative, but aims to reduce or maintain oedema through reducing excessive capillary filtration and maximizing lymphatic drainage.[73] Conservative treatment is nurse- or therapist-driven throughout Europe, and consists of the application of external compression administered as either compression garments or multi-layer lymphoedema bandaging, exercise, skin care and manual or simple lymphatic drainage massage.[27] The role of the nurse or therapist in providing information and support to empower the patient in self-care of this chronic condition is an important aspect of lymphoedema management.

Other non-mainstream treatments include surgical treatments such as liposuction and controlled compression,[74] which have demonstrated good results in long-term maintenance of limb volume reduction without further damage to the structure of the lymphatic vessels. The use of hyperbaric oxygen treatments is showing promising results in reduction of lymphoedema and softening of radiation fibrosis.[75,76]

The literature identifies several studies in lymphoedema management which tend to focus upon either the intensive phase of treatment, where multi-layered lymphoedema bandaging (MLLB) and manual lymphatic drainage (MLD) are the compression and massage modalities of choice, or the maintenance phase, where bandages and MLD are substituted for compression hosiery and simple lymphatic drainage. It can be difficult where treatment relies on a quartet of modalities to tease out the exact contribution of each modality; therefore, where research is not forthcoming, a theoretical rationale for treatment use will be offered.

Complex decongestive therapy

CDT refers to an intensive system of lymphoedema management that utilizes all four cornerstones of treatment: namely, the application of MLLB, skin hygiene measures, exercise and MLD.[77–79] Treatment is provided (usually as an inpatient) for a period of 2–4 weeks, making this a costly and manpower-intensive treatment modality.

CDT is usually reserved for patients with complex lymphoedemas, which, due to poor shaping, gross size, tissue fibrosis or skin damage, are unable to be fitted with or tolerate compression hosiery.[80–82] Studies investigating the combined effect of CDT generally demonstrate significant but short-term effectiveness of this treatment regimen in gaining control of or palliating lymphoedema.[80,81] The efficacy of CDT in comparison to treatment with compression hosiery (as maintenance phase treatment) has been demonstrated for both upper and lower limbs, in a randomized controlled study.[82] However, CDT should not be used in isolation from maintenance therapies, which replace lymphoedema bandaging with compression garments, and MLD with simpler lymphatic drainage techniques, as these form an important component of ongoing self-care for patients.

In many treatment centres, pneumatic compression is used as an adjunct to CDT.[83] In addition to daily multi-layer lymphoedema bandaging and MLLB, the patient also receives treatment using a pneumatic pump device, which has been shown to reduce oedema volume through enhancing venous return, rather than through removal of protein or lymph.[84] Other centres substitute MLLB for the use of pneumatic or sequential compression devices, in both CDT and maintenance phases of treatment.[85,86] Limb volume reductions (both upper and lower limb) of 33–43% in mild or moderate and 19% in cases of severe, long-standing lymphoedema have been documented.[85].

It is possible that provision of CDT alone may not provide the full picture in determining its effectiveness. The extent of swelling on commencement of CDT has been shown to be a more reliable indicator of volume reduction than the time after onset of lymphoedema when the patient presents for treatment.[81] Patients with the least volume of lymphoedema do not have extensive fibrotic skin changes, loss of elasticity or other pathological skin or tissue changes that complicate treatment.[81].

Application of compression

The application of compression to a lymphoedematous limb is the mainstay of lymphoedema treatment. Although not all cancer nurses will be involved in the prescription or application of compression bandaging or garments, it is conceivable that every cancer nurse or therapist will have some contact with patients requiring assistance or advice regarding this treatment modality. Compression is applied though the use of low-stretch bandages and graduated compression garments, although there are an increasing number of rigid support devices now available to provide patient-friendly alternatives or adjuncts to these means of compression.[87]

Low-stretch bandages and rigid hosiery are preferable options in providing compression for lymphoedema treatment. A low resting pressure and a high working pressure allow minimal application of compression at rest, and substantial increases in compression during exercise or limb movement, allowing the bandage/hosiery to be worn comfortably all day.[78] Compression garments are generally removed at night, as capillary filtration reduces with prolonged rest, whereas bandages remain in situ for 24 hours before being renewed by the therapist.

Contraindications for the application of compression include the presence of thrombosis, infection, superior vena cava obstruction (SVCO), severe cardiac failure and arterial insufficiency.[78]

Multi-layer lymphoedema bandaging

MLLB is used during the intensive phase of treatment, with aims to reduce limb volume, improve limb shape and protect fragile skin (Box 25.2).[78,82,88] Oedema is reduced through enhancement of lymphatic formation from the interstitium, and its take-up by the initial or superficial lymphatics. Providing a firm casing against which the muscle can squeeze the superficial lymphatics during activity serves to improve lymphatic drainage, reverse fibrotic and inflammatory skin changes and provide impetus to propel lymph toward the root of the limb.[78] MLLB also has benefits over compression garments where skin folds are present, as garments can gather and tourniquet around skin folds, increasing the risk of thrombosis formation.[78]

Lymphorrhoea may be treated through the gentle application of short-stretch compression bandages (discussed later) over non-adhesive absorbent dressings, and padding of skin folds, and bony prominences. Bandages need replacing whenever exudate strikes through the bandaging, with treatment for 24–48 hours able to control most episodes of lymphoedema.[88–90] Where pain is present, bandaging may not be tolerated. Occasionally, application of compression may be anatomically impossible.[79,91]

Compression garments

Compression through application of an elasticated garment is an essential element in the maintenance phase of lymphoedema management. Any improvement gained through intensive bandaging, exercise or lymphatic drainage is lost if the patient does not wear an appropriate compression garment, as oedema bulk will reaccumulate into the overstretched tissues of the swollen limb.[78] As such, compression garments form an integral cornerstone of treatment.[92]

Compression garments for both arms and legs are available in a wide variety of styles, sizes and compression classes, with off-the-shelf and made-to-measure varieties available for both limb and head and neck oedema. Compression classes for garments are not standardized internationally, with compression garments made to British standards providing less compression than European-manufactured garments.

Box 25.2

Indications for multi-layered lymphoedema bandaging[72,76,82]

- Long-standing or severe lymphoedema
- Awkwardly shaped limbs or skin folds
- Lymphorrhoea (weeping of lymph from affected limb) or fragile skin
- Hardened fibrotic skin conditions
- Excess limb volume greater than 20%

All grades of compression garment have a potential use in the management of lymphoedema, with lower compression class garments providing gentle support or compression in the palliative care setting, or for patients who are unable to tolerate or apply firmer varieties. The use of antiembolism stockings within hospitals to treat lymphoedema should also be avoided, as they do not provide graduated external compression and therefore do not reduce or control swelling.[78]

Compression sleeves work by exerting sufficient compression to the swollen tissues to effect a raise in interstitial fluid pressure, with arm swelling controlled through the subsequent reduction of fluid filtration rate and/or raising the fluid drainage rate from the swollen arm.[93] A similar effect has been noted in compression garments for the lower limbs, where calf muscle pump exercises in patients wearing compression stockings produces a similar effect in raising tissue fluid and lymphatic pressure.[94] The use of padding within the gusset of undergarments may provide sufficient compression to treat vulvar, perineal or scrotal swelling, although few garments are available commercially with this intent.

Other garments which may be used to treat limb oedema fall into the category of 'adjustable compression gradient wrap garments'.[87,95,96] These garments may be worn in conjunction with regular compression garments, or may be available as garments to be worn overnight. Patient education is paramount in the safe use of such garments, as there are limited studies documenting their use.

Promoting skin hygiene

The evidence for most skin care advice in lymphoedema management is either anecdotal or based upon physiological principles rather than clinical trial data.[33] The main aims of intervention are to maintain or improve the integrity of the skin, promote comfort from tautness or stretching of the skin, to reverse dry skin and thickened skin changes where possible and to prevent acute inflammatory episodes from developing.[30,79,89,90,97,98,99]

The nursing role in skin care for lymphoedema is based around advice to the patient regarding appropriate skin hygiene measures, and providing this care for patients who are unable to do so for themselves. It proves to be an area of care which can afford the patient a great deal of comfort, yet is often overlooked in importance,[98] despite being an area of care that all nurses in cancer or community care can be involved in.

Current advice to patients is based upon careful washing of the affected area with a gentle, non-perfumed soap, cleanser or aqueous cream. The skin should be carefully dried, before application of suitable emollients. Emollients should be chosen according to the condition of the skin, with simple unperfumed cream preparations suitable for soft, supple skin, and ointment and oil-based preparations necessary for dry and hardened skin conditions.[90] Treatment of hyperkeratosis and papillomatosis (hardened skin conditions) should be undertaken on direction of a dermatologist.[30,90]

Skin folds or creases between digits can harbour fungal infections such as *Candida* sp. (thrush) or tinea pedis.[98] Patients should be advised that these conditions may be recurrent and need treating with appropriate topical antifungal preparations which can generally be bought without prescription at a pharmacy. If the feet are affected, then shoes and other footwear should also be treated to prevent continual reinfection. Patients with fungal infections resistant to simple antifungal applications should be referred to either a general practitioner or practice nurse for further pharmaceutical intervention.

Infection

Where infection or acute inflammatory episodes (AIE) occur, patients should be advised to seek medical advice, as intervention with antibiotics is recommended, as is bedrest and increase in fluid intake until symptoms of raised temperature, rigor, redness, pain and increased swelling subside. Repeated AIE is common in lymphoedema, and swelling may worsen with each episode due to cumulative intraluminal lymph vessel damage.[99] Long-term or prophylactic treatment with antibiotics may prove necessary in patients who have repeated attacks of AIE, although basic skin care advice should still be followed wherever possible to minimize soreness and promote skin repair.[100]

EXERCISE AND MOVEMENT

Muscular contraction and relaxation in the foot, calf and arm not only enhance venous and lymphatic return[48] but also provide a massaging effect to the overlying tissues, stimulating the superficial lymphatic network within the skin. These are also the main factors influencing working and resting pressure of compression bandaging and compression garments, which in turn influence lymphatic return.[46] Maintenance of good limb function is essential for quality of life, as immobility of a limb can reduce lymphatic drainage and lead to joint stiffness, reduced function and discomfort[48] and may be further compromised by tissue fibrosis or advanced local disease.[101]

Prevention of joint stiffness needs to be addressed at an early stage of cancer treatment, with clinical initiatives such as exercise classes and information booklets providing clear instruction on interventions and self-care for a population which may not be used to such activity.[102,103] Patients developing lymphoedema of the arm following breast cancer intervention tend to have a higher preoperative body mass index (BMI)[104,105] and significant reduction of their arm activity following surgery, in comparison to those who had not developed arm swelling and whose activity schedule remained largely unaltered.[105]

Strenuous exercise

Although exercise and movement are considered essential for maintenance of limb function and mobility, assessment of the fitness level of the patient must be undertaken, and avoidance of overly strenuous exercise for their ability level stressed. Vigorous exercise requires a sudden increase in blood supply, therefore leading to an increased capillary filtration rate, and thus increased production of lymph with a potential for further swelling.[31] No published data look at the level or intensity of exercise that can be performed safely by all following axillary or inguinal dissection,[46] although where patients are engaged in a gradual return to exercise activity and fitness training regimens, positive benefits in terms of increased stamina, strength, flexibility, well-being and morale are documented with no adverse effect on volume of lymphoedema.[6,46,106,107]

The patient needs to be aware of the effects exercise has on their oedema, so that activities may be modified for future use. The impact of everyday activities should also be considered as part of the activity profile of each individual. Residual disease and morbidities must also be accounted for in the preparation of any such exercise programme.

Elevation of the resting limb has long been recommended as an aid to volume reduction or maintenance. Elevation of the limb above the level of the heart will force hydrostatic pressure to act in the direction of blood flow and aid venous return, reduce capillary filtration rate and reduce the need for a muscle pump.[31] Although this may be useful for lower limbs, especially where limb dependency is present, its use to reduce arm lymphoedema is questionable and, where used excessively, may exacerbate shoulder stiffness and discomfort,[108,109] and may only be of use to promote comfort and aid venous return during infection or AIE where additional, transient swelling may be present.[100]

Lymphatic drainage

Lymphatic drainage techniques are based upon the technique of MLD, a series of gentle, rhythmical skin movements first developed in the 1930s by Dr Emil Vodder as a tool for facial cosmetic treatment.[110] MLD techniques are designed to move the skin over the underlying tissues, in order to increase evacuation of extracellular fluid from the interstitium and aid its reabsorption by deeper lymphatics without increasing capillary filtration.[83,84,92] Lymph is channelled away from oedematous areas, encouraging the development of anastomoses and collateral lymphatic routes to further improve lymphatic drainage.[111] This technique is directed toward the lymph nodes of the neck, where lymph is filtered into the general circulation.[112] Aside from its effects on lymphoedema, MLD has been claimed to have effects on the nervous, muscular and immune system.[112]

Although recognized as an integral component of lymphoedema management, its efficacy in the context of CDT has been limited to small-scale studies demonstrating its effect on volume reduction. This finding has been counterbalanced by those who have found no significant difference in comparison with a control group not receiving MLD.[57,113,114] Positive outcomes reported include reduction in limb volume, reduced dermal thickness and improved quality of life in the areas of emotional function, sleep disturbance and altered sensation.[114]

Where methods of applying compression are difficult, e.g. in head, neck or truncal lymphoedema, MLD is often the only viable conservative treatment option. Improvements in swelling, swallowing and speaking and improvement in feelings of tension have been documented as a result of MLD treatment with or without made-to-measure compression garments for the head and neck.[24,115]

The use of lymphatic drainage techniques in the presence of active disease is controversial, due to the potential for metastatic spread via the lymphatics.[110] Clinical research, however, reports no increase in local cancer recurrence rates for patients receiving and demonstrable improvements in quality of life.[23] Other contraindications for the use of MLD include acute inflammation (due to infection or allergy), recent thrombosis and oedema caused by congestive cardiac failure or SVCO.[110]

Several schools of MLD are currently in existence, all of which have developed from the original technique of Dr Vodder. Despite similarities in practice, standardization of treatment is yet to become a reality, with discussion about the optimum length of treatment time and possible contraindications to treatment.

Simple lymphatic drainage

Simple lymphatic drainage (SLD) is a simplified and self-administered form of MLD designed to be easily performed by patients, relatives or carers.[114,116] Although no research has specifically explored its efficacy, it is in common use and is advocated by therapists in view of anecdotal reports of good results.[114,116] It does not replace the need for MLD in many patients, but is a useful adjunct to a treatment programme, particularly in the maintenance phase.[92] Uptake and effectiveness of SLD are thought to be related to the ability of the patient to physically perform the massage, whether the patient has had previous experience of MLD, the quality of instruction and their motivation to perform this massage daily.[116]

CONCLUSION AND IMPLICATIONS FOR PRACTICE

Thousands of patients yearly receive appropriate care for lymphoedema. As a complex chronic condition arising from the treatment or advancement of cancer, this requires specialist intervention and dedicated self-care in its control and treatment. The large numbers of patients with a lifelong risk of developing lymphoedema by nature of their disease process or treatment point to a role for all nurses and therapists involved in cancer care.

The pathophysiology of lymphoedema provides the key to appropriate treatment. However, this is reliant on accurate diagnosis of the condition, and recognition of triggers and patterns of swelling. Assessment needs to consider the extent and impact of lymphoedema on patient well-being and quality of life.

The use of compression, exercise, skin hygiene measures and lymphatic drainage techniques have become common throughout Europe and beyond, for the management of lymphoedematous limbs. The challenge is now to standardize their implementation, while remaining open-minded about novel treatments and alternatives. Much currently available research is on a small scale and lacking in generalizability. Further and larger-scale research needs to be funded to explore the experience of the patient with lymphoedema and the efficacy of treatment combinations. A more overt recognition of the problem of lymphoedema needs to be incorporated into cancer nursing curricula to ensure widespread recognition of lymphoedema by both healthcare professionals and patients. Cancer nurses are ideally placed to facilitate appropriate referral, and support self-care by patients, relatives and carers. However, nurses must also be involved in service design and the development of specialist practice roles in order to influence policy, treatment and outcomes.

REFERENCES

1. Williams A. Lymphoedema. In: Corner J, Bailey C, eds. Cancer nursing: care in context, Oxford: Blackwell Science; 2001:383–390.

2. Bianchi J, Todd M. The management of a patient with lymphoedema of the legs. Nurs Stand 2000; 14: 40, 51–56.

3. Keeley V. Classification of lymphoedema. In: Twycross R, Jenns K, Todd J, eds. Lymphoedema. Abingdon, Oxon: Radcliffe Medical Press; 2000:22–43.

4. Oliver G. Lymphoedema: the hidden side effect of cancer. Cancer Nurs Pract 2002: 1(8):8–9.

5. Steen-Zupanc U. pers comm; 2002.

6. Damstra R, de Groot LJ, Hengst-Oppenhuizen, et al. Lymfoedeem in de Practijk. Drachten: Stichting Lymfologie Centrum Noord Nederland; 2000.

7. Mortimer PS. Lymphoedema. Vasc Surg 1996:73–77.

8. Kissin MW, Querci della Rovere G, Easton D, et al. Risk of lymphoedema following the treatment of breast cancer. Br J Surg 1986; 73:589–584.

9. Brennan MJ. Lymphedema following the surgical treatment of breast cancer: a review of pathophysiology and treatment. J Pain Symptom Manage 1992; 7 (2):110–116.

10. Hoe AL, Iven D, Royle GT, et al. Incidence of arm swelling following axillary clearance for breast cancer. Br J Surg 1992; 79:261–262.

11. Paci E, Cariddi A, Barchielli A, et al. Long term sequelae of breast cancer surgery. Tumori 1996; 82:321–324.

12. Petrek JA, Pressman PI, Smith RA. Lymphedema: current issues in research and management. CA Cancer J Clin 2000; 50:292–307.

13. Logan V. Incidence and prevalence of lymphoedema. J Clin Nurs 1995; 4(4):213–219.

14. Suneson BL, Lindholm C, Hamrin E. Clinical incidence of lymphedema in breast cancer patients in Jonkoping County, Sweden. Eur J Cancer Care 1996; 5:7–12.

15. Stanton AWB, Levick JR, Mortimer PS. Current puzzles presented by postmastectomy oedema (breast cancer related lymphoedema). Vasc Med 1996, 1:213–225.

16. Kwan W, Jackson J, Weir LM, et al. Chronic arm morbidity after curative breast cancer treatment: prevalence and impact on quality of life. J Clin Oncol 2002; 20(20):4242–4248.

17. Moffatt C, Franks PJ, Doherty DC, et al Lymphoedema: an underestimated health problem. QJM 2003; 96(10):731–738.

18. Petlund CF. Prevalence and incidence of chronic lymphoedema in a western European country. In Nishi M, Uchino S, Yabuki S, eds. Progress in Lymphology XII, Amsterdam: Excerpta Medical International Congress Service; 1990; 887:391–394

19. Badger C, Seers K, Preston N, et al. Benzo-pyrones for reducing and controlling lymphoedema of the limbs. The Cochrane Database of Systematic Reviews 2002; No. 4.

20. Smith AK, Coakley FV, Jackson R, et al. CT and MRI of retroperitoneal edema associated with large uterine leimyomas. J Comput Assist Tomogr 2002; 26(3):459–461.

21. Spratt J. Groin dissection. J Surg Oncol 2000; 73:243–262.

22. Coleman RL. Vulvar lymphatic mapping: coming of age? Ann Surg Oncol 2002; 9(9):823–825.

23. Preisler VK, Hagen R, Hoppe F. [Indications and risks of manual lymph drainage in head-neck tumors.] Laryngorhinootologie 1998; 77(4):207-212. [in German]

24. Piso DU, Eckardt A, Liebermann A, et al. Early rehabilitation of head-neck edema after curative surgery for orofacial tumors. Am J Phys Med Rehabil 2001; 80(4):261–269.

25. Withey S, Pracey P, Rhys-Evans P. Lymphoedema of the head and neck. In: Twycross R, Jenns K, Todd J, eds. Lymphoedema. Abingdon, Oxon: Radcliffe Medical Press; 2000;306–320.

26. Stanton AW, Holroyd B, Mortimer PS, et al. Comparison of microvascular filtration in human arms with and without postmastectomy oedema. Exp Physiol 1999; 84(2):405–419.

27. Mortimer PS. Investigation and management of lymphoedema. Vasc Med Rev 1990; 1:1–20.

28. Stanton A . How does tissue swelling occur? The physiology and pathophysiology of interstitial fluid formation. In: Twycross R, Jenns K, Todd J, eds. Lymphoedema. Abingdon, Oxon: Radcliffe Medical Press; 2000:11–21.

29. Földi E, Foldi M, Weissleder H. Conservative treatment of lymphoedema of the limbs. Angiology 1985; 36:171–180.

30. Williams A., Venables J. Skin care in patients with uncomplicated lymphoedema. J Wound Care 1996: 5(5):223–226.

31. Hughes K. Exercise and lymphoedema. In: Twycross R, Jenns K, Todd J, eds. Lymphoedema. Abingdon, Oxon: Radcliffe Medical Press; 2000:22–43.

32. Woods M. Using philosophy, knowledge and theory to assess a patient with lymphoedema. Int J Palliat Nurs 2002;, 8 (4):176–181.

33. Harris SR, Hugi MR, Olivotto IA, et al. Clinical practice guidelines for the care and treatment of

breast cancer: 11. Lymphedema. CMAJ 2001; 164(2):191–199.

34. Cole T. Risk factors associated with lymphoedema, British Lymphology Society Annual Conference Proceedings 2000; online at: http://www.lymphoedema.org/bls/blsc0035.htm -COLE

35. Gomes PJ, Long V, Barker P. Implementation of a policy to reduce the incidence and severity of lymphoedema following the treatment of breast cancer. J Clin Excellence 2000; 1(4):243–245.

36. Smith J. The practice of venepuncture in lymphoedema. Eur J Cancer Care 1998; 7:97–98.

37. Joffe HV, Goldhaber SZ. Upper-extremity deep vein thrombosis. Circulation 2002; 106:1874–1880.

38. Naylor W, Laverty D, Mallett J. The Royal Marsden Hospital handbook of wound management in cancer care. Oxford: Blackwell Science; 2000.

39. Tengrup I, Tennvall-Nittby L, Christiansson I, Laurin M. Arm morbidity after breast conserving therapy for breast cancer. Acta Oncol 2001; 39(3):393–397.

40. Hojris I, Andersen J, Overgaard M, et al. Late treatment-related morbidity in breast cancer patients randomised to postmastectomy radiotherapy and systemic treatment versus systemic treatment alone. Acta Oncol 2000; 39:355–372.

41. Mason W. Exploring rehabilitation within lymphoedema management. Int J Palliat Nurs 2000; 6(6):265–273.

42. Bowling A. Measuring health. 2nd edn. Buckingham: Open University Press;1997.

43. Woods M. An audit of swollen limb measurements. Nurs Stand 1994; 9(5):24–26.

44. Piller N. Gaining an accurate assessment of the stages of lymphoedema subsequent to cancer: the role of objective and subjective information, when to make measurements and their optimal use. Eur J Lymphol 1999; 7(25):1–9.

45. Johansson K. Lymphoedema: a physiotherapeutic approach. Lund: Lund University; 2002.

46. Miller LT. Management of breast cancer related lymphedema. In: Mackin EJ, Callahan AD, Osterman AL, et al, eds. Rehabilitation of the hand and upper extremity. 5th edn. Vol. 1. St Louis: Mosby; 2002:914–928.

47. Bumpers H, Best IM, Norman D, et al. Debilitating lymphedema of the upper extremity after treatment of breast cancer. Am J Clin Oncol 2002; 25(4):365–367.

48. Robertson-Squire M. The patients perspective. In: Twycross R, Jenns K, Todd J, eds. Lymphoedema. Abingdon, Oxon: Radcliffe Medical Press; 2000:22–43.

49. Swedborg I, Wallgren A. The effect of pre- and postmastectomy radiotherapy on the degree of edema, shoulder-joint mobility, and gripping force. Cancer 1981; 47(5):877–881.

50. Newman ML, Brennan M, Passik S. Lymphoedema complicated by pain and psychological distress: a case with complex treatment needs. J Pain Symptom Manage 1996; 12(6):376–379.

51. Twycross R. Pain in lymphoedema. In: Twycross R, Jenns K, Todd J, eds. Lymphoedema. Abingdon, Oxon: Radcliffe Medical Press; 2000:68–88.

52. Badger C. Pain in the chronically swollen limb. In: Partsch H, ed. Progress in lymphology. Amsterdam: Elsevier Science; 1988:243–246.

53. Vecht CJ. Arm pain in the patient with breast cancer. J Pain Symptom Manage 1990; 5(2):109–117.

54. Johansson S, Svensson H, Larsson LG, et al. Brachial plexopathy after postoperative radiotherapy of breast cancer patients. Acta Oncol 2000; 39(3):373–382.

55. Bozentka DJ, Beredjiklian PK, Chan PSH, et al. Hand disorders following axillary dissection for breast cancer. The University of Pennsylvania Orthopaed J 2001; 14:35–37.

56. Keeley V. Oedema in advanced cancer. In: Twycross R, Jenns K, Todd J, eds. Lymphoedema. Abingdon, Oxon: Radcliffe Medical Press; 2000:338–358.

57. Johansson K, Albertsson M, Ingvar M, et al. Effects of compression bandaging with or without manual lymph drainage treatment in patients with post operative arm lymphedema. Lymphology 1999; 32(3):103–110.

58. Tobin MB, Lacey HJ, Meyer L, et al. The psychological morbidity of breast cancer-related arm swelling. Cancer 1993; 72:3248–3252.

59. Passik SD, Macdonald MV. Psychosocial aspects of upper extremity lymphedema in women treated for breast cancer. Cancer 1995; 83:2817–2820.

60. Potter S. An investigation into the problems and needs of patients with secondary lymphoedema of the leg. Unpublished MSc Dissertation, Surrey University; 1996.

61. Hewson D. Coping with loss of ability: "good grief" or episodic stress responses? Soc Sci Med 1997; 44(8):1129–1139.

62. Cella DF, Tross S. Psychological adjustment to survival from Hodgkin's disease. J Consult Clin Psychol 1986; 54(5):616–622.

63. Lee-Jones C, Humphris G, Dixon R, et al. Fear of cancer recurrence – a literature review and proposed cognitive formulation to explain exacerbation of recurrence fears. Psychooncology 1997; 6:95–105.

64. Price, B. Body image, nursing concepts and care. London: Prentice Hall; 1990.

65. Woods M. Patients perceptions of breast cancer related lymphoedema. Eur J Cancer Care 1993; 2:125–128.

66. Woods M, Tobin M, Mortimer P. The psychosocial morbidity of breast cancer patients

with lymphoedema. Cancer Nur 1994; 18(6):467–471.

67. Dunkel-Schetter C, Feinstein LG, Taylor SE, et al. Patterns of coping with cancer. Health Psychol 1992; 11(2):79–87.

68. Bergman R. Understanding the patient in all his human needs. J Adv Nurs 1982; 8:185–190.

69. Hare M. The lived experience of breast cancer-related lymphoedema. Cancer Nurs Pract 2000; 15(7):36–43.

70. Derogatis LR. The psychosocial adjustment to illness scale (PAIS). J Psychosom Res 1986; 30:77–91.

71. Sitzia J, Sobrido J. Measurement of health-related quality of life of patients receiving conservative treatment for limb lymphoedema using the Nottingham Health Profile. Qual Life Res 1997; 6:373–384.

72. Coster S, Poole K, Fallowfield LJ. The validation of a quality of life scale to assess the impact of arm morbidity in breast cancer patients post-operatively. Breast Cancer Res Treat 2001; 68(3):273–282.

73. Casley-Smith JR. Casley-Smith JR. Modern treatment for lymphoedema. Adelaide: Terrace Printing; 1997.

74. Brorson H, Svensson H. Liposuction combined with controlled compression therapy reduces arm lymphedema more effectively than controlled compression alone. Plastic Reconstruct Surg 1998; 102:1058–1067.

75. Gothard L, Stanton A, MacLaren J et al. Non-randomised phase II trial of hyperbaric oxygen therapy in patients with chronic arm lymphoedema and tissue fibrosis after radiotherapy for early breast cancer. Radiother Oncol 2004; 70:217-224.

76. Pritchard J, Anand P, Broome J, et al. Double-blind randomized phase II study of hyperbaric oxygen in patients with radiation-induced brachial plexopathy. Radiother Oncol 2001; 58:279–286.

77. MacLaren J, Harmer V. Breast cancer related lymphoedema: a review of evidence based management. CME Cancer Med 2002; 1(2):56–60.

78. Todd J. Containment in the management of lymphoedema. In: Twycross R, Jenns K, Todd J, eds. Lymphoedema. Abingdon, Oxon: Radcliffe Medical Press; 2000:165–202.

79. Gilbert J, Mortimer P. Current views on the management of breast cancer lymphoedema. CME Breast 2001; 1(1):14–17.

80. Kirshbaum M. The development, implementation and evaluation of guidelines for the management of breast cancer related lymphoedema. Eur J Cancer Care 1996; 5:246–251.

81. Ramos SM, O'Donnell LS, Knight G. Edema volume, not timing is the key to success in lymphedema treatment. Am J Surg 1999; 178(4):311–315.

82. Badger CMA, Peacock JL, Mortimer PS. A randomized, controlled, parallel-group clinical trial comparing multi-layer bandaging followed by hosiery versus hosiery alone in the treatment of patients with lymphoedema of the limb. Cancer 2000; 88(12):2832–2837.

83. Leduc A, Leduc O. Manual lymphatic drainage. In: Twycross R, Jenns K, Todd J, eds. Lymphoedema. Abingdon, Oxon: Radcliffe Medical Press; 2000:203–216.

84. Leduc A, Leduc O. Physical treatment of oedema. Eur J Lymphol 1990; 1:8.

85. Wozniewski M, Jasinski R, Pilch U. Complex physical therapy for lymphoedema of the limbs. Physiotherapy 2000; 87(5):252–256.

86. Waller A, Bercovitch M. Transcutaneous electrical nerve stimulation. In: Twycross R, Jenns K, Todd J, eds. Lymphoedema. Abingdon, Oxon: Radcliffe Medical Press; 2000:271–282.

87. Haslett ML, Aitken MJ. Evaluating the effectiveness of a compression sleeve in managing secondary lymphoedema. J Wound Care 2002; 11(10):401–404.

88. Mallett J, Dougherty L, eds. The Royal Marsden Hospital manual of clinical nursing procedures. 5th edn. Oxford: Blackwell Science; 2000.

89. Veitch J. Problems in lymphoedema. Wound Manage 1993: 4(2):42–45.

90. Linnitt N. Skin management in lymphoedema. In: Twycross R, Jenns K, Todd J, eds. Lymphoedema. Abingdon, Oxon: Radcliffe Medical Press; 2000:22–43.

91. Ling J, Duncan A, Laverty D, et al. Lymphorrhoea in palliative care. Int J Palliat Nurs 1997; 4:50–52.

92. British Lymphology Society. Strategy for lymphoedema care. Sevenoaks: BLS; 2001.

93. Bates DO, Stanton WB, Levick JR, et al. The effect of hosiery on interstitial fluid pressure and arm volume fluctuations in breast cancer related lymphoedema. Phlebology 1995; 10:46–50.

94. Olszewski WL, Bryla P. Lymph and tissue pressures in patients with lymphedema, during massage and walking with elastic support. Lymphology 1994; 27(Suppl):81–93.

95. Bergan J, Sparks SR. Non-elastic compression: an alternative in management of chronic venous insufficiency. J Wound Ostomy Continence Nurs 2000; 27(2):83–89.

96. Davis BS. Lymphedema after breast cancer. Am J Nurs 2001; 101(4):24AAAA–24DDDD.

97. Kubik S. Lymphatics of the skin. In: Cluzan RV, Pecking AP, Lokiec FM, eds. Progress in lymphology –XIII. Int Cong Ser 994, Zurich: Elsevier Science; 1992:11–14.

98. MacLaren J. Skin changes in lymphoedema: pathophysiology and treatment options. Int J Palliat Nurs 2001; 7(8):381–389.

99. Mortimer PS. The dermatologist's contribution to lymphedema management. Scope on Phlebology and Lymphology 1995:17–19.

100. Jeffs E. The effect of acute inflammatory episodes (cellulitis) on the treatment of lymphoedema. J Tissue Viability 1993; 3(2):51–55.

101. Jenns K. Management strategies. In: Twycross R, Jenns K, Todd J, eds. Lymphoedema. Abingdon, Oxon: Radcliffe Medical Press; 2000:97–117.

102. Hammick M, Howard E, Macleod H, et al. Multidisciplinary symptom control class for breast cancer patients. Br J Ther Rehabil 1996; 3(6):333–336.

103. Box R, Reul-Hirche HM, Bullock-Saxton JE, et al. Shoulder movement after breast cancer surgery: results of a randomised controlled study of postoperative physiotherapy. Breast Cancer Res Treat 2002; 75(1):35–50.

104. Meric F, Buchholz TA, Mirza NQ,et al. Long-term complications associated with breast-conservation surgery and radiotherapy. Ann Surg Oncol 2002; 9(6):543–549.

105. Johansson K, Ingvar C, Albertson M, et al. Arm lymphoedema, shoulder mobility and muscle strength after breast cancer treatment. Adv Physiother 2001; 3:55–66.

106. Harris SR, Niesen -Vertommen SL. Challenging the myth of exercise-induced lymphedema following breast cancer: a series of case reports. J Surg Oncol 2000; 74:95–99.

107. Miller L. Postsurgery breast cancer outpatient program. Clin Manage 1992; 12(4):50–56.

108. Boland RA, Adams RD. Acute angles of head-up tilt do not affect forearm and hand volume. Aust J Physiother 2000; 46:123–131.

109. Swedborg I, Norrefalk JR, Piller NB, Asard C. Lymphoedema post-mastectomy: is elevation alone an effective treatment? Scand J Rehabil Med1993; 25(2):79–82.

110. Wittlinger H, Wittlinger G. Textbook of Doctor Vodder's manual lymph drainage. Vol 1: basic course. 6th revised English edn. Heidelberg: Haug; 1998.

111. Tribe K. Treatment of lymphoedema: the central importance of manual lymph drainage. Physiotherapy 1995: 81(3):154–156.

112. Kurz I. Textbook of Dr Vodder's manual lymph drainage. Vol 2. 3rd edn. Brussels: Haug; 1986.

113. Andersen L, Hojris I, Erlandsen M, et al. Treatment of breast-cancer-related lymphedema with or without manual lymphatic drainage. Acta Oncolog 2000: 39(3):399–405.

114. Williams A, Vadgama A, Franks P, et al. A randomized controlled crossover study of manual lymphatic drainage therapy in women with breast cancer-related lymphoedema. Eur J Cancer Care 2002; 11(4):254–261.

115. Koscielny S, Brauer B, Sonnefeld U. Effect of manual lymph drainage treatment for quality of life in head and neck cancer patients. Eur J Lymphol Rel Probl 1999; 7(28):112–114.

116. Bellhouse S. Simple lymphatic drainage. In: Twycross R, Jenns K, Todd J, eds. Lymphoedema. Abingdon, Oxon: Radcliffe Medical Press; 2000:217–235.

CHAPTER 26

Oral Complications in Patients with Cancer

KARIS KF CHENG

CHAPTER CONTENTS

Introduction	575	Mechanism and clinical manifestations of xerostomia	590	
Types and consequences of oral complications	575	Assessment	590	
		Management	591	
Oral mucositis	576	Taste dysfunctions	594	
Mechanism and clinical manifestations of oral mucositis	576	Conclusion	595	
Assessment	579	Resources	596	
Management	580	References	596	
Xerostomia and salivary gland hypofunction	589			

INTRODUCTION

Patients treated with systemic chemotherapy and/or head and neck irradiation for malignant diseases suffer from a multitude of intense and debilitating oral complications. Oral mucositis, xerostomia and taste changes are among the most common oral complications that may cause significant physical and psychological consequences. To alleviate these distressing oral complications is of high priority in the cancer care setting. This chapter covers several key aspects of nursing care of patients with common oral complications, including the mechanism and clinical manifestation, nursing assessment, multidisciplinary approach with emphasis on symptom control, oral care, nutritional management and patient education.

TYPES AND CONSEQUENCES OF ORAL COMPLICATIONS

Numerous oral sequelae, including mucositis, xerostomia (hyposalivation), taste changes (absence, partial loss or impairment of the sense of taste), oral infection and hemorrhage (Table 26.1) occur due to chemotherapy and radiotherapy. Although these oral conditions are not life-threatening complications, they cause a number of severe consequences that negatively impacts on patients' treatment outcome, daily living and functioning, as well as quality of life. Not only are the ulcerative lesion and altered salivation painful, resulting in significant discomfort, but they also often cause profound difficulties with chewing, swallowing, smiling and communicating verbally.[1-3] For some patients, it becomes impossible to eat, drink or even to swallow their own saliva.[2] Patients are often unable to sleep because of mouth pain and dryness.[1,4] The chewing and swallowing problems, combined with damaged taste buds or diminished taste sensitivity, appear to increase patients' reluctance to eat, resulting in compromised nutritional intake with significant weight loss and malnutrition.[3,5,6] It has been reported that 88%[5] and 37%[6] of patients with head and neck cancer developed oral mucositis and transient taste changes, respectively, that interfered with oral intake. In addition to malnutrition, eating problems often lead to feelings of social isolation.[2] For some patients with mouth pain and oral dysfunction, the condition is of such severity as to require the use of opioid analgesics, supplemental nutrition (including total parenteral nutrition), nasogastric tube feeding and percutaneous endoscopic gastrostomy, or the need for interruption or modification of the cancer treatment.[5,7] Moreover, the resulting low salivary pH and buffering capacity and ulcerative lesions can even render patients susceptible to dental caries and potentially fatal septicaemia in myelosuppressed individuals.[8,9] The incidence of an oral focus in septicaemia has been reported in 32–54% of patients despite the frequent use of antibacterial prophylaxis for patients with prolonged neutropenia.[10,11] All these conditions may increase treatment cost, prolong hospital stay, preclude further cancer treatment, jeopardize survival or irrevocably alter quality of life.[7,12–14]

ORAL MUCOSITIS

The terms 'oral mucositis' and 'stomatitis' have been used interchangeably in the literature to describe the inflammatory response of oral mucosal epithelial cells. Oral mucositis is a more specific definition, in which an inflammatory and ulcerative condition of the oral mucosal membrane has been clinically documented in association with chemotherapy or head and neck irradiation. The prevalence of oral mucositis ranges from 12% in patients receiving adjuvant chemotherapy to 99% in patients subjected to high-dose myeloablative chemotherapy for bone marrow transplant (BMT).[15,16] The prevalence of oral mucositis in patients undergoing standard- and high-dose chemotherapy is approximately 40%[17] and 50%,[18] respectively. Approximately 60% and 90% of patients with head and neck cancer receiving standard radiotherapy and chemoradiotherapy, respectively, will develop oral mucositis[19] (Table 26.2).

Mechanism and clinical manifestations of oral mucositis

The vast majority of research data supports the view that multiple mechanisms account for the development and progression of oral mucositis. This involves a complex interaction of chemotherapeutic drugs or irradiation on mitosis of rapidly proliferating mucosal cells,

Table 26.1: Oral complication of chemotherapy and radiotherapy		
Oral complication	Chemotherapy	Radiotherapy
Mucositis	✓	✓
Xerostomia	✓	✓
Xerostomia-associated caries		✓
Taste alterations	✓	✓
Infection	✓	✓
Bleeding	✓	✓
Osteonecrosis		✓
Trismus		✓

Table 26.2: Prevalence of oral mucositis

Type of cancer treatment/malignancy	Prevalence rate
Adjuvant CT	12%
Standard-dose CT	40%
High-dose CT	50%
High-dose CT for BMT	76–99%
CT for solid tumors	21–31%
CT for leukemia	50%
Standard RT for head and neck cancer	60%
Chemoradiotherapy for head and neck cancer	90%

BMT = bone marrow transplant; CT = chemotherapy; RT = radiotherapy.
Source: data complied from References 15–21.

local tissue cytokine and elements of oral microbial environment.[20] Another proposed mechanism involves the alteration of salivary immunoglobulins, proteins, electrolytes and non-specific host defence in saliva, as well as apoptosis. The underlying aetiophysiological mechanism of chemotherapy- and radiotherapy-induced mucositis is similar. However, differences exist and are related particularly to the systemic effects and resultant myelosuppression of chemotherapy, in which neutropenia and thrombocytopenia can influence oral mucositis indirectly through secondary infection and haemorrhage.[17,19]

Currently, the four interdependent phases – namely, the inflammatory/vascular phase, the epithelial phase, the ulcerative/bacterial phase and the healing phase – proposed by Sonis underpin the sequential events, resulting in oral mucositis (Fig. 26.1).[20] Initially, chemotherapeutic agents or ionizing radiation insults will cause the release of inflammatory cytokines (tumor necrosis factor-α, interleukin-1 and perhaps interleukin-6) from the mucosal epithelial and adjacent connective tissue shortly after administration, resulting in mucosal tissue damage and increased submucosal vascularity. In the epithelial phase, both chemotherapeutic agents and ionizing irradiation disrupt the proliferating (S) phase of the cell cycle and thus cell division, leading to reduced epithelial proliferation and

differentiation and decreased replacement of cell loss from the mucosal surface. In the ulcerative/bacterial phase, localized areas of erosions occur that are often covered with a fibrinous pseudomembrane. Secondary oral bacterial colonization, involving primarily Gram-negative microorganisms, provides a source of endotoxin, further stimulating cytokine release and intensifying inflammatory response and mucosal injury. In the final phase, healing of the oral mucosa represents complex interactions of epithelial cell proliferation and maturation, and hematological recovery, as well as local microflora re-establishment.[20]

Numerous factors can contribute to the development of oral mucositis in patients with cancer (Box 26.1). A meticulous assessment of all possible risk factors will facilitate the identification of patients at increased risk for the development of more severe oral mucositis so that nurses can make pretreatment assessment and plan effective interventions to diminish the severity of oral mucositis.

The risk of oral mucositis varies with the cytotoxic regimen and the individual.[21,22] Chemotherapeutic drugs that are cell-cycle specific, interfering with either DNA, RNA or protein synthesis, have been reported to produce a high incidence and severity of oral mucositis.[23] Patients receiving myelosuppressive chemotherapy resulting in prolonged

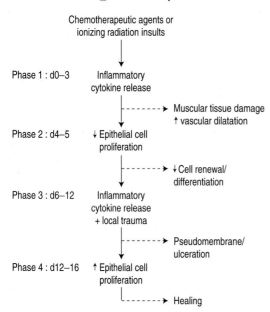

Phase 1 : d0–3   Inflammatory
                  cytokine release

                  - - - - - - → Muscular tissue damage
                                ↑ vascular dilatation

Phase 2 : d4–5   ↓ Epithelial cell
                  proliferation

                  - - - - - - → ↓ Cell renewal/
                                differentiation

Phase 3 : d6–12   Inflammatory
                  cytokine release
                  + local trauma

                  - - - - - - → Pseudomembrane/
                                ulceration

Phase 4 : d12–16 ↑ Epithelial cell
                  proliferation

                  - - - - - - → Healing

Figure 26.1: Sonis's model of oral mucositis. (Adapted from Sonis[20] with permission.)

Box 26.1

Potential risk factors contributing to oral mucositis

Patient-related
Age
Gender
Pre-existing periodontal and dental problem
Ill-fitting dental prostheses
Oral hygienic status
Oral microbial environment
Mucosal trauma: physical, chemical, thermal
Alcohol and tobacco use
Nutritional status
Liver and renal functional status
Type of malignant disease
Genetic influence on inflammatory response

Cancer treatment-related
Chemotherapy
Radiotherapy
Myelo- and immunosuppression
Salivary dysfunction:

- Reduced secretory IgA
- Reduced salivary flow

Data compiled from References 16, 17, 21, 22 and 26.

neutropenia also increase the risk of developing oral mucositis.[24] Certain chemotherapeutic agents such as methotrexate and etoposide, which may be secreted in the saliva, have been reported to correlate with increased prevalence of oral mucositis.[25,26] Patients treated with combinations of agents that are known to cause oral mucositis are more likely to suffer from such toxicity.[27] Oral mucositis can also occur when two agents, such as 5-fluorouracil (5-FU) and leucovorin (folinic acid), are used concurrently, even though the latter does not usually induce oral mucositis on its own.[28] Majorana et al indicated that multiple-agent chemotherapy protocols, especially those with multiple alkylating agents, will induce severe oral mucositis, unlike single-drug protocols.[29] There is evidence to suggest that high-dose methotrexate, etoposide and melphalan cause the most serious forms of oral mucositis.[16,28] Oral mucositis is common when the irradiated fields include the salivary glands or metallic dental restorations, and include a larger blood supply or a higher cell turnover rate, e.g. in the uvula and soft palate.[30] The severity of oral mucositis increases when the total dose of irradiation cumulates to 50–60 Gy, and when a hyperfractionation schedule of two irradiated treatments per day is used.[31] The concomitant administration of chemotherapy contributes to the earlier development and more severe irradiation mucositis[32] (Box 26.2).

Numerous patient-related factors have been reported to produce oral mucositis. While few multivariate studies has specifically analysed these host factors, evidence suggests that age, oral hygiene level, nutritional status and xerostomia condition are contributory factors to the susceptibility of mucositis.[16,33] In general, children and older adult patients are at increased risk of developing oral mucositis. Such a high risk may be related to the high proliferating rate of epithelial basal cells, variations in resistance and immunological status in children and the physiological decline in renal function associated with ageing in older patients.[17,34] Poor oral hygiene and pre-existing dental problems often increase the severity of oral mucositis because of the pathogenicity of oral microflora. It has been reported that the correction of the pre-existing dental condition and effective oral hygiene during cancer therapy can diminish the incidence and severity of mucositis.[35,36] The

Box 26.2

Risk factors related to chemotherapy and radiotherapy

Chemotherapy

Cell-cycle specific, interfering with either DNA, RNA or protein synthesis:

- Antimetabolites
- Antitumour antibiotics

Agents secreted in the saliva:

- Etoposide, methotrexate

Combination of agents that are known to cause oral mucositis

Multiple alkylating agents

Radiotherapy

High cumulative dose of radiotherapy:

- Total dose of 50–60 Gy

Hyperfractionation schedule:

- Two irradiated treatments per day

Concurrent use of chemotherapy

Mucosal tissue with fine vasculature and higher cell turnover rate:

- Uvula
- Soft palates

Irradiated field:

- Salivary glands
- Sites near dental fillings with metallic restoration

Data compiled from references 23–32.

toxicity from chemotherapy and radiotherapy has been reported to be influenced by the nutritional status of the patient.[37] Patients may develop more severe mucositis if their nutrition is poor, through malnourished host immune responses and impairment of mucosal regeneration. Xerostomia that develops as a result of irradiation of the salivary glands or drug use leads to a decline in glycoprotein production, especially immunoglobulin, and an increase in acidity (pH 5.5 or less), which render the epithelial cells more vulnerable to opportunistic bacterial and fungal infection and thus increase the risk for oral mucositis.[38]

Clinically, the manifestations of oral mucositis may range from generalized erythema, atrophy and oedema to pseudomembranous degeneration, frank ulceration and haemorrhage. The non-keratinized mucosa is mostly affected, as it lacks a cornified layer to resist local trauma and has a higher cell turnover rate and greater blood flow than keratinized mucosa. The oral ulcerative lesions are mostly presented in a bilateral pattern. While labial and buccal mucosa are most commonly affected in chemotherapy,[39] uvula and soft palate respond more intensely to irradiation.[40]

Owing to superficial epithelium being replaced completely every 7–14 days, the cytotoxic effect of chemotherapeutic agents and irradiation on the epithelium of the oral cavity may not therefore be immediately noticeable. Clinically, oral mucositis is usually observed 3–5 days after the initiation of chemotherapy[17,41] or by the end of the first week of irradiation (after 10 Gy).[32] Chemotherapy-induced oral mucositis reaches peak intensity at 7–14 days and slowly resolves unless complicated by infections or repeated drug administration. More than 90% of patients recover from oral mucositis within 1–2 weeks.[15,41] Woo et al indicated that oral ulcerative lesions typically last for a median of 6 days, with resolution of ulcers in most patients by 15 days.[42] Irradiation-induced oral mucositis reaches maximum intensity by the end of the treatment (during week 4 and week 5). Healing then takes approximately 2–3 weeks.[32]

Assessment

Accurate and reliable assessment of oral mucositis is necessary to monitor the degree of oral mucosal reaction to chemotherapy or radiotherapy. This will assist in planning care and therapeutic measures, and in evaluating patients' responsiveness to treatment. The oral mucositis assessment should include the description of oral mucosal change and its severity. Additionally, oral symptoms such as painful mouth and throat, difficulty in chewing, swallowing and speaking, as well as dry mouth, should be assessed to evaluate the extent of oral mucositis. Nutritional status and psychosocial morbidity, such as weight loss and/or psychological distress, may vary with the severity of oral mucositis and thus also need to be evaluated. The assessment of oral symptoms can be made using a 4- or 5-point Likert scale and visual analogue scales. Nurses can devise patient diaries or other patient recording methods to enable patients to track daily oral symptoms. This may provide nurses with more precise information to plan interventions.

Currently, there is a multitude of oral mucositis grading scales, but there is no one widely accepted assessment instrument. In general, the scoring systems that have appeared in the literature, to date, can be divided into two categories: those that describe and quantify the general appearance of the oral cavity using 4 or 5 grades and those that use a scoring system to evaluate parameters relating to physical changes in the oral mucosa, subjective complaints (e.g. pain, taste, dryness) and/or functional performance (e.g. talking, swallowing). The most commonly used oral mucositis scoring systems are listed in Table 26.3, including the World Health Organization (WHO) Mucositis Scale,[43] National Cancer Institute Common Toxicity Criteria (NCI-CTC) scale,[14] Western Consortium for Cancer Nursing Research Staging System for stomatitis (WCCNR Staging System),[44] Oral Mucositis Index (OMI)[45] and Oral Assessment Guide (OAG).[46]

Management

Approaches for the prevention and treatment of oral mucositis range from altering the mucosal exposure to chemotherapeutic agents and irradiation, modifying the epithelial proliferative capabilities, altering the potential for infectious or inflammatory complications and providing supportive care (Table 26.4). Until now, no intervention has been shown to be uniformly efficacious and can be accepted as evidence-based standard therapy. Although some approaches seem to be quite promising for prophylaxis or treatment of oral mucositis, they are limited to patients who have received selected cancer treatments, e.g. local application of ice-chips (cryotherapy) in bolus 5-FU or propantheline for etoposide. Recently, several biologically active factors and immunomodulatory therapy are being considered for their potential efficacy in controlling oral mucositis.[47–49] Although these special therapies should bring new challenges and insight in oral mucositis management, they are expensive, which may limit their widespread application. Currently, the most acceptable forms of interventions are reduction of patient risk factors, prophylactic elimination of dental and periodontal foci of pathological conditions before cancer treatment, systematic oral hygienic care, pain relief and nutritional support.

Collaborative multidisciplinary approaches on oral mucositis care

Collaborative multidisciplinary team approaches involving nurses, physician, dentists, nutritionists, patients and families with multidimensional interventions has recently been advocated to manage the complex nature of oral mucositis. In multidisciplinary care, responsibilities for oral mucositis care should be clarified and aligned with the expertise and scope of practice of the team members. Outcome evaluation and quality monitoring are needed, and will be greatly facilitated by the use of consistent assessment parameters.[50] Cancer nurses undoubtedly play a central role in performing meticulous assessment, such as helping patients to develop their oral self-care practice and providing supportive and psychosocial care, as well as making appropriate referrals. Table 26.5 highlights the main principles and areas of oral mucositis management by different multidisciplinary team members.

Oral care

Considerable work has addressed the potential role of oral microflora in the pathogenesis of oral mucositis, and suggested the potential of oral hygiene measures to reduce oral mucositis.[51,52] Many cancer teams consider an oral care protocol an important adjunct to the prophylaxis and management of oral mucositis; however, variability continues to exist in clinical practice among institutions and few are supported by adequate research evidence.[53] In general, the regimen of oral care should include tooth-brushing and mouth-rinsing, thereby minimizing the risk of developing oral complications.[30,54] In addition, any protocol for oral care should be simple, realistic and acceptable for the patients and family members in order to ensure proper implementation and patient compliance in both clinical and home settings.

Evidence suggests that the frequency and consistency of oral care are more important than the use of a particular device or agent in

Table 26.3: Oral mucositis assessment scales

Name	Characteristics	Validity & reliability	Strengths	Drawbacks
General or gross variables assessment scale				
World Health Organization Mucositis Scale[43]	Grade 0: no change Grade 1 sore mouth/no ulcers Grade 2: sore mouth with ulcers Grade 3: liquid diet only Grade 4: unable to eat or drink	No data	Simple and easy to use	Cannot capture the variety of oral changes that occur with cancer therapy, e.g. erythema and ulcerative changes
National Cancer Institute Common Toxicity Criteria[14]	Grade 0: none Grade 1: painless ulcer Grade 2: painful ulcer, can eat Grade 3: painful ulcer, cannot eat Grade 4: requires parenteral/enteral support	No data	Simple and easy to use	Cannot capture the variety of oral changes that occur with cancer therapy, e.g. erythema and ulcerative changes
Multiple oral mucositis component variables assessment scale				
Western Consortium for Cancer Nursing Research Staging System for stomatitis[44]	Holistic assessment Three-stage system to address functional (ability to eat, drink and talk) and the observable dimension (erythema, oedema, lesions, bleeding and infection)	Concurrent validity: 0.57–0.76 Content validity supported	More emphasis on overall oral status and deviations from normal	Less emphasis on specific anatomical sites

(continues)

Table 26.3: Oral mucositis assessment scales—cont'd

Name	Characteristics	Validity & reliability	Strengths	Drawbacks
Oral Mucositis Index[45]	34 items with a scale ranging from 0 to 3 (normal to severe): atrophy, erythema, pseudomembranous ulceration, hyperkeratosis, lichenoid and oedema items over different anatomical areas of the oral cavity	Cronbach's alpha & Guttman split-half coefficient: (0.84–0.93) Content validity supported	More emphasis on specific anatomical sites	Less emphasis on functional dimension Too complex for clinical use
Oral Assessment Guide[46]	Eight subscales: voice, swallow, lips, tongue, saliva, mucous membrane, gingiva and teeth-denture with 3 levels of descriptors: 1 normal 2 mild alteration 3 definite compromise of either epithelial integrity or system function	Nurse-to-nurse interrater reliability: 0.912 Content validity supported	Clinical usefulness	Functional parameters in less detail All oral mucosal surfaces are scored by a single score simultaneously for several descriptive variables

Table 26.4: Approaches for the prevention and treatment of oral mucositis

Preventative interventions	Antiseptic/anti-inflammatory interventions
Mucosal exposure alteration Allopurinol Chronomodulation of chemotherapy Cryotherapy Folinic acid (leucovorin) Midline mucosa-sparing blocks Modification in cancer treatment protocol Propantheline	*Antibacterial/anti-inflammatory mouthwash:* • Benzydamine hydrochloride • Chamomile • Chlorhexidine gluconate • Corticosteriods • Honey • Lozenges composed of bacitracin, clotrimazole, gentamicin • Lozenges composed of polymyxin B, tobramycin, amphotericin B • Povidone-iodine
Mucosal proliferation & maturation modifiers Amifostine Beta-carotene Cytokines: • Granulocyte-CSF/ macrophage-CSF • Epidermal growth factor • Transforming growth factor β3 • Interleukin-1/-11 • Keratinocyte growth factor Glutamine	• Tetrachlorodecaoxide Bland rinses: • Saline or bicarbonate solutions Oral/dental care Pretreatment oral/dental stabilization *Miscellaneous approaches* Antioxidant (azelastine) Pilocarpine
Immunomodulatory agents: • Pentoxifylline • Immunoglobulin Low-energy lasers (helium-neon) Prostaglandins 1 and 2	**Treatment of established oral mucositis**
	Oral care Dietary modification/supplements Vitamin supplements Topical mucosal-coating agents: • Sucralfate • Magnesium hydroxide • Hydroxypropyl cellulose films Topical anaesthetics Systemic analgesics Capsaicin

Data compiled from references [38, 84, 110, 112, 133–135].
CSF = colony-stimulating factor.

managing oral mucositis.[55,56] Oral care should be performed at least after meals, in the morning and at bedtime, and the frequency should be increased as the severity of oral mucositis increases.[54] For patients with mild mucositis, oral care should be performed every 2–4 hours and patients with moderate to severe mucositis should perform oral care every 1–2 hours.[57] In one study, the frequency of oral care protocol based on the anticipated clinical time course was found to be effective in reducing the incidence and severity of chemotherapy-induced oral mucositis (Box 26.3).[58] Low neutrophil count could also be an indicator to increase the frequency of oral care, as research studies show an inverse relationship between the degree of

Table 26.5: Collaborative multidisciplinary approaches on oral mucositis

Principles of oral mucositis management	Areas of oral mucositis management	Multidisciplinary team
Achieve optimal precancer treatment dental condition	Assess pre-existing dental and periodontal condition, possible sites of infection and irritation in the mouth Eliminate acute and potential dental and periodontal foci of pathogenic conditions	Dentistry
Minimize stomatoxicity (prior cancer treatment)	Assess risk factors and identify patients at increased risk Assess patients' tolerance to cancer treatment: anticipated stomatotoxicity, myelosuppression, liver and renal toxicity Avoidance of medication that alters renal function	Nursing and medicine
Maintain optimal oral hygiene status	Implement evidenced-based oral care protocol	Nursing, dentistry, patient and family
Minimize stomatoxicity (during and after cancer treatment)	Monitor anticipated stomatotoxicity, myelosuppression, liver and renal toxicity Modification of cancer treatment	Nursing and medicine
Prevent oral or systemic infection	Monitor signs and symptoms of infection, myelosuppression state Obtain surveillance culture from suspected regions Implement antibiotic, antifungal and antiviral therapy	Nursing and medicine
Achieve optimal oral symptoms control	Assess and monitor oral symptoms Implement supportive care: topical or systemic analgesic according to WHO's analgesic ladder, psychotherapeutic intervention, bland rinsing and ice chips	Nursing, medicine, patient and family
Achieve optimal nutritional status	Assess and monitor nutrition status Modify diet and count calorie intake Implement fluid resuscitation, nutritional supplements	Nursing, medicine and nutritionist
Prevention of oral trauma	Minimize physical, chemical and thermal insults	Patient and family
Patient and family education	Provide information/instruction on the causes and risk factors and clinical course of oral mucositis, systematic oral hygienic care, diet selection/modification, tobacco smoking and alcohol drinking cessation	Nursing
Minimize emotional distress	Provide psychosocial support	Nursing and family

oral mucositis and the level of absolute neutrophil count.[42,56,58]

Brushing is one of the most effective ways to remove dental plaque and debris on tooth enamel.[30] In one study involving children treated with chemotherapy for malignant diseases, tooth-brushing was significantly effective in reducing oral lesions as compared to a control group not using tooth-brushing.[59] It has also been suggested that the use of an extra-soft toothbrush may help to reduce the risk of trauma to gingival and other soft tissues, as well as promote healing of the epithelium.[29,60] According to the American Dental Association, effective brushing can be achieved by using the Bass sulcular technique in which short, horizontal or circular strokes are applied with gentle pressure to the junction of the gums and teeth (45°). The biting surfaces are scrubbed with longer strokes; the tongue is gently brushed to stimulate circulation and remove debris.[54] Majorana et al suggested that gentle tongue-brushing could further help in the reduction of bacteria and possible

Candida levels on the tongue.[29] Several authors recommended that patients treated for acute leukaemia discontinue tooth-brushing when the platelet count drops below 20 $\times 10^9$/L in order to reduce the risk of oral bleeding.[61,62] However, other investigators have continued to argue that plaque accumulation and gingival inflammation may be more detrimental than the risk of haemorrhage inherent in oral hygiene measures.[60,63] Flossing is another important aspect of oral hygiene, as it allows a patient to clean the surfaces between the teeth. However, patients should avoid flossing if it causes pain or if their platelet levels are less than 40 $\times 10^9$/L.[63]

Sodium chloride solution 0.9% (normal saline), an isotonic solution, is generally supported in the literature as part of the oral hygiene measure to rinse off debris, moisturize mucosal surface and reduce mild to moderate mouth pain for individuals undergoing cancer treatment.[29,30] In Tombes and Gallucci's study, normal saline was shown to be chemically therapeutic in promoting healing and tissue

---

Box 26.3
Oral care protocol for patients in chemotherapy

Perform oral care according to the following procedures at the 1st, 2nd and 3rd week after the initiation of chemotherapy (days 1–21)
After waking up • Brush the teeth with a soft toothbrush and toothpaste using the Bass technique for 90 seconds, and then rinse the mouth thoroughly with water • Rinse the mouth with 60–80 ml sodium chloride solution for 30 seconds • Moisten the toothbrush with the sodium chloride solution. Gently clean and massage the gums, tongue and soft tissue with the toothbrush. • Rinse the mouth with 10–20 ml oral rinse agent for 30 seconds. Swish thoroughly and spit out.
Every 4 hours and within 30 minutes after each meal (for the 1st and 3rd weeks) • Rinse the mouth with 60–80 ml sodium chloride solution for 30 seconds
Every 2 hours and within 30 minutes after each meal (for the 2nd week only; days 7–14) • Rinse the mouth with 60–80 ml sodium chloride solution for 30 seconds
Before bedtime • Do the same oral care procedures as after waking up
Source: Modified from Cheng KKF, Molassiotis A, Chang AM. An oral care protocol intervention to prevent chemotherapy-induced oral mucositis in paediatric cancer patients: a pilot study. Eur J Oncol Nurs 2002; 6(2):66–73l, with permission.

granulation.[64] Rosenberg indicated that rinsing with normal saline after meals and at bedtime could be soothing and aid in diluting mouth acids and plaque toxins.[27] Several reports also indicated that frequent oral rinsing with normal saline was beneficial in diminishing oral mucositis.[30,58,65,66] Patients should be encouraged to rinse for 30 seconds to 1 minute using an alternating ballooning and sucking cheek motion to force solution between the teeth.[30] As labial surfaces may not be well irrigated during the sucking cheek motion, nurses need to instruct patients specifically to direct the rinse into the labial vestibule as part of the rinsing action.[58]

Currently, the range of mouthwashes that have been used and studied for oral mucositis is extensive, including sodium bicarbonate, hydrogen peroxide, glycerin thymole, glycerin lemon, and antibacterial mouthwashes such as chamomile, honey, benzydamine hydrochloride, chlorhexidine gluconate, povidone-iodine, lozenges with polymyxin, tobramycin, amphotericin (PTA) and bacitracin, clotrimazole and gentamicin (BcoG). From the evidence to date, sodium bicarbonate and hydrogen peroxide seem inappropriate for the treatment of oral mucositis due to the alteration of the pH, resulting in disturbance of mucosal regeneration.[64,67] Glycerin thymole or glycerin lemon rinses have been reported to be less effective than saline solution.[68] Chamomile has known anti-inflammatory, antibacterial and antifungal properties. In an initial uncontrolled study of patients treated with chemotherapy or radiotherapy, chamomile mouthwash applied prophylactically delayed the onset and reduced the severity of oral mucositis.[66] The results of a randomized controlled trial, however, did not show any benefit of chamomile to ameliorate 5-FU-induced oral mucositis and dysphagia.[69] Honey is the byproduct of flower nectar, and has antibacterial properties. A randomized controlled trial compared the efficacy of topical pure honey with normal medical care provided for patients treated with head and neck irradiation. In this preliminary study the honey group experienced significant reduction in grade 3 and 4 mucositis and had significant positive weight gain comapred to the 'normal medical care group'.[70]

Benzydamine hydrochloride is a nonsteroidal drug with anti-inflammatory, pain relieving and antimicrobial properties.[71] Earlier clinical studies reported not only a trend towards reduction in mouth pain but also a reduction in oral ulceration when patients used benzydamine prophylactically in radiotherapy.[71–73] In a recent multicentre study, benzydamine hydrochloride significantly reduced erythema and ulceration in patients receiving head and neck irradiation.[74] Chlorhexidine gluconate is a broad-spectrum antimicrobial and antiseptic,[75] and is the most commonly used agent in clinical settings in treating oral mucositis.[76] However, the relative efficacy of chlorhexidine varied in different studies. Although several clinical trials of patients receiving chemotherapy and BMT showed reduced oral mucositis,[58,75,77–80] Foote et al found that patients treated with oral irradiation using chlorhexidine experienced significantly more oral mucositis than a placebo group.[81] Another four studies compared the efficacy of chlorhexidine with placebo rinse or sterile water in patients undergoing chemotherapy or BMT.[62,82,83] One of the studies that compared the effects of chlorhexidine to salt and soda mouth rinse on chemotherapy-induced mucositis[55] failed to yield significant results. Since chlorhexidine has been shown to reduce oral bacterial and fungal colonization, the prophylactic use of chlorhexidine in patients receiving myelosuppressive therapy has been advocated by some studies.[75,84] Nevertheless, some patients may not tolerate chlorhexidine, as the alcohol content of chlorhexidine can cause oral stinging, and the solution can leave brown stains on teeth and soft tissues. Chlorhexidine diluted with an equal volume of water will help to minimize stinging with no loss of efficacy.[85] Patients need to avoid tannin-containing substances such as tea or red wine in order to decrease discolorations.[86] In addition, chlorhexidine should be administered 1 hour apart with nystatin to avoid their competition for the same binding sites.[87]

In two studies involving patients with head and neck cancer treated with radiotherapy and carboplatin, povidone-iodine has shown significant effect in reducing oral mucositis.[88,89] Spijkervet et al compared 15 patients using

PTA lozenges with patients given chlorhexidine and water rinses, and reported less severe irradiation mucositis in the PTA group.[90] Symonds et al reported a significant reduction in the worst grade and distribution of oral mucositis when patients used PTA lozenges.[91] In contrast, none of the outcome measures yielded significant results except patients' self-rating of mucositis in Okuno et al's study.[92] El-Sayed et al, using a multicentre clinical trial design, evaluated the efficacy of an economically viable antimicrobial lozenge BcoG in the alleviation of irradiation mucositis. The antimicrobial activity of BcoG is similar to PTA lozenge, which can suppress the Gram-negative bacteria and yeast counts. However, no differences were found in the severity of mucositis among the groups[51] (Table 26.6).

Table 26.6: Studies for antibacterial mouthwashes on oral mucositis					
Study	Mouthwash	No. of patients (study/control)	Cancer treatment	Study design	Results
Carl et al[66]	Chamomile	98	CT or RT	Descriptive	Delayed onset and reduced severity of mucositis
Fidler et al[69]	Chamomile	164 (82/82)	CT	r, db, pc	No benefit
Biswal et al[70]	Honey	40 (20/20)	RT	r, c	Reduced grade 3/4 mucositis
Sonis et al[72]	Benzydamine	9	CT	Descriptive	Reduced ulceration and erythema
Kim and Lakshmi[71]	Benzydamine	67 (37/30)	RT	r, db, c	Reduced severity of mucositis
Epstein et al[73]	Benzydamine	27	RT	r, c	Reduced total area and size of ulceration
Epstein et al[74]	Benzydamine	172 (84/88)	RT	r, pc	Reduced erythema / ulceration during conventional RT (<50 Gy)
McGaw and Belch[79]	Chlorhexidine	16 (8/8)	CT	r, db, pc	Reduced mucositis
Ferretti et al[78]	Chlorhexidine	48 (24/24)	CT for BMT	r, db, pc	Reduced mucositis
Ferretti et al[77]	Chlorhexidine	51 (24/27)	CT for BMT	r, db, pc	Reduced incidence and severity of mucositis
Wahlin[63]	Chlorhexidine	28 (14/14)	CT	r, c	No benefit
Weisdorf et al[83]	Chlorhexidine	100 (50/50)	CT for BMT	r, db, pc	No benefit

(continues)

Table 26.6: Studies for antibacterial mouthwashes on oral mucositis—cont'd

Study	Mouthwash	No. of patients (study/control)	Cancer treatment	Study design	Results
Ferretti et al[75]	Chlorhexidine	31 (10/21) 30 (16/14)	CT alone CT + RT	r, db, pc	Reduced mucositis in CT group only
Epstein et al[11]	Chlorhexidine	99 (18/34/16/18)	CT for BMT	r, c	No benefit
Rutkauskas and Davis[80]	Chlorhexidine	13 (6/7)	CT for BMT	r, db, c	Exhibited fewer and less painful mucositis lesions
Foote et al[81]	Chlorhexidine	52 (25/27)	RT	r, db, pc	No benefit
Dodd et al[82]	Chlorhexidine	222 (110/112)	CT	r, db, pc	No benefit
Dodd et al[12]	Chlorhexidine	142 (51/49/42)	CT	r, db, c	No benefit
Adamietz et al[88]	Povidone-iodine	40 (20/20)	CT + RT	r, c	Delay onset, reduced incidence and total duration, worst grade of mucositis
Rahn et al[89]	Povidone-iodine	40 (20/20)	CT + RT	r, c	Delay onset, reduced incidence and total duration, worst grade of mucositis
Spijkervet et al[90]	PTA lozenge	15 (7/8)	RT	r, c	Less severe mucositis
Symonds et al[91]	PTA lozenge	275 (136/139)	RT	r, db, pc	Reduced worst grade and distribution of mucositis
Okuno et al[92]	PTA lozenge	112 (54/58)	RT	r, db, pc	No benefit
El-Sayed et al[51]	BcoG lozenge	137 (69/68)	RT	r, pc	No benefit

BMT = bone marrow transplant; CT = chemotherapy; db = double-blind; pc = placebo controlled; r = randomized; RT = radiotherapy.

Supportive care

Analgesic support has been the key focus of supportive care for the management of mucositis pain and oral symptoms. Topical analgesics and anaesthetic agents may be helpful when they are applied to localized areas or used as a rinse when mucosal involvement is widespread.[7,93] Viscous lidocaine and Xylocaine in mouth rinses are frequently recommended on clinical grounds, but currently there is no evidence to support their use. Lidocaine solution as a topical anaesthetic mouthwash to manage mucositis pain has been suggested but its degree of anaesthesia may cause loss of the gag reflex, increasing the risk of aspiration.[94] Clinical trials using benzydamine have been shown to be effective in treating mucositis pain resulting from cancer chemotherapy or radiotherapy.[71,73,95] Dyclomine hydrochloride, a topical anaesthetic, has been shown to provide better pain relief than viscous lidocaine with 1% cocaine and a solution containing kaolin-pectin, diphenhydramine and saline.[96] Systemic narcotic therapy or patient-controlled administration of opioids may be needed if the oral mucositis is severe and interferes with nutritional intake and quality of life. However, there is limited evidence to establish its efficacy and evaluate its effectiveness in the control of mucositis pain. Capsaicin-containing chilli peppers have been said to desensitize neurons and thus mucositis pain. Results reported from a study with capsaicin, however, showed no significant positive effects in mucositis pain.[97] In a systematic review, Pan et al reported that relaxation and imagery could improve mucositis pain.[98]

Ulceration of the oropharynx will make eating and swallowing painful and unpleasant.[1,38] Diet modification and nutritional support intervention can help to maintain adequate dietary intake and prevent malnourishment. The texture and consistency of a patient's food may have to be adjusted. Patients should be instructed to avoid dry, salty, spicy, acidic and hot foods as they can potentially damage oral mucosa. Cold, soft and liquid-form foods may help to decrease oral comfort and enhance swallowing[38] (Box 26.4). In severe oral mucositis, nutritional support in the form of liquid preparations, such as fluid replacement and parenteral nutrition, is essential to maintain an optimal nutritional status.[1,38] Daily supplementary vitamins and minerals may be helpful.[99] Collaboration with nutritionists is strongly recommended to help patients maintain a well-balanced diet.

Patient and family education is crucial in any aspect of oral mucositis care. Table 26.5 lists the information that nurses can provide to their patients in order to help them to understand and cope with oral mucositis. Zerbe et al point out that the psychological preparation of patients and their families is essential, particularly in assuring them that discomfort is

---

Box 26.4

Dietary guidelines for patients with oral mucositis

General measures
Cook food until tender
Cut food into small pieces
Mix food with liquids (mild gravies, sauces)
Use a straw for liquids

Encourage
Liquids
High-moisture foods
Puréed meats and vegetables
Cooked cereals (oatmeal)
Scrambled eggs
Puddings, custards, gelatins
Cottage cheese
Soft low-acid fruits (watermelon, bananas, peaches, apple sauce)
Milkshakes
Cold items (Popsicles, ice cubes)

Avoid
Coarse or dry foods (crackers, toast, raw vegetables)
Spicy foods
Salty foods
Hot or warm foods
Citrus fruits (oranges, tangerines, grapefruits)

Source: adapted from Wilkes JD. Prevention and treatment of oral mucositis following cancer chemotherapy. Semin Oncol 1998; 25(5):538–551, with permission.

---

temporary and that resolution of oral mucositis usually takes a predictable course.[93] The National Institute of Health report stressed that systematic patient and family education is paramount to enhance patient compliance to the recommended preventative measures.[14] In Cheng et al[58] and Kenny's[56] studies, pretreatment patient education on oral self-care measures and reinforcement of instructions by the nurses and the family were found to enhance patient compliance to the oral care regimen.

XEROSTOMIA AND SALIVARY GLAND HYPOFUNCTION

Xerostomia can be an acute and a chronic condition characterized by a subjective feeling/perception of oral dryness. Although the perception of dry mouth is poorly correlated with salivary flow rate, this adverse condition is always accompanied by salivary gland hypofunction and a dramatic reduction in the secretion of resting saliva arising from head and neck irradiation.[100] Xerostomia is the most prevalent long-term complication (approaching 100%) associated with head and neck irradiation.[101] Although xerostomia has not been reported as a sequela in patients treated with chemotherapy alone,[102] xerostomia secondary to neoadjuvant chemotherapy in treating head and neck cancer occurs in 25% of patients.[6]

Xerostomia is an intensely distressing condition that negatively impacts on patients' daily functioning and quality of life.[9,100,103] With an inability to lubricate and form food bolus, patients often complain of difficulty in chewing and swallowing, as well as the food continually sticking to the teeth. Patients often have abnormal swallowing patterns, in which the movement of a bolus from mouth to pharynx is slowed.[9,100] The oral microbial environment may predispose to bacterial and fungal overgrowth as a result of low salivary pH and buffering capacity. In a recent study, Torres et al indicated an inverse relationship between salivary flow and the occurrence of *Candida albicans*.[104] Papas reported that the concentrations of *Lactobacillus* and *Streptococcus mutans* were often elevated 1000-fold in patients who had undergone radiotherapy as compared to their preradiation levels.[100] These alterations render a patient highly susceptible to dental caries and oral infection, particularly if accompanied with immunosuppression, mucositis, poor oral hygiene and malnutrition.[9,54]

Mechanism and clinical manifestations of xerostomia

There is a suggestion in recent literature that xerostomia is caused by early apoptotic (programmed cell death) and late necrotic action (passive form of cell death) during irradiation on salivary glands, causing atrophy, chronic inflammation, fibrosis and necrosis in both acinar and ductal cells.[105] The acinar cells atrophy and chronic inflammation of the gland tissue induces profound functional changes in saliva flow rate and composition. The magnitude of xerostomia depends on field, dosage, location and volume of glandular tissue irradiated.[105–107] The irradiation field, particularly the parotid glands, has a higher mitotic rate and the prevalence of serous cells is an important determinant of xerostomia.[105] Patients with tumours of the nasopharynx, oropharynx and unknown primary sites are generally irradiated in a bilateral manner. Thus, the parotid gland is often entirely covered within the irradiation field, and results in severe xerostomia. Individuals whose tumour location allows a portion of the parotid gland to be spared (such as laryngeal tumours, Hodgkin's disease or non-Hodgkin's lymphoma) have lesser salivary gland hypofunction and xerostomia.[105]

Salivary gland hypofunction and xerostomia occur predictably in a radiation dose-dependent manner.[105,108] Guchelaar et al indicated that a 50–60% decrease in salivary flow occurred after a fractionated dose of 10 Gy during the first week of radiotherapy. The saliva might become viscous or ropy in consistency, and most patients experienced the first signs of xerostomia at this stage.[105] Above 15 Gy, the salivary glands would become damaged irreversibly, resulting in a progressive worsening of the hyposalivation.[109] Reddy et al indicated that after a fractionated dose of 30 Gy, measurable salivary flow is eliminated from half of all parotid glands. Therefore, significant flow reduction would commonly be observed in patients receiving 30 Gy onwards.[110] An irreversible or permanent loss of function has been suggested with the doses of 40 Gy by Momm and Guttenberger,[111] and ≥50Gy by Brizel et al.[112] Nauntofte pointed out that fully irradiated parotid glands receiving doses higher than 60 Gy underwent permanent damage, resulting in hypofunction without recovery of gland function.[113]

Assessment

A thorough assessment for the quality of saliva and the extent of xerostomia is of paramount importance before initiating, and throughout treatment, as well as in follow-up visits. In addition, patients' comfort while chewing, swallowing and eating; nutritional status; and psychosocial functioning such as social contact or social eating should be assessed. Currently,

Table 26.8 Xerostomia interventions—cont'd

Approaches	Mechanism and benefits	Drawbacks
Sialogogues: e.g. oral pilocarpine, neostigmine, nicotinic acid, potassium iodide, bromhexine, carbacholine, anetholetritione	Cholinergic drugs Hyperstimulation of small residual volumes of salivary gland Palliate symptoms of xerostomia	Cholinergic side-effects (e.g. bradycardia, hypertension, gastrointestinal upset) Lifelong treatment
Parotid-sparing technique	Sparing at least one parotid gland during the process of irradiation Preserve parotid function and prevent xerostomia	Inappropriate for patients with cancer of the nasopharynx, base of the tongue, glossoepiglottis and pyriform sinus, because the rates of opposite neck node metastasis in these patients are high
Radioprotective medications: e.g. amifostine (before every fraction)	Scavenging of radiation-induced free radicals Protect against radiation-induced xerostomia	Associate with several side-effects: nausea, vomiting, hypotension and allergic reactions
Acupuncture	Autonomic stimulation of salivary tissue by needles	Temporary relief Requires experienced practitioner Difficult to optimize technique

It is rare for all the minor and major glands to be totally compromised in radiotherapy.[105] Conceivably, the minimal residual salivary glands can be stimulated by masticatory or gustatory stimuli to enhance salivary flow and thus produce symptomatic relief for xerostomic patients. Amerongen[109] and Holmes[9] have indicated that chewing can potentiate salivation. Chewing gum containing monocalcium phosphate monohydrate has been shown to be effective in stimulating salivary flow in several studies.[121] In addition, a variety of substances, including ascorbic acid, malic acid and citric acid, can be used to stimulate salivary flow. However, they are not recommended for long-term use, as those organic acids may cause demineralization of the dental enamel and so potentiate carcinogenesis. Sialogogue therapy, including neostigmine,

nicotinic acid, potassium iodide, bromhexine and pilocarpine, has recently been suggested and investigated to stimulate residual salivary glands. Several studies reported that taking oral pilocarpine 5–10 mg three times per day is effective in increasing salivary flow and improving the symptoms of xerostomia, including difficulty in swallowing, chewing and speaking.[122,123] Nevertheless, extreme caution in the use of pilocarpine is important due to reported cholinergic side-effects of sweating, gastrointestinal disturbance, cardiac problems, glaucoma, headache and flushing.

Recently, considerable efforts have been made to use sparing techniques to preserve contralateral parotid function and to develop radioprotective medications to reduce irradiation xerostomia. Reddy et al studied 114 patients with cancer of the oral cavity irradiated with parotid-sparing technique vs bilateral opposed photon beams.[110] The authors demonstrated that the parotid-sparing irradiation technique has a protective effect on the salivary gland as well as helping patients to maintain their oral nutrition and baseline body weight during and after irradiation. However, this technique is limited to patients who have a low risk of contralateral neck node metastases. In a randomized controlled trial, amifostine (200 mg/m² intravenous) was used as a radioprotector; it was administered daily 15–30 minutes before irradiation. The results demonstrated that amifostine was effective in reducing xerostomia. However, the use of amifostine has been associated with a number of side-effects, including nausea, vomiting, hypotension and allergic reactions.[112]

Dental caries and oral infection prevention

Prevention and early detection of dental caries and oral infection are of paramount consideration in the management of xerostomia. It is important that prophylactic elimination of acute and potential dental and periodontal foci of pathological conditions should be made before starting radiotherapy, so that the detrimental effects of irradiation can be minimized. In addition, regular oral and dental assessment is necessary to assist in early detection of caries and infection. Feber indicated that dentate patients should be monitored closely every 3 months after radiotherapy to detect dental decay and oral infection.[124] Oral hygiene instructions should be reinforced regularly. Patients should also be instructed to use home fluoride treatment frequently on a daily basis, including fluoride rinse or fluoride gel, to prevent xerostomia-associated caries. In Joyston-Bechal et al's study, a regimen using fluoride and chlorhexidine gel applied daily was shown to be effective in reducing xerostomia-associated caries.[125] Patients with xerostomia may increase their desire for sweet foods as a result of alteration of the sugar concentration gradient in saliva.[107] Nurses should advise the patients to avoid sugary sweets and acidic foods and drinks in order to lower the risk of dental caries and teeth erosion.

Food selection and nutrition

With a reduction or loss of saliva, chewing and swallowing can become very difficult and unpleasant. It is essential for nurses to monitor closely a patient's nutritional and hydration status, as well as to provide advice to patients and their families on food selection and nutrition maintenance. When helping patients with xerostomia to select food, nurses should take into consideration several factors, such as texture, potential irritability to oral mucosa, tolerability to patients and nutritional values. Patients with xerostomia may not tolerate solid foods that require a large amount of water to dissolve. Instead, liquid form of foods may be a better choice for patients. Increasing fluid intake during meals and snacks and softening or moistening food with milk or gravy may be helpful to lubricate food and ease swallowing.[126] Nurses should also advise patients to maintain a balanced diet and avoid foods that can cause irritation to oral mucosa. Dry foods such as bread and biscuits and sticky foods such as peanut butter should be avoided. In addition, carbonated and caffeine-containing beverages, which can cause dehydration, and spicy and acidic foods, which can cause a burning sensation, should be avoided.[9,126]

TASTE DYSFUNCTIONS

Taste dysfunctions, including partial (hypogeusia), complete loss of taste (ageusia) and distorted tastes (dysgeusia) with changes in bitter, sweet and metallic tastes, are significant eating problems associated with cancer treatments.[2] They affect 68%[127] and 90%[5] of patients receiving some forms of chemotherapy and head and neck irradiation, respectively. Cytotoxic drugs that have been associated with taste changes include carboplatin, cisplatin, cyclophosphamide, doxorubicin, 5-FU, levamisole and methotrexate.[128,129] In particular, single-agent or combination chemotherapy with doxorubicin and cisplatin are most likely to be associated with more frequent and intense taste changes.[127] The causes of taste dysfunction include damage to taste receptors and neurons and damage to salivary glands, resulting in reduced saliva flow so that tastants do not dissolve and reach the receptor to initiate the taste response.[6] Other factors inducing taste change in patients with cancer are progressive malignant disease, zinc deficiency, environmental factors and other non-chemotherapy drugs such as antiemetics, antidepressants and antihypertensives.[128–131] Taste changes usually occur during or shortly after chemotherapy administration and last for a few hours to several months.[6,129] Taste change begins with a cumulative dose of 10–20 Gy and progresses as doses reach 40 Gy. Taste sensation is generally improved within 20–60 days after radiotherapy, and fully recovered 6–12 months after the completion of radiotherapy. Some patients who have had their major salivary glands treated with high-dose chemotherapy report a permanent sense of dryness with associated taste loss.[102]

Loss of taste or changes in taste are associated with loss of pleasure in eating and food aversions, leading to inadequate food intake and subsequent weight loss. Currently, there is no instrument to measure subjective taste changes in patients with cancer. The management of taste change is complex, requiring strategies to improve taste and enhance food intake; to maintain oral hygiene; and to monitor taste perception and body weight (Box 26.5). Nurses can work collaboratively with nutritionists to help their patients and families to determine the best method to ensure adequate intake of food.[102] The identification of rejected foods and the planning of an appropriate, nutrient-equivalent food to substitute rejected foods can help patients to maintain food consumption.[132] Increased salt and seasoning, e.g. spices, seasonings, condiments and hot peppers, are also helpful in improving taste change and thus food intake.[127] Because a dry mouth and decreased salivation may contribute to taste abnormalities, encouraging the intake of liquids and provision of moist food may help to enhance food intake.[132] The use of artificial saliva, or sucking hard candies, can be effective in increasing saliva flow and hence taste sensation.[119] Continuous assessment of taste perception and body weight may provide a clearer understanding of the problem and may lead to

---

Box 26.5

Strategies to manage taste dysfunction

Taste perceptions assessment

Caloric count

Body weight measurement

Identify rejected foods and explore other foods with similar nutrient value

Improve taste:

- Increase seasoning
- Increase salt
- Change cooking methods

Provision of moist food

Encourage the intake of liquids

Use of artificial saliva

Use of other agents to increase salivary flow

Sucking on hard candy

Frequent oral care

Source: information compiled from references 102, 127, 132

---

interventions that minimize negative effects from taste changes.[127]

CONCLUSION

Chemotherapy and head and neck irradiation are frequently associated with extensive injuries on oral mucosal and glandular tissues; however, the actual problem of oral sequelae experienced by a patient results from a complex interaction between the perception of pain/discomfort and the altered oral function. In cancer care the alleviation of these distressing oral complications involving multidisciplinary effort is paramount. Nurses should take a significant leadership role in helping their patients to understand and cope with oral complications, in dealing with the complexities of oral complications and their associated consequences and in promoting multidisciplinary collaboration among healthcare providers to achieve optimal patient care. Nurses should also continue to be involved in clinical research, with emphasis on further development of nursing interventions to provide the basis of best practice for oral complications. The psychosocial aspects of oral complications need to be identified, and interventions should be planned, especially for patients with persisting oral symptoms and functional impairment. Another challenge for the future study is to determine how oral care and nutritional and psychotherapeutic interventions can be linked to the use of new biological agents to create a comprehensive or integrated approach of care for oral complications.

RESOURCES

The following resources on the management and study of oral complications associated with chemotherapy and radiotherapy provide useful educational and clinical trials information for nurses:

- National Cancer Institute's Cancer Information Service
  (http://www.cancernet.nci.nih.gov)
- National Library of Medicine
  (http://clinicaltrials.gov/)
- National Oral Health Information Clearinghouse
  (http://www.nohic.nidcr.nih.gov)

REFERENCES

1. Bellm LA, Epstein JB, Rose-Ped P, et al. Patient reports of complications of bone marrow transplantation. Support Care Cancer 2000; 8:33–39.

2. Larsson M, Hedelin B, Athlin E. Lived experiences of eating problems for patients with head and neck cancer during radiotherapy. J Clin Nurs 2003; 12:562–570.

3. Ohrn KEO, Wahlin YB, Sjoden PO. Oral status during radiotherapy and chemotherapy: a descriptive study of patient experiences and the occurrence of oral complications. Support Care Cancer 2001; 9:247–257.

4. Vissink A, Gravenmade EJ, Panders AK, et al. A clinical comparison between commercially available mucin- and CMC-containing saliva substitutes. Int J Oral Surg 1983; 12:232–238.

5. Rose-Ped AM, Bellm LA, Epstein JB, et al. Complications of radiation therapy for head and neck cancers: the patient's perspective. Cancer Nurs 2002; 25(6):461–467.

6. Lockhart PB, Clark JR. Oral complications following neoadjuvant chemotherapy in patients with head and neck cancer. NCI Monogr 1990; 9:99–101.

7. Sonis ST, Oster G, Fuchs H, et al. Oral mucositis and the clinical and economic outcomes of hematopoietic stem-cell transplantation. J Clin Oncol 2001; 19(8):2201–2205.

8. Heimdahl A. Prevention and management of oral infections in cancer patients. Support Care Cancer 1999; 7:224–228.

9. Holmes S. Xerostomia: aetiology and management in cancer patients. Support Care Cancer 1998; 6:348–355.

10. Bergmann OJ. Oral infections and septicemia in immuno-compromised patients with hematologic malignancies. J Clin Microbiol 1988; 26:2105–2109.

11. Epstein JB, Vickars L, Spinelli J, Reece D. Efficacy of chlorhexidine and nystatin rinses in prevention of oral complications in leukemia and bone marrow transplantation. Oral Surg Oral Med Oral Path 1992; 73:682–689.

12. Dodd MJ, Dibble S, Miaskowski C, et al. A comparison of the affective state and quality of life of chemotherapy patients who do and do not develop chemotherapy-induced oral mucositis. J Pain Symptom Manage 2001; 21(6):498–505.

13. Lin A, Kim HM, Terrell JE. Quality of life after parotid-sparing IMRT for head and neck cancer: a prospective longitudinal study. Int J Radiat Oncol Biol Phys 2003; 57(1):61–70.

14. National Institutes of Health. Consensus development conference statement on oral complications of cancer therapies: diagnosis, prevention, and treatment. National Institutes of Health 1987; 7(17):1–12.

15. Dreizen S. Description and incidence of oral complications. Antl Cancer Inst Monogr 1990; 9:11–15.

16. Wardley AM, Jayson GC, Swindell R, et al. Prospective evaluation of oral mucositis in patients receiving myeloablative conditioning regimens and haemopoietic progenitor rescue. Br J Haematol 2000; 110:292–299.

17. Sonis S, Clark J. Prevention and management of oral mucositis induced by antineoplastic therapy. Oncology 1991; 5(12):11–17.

18. Karthaus M, Rosenthal C, Ganse RA. Prophylaxis and treatment of chemo- and radiotherapy-induced oral mucositis – are there new strategies? Bone Marrow Transplant 1999; 24:1095–1108.

19. Sutherland SE, Browman GP. Prophylaxis of oral mucositis in irradiated head-and-neck cancer patients: a proposed classification scheme of interventions and meta-analysis of randomised controlled trials. Int J Radiat Oncol Biol Phys 2001; 49(4):917–930.

20. Sonis ST. Mucositis as a biological process: a new hypothesis for the development of chemotherapy-induced stomatotoxicity. Oral Oncol 1998; 34:39–43.

21. Barasch A, Peterson DE. Risk factors for ulcerative oral mucositis in cancer patients:

unanswered questions. Oral Oncol 2003; 39:91–100.

22. Bolwell BJ, Kalaycio M, Sobecks R, et al. A multivariable analysis of factors influencing mucositis after autologous progenitor cell transplantation. Bone Marrow Transplant 2002; 30:587–591.

23. Peterson DE, Schubert MM. Oral toxicity. In: Perry MC, ed. The chemotherapy source book. 2nd edn. Baltimore: Williams and Wilkins; 1996:571–594.

24. McCarthy GM, Awde JD, Ghandi H, et al. Risk factors associated with mucositis in cancer patients receiving 5-fluorouracil. Oral Oncol 1998; 34:489–490.

25. Brown RA, Herzig RH, Wolff SN. High dose etoposide and cyclosphamide without bone marrow transplantation for resistant hematologic malignancies. Blood 1990; 76:473–479.

26. Oliff A, Bleyerm WA, Poplack, DG. Methotrexate-induced oral mucositis and salivary methotrexate concentrations. Cancer Chemo Pharm 1997; 2:225–226.

27. Rosenberg SW. Oral care of chemotherapy patients. Dental Clin North Am 1990; 34:239–250.

28. Poon MA, O'Connel MJ, Moertel CG. Biochemical modulations of fluorouracil: evidence of significant improvement of surveillance and quality of life in patients with advanced colorectal carcinoma. J Clin Oncol 1989; 7:1407–1418.

29. Majorana A, Schubert MM, Porta F, et al. Oral complications of pediatric hematopoietic cell transplantation: diagnosis and management. Support Care Cancer 2000; 8:353–365.

30. Madeya ML. Oral complications from cancer therapy: part 2 – nursing implications for assessment and treatment. Oncol Nurs Forum 1996; 23(5):808–819.

31. Horiot JC, Le Fur R, N'Guyen T, et al. Hyperfractionation versus conventional fractionation in oropharyngeal carcinoma: final analysis of a randomised trial of the EORTC cooperative group of radiotherapy. Radiother Oncol 1992; 25:231–241.

32. Stokman MA, Spijkervet FKL, Wymenga ANM, et al. Quantification of oral mucositis due to radiotherapy by determining viability and maturation of epithelial cells. J Oral Pathol Med 2002; 31:153–157.

33. Berger AM, Eilers J. Factors influencing oral cavity status during high-dose antineoplastic therapy: a secondary data analysis. Oncol Nurs Forum 1998; 25(9):1623–1626.

34. Lichtman SM. Physiological aspects of aging: implications for the treatment of cancer. Drugs Aging 1995; 7:212–225.

35. Borowski B, Benhamou E, Pico JL, et al. Prevention of oral mucositis in patients treated with high-dose chemotherapy and bone marrow transplantation: a randomised controlled trial comparing two protocols of dental care. Oral Oncol Eur J Cancer 1994; 30B(2):93–97.

36. Overholser CD. Oral care for cancer patient. In: Klastersky J, ed. Supportive care. New York: Marcel Dekker; 1996:125–146.

37. Hickey AJ, Toth B, Lindquist SB. Effect of intravenous hyperalimentation and oral care on the development of oral stomatitis during cancer chemotherapy. J Prosthet Dent 1982; 47:188–193.

38. Wilkes JD. Prevention and treatment of oral mucositis following cancer chemotherapy. Semin Oncol 1998; 25(5):538–551.

39. Ramirez-Amador V, Esquivel-Pedraza L, Mohar A, et al. Chemotherapy-associated oral mucosal lesions in patients with leukemia or lymphoma. Oral Oncol Eur J Cancer 1996; 32B(5):322–327.

40. Whitmyer CC, Waskowski JC, Iffland HA. Radiotherapy and oral sequelae: preventive and management protocols. J Dent Hyg 1997; 71(1):23–39.

41. Loprinzi CL, Gastineau DA, Foote RL. Oral complications. In: Abeloff MD, Armitage JO, Lichter AS, Niederhuber JE, eds. Clinical oncology. New York: Churchill Livingstone; 1995:741–754.

42. Woo SW, Sonis ST, Monopoli MM, Sonis AL. A longitudinal study of ulcerative mucositis in bone marrow transplant recipients. Cancer 1993; 72:1612–1617.

43. World Health Organization. Handbook for reporting results of cancer treatment. Geneva: Offset publication; 1979; 48:15–22.

44. Western Consortium for Cancer Nursing Research. Priorities for cancer nursing research: a Canadian replication. Cancer Nurs 1987; 10(6):319–326.

45. Schubert MM, Williams BE, Lloid ME, et al. Clinical assessment scale for the rating of oral mucosal changes associated with bone marrow transplantation. Cancer 1992; 69:2469–2477.

46. Eilers J, Berger AM, Peterson MC. Development, testing, and application of the oral assessment. Oncol Nurs Forum 1988; 15:325–330.

47. Plevova P, Blazek B. Intravenous immunogloblin as prophylaxis of chemotherapy-induced oral mucositis. J Natl Cancer Inst 1997; 89:326–327.

48. Sprinzl GM, Galvan O, de Vries A, et al. Local application of granulocyte-macrophage colony stimulating factor (GM-CSF) for the treatment of oral mucositis. Eur J Cancer 2001; 37:2003–2009.

49. Sonis ST, van Vugt AG, McDonald J, et al. Mitigating effects of interleukin 11 on consecutive courses of 5-fluorouracil-induced ulcerative mucositis in hamsters. Cytokine 1997; 9:605–612.

50. Fulton JS, Middleton GJ, McPhail JT. Management of oral complications. Sem Oncol Nur 2002; 18(1):28–35.

51. El-Sayed S, Nabid A, Shelley W, et al. Prophylaxis of radiation-associated mucositis in conventionally treated patients with head and neck cancer: a double-blind, phase III, randomised, controlled trial evaluating the clinical efficacy of an antimicrobial lozenge using a validated mucositis scoring system. J Clin Oncol 2002; 20:3956–3963.

52. Shieh SH, Wang ST, Tsai ST, Tseng CC. Mouth care for nasopharyngeal cancer patients undergoing radiotherapy. Oral Oncol 1997; 33:36–41.

53. Mueller BA, Millheim ET, Farrington EA, et al. Mucositis management practices for hospitalised patients: national survey results. J Pain Symptom Manage 1995; 10(7):510–520.

54. Beck S. Mucositis. In Groenwald SL, Frogge MH, Goodman M, Yarbro CH, eds. Cancer symptom management. Boston: Jones and Bartlett; 1996:308–323.

55. Dodd MJ, Dibble SL, Miaskowski C, et al. Randomized clinical trial of the effectiveness of 3 commonly used mouthwashes to treat chemotherapy-induced mucositis. Oral Surg Oral Med Oral Path 2000; 90(1): 39–47.

56. Kenny SA. Effects of two oral care protocols on the incidence of stomatitis in hematology patients. Cancer Nurs 1990; 13(6):345–353.

57. Iwamoto RR. Alterations in oral status. In: McCorkle R, ed. Cancer nursing: a comprehensive textbook. 2nd edn. Philadelphia: WB Saunders; 1996.

58. Cheng KKF, Molassiotis A, Chang AM, et al. Evaluation of an oral care protocol intervention in the prevention of chemotherapy-induced oral mucositis in pediatric cancer patients. Eur J Cancer 2001; 37:2056–2063.

59. Bonnaure-Mallet M, Bunetel L, Tricot-Doleux S, et al. Oral complcations during treatment of malignant diseases in childhood: effects of tooth brushing. Eur J Cancer 1998; 34(10):1588–1591.

60. Biron P, Sebban C, Gourmet R, et al. Research controversies in management of oral mucositis. Support Care Cancer 2000; 8:68–71.

61. Vuolo SJ. Oral complications of cancer chemotherapy and dental care for the cancer patient receiving antineoplastic drug therapy: a literature review. J Dent 1987; 57:50–59.

62. Wright WE, Haller JM, Harlow SA, Pizzo PA. An oral disease prevention program for patients receiving radiation and chemotherapy. J Am Dent Assoc 1985; 110:43–47.

63. Wahlin YB. Effects of chlorhexidine mouthrinse on oral health in patients with acute leukemia. Oral Surg Oral Med Oral Path 1989; 68:279–287.

64. Tomebes MB, Gallucci B. The effects of hydrogen peroxide rinses on the normal oral mucosa. Nurs Res 1993; 42(6):332–337.

65. Carl W. Oral complications of local and systemic cancer treatment. Curr Opin Oncol 1995; 7:320–324.

66. Carl W, Emrich L. Management of oral mucositis during local radiation and systemic chemotherapy: a study of 98 patients. J Prosthet Dent 1991; 66:361–369.

67. Feber T. Management of oral mucositis in oral irradiation. Clin Oncol 1996; 8:106–111.

68. Hatton Smith CK. A last bastion of ritualized practice? A review of nurses' knowledge of healthcare. Prof Nurse 1994; (304):306–308.

69. Fidler P, Loprinzi CL, O'Fallon JR, et al. Prospective evaluation of a chamomile mouthwash for prevention of 5-FU induced oral mucositis. Cancer 1996; 77:522–525.

70. Biswal BM, Zakaria A, Ahmad NM. Topical application of honey in the management of radiation mucositis: a preliminary study. Support Care Cancer 2003; 11:242–248.

71. Kim JH, Lakshmi V. Benzydamine HCI, a new agent for the treatment of radiation mucositis of the oropharynx. Am J Clin Oncol 1986; 9(2):132–134.

72. Sonis ST, Clairmont F, Lockhart PB, Connolly SF. Benzydamine HCL in the management of chemotherapy-induced mucositis. J Oral Med 1985; 40:67–71.

73. Epstein JB, Stevenson-Moore P, Jackson S, et al. Prevention of oral mucositis in radiation therapy: a controlled study with benzydamine hydrochloride rinse. Int J Radiat Oncol Biol Phy 1989; 16:1571–1575.

74. Epstein JB, Silverman S, Paggiarino DA, et al. Benzydamine HCL for prophylaxis of radiation-induced oral mucositis: results from a multicenter, randomised, double-blind, placebo-controlled clinical trial. Cancer 2001; 92:875–885.

75. Ferretti GA, Raybould TP, Brown AT, et al. Chlorhexidine prophylaxis for chemotherapy- and radiotherapy-induced stomatitis: a randomized double-blind trial. Oral Surg Oral Med Oral Pathol 1990; 69:331–338.

76. Ezzone S, Jolly D, Replogle K, et al. Survey of oral hygiene regimens among bone marrow transplant centers. Oncol Nurs Forum 1993; 20(9):1375–1381.

77. Ferretti GA, Ash RC, Brown AT, et al. Control of oral mucositis and candidiasis in marrow transplantation: a prospective, double-blind trial of chlorhexidine digluconate oral rinse. Bone Marrow Transplant 1988; 3:483–493.

78. Ferretti GA, Largent BM, Ash RC, et al. Chlorhexidine for prophylaxis against oral infections and associated complications in patients receiving bone marrow transplants. J Am Dent Assoc 1987; 114\;461–471.

79. McGaw WT, Belch A. Oral complications of acute leukemia: prophylactic impact of a chlorhexidine mouth rinse regimen. Oral Surg Oral Med Oral Pathol 1985; 60(3):275–280.

80. Rutkauskas JS, Davis JW. Effects of chlorhexidine during immunosuppressive chemotherapy: a preliminary report. Oral Surg Oral Med Oral Path 1993; 76(4):441–448.

81. Foote RL, Loprinzi CL, Frank AR, et al. Randomized trial of a chlorhexidine mouthwash for alleviation of radiation-induced mucositis. J Clin Oncol 1994; 12:2630–2633.

82. Dodd MJ, Larson PJ, Dibble SL, et al. Randomized clinical trial of chlorhexidine versus placebo for prevention of oral mucositis in patients receiving chemotherapy. Oncol Nurs Forum 1996; 23(6):921–927.

83. Weisdorf DJ, Bostrum B, Raether D, et al. Oropharyngeal mucositis complicating bone marrow transplantation: prognostic factors and the effect of chlorhexidine mouth rinse. Bone Marrow Transplant 1989; 4:89–95.

84. Shaw MJ, Kumar NDK, Duggal M, et al. Oral management of patients following oncology treatment: literature review. Br J Oral Max Surg 2000; 38:519–524.

85. Ernst CP, Prockl K, Willerhausen B. The effectiveness and side effects of 0.1% and 0.2% chlorhexidine mouthrinse: a clinical study. Quintessence Int 1998; 29(7):443–448.

86. Prayitno S, Taylor L, Cadogan S, Addy M. An in vivo study of dietary factors in the etiology of tooth staining associated with the use of chlorhexidine. J Periodontal Res1979; 14:411–417.

87. Barkvoll P, Attramadal A. Effect of nystatin and chlorhexidine digluconate on *Candida albicans*. Oral Surg Oral Med Oral Path 1989; 67:279–281.

88. Adamietz IA, Rahn R, Bottcher HD, et al. Prophylaxis with povidone-iodine against induction of oral mucositis by radiochemotherapy. Support Care Cancer 1998; 6:373–377.

89. Rahn R, Adamietz IA, Boettcher HD, et al. Povidone-iodine to prevent mucositis in patients during antineoplastic radiochemotherapy. Dermatology 1997; 2:57–61.

90. Spijkervet FK, Van Saene HK, Van Saene JJ, et al. Mucositis prevention by selective elimination of the oral flora in irradiated head and neck cancer patients. J Oral Pathol Med 1990; 19:486–489.

91. Symonds RP, McIlroy P, Khorrami J, et al. The reduction of radiation mucositis by selective decontamination antibiotic pastilles: a placebo-controlled double-blind trial. Br J Cancer 1996; 74:312–317.

92. Okuno SH, Foote RL, Loprinzi, CL, et al. A randomised trial of a nonabsorable antibiotic lozenge given to alleviate radiation-induced mucositis. Cancer 1997; 79:2193–2199.

93. Zerbe MB, Parkerson SG, Ortlieb ML, Spitzer T. Relationships between oral mucositis and treatment variables in bone marrow transplant patients. Cancer Nurs 1992; 15(3):196–205.

94. Beck S. Prevention and management of oral complications in cancer patients. Curr Issues Cancer Nurs Pract Updates 1992; 1:1–12.

95. Schubert MM, Newton RE. The use benzydamine HCl for the management of cancer therapy-induced mucositis: preliminary report of a multicentre study. Int J Tissue React 1987; 4(2):99–103.

96. Carnel SB, Blakesless DB, Oswald SG, Barnes M. Treatment of radiation- and chemotherapy-induced stomatitis. Otolaryngol Head Neck Surg 1990; 102(4):326–330.

97. Berger AM, Henderson M, Nadoolman W, et al. Oral capsaicin provides temporary relief for oral mucositis pain secondary to chemotherapy/radiation therapy. J Pain Symptom Manage 1995; 10(3):243.

98. Pan CX, Morrison S, Ness J, et al. Complementary and alternative medicine in the management of pain, dyspnea, and nausea and vomiting near the end of life: a systematic review. J Pain Symptom Manage 2000; 20(5):374–387.

99. Wadleigh RG, Redman RS, Graham ML, et al. Vitamin E in the treatment of chemo-induced mucositis. Am J Med 1992; 92:481.

100. Papas A. Consequence of xerostomia and salivary gland hypofunction. Proc MASCC/ISOO 14th International Symposium Supportive Care in Cancer; 2002.

101. Makkonen TA, Edelman L, Forsten L. Salivary flow and caries prevention in patients receiving radiotherapy. Proc Finn Dent Soc 1986, 82:93–100.

102. Zlotolow IM, Berger AM. Oral manifestations and complications of cancer therapy. In: Berger AM, Portenoy RK, Weissman DE, eds. Principles and practice of palliative care and supportive oncology. 2nd edn. Philadelphia: Lippincott, Williams and Wilkins; 2002:282–298.

103. Atkinson JC, Fox, PC. Salivary gland dysfunction. Clin Geriatr Med 1992; 8:499–511.

104. Torres SR, Peixoto CB, Caldas DM, et al. Relationship between salivary flow rates and *Candida* counts in subjects with xerostomia.. Oral Surg Oral Med Oral Path 2002; 93(2):149–54.

105. Guchelaar HJ, Vermes A, Meerwaldt JH. Radiation-induced xerostomia: pathophysiology, clinical course and supportive treatment. Support Care Cancer 1997; 5:281–288.

106. Ghalichabaf M, DeBiase C, Stodey CK. A new technique for the fabrication of fluoride carriers in patients receiving radiotherapy to the head and neck. Compend Contin Educ Dent 1994; 470:473–476.

107. Mira JG, Wescott WB, Starcke, EN, Shannon IL. Some factors influencing salivary function when treating with radiotherapy. Int J Radiat Oncol Biol Phy 1981; 7:535–541.

108. Valdez HI, Wolff A, Atkinson JC, Macynski AA, Fox PC. Use of pilocarpine during head and neck radiation therapy to reduce xerostomia and

salivary dysfunction. Cancer 1993; 71:1848–1851.

109. Amerongen A, van N. Current therapies for xerostomia and salivary gland hypofunction associated with cancer therapies. Proc MASCC/ISOO 14th International Symposium Supportive Care in Cancer; 2002.

110. Reddy SP, Leman CR, Marks JE, Emami B. Parotid-sparing irradiation for cancer of the oral cavity: maintenance of oral nutrition and body weight by preserving parotid function. Am J Clin Oncol 2001; 24(4):341–346.

111. Momm F, Guttenberger R. Treatment of xerostomia following radiotherapy: does age matter? Support Care Cancer 2002; 10:505–508.

112. Brizel DM, Wasserman TH, Henke M, et al. Phase III randomized trial of amifostine as a radioprotector in head and neck cancer. J Clin Oncol 2000; 18(19):3339–3345.

113. Nauntofte B. Mechanisms of xerostomia and salivary gland hypofunction associated with cancer therapies. Proc MASCC/ISOO 14th International Symposium Supportive Care in Cancer; 2002.

114. Eisbruch A, Rhodus N, Rosenthal D, et al. How should we measure and report radiotherapy-induced xerostomia. Semin Rad Oncol 2003; 13(3):226–234.

115. Johnstone PAS, Peng YP, May BC, et al. Acupuncture for pilocarpine-resistant xerostomia following radiotherapy for head and neck malignancies. Int J Rad Oncol Biol Phys 2001; 50(2):353–357.

116. Pai S, Ghezzi EM, Ship JA, Mich A. Development of a visual analogue scale questionnaire for subjective assessment of a salivary dysfunction. Oral Surg Oral Med Oral Pathol Oral Radiol Endod 2001; 91:311–316.

117. Radiation Therapy Oncology Group (RTOG). http://www.rtog.org/members/toxicity.

118. Duxbury AJ, Thakker NS, Wastell DG. A double blind crossover trial of a mucin-containing artificial saliva. Br Dent J 1989; 166(4):115–120.

119. Olsson H, Axell T. Objective and subjective efficacy of saliva substitutes containing mucin and carboxymethylcellulose. Scand J Dent Res 1991; 94:316–319.

120. Kusler DL, Rambur BA. Treatment for radiation-induced xerostomia. Cancer Nurs 1992; 15:191–195.

121. Abelson DC, Barton J, Mendel ID. The effect of chewing sorbitol-sweetened gum on salivary flow and cemental plaque in subjects with low salivary flow. J Clin Dent 1990; 2:3–5.

122. Johnson JT, Ferretti GA, Nethry WJ, et al. Oral pilocarpine for post-irradiation xerostomia in patients with head and neck cancer. N Engl J Med 1993; 329:390–395.

123. Rieke JW, Hafermann MD, Johnson JJ, et al. Oral pilocarpine for radiation-induced xerostomia: integrated efficacy and safety results from two prospective randomized clinical trials. Int J Radiol Oncol Biol Phys 1995; 31:661–669.

124. Feber T. Head and neck oncology nursing. Philadelphia: Whurr Publishers; 2000.

125. Joyston-Bechal S, Hayes K, Davenport ES, Hardie JM. Caries incidence, mutans streptococci and lactobacilli in irradiated patients during a 12 month preventative programme using chlorhexidine and fluoride. Caries Res 1992; 26:384–90.

126. Iwamoto RR. Xerostomia. In: Yarbro CH, Frogge MH, Goodman M, eds. Cancer symptom management. 2nd edn. London: Jones and Barlett; 1999:264–271.

127. Wickham RS, Rehwaldt M, Kefer C, et al. Taste changes experienced by patients receiving chemotherapy. Oncol Nurs Forum 1999; 26(4):697–706.

128. Fanning J, Hilgers RD. High-dose cisplatin carboplatin chemotherapy in primary advanced epithelial ovarian cancer. Gynecologic Oncol 1993; 51:182–186.

129. Rhodes VA, McDaniel R, Hanson B, et al. Sensory perception of patients on selected antineoplastic chemotherapy protocols. Cancer Nurs 1994; 17:45–51.

130. Ruz S, Cavan K, Bettger W, et al. Development of a dietary model for the study of mild zinc deficiency in humans and evaluation of biochemical and functional indices of zinc status, J Clin Nutr 1991; 53:1295–1303.

131. Ackerman BH, Kasbekar N. Disturbances of taste and smell induced by drugs. Pharmacotherapy 1997; 17:482–496.

132. Holmes S. Food avoidance in patients undergoing cancer chemotherapy. Support Care Cancer 1993; 1:326–330.

133. Cheng KKF. Prevention and treatment of oropharyngeal mucositis following cancer therapy: are there new approaches? Cancer Nurs 2004; 27(3):183–205.

134. Knox JJ, Puodziunas ALV, Feld R. Chemotherapy-induced oral mucositis: prevention and management. Drug Aging 2000; 17(4):257–267.

135. Plevova P. Prevention and treatment of chemotherapy- and radiotherapy-induced oral mucositis: a review. Oral Oncol 1999; 35:453–470.

CHAPTER 27

Alopecia

DIANE BATCHELOR

CHAPTER CONTENTS

Introduction	601	Body image, self-esteem and sexuality	610
Hair	602	Nursing management of the patient with complete or incomplete hair loss	611
Anatomy and physiology of hair/ hair follicle	602	Self-care strategies to cope with alopecia: teaching and information	611
Hair growth	602	Self-care strategies to minimize alopecia	612
Hair loss	603	Self-care strategies to protect the scalp	612
Chemotherapy-induced alopecia	603	Head shaving or wearing a wig	612
Patterns of hair loss and regrowth	605	Supportive programmes	614
Radiotherapy	606		
Hormonal therapy and biotherapy	606	Conclusion	614
Prevention of alopecia	606	References	614
Mechanical measures	606		
Physical methods	607		
Biological measures	608		
The impact of alopecia	609		

INTRODUCTION

Throughout history, hair has been symbolic of the social, cultural, sexual, moral and political climate.[1,2] Many aspects of life are reflected in hairstyles, such as occupation, age, religion, ethnicity, socioeconomic status and political orientation as well as more individual identities – moods, personal states and fun. Therefore, hair is one of our most powerful public and physical symbols of individual and group/cultural identity or status. It can be used as a marker of social/sexual status, social expression and social control.[2]

Hair is a symbol of gender and mirrors its opposition. The two genders have slightly dif-ferent patterns of hair distribution due to hormonal differences. Men maximize their body hair and minimize head and facial hair, whereas the opposite is true for women. Masculinity can be symbolized by facial and chest hair. Hair symbolizes the person. Its style can communicate self and can therefore provoke social reactions.[3] It is associated with personal growth, maturity and life or life processes. Furthermore, it is immortal, because it survives death, and while the body decomposes, the hair does not, giving it richness and power.[2]

Present-day views of the body in Western society seem to reflect a growing relaxation with the symbolism of hair. An increased acceptance is seen for persons with physical disabilities and the limitations of the body.

Alopecia is a frequent side-effect of cancer treatments and ranges from sporadic thinning to complete hair loss. Patients themselves may vary in the amount of distress they experience with hair loss, as it is entirely dependent on the individual concerned.[4] In order to fully understand this phenomenon, the following key points will be addressed in this chapter:

- hair and its function
- effects of common treatments
- methods of prevention
- physical, psychosocial and spiritual impact
- nursing care
- self-care activities.

HAIR

Anatomy and physiology of hair/hair follicle

Skin functions as a protector, temperature regulator and multiple sensing device. The skin has several appendages, of which the most important is hair.[5] Hair follicles are invaginations of the epidermis, which contain hair. Each hair develops from the lowermost portion of the hair follicle from compacted, keratinized cells and becomes a hair shaft of different layers.[6] Each follicle has its own microcirculation, which supplies it with nourishment.[5] Hair colour is caused by the activity of melanocytes that produce the pigment present in the cells of the hair shaft. Human hairs are endowed with a network of nerves surrounding the follicle.[7] These nerves cause goose pimples, hair that stands on end and can be responsible for hair pain.[5]

Scalp hair, in particular, participates in the body's thermoregulatory mechanisms by preserving heat.[8] In addition, hair provides some protection against injury, and the harmful effects of solar radiation as well as having a sensory function.[6,9] The presence or absence, distribution and relative abundance of hair in certain regions (face, scalp, pubis, axillae) are secondary sexual characteristics that play subtle roles in visual appeal, i.e. socio-sexual communication.[6] Less apparent but equally important is the role of hair in the dissemination of scent from the skin. The axillary and pubic hair possessed by both males and females play an important role in this function of the skin.[7,9,10]

Hair growth

The scalp has about 100,000 hairs; of these 85–90% are actively growing at any one time. Growing hair follicles have been described as the most rapidly proliferating cells in the body. A hair shaft elongates as a result of cellular proliferation in the hair follicle, and gradual extrusion of the shaft from the follicle occurs. Increase of scalp hair length has been accurately averaged at 0.37 mm daily.[11]

The follicle has cycles involving growth, rest and loss of hair (moulting). Approximately 100 hairs are shed every day.[13] Each hair follicle has a period of active growth, called anagen, followed by a transitional phase called catagen (approximately 2–3 weeks), and then by a resting phase called telogen. Hair growth on the scalp during anagen may be quite long lasting (range 2–10 years), whereas the transition phase of catagen is short, followed by the telogen phase, which lasts between 1 and 3 months.[12] During telogen, hair is retained in the upper portion of the follicle and shed after 3 months, when the new anagen hair starts to grow in the depth of the follicle and push the old hairs out. Approximately 10% of our hair is at any one time in the telogen phase. In addition, the proportion of follicles in anagen fluctuates seasonally, the peak being in March and falling steadily to a trough in September.[10] In contrast to scalp hair, hairs elsewhere on the body, such as legs, eyelashes, eyebrows and the pubic area, have a shorter anagen phase and longer catagen and telogen phases.[14]

In a healthy individual, the pattern of hair growth – i.e. distribution, density, thickness and colour – is essentially dependent on hereditary factors that determine the response of embryonic hair-forming tissue to regulating hormonal influences. In addition, the phases of hair growth are dependent on age and body region; they can also be affected by physiological and psychological events.[15] Hair growth can vary with the season.[7] Their colour, size and disposition can vary according to race, age, sex and region of the body. In addition, neural stimuli, circulatory conditions, metabolism and general health have an influence on the quality and the quantity of hair shafts produced.[10,16] Hair growth on the scalp, face and pubis are strongly influenced by sex hormones, especially androgens, but also by adrenal cortex, thyroid, pituitary and pineal hormones.[16] The actions of these hormones on hair growth are complex and not well known.

HAIR LOSS

Alopecia connotes the diffuse shedding of hair, and to be noticeable, at least 50% of hair must be lost.[15] Alopecia can range from sporadic thinning to complete baldness.[17,18] Chemotherapy, radiation therapy or hormonal therapy in patients with cancer can all cause complete or partial alopecia.

Chemotherapy-induced alopecia

Drug therapy has the ability to influence hair growth, with the most common cutaneous side-effect of chemotherapy being alopecia.[19] Structural damage of human scalp hairs occurs following the administration of a variety of cancer chemotherapeutic drugs.[20] Most of the drugs used in cancer chemotherapy affect the growth and metabolism of not only malignant cells but also certain normal tissues as well. Tissues with rapid metabolic and mitotic rates such as the roots of scalp hairs are most noticeably affected.[20] The effect on the hair follicle may be decreased rate of hair growth, and partial or complete hair loss.[21] One explanation for this phenomena is that up to 90% of all hair follicles are in a phase of rapid growth and the high blood flow rate around the hair bulbs results in an optimal bioavailability of many compounds to this area.[16] In addition, studies have shown that human hair follicles possess an armament of enzymes necessary to toxify and detoxify drugs or other potentially toxic environmental compounds.[22]

It is while they are growing, the anagen phase, that hair follicles are subject to the disruptive effect of chemotherapy drugs. Hairs that are in the telogen phase are not affected by antineoplastic agents.[23] Alopecia can be the result of atrophy to the hair root, causing hair to be lost readily, either falling out spontaneously or being removed by casual procedures such as combing the hair. Alopecia can also be the result of diminution of the diameter of the hair bulb. This causes hair shaft constriction, which results in hair breaking off at the point of constriction.[20] Telogen effluvium is another mechanism; this is characterized by an accelerated entering of hairs into the telogen phase, followed by increased hair loss several months later.[24] Therefore, there are three mechanisms whereby alopecia can occur.

The incidence and severity of chemotherapy-induced alopecia appear to be dependent on many factors such as the half-life of the active metabolite of the chemotherapy agent(s), mono- or combination therapy, the dose, the length of the infusion and schedule and possibly the condition of the hair.[15,25] The literature varies greatly in the categorization of which agents cause severe, moderate or mild alopecia. Table 27.1 describes a compilation of frequently administered chemotherapy agents and the severity of hair loss experienced. As with most chemotherapy-related toxicity, the severity of the side-effect is also route-, dose- and schedule-dependent.[15] In addition, there may be marked differences in the potential for alopecia between drugs belonging to the same generic class.[18] Some chemotherapy agents do not cause alopecia at all such as fludarabine, estramustine, lomustine, methotrexate and cladribine.

Hair loss usually begins 7–10 days following the initiation of chemotherapy and may be quite prominent within 1 or 2 months of treatment[26] or within 2–3 weeks following chemotherapy[15,27,28] and may be rapid.[15] Hair loss can continue for the next 3–4 weeks.[15] The toxic effects on the hair are almost always reversible after treatment is completed. A delay of 4–6 weeks is common before regrowth begins.[28] These descriptions are general and do not apply to all agents. In general, hair loss has been insufficiently described per cytostatic agent and comparisons need to be made between hair loss caused by monotherapy and hair loss from combination therapy.

Early reports on the incidence of alopecia show that practically every alkylating agent when

Table 27.1: Drugs that cause alopecia and their severity

Mild alopecia	Moderate alopecia	Severe alopecia
Amsacrine	Actinomycin	Adriamycin (doxorubicin)
Bleomycin	Busulfan	Cyclophosphamide
Capecitabine	CPT 11	Daunorubicin
Carmustine	Floxuridine	Epirubicin
Chlorambucil	Methotrexate	Etoposide
Cisplatin	Mitomycin	Ifosfamide
Cytosine arabinoside	Nitrogen mustard	Taxol (paclitaxel)
Dacarbazine	Teniposide	Taxotere (docetaxel)
Fluorouracil	Topotecan	Vinblastine
Hexamethylmelanine	Vinorelbine	Vincristine
Hydroxyurea		Vindesine
L-asparaginase		
Melphalan		
Mercaptopurine		
Streptozocin		
Tioguanine		
Thiotepa		

Source: from References 14, 17 and 18.
NB. In general, mild and moderate hair loss would refer to incomplete hair loss that may not always occur in each patient and severe alopecia would be complete hair loss that occurs in the majority of patients.

given in large enough doses will result in alopecia.[29] Alopecia probably occurs with vincristine (42–65%), cyclophosphamide (0–100%) and 5-fluorouracil (5-FU) (10%) than with other agents.[29,30] Hennessey[31] reports that hair loss does not occur in patients receiving intraperitoneal cyclophosphamide, indicating that exposure of the drug to the hair roots is necessary to produce this effect and that possibly low doses given locally will not penetrate the bloodstream, protecting the roots from harm. Fulton[32] states that hair loss is uncommon with 5-FU, although partial hair loss or hair thinning can be expected. Taplin et al[33] specify that grade 1 alopecia is a common side-effect of 5-FU therapy, which causes little concern. Cyclophosphamide, methotrexate and 5-FU (CMF), which is given for breast cancer, is associated with a gradual rise in both the incidence and severity of alopecia throughout the treatment period. By cycle 4, 95% of patients reported hair loss in one study.[34] Sufficient data on patient experiences with newer chemotherapy agents are not yet available.

High-dose intermittent intravenous therapy is commonly associated with sudden and almost complete hair loss.[35] Anecdotal reports suggest that irreversible hair loss may occur in patients who undergo conditioning prior to stem cell transplantation and permanent hair loss with Taxotere (docetaxel) has been reported. Drugs given orally, daily or on a weekly schedule at lower doses cause significantly less hair loss, even though the total dose may be large.[18]

Treatment for testis cancer, using either bleomycin, etoposide and cisplatin (BEP) or cisplatin, vincristine and bleomycin (PVB), resulted in alopecia 2–3 weeks after the first treatment. Hair regrowth should begin within 1 month following completion of therapy and may not resemble the original shade and structure.[36] In a study of side-effects of the cyclophosphamide, doxorubicin, Oncovin (vincristine) and prednisolone (CHOP) schedule, alopecia was the most common problem noted in >90% of patients by cycle 3 (range 61–98%). From cycle 3 to the end of therapy, all patients experienced hair loss. The severity was assessed as a percentage loss. The mean severity after cycle 1 was 50% and became a peak of 95% after cycle 5.[37] In a study comparing CHOP to CNOP (mitoxantrone replacing doxorubicin), significantly less hair loss was seen (61% vs 14%, respectively), whereas both regimens had equal effectiveness.[38]

Patients with lung cancer experience problems related to the disease and treatment. Alopecia is associated with some of the common agents used to treat this disease: i.e. cyclophosphamide, doxorubicin and etoposide (CDE).[39] Doxorubicin causes alopecia in 80% of patients. Cyclophosphamide-induced alopecia depends on the dose.[35] Certain regimens in the treatment of breast cancer, ovarian cancer, lung cancer and lymphoma can cause 100% hair loss.[40]

In a study by Batchelor,[41] in women with breast cancer treated with Adriamycin (doxorubicin) (Doxorubin Rapid Dissolution) and cyclophosphamide, hair loss began 12.5 days (SD = 5.0) following day 1 of chemotherapy and was most severe on day 17 (SD = 1.9) of the first treatment.[41] Due to the rapid onset of hair loss, the exact location from where it occurred could not be established. Only 18% of the sample stated they could establish where it started on day 17. Hair pain was the most frequently occurring complaint and it began an average of 1 day prior to the onset of hair loss. Maximal hair loss on the head was 89% following the 3rd treatment, and 81% for other areas (axilla, pubic hair, arms and legs) following the 4th treatment.

Patterns of hair loss and regrowth

Hair loss can be either complete or incomplete and occur on any hair-bearing area of the body. Studies by Orfanos et al[22] showed that in more that 50% of all cases of hair loss due to chemotherapy, it occurred not only on the scalp but also on other regions of the body. Long-term therapy may result in the loss of pubic, axillary and facial hair in addition to scalp hair.[15,42] Many patients report scalp sensitivity, losses of body heat through the scalp and hair pain.[41,43] Male patients may lose facial hair or reduce the frequency of their shaving from daily to between 1 and 3 times per week. The rate of hair growth can be reduced to 0.004–0.1 mm/day as opposed to the normal value of 0.37 mm/day.

Complete hair loss

Complete hair loss encompasses losing all the hair and is associated with severely epilating agents and radiotherapy >500 cGy. Since 90% of the hair is in the growth phase at any one time, complete hair loss on the scalp will encompass 90% of all hair, except with radiotherapy, which will cause 100% hair loss on the area that has been treated. With complete hair loss, a large percentage of hair falls out in a short period of time. Complete hair loss is usually associated with hair loss on other parts of the body. In a recent study,[41] it was shown that the majority of women who experienced chemotherapy-induced hair loss lost a maximum of 89% on the scalp. Hair loss on the rest of the body continued until the end of the 4th cycle and included the axilla, pubic hair, eyebrows, eyelashes, arm and leg hair.[41]

Incomplete hair loss

Incomplete hair loss is usually related to treatment with moderately or mildly epilating agents and is not well described in the literature. In addition, hormonal and biotherapy agents can have this type of hair loss. It can be characterized by light hair loss following each treatment that remains undetectable by others or it could progress slowly to patchy alopecia that is noticeable. The hair that remains is usually described as being lifeless and difficult to manage.

Hair growth

When hair grows following chemotherapy, approximately 65% of patients experience a change from their previous hair, but this has not been documented with any regularity.[44] Some authors report that alteration in colour and texture of hair can occur, with a colour difference as the most common change. Some patients notice that their hair has greyed, ageing them considerably, and approximately 33–35% of patients experience a change in hair structure and texture.[45,46] It has been reported that hair grows back about 1/4 inch per month and in general is coarser. Gradually, it returns to its normal character.[47,48] Hair may feel thinner than prior to chemotherapy.[25] Data on alterations of hair characteristics following chemotherapy for testicular cancer include 28% alteration in hair colour, 41% change in hair texture and 53% change in hair type.[36]

Radiotherapy

Radiation-induced hair loss is more variable and less predictable than chemotherapy-induced hair loss.[49] There is, unfortunately, limited literature on this topic. Hair loss, if it occurs, takes place at the area of radiation. Permanent hair loss and changed quality of hair growth occurs with higher doses of radiotherapy (>500 cGy). If appropriate, patients can be encouraged to grow their hair longer over the places of baldness.

Hormonal therapy and biotherapy

Hair growth is influenced by hormones, as demonstrated by hair development in genital areas during puberty or accentuated hair growth (virilization) in women on androgen therapies. Accentuated (>100 hairs/day) hair loss can occur after initiating hormonal therapy, although this has not been accurately

studied. For example, the antioestrogenic effect of tamoxifen could drive hair follicles towards a resting phase. There have been incidental reports of complete hair loss with tamoxifen.[50] This antioestrogen effect may enhance androgen action on follicles, causing alopecia in genetically susceptible patients. An accurate description of hair loss with other agents is lacking. Immunotherapy with interferon and interleukin-2 can cause delayed, incomplete light hair loss, which starts 3 months after therapy begins. Hair loss is incomplete, usually unnoticeable to others and is short-lived. Replacement hairs can be seen growing where the old hairs have fallen out.

PREVENTION OF ALOPECIA

Since the late 1960s, oncologists and oncology nurses have used methods that attempt to prevent chemotherapy-induced scalp alopecia with varying success. These methods have included mechanical methods such as scalp tourniquets to physical devices such as hypothermia and biological agents such as folic acid or α-tocopherol (AT) or more recently cytokines.[51,52] The goals of preventative techniques are to prevent hair loss, improve physical appearance and preserve body image.

Mechanical measures

Scalp tourniquet methods with successes and failures have been described by a number of authors.[4,31,53–59] Scalp tourniquets are the application of bands around the head, which are applied under pressure. They work by temporarily decreasing blood flow to the scalp and limiting follicle exposure to chemotherapy agents.[30] Although authors described mild to moderate hair preservation with this technique, the studies were either performed in small numbers of patients or patients were excluded from final data collection due to refusals to use the tourniquet. In addition, the methodology was often inconsistent and/or control groups were absent. The chemotherapy types and doses varied, as well as the tourniquet pressures used.[60] With the advent of scalp hypothermia techniques, this rather time-consuming, cumbersome and uncomfortable method became obsolete.

Physical methods

Hypothermia for prevention of alopecia is the application of cold to the scalp. Hypothermia works by three mechanisms:

- reduced scalp perfusion of hair follicles by means of vasoconstriction, thereby limiting the amount of exposure to the chemotherapy agent (with a reduction of intradermal scalp temperature to 30°C; scalp blood flow decreased to 25%)
- reduced temperature-dependent cellular uptake of chemotherapy
- a reduced intrafollicular drug metabolic rate.[40,61]

Hair conservation can be obtained when scalp temperature is reduced to a level ≤24°C.[62,63]

The earliest report of scalp hypothermia found in the literature was in 1973. Luce et al[64] reported that patients who received Adriamycin (doxorubicin) (Doxorubin Rapid Dissolution) as a single injection every 3 weeks, underwent scalp cooling for a period lasting from 5 minutes before chemotherapy until 10–20 minutes after each Adriamycin (doxorubicin) (Doxorubin Rapid Dissolution) injection. This randomized study showed that the 16 patients without scalp cooling lost an average of 80% of their hair and the 12 patients who had scalp cooling lost an average of 30%. This study demonstrated that scalp hypothermia could offer benefit to patients who receive epilating chemotherapy. Since then, many other studies have shown that the effectiveness of the various techniques employing hypothermia can range from 0 to 90%. Several cooling systems have been devised, such as the application of the ice turban, cooling fluid ring turbans, cold air hoods and cryogel caps.[41] The ice and cooling fluid turban have been less popular since the development of cryogel caps. In general, gel caps for ease of use are superior to ice packs because they are simpler to prepare, less uncomfortable and cause no problem such as melting during treatment. In terms of effectiveness, it cannot be ascertained from these studies which method is the most effective. The exception is the use of cold air to achieve an epidermal scalp temperature of <15°C. This method seems more effective than cryogel caps in controlling alopecia related to treatments with doxorubicin.[40,65]

Factors that influence the success of hypothermia

Hypothermia is not 100% effective. The effectiveness of scalp cooling is dependent on a number of factors, such as the presence of liver metastases or liver dysfunction, which can prolong the half-life of certain chemotherapy agents.[60,62,66–73] Only patients treated with drug combinations that are rapidly administered (<60 minutes) seem to benefit from scalp hypothermia.[74] Dose has been considered an issue for the success of hypothermia. Several reports suggest that doxorubicin causes significantly more hair loss at doses >50 mg/m^2.[15]

The degree of scalp cooling can also influence the success of hypothermia. It has been suggested that temperatures <22°C are necessary to obtain a hair-preserving effect.[61,62,75] Maximal cooling is usually accomplished following 20–30 minutes of hypothermia[75] but must be maintained until the half-time of the active drug is complete or the scalp is sufficiently cooled.[63] The application of the cooling device, i.e. how close it is to the scalp, the presence of air preventing contact and how long it remains in place may be other success factors. Many investigators wet the hair to increase conduction of the cold.[67,68,70,76] If the scalp cooling apparatus is ill-fitting, the cooling will be non-uniform.[77] The cooling apparatus is often very heavy and uncomfortable: due to its size and weight, it is difficult to keep it in position. Its application takes time, is expensive and constant temperatures are difficult to achieve.

Scalp metastases have been reported in the literature and their development has been a major limitation for the broad-scale application of hypothermia until recently. Theoretically, tumour cells that have seeded in the scalp might not receive adequate treatment, allowing them to grow at a later date.[4,78] Various authors have reported an incidence of scalp metastases occurring in 0.25–11% of patients.[79–83] It is advised that scalp hypothermia should not be used in patients with leukaemia or other neoplastic diseases in which numerous stem cells may be present in the scalp.[84] On the basis of these data, the use of scalp hypothermia was halted by the Food and Drug Administration (FDA) in the USA.[42] Some authors have reported no occurrence of scalp metastases and feel that the need for hair preservation far outweighs the risks.[73,85,86] Other workers have stated that hypothermia could be made available to patients with advanced disease where there would be no detriment to hindering the curative process, although it is contraindicated in patients presenting with scalp metastases.[68,70,78] If the treatment is palliative, the possibility of scalp metastases should not present a serious obstacle. However, if treatment is curative, this risk may be enough to rule out use of scalp hypothermia.[81] Patients should be made aware of this risk when making the choice for hypothermia.

The side-effects of hypothermia are uncomfortable. The most common side-effects reported include headache, dizziness, aversion for ice, nausea and vomiting, cold feeling on the scalp and/or throughout the body, a heavy feeling on the head, scalp metastases and transient light-headedness following cap removal.[87] A more thorough report of side-effects is given by Peck et al,[88] who suggest that tolerance and sensitivity to scalp cooling increases with each cycle or cold intolerance can develop by the 3rd, 4th and 5th cycles. Side-effects are more distressing when experienced outside the duration of treatment. Anticipatory anxiety has been noted as well as increasing needle phobia, nausea and anxiety. Patients have stated the length of time for the procedure was worse than the procedure itself.[89]

Despite the large number of studies on hypothermia, they are difficult to compare with one another due to the plethora of uncontrolled variables that may affect the outcome. In addition, many studies had small sample sizes and were non-randomized or had no control group. Assessment parameters for measuring alopecia also varied per study, as well as the definition of clinically relevant alopecia. A degree of success was seen in most studies but was dependent on the different types of chemotherapy regimens used, the dose and how hypothermia was administered. In addition, the patient's reactions were underreported as well as the details of the hypothermia procedure Efficiency of the appli-

ances in terms of patient comfort and their invested time, staff time/effort ratio and costs vary with the methods employed. Many studies have not addressed these issues.[8,40,60,90,91] Acquiring consensus on the effectiveness of hypothermia remains difficult. Therefore, this modality cannot be used as a standard preventative treatment.[78] Recent developments show that the new-generation cryogel cap, tested in Israel, showed moderate effectiveness in patients with adjuvant breast cancer. The incidence of alopecia in the hypothermia group was 48%, whereas it was 81% in the group who had not undergone cooling.[85]

Some studies have looked at the effects of hypothermia on Taxotere (docetaxel)-induced hair loss. Lemenagere et al,[92] Katsimbri et al[93] and MacDuff et al[94] have shown varied effectiveness in diminishing Taxotere (docetaxel)-related hair loss, respectively WHO ≤2 grade in 86%, grade 0–2 in 88%, and marginal protective effects. It is important to define particular patient populations that could derive benefit from hypothermia without the possible risk for scalp metastases and minimal side-effects and maximum effectiveness.

Biological measures

Biological methods of hair preservation focus on promoting hair growth or protecting the hair follicle. Two agents have been studied in men. Minoxidil 2%, a biological agent that promotes hair growth, as topical solution applied twice daily, is known to induce hair growth and prevent hair loss in normal male pattern baldness. Clinical investigation has demonstrated that minoxidil is most effective if some hair is present and stimulates suboptimal follicles.[95] The side-effects are few and present in <2% of patients.[96] In a study involving women who underwent chemotherapy with Cytoxan (cyclophosphamide), Adriamycin (doxorubicin) (Doxorubin Rapid Dissolution) and cisplatin or vincristine, mitomycin C and cisplatin, no benefit was reported from twice-daily applications of a 2% solution of minoxidil.[97]

Folic acid when administered with methotrexate can prevent alopecia.[78] Large doses of the vitamin α-tocopherol were administered to patients who received doxorubicin and 69% did not experience alopecia.[51] Perez et al[98] and Martin-Jimenez et al,[52] who repeated this study and demonstrated that AT had no effect in preventing doxorubicin-induced alopecia, have challenged these results. Powis et al[99] stated that in both studies other agents were added to the doxorubicin that could have negated the effects of AT. He demonstrated that supplementation of the diet in animal models was effective. Other measures use biological substances derived from the body to combat hair loss. These are in a very early stage of development. Although studies are ongoing to develop new biological agents to prevent hair loss and some effectiveness has been seen, the use of these agents remains unclear and application in the clinical setting is not recommended.

THE IMPACT OF ALOPECIA

Therapies for cancer have side-effects and each side-effect has a physical, psychosocial and spiritual impact. Alopecia is not different. Already overwhelmed with all the inherent issues of a newly diagnosed cancer or a cancer recurrence, issues around hair loss are significant.[41,100] The loss of body hair means a loss of protection from injury and the sun. Loss of the eyelashes permits foreign matter to enter the eyes more easily. Loss of nasal hair can contribute to more dust entering the nasal cavity. Complete hair loss on the head can have an effect on temperature regulation, whereby the head becomes cooler, giving a general sensation of feeling cold on other parts of the body. Loss of pubic hair can be uncomfortable and the skin may become easily chaffed.

One physician who underwent chemotherapy described her experience with chemotherapy:[101]

> Mentally I had prepared myself for the likelihood of losing my hair and having to wear a wig; but the physical reality of the hair falling out posed emotional and practical problems which I had not anticipated. For 2 weeks I was in tears every morning, plucking the clumps of hair from all over the bedclothes. Intellectually I understood what was happening, but emotionally it reinforced my feelings that I was losing a part of myself.

The psychological and social impact of hair loss, as summarized from current literature, are the following: a symbol of cancer (for self),

symbol of cancer (for others), personal confrontation with being ill or mortality, vulnerability, powerlessness, shame, loss of privacy, punishment, a change in self-perception (for self) or a change in sexual attractiveness (for others).[1] Coates et al[102] demonstrated that alopecia ranked third in the list of distressing symptoms, after nausea and vomiting. This varied only slightly between women and men.

In a study performed by Gallagher,[103] a detailed examination was given of the meaning of hair loss over time in a sample of women receiving alopecia-inducing cancer chemotherapy. Personal history, experiences as well as meanings of cancer images and one's hair shape symptom responses.

Analysis revealed three processes:

- affective anticipation rehearsal, which begins when one learns that hair loss will probably occur
- confronting the hair loss, which is acknowledging real hair loss
- management of the hair loss experience, which involves a number of appraisals and strategies intended to construct a new self.[103,104]

These processes are similar to the common themes identified in a narrative analysis of 15 women participating in a descriptive study of alopecia.[105] The common themes identified were preparing for hair loss, experiencing hair falling out, realising an altered sense of self, trying to look normal, being reminded of the disease, joking about alopecia, sharing being bald, having problems with wigs, taking control and experiencing hair growing back.

Although hair loss is usually reversible, it often has a dramatic psychological impact on the acceptance of treatment.[106] Patients have refused chemotherapy for fear of losing their hair.[51,73,88,107–109] However, the drive for survival is often the most important goal, which inhibits refusal of treatment. For many subjects, physical characteristics may become less important as measures of worth and living becomes more important.[24] In addition, it is not the mere occurrence of adverse events but the difficulty in managing them that contribute to non-compliance.[110]

In a study by Tierney et al,[111] 58% of patients expected hair loss to be the worst side-effect of all, but 21.7% rated it as such. Furthermore, another study reported that although patients found hair loss disturbing, it was tolerable provided wigs are available and preparation is given.[112] Subjects also stated that alopecia bothered them very little because they had been told about it and expected it.[113] Kiebert et al[114] reported that patients with breast cancer receiving adjuvant chemotherapy considered hair loss a severe side-effect although it was not prominent enough to cause a significant change in well-being. Also, in a study involving 55 women with breast cancer receiving adjuvant treatment with Adriamycin (doxorubicin) (Doxorubin Rapid Dissolution) and cyclophosphamide, 24% of the women reported hair loss having a clinically significant impact, whereas 40% experienced no impact at all.[41] In addition, 58% of the sample was active in deciding to shave their heads once hair loss occurred. The most stressful moment of hair loss was identified as when it began. Once hair loss began, most women stated that any hopes that they might be spared this side-effect waned and the acceptance process began.

Body image, self-esteem and sexuality

Most individuals consider their hairstyle an important part of their personal identity, and hair plays an important role in social and sexual communication. If we are aware of the relationship between a patient's hairstyle and overall appearance, then the relationship becomes clear between the presence of one's hair, self-concept and body image.[115] Body image is one component of self-concept, involving the picture of one's own body which we form in our mind, the way in which our body appears to ourselves (see Ch.32 on altered body image).[116] Hair changes place one at risk for an altered body image and can have an effect on significant others.[117] These changes can be reflected in the three aspects of the body:

- the body as a way of being in the world, which includes sensations and symptoms

- the body as a symbol or social expression
- the body as a necessary expression of existence.[118]

Two studies have established the influence of alopecia on body image. The first study was carried out by Wagner and Gorely[21] in a group of patients who received chemotherapy for haematological malignancies and solid tumours, of which 43 had observable alopecia and 34 did not. Although subjects with alopecia decreased their social activities, it was not significant, and this study did not confirm a negative association between alopecia and body image. Only those patients who had reported that their hair was important to them had demonstrated significantly different scores in body image between the alopecia group as opposed to the group without alopecia. The authors stated that many patients reformulate body image by focusing not on physical appearance but on spiritual issues, a sense of inner worth and strengthened family relationships.[21] The second study by Baxley et al[115] was carried out to re-examine the relationship between body image and hair loss in 40 patients receiving varying types of chemotherapy on an in- and outpatient basis. Twenty patients experienced hair loss and 20 did not. The results demonstrated that alopecia could negatively influence body image. These two studies have limitations in design and outcomes and denote a need for further studies to establish positive or negative associations between hair loss and body image.

Individuals who lose their hair may lose important aspects of their self, such as symbols of femininity, which places them at risk for lowered self-esteem.[119] Alopecia has a very negative psychological effect, particularly on female and young patients, conditioning the patient's quality of life with serious consequences.[80,108] Although the male self-image is just as affected by alopecia, men seem to deal with it more easily because male baldness is more socially acceptable.[120] Younger patients have more difficulty with the side-effects of chemotherapy.[110] In children, hair loss may block opportunities to interact successfully with the environment and thus prevent the development of self-image or self-esteem.[121]

As hair loss can have an effect on sexuality (see Ch. 31), it is important to realize that the patient's partner may not want to have sexual contact because alopecia may be a daily reminder of the partner's cancer. Loss of pubic hair may be sexually exciting, or it may remind the patient or partner of being a child so that sex is avoided because it may feel like incest. Single patients may be reluctant to date and/or initiate sexual contact because of the effect of alopecia on body image.[122] Furthermore, hair may be a symbol of religious affiliation (i.e. Hindu) and, as such, hair loss may have spiritual implications. However, data around this topic do not exist.

NURSING MANAGEMENT OF THE PATIENT WITH COMPLETE OR INCOMPLETE HAIR LOSS

Because alopecia is unavoidable in many patients, even though it is considered as a minor toxicity in treatment evaluations, nurses and physicians should try to help the patient prepare for the sudden loss of hair, thus minimizing the negative impact on the patient's self-image.[21,27] Understanding the meaning and the level of importance of hair to a particular person is the first step to creating meaningful interventions.[1] In addition, nurses should help patients control symptoms and identify and use more, coping mechanisms. The significance for the partner and family/friends is also important.[14] Therefore, an individualized approach is necessary. Women may need more accurate expectations about the physical changes during hair loss. The positive value of specific information and its impact on hopefulness is well recognized and the positive value of side-effect management information in self-care for patients receiving chemotherapy has been repeatedly shown.[123-126] As patients often have to deal with alopecia at home, it becomes important that a variety of self-care interventions be taught so that patients can choose which interventions will be appropriate for them. Providing the patient with cancer information about side-effect management techniques clearly has many advantages. The patient can identify the side-effect and be prompt in resorting to self-care that will alleviate it.[124]

The change from inpatient to outpatient administration of chemotherapy in the past few years has shifted the responsibility for managing the treatment of side-effects from health-care providers to patients and their families.[28] Therefore, patients should be instructed how to initiate self-care activities and health professionals should audit these self-care interventions and, when necessary, adapt them to the individual patient.

Patient teaching and emotional support help the patient anticipate hair loss, realize its impact, verbalize an understanding of factors that cause alopecia and learn self-care techniques.[35] Patients and their families should be informed as soon as possible, preferably before their treatments.[120] Patients have stated that hair loss bothered them very little because they had been told about it and expected it.[113]

Self-care strategies to cope with alopecia: teaching and information

Self-care strategies to cope with hair loss may be taught, which will hopefully contribute to diminishing the distress over this side-effect. It is important to explore past experiences and feelings with illness, treatment and hair loss before teaching self-care strategies to cope with hair loss. In addition, it is important to explore the meaning of hair loss for both patients and their significant others.[103] Professional care providers should pay attention to the degree of perceived support of patients and changes in the social environment and the role of significant others.[128] This gives the nurses necessary information to be able to provide the patient with individualized self-care strategies to cope with hair loss. Many patients find comfort in talking with others or discussing responses to alopecia with other patients.[117,127] Patients who are undergoing chemotherapy-induced alopecia should receive both written and verbal information, as shown in Box 27.1. In an interview session, feelings about hair loss can be validated and self-image addressed. During the interview it is important to find out how the individual or others thinks about him/herself without hair, how she/he anticipates thinking and experiencing self without hair and what other people will do or think.

611

Self-care strategies to minimize alopecia

Patients should receive information regarding how to minimize hair loss, although insufficient testing or evidence is available on the efficacy of such interventions. Minimizing interventions could include encouraging individuals with long hair to try a shorter style. Short hair tends to disguise hair thinning and also minimize the problem of shedding long hair, which may create anxiety. However, Chernecky[136] states that keeping the hair long if possible can be arranged to cover areas of baldness.[8,28,32,35,45, 134, 135] It is also recom-

mended to avoid daily shampooing. Patients can use a protein-rich shampoo or one that is pH balanced with conditioner every 4–7 days.[17,28,118,134] Baby shampoo has also been suggested.[45,126,136] Patients should rinse thoroughly with lukewarm water, pat dry and let it dry naturally or use a soft towel.[17,28,117,134] A wide-toothed comb or a soft-bristled brush should be used.[18,45, 117,126,132,134] However, two studies have actually challenged the effect of minimizing interventions. No relationship has been found between the extent of hair loss post chemotherapy and hair care practices including shampooing, blow-drying, teasing, combing, brushing, washing and setting, history of permanents, or colouring use of hair spray or curling irons.[41,137] In addition, self-care activities listed for hair loss, such as shampoo and brush choice, were chosen by fewer than 25% of patients in one study, and of those only two patients felt that using a soft brush was effective.[137]

Self-care strategies to protect the scalp

Since hair has a protective function, it is important to teach patients how to protect the scalp and other affected areas such as the eyes from cold, heat, the sun and mechanical irritation. Avoiding exposure to the sun and using sun protection factors are deemed important.[8,15,17,18,36,45,117,126,127,132,134] Eye glasses or sunglasses should be used to protect eyes.[18,35,45,127] In addition, cleansing eye drops to remove foreign particles from the eyes could provide soothing relief.[8] Head coverings to prevent scalp irritation or heat loss and conserve warmth and wearing a wig are advised.[18,35,36,42,47,117,127,134] The nurse should ensure the wig lining is comfortable and non-irritating.[128] Massaging and applying creme to the scalp may keep it soft, e.g. with baby oil and mineral oil or vitamin A&D ointment may used to reduce itching.[17, 35,45,47, 126]

Head shaving or wearing a wig

Increasingly, individuals with cancer are taking control of events they are confronted with, e.g. once hair loss becomes pronounced, more

---

Box 27.1

Information for patients who may experience hair loss

What is hair loss?

Why hair loss occurs

Risk of undergoing hair loss

How hair will fall out (quickly or over time)

When hair loss begins and ends

Where does it begin and the degree of hair loss

Symptoms or complaints associated with hair loss

How to minimize hair loss

How it will grow back, (ir)reversibility of hair loss

Changes in hair following hair loss

The impact of hair loss; psychosocial implications

Possible effects on body image and sexuality

Altered sense of self/appearance

What to do about hair loss

How to cope with hair loss

Shaving the head

Scalp care following hair loss

How to use protective measures

When, where and how to purchase wigs

Information about wigs: activity limitation, what to watch out for

Wig care

Details on insurance coverage (not all wigs are fully reimbursed in all countries)

Available resources for support such as the programme: 'Look good, feel better'

Source: references 8, 17, 18, 28, 36, 45, 47, 78, 103, 105, 109, 120, 126–133.

patients are shaving their heads. Patients seem to experience less scalp discomfort and pain compared to those who do not.[47] In addition, it promotes even regrowth, often permitting the patient to go without a wig sooner.[28] In one study, 58% of all women were active in removing their hair, either cutting it very short (1–2 cm) or shaving it off.[41] Beginning hair loss, especially when dramatic, is physically disturbing. Falling hair is cumbersome as it falls on clothing, furniture and food. Emotionally, it can be very disturbing to the patient and those around the patient.

This intervention has not been routinely offered to people who will experience complete hair loss. Nurses should inform patients about this option early on before treatment has begun. There are advantages and disadvantages to shaving. Advantages may include preventing confrontation with falling hair, giving a sense of control as hair loss begins, assisting in even regrowth of hair, assisting in fitting and fixating the wig and hair regrowth can be recognized earlier. However, disadvantages may be that head shaving can be very confronting. If the head is not shaven to the skin, the remaining short hairs will still fall out. The remaining short hairs can also be uncomfortable under the wig or, if completely shaven to the skin, the skin could become irritated. Once hair falls out, individuals are faced with two choices: going bald or wearing a wig or headpiece.

Going bald without a wig as creation of a new social identity[41] could be another way to cope with hair loss or be the symbol of the patient's new identity. Highlighting other features to distract from hair loss or emphasizing other fine qualities that the patient has is also a strategy for dealing with hair loss.[45] A person may make changes to convey different messages to others.[118] Patients should be encouraged to express positive and negative feelings about hair loss.[28]

When the patient decides to use a wig, it is preferable to buy a wig from a well-known salon that deals with quality wigs and that can provide a measure of support and privacy to patients during fittings. Patients can be encouraged to bring friends or family to help them chose. Wigs should be selected before the patient has lost his/her hair in order to match the colour, style and hair texture.[8,18,42,127] Alternatively, a photo should be made and a snip of hair taken before hair loss occurs and used as a basis for purchasing the wig.[43,127]

Wigs can be purchased from human or synthetic hair. Synthetic and human hair wigs are equally durable and can both be matched to the patient's own hair colour and desired cut. Human hair is more expensive but has a natural feel and versatility. Many women favour synthetic wigs, since they are easier to maintain, hold their set longer, dry faster after washing, and are far less expensive than 'real hair' (wigs. www.lookgoodfeelbetter.org/). It is suggested to buy a wig that is slightly lighter in colour, as darker colours tend to drain colour from the face. Information on financial assistance or third-party coverage for wigs should be provided.[18,36] Consideration should be given to the provision of a second wig for patients who need to wash it and use it again within a certain time frame.[109] When hair starts to grow, it may be 3–6 months after therapy before there is enough hair on the head before one considers removing the wig. When hair grows back, it does not all grow evenly and the first hairs are rather downy. One may consider cutting the hair evenly when the hair is 3–4 cm long.

The salon usually provides washing instructions or wig care. Wig care is important and consists of storing the wig in a cool dry place on a stand or head. Generally, a wig should be washed after every 6–8 wearings in warm climates or after every 12–15 wearings in coolers ones (www.lookgoodfeelbetter.org/). Washing instructions are usually given with the wig. After washing, patients need to tightly finger squeeze each curl on curly styles while the wig is still wet. On both straight and curly styles, gentle towel blot to remove excess water is recommended. Wigs could be air-dried on a clean, dry towel or a wire head form that allows air circulation. The wig stand should not be situated near heat sources or in direct sunlight and blow dryers or other heat appliances should not be used on synthetic wigs. Also, combing, brushing or picking a wet wig is not advisable.

Supportive programmes

Suggesting that patients participate in programmes or support groups such as 'Look Good, Feel Better' offered in many countries throughout the world can help patients optimize their appearance during hair loss.[15,42,117,135] This programme can assist patients to accept a different, perhaps transient, view of themselves until they can recover from this obvious effect of their treatment.[49] Patients in various stages of treatment receive makeover tips and personal attention from professionals trained to meet their needs. Professional advice is provided on wigs, scarves and accessories. Teen sessions also include social and health tips. The contact with other people who are experiencing the same problem validates emotional experiences and offers support.

CONCLUSION

Nurses rely on traditional sources of information about alopecia, and much of the information is not research-based. For example, we suggest to patients that there are interventions that will minimize alopecia, although it is unknown if and how that will help. In addition, it creates false hope that hair loss might be kept under control, and this may be detrimental to the patient's ability to cope if it does occur. It might be more feasible to use an intervention employing guided imagery and coping with anticipatory grief to desensitize patients to the hair loss experience and maintain coping.[138] The issue of prevention of hair loss needs to be explored further. There is evidence of some side-effects of the use of hypothermia techniques with cold caps, and research is needed to quantify the distress, as well as the long-term benefits, such as quality of the hair, after chemotherapy is complete. The effect of this intervention on nursing time is essential if this is to be adopted as standard therapy.

REFERENCES

1. Freedman TG. Social and cultural dimensions of hair loss in women treated for breast cancer. Cancer Nurs 1994; 17(4):334–341.

2. Firth RW. Hair as private asset and public symbol. In: Symbols – public and private. London: George Allen & Unwin; 1973:262–298.

3. Harre J. A matter of the length of hair: beliefs and symbols in social studies No. 10. New Zealand: National Education; 1968.

4. Holmes W. Alopecia from chemotherapy: can nursing measures help? In: Clinical and scientific sessions. Am Nurs Assoc 1979:223–233

5. Antoni CP, Thibodeau GA. Skin and the appendages. In: The textbook of anatomy and physiology. 11th edn. St. Louis: Mosby; 1983:82–83.

6. Williams P. Appendages of skin – hairs. In: Bannister LH, Berry MM, Collins P et al, eds. Gray's anatomy – the anatomical basis of medicine and surgery. 38th edn. London: Churchill Livingstone; 1995:400–405.

7. Orfanos CE. Hair and hair growth. In: Orfanos CE, Happle R, eds. Hair and hair diseases. Berlin: Springer-Verlag; 1991:485–529

8. Keller JF, Blausey LA. Nursing issues and management in chemotherapy-induced alopecia. Oncol Nurs Forum 1988; 15(5):603–607.

9. Messenger AG. The control of hair growth: an overview. J Invest Derm 1993; 101(1 Suppl): 4S–9S.

10. Randall VA, Eblin FJG. Seasonal changes in human hair growth. Br J Dermatol 1991; 124:146–151.

11. Munro DD. Disorders of hair. In: Fitzpatrick TB, Arndt KA, Clard WH, et al, eds. Dermatology in general medicine. New York: McGraw-Hill; 1971:297–331.

12. Orfanos CE, Hair and hair growth. In: Orfanos CE, Happle R, eds. Hair and hair diseases. Berlin: Springer-Verlag; 1991:485–529.

13. Bekhor PS. Common hair disorders. Austr Fam Phys 1986; 15(7):868–874.

14. Goodman M, Ladd L, Purl S. Integumentary and mucous membrane alternations. In: Groenwald SL, Frogge MH, Goodman M, Yarbro CH, eds. Cancer nursing: principles and practice. Boston: Jones and Bartlett; 1996:785–788.

15. Howser DM. Alopecia – the problem of alopecia in cancer. In: Groenwald SL, Frogge MH, Goodman M, Yarbro CH, eds. Cancer symptom management. Boston: Jones and Bartlett; 1996:261–268.

16. Junqueira LC, Carneiro J, Kelly RO, eds. Subcutaneous tissue – hairs. In: Basic histology. 8th edn. Stamford, Connecticut: Appleton & Lange; 1995:352–355.

17. Schlesselman SM. Helping your cancer patient cope with alopecia. Nursing 1988; December:43–45.

18. Joss RA, Kiser J, Weston S, Brunner KW. Fighting alopecia in cancer chemotherapy. Recent Results Cancer Res 1988; 108:117–126.

19. Dunagin WG. Clinical toxicity of chemotherapeutic agents: dermatologic toxicity. Semin Oncol 1982; 9(1):14–22.

20. Crounse RG, Van Scott EJ. Changes in scalp hair roots as a measure of toxicity from cancer chemotherapeutic drugs. J Invest Dermatol 1960; 35:83–90.

21. Wagner L, Gorely M. Body image and patients experiencing alopecia as a result of cancer chemotherapy. Cancer Nurs 1979; 2(5):365–369.

22. Orfanos CE, Imcke E. Hair and hair cosmetics. In: Orfanos CE, Happle R, eds. Hair and hair diseases. Berlin: Springer-Verlag; 1991:887–921.

23. Dunagin WG. Dermatologic toxicity. In: Perry MC, Yarbro JW, eds. Toxicity of chemotherapy. New York: Grune & Stratton; 1984:125–145.

24. Kligman AM. Pathologic dynamics of human hair loss. Telogen effluvium. Arch Dermatol 1961; 83:175–198.

25. Hood AF. Cutaneous side effects of cancer chemotherapy. Med Clin North Am 1986; 70(1):187–209.

26. DeSpain JD. Dermatologic toxicity of chemotherapy. Semin Oncol 1992; 19(5):501–507.

27. Villani C, Inghirami P, Pjetrangeli D, Tomao S, Pucci G. Prevention by hypothermic cap of antiblastic induced-alopecia. Eur J Gynaecol Oncol 1986; VII(1):15–17.

28. Camp-Sorrell D. Chemotherapy: toxicity management. In: Henke Yarbo C, Goodman B, Hansen Frogge M, Groenwald SL, eds. Cancer nursing: principles and practice. 5th edn. Boston: Jones and Bartlett; 2000: 470–471.

29. Whitshaw E. Cyclophosphamide. Proc Symp Royal College of Surgeons, Bristol; 1963:97.

30. Simister JM. Alopecia and cytotoxic drugs. Br Med J 1966; 2(522):1138.

31. Hennessey JD. Alopecia and cytotoxic drugs. Br Med J 1966; 2:1138.

32. Fulton JS. Chemotherapeutic treatment of colorectal cancer: rationale, trends, and nursing care. J Wound Ostom Contin Nurs 1994; 21(1):12–21.

33. Taplin SC, Blanke CD, Baughman C. Nursing care strategies for the management of side effects in patients treated for colorectal cancer. Semin Oncol 1997; 24(5):S18–64 and S18–70.

34. Sitzia J. Higgins L. Side effects of cyclophosphamide, methotrexate, and 5-fluorouracil (CMF) chemotherapy for breast cancer. Cancer Pract 1998: 6(1):13–21.

35. Wilkes GM. Potential toxicities and nursing management. In: Barton Burke M, Wilkes GM, Inguersen K, eds. Cancer chemotherapy: a nursing process approach. 2nd edn. Boston: Jones and Bartlett; 1996:130–135.

36. Higgs DJ. The Patient with testicular cancer: nursing management of chemotherapy. Oncol Nurs Forum 1990; 17(2):243–249.

37. Sitzia J, North C, Stanley J, Winterberg N. Side effects of CHOP in the treatment of non-Hodgkin's lymphoma. Cancer Nurs 1997; 20(6):430–439.

38. Bezwoda W, Rastogi RB, Erazo Valla A, et al. Long-term results of a multicentre randomised, comparative phase III trial of CHOP versus CNOP regimens in patients with intermediate- and high-grade non-Hodgkin's lymphomas. Eur J Canc Care 1995; 31A(6):911–916.

39. Moseley J. Nursing management of toxicities associated with chemotherapy for lung cancer. Semin Oncol Nurs 1987; 3(3):202–210.

40. Hillen HFP, Breed WPM, Botman CJ. Scalp cooling by cold air for the prevention of chemotherapy-induced alopecia. Neth J Med 1990; 37:231–235.

41. Batchelor D. Hair and cancer chemotherapy: consequences and nursing care – a literature study. Eur J Cancer Care 2001; (10):147–163.

42. Seipp CA. Hair loss. In: DeVita VT, Hellman S, Rosenberg SA, eds. Cancer: principles and practice of oncology, Vol 2. 5th edn. Philadelphia: Lippencott-Raven; 1997:27–57.

43. Ehmann Lombardo J, Sheehan A, Decker GM. Intervening with alopecia: exploring an entrepreneurial role for oncology nurses. Oncol Nurs Forum 1991; 18(4):769–773.

44. Robinson A, Jones W. Changes in scalp hair after cancer chemotherapy. Eur J Cancer Clin Oncol 1989; 25 (1):155–156.

45. Didonato K. Standards of clinical nursing practice: alopecia. Cancer Nurs 1985; 8(1):76–77.

46. Fairlamb DJ. Hair changes following cytotoxic drug induced alopecia. Postgrad Med J 1988; 64:907.

47. Goodman MS. Chemotherapy toxicities. In: Cancer: chemotherapy and care. 3rd edn. Princeton, NJ: Bristol-Meyers Squibb; 1992:45.

48. Wilkes GM. Potential toxicities and nursing management. In: Barton Burke M, Wilkes GM, Inguersen K, eds. Cancer chemotherapy: a nursing process approach. 2nd ed. Boston: Jones and Bartlett; 1996:130–135.

49. Reeves D. Alopecia. In: Yarbro, CH, Frogge MH, Goodman M, eds. Cancer symptom management. 2nd edn. Boston: Jones and Bartlett; 1999:275–285.

50. Puglisi F, Aprile G, Sobrero A. Tamoxifen-induced total alopecia. Ann Intern Med. 2001; 134(12):1154–1155.

51. Wood LA. Possible prevention of adriamycin-induced alopecia by tocopherol. N Engl J Med 1985; 312:1060.

52. Martin-Jimenez M, Diaz-Rubio E, Gonzales Larriba JL, Sangro B. Failure of high-dose tocopherol to prevent alopecia induced by doxorubicin. N Engl J Med 1986; 315(14):894–895.

53. O'Brien R, Zelson JH, Schwartz AD, Pearson HA. Scalp tourniquet to lessen alopecia after vincristine. N Engl J Med 1970; 283:1469.

54. Lyons AR. Prevention of hair loss by head-band during cytotoxic therapy. Lancet 1974; 1:354.

55. Pesce A, Cassuto JP, Joyner MV, DuJardin P, Audoly P. Scalp tourniquet in the prevention of chemotherapy-induced alopecia. N Engl J Med 1978; 298:1204–1205.

56. Soukoup M, Campbell A, Gray M, et al. Adriamycin, alopecia and scalp tourniquet. Cancer Treat Rep 1978; 62(2):489–490.

57. Lovejoy NC. Preventing hair loss during adriamycin therapy. Cancer Nurs 1979; 2(2):117–121.

58. Maxwell M. Scalp tourniquets for chemotherapy-induced alopecia. Am J Nurs 1980; 80:900–903.

59. Kennedy M, Packard R, Grant M, et al. The effects of using Chemocap® on occurrence of chemotherapy-induced alopecia. Oncol Nurs Forum 1982; 10(1):19–24.

60. Cline BW. Prevention of chemotherapy-induced alopecia: a review of the literature. Cancer Nurs 1984; 7(3):221–228.

61. Bülow J, Friberg L, Gaardsting O, Hansen M. Frontal subcutaneous blood flow, and epi- and subcutaneous temperatures during scalp cooling in normal man. Scand J Clin Lab Invest 1985; 45:505–508.

62. Cooke T, Gregory RP, Middleton J, Williams C. Prevention of doxorubicin-induced alopecia. Br Med J 1981; 282:734–735.

63. Gregory RP, Buchanan RB, Grace A, Cooke T. Prevention of Adriamycin-induced alopecia by scalp hypothermia: the relationship to the degree of cooling. Surg Res Soc Abstracts 1981; 86:813.

64. Luce JT, Raffetto TJ, Crisp IA, Grief GC. Prevention of alopecia by scalp cooling of patients receiving Adriamycin. Cancer Chemother Rep 1973; 57(1):108–109.

65. Tollenaar RAEM, Liefers GJ, Repelaer van Driel OJ, Van de Velde CJH. Scalp cooling has no place in the prevention of alopecia in adjuvant chemotherapy for breast cancer. Eur J Cancer 1994; 30A(10):1448–1453.

66. Anderson JE, Hunt JM, Smith IE. Prevention of doxorubin-induced alopecia by scalp cooling in patients with advanced breast cancer. Br Med J 1981; 282:423–424.

67. Guy R, Parker H, Shah S, Geddes D. Scalp cooling by thermocirculator. Lancet 1982; 1(8278):937–938.

68. Hunt J, Anderson JE, Smith IE. Scalp hypothermia to prevent adriamycin-induced hair loss. Cancer Nurs 1982;5(1):25–31.

69. Di Giulio F, Giaccone G, Morandini MP. Scalp hypothermia in the prevention of alopecia induced by doxorubicin. Proc ECCO 1983;4: abstract No. 725:192.

70. Johansen Vendelbo L. Scalp hypothermia in the prevention of chemo-induced alopecia. Acta Radiol 1985; 24(3):113–116.

71. Parker R. The effectiveness of scalp hypothermia in preventing cyclophosphamide-induced alopecia. Oncol Nurs Forum 1987; 14(6):49–53.

72. Robinson MH, Jones AC, Durrant KD. Effectiveness of scalp cooling in reducing alopecia caused by epirubicin treatment of advanced breast cancer. Cancer Treat Rep 1987; 71(10):913–914.

73. Giacconne G, Di Giulio F, Morandini MP, Calciati A. Scalp hypothermia in the prevention of doxorubicin-induced hair loss. Cancer Nurs 1988; 11(3):170–173.

74. Belpomme D, Mignot L, Grandjean M, et al. Prévention de l'alopécie des chimiothérapies anticancéreuses par hypothermie du cuir chevelu. La Nouvelle Presse Médicale 1982; 11(12):929–931.

75. Gregory RP, Cooke T, Middleton J, Buchanan RB, Williams CJ. Prevention of doxorubicin-induced alopecia by scalp hypothermia: relation to degree of cooling. Br Med J 1982; 284:1674.

76. Dougherty L. Patients' views on scalp cooling in chemotherapy. Prof Nurse 1996; 11(12):785.

77. Adams L, Lawson N, Maxted KJ, Symonds RP. The prevention of hair loss from chemotherapy by the use of cold-air scalp-cooling. Eur J Cancer Care 1992; 1:5:16–18

78. Franssen CFM, Hillen HFP. Haaruitval door cytostatica. Ned Tijdschr Geneeskd 1991; 135(24):1070–1073.

79. Seipp CA. Scalp hypothermia: indications for precaution. Oncol Nurs Forum 1983; 10(1):12.

80. Dean JC, Griffith KS, Cetas TC, et al. Scalp hypothermia: a comparison of ice packs and the Kold Kap in the prevention of doxorubicin-induced alopecia. J Clin Oncol 1983; 1(1):33–37.

81. Smith F, McCabe MS. Preventing chemotherapy-induced alopecia. Am Fam Phys 1984; 28(1):182–184.

82. Middleton J, Franks D, Buchanan RB, et al. Failure of scalp hypothermia to prevent hair loss when cyclophosphamide is added to doxorubicin and vincristine. Cancer Treat Rep 1985; 69(4);373–375.

83. Peck HJ, Mitchell H, Stewart AL. Evaluating the efficacy of scalp cooling using the Penguin cold cap system to reduce alopecia in patients undergoing chemotherapy for breast cancer. Eur J Oncol Nurs. 2000 Dec;4(4):246–8.

84. Dean JC, Salmon SE, Griffith KS. Prevention of doxorubin-induced hair loss with scalp hypothermia. N Engl J Med 1979; 301(26):1427–1429.

85. Ron IG, Kalmus Y, Kalmus Z, Inbar M, Chaitchik S. Scalp cooling in the prevention of alopecia in patients receiving depilating

chemotherapy. Support Care Cancer 1997; 5:136–138.

86. Protiere C, Evans K, Camerlo J, et al. Efficacy and tolerance of a scalp-cooling system for prevention of hair loss and the experience of breast cancer patients treated by adjuvant chemotherapy. Support Care Cancer 2002;10(7):529–537. Epub 2002 Aug 15.

87. Satterwhite B. The use of scalp hypothermia in the prevention of doxorubicin-induced hair loss. Cancer 1984; 54:34–37.

88. Peck HJ, Mitchell H, Stewart AL. Evaluating the efficacy of scalp cooling using the Penguin cold cap system to reduce alopecia in patients undergoing chemotherapy for breast cancer. Eur J Oncol Nurs 2000; 4(4):246–248.

89. Dougherty L. Patients' views on scalp cooling in chemotherapy. Prof Nurse 1996; 11(12):785.

90. Tigges FJ. Prophylaxe der Adriamycin bedingten Alopezie. Munch.Med WSChr 1981; 123(18):737–738.

91. Tierney A. Preventing chemotherapy-induced alopecia in cancer patients: is scalp cooling worthwhile? J Adv Nurs 1987; 12:303–310.

92. Lemenager M, Lecomte S, Bonneterre ME, et al. Effectiveness of cold cap in the prevention of docetaxel-induced alopecia. Eur J Cancer 1997; 33(2):297–300.

93. Katsimbri P, Bamias A, Pavlidis N. Prevention of chemotherapy-induced alopecia using an effective scalp cooling system. Eur J Cancer 2000; 36(6):766–771.

94. Macduff C, Mackenzie T, Hutcheon A, Melville L, Archibald H. The effectiveness of scalp cooling in preventing alopecia for patients receiving epirubicin and docetaxel. Eur J Cancer Care 2003; 12(2):154–161.

95. Shapiro J, Price VH. Hair regrowth: therapeutic agents. Dermatol Clin 1998; 16(2):341–356.

96. Burnett JW. Dermatology days. Proc Dermatology Days Symp 1990; 45:155.

97. Granai CO, Frederickson H, Gajewski W, et al. The use of minoxidil to attempt to prevent alopecia during chemotherapy for gynecologic malignancies. Eur J Gynaec Oncol 1991; XII(2):129–132.

98. Perez JE, Macchiavelli M, Leone BA, et al. High-dose alpha-tocopherol as a preventive of doxorubicin-induced alopecia. Cancer Treat Rep 1986; 70(10):1213–1214.

99. Powis G, Kooistra KL. Doxorubicin-induced hair loss in the Angora rabbit: a study of treatments to protects against the hair loss. Cancer Chemother Pharmacol 1987; 20:291–296.

100. Munstedt K, Manthey N, Sachsse S, Vahrson H. Changes in self-concept and body image during alopecia-induced cancer chemotherapy. Support Care Cancer 1997; 5(2):139–143.

101. Clement-Jones V. Cancer and beyond: the formation of BACUP. Br Med. J 1985; 291:1021–1023.

102. Coates A, Abraham S, Kaye SB, et al. On the receiving end – patient perception of the side-effects of cancer chemotherapy. Eur J Cancer 1983; 19(2):203–208.

103. Gallagher J. Women's experience of hair loss associated with cancer chemotherapy: a qualitative study. Dissertation, University of Massachusetts; 1992.

104. Gallagher J. Chemotherapy-induced hair loss. Impact on women's quality of life. In: Cohen, MZ, ed. Quality of life: a nursing challenge. Philadelphia: Meniscus Health Care Communications; 1997:75–78.

105. Williams J, Wood C, Cunningham-Warburton P. A Narrative Study of Chemotherapy-Induced Alopecia. Oncol Nurs Forum 1999;26(9):1463–8.

106. Arzouman JMR, Dudas S, Estwing Ferrans C, Holm K. Quality of life of patients with sarcoma postchemotherapy. Oncol Nurs Forum 1991;18(5):889–894.

107. Kennedy M, Packard R, Grant M, Padilla G, Presant C, Chillar R. The Effects of Using Chemocap® on Occurence of Chemotherapy-Induced Alopecia. Oncol Nurs Forum 1982;10(1):19–24.

108. Wheelock JB, Myers MB, Krebs HB, Goplerud DR. Ineffectiveness of scalp hypothermia in the prevention of alopecia in patients treated with doxorubicin and cisplatin combinations. Cancer Treat Rep 1984; 68(11):1387–1388.

109. Tierney A, Taylor J. Chemotherapy-induced hair loss. Nurs Stand 1991; 5(38):29–31.

110. Richardson JL, Marks G, Levine A. The influence of symptoms of disease and side effects of treatment on compliance with cancer therapy. J Clin Oncol 1988; 6(11):1746–1752.

111. Tierney A, Taylor J, Closs SJ. Knowledge, expectations and experiences of patients receiving chemotherapy for breast cancer. Scand J Caring Sci 1992; 6(2):75–80.

112. Edelstyn GA, MacRae KD, MacDonald FM. Improvement of life quality in cancer patients undergoing chemotherapy. Clin Oncol 1979; 5:43–49.

113. Richards ME, Martinson IM. Patients' perceptions of the impact of chemotherapy side effects and their methods of coping with this impact. In: Debellis R, Hyman GA, Seeland IB, et al, eds. Psychosocial aspects of chemotherapy in cancer care: the patient, family and staff. New York: Hawthorn Press; 1987:53–78.

114. Kiebert GM, de Haes JHCJM, Kievit J, van de Velde CJH. Effect of peri-operative chemotherapy on the quality of life of patients with early breast cancer. Eur J Cancer 1990; 26(10):1038–1042.

115. Baxley KO, Erdman LK, Henry EB, Roof JB. Alopecia: effect on cancer patients' body image. Cancer Nurs 1984; 7(6):499–503.

116. Schindler P. Image and appearance of the human body. London: Kegan Paul; 1935.

117. Freitas BA. Coping: altered body image and alopecia. In: Itano FK, Taoka KN, eds. Core curriculum for oncology nursing. 3rd edn. Philadelphia: WB Saunders; 1998:54–59.

118. Cohen Zichi M, Kahn DL, Steeves RH. Beyond body image: the experience of breast cancer. Oncol Nurs Forum 1998; 25 (5):835–841.

119. Carpenter Sharkey J, Brockopp DY. Evaluation of self-esteem of women with cancer receiving chemotherapy. Oncol Nurs Forum 1994; 21(4):751–757.

120. Vandegrift KV. The development of an oncology alopecia wig program. J Intravenous Nurs 1994; 17(2):78–82.

121. Reid U. Stigma of hair loss after chemotherapy. Paediatr Nurs 1997; 9(3):16–18.

122. Gates RA, Fink RM. Symptom effect on sexuality. In: Gates RA, Fink RM, eds. Oncology nursing secrets. Philadephia: Hanley & Belfus; 1997:316.

123. Cassileth BR, Zupkis RV, Sutton-Smith K, March V. Information and participation preferences amongst cancer patients. Ann Intern Med 1980; 92:832–836.

124. Dodd MJ. Self-care for side effects in cancer chemotherapy: an assessment of nursing interventions – Part II. Cancer Nurs 1983; 6(1):63–67.

125. Dodd MJ. Assessing patient self-care for side effects of cancer chemotherapy – Part I. Cancer Nurs 1982; 5(6):447–451.

126. Rhodes VA, McDaniel RW, Johnson MH. Patient education: self-care guides. Semin Oncol Nurs 1995; 11(4):298–304.

127. Goodman M, Hildesley LJ, Purl S. Integumentary and mucous membrane alternations. In: Groenwald SL, Frogge MH, Goodman M, Yarbro CH, eds. Cancer nursing: principles and practice. Boston: Jones and Bartlett; 1997:785–788.

128. Rose K. The stress of chemotherapy. Can Nurse 1978; 74(5):18–21.

129. Freitas BA. Coping: Altered body image and alopecia. In: Itano FK, Taoka KN, eds. Core curriculum for oncology nursing. 3rd edn. Philadelphia: WB Saunders; 1998:54–59.

130. Lilley LL. Side effects associated with pediatric chemotherapy: management and patient education issues. Pediatr Nurs 1990; 16(3):252–255.

131. Fulton JS. Chemotherapeutic treatment of colorectal cancer: rationale, trends, and nursing care. J Wound Ostom Contin Nurs 1994; 21(1):12–21.

132. Gross J, Johnson BL. Protective mechanisms: alopecia. In: Gross J, Johnson BL, eds. Handbook of oncology nursing. 2nd edn. Boston: Jones and Bartlett; 1994:450 and 455.

133. Irwin E, Arnold A, Whelan TJ, Reyno LM, Cranton P. Offering a choice between two adjuvant chemotherapy regimens: a pilot study to develop a decision aid for women with breast cancer. Patient Educ Couns 1999; 37(3):283–291.

134. Davidhizar R, Bartlett D. When your patients lose their hair. Today's OR Nurse 1993; 15(3):39–42.

135. Kaderman C, Kaderman RA, Toonkel R. The psychosocial aspects of beast cancer. Nurs Practit Forum 1999; 10(3):165–174.

136. Chernecky CC. Alopecia. In: Yasko, JM, ed. Guidelines for care in symptom management. Virginia: Reston Publishing; 1983:104–117.

137. Foltz AT, Gaines G, Gullatte M. Recalled side effects and self-care actions of patients receiving inpatient chemotherapy. Oncol Nurs Forum 1996; 23(4):679–683.

138. McGarvey EL, Baum LD, Pinkerton RC, Rogers LM. Psychological sequelae and alopecia among women with cancer. Cancer Pract 2001; 9(6):283–289.

CHAPTER 28

Malignant Effusions

SHELLEY DOLAN AND NANCY J PRESTON

CHAPTER CONTENTS

Introduction	619	Thoracic/pleural effusions	624
Anatomy and physiology	619	The aetiology of malignant pleural effusion	624
		Epidemiology	624
Malignant ascites	620	Pathophysiology	625
The natural history of malignant ascites	620	Diagnosis	625
Aetiology of malignant ascites	620	Therapeutic interventions for malignant pleural effusion	626
Incidence and prevalence of malignant ascites	621	Conclusion	628
Symptoms associated with malignant ascites	622	References	629
Current therapies for malignant ascites	622		

INTRODUCTION

Malignant effusions are abnormal collections of fluid which can collect in a number of places in the body, but most commonly in either the peritoneal or pleural space. In the peritoneal space, the effusion is called malignant ascites (MA) and in the pleural space it is called a malignant pleural effusion (MPE). The diagnosis of a malignant effusion is usually made by the patient's history and then, in the case of an MPE, a chest X-ray, and in both cases drainage and cytological examination of the fluid. The differential diagnosis would be fluid caused by infection, inflammation or in the lungs by cardiac failure. Malignant effusions are generally associated with cancer that has progressed to a metastatic stage. Both types of effusion can be managed using a variety of methods, but the fluid will often reaccumulate.[1]

ANATOMY AND PHYSIOLOGY

The peritoneal and pleural linings consist of double membranes. The peritoneal cavity surrounds the abdominal organs and the pleural linings surround the lungs. Both are moistened with a small amount of fluid, which reduces friction during movement and respiration. As the membranes of the linings are permeable, fluid enters and exits through capillaries and the lymphatic system. The lymphatic vessels in the pleural cavity are connected to the thoracic duct. The lymphatic vessels draining free fluid into the peritoneal cavity are connected to the right lymphatic duct.

When fluid accumulates in a space like the peritoneal cavity or pleural cavity, it is called central oedema. Fluid collects due to two primary sources: overproduction or obstruction. When too much fluid is produced, this results in 'high-output failure' of the lymphatic system.[2]

High-output failure is characterized by a lymphatic system that has become overwhelmed and cannot manage the increased volume of circulating fluid. This increased fluid collects in the available space where it is produced. Obstruction of the lymphatic system results in 'low-output failure', where the lymphatic system is impaired in its ability to move the fluid. Once again, fluid accumulates because it cannot move out of the cavity. Obstruction of the lymphatic system with tumour is the most common cause, but also removal of lymphatic vessels during cancer surgery will impair drainage.[3,4] It is not uncommon for both factors to play a role in the development of any central oedema.

MALIGNANT ASCITES

Ascites is the accumulation of fluid in the peritoneal cavity. It can develop from a variety of causes, both malignant and non-malignant. In this chapter, only ascites resulting from a malignancy, i.e. MA, will be described. As fluid accumulates, the abdomen is pushed forward to accommodate the fluid, distorting the appearance of the patient's body.

The following section will describe the natural history of MA, its aetiology, incidence, associated symptoms and their effect upon well-being, and treatments used in the management of MA. Unfortunately, there is a dearth of good-quality research assessing either treatments for the management of ascites or the impact of ascites upon patients' well-being.

The natural history of malignant ascites

The organs of the peritoneal cavity push into the peritoneal lining. There are two membranes that make up the peritoneal lining, called the parietal and the visceral linings. Between the two linings is a small volume of fluid whose purpose is to prevent the two linings adhering to each other. As a result of changes in pressure exerted during respiration, fluid drains out of the peritoneal cavity in an upwards direction through the diaphragmatic lymphatic vessels. In a patient with MA, either the volume of fluid is too great to drain or the drainage pathways are blocked and large volumes of fluid collect inside the lining.

There are no historical studies that describe the natural history of the development of MA and its treatment. How much ascitic fluid builds up before the patient seeks treatment is variable. Paracentesis (abdominal drainage) is the commonest treatment for ascites.[5] The literature demonstrates that investigators rarely include the volume of ascites present when patients are referred for any intervention. However, the volume drained in four studies ranged from 0.1 L to 9 L, with the average volume being 4 L (Table 28.1).

Many patients require frequent drainage procedures, as the fluid reaccumulates, but the frequency of drainage procedures is unknown. A common clinical picture is one of patients developing large volumes of MA requiring frequent drainage.

Aetiology of malignant ascites

The aetiology of MA is still unclear; however, the two primary causes that are thought to be involved in its development are overproduction of fluid in the peritoneal cavity and/or lymphatic obstruction of the diaphragmatic lymphatic vessels. Overproduction of fluid in the peritoneal cavity results from two primary causes:

- tumour compression of the hepatobiliary blood vessels, forcing extra fluid out of the general circulation
- increased permeability of the peritoneal lining, thereby increasing the amount of fluid in the peritoneal cavity.

In the 1940s and 1950s, ascites was classified into either transudative or exudative, by testing its protein content; this classification was then used to differentiate the cause of the ascites. If fluid is forced out of the circulation as a result of tumour pressure, the fluid will be low in protein and classified as a transudate. If the fluid has developed by vessels becoming more permeable, then the fluid will have a high protein content and is an exudate. From the late 1980s, however, this classification has been challenged, with authors claiming a superiority for the serum–ascites albumin gradient.[6–9] Most ascites

Table 28.1: Four studies showing the mean volume of ascitic fluid drained

Study authors	Mean volume drained	Range
Bronskill et al 1977[87]	4.12 L	1.09–8.47 L
Ross et al 1989[88]	3.5 L	0.1–9.0 L
Richard et al 2001[24]	Not given	1.5–3 L
Preston 2004[15]	4.7 L	0.8–8.25 L

arising from a malignancy is an exudate.[7] For a transudate to develop, there would be a tumour in the liver, which is more common in some cancers. Assessing the cause of MA is an important part of the assessment of the patient, the diagnosis and treatment plans.

Tumours as a source of fluid

Tumours themselves can either directly or indirectly produce fluid in the peritoneal cavity. Hirabayashi and Graham[10] showed that the peritoneal cavity increases in permeability in the presence of tumour that has implanted on the peritoneal lining. They measured fluid production at a variety of sites around the peritoneal cavity and found that the tumours themselves produced fluid. They also found that the tumour's greatest impact was upon the surrounding lining, especially around the omentum, making it extremely permeable. The omentum or fatty apron is a double fold of peritoneum connecting the stomach with other abdominal organs. Garrison et al[11] also found an increased vascular permeability in the peritoneal cavity in people with MA, allowing the passage of large molecules such as protein into the peritoneal cavity. They hypothesized that a tumour must produce a substance that causes this increased permeability. Tamsma et al, in their review of the pathogenesis of MA, describe the net increase of fluid as being due to an increase in overall capillary membrane surface, increased capillary permeability and an increase of intraperitoneal protein, leading to increased oncotic pressure.[12] Tamsma et al hypothesize that this sequence may be the result of biologically active peptides produced by tumour cells and that future therapy may be targeted against these peptides.

Obstruction of the vessels that drain the peritoneal cavity

Obstruction of the diaphragmatic lymphatic vessels is also involved in the development of MA. Lymphatic obstruction of the diaphragmatic lymphatic vessels was demonstrated by Feldman et al in 1972.[13] They injected mice with a murine cancer cell line known to be associated with the development of MA. They then labelled erythrocytes with a radioactive tracer and injected them into the peritoneal cavity and traced their movement. Erythrocytes are too large to leave the peritoneal cavity by any other route than the diaphragmatic lymphatic vessels. They were able to show a blockage of the lymphatic vessels by the clumping of erythrocytes around their entrance. Blockage of lymphatic vessels was followed by accumulation of ascites, as the fluid had no exit from the peritoneal cavity.

Incidence and prevalence of malignant ascites

No studies have been conducted to measure the incidence or prevalence of ascites. Regnard and Mannix[14] reviewed the primary reasons for admission to their hospice and found 6% of admissions could be accounted for by MA. This figure only represents those patients for whom MA was the primary reason for admission and is therefore likely to be an underrepresentation of the problem.

Although it is unclear how common MA is, there is some evidence to suggest which patients are more likely to develop it. Preston[15] collated 31 research papers showing the tumour of origin for 1102 people with MA. These papers were predominantly intervention trials. None of the studies reported their sampling techniques to derive their patient population. Some centres may not have had access to patients with a broad range of tumour types; therefore, a note of caution is needed when interpreting such data. However, the author found that the most common tumour was ovarian cancer, accounting for 321 cases (30%). The next most common tumours included were colon cancer, breast cancer, pancreatic cancer and adenocarcinoma of unknown origin (Fig. 28.1). MA was shown to result from 26 possible tumour types.

Because of the high numbers of female cancers that result in MA, it is not surprising that the ratio of females to males in this review was 2.5 to 1. The average age of the patients in the studies was 58 years old.

Symptoms associated with malignant ascites

Symptoms associated with MA are similar to those of any group of patients with advanced cancer. The most common symptom is abdominal discomfort, which goes on to cause problems such as difficulty with bending and sitting, feeling bloated and feeling uncomfortable. Other common symptoms are loss of appetite, fatigue, indigestion, pain and emotional distress.[16,17] A further area of concern for patients is body image. Many of these symptoms can be addressed individually but others are difficult to reverse or relieve. Drainage alone offers some symptomatic relief;[18] however, more research is needed to quantify the distress caused by these symptoms. Nurses need to address basic concepts such as information-giving to help relieve anxieties and not assume that they have already been addressed.

Current therapies for malignant ascites

There are six main approaches to the management of MA:

- paracentesis
- indwelling catheter
- diuretic therapy
- peritoneovenous shunt
- intraperitoneal pharmacological or biological therapy
- breathing exercises.

Two surveys of practice have been conducted. Lee et al[19] reported the practice of 44 physicians in Canada, wheras Preston[15] reported the findings from 195 palliative care units in the United Kingdom. The most common treatment in both was paracentesis followed by diuretic therapy. The attitude towards therapy, however, was different. Lee et al reported a greater acceptance of using paracentesis than diuretic therapy. Preston found views towards paracentesis and diuretic therapy were often in opposition. A picture emerged from Preston's survey showing a lack of clarity in practice and a lack of information on how best to manage MA.

There are few high-quality trials investigating treatments associated with MA. A summary of treatment gives the most useful information based upon the best possible evidence from which to make management decisions.

Paracentesis

Paracentesis is the drainage of fluid from the peritoneal cavity using a catheter. This appears to be common practice in palliative care units.[15,20] However, there are many questions relating to the drainage of MA that are unanswered. Key questions are:

- Which drain to use?
- Should drainage be carried out under ultrasound guidance?

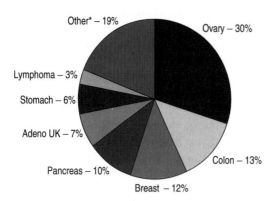

Figure 28.1: Number of primary tumour sites for ascites (*n* = 1102).

Other* – 19%
Ovary – 30%
Lymphoma – 3%
Stomach – 6%
Adeno UK – 7%
Pancreas – 10%
Breast – 12%
Colon – 13%

- How fast to drain?
- Should albumin be used to supplement protein loss?

There is no direct research evaluating these management issues. Patient preference regarding which type of drainage catheter to use may guide practice. For example, patients in Preston's study[15] preferred suprapubic catheter (soft) as opposed to the peritoneal dialysis catheter (rigid).

However, two problems arise with using the suprapubic catheter: first, it is not licensed for use as a peritoneal drainage catheter; secondly, the catheter is expensive. Other catheters used are paediatric chest catheters and large-bore cannulas.

Preston interviewed 32 patients about the use of paracentesis. Although all the patients were apprehensive prior to their first drainage procedure, they all said that they would welcome a subsequent drain when required. The procedure was well tolerated. As stated previously, all symptoms improved after drainage, except emotional discomfort.

Indwelling catheter

In an attempt to reduce hospital admissions, studies have evaluated a semi-permanent drainage catheter, which is left in situ so that the patient can have drainage at home. The patient shares the management of the catheter with a stoma nurse or community nurse. Belfort et al[21] conducted the principal study and, with three subsequent studies, modified their approach.[22–24] None of these studies compared patient satisfaction or concomitant side-effects of an indwelling shunt with paracentesis alone. The infection rates from indwelling shunts are higher than for paracentesis alone and the use of semi-permanent catheters needs further exploration. The additional burden of caring for a catheter and the obvious problems with body image distortion may make it less acceptable to patients than the research suggests.

The use of ultrasound to guide drainage was recommended in the drainage protocol drawn up at the Royal Marsden Hospital, London. However, ultrasound facilities are less available in palliative care settings. Preston found that hospices were more likely to carry out an ultrasound if they had one on site. Furthermore, most centres pointed to the usefulness of ultrasound in preventing bowel perforation by the drainage catheter.

Speed of drainage has only been assessed in case studies. In non-malignant ascites, large-volume drainage procedures are recommended. However, given the poor physical state of many patients with MA, caution is advised and the longer the drain is left in place the greater the likelihood of infection.[21,25] Drainage regimens vary from institution to institution, but a drainage rate of 1 L every 2 hours has been recommended.[26] The use of albumin to act as a plasma expander following drainage to prevent hypovolaemic shock and to compensate for the loss of protein following drainage has not been evaluated. However, a systematic review of the use of albumin in critically ill patients following shock found no evidence that albumin administration reduces mortality in critically ill patients with hypovolaemia. Given its expense, it was recommended that future use of albumin should only be carried out in randomized controlled trials.[27]

Diuretic therapy

Diuretic therapy is used by 98% of palliative care physicians in the United Kingdom at least for some of the time to manage MA;[15] by contrast, only 61% of Canadian palliative care physicians used diuretic therapy. From comments in the survey by Preston,[15] it was clear that there was some confusion about the efficacy of diuretic therapy, yet it was generally seen as less intrusive than paracentesis. With a lack of clear guidance from research studies, it is not surprising that there is confusion in clinical practice.

The use of diuretic therapies has not been fully evaluated. Greenway et al supported its use from a prospective study of 17 patients with ascites,[28] whereas Pockros et al found diuretic therapy simply dehydrated patients.[29] They found that there was no movement of fluid from the peritoneal space, apparently due to lymphatic obstruction. Therefore, more research is needed in the use of diuretic therapy with MA.

Peritoneovenous shunts

The majority of research about the treatment for MA relates to the use of peritoneovenous shunts. A shunt is placed in the peritoneal cavity and tunnels under the skin and enters the vena cava. Fluid moves along the shunt as a result of changes in pressure during breathing. Peritoneovenous shunts were used more in the 1970s and 1980s; they then diminished in popularity, but more recently have been shown to be effective and easier to insert in the hands of interventional radiologists.[30–32] In the past, these shunts were often placed under general anaesthetic, but now using a percutaneous approach local anaesthetic is used. All devices left in situ are associated with problems such as infection and blockage; however, several studies have demonstrated relief of symptoms and a lessening of patient risk.

There are two types of shunt: Leveen and Denver. The Leveen shunt is a simple shunt where fluid is moved through changes in pressure exerted through breathing exercises. Leveen et al[33] recommended the use of breathing exercises and wearing an abdominal binder to assist flow. Thick or bloody ascites is likely to block peritoneovenous shunts and so they are contraindicated. The Denver shunt has a chamber that can be pressed to encourage flow and to remove any debris that might be blocking the catheter. Although a shunt prevents the need for repeated paracentesis, blockage occurs in 25% of shunts.[30]

Intraperitoneal therapy

Drainage of the MA provides the opportunity to instil pharmacological or biological agents to treat the underlying cancer. Unfortunately, any agent instilled into the peritoneal cavity has difficulty being reabsorbed if the molecular size of the particles means it can only be removed by the lymphatic system, which is generally impaired. As substances accumulate in the peritoneal cavity, bowel obstruction can be a problem for any patients undergoing intraperitoneal therapy. Although many trials have been conducted, there are as yet no proven therapies. Tumour necrosis factor was initially thought to be beneficial;[34] however, compared to drainage alone, it has been found to be ineffective. More recently, studies have

been conducted looking at other agents such as the bispecific antibody (HEA125xOKT3) and a streptococcal preparation OK-432. Although in the early stages of research, both studies were able to demonstrate a positive clinical response in the majority of patients, although the sample sizes were small: 10 and 51 patients, respectively.[35,36]

THORACIC/PLEURAL EFFUSIONS

This section will firstly describe the aetiology, epidemiology and pathogenesis of malignant pleural effusion (MPE) and then will go on to describe the specific patient issues of diagnosis, treatment and supportive care.

Pleural effusion is the accumulation of fluid, either an exudate or rarely a transudate, in the pleural space. Pleural effusions can result from non-malignant causes such as infection, trauma or severe burns, pulmonary embolus, severe lung injury and congestive cardiac failure. The most common cause, thought to be responsible for 50% of pleural effusions, is cancer, and these effusions are known as MPEs. For people over 60 years old, cancer is the most common cause of pleural effusion.[37] MPEs are associated with significant morbidity, with patients experiencing pain, a dry cough, decreased exercise tolerance and progressive shortness of breath.[38,39]

The aetiology of malignant pleural effusion

Although all cancers have been reported to involve the pleura,[40,41] the most common aetiologies for the development of MPE are cancers of the lung, breast, lymphoma (Hodgkin's and non-Hodgkin's) and, to a much lesser extent, ovarian, gastrointestinal and genitourinary cancers.[42] Lung cancer is the most common cause of MPE, accounting for approximately one-third of the total, with breast cancer the second most common cause.[41]

Epidemiology

Although there are no reported epidemiological studies, the annual incidence of MPE in the United States is estimated to be greater than

150,000 cases per year.[43] Studies indicate that 42–77% of all exudative effusions are secondary to cancer.[44,45] Approximately 30% of patients with effusions present with bilateral effusions at diagnosis and about half of patients with lung or breast cancer will develop MPE during their lifetime.[46] In one postmortem study, MPEs were found in 15% of all patients who died with cancer.[47] It is also important to note that MPE may exist and the primary cancer may not be identified.[48] Finally, mesothelioma is also associated with the development of MPE and the incidence of this disease is associated with patterns of geography and occupation but also occurs independently of asbestos contamination.[49]

Pathophysiology

The pleura encasing the lungs is composed of two layers: the parietal (outer layer) and visceral (inner layer); both are composed of a thin layer of mesothelium that encases the lungs on one side and the thoracic cavity on the other. Between the parietal and visceral pleura is the pleural space. The parietal pleura lines the thorax, diaphragm and mediastinum with capillaries, which are supplied by the intercostal arteries. The parietal pleura also contains nerve endings, whereas the visceral pleura contains no nerve endings.[46]

The pleural space has a dynamic quality, with constant changes in the composition of pleural fluid. Normally the pleura contains between 10 and 40 ml of hypoproteinaemic filtrate from the plasma, originating from the capillary bed of the parietal pleura.[50] Every day about 5–10 L of fluid is produced, with all but 30 ml being reabsorbed by the subpleural pulmonary capillaries and to a lesser extent by the pleural lymphatic system.[51]

Cancer can cause MPE directly or indirectly, by a tumour directly infiltrating the pleura itself or by the cancer changing the integrity of the lymphatic system anywhere between the parietal pleura and the lymph nodes of the mediastinum. In the largest proportion of cases, MPE is associated with metastatic spread of the cancer by tumour emboli to the visceral pleural surface or secondary seeding to the parietal pleura.[41] The presence of tumour increases the capillary permeability due to inflammation or to the endothelial damage. As cancer is predominantly a disease of later life, it is important to remember that co-morbid conditions can increase pleural effusions such as pneumonia, ascites, congestive cardiac failure, renal failure, hypoalbuminaemia, pulmonary embolus and rheumatological disorders.[50]

As stated, the fluid of MPE can be an exudate or transudate, but is most commonly an exudate with a fluid to serum protein ratio of >0.5 and lactate dehydrogenase ratio >0.6.[52]

Diagnosis

Most people who have developed MPE present with symptoms, the most common being breathlessness, particularly breathlessness following exertion, followed by cough, chest pain and a flu-like illness.[41,50,53] The chest pain of MPE varies from a dull ache to a sharp pain pleuritic in nature. These specific chest symptoms may be accompanied by more general symptoms such as anorexia, weight loss and malaise related to the existence of advanced cancer. On clinical examination, auscultation will usually reveal decreased breath sounds in the affected area with dullness to percussion and decreased fremitus. If effusions are large, tracheal deviation may be observed.[50] The diagnosis will usually be confirmed radiologically by a chest X-ray with posteroanterior and more accurately lateral decubitus X-rays able to detect effusions as small as 200 ml.[46,54] Most patients who present symptomatically will have pleural effusions ranging from 500 to 2000 ml in volume.[55] Further radiological imaging may be necessary to define the MPE, with ultrasound and computed tomography (CT) scan being particularly helpful in smaller effusions or where the fluid is loculated.[50] Magnetic resonance imaging (MRI) has not been shown to be useful, although it may be useful in demonstrating the extent of tumour invasion.[56–58] Finally, positron emission tomography (PET) has currently been shown to be of limited use in MPE, except in evaluating mesothelioma.[59]

Having established that there is an effusion in the absence of an enlarged heart size, or where there is an enlarged heart but good reason to suspect cancer, a diagnostic thoracocentesis should be performed.[41,50] The fluid obtained should be sent for cytology, nucleated cell count and differential, total protein, lactate dehydrogenase, glucose, pH and amylase (see Table 28.2 for tests and diagnostic application).[41] The complications associated with thoracocentesis are pneumothorax, haemorrhage, infection and trauma to the liver or spleen.

If thoracocentesis is unable to provide the diagnosis, the following tests may be used in order of safe application:

- thoracoscopy
- pleuroscopy
- closed pleural biopsy
- bronchoscopy
- surgical biopsy.

Therapeutic interventions for malignant pleural effusion

Decisions on the treatment plan must be based on a global assessment of the patient's condition. Many patients with MPE will have advanced or metastatic disease and will therefore require a treatment plan that addresses all their needs and takes into account the primary tumour (if known), the extent of their disease, performance status, their prognosis and any

co-morbid conditions. It is important to note that some MPEs will have been an incidental finding in patients who are not symptomatic; in these patients, surveillance alone is recommended.[38,39] If the primary malignancy is amenable to treatment, then systemic chemotherapy, radiotherapy or surgery may be used in the first instance. For many patients, however, the symptom that most directly affects their quality of life is breathlessness and the fear and physical limitations this causes. Therefore, the most immediate requirement will be the relief of their breathlessness. The following therapeutic interventions are those that may be offered (in order of the most commonly used interventions):

- thoracocentesis and tube drainage
- sclerotherapy
- systemic treatment
- tunnelled long-term catheters and drainage
- thoracoscopy
- pleuroperitoneal shunting
- pleurectomy.

In determining the treatment plan and selecting from the above options, careful consideration and discussion with the patient will need to determine probable prognosis and perform-

Table 28.2: Diagnostic tests performed on pleural fluid obtained from thoracocentesis	
Test	**Diagnostic significance**
Cytology	The simplest definitive test for confirming MPE; however, diagnostic success is variable, being dependent on the extent of the disease and the cancer primary[60]
pH	One-third of MPE have a pH <7.30 in the presence of a low glucose; however, also seen with infection and haemorrhage[50]
Amylase	Elevated amylase levels (without oesophageal rupture) are indicative of an MPE – typically adenocarcinoma of the lung[61,62]
Nucleated cell count	MPE typically shows a concentration of lymphocytes or mononuclear cells[63,64]
Cytogenetic analysis	Useful in cases that are difficult to diagnose, and has been used particularly to diagnose mesothelioma[50,53]

ance status. Where the patient's prognosis is limited or performance status is poor, then repeated MPE aspiration will improve breathlessness and avoid lengthy hospitalization. Where the patient is thought to have a better prognosis and has a good performance status, the emphasis of treatment should be on drainage and then prevention of recurrence of the MPE.[39]

Tube drainage

Traditionally, large-bore intercostal tubes (24–32F) were used in the drainage of MPE. These tubes are, however, very uncomfortable for patients, and this discomfort is important to avoid, especially where repeated drainage may be necessary. Therefore, over the last 10 years, clinicians have sought to use smaller-bore tubes (8–14F) and have been able to demonstrate similar efficacy with greatly improved patient comfort.[38,65–68] These small-bore catheters are typically introduced under ultrasound or CT guidance. Placement is usually in the midaxillary line at the sixth or seventh intercostal space. The technique used following instillation of local anaesthetic is a Seldinger technique using a guide wire and then sequential dilators, and finally a pigtail catheter inserted and affixed to the skin using an adherent disc.[38] Following successful insertion, position and absence of pneumothorax checked by chest X-ray, the tube is aspirated and then attached to low suction (10–20 cmH_2O). There is a high rate of MPE reaccumulation following drainage, and therefore once successful drainage and complete lung expansion has been demonstrated, sclerosis will usually be attempted.[68]

Pleurodesis or sclerosis

The aim of pleurodesis is to prevent reaccumulation of the MPE and therefore reduce symptoms and the need for hospitalization. To achieve this aim, the pleural space needs to be obliterated by the instillation of an agent that causes adhesions. Before attempting pleurodesis, it is essential that all the pleural fluid has been drained.[46] The technique used is to instil a sclerotic agent into the pleural space through the thoracic tube or during thoracoscopy.[69] The ideal sclerosing substance will have a high

molecular weight, be well tolerated with minimal side-effects, have a low regional and rapid systemic clearance and have a steep dose–response curve.[39] Many agents have been tried (see below), but despite many trials, the small sample sizes, poor study design and different criteria for the measurement of response mean that it remains difficult to decide upon the ideal sclerosing agent.[39,69]

The following sclerotic agents are used in the treatment of MPE:

- tetracycline
- doxycycline
- minocycline
- bleomycin
- cytarabine
- cisplatin
- sterile talc.

Until 1998, tetracycline was the most common sclerotic agent until its production ceased in the United States. Tetracycline has been shown to be effective in approximately 65% of cases, is well tolerated and is inexpensive. Tetracycline derivatives such as doxycycline and minocycline have been studied in small numbers, but neither agent is easily available. Bleomycin is the most widely used anticancer drug for sclerosis. Bleomycin has a similar efficacy to tetracycline, being effective in approximately 60% of cases and has an acceptable side-effect profile; however, it is a more expensive treatment.[70] Talc was first used as a sclerotic agent in 1935, but has been developed to be used either as talc poudrage used at thoracoscopy using an atomizer[71–73] or as a talc slurry instilled via the chest tube. Talc in either form has a high efficacy rate of 80-100%, and is usually well tolerated and inexpensive. Talc pneumonitis, or talc acute respiratory distress syndrome (ARDS), has, however, been reported in a small percentage of patients and it is thought that this may be dose-related.[74]

Important considerations in preparing the patient for this procedure are the likely symptoms following the procedure and the need for regular repositioning to allow distribution of the sclerosing agent. Following pleurodesis, it is important that the patient is monitored and prompt action taken to relieve any pain or discomfort or any sign of respiratory distress. The most common symptom immediately following pleurodesis is pain, which is often described as pleuritic in nature.[46]

Tunnelled long-term catheters and drainage

The placement of a long-term tunnelled pleural catheter (TPC) has been demonstrated in several studies to achieve effective control of MPE, with limited problems, and has been effective in the outpatient setting.[37,38,75–80] The catheter can be inserted at a clinic appointment and the patient and their 'family' taught how to drain the catheter at home. The use of a TPC has also been coupled with sclerotic therapy in the outpatient setting. The only exclusion to TPC is where the MPE is multiloculated and is therefore not amenable to drainage.[37] Long-term pleural catheters do seem therefore to represent a significant patient advantage in effectively controlling symptoms, with the added advantage of less hospital admissions; this is of course particularly important in patients who may have a limited prognosis.

Surgical treatment – pleurectomy

An open pleurectomy involves the operative removal of the parietal pleura under general anaesthesia in the operating theatre. The surgery effectively achieves pleurodesis but carries a high morbidity and mortality rate and is therefore rarely performed.[39] Video-assisted thoracoscopic surgery (VATS) is, however, a much safer technique and has demonstrated efficacy in both diagnosis and therapeutic intervention. This technique has been developed relatively recently and is therefore not available in all centres but it has been shown to be successful and a much safer technique than open pleurectomy.[39,81–83]

Pleuroperitoneal shunting

Pleuroperitoneal shunting is an intervention used when pleurodesis is not possible or has not been successful, usually because of a 'trapped lung' condition. Patients with 'trapped lung' have a dense layer of malignant tissue encasing the visceral pleura, which prevents complete re-expansion of the lung following drainage of a MPE. This means that apposition of the two surfaces of the pleura cannot be achieved and sclerosis will therefore be ineffective.[84] The shunt is inserted by thoracoscopy or mini-thoracotomy and shunts the fluid from the pleural space to the peritoneal cavity. Compression of the shunt is necessary to activate fluid movement. Shunt occlusion has been demonstrated in 12% of patients, necessitating shunt replacement;[85] infection is also seen and may necessitate removal of the shunt and replacement with a long-term catheter. There is a potential risk of causing peritoneal tumour seeding but currently this has not been convincingly proven.[41]

CONCLUSION

Malignant ascites and malignant pleural effusions are common and debilitating conditions associated in many cases with advanced or metastatic disease. Some patients are asymptomatic and, in their case, surveillance coupled with systemic treatment of their cancer is indicated. The majority of patients who develop either MA or MPE are symptomatic, with abdominal discomfort and fatigue being the most common symptoms of MA and breathlessness, particularly on exertion, being the most common symptom of MPE. These symptoms are both frightening and physically debilitating and the patient needs skilled interdisciplinary intervention. Nurses can work with patients and their families to develop ways to live with MA or MPE and still achieve their personal priorities for living. Chronic pain and fatigue are symptoms where the management strategies need to be proactively discussed and planned with the patient and their family.[86] It is important that a good relationship is developed between the clinical team and the patient and that the patient understands the nature of the disease. MA is an area that is underresearched and current therapies need further evaluation in controlled trials. Currently, the main, and safest, treatment approach is intermittent drainage; however, the effect of MA and its treatment on patients' well-being needs further exploration. Areas for research have been highlighted throughout this chapter.

There is an increasing role for nurses as therapists in this area, with one of the nurse's primary roles being to help patients understand what is happening to them, with the aim of reducing the their anxiety. Nurses also need to take a role in assessing the patient's symptoms and offering advice.

In most cases the patient will be treated eventually in the outpatient setting, and it is therefore imperative that effective communication exists between the hospital and primary care setting. Nurses working in gynaecological, lung and breast cancer settings need to ensure that they are familiar both with the aetiology of MA and MPE, its diagnosis and the various treatment interventions possible. All cancer nurses need to be aware that MA and MPE can occur with many malignancies.

Finally, it is important that all of the above interventions are coupled with the highest standards of therapeutic nursing and supportive care from the multidisciplinary team. In most cases, the person with cancer who has developed recurrent MA or MPE has less time to live. How that person is enabled to live relies on the support and effective communication of the interdisciplinary team across all care settings.

REFERENCES

1. Cancerbacup. Management of a pleural effusion, www.cancerbacup.org.uk.
2. Witte CL, Witte MH. Splanchnic circulatory and tissue fluid dynamics in portal hypertension. Fed Proc 1983; 42(6):1685–1689.
3. Weiser AC, Lindgren BW, Ritchey ML. Chylous ascites following surgical treatment for Wilms tumor. J Urol 2003;170(4 Pt 2):1667–1669; discussion 1669.
4. Inaba Y, Arai Y, Matsueda K. Intractable massive ascites following radical gastrectomy, treatment with local intraperitoneal administration of OK-432 using a unified CT and fluoroscopy system. Australas Radiol 2003;47(4):465–467.
5. Parsons SL, Watson SA, Steele RJC. Malignant ascites. Br J Surg 1996; 83(1):6–14.
6. Rector WG, Reynolds TB. Superiority of the serum-ascites albumin difference over the ascites total protein concentration in separation of transudative and exudative ascites. Am J Med 1984; 77:83–85.
7. Runyon BA, Montano AA, Akriviadis EA, et al. The serum-ascites albumin gradient is superior to the exudate-transudate concept in the differential diagnosis of ascites. Ann Intern Med 1992; 117(3):215–220.
8. Gupta R, Misra SP, Dwivedi M, et al. Diagnostic ascites: value of total protein albumin, cholesterol their ratios serum ascites albumin and cholesterol gradient. J Gastroenterol Hepatol 1995; 10(3):295–299.
9. Beg, M, Husain, S, Ahmed N. Serum/ascites albumin gradient in differential diagnosis of ascites. J Indian Acad Clin Med 2001; 2(1&2):51–54.
10. Hirabayashi K, Graham J. Genesis of ascites in ovarian cancer. Am J Obstet Gynecol 1970; 106(4):492–497.
11. Garrison RN, Kaelin, LD, Galloway, RH. et al. Malignant ascites. Clinical and experimental observations. Ann Surg 1986; 203(6):644–651.
12. Tamsma JT, Keizer HJ, Meinders AE. Pathogenesis of malignant ascites: Starling's law of capillary hemodynamics revisited. Ann Oncol 2001; 12(10):1353–1357.
13. Feldman GB, Knapp RC, Order SE. The role of lymphatic obstruction in the formation of ascites in a murine ovarian carcinoma. Cancer Res 1972; 32(8):1663–1666.
14. Regnard C, Mannix K. Management of ascites in advanced cancer – a flow diagram. Palliat Med 1972; 4:45–57.
15. Preston N. The development of a novel nursing intervention for malignant ascites. PhD Thesis. University of London. 2004
16. Kehoe C. Malignant ascites: etiology, diagnosis and treatment. Oncol Nurs Forum 1991; 18(3):523–530.
17. Preston N. New strategies for the management of malignant ascites. Eur J Cancer Care 1995; 4(4):178–183.
18. McNamara P. Paracentesis – an effective method of symptom control in the palliative care setting. Palliat Med 2000; 14(1):62–64.
19. Lee CW, Bociek G, Faught W. A survey of practice in management of malignant ascites. J Pain Symptom Manage 1998; 16(2):96–101.
20. Johnson IS, Rogers C, Biswas B, Ahmedzai S. What do hospices do? A survey of hospices in the United Kingdom and Republic of Ireland. BMJ 1990; 300(6727):791–793.
21. Belfort MA, Stevens PJ, DeHaek K, Soeters R, Krige JE. A new approach to the management of malignant ascites: a permanently implanted abdominal drain. Eur J Surg Oncol 1990; 16(1):47–53.
22. Lee DH, Yu JS, Hwang JC, et al. Percutaneous placement of self-expandable metallic biliary stents in malignant extrahepatic strictures: indications of transpapillary and suprapapillary methods. Korean J Radiol 2000; 1(2):65–72.
23. O'Neill MR, Weissleder R. Tunneled peritoneal catheter placement under sonographic and fluoroscopic guidance in the palliative treatment

of malignant ascites. Am J Roentgenol 2001; 177(3):615–618.

24. Richard HM 3rd, Coldwell DM, Boyd-Kranis RL, Murthy R, Van Echo DA. Pleura tunnelled catheter in the management of malignant ascites. J Vasc Interv Radiol 2001; 12(3):373–375.

25. Appelqvist P, Silvo J, Samela L, et al. On the treatment and prognosis of malignant ascites: is the survival time determined when the abdominal paracentesis is needed?. J Surg Oncol 1982; 20(4):238–242.

26. Mallett J, Dougherty L. The Royal Marsden manual of clinical nursing procedures. Oxford: Blackwell Science; 2000:33–38.

27. Cochrane Injuries Group. Human albumin administration in critically ill patients: systematic review of randomised controlled trials. BMJ 1998; 317(7153):235–240.

28. Greenway B, Johnson PJ, Williams R. Control of malignant ascites with spironolactone. Br J Surg 1982; 69:441–442.

29. Pockros PJ, Esrason KT, Nguyen C, Duque J, Woods S. Mobilization of malignant ascites with diuretics is dependent on ascitic fluid characteristics. Gastroenterology 1992; 103(4):1302–1306.

30. Smith EM, Jayson GC. The current and future management of malignant ascites. Clin Oncol 2003; 15(2):59–72.

31. Zanon C, Grosso M, Apra F, et al. Palliative treatment of malignant refractory ascites by positioning of Denver peritoneovenus shunt. Tumori 2002; 88(2):123–127.

32. Park JS, Won JY, Park SI, et al. Percutaneous peritoneovenus shunt creation for the treatment of benign and malignant refractory ascites. J Vasc Interv Radiol 2001; 12(12):1445–1448.

33. Leveen HH, Christoudias G, Ip M, et al. Peritoneo-venous shunting for ascites. Ann Surg 1974; 180(4):580–591.

34. Del Mastro L, Venturini M, Giannessi PG, et al. Intraperitoneal infusion of recombinant human tumor necrosis factor and mitoxantrone in neoplastic ascites: a feasibility study. Anticancer Res 1995; 15(5B):2207–2212.

35. Marme A, Strauss G, Bastert G, et al. Intraperitoneal bispecific antibody (HEA125xOKT3) therapy inhibits malignant ascites production in advanced ovarian carcinoma. Int J Cancer 2002; 101(2):183–189.

36. Yamaguchi Y, Oshita A, Kawabuchi Y, et al. Locoregional immunotherapy of malignant ascites from gastric cancer using DTH-oriented doses of the steptococcal preparation OK-432: treatment of Th1 dysfunction in the ascites microenvironment. Int J Oncol 2004; 24(4):959–966.

37. Pollack JS, Burdge CM, Rosenblatt M, et al. Treatment of malignant pleural effusions with tunneled long-term drainage catheters. J Vasc Interv Radiol 2001;12(2):201–208.

38. Erasmus JJ, Patz EF. Treatment of malignant pleural effusions. Curr Opin Pulm Med 1999; 5(4):250–255.

39. Antunes G, Neville E. Management of malignant pleural effusions. Thorax 2000; 55:981–983.

40. Hausheer FH, Yarbro JW. Diagnosis and treatment of malignant pleural effusion. Semin Oncol 1985; 12:54–75.

41. American Thoracic Society. Management of malignant pleural effusions. Am J Respir Crit Care Med 2000; 162:1987–2001.

42. Sahn SA. Malignancy metastatic to the pleura. Clin Chest Med 1998; 19:351–361.

43. Cancer Statistics. CA Cancer J Clin 1997; 47:8–12.

44. Marel M, Zrustova M, Stasny B, et al. The incidence of pleural effusion in a well-defined region: epidemiologic study in central Bohemia. Chest 1993; 104:1486–1489.

45. Valdes L, Alvarez D, Valle JM, et al. The etiology of pleural effusions in an area with high incidence of tuberculosis. Chest 1996; 109:158–162.

46. Taubert J. Management of malignant pleural effusions. Nurs Clin North Am 2001; 36(4):665–683.

47. Rodriguez-Panadero F, Borderas Naranjo F, Lopez Mejias J. Pleural metastatic tumours and effusions. Frequency and pathogenic mechanisms in a post-mortem series. Eur Respir J 1989; 2:366–369.

48. Johnston WW. The malignant pleural effusion: a review of cytopathological diagnoses of 584 specimens from 472 consecutive patients. Cancer 1985; 56:905–909.

49. Peterson JT, Greenberg DS, Buffler PA. Non-asbestos related malignant mesothelioma: a review. Cancer 1984;, 54:951–960.

50. Decamp MM, Mentzer SJ, Swanson SJ, Sugarbaker DJ. Malignant effusive disease of the pleura and pericardium. Chest 1997; 112, 4(Suppl):291S–295S.

51. Stewart PB. The rate of formation and lymphatic removal of fluid in pleural effusions. J Clin Invest 1963; 42(2):258–262.

52. Zimmerman LH. Pleural effusions. In: Goldstein RH, O'Connell JJ, Karlinsky JB, eds. A practical approach to pulmonary medicine. Philadelphia: Lippincott-Raven; 1997:195–205.

53. Wick MR, Moran CA, Mills SE, Suster S. Immunohistochemical differential diagnosis of pleural effusions, with emphasis on malignant mesothelioma. Curr Opin Pulm Med 2001; 7(4):187–192.

54. Woodring JH. Recognition of pleural effusion on supine radiographs: How much fluid is required? Am J Radiol 1984; 142:59–64.

55. Chernow B, Sahn SA. Carcinomatous involvement of the pleura: an analysis of 96 patients. Am J Med 1977; 63:695–702.

56. Patz EF, Shaffer K, Piwnica-Worms DR, et al. Malignant pleural mesothelioma: value of CT and MRI imaging in predicting respectability. Am J Roentgenol 1992; 159:961–966.

57. Carlsen SE, Bergin CJ, Hoppe RT. MR imaging to detect chest wall and pleural involvement in patients with lymphoma: effect on radiation therapy planning. Am J Roentgenol 1993; 160:191–195.

58. Bittner RC, Felix R. Magnetic resonance (MR) imaging of the chest: state of the art. Eur Respir J 1998; 11:1392–1404.

59. Bernard F, Sterman D, Smith RJ, et al. Metabolic imaging of malignant pleural mesothelioma with fluorodeoxyglucose positron emission tomography. Chest 1998; 144:713–722.

60. Starr RL, Sherman ME. The value of multiple preparations in the diagnosis of malignant pleural effusions. Acta Cytol 1991; 35:533–537.

61. Hillerdal G, Lindqvist U, Engstrom-Laurent A. Hyaluronan in pleural effusions and in serum. Cancer 1991; 67:2410–2414.

62. Joseph J, Vuney S, Beck P, et al. A prospective study of amylase-rich pleural effusions with special reference to amylase isoenzyme analysis. Chest 1992; 102:1455–1459.

63. Rubins JB, Rubins HB. Etiology and prognostic significance of eosinophilic pleural effusions. Chest 1996; 110:1271–1274.

64. Villena V, Perez V, Pozo F, et al. Amylase levels in pleural effusions: a consecutive unselected series of 841 patients. Chest 2002; 121(2):470–474.

65. Reinhold C, Illescas FF, Atri M, et al. Treatment of pleural effusions and pneumothorax with catheters placed percutaneously under image guidance. Am J Roentgenol 1989; 152:1189–1191.

66. Parker LA, Charnock GC, Delany DJ. Small bore catheter drainage and sclerotherapy for malignant effusions. Cancer 1989; 64:1218–1221.

67. Morrison MC, Mueller PR, Lee MJ, et al. Sclerotherapy of malignant pleural effusion through sonographically placed small bore catheters. Am J Roentgenol 1992; 158:41–43.

68. Parulekar W, Di Primio G, Matzinger F. et al. Use of small-bore vs large-bore chest tubes for treatment of malignant pleural effusions. Chest, 2001; 120(1):19–25.

69. Agarwal R, Shaw P. Pleurodesis for malignant pleural effusions (Protocol for a Cochrane Review). In: The Cochrane Library, Issue 4. Oxford: Update Software; 2000:1–6.

70. Walker-Renard PB, Vaughan LM, Sahn SA. Chemical pleurodesis for malignant pleural effusions. Ann Intern Med 1994; 120:56–64.

71. Viallat JR, Rey F, Astoul P, et al. Thoracoscopic talc poudrage pleurodesis for malignant effusions. A review of 360 cases. Chest 1996; 110(6):1387–1393.

72. Diacon AH, Wyser C, Bolliger CT, et al. Prospective randomized comparison of thoracoscopic talc poudrage under local anesthesia versus bleomycin instillation for pleurodesis in malignant pleural effusions. Am J Respir Crit Care Med 2000; 162:1445–1449.

73. Milanez de Campos JR, Vargas FS, de Campos Werebe E, et al. Thoracoscopy talc poudrage: a 15-year experience. Chest 2001; 113(3):801–806.

74. York A, Bondoc P, Bach P, et al. Talc pneumonitis: incidence, clinical features and outcome. Chest 1999; 116(Suppl):358–359S.

75. Leff RS, Eisenberg B, Baisden CE, et al. Drainage of recurrent pleural effusion via an implanted port and intrapleural catheter. Ann Intern Med 1986; 104:208–209.

76. Hewitt JB, Janssen WR. A management strategy for malignancy-induced pleural effusion: long-term thoracostomy drainage. Oncol Nurse Forum 1987; 14:17–22.

77. Zeldin DC, Rodriguez RM, Glassford DM. Management of refractory MPEs with a chronic indwelling pleural catheter. Chest 1991; 100:87S.

78. Robinson RD, Fullerton DA, Albert JD, et al. Use of pleural Tenckhoff catheter to palliate malignant pleural effusion. Ann Thorac Surg 1994; 57:286–288.

79. Driesen P, Boutin C, Viallat JR. Implantable access system for prolonged intrapleural immunotherapy. Eur Respir J 1994; 7:1889–1892.

80. Pien GW, Gant MJ, Washam CL, et al. Use of an implantable pleural catheter for trapped lung syndrome in patients with malignant pleural effusion. Chest 2001; 119(6):1641–1646.

81. Waller DA, Morritt GN, Forty J. Video-assisted thoracoscopic pleurectomy in the management of malignant pleural effusion. Chest 1995; 107:1454–1456.

82. Yim APC, Chung SS, Lee TW, et al. Thorascopic management of malignant pleural effusions. Chest 1996; 109:1234–1238.

83. Loddenkemper R. Thoracoscopy: state of the art. Eur Respir J 1998; 11:213–221.

84. Light RW. Pleural effusion due to miscellaneous diseases. In: Light RW, ed. Pleural diseases. Philadelphia: Williams and Wilkins; 1995:224–241.

85. al-Kattan KM, Kaplan DK, Goldstraw P. The non-functioning pleuroperitoneal shunt: revise or replace? Thorac Cardiovasc Surg 1994; 42(5):310–312.

86. Cella D, Peterman A, Passik S, et al. Progress toward guidelines for the management of fatigue. Oncology 1998; 12:369–377.

CHAPTER 29

Anorexia, Cachexia and Malnutrition

ALEXANDER MOLASSIOTIS AND JAN FOUBERT

CHAPTER CONTENTS

Introduction	633
Development of anorexia and cachexia	633
Anorexia	633
Factors contributing to anorexia	634
Cachexia	634
Incidence of malnutrition and cachexia	635
Factors contributing to cancer cachexia	635
Metabolic alterations	637
Cancer-specific cachectic factors (or tumour-derived catabolic factors)	637
Reasons affecting progression of malnutrition	639
Consequences of malnutrition	639
Nutritional assessment	640
Clinical assessment	640
Anthropometric measurements	641
Laboratory measurements	642
Identification of nutritional risk	643

Patient-Generated Subjective Global Assessment	643
Oncology Screening Tool	643
Other malnutrition screening and assessment tools	644
Nutritional support in patients with cancer	644
Dietary advice and counselling	645
Enteral and parenteral nutrition	647
Effective pharmacological therapies	647
Promising pharmacological approaches	648
Fish oil, n-3 fatty acids and eicosapentaenoic acid	648
Non-pharmacological approaches	648
General guidelines for nutritional support	649
Quality of life issues	649
Conclusion	650
References	651

INTRODUCTION

This chapter discusses the pertinent issues around anorexia and cachexia in patients with cancer and the factors related to these syndromes and addresses the issue of malnutrition. A section of the chapter is devoted to the different ways of assessing the nutritional status of patients with cancer and the importance of regular assessment. A large part of the chapter also deals with the management of nutritional problems, be it pharmacological or non-pharmacological in nature, presenting critically the available evidence. The effects of malnutrition, anorexia and cachexia on quality of life are also discussed. Overall, the aim of this chapter is to enhance the health professionals' understanding of anorexia and cachexia, two complex conditions that so far have received little attention in the cancer literature.

DEVELOPMENT OF ANOREXIA AND CACHEXIA

Anorexia

Anorexia or lack of appetite is a common symptom of many illnesses. Anorexia is also a contributing factor for cachexia. It is estimated that as many as 40% of patients with cancer experience anorexia at diagnosis and up to 70% in more advanced stages of the disease.[1] When anorexia is prolonged, as in the case of many advanced cancers, the patient experiences protein calorie malnutrition, losing simultaneously lean muscle mass and experiencing as much as 20–30% decrease in metabolic rate.[2,3] Many authors talk about the syndrome of anorexia–cachexia, as many times it is difficult to separate anorexia (symptom) from cachexia (sign). This is a dynamic continuum starting with anorexia (sometimes appearing long before the patient is diagnosed with cancer), and finishing with death accompanied with profound cachexia, malnourishment and weight loss.[1] However, it is now established that, although anorexia is often associated with cachexia, it is unlikely that the weight loss experienced by patients with cancer arises primarily from the reduction in food intake.[4]

Factors contributing to anorexia

Tisdale[4] and Davis and Dickerson[5] describe in their review articles a number of factors contributing to anorexia, detailed below. For example, patients with cancer often complain of decreased taste and smell of food, resulting in increased sweet and decreased bitter thresholds. In some cases, the loss of appetite is due to depression or stress; depression-induced anorexia can be misdiagnosed, especially in advancing cancers. Depression has long been associated with weight loss and anorexia. Further, radiation and chemotherapy are some of the possible factors contributing to cancer malnutrition. Nausea and vomiting, particularly with chemotherapy, bowel obstruction and dysphagia (difficulty with swallowing) complicate matters further. Early satiety is commonly reported in patients with anorexia, feeling full after eating even small amounts of food. Mucositis can result in dysphagia and odynophagia (sensation of pain behind sternum as food or fluid is swallowed), making eating food or drinking fluids undesirable. Furthermore, social factors may be responsible, such as change in eating environment or companions.[6,7]

The pathophysiological mechanisms of anorexia are not clearly understood, but evidence from a number of studies (including some animal studies) suggest that neuropeptides, amino acids or cytokines may be involved. Chance et al[8] have shown that anorexia in tumour-bearing rats was caused probably by a dysfunction in the hypothalamic membrane adenylate cyclase system, as determined by reduced responsiveness to the inhibitory effect of neuropeptide Y and the stimulatory effect of isoprenaline. Further, an amino acid called tryptophan, a precursor of serotonin, is involved in the pathogenesis of cancer anorexia by increasing ventromedial hypothalamic serotoninergic activity.[9] Also, release of chemicals by the tumour or the host immune system may cause anorexia, as certain cytokines, including tumour necrosis factor-α (TNF-α) and interleukin-1 (IL-1), act directly on the brain to produce anorexia.[10,11]

Cachexia

Cancer cachexia is a complex, multifactorial syndrome characterized by progressive, involuntary weight loss. It is a life-threatening muscle-wasting syndrome. Clinical features include anorexia, early satiety, depletion of lean body mass, muscle weakness (asthenia), oedema, fatigue, impaired immune function, possible decreased motor and mental skills and declines in attention span and concentration. Accelerated mobilization and consumption of host protein stores from peripheral tissues occur to support gluconeogenesis and acute phase protein synthesis. Cachexia should be distinguished from simple starvation, as the latter is associated with a relative sparing of lean tissue with the preferential consumption of fat.[12,13]

The clinical appearance of patients affected by cancer cachexia is characteristic: patients have pale and atrophic skin and wasted faces, and suffer from severe skeletal muscle wasting and a considerable loss of subcutaneous fat stores, sometimes hidden by the presence of oedema. Unlike patients with anorexia nervosa in whom weight loss is due to a more or less proportional decrease in the size of all organs, patients with malignant cachexia have an increase in the size of the liver, kidney and spleen.[12,13]

As progressive weight loss is a major characteristic of cancer cachexia, the terms cachexia and disease-related malnutrition are often used interchangeably. This is not completely correct. Disease-related malnutrition arises if intake of energy and nutrients is insufficient to meet an individual's requirements. However, inadequate intake of energy and nutrients alone is unable to account for the changes in body composition seen in patients with cancer who have cachexia.

Incidence of malnutrition and cachexia

The global incidence of malnutrition during the course of cancer ranges from 30% to 90%, and is not only dependent on the type, location, grade, stage and spread of the tumour but also on anticancer treatments as well as on age, gender and individual susceptibilities.[7,14,15] During the course of disease, a weight loss of greater than 10% of pre-illness body weight may occur in up to 45% of patients with cancer.[12,16] Highest rates are seen in stomach (83%) and pancreatic cancer (83%), followed by upper gastrointestinal cancers (i.e. oesophagus, 79%; head and neck, 72%), lung and colorectal cancers (40–61%), with a considerably lower incidence in breast cancer; the mean incidence in the general cancer population is around 60–63%.[12,14]

Studies have shown that at the time of diagnosis, all patients with unresectable pancreatic cancer had lost weight (median 14.2%), and 35% of them had a body mass index (BMI) <20.[17] Further, Lees[18] reported that 57% of patients with head and neck cancer had lost weight on commencing treatment and Daly et al[19] found that 57% of patients with oesophageal cancer reported weight loss. Similarly, Hammerlid et al[20] found that 51% of patients with head and neck cancer were malnourished. In a study by Magné et al,[21] one-third of patients with advanced head and neck cancer undergoing chemotherapy and radiotherapy were found to be malnourished. Collins et al[22] reported that 13% of patients with laryngeal carcinoma were malnourished at presentation (BMI <20) and 26% of patients complained of weight loss (mean 5.35%). During radiation treatment, 49% had a documented weight loss (mean 6.4%), with 13.3% of patients losing >10% of their body weight during treatment. The BMI at the end of treatment was significantly lower than at presentation (despite dietary counselling and/or oral supplementation). Finally, mean body weight loss in dysphagic patients with cancer of the oesophagus prior to nutritional support was 18.8%.[23] Also, patients with acute leukaemia have been reported to experience a median weight loss of 8% during treatment, with one-third of patients losing more than 10% of body weight.[24] Reported incidence of malnutrition in children with cancer ranges from 5 to 30% at diagnosis to over 50% during therapy.[25–28]

Gender has recently emerged as a discriminating factor in patients with non-small cell lung carcinoma (NSCLC). Palomares et al[15] evaluated the role of gender and weight-loss patterns in predicting clinical outcomes in a balanced population of men and women presenting with NSCLC. Overall median survival after diagnosis was significantly shorter for men with NSCLC than for women with the disease. Men lost significantly more weight over their disease course than women and experienced an eight-fold faster rate of initial weight loss. In multivariate analysis, the strongest independent predictors of NSCLC patient survival were stage of disease, initial weight-loss rate and gender. These results suggest that weight loss may play a role in mediating gender-related differences in NSCLC patient survival.

Factors contributing to cancer cachexia

Patients with cancer cachexia experience a profound wasting of adipose tissue and lean body mass. Our understanding of the aetiology of cancer cachexia is still rather limited. It is believed that malnutrition and cachexia occur through a variety of mechanisms, having to do with both the tumour itself and its treatment.

Although anorexia is common, a decreased food intake alone is unable to account for the changes in body composition seen in patients with cancer because:[4,29]

635

- cachexia involves massive depletion of skeletal muscle that does not occur during anorexia
- increasing nutrient intake is unable to completely reverse the wasting syndrome
- cachexia can occur without anorexia
- food intake might be normal for the lower-weight patients with cancer
- appetite stimulants (such as megestrol acetate) do not significantly improve lean body mass.

Although energy expenditure is increased in some patients, cachexia can occur even with normal energy expenditure. Various factors are believed to act as mediators of anorexia and metabolic disturbances of patients with cancer. These include proinflammatory cytokines, such as TNF-α, interleukins IL-1 and IL-6 and interferon-gamma (IFN-γ), as well as tumour-derived factors such as lipid mobilizing factor (LMF) and protein mobilizing factor (PMF), which can directly mobilize fatty acids and amino acids from adipose tissue and skeletal muscle, respectively.[29] The factors thought to be important in the development of malnutrition and cachexia are related to the systemic effects of the disease, the local effects of the tumour, psychological factors and side-effects of treatments, which lead to reduced food intake and/or metabolic disturbances.[4,7,30–32]

Systemic effects of disease

Diminished food intake is very common in patients with cancer. Anorexia, nausea, vomiting, altered perceptions of taste and smell or pain are all systemic effects of the disease, which may contribute to the reduction in oral intake of patients with cancer. Taste changes are a frequent and significant problem in patients with cancer. Cancer-related taste alterations are postulated to be (at least partly) the result of the influence of factors excreted by tumour cells.[6] Pain on eating or pain in general may also contribute to a reduction in food intake.

Local effects of tumour

Local effects of the tumour include odynophagia, dysphagia, intestinal or gastric obstruction, early satiety, malabsorption and pain.

Dysphagia and odynophagia are particularly marked in patients with head and neck cancer and oesophageal cancer. Dysphagia is seen in up to 74% of patients with oesophageal cancer and 32% of patients with cancer of the larynx.[19,33] Tumours in the gastrointestinal and hepatobiliary tract, but also metastatic cancers outside the gastrointestinal tract pressing on gastrointestinal structures, are often complicated by partial or total digestive obstruction, leading to nausea, vomiting and early satiety. In some patients, relapsing episodes of obstruction or blind-loop syndromes can seriously affect nutrient absorption.[7] Anorexia, early satiety, dry mouth, pain and nausea are the most frequent symptoms affecting nutritional intake.[34]

Psychological factors

Fear, depression and anxiety, which are not uncommon in patients with cancer, can also negatively affect nutrient intake. These psychological responses often alter the behaviour and attitude of the patient. One response to a devastating illness is rejection of things that 'nourish and nurture'.[35] Patients may also complain of general weakness and fatigue or report diminished energy levels, and one probable cause for that may be the inability to eat and early satiety.[2] A link between fatigue and cachexia is implied in an editorial by Glaus,[36] but there is a lack of understanding of how these symptoms work synergistically. Cachexia may be another example where psychosocial and physical aspects of a condition are interwoven.

Effects of cancer treatments

Side-effects of treatments can also be a major cause of malnutrition in patients with cancer. Each cancer treatment may induce acute and delayed gastrointestinal symptoms and exert negative effects on the patient's nutritional status. Chemotherapeutic agents contribute to host malnutrition by a variety of mechanisms, including nausea and vomiting, mucositis, gastrointestinal dysfunction and learned food aversions. In a study of patients with acute leukaemia,[24] food intake of patients was diminished during those periods in which they suffered most intensively from the side-effects of chemotherapy. Radiation therapy also contributes to the cancer patient's malnourished state. The severity and incidence of malnutrition are determined by the body region undergoing radiation, dose, duration and volume of therapy. Nutritional alterations may result from local therapy to the central nervous system (nausea and vomiting), head and neck (mucositis, dysphagia, xerostomia, trismus), thorax (dysphagia, fibrosis, fistulae) and abdomen/pelvis (diarrhoea, enteritis, malabsorption). Surgical treatment has an effect on nutritional intake and status if it involves oral, oesophageal and/or gastrointestinal resections.[30,37,38]

Metabolic alterations

Although metabolic changes are known to occur as part of the cancer process, the mechanisms are still not fully understood. Metabolic disturbances associated with cancer affect both energy expenditure and the metabolism of protein, fat and carbohydrate.[7] The progressive weight loss of patients with cancer has proven difficult to reverse, and it has been suggested that the metabolic response to cancer prevents the efficient use of nutrition.[39] Part of this metabolic response is the hepatic acute-phase protein response. The acute-phase protein response has been shown to be associated with hypermetabolism, accelerated weight loss[17,40,41] and poor survival in patients with advanced cancer.[42,43]

Alterations in energy expenditure

There has been major controversy over whether patients with cancer have elevated energy expenditure relative to (weight-losing) patients with other illnesses. Several studies of energy expenditure have been reported with varied results. Although initial studies mostly reported markedly elevated resting energy expenditure in patients with cancer, several more recent studies (based on indirect calorimetry) have reported only slightly increased, unchanged or even decreased resting energy expenditure.[7,12] According to Bozzetti,[12] it is now generally accepted that many patients with cancer are mildly hypermetabolic, with an increase in energy expenditure

ranging between 140 and 290 kcal/day. Energy expenditure of patients with cancer appears to depend on presence or absence of an acute-phase protein response, type of cancer, response to treatment/presence of tumour and duration of the disease. Other alterations are seen in the protein metabolism, carbohydrate metabolism and lipid metabolism.

Specific humoral and inflammatory responses

Over the past three decades, explanations of how tumours modulate host metabolism have been sought. In recent years, interest has focused on the role that the immune system plays in the development of cachexia. Investigators initially hypothesized that the chronic production of two inflammatory cytokines, TNF-α and/or IL-1, could explain the host non-specific responses that resulted in cachexia. Other pro-inflammatory cytokines, including IL-6 and IFN-γ, have been more recently proposed to be involved in this complex process.[44] Furthermore, tumour-derived factors (such as PMF and LMF) are now believed to play a role in the development of cancer cachexia. Some of these factors and their effects are presented in Table 29.1.

Cancer-specific cachectic factors (or tumour-derived catabolic factors)

Protein mobilizing factor

A newly described tumour-specific 24-kDa glycoprotein, called protein mobilizing factor (PMF or proteolysis-inducing factor), has been identified in the urine of cachectic patients with cancer. PMF has been shown to cause enhanced skeletal muscle proteolysis when given to mice.[4,45]

Lipid mobilizing factor

Evidence suggests that cachexia-inducing tumours also produce a lipid mobilizing factor. This LMF is a 43 kDa glycoprotein (similar to zinc-α2-glycoprotein, an acute phase protein), and was recently isolated from a cachexia-inducing murine tumour and from the urine of cachectic patients with unresectable pancreatic carcinoma.[4] LMF directly stimulates lipolysis in a cyclic AMP-dependent manner and increases energy expenditure.[4]

Table 29.1: Metabolic effects of cytokines involved in cachexia

Cytokine or cachexia	Production	Effects related to anorexia
Tumour necrosis factor-α (TNF-α)	Increased in tumour-bearing hosts Serum levels not increased in most studies Levels do not seem to correlate with malnutrition Produced by macrophages	Injection into animals induces anorexia and weight loss May increase resting energy expenditure May have local GI effects (e.g. delay of gastric emptying) Inhibits lipoprotein lipase Causes hypertriglyceridaemia Depletes total body fat stores Increases muscle protein breakdown Increases synthesis of APP Increases hepatic glucose output and glyconeogenesis Inhibition by antibodies reverses some of the above effects
Interleukin-1 (IL-1)	Serum levels not increased in most studies Serum levels do not correlate with malnutrition Produced by macrophages	Injection induces anorexia and weight loss, more so than TNF-α May increase resting energy expenditure Causes similar effects on fat and carbohydrate metabolism as TNF-α Inhibition by antibodies reverses some of the above effects
Interleukin-6 (IL-6)	Increased in tumour-bearing hosts Production induced by TNF-α and IL-1 Levels correlate with extent of tumour burden in animal models Produced by macrophages and fibroblasts	Induces hepatic glyconeogenesis Increases synthesis of APP Increases lipolysis Inhibition by antibodies reverses anorexia and APPR in animals
Interferon-γ (IFN-γ)	Produced by activated T lymphocytes	Augments effects of TNF-α on lipid metabolism Inhibits lipoprotein lipase Inhibition by antibodies in tumour-bearing animals reduces weight loss

GI, gastrointestinal; APP, amyloid precursor protein; APPR, acute-phase protein response.

Antagonists of tumour catabolic factors will provide important new agents in the treatment of cancer cachexia.[4] For example, the biological activity of both the LMF and PMF is attenuated by eicosapentaenoic acid.[29] Other factors which may have a role in malnutrition and cachexia of patients with cancer include recently identified peptides (e.g. leptin and its receptors, melanin-concentrating hormones), changes in cytokine concentrations in the central nervous system and alterations in other neuroregulators of appetite. However, data in this area are minimal (reviewed by Mutlu and Mobarhan[31]).

Cancer-specific pathway modulations

Recent biochemical evidence has shown that up-regulation of the ATP–ubiquitin–proteasome pathway, perhaps modulated by TNF-α or IL-6, may be (at least partly) responsible for the continual protein breakdown seen in patients with cancer.[4,29] In this ATP-dependent process, proteins are marked for degradation by attachment to ubiquitin (Ub) molecules, undergo proteolysis to peptides by a 26S proteasome complex and are then rapidly degraded into amino-acids in the cytosol.[46] Activation of the Ub–proteasome pathway has been demonstrated in the bodies of tumour-bearing rats and human cell lines, and although its role in human cachexia needs to be further delineated, it may be a target for future therapies for cachexia.[47]

REASONS AFFECTING PROGRESSION OF MALNUTRITION

A comprehensive review by Greene[48] has provided a detailed summary of potential reasons for progression of disease-related malnutrition in the hospital as well as in the community. The key points with regard to the progression of disease-related malnutrition are:

- disease- and treatment-associated factors
- inadequate provision of nutrition to patients in hospital and community settings (poor palatability; inadequate presentation and serving of food; inflexible catering systems; lack of assistance with shopping, cooking or eating meals)
- lack of awareness and recognition of problem by medical and nursing staff (lack of training, knowledge and/or interest or poor organization of nutritional services).

Furthermore, Grosvenor et al[49] undertook a study to determine which symptoms influ-

enced weight loss in an advanced cancer population. Energy intake was surprisingly similar in patients with weight loss compared with those without weight loss. However, symptoms occurring significantly more frequently in patients with weight loss included abdominal fullness, taste changes, vomiting and mouth dryness.

CONSEQUENCES OF MALNUTRITION

Weight loss is a major cause of morbidity and mortality in advanced cancer.[50,51] Progressive weight loss is a common feature of many types of cancer and is associated not only with a poor quality of life and poor response to chemotherapy but also with a shorter survival time than found in patients with comparable tumours without weight loss.[29] One of the most significant studies on the consequences of malnutrition in patients with cancer is the one by Andreyev et al.[52] The investigators carried out a retrospective investigation of whether weight loss at presentation influences outcomes of patients who are to receive chemotherapy for gastrointestinal cancers. In 1555 patients treated over a 6-year period, weight loss at presentation was reported more commonly by men than women. Although patients with weight loss received lower chemotherapy doses initially, they developed more frequent and more severe dose-limiting toxicity than patients without weight loss. Consequently, patients with weight loss on average received 1 month less treatment. Weight loss correlated with shorter survival, decreased response to treatment, decreased quality of life and impaired performance status.

Reported consequences of disease-related malnutrition in adult patients with cancer include the following:

- lower quality of life (lower general health, lower social functioning, lower outlook/happiness) [51,52]
- reduced response to chemotherapy[50,52]
- increased risk of chemotherapy-induced toxicity[52]
- higher risk of postoperative complications[53,54]

- reduced functional capacity/performance status[50,52,55]

- reduced muscle function[56]

- longer hospital stay (with hospitals stays in malnourished patients being 50–100% longer than in well-nourished patients)[57–59]

- higher prescription rates and consultation rates[60]

- higher costs[59]

- higher mortality, especially in patients with gastrointestinal cancer[61,62] and in patients undergoing bone marrow transplantation[63,64]

- severe psychosocial distress in many patients and their families (as malnutrition may have profound philosophical and sometimes religious connotations)[65]

- Shorter survival, perhaps as a result of malnourished patients receiving less chemotherapy and developing more toxicity than well-nourished patients.[50,52,66]

In paediatric patients with cancer, malnutrition is also associated with poorer outcomes, reduced tolerance to therapy, more relapses and higher risk of infections.[67,68]

NUTRITIONAL ASSESSMENT

The first step in the nutritional care of a cancer patient is a thorough nutritional assessment. All patients with cancer should have a regular evaluation of nutritional status, starting at the time of diagnosis, and continuing during treatment. The importance of a standardized and systematic nutritional assessment cannot be overemphasized. Bloch[69] emphasized that nurses are in a key position to provide support to patients and their families with regard to nutritional issues, and that their contribution to ongoing assessment of nutritional status and early intervention to meet nutritional needs is of paramount importance.

The aims of nutritional assessment are:

- to determine if a patient has, or is at risk of developing malnutrition or specific nutrient deficiencies

- to quantify a patient's risk of developing malnutrition-related complications

- to provide guidelines for short- and longer-term nutritional support

- to monitor the adequacy of nutritional therapy.[13,37,31,70]

Nutritional assessment of a cancer patient should preferably consist of a clinical assessment and of anthropometric measurements. Patients who are identified at nutritional risk may require more detailed assessments, including body composition and biochemical measurements. Whenever possible, patient-reported data should be compared with objective medical (and non-medical) information. Relying solely on a patient's recall can lead to over- or underdiagnosis, especially in the case of weight changes.[31] Nutritional assessment should preferably be combined with a careful evaluation of functional capacity and quality of life, to ensure that nutritional support is tailored to the patient's needs and requires a minimum of constraints.[7]

Clinical assessment

The clinical assessment of the patient with cancer should ideally consist of a medical history, dietary history, social history and a physical examination.[13,31,37,70]

Medical history

A medical history, which includes assessment of past and present medical problems and (anticancer) treatments, may provide clues to nutritional deficiencies. Special attention should be given to conditions that interfere with adequate intake, increase losses and/or affect nutrient needs. For example, previous gastrectomy may lead to dumping syndrome, diarrhoea or folate deficiency, whereas ileal resection or chronic pancreatitis may be associated with steatorrhoea and deficiencies in fat-soluble vitamins. Furthermore, patients with cancer may have diabetes, hypertension or cardiovascular, renal or respiratory problems that predispose to nutrition deficits. A careful review of tumour- and therapy-related problems should focus on recent weight loss, weakness, fatigue, anorexia, nausea, vomiting, early satiety, pain, xerostomia, stomatitis, dysphagia, odynophagia, oesophagitis, abdominal pain, bloating, diarrhoea and constipation. Furthermore, the psychological response to disease should be assessed (e.g. depression, anxiety).[13,31,37,70] It should be remembered that elderly patients may have impaired digestive and absorptive functions such as oesophageal and gastric dysmotility, atrophic gastritis and achlorhydria.[35] Use of medications (other than chemotherapeutic agents) should also be evaluated to determine whether they may influence nutrient intake, gastrointestinal function and/or have catabolic properties.

Dietary history

Analysis of the dietary pattern of the patient may range from an estimate of actual food consumption, as distinguished from the amount of food prepared or eaten from a plate, or a simple screening by food groups of a 24-hour dietary recall to a computer-facilitated nutrient analysis of a record kept for 3 days. Other information important to the dietary history includes level of activity, ability to eat without assistance, use of dietary supplements, (changes in) food aversions and preferences, taste and smell changes, unusual food habits, fear of undesirable effects after eating (e.g. pain, cramping, nausea, distension, flatus), possible religious/cultural constraints to the diet and psychological response to previous nutritional support.

Social and psychological history

The social history provides information about the structure of the family, past and present lifestyle, social support systems as well as cultural and religious background, education and economic status of the family.[31] Psychological history can include information on how the patient is coping with the illness, adjustment difficulties, anxiety or depression.

Physical examination

The physical examination includes a careful examination of the patient, looking for signs of general malnutrition (e.g. loss of subcutaneous adipose tissue, peripheral oedema, ascites, skin lesions, poor hair and nail quality and loss of skin turgor) and of specific micronutrient deficiencies (e.g. anaemia, vitamin deficiencies,

rickets). It should be remembered that ascites may also be due to the tumour or infiltration of the liver in end-stage renal cancer and that hair and nail problems may be the result of chemotherapy or radiation therapy.

Anthropometric measurements

Weight changes

Weight is still the most meaningful parameter in nutritional status. DeWys et al, in their 1980 classic article,[50] highlight the importance of a history of weight loss of more than 6% of premorbid body weight at the time of treatment initiation. Weight measurements are the easiest measures to obtain and should be made frequently in patients with cancer. However, body weight is not always a reliable indicator of nutritional status in patients with cancer. Weight depends greatly on the patient's hydration status. Many treatments and conditions in patients with cancer lead to oedema and changes in the normal intracellular fluid-to-protein ratio. This may lead to underestimation of the patient's protein losses. Therefore, every effort should be made to determine hydration status in conjunction with weight. Furthermore, tumour mass may contribute up to 10% of body weight in children[71] and up to 4–5% in adults.[7,12]

A variety of weight indices have been developed to standardize weight measurements, including weight-to-height ratios, per cent weight loss and per cent ideal body weight, but these indices are subject to errors associated with establishing normal or standard values. Serial weight determinations over a sufficient time provide a more reliable indicator of lean body mass gain or loss. Involuntary weight loss of 5–10% or more over the last 3–6 months places a person at nutritional risk, and such risk should be identified as early as possible.[7,35,72] In Tables 29.2 and 29.3, two different classifications of nutritional status are given on the basis of recent, unintentional weight loss. In the first classification (adapted from Elia[72]) only the percentage of weight loss is taken into account. The second classification (adapted from Ottery[73] and Nitenberg and Raynard[7]) also considers the rate of recent weight loss.

Table 29.2: Classification of nutritional status on the basis of the percentage of recent weight loss

Weight loss in the last 3–6 months	Severity of malnutrition
<5%	Mild
5–10%	Moderate
>10%	Severe

Source: adapted from Elia.[72]

Body composition

In addition to weight changes, malnourished patients with cancer exhibit alterations in body composition, loss of subcutaneous fat stores and lean body mass. Body composition can be roughly estimated using a combination of skin-fold and mid arm circumference measurements.

The thickness of subscapular and triceps skinfolds provides an index of body fat. Furthermore, mid-upper arm circumference (MUAC) is an anthropometric indicator of muscle mass. Increases in MUAC are more likely to comprise muscle and less likely to be affected by oedema than body weight. In order to fully differentiate between lean body mass and fat mass, triceps skinfold and MUAC measurements can be combined mathematically to obtain an estimate of arm muscle area and arm fat area. Interpretation of data derived from skinfold and MUAC measurements is limited, however, as these techniques are only indirect measurements of body composition, normal values are population-specific, inter-observer errors may be large, values may vary with hydration status and values have not been validated in patients with cancer.[7] In addition, subcutaneous fat distribution appears not to be symmetric.

More sophisticated and precise methods of assessing body composition, which are mostly used for research purposes, include isotope dilution, bioelectrical and absorptiometry methods. These methods measure whole-tissue compartments, mostly using either a two-com-partment model (fat and fat-free mass) or a three-compartment model (fat, lean body mass and bone). More information on these methods can be found in Reilly[74] and Zemel et al.[75]

Bioelectrical impedance analysis (BIA) is currently becoming more popular for use in the clinical setting, as it is relatively cheap and easy to use, shows a good correlation with isotopic dilution and is able to discriminate between malnourished and well-nourished patients even in case of oedema.[7] Fredrix et al[76] validated the BIA method for body composition estimation in elderly patients with cancer using the deuterium dilution technique as the reference method. They concluded that this is a useful measure for the assessment of body composition in patients with cancer.

Laboratory measurements

Biochemical measurements have only limited value in the assessment of the nutritional status of a patient with cancer, as they are non-specific for malnutrition, and many of these parameters are dynamic and change on a daily basis, compensated by homeostatic mechanisms and/or influenced by the disease process.[77] The choice of biochemical parameters to evaluate and monitor the patient's nutritional status depends on

Table 29.3: Classification of nutritional status on the basis of the percentage and rate of recent weight loss

Time	Mild malnutrition Weight loss (% of usual weight)	Severe malnutrition
1 week	1–2%	>2%
1 month	5%	>5%
3 months	7.5%	>7.5%
6 months	10%	>10%

Source: adapted from Ottery[73] and Nitenberg and Raynard.[7]

the patient's medical condition and suspected nutrient deficiencies, and on the availability, cost, predictive values, sensitivity, specificity, reliability and validity of biochemical tests. Usual tests include serum protein concentrations (i.e. albumin, transferrin, prealbumin or retino-binding proteins) and haematological tests (i.e. tests suggestive of iron-deficiency anaemia or microcytic anaemia) as well as tests of immune function (as it is affected by malnutrition), electrolyte levels and minerals (Ca, Mg, P) and vitamins (i.e. vitamin B_6 in Hodgkin's disease patients or folate status in gastrectomy patients).

In patients with cancer, serum protein values may lead, however, to false conclusions. For instance, Shike et al[78] found serum albumin and total serum protein values to be normal in patients with small-cell lung cancer who were diagnosed as being malnourished on the basis of their weight loss, creatinine index, negative nitrogen balance and low potassium and fat stores. Thus, decreased lean body mass may not necessarily correlate with low circulating proteins in patients with cancer. Shortcomings also exist with the interpretation of other haematological and biochemical measurements.

IDENTIFICATION OF NUTRITIONAL RISK

The initial nutritional screening and assessment of oncology patients should provide data that will clarify the nutritional risk category in which the patient should be placed. In order to clearly define the role of nutritional support and the maintenance of body composition (both within the setting of clinical trials and in clinical practice), healthcare professionals should have access to an effective, reproducible and easy-to-use screening and assessment tool. The use of a standardized, validated instrument facilitates ongoing assessment of nutritional status and guides appropriate interventions.[13]

Patient-Generated Subjective Global Assessment

The Patient-Generated Subjective Global Assessment (PG-SGA) has been modified and tested for patients with cancer by Ottery.[79] The PG-SGA has been accepted by the Oncology Nutrition Dietetic Practice Group of the American Dietetic Association as the standard for nutritional assessment of patients with cancer.[13] The PG-SGA should assist the clinician with assessing a patient's nutritional status at baseline or soon after initial presentation. For this assessment, a simple, one-page form is used. The patient completes more than half of the page, with questions about weight changes over time (1 year, 6 months and within the past 2 weeks), food intake within the past month, symptoms that would affect eating and functional capacity. A staff member should complete the remaining questions, with information on diagnosis and staging, metabolic stress levels (if known) and physical findings of fat and muscle wasting, oedema and ascites. A three-level rating is then determined.[79] Based upon the PG-SGA stratification, the appropriate level of nutritional intervention can be determined, as shown in Table 29.4.[13] The PG-SGA is an economical and easy screening methods that does not need special training as some of the previous methods described. Also, it has been shown to be a valid method of screening, as compared to objective criteria, with sensitivity (false negatives) of 96% and specificity (false positives) of 83%.[34] The complete scale and scoring instructions can also be seen in Finley[80] and Thoresen et al.[34]

Oncology Screening Tool

In the Oncology Screening Tool, developed at the Memorial Sloan-Kettering Cancer Center, the initial screening is performed by a nurse, dietitian or other qualified person (reviewed by Bloch[35]). This screening tool is based on weight loss and a 2-week or longer history of decreased food intake from normal, nausea and vomiting, diarrhoea, mouth sores and chewing or swallowing difficulty. Based on these factors, a patient's risk is classified as (1) low risk or (2) moderate to high risk. Only the moderate- to high-risk patients are seen by a dietitian within 24 hours, at which time a comprehensive nutritional assessment is performed.

Table 29.4: Guidelines for Subjective Global Assessment categories for patients with cancer

	Stage A	Stage B	Stage C
Category	Well-nourished	Moderately malnourished or suspected malnutrition	Severely malnourished
Weight	No weight loss or recent non-fluid weight gain	± 5% weight loss within 1 month (or 10% in 6 months) No weight stabilization or weight gain	> 5% weight loss within 1 month (or > 10% in 6 months) No weight stabilization or weight gain
Nutrient intake	No deficit or significant recent improvement	Definite decrease in intake	Severe deficit in intake
Symptoms affecting nutrient intake	None or significant recent improvement allowing adequate intake	Presence of symptoms affecting intake	Presence of symptoms affecting intake
Functioning	No deficit or significant recent improvement	Moderate functional deficit or recent deterioration	Severe functional deficit or significant recent deterioration
Physical examination	No deficit or chronic deficit but with recent clinical improvement	Evidence of mild to moderate loss of fat and/or muscle mass and/or muscle tone on palpation	Obvious signs of malnutrition (e.g. severe loss of fat and/or muscle mass, possible oedema)

This assessment includes general appearance, fluid status, height and weight (pre-illness; usual; current, considering hydration status), medical history, diet history, medications, laboratory values, mechanical and physical limitations affecting intake, mental status, malabsorption status, cancer treatment plans, cultural influences to dietary practices and ability to self-feed. From this assessment, a nutrition care plan is developed. The final classification of the patient into either moderate or high nutritional risk is based on diagnosis, complications, treatment and weight status. Moderate-risk patients are reassessed by the dietician within 5 days, and high-risk patients within 3 days. Low-risk patients are rescreened by the dietician on the 6th day to verify their initial risk level or to recategorize them if their status has changed.

Other malnutrition screening and assessment tools

Harrison and Fong[70] suggest to use a scale of malnutrition based on weight loss, serum albumin and transferrin, and hypersensitivity skin testing (Table 29.5).

NUTRITIONAL SUPPORT IN PATIENTS WITH CANCER

Nutritional support is a vital adjunct to cancer treatment. The main goal of nutritional sup-

Table 29.5: Clinical evaluation of malnutrition

Degree of malnutrition	Clinical findings	Laboratory findings
None	No weight loss	Normal albumin Normal transferrin Reactive delayed hypersensitivity skin test
Mild	<5% weight loss	Albumin <3.5 g/dl Decreased transferrin level
Moderate	5–10% weight loss	Albumin <3.2 g/dl Less than 5 mm reactivity on skin test
Severe	10% weight loss Muscle weakness	Albumin <2.7 g/dl Non-reactive skin test

port in patients with cancer is to provide adequate amounts of energy and nutrients, to maintain or improve nutritional status and to support immune function, while minimizing gastrointestinal symptoms and maximizing quality of life. In this respect, nutritional support can be seen as supportive therapy.[13,38,70,78] Mercadante[81] has phrased this as follows: '. . . there is no disease during which patients benefit from prolonged wasting'.

Dietary advice and counselling

Even if no nutritional problems are identified, the importance of good nutrition should be stressed and oncology patients should be encouraged to meet their needs via a healthy, well-balanced diet.[77] If nutritional intake is inadequate, attempting to improve intake of patients with cancer via normal foods and beverages is mostly the first step in the process of providing nutritional support. Simple dietary advice focused on food quality and quantity may be sufficient to correct the problem. The first nutritional objectives for oncology patients with a poor food intake are to increase the frequency of consumption of food and beverages, and to increase the energy and nutrient content of foods and fluids consumed. Patients should be encouraged to take small meals, snacks or nourishing drinks at regular intervals, e.g. every 2–3 hours. Furthermore, they should be motivated to consume foods and drinks, which provide concentrated sources of energy, protein and micronutrients in a relatively small volume (e.g. meat, cheese, full-fat yoghurt, milk-based drink or cream soup). Patients with cancer may also benefit from food-enrichment strategies which boost the energy content of foods without significantly affecting their volume (e.g. adding cheese and/or cream to soup and savoury dishes).[35,38,77] Patients may have to be re-educated about food choices. Information given previously about healthy eating may no longer be appropriate. Many patients try to avoid fat and eat lots of fruits, vegetables and fibre.[35]

Special guidance to help in alleviating problems which affect food intake – such as anorexia, nausea, sore or dry mouth and swallowing difficulties – may also result in considerable improvements in oral intake. As both disease and antineoplastic therapy may be associated with gastrointestinal disorders and other side-effects affecting food intake, modifications in texture and types of diets offered and other dietary measures may be necessary. In Box 29.1, a summary is given of guidelines for dietary management of common nutritional problems in oncology patients (summarizing work in Refs 6, 31, 38, 68, 77 and 80). Similarly, nausea and vomiting, mucositis and xerostomia, or diarrhoea and constipation need to be corrected, and useful information is discussed in Chapters 20, 26 and 22, respectively.

The psychological aspects of anorexia and cachexia can be very important for patients and their carers. Feeding a dependant is the essence of nature and this fundamental breakdown must be addressed with both patients and their families/carers.[82] Dietary advice should extend to the family members of the patients with cancer

---

Box 29.1

Dietary management of common nutritional problems

Anorexia
- Offer small, frequent meals/snacks high in energy and protein (5–6/day)
- If a main mail is not eaten, give a snack (e.g. a sandwich, yoghurt, biscuits, crackers and cheese, fruit) or a nourishing drink (e.g. a milky drink, cream soup) instead
- Stimulate to eat most at times when appetite is best (i.e. many people have a better appetite in the morning)
- Avoid drinking just before and during meals. Give beverages at least half an hour before or at the end of the meal
- Create a pleasant mealtime atmosphere (e.g. enhancing food aromas, varied colours and textures of foods, soft music, avoiding noxious odours)
- Relaxation techniques and light exercise before meals may help to improve appetite
- If allowed, a glass of wine may serve as an appetite stimulant
- Consider the use of appetite-enhancing agents
- Increase calories and protein in diet
- Find a nutritional supplement which is appealing
- Soft, cool, frozen foods may be more appealing
- Keep healthy snacks handy

Taste changes
- Identify taste changes and offer foods that are still appealing
- Reduce exposure to odours
- Maintain good oral hygiene, especially before and after meals
- Encourage fluid intake
- Use lemon drops and gum to promote salivation and enhance taste sensation before meals
- Herbs, spices, flavour extracts and marinades may enhance food taste
- Offer poultry, fish, eggs and dairy products (especially in case of 'metallic' taste)
- Cold foods may be better accepted
- Offer highly aromatic foods
- Vary the colour and texture of the foods
- Offer fruit-flavoured beverages
- Avoid tobacco and alcohol
- Avoid commercial mouthwashes

Food aversions
- Avoid intake of favourite foods prior to treatment
- Offer carbohydrate-based meals rather than protein-based meals (of no important social significance) prior to treatment

Thick, viscous saliva
- Encourage fluid intake
- Use clear fluids (e.g. tea, popsicles, slushes)
- Maintain good oral hygiene

Dysphagia
- Use liquid, blenderized or soft foods

Source: from Refs 6, 31, 38, 68, 77 and 80.

and help them understand that their loved one is not starving to death but there are metabolic abnormalities due to cancer and that administration of more food will not result in the expected outcomes.[65] This, in turn, will help both patients and families to decrease their emotional distress and maintain the social benefits of mealtimes.[65] Family involvement usually improves the patient's food intake (as they bring favourite foods) and family bonds are strengthened.[83]

Furthermore, two well-designed randomized trials have examined the role of oral nutritional supplements in patients with advanced cancer receiving chemotherapy.[51,84] In these studies, patients were randomized to receive nutritional counselling to raise their energy levels and protein intake or to remain on ad-lib intake. In both studies it was shown that a significant increase in nutritional intake took place in the intervention group for over 3 months. However, no benefit was established in terms of weight gain, anthropometric measures, response rate, survival or quality of life between the experimental and control groups. Dietary counselling combined with other nutritional interventions may, however, be more appropriate.[85]

Enteral and parenteral nutrition

It was hoped that enteral or parenteral feeding would improve cancer malnutrition. However, the inability of hypercaloric nutritional support to increase lean mass, especially skeletal mass, and improve patients' survival or quality of life have been repeatedly reported in the literature.[82,83,86] A number of studies were carried out in the 1980s and meta-analysis of these studies has shown no improvement in survival (and perhaps reduced survival), poor tumour response and significant infectious complications.[51,84] More recent reviews also support the ineffectiveness of enteral or parenteral nutrition.[1,5] Some older studies, reviewed by Kotler[86] in patients with AIDS and patients with lymphoma, show that weight gain may occur, but it leads almost solely to fat accumulation. Nevertheless, in certain clinical situations (i.e. patients recovering from surgery or patients with complications from treatment for a responsive tumour), intensive nutrition of this kind may be appropriate, balancing the risks and benefits.[1,82]

Effective pharmacological therapies

Appetite stimulants and anabolic therapies have been tried extensively as supportive measures in cancer anorexia–cachexia and some also have effects on patients' nutritional status. The medical use of marijuana and other cannabinoids has been recently advocated.[1,86] Dronabinol is the most commonly used cannabinoid, has appetite-stimulating effects and can increase weight in both patients with advanced cancer and AIDS.[1,87] However, a recent large randomized trial of patients with advanced cancer ($n = 469$) provides evidence of inferior anorexia palliation for dronabinol compared to megestrol acetate.[88] Megestrol acetate (a progesterone) has been studied in at least 15 studies (more than 2000 patients) and a systematic review concluded that the effects of high-dose progestins on appetite and body weight are clearly demonstrated, even though it was noted that further research is necessary to establish the best therapeutic index of progestin activity.[89] Lower doses of megestrol have also been shown to alleviate fatigue and nausea, and also improve activity and general well-being, although it may not improve quality of life.[5]

At least six randomized trials have tested the effects of corticosteroids for cancer cachexia. Most research has shown a limited effect (of up to 4 weeks) on appetite, food intake, perception of well-being and performance status, although significant weight gain was not shown.[65] Dexamethasone seems equal to megestrol as an appetite stimulant. Anabolic corticosteroids may have some benefits, as they increase muscle mass in individuals (i.e. athletes), but little research exists in patients with cancer. Other treatments that have shown some improvements, mostly as appetite stimulants but also in terms of weight gain and performance, include serotonin antagonists, growth factors, non-steroidal anti-inflammatory drugs (NSAIDs), anticytokines, metoclopramide or pentoxifylline.[1,5,65,86,90,91] Furthermore, depression can be the result of anorexia and cachexia, but also can itself lead to anorexia and weight loss, and anxiolytic or antidepressant drugs may improve such a situation.[83]

Promising pharmacological approaches

A number of drugs are currently in phase II and phase III trials with patients with cancer, as preliminary evidence suggests efficacy in relation to some of the mechanisms associated with cachexia. Thalidomide, an old hypnotic and antiemetic drug which was withdrawn in the 1960s due to its teratogenic effects, is now reappearing as a drug in the management of cachexia, due to the observed effects it has on appetite and weight gain in both HIV and patients with cancer.[65] Thalidomide may be particularly effective in improving appetite and perception of well-being.[92] Several studies have also shown effects on other variables such as fatigue, well-being, insomnia and chronic nausea.[93] Complex immunomodulatory effects may be responsible for the effects shown with the use of thalidomide. Furthermore, another drug, melatonin, has been shown, in small studies of a single team of investigators, to improve survival and nutritional status (i.e. cachexia rate of 26% in best supportive care vs 5% in best supportive care plus melatonin), although replication of these studies is necessary.[94,95] Another promising intervention is the infusion of a molecule called adenosine triphosphate (ATP), which has been tested in a study of 58 patients with lung cancer and weight-loss inhibition was clearly demonstrated.[96] However, potential side-effects and a number of methodological limitations (i.e. lack of blinded allocation of subjects) suggest that more work is needed in this area before ATP is introduced as a drug against cachexia and weight loss.

Fish oil, *n*-3 fatty acids and eicosapentaenoic acid

Fish oil, rich in the *n*-3 fatty acid eicosapentaenoic acid (EPA), has shown marked attenuation in cachexia in patients with pancreatic cancer.[97] This study used fish oil capsules containing 18% EPA. The same team reported that EPA supplementation in weight-losing patients with pancreatic cancer (*n* = 26) stabilized weight loss, patients had a median weight gain of 0.5 kg, and this stabilization of weight was maintained for 3 months.[98] A large randomized study of 200 patients with pancreatic cancer using supplements enriched with fish oil has also been carried out. It was shown that those who managed the target of around 2 g of EPA and 600 kcal per day (through a nutritional supplement) achieved a significant increase in weight and lean body mass.[91] Barber[99] reviewed the available literature on the use of fish oil-enriched nutritional supplementation and concluded that fish oil and EPA have the potential of normalizing the metabolic alterations that take place in cachexia and may allow the supply of additional nutrition to produce anabolism. EPA-containing nutritional supplements have recently appeared on the market with the trade name ProSure™, as dietary supplements that can improve appetite and weight, increase lean body mass and have positive effects on patients' quality of life, and they may be extremely useful in the management of anorexia–cachexia. However, a large randomized trial with the full results of the study by Fearon et al[91] is eagerly awaited, which will inform whether this new product is effective in the treatment of cancer weight loss and malnutrition.

Non-pharmacological approaches

Resistance exercise training has been tested in various clinical populations, and improvements in the nutritional status has been reported in patients with congestive heart failure and HIV illness:[100,101] this is an approach that also needs to be investigated for patients with cancer. Nevertheless, the literature suggests that combination of resistance exercise with medication may produce better results.[102] Further, interventions such as hypnosis, relaxation and short-term group psychotherapy indicate that there is some benefit in relation to anorexia and fatigue, although which subgroup of patients with cancer is more likely to benefit needs to be determined.[103] The use of medicinal herbs may be another area of future research endeavour in the management of cachexia, as animal studies have shown that a specific herb (*Coptidis rhizoma*) may have anti-cachectic effects.[104] Many patients in the qualitative study by McGrath[105] reported using complementary therapies for their eating problems (i.e. use of ginger for nausea), although the effectiveness of such methods has not been evaluated to date.

A systematic review of the literature further confirms that non-pharmacological methods increased caloric and protein intake but resulted in no improvement in nutritional status, significant weight gain, tumour response, survival or quality of life.[106] Furthermore, weight, appetite and quality of life were improved when megestrol acetate was given, but the nutritional status was not improved.[106] The same review reports that some exercise studies did show improvements in nutrition-related outcomes, but these were not primary research outcomes, and thus further research is needed in this area.

General guidelines for nutritional support

A number of expert publications, some reviewed briefly above, have included recommendations for nutritional support in patients with cancer. These guidelines have been summarized in Box 29.2.

QUALITY OF LIFE ISSUES

Anorexia and cachexia produce disruptions in the daily life of patients with cancer and affect them both at a physical and psychosocial level. These disruptions and experiences are subjective in nature and different from person to person. Little work, however, has been directed to this area. Severe weight loss involves deterioration of muscle function and this is associated with a decline in physical functioning, body image disturbances and loss of control over bodily functions.[51,79] Significantly better quality of life scores have been reported in patients with oesophageal, gastric, colorectal and pancreatic cancer without weight loss than those with weight loss.[52] Past research also suggests that albumin, appetite and performance status are factors associated with weight loss and reduced quality of life in patients with gastrointestinal cancer.[108] Differences in performance

---

Box 29.2

Guidelines for nutritional support in patients with cancer

- As patients with cancer are at nutrition risk, all patients with cancer should undergo nutritional screening to identify those who require formal nutritional assessment with development of a nutrition care plan[70,107]
- Enteral nutrition should be given priority over total parenteral nutrition (TPN), as long as feeding through the gut is not contraindicated.[70]
- Eicosapentaenoic acid (EPA) (found in fish oil) has demonstarted potential in decreasing weight loss, lean body mass, survival and improving quality of life in weight-losing patients with cancer.[99]
- Routine use of nutritional support is not indicated in previously well-nourished patients undergoing surgery. Patients who are moderately to severely malnourished may benefit from preoperative nutritional support if administered for 7–14 days perioperatively.[70,107]
- Nutritional support should not be used routinely in well-nourished patients receiving chemotherapy or radiotherapy.[70,107]
- Nutritional support is appropriate in patients receiving active anticancer treatment who are malnourished and who are anticipated to have an inadequate oral intake for at least 5 days.[14,70,107]
- Nutritional support is appropriate in patients undergoing haemopoietic stem cell transplantation in whom oral intake is inadequate to meet requirements, or who develop moderate to severe graft versus host disease (GvHD) accompanied by poor oral intake.[107]
- Patients who are candidates for nutritional support should receive it prior to or in conjunction with the start of therapy.[14]
- Patients undergoing haemopoietic stem cell transplant should receive dietary counselling regarding high-risk foods and safe food handling during the period of immunosuppression.[107]
- The palliative use of nutritional support in terminally ill patients with cancer is rarely indicated.[107]

status between weight-losing and weight-gaining patients are reported in the literature, suggesting that weight loss or gain >2.5 kg over a 6- to 8-week period is necessary to produce significant alterations in the performance status.[109] Furthermore, certain pharmacological treatments for anorexia–cachexia have also been shown to improve quality of life (i.e. megestrol acetate).[110]

The only qualitative work to date is a recent Australian study which examined the perceptions on nutritional issues in 22 patients with haematological malignancies and 10 of their carers.[105] In this study it was shown that both patients and carers placed high significance on their nutritional status, and they mentioned problems with hospital food, lack of cultural understanding around nutrition, the important role of dieticians (even if their role was not so creative) and the key role of the medical staff in providing advice and medication for their eating difficulties. Also, the caregiver's role was emphasized.

Not only patients with advanced disease suffer from anorexia and cachexia. Re-analysing data from two older quality of life studies in patients with haematological malignancies,[111] it was observed that even long-term survivors may experience these distressing symptoms. Results indicated that 6.7% of patients at a mean post-treatment time of 39.6 months complained of lack of appetite ($n = 164$). Correlations were observed with 'appetite loss' and all psychosocial adjustment variables (i.e. social adjustment, vocational adjustment or adjustment with domestic environment), psychological variables such as depression ($r = 0.59$, $p<0.001$), anxiety ($r = 0.36$, $p<0.001$), the Rotterdam Symptom Checklist psychological symptom subscale ($r = 0.49$, $p<0.001$) or the Rotterdam Symptom Checklist physical symptom subscale ($r = 0.70$, $p<0.001$). In the same study, multivariate analysis showed that symptoms predictive of loss of appetite included constipation, dry mouth, shivering, nervousness, nausea and difficulty sleeping, explaining almost 59% of the variance in the independent variable ($r^2 = 0.588$, $p<0.001$). In the second study using the EORTC QOL-C30 scale in 28 long-term survivors of haematological cancers after bone marrow transplantation (mean time post-transplant = 41.2 months), 7.1% complained of 'quite a bit' lack of appetite and 25% for weight loss during the past month. Multivariate analysis of symptoms predicting lack of appetite showed that only one variable, having trouble sleeping, was a predictor explaining almost 50% of the variance. Predictors for weight loss included fatigue, presence of infections, lack of appetite and cognitive functioning, explaining 58% of the variance. Difficulty with sleeping is a prognostic factor of lack of appetite that has not been identified before and merits further investigation.

Currently, there is a limited range of choices for measuring the impact of anorexia and cachexia on the quality of life in patients with cancer. A brief questionnaire developed in the mid-1990s, the Bristol-Myers Anorexia/Cachexia Instrument, can be very useful in determining the value of treatment for anorexia–cachexia.[112] However, it is difficult to use it outside a trial setting. More recently, a shorter version of the Functional Assessment of Anorexia/Cachexia Therapy (FAACT) questionnaire has been validated with a large cancer population, and this could be a useful tool to quantify the experiences of cancer patients with anorexia–cachexia in their lives.[113]

CONCLUSION

It is clear that our understanding of anorexia and cachexia is still limited (but increasing), and that a multidisciplinary team effort is required in the management of anorexia, cachexia and weight loss. The field of nutritional oncology is just appearing and there are many things to be done in the future. Besides awareness, patient advocacy and ongoing nutritional assessment in patients with cancer, patient (and family) education are important. This will be challenging, as nurses traditionally are not well equipped through their training to deal with nutritional problems; therefore, a nutritionist should be a key member of the multidisciplinary team. There are a lot of questions around anorexia and cachexia that we will need to answer in the future: Is EPA (or fish oil) and any other of the emerging drugs the answer to the difficult management of cachexia and weight loss? Is it correct to put together anorexia and cachexia, or they are two different but related symptoms? What is the relationship between fatigue and anorexia–cachexia?

We need to base our practice in evidence, and as the evidence in the management of anorexia–cachexia is limited, we need to focus more on evaluating the best therapeutic approaches. It is also vital to develop better and clear criteria for diagnosing and staging cachexia. For all these factors, a deeper understanding of the mechanisms behind anorexia and cachexia will be imperative if we are to develop clear models to manage patients effectively. Some cancer centres have developed a more standardized approach to nutritional issues, developing nutrition protocols for the multidisciplinary team (i.e. Christie Hospital in Manchester, UK[115]), and this may be a way forward in addressing some of the issues around cancer and nutrition. Validated tools measuring anorexia and cachexia are needed, in order to encourage consistency across settings and across patients' experiences. There is minimal literature to date on issues around family care in patients with cachexia or the psychosocial needs of cachectic/weight-losing patients. Qualitative research in this area is lacking. Quality of life research will not only be vital in determining the effects of the various treatments for cachexia but also in assessing the individual experiences of cachectic patients throught their cancer trajectories.

REFERENCES

1. Nelson KA. Modern management of the cancer anorexia–cachexia syndrome. Curr Oncol Rep 2000; 2:362–368.

2. Stepp L, Pakiz TS. Anorexia and cachexia in advanced cancer. Nurs Clin North Am 2001; 36:735–744.

3. Guyton AC. Textbook of medical physiology. 8th edn. Philadelphia: WB Saunders; 1991:782.

4. Tisdale MJ. Cancer anorexia and cachexia. Nutrition 2001; 17: 438–442.

5. Davis MP, Dickerson D. Cachexia and anorexia: cancer's covert killer. Support Care Cancer 2000; 8:180–187.

6. Grant M, Kravits K. Symptoms and their impact on nutrition. Semin Oncol Nurs 2000; 16:113–121.

7. Nitenberg G, Raynard B. Nutritional support of the cancer patient: issues and dilemmas. Crit Rev Oncol Hematol 2000; 34:137–168.

8. Chance WT, Balasubramaniam A, Borchero M, Fischer JE. Refractory hypothalamic adenylate cyclase in anorectic tumour bearing rats. Implications for NPY-induced feeding. Brain Res 1995;, 691:180–184.

9. Cangiano C, Laviano A, Meguid MM, et al. Effects of administration of oral branched-chain amino acids on anorexia and caloric intake in patients with cancer. J Natl Cancer Inst 1996; 88:550–552.

10. Tracey KJ, Morgello S, Koplin B, et al. Metabolic effects of cachectin/tumor necrosis factor are modified by site of production. J Clin Invest 1990; 86:2014–2024.

11. Plata-Salaman CR. Cytokine-induced anorexia. Behavioral, cellular, and molecular mechanisms. Ann N Y Acad Sci 1998; 856:160–170.

12. Bozzetti F. Nutrition and gastrointestinal cancer. Curr Opin Nutr Metab Care 2001; 4:541–546.

13. Langer CJ, Hoffman JP, Ottery FD. Clinical significance of weight loss in patients with cancer: rationale for the use of anabolic agents in the treatment of cancer-related cachexia. Nutrition 2001; 17:S1–20.

14. Laviano A, Meguid MM. Nutritional issues in cancer management. Nutrition 1996; 12:358–371.

15. Palomares MR, Sayre JW, Shekar KC, Lillington LM, Chlebowski RT. Gender influence on weight-loss pattern and survival of nonsmall cell lung carcinoma patients. Cancer 1996; 78:2119–2126.

16. Bosaeus I, Daneryd P, Svanberg E, Lundholm K. Dietary intake and resting energy expenditure in relation to weight loss in unselected patients with cancer. Int J Cancer 2001; 93:380–383.

17. Wigmore SJ, Plester CE, Richardson RA, Fearon KC. Changes in nutritional status associated with unresectable pancreatic cancer. Br J Cancer 1997; 75:106–109.

18. Lees J. Incidence of weight loss in head and neck patients with cancer on commencing radiotherapy treatment at a regional oncology centre. Eur J Cancer Care 1999; 8:133–136.

19. Daly JM, Fry WA, Little AG, et al. Esophageal cancer: results of an American College of Surgeons Patient Care Evaluation Study. J Am Coll Surg 2000; 190:562–72; discussion 572–573.

20. Hammerlid E, Wirblad B, Sandin C, et al. Malnutrition and food intake in relation to quality of life in head and neck patients with cancer. Head Neck 1998; 20:540–548.

21. Magné N, Marcy PY, Chamorey E, et al. Concomitant twice-a-day radiotherapy and chemotherapy in unresectable head and neck patients with cancer: a long-term quality of life analysis. Head Neck 2001; 23:678–682.

22. Collins MM, Wight RG, Partridge G. Nutritional consequences of radiotherapy in early laryngeal carcinoma. Ann R Coll Surg Engl 1999; 81:376–381.

23. Bozzetti F, Cozzaglio L, Gavazzi C, et al.. Nutritional support in patients with cancer of the esophagus: impact on nutritional status, patient compliance to therapy, and survival. Tumori 1998; 84:681–686.

24. Ollenschläger G, Thomas W, Konkol K, Diehl V, Roth E. Nutritional behaviour and quality of life during oncological polychemotherapy: results of a prospective study on the efficacy of oral nutrition therapy in patients with acute leukaemia. Eur J Clin Invest 1992; 22:546–553.

25. Kurugöl Z, Egemen A, Çetingül N, et al. Early determination of nutritional problems in pediatric patients with cancer. Turkish J Pediatr 1997; 39:325–334.

26. Reilly JJ, Weir J, McColl JH, Gibson BE. Prevalence of protein–energy malnutrition at diagnosis in children with acute lymphoblastic leukemia. J Pediatr Gastroenterol Nutr 1999; 29:194–197.

27. Pietsch JB, Ford C. Children with cancer: measurements of nutritional status at diagnosis. Nutr Clin Pract 2000; 15:185–188.

28. Yaris N, Akyuz C, Coskun T, Buyukpamukcu M. Serum carnitine levels of pediatric patients with cancer. Pediatr Hematol Oncol 2002; 19:1–8.

29. Tisdale MJ. Wasting in cancer. J Nutr 1999; 129:243S–246S.

30. Rivadeneira DE, Evoy D, Faley III TJ, et al. Nutritional support of the cancer patient. Ca Cancer J Clin 1998; 48:69–80.

31. Mutlu EA, Mobarhan S. Nutrition in the care of the cancer patient. Nutr Clin Care 2000; 3:3–23.

32. Fearon KCH, Barber MD, Moses AGW. The cancer cachexia syndrome. Surg Oncol Clin North Am 2001; 10:109–126.

33. Miziara ID, Cahali MB, Murakami MS, Figueiredo LA, Guimaraes JR. Cancer of the larynx: correlation of clinical characteristics, site of origin, stage, histology and diagnostic delay. Rev Laryngol Otol Rhinol 1998; 119:101–104.

34. Thoresen L, Fjeldstad I, Krogstad K, Kaasa S, Falkmer UG. Nutritional status of patients with advanced cancer: the value of using the subjective global assessment of nutritional status as a screening tool. Palliat Med 2002; 16:33–42.

35. Bloch AS. Cancer. In: Matarese LE, Gottschlich MM, eds. Contemporary nutrition support practice. A clinical guide. Philadelphia: WB Saunders; 1998:475–495.

36. Glaus A. Fatigue and cachexia in patients with cancer. Support Care Cancer 1998, 6:77–78.

37. Bloch AS. Cancer. In: Gottschlich MM, Matarese LE, Shronts EP, eds. Nutrition support dietetics. Core curriculum. 2nd edn. Silver Springs, MD: Aspen; 1993:213–227.

38. Parkman Williams C. Nutrition management of cancer. In: Pediatric manual of clinical dietetics. The American Dietetic Association, Library of Congress, 1998:151–160.

39. Moldawer LL, Copeland EM 3rd. Proinflammatory cytokines, nutritional support, and the cachexia syndrome: interactions and therapeutic options. Cancer 1997; 79:1828–1839.

40. Falconer JS, Fearon KC, Plester CE, Ross JA, Carter DC. Cytokines, the acute-phase response, and resting energy expenditure in cachectic patients with pancreatic cancer. Ann Surg 1994; 219:325–331.

41. Staal-van den Brekel AJ, Dentener MA, Schols AM, Buurman WA, Wouters EF. Increased resting energy expenditure and weight loss are related to a systemic inflammatory response in lung patients with cancer. J Clin Oncol 1995; 13:2600–2605.

42. Blay JY, Negrier S, Combaret V, et al. Serum level of interleukin 6 as a prognosis factor in metastatic renal cell carcinoma. Cancer Res 1992; 52:3317–3322.

43. Falconer JS, Fearon KC, Ross JA. Acute-phase protein response and survival duration of patients with pancreatic cancer. Cancer 1995; 75:2077–2082.

44. Espat NJ, Copeland EM, Moldawer LL. Tumor necrosis factor and cachexia: a current perspective. Surg Oncol 1994; 3:255–262.

45. Barber MD, Ross JA, Fearon KC. The anti-cachectic effect of fatty acids. Proc Nutr Soc 1998; 57:571–576.

46. Lecker SH, Solomon V, Mitch WE, Goldberg AL. Muscle protein breakdown and the critical role of the ubiquitin–proteasome pathway in normal and disease states. J Nutr 1999; 129:227S–237S.

47. Baracos VE, DeVivo C, Hoyle DH, Goldberg AL. Activation of the ATP–ubiquitin–proteasome pathway in skeletal muscle of cachectic rats bearing a hepatoma. Am J Physiol 1995; 268:E996–1006.

48. Green CJ. Existence, causes and consequences of disease-related malnutrition in the hospital and the community, and clinical and financial benefits of nutritional intervention. Clin Nutr 1999; 18:3–28.

49. Grosvenor M, Bulcavage L, Chlebowski RT. Symptoms potentially influencing weight loss in a cancer population. Cancer 1989; 15:330–334.

50. DeWys WD, Begg C, Lavin PT, et al. Prosnostic effect of weight loss prior to chemotherapy in patients with cancer. Am J Med 1980; 69:491–497.

51. Ovesen L, Allingstrum L, Hannibal J, Mortensen EL, Hansen O. Effect of dietary counselling on food intake, bodyweight, response rate, survival and quality of life in patients with cancer undergoing chemotherapy: a prospective, randomized study. J Clin Oncol 1993;, 11:2043–2049.

52. Andreyev HJN, Norman AR, Oates J, Cunningham D. Why do patients with weight loss have a worse outcome when undergoing chemotherapy for gastrointestinal malignancies? Eur J Cancer 1998; 34:503–509.

53. van Bokhorst-de van der Schueren MA, van Leeuwen PA, Sauerwein HP, et al. Assessment of malnutrition parameters in head and neck cancer and their relation to postoperative complications. Head Neck 1997; 19:419–425.

54. Jagoe RT, Goodship THJ, Gibson GJ. The influence of nutritional status on complications after operations for lung cancer. Ann Thorac Surg 2001; 71:936–943.

55. Barber MD, Ross JA, Voss AC, Tisdale MJ, Fearon KC. The effect of an oral nutritional supplement enriched with fish oil on weight-loss in patients with pancreatic cancer. Br J Cancer 1999; 81:80–86.

56. Zeiderman MR, McMahon MJ. The role of objective measurement of skeletal muscle function in the pre-operative patient. Clin Nutr 1989; 8:161–166.

57. Shaw-Stiffel TA, Zarny LA, Pleban WE, et al. Effect of nutrition status and other factors on length of hospital stay after major gastrointestinal surgery. Nutrition 1993; 9:140–145.

58. Edington J, Boorman J, Durrant ER, et al. The Malnutrition Prevalence Group. Prevalence of malnutrition on admission to four hospitals in England. Clin Nutr 2000; 19:191–195.

59. Braunschweig C, Gomez S, Sheean PM. Impact of declines in nutritional status on outcomes in adult patients hospitalized for more than 7 days. JADA 2000; 100:1316–1322.

60. Edington J, Winter PD, Coles SJ, Gale CR, Martyn CN. Outcomes of undernutrition in patients in the community with cancer or cardiovascular disease. Proc Nutr Soc 1999; 58:655–661.

61. Rey-Ferro M, Castaño R, Orozco O, Serna A, Moreno A. Nutritional and immunologic evaluation of patients with gastric cancer before and after surgery. Nutrition 1997; 13:878–881.

62. Persson C, Sjoden PO, Glimelius B. The Swedish version of the patient-generated subjective global assessment of nutritional status: gastrointestinal vs urological cancers. Clin Nutr 1999; 18:71–77.

63. Deeg HJ, Seidel K, Bruemmer B, Pepe MS, Appelbaum FR. Impact of patient weight on non-relapse mortality after marrow transplantation. Bone Marrow Transplant 1995; 15:461–468.

64. Dickson TM, Kusnierz-Glaz CR, Blume KG, et al. Impact of admission body weight and chemotherapy dose adjustment on the outcome of autologous bone marrow transplantation. Biol Blood Marrow Transplant 1999; 5:299–305.

65. Bruera E, Sweeney C. Cachexia and asthenia in patients with cancer. Lancet Oncol 2000; 1:138–147.

66. Gogos CA, Ginopoulos P, Salsa B, et al. Dietary omega-3 polyunsaturated fatty acids plus vitamin E restore immunodeficiency and prolong survival for severely ill patients with generalized malignancy: a randomized control trial. Cancer 1998; 15:395–402.

67. Taj MM, Pearson AD, Mumford DB, Price L. Effect of nutritional status on the incidence of infection in childhood cancer. Pediatr Hematol Oncol 1993; 10:283–287.

68. Shaw V, Lawson M. Clinical paediatric dietetics. 2nd edn. London: Blackwell Science; 2001.

69. Bloch A. Nutrition support in cancer. Semin Oncol Nurs 2000; 16:122–127.

70. Harrison LE, Fong Y. Enteral nutrition in the cancer patient. In: Rombeau JL, Rolandelli RH, eds. Enteral and tube feeding. 3rd edn. Philadelphia: WB Saunders; 1997:300–323.

71. Oguz A, Karadeniz C, Pelit M, Hasanoglu A. Arm anthropometry in evaluation of malnutrition in children with cancer. Pediatr Hematol Oncol 1999; 16:35–41.

72. Elia M, ed. Maidenhead: Malnutrition Advisory Group (MAG), Standing Committee of BAPEN; 2000.

73. Ottery FD. Supportive nutrition to prevent cachexia and improve quality of life. Semin Oncol 1995; 22(2 Suppl 3):98–111.

74. Reilly JJ. Assessment of body composition in infants and children. Nutrition 1998; 14:821–825.

75. Zemel BS, Riley EM, Stallings VA. Evaluation of methodology for nutritional assessment in children: anthropometry, body composition, and energy expenditure. Ann Rev Nutr 1997; 17:211–235.

76. Fredrix EW, Soeters PB, Wouters EF, et al. Effect of different tumor types on resting energy expenditure. Cancer Res 1991; 51:6138–6141.

77. Thomas B. Manual of dietetic practice. 3rd edn. Oxford: Blackwell Scientific Publications; 2001:637–647.

78. Shike M, Russel DM, Detsky AS, et al. Changes in body composition in patients with small-cell lung cancer. The effect of total parenteral nutrition as an adjunct to chemotherapy. Ann Intern Med 1984; 101:303–309.

79. Ottery FD. Cancer cachexia: prevention, early diagnosis, and management. Cancer Pract 1994; 2:123–131.

80. Finley JP. Management of cancer cachexia. AACN Clin Issues 2000; 11:590–603.

81. Mercadante S. Parenteral versus enteral nutrition in patients with cancer: indications and practice. Support Care Cancer 1998; 6:85–93.

82. Bruera E. ABC of palliative care: anorexia, cachexia, and nutrition. BMJ 1997, 315:1219–1222.

83. Inui A. Cancer anorexia–cachexia syndrome: current issues in research and management. CA Cancer J Clin 2002; 52:72–91.

84. Evans WK, Nixon DW, Daly JM, et al. A randomized study of oral nutritional support versus ad lib nutritional intake during chemotherapy for advanced colorectal and non-small-cell lung cancer. J Clin Oncol 1987; 5:113–124.

85. Whitman MM. The starving patient: supportive care for people with cancer. Clin J Oncol Nurs 2000; 4:121–125.

86. Kotler DP. Cachexia. Ann Intern Med 2000; 133:622–634.

87. Beal JE, Olson R, Laubenstein L, et al. Dronabinol as a treatment for anorexia associated with weight loss in patients with AIDS. J Pain Symptom Manage 1995; 10:89–97.

88. Jatoi A, Windschitl HE, Loprinzi CL, et al. Dronabinol versus megestrol acetate versus combination therapy for cancer-associated anorexia: a North Central Cancer Treatment Group study. J Clin Oncol 2002; 20:567–573.

89. Maltoni M, Nanni O, Scarpi E, et al. High-dose progestins for the treatment of cancer anorexia–cachexia syndrome: a systematic review of randomised clinical trials. Ann Oncol 2001; 12:289–300.

90. Davis MP. New drugs for the anorexia–cachexia syndrome. Curr Oncol Rep 2002; 4:264–274.

91. Fearon KCH, von Meyenfeldt M, Moses AGW, et al. An energy and protein dense, high 3-fatty acid oral supplement promotes weight gain in cancer cachexia. Eur J Cancer 2001; 37(Suppl.6):S27–28.

92. Bruera E, Neumann CM, Pituskin E, et al. Thalidomide in patients with cachexia due to terminal cancer: preliminary report. Ann Oncol 1999; 10:857–859.

93. Peuckmann V, Fisch M, Bruera E. Potential novel uses of thalidomide: focus on palliative care. Drugs 2000; 60:273–292.

94. Lissoni P, Paolorossi F, Ardizzoia A, et al. A randomized study of chemotherapy with cisplatin plus etoposide versus chemoendocrine therapy with cisplatin, etoposide and the pineal hormone melatonin as a first-line treatment of advanced non-small cell lung patients with cancer in a poor clinical state. J Pineal Res 1997; 23:15–19.

95. Lissoni P. Is there a role for melatonin in supportive care? Support Care Cancer 2002; 10:110–116.

96. Agteresch HJ, Rietveld T, Kerkhofs LGM, et al. Beneficial effects of adenosine triphosphate on nutritional status in advanced lung patients with cancer: a randomized clinical trial. J Clin Oncol 2002; 20:371–378.

97. Wigmore SJ, Ross JA, Falconer JS, et al. The effect of polyunsaturated fatty acids on the progress of cachexia in patients with pancreatic cancer. Nutrition 1996; 12(Suppl):S27–30.

98. Wigmore SJ, Barber MD, Ross JA, Tisdale MJ, Fearon KCH. Effect of oral eicosapentaenoic acid on weight loss in patients with pancreatic cancer. Nutr Cancer 2000; 36:177–184.

99. Barber MD. Cancer cachexia and its treatment with fish-oil-enriched nutritional supplementation. Nutrition 2001; 17:751–755.

100. Belardinelli R, Georgiou D, Cianci G, Purcaro A. Randomized, controlled trial of long-term moderate exercise training in chronic heart failure: effects on functional capacity, quality of life, and clinical outcome. Circulation 1999; 99:1173–1182.

101. Roubenoff R, McDermott A, Weis L, et al. Short-term progressive resistance training increases strength and lean body mass in adults infected with human immunodeficiency virus. AIDS 1999; 13:231–239.

102. Strawford A, Barbieri T, Van Loan M, et al. Resistance exercise and supraphysiologic androgen therapy in eugonadal men with HIV-related weight loss: a randomized controlled trial. JAMA 1999; 281:1282–1290.

103. Higginson I, Winget C. Psychological impact of cancer cachexia on the patient and family. In: Bruera E, Higginson I, eds. Cachexia–anorexia in patients with cancer. Oxford: Oxford University Press; 1996:172–183.

104. Iizuka N, Miyamoto K, Hazama S, et al. Anticachectic effects of Coptidis rhizoma, an anti-inflammatory herb, on esophageal cancer cells that produce interleukin 6. Cancer Letters 2000; 158:35–41.

105. McGrath P. Reflections on nutritional issues associated with cancer therapy. Cancer Pract 2002; 10:94–101.

106. Brown JK. A systematic review of the evidence on symptom management of cancer-related anorexia and cachexia. Oncol Nurs Forum 2002; 29:517–532.

107. A.S.P.E.N. Board of Directors and The Clinical Guidelines Task Force. Guidelines for the use of parenteral and enteral nutrition in adult and pediatric patients. JPEN 2002; 26:82SA–85SA.

108. O'Gorman P, McMillan DC, McArdle CS. Impact of weight loss, appetite, and the inflammatory response on quality of life in gastrointestinal patients with cancer. Nutr Cancer 1998; 32:76–80.

109. O'Gorman P, McMillan DC, McArdle CS. Longitudinal study of weight, appetite, performance status, and inflammation in advanced gastrointestinal cancer. Nutr Cancer 1999; 35:127–129.

110. Yeh SS, Wy SY, Lee TP, et al. Improvement in quality-of-life measures and stimulation of weight gain after treatment with megestrol acetate oral suspension in geriatric cachexia: results of a double-blind, placebo-controlled study. J Am Geriatr Soc 2000; 48:485–492.

111. Molassiotis A, van den Akker OBA, Milligan DW, et al. Quality of life in bone marrow transplant long-term survivors: comparison with a matched group of patients treated with maintenance chemotherapy. Bone Marrow Transplant 1996; 17:249–258.

112. Molassiotis A, Morris PJ. Quality of life in patients with chronic myeloid leukemia after unrelated donor bone marrow transplantation. Cancer Nurs 1999; 22:340–349.

113. Cella DF, VonRoenn J, Lloyd S, Browder HP. The Bristol-Myers Anorexia/Cachexia Recovery Instrument (BACRI): a brief assessment of patients' subjective response to treatment for anorexia/cachexia. Qual Life Res 1995; 4:221–231.

114. Ribaudo JM, Cella D, Hahn EA, et al. Re-validation and shortening of the Functional Assessment of Anorexia/Cachexia Therapy (FAACT) questionnaire. Qual Life Res 2001; 9:1137–1146.

115. http://www.christie.nhs.uk/profinfo/departments/nursing/nursing-developments/developments/nutrition.pdf.

CHAPTER 30

Cancer-related Fatigue

KARIN AHLBERG

CHAPTER CONTENTS

Introduction	657	The outcomes of fatigue	663
The concept of fatigue	657	Assessment of cancer-related fatigue	663
Theoretical models for understanding cancer-related fatigue	658	Instruments to measure cancer-related fatigue	664
The function of fatigue	659	Management	664
		Non-pharmacological interventions	666
Incidence	659	Pharmacological therapy	667
The patient perspective of cancer-related fatigue	659	Cancer-related therapy from the caregivers' perspective	668
Aetiology	660	Conclusion	668
Physiological factors	660	References	669
Psychosocial factors	662		
Physical activity	662		
Demographic characteristics	662		

INTRODUCTION

Cancer-related fatigue (CRF) is a subjectively experienced symptom that is multidimensional and multifactorial. It has emerged as one of the major concomitants of cancer and its treatment, as it has a profound impact on health-related quality of life and the patient's situation in general. Although most patients with cancer report that fatigue is a major obstacle in maintaining normal daily activities and quality of life, it is seldom assessed and/or treated in clinical practice.

CRF affects 70–100% of patients with cancer, and depends on the specific site/organ involvement, the treatment modalities used and the presence of other symptoms.[1–6] The mechanisms responsible for the development of CRF are poorly understood.[7] Psychological, social

and physiological factors are involved as are therapy-related side-effects such as anaemia, pain, depression, dyspnoea, nausea, vomiting, infection and malnutrition.[8] Since fatigue changes over time, evaluations must be carried out repeatedly in relation to the disease, cancer therapy and the patient's situation.[9] This chapter describes the concept of fatigue, including symptoms, prevalence and aetiology. Further, the evaluation and management of CRF are described. The distress associated with CRF and consequences of CRF are also discussed.

THE CONCEPT OF FATIGUE

Fatigue is symptomatic of a variety of conditions in patients with cancer. CRF occurs over a continuum, ranging from tiredness to exhaustion. But in contrast to 'normal tiredness', CRF is perceived as being of greater magnitude, disproportionate to activity or exertion, and not completely relieved by rest. CRF is a condition in which a person with cancer experiences an overwhelming and sustained sense of exhaustion, and has a decreased capacity for physical and mental work.[10] Fatigue refers broadly to a sense of malaise, tiredness, exhaustion or feeling sick. CRF may include a variety of sensations or feelings and a variety of expressions of reduced capacity at physical, mental, emotional or social levels.[11] A major challenge in classifying fatigue is differentiating among its causes, indicators and effects. Fatigue has been identified by patients with cancer as a major obstacle to normal functioning and a good quality of life.[12] The term 'asthenia' has been used to describe fatigue in oncology patients but has no specific meaning apart from the more common term.

In the literature, definitions of fatigue primarily based on the perspective of nursing are found. Definitions include a multidimensional perspective and are based on subjective experiences. Ream and Richardson[13] state that:

fatigue is a subjective, unpleasant symptom which incorporates total body feelings ranging from tiredness to exhaustion creating an unrelenting overall condition which interferes with individuals' ability to function to their normal capacity.

Mock and colleagues[8] define CRF as:

a persistent, subjective sense of tiredness related to cancer or cancer treatment that interferes with usual functioning.

Theoretical models for understanding cancer-related fatigue

Within the area of cancer-related fatigue, there are few theoretical models. The most established is the Integrated Fatigue Model (IFM) by Piper and colleagues[14] (Fig. 30.1). The IFM has a deductive approach based on the five primary areas where fatigue has been studied: psychology, physiology, ergonomics, medicine and care. The IFM functions primarily as an explanatory model for the aetiology of fatigue, as well as the scope of the symptom and the factors that can affect how a patient experiences fatigue. This model addresses many potential causes of CRF but there is limited guidance for

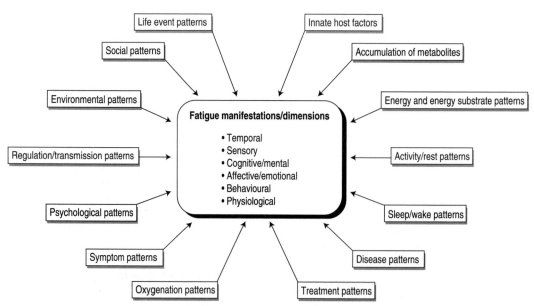

Figure 30.1: Integrated Fatigue Model (IFM) by Piper and colleagues. (© 1997 Reproduced with permission from Barbara F Piper DNSc, RN, AOCN, FAAN.)

management of fatigue. Examples of other cancer-oriented theoretical models are Aistar's 'Organizing Framework',[15] Winningham et al's Psychobiologic-Entropy Hypothesis'[16] and Cimprich's' 'Attentional Theory'.[17–19]

The Conceptual Model of Symptom Management[20,21] is a broad and extensive model that can be used for understanding symptoms, designing and testing management strategies and for evaluating outcomes. The model makes it possible to study a phenomenon from both a subjective and an objective perspective. When both the underlying cause and presenting symptoms are concurrently managed, patients are more likely to remain in treatment and to benefit from the expertise of healthcare professionals. The model includes three dimensions:

1 symptom experience
2 symptom management strategies
3 symptom outcome.

The model is based on the relation between these three dimensions and the result in this case is that fatigue in a patient can be mapped, evaluated and treated. In the model, the recognized domains of nursing science – environment and health and illness – are variables believed to influence all the dimensions and reflect demographic and biopsychosocial factors. Environment is the aggregate of conditions or circumstances within which a symptom occurs. Health and illness are composed of variables, including health status, disease and injury.[21] Within a nursing perspective, managing symptoms requires an understanding of the patient's experience of the symptom as well as the responses and the outcomes from the symptom experience. Healthcare professionals have difficulty developing symptom management strategies that can be applied across acute and home-care settings because few models of symptom management have been tested empirically.[21] The Conceptual Model of Symptom Management is applicable to practice and to research. The model may provide direction for selecting clinical interventions, performing research and bridging an array of cancer-related fatigue symptoms.

THE FUNCTION OF FATIGUE

Whether fatigue as a symptom has any function at all is unclear. In healthy individuals, fatigue may function as a defensive and/or pleasant response following physical or mental exertion. For patients with a chronic disease, fatigue may become a major distressing symptom[16] that may impair daily functioning and lead to negative effects on their quality of life.[22] For individuals with a difficult and/or chronic illness, the experience may cause frustration and stress.[23]

INCIDENCE

It seems that fatigue is a universal complaint that may or may not be related to medical diagnosis or to therapeutic treatment. In epidemiological studies of healthy populations, about 20% report fatigue,[24,25] and this fatigue correlates to psychological morbidity.[25] CRF is considered to be one of the most frequently reported symptoms in patients with cancer and is the most prevalent symptom of individuals receiving cancer treatment with radiation therapy, cytotoxic chemotherapy or biological response modifiers, affecting 70–100% of patients.[2,5,26–29] Cancer survivors report fatigue to be a problem months to years after treatment ends.[3] In a study designed to confirm the prevalence and duration of fatigue in patients with cancer having a prior history of chemotherapy ($n = 379$), 76% of patients experienced fatigue at least a few days each month during their most recent chemotherapy; 30% experienced fatigue on a daily basis.[22]

THE PATIENT PERSPECTIVE OF CANCER-RELATED FATIGUE

Several qualitative studies have been conducted exploring the experience of fatigue from the patient's perspective.[10,30–32] These studies indicate that fatigue is an experience of the whole person, i.e. body and mind; it is a complex phenomenon with physical, emotional and mental sensations, and has a great impact on everyday function and perception of control.

The respondents in the study by Magnusson et al[32] tried to explain the experience of fatigue but not everybody could find a word for it. The words used as descriptions of fatigue were, for example, 'listless', 'sluggish', 'faint', 'despondent', 'apathetic', 'tired', 'slack', 'indifferent', and 'paralysing fatigue'. The use of metaphors, instead of the term fatigue, is also common: e.g. 'my feet feel like lead' or 'I couldn't run, my legs felt like spaghetti'.[32]

AETIOLOGY

The specific mechanisms responsible for the development of CRF are not completely known. Further studies on the identification of the mechanism(s) of fatigue associated with cancer and its treatment requires studies that both characterize the phenomenon of fatigue, supplemented by measurements of a range of physiological, biochemical, psychosocial and demographic factors. It is unlikely that a single cause can be isolated and there are probably a number of factors that for each individual patient cause the fatigue experienced.

Physiological factors

Anaemia

Anaemia is one of the most studied contributing factors in fatigue related to cancer and cancer therapy.[29] Numerous multifactorial mechanisms underlie the anaemia of cancer. Potential causes include haemorrhage, haemolysis and nutritional deficiencies, as well as the increased production of cytokines which counteract the differentiation of erythroid precursors, reducing the production of erythropoietin and contributing to impaired iron utilization.[33] Anaemia is a deficiency of red blood cells or haemoglobin, which leads to a reduction in the oxygen-carrying capacity of blood.[34] Anaemia, commonly defined as a haemoglobin level of <12 g/dl, occurs in over 30% of patients with cancer at any point in time, and its incidence increases with treatment and progressive disease.[35] Untreated anaemia negatively affects the success of radia-

tion therapy, activities of daily living and morbidity and mortality.[36] Anaemia is also associated with impaired health-related quality of life.[37] It would seem reasonable to assume that the degree of anaemia correlates with the intensity of fatigue in patients with cancer. In a study by Glaus and Muller,[38] haemoglobin was measured in 444 patients with cancer with different types and stages of cancer and treatment modalities. The results of this study suggested that patients with cancer with a haemoglobin level below 11 g/dl had higher levels of fatigue than patients with higher haemoglobin levels, indicating that fatigue was a function of the grade of anaemia. The correlation between fatigue and anaemia was most prominent with respect to physical fatigue, such as reduced physical performance or weakness. Only prospective studies can define whether the degree of fatigue depends on the degree of anaemia or if there is simply a correlation between the two that is dependent on mutual factors such as disease stage.

Cancer therapy

The mechanisms of fatigue related to cancer treatment are multifactorial and also include other factors such as other parallel existing symptoms. Studies have demonstrated that fatigue increases during radiation therapy.[6,39,40] Similarly, fatigue increases during chemotherapy[28] and hormonal therapy.[5] Fatigue is a dose-limiting side-effect of interferon therapy; it is reported by almost 100% of patients and is mediated by neurendrocrine dysfunction.[41] Postoperative fatigue has frequently been observed in patients who undergo surgery as a part of their cancer treatment, but there is little research that has examined the causes and correlates of this fatigue.[42]

The incidence and severity of fatigue in patients receiving radiotherapy depend on the irradiated volume and involved organs and/or the length of radiation therapy. Fatigue usually develops during the first week of treatment and then diminishes 2–4 weeks after completing treatment. In a study by Magnan and Mood,[43] the fatigue onset varied widely; patients reported fatigue onset as early as the 1st and as late as the 38th day of treatment. Several studies have shown that fatigue is felt to be the worst side-effect during the last week of treatment.[6,44,45] The level of fatigue slowly decreases to pre-treatment levels by 3 months after treatment.[46,47]

Generally, the presence and severity of side-effects in chemotherapy treatment varies, depending on the type of drug(s) and their dosage. The presence of fatigue in a patient who is being treated with chemotherapy is well documented. The patient often relates the fatigue directly to the treatment and exhibits increased energy just before the next cycle of treatments. The patient usually experiences fatigue during the first 3–4 days after receiving treatment; it reaches its maximum on about the 10th day of treatment and then declines again.[16]

Tumour burden

Although it seems reasonable to assume that the extent of tumour bulk or presence of metastatic disease will influence the degree of fatigue, in several studies no correlation was found with either type of tumour or the presence of metastasis.[48,49] This may have been because of the small number of patients of each type and stage in these studies. Two studies have reported an effect of disease burden upon the degree of fatigue[5,11] when patients with different types of tumours were collectively analysed. In one of these, comparing four groups of patients recently diagnosed with breast, prostatic, inoperable non-small cell lung cancer or receiving inpatient palliative care, the two latter groups experienced a higher degree of fatigue.[5] One study of elderly patients newly diagnosed with different cancers has reported an effect of disease burden (early vs late clinical stage) upon the degree of fatigue.[50] In patients with metastatic disease, the prevalence of cancer-related fatigue exceeds 75%, and cancer survivors report that fatigue is a disruptive symptom months or even years after treatment ends.[3,51] Overall, these studies lend support to the hypothesis that tumour stage is correlated with the degree of fatigue.

Cytokines

One possible explanation for the development of fatigue in patients with cancer is the increased secretion of pro-inflammatory cytokines.[52,53]

Pro-inflammatory cytokines, e.g. interleukins (ILs), interferon or tumour necrosis factor (TNF), are proteins that mediate cell-to-cell communication and have been reported to be released in greater amounts in patients with cancer as part of the host response to the tumour, in response to tissue damage, or due to depletion of immune cell subsets associated with treatment for the disease.[54] This cytokine release may contribute to the development of fatigue by effects on the endocrine system and neurotransmitters,[55] for example, as suggested in chronic fatigue syndrome.[56] High levels of TNF-α, IL-1 and IL-6 have been described in a variety of cancers and may contribute to the experience of being fatigued.[53]

Other symptoms: anorexia, pain and insomnia

Anorexia is often a contributory factor for the development of fatigue. Involuntary weight loss may be a result of anorexia: correlations between fatigue and weight loss in patients with cancer have been documented, but conflicting data exist. It has been proposed that cytokines interfere with the hypothalamic control of hunger sensation, and mediate the development of cachexia.[57] Anorexia has a complex pathophysiology that correlates with poor outcomes and compromises the patient's quality of life. If there is a correlation between anorexia and fatigue, efforts to maintain nutritional status can decrease or prevent some of the fatigue associated with cancer and its treatment.[58]

Pain is recognized as a personal experience and a symptom that has great impact on a patient's quality of life. Pain is one of the most common problems experienced by oncology patients. Of patients receiving active treatment, 30–50% experience pain on a daily basis.[59-61] Pain and fatigue have several components in common, such as being subjective, being prevalent in most patients with cancer and being caused by multiple factors of both a physical and psychological nature.[62] A significant positive correlation between pain and fatigue has been reported in patients with cancer.[63] Burrows and colleagues[64] found in their study that patients with pain, in this case somatic and visceral pain, had significantly higher fatigue scores than pain-free patients. In addition, patients with pain had significantly more symptom distress, lower levels of physical and psychological well-being and total quality of life than pain-free patients.[64]

There is limited research on insomnia in patients with cancer, but evidence is accumulating that sleep is often disturbed in these patients, probably owing to a variety of causes.[65] The bulk of research on insomnia has been performed in general populations rather than in patients who are ill. Clinical experience suggests that cancer, as well as cancer treatment and associated symptoms, results in sleep disturbances.[21] A study by Berger and Farr,[66] the aim of which was to identify indicators involving circadian activity/rest cycles associated with higher levels of CRF, showed that women who had increased night awakenings reported higher CRF levels, with the strongest association being number of night awakenings. In a study that evaluated pain, fatigue and sleep disturbances in 24 outpatients with cancer who were receiving radiation therapy,[61] patients reported significantly lower fatigue scores in the morning as compared to the evening. In addition, patients experienced significant sleep disturbances. Patients who had received a higher percentage of their radiation treatments reported more sleep disturbances. Ancoli-Israel and colleagues[65] reported that some degree of CRF experienced during the day may be related to sleep/wake cycles or to the quality and quantity of sleep obtained at night. In women with breast cancer who are undergoing radiotherapy, fatigue and difficulty sleeping were positively correlated.[67]

Psychosocial factors

CRF has been consistently correlated with psychosocial factors such as anxiety and depression,[67-69] difficulty sleeping,[66] full-time employment status[70] and low levels of physical functioning.[71] It is unclear whether fatigue results from prolonged emotional distress characterized by anxiety, depression and difficulty sleeping or whether high levels of fatigue lead patients to feel anxious and depressed about their reduced ability to conduct usual activities. Both mechanisms seem possible.[29] Fatigue and depression do not follow the same clinical course; the cause-and-effect relationship between these two variables has not yet been established. It has to be remembered that fatigue is not only a symptom of many somatic illnesses but also one of the key symptoms of depression.[72]

Physical activity

In healthy individuals, physical activity has been associated with fatigue[73] and may also be a cause of CRF. One reason for this may be that the natural response to feeling fatigued is to decrease physical activity.[15] Fatigue is inversely correlated with activity levels and with functional capacity. A consistent decrease in the level of daily activity over the often lengthy period of cancer treatment may eventually lead to a reduced tolerance for normal activity and high levels of fatigue.[66] Chen[73] showed that inactive people have more than twice the risk of those who were active of being afflicted with fatigue.

Demographic characteristics

The relationship between fatigue and demographic characteristics is not well defined, and conflicting data exists. Age may be a risk factor for developing fatigue. Many conditions that would not be considered normal in a younger population are routinely accepted in older people as part of 'normal' ageing; among these conditions are many chronic and debilitating conditions such as pain, insomnia, weakness and fatigue.[74] Schwarz and Hinz[75] state that higher age is associated with lower fatigue levels. Liao and Ferrell[76] suggest that fatigue is a symptom often found among older people. Gender may be a risk factor, as female patients report fatigue more often than men.[77] Glaus[23] has shown that women have higher mean levels of fatigue compared to men. Thus the impact of age and gender may be of great importance in the interpretation of available data regarding prevalence and severity of fatigue in connection with cancer and cancer therapy. A higher level of fatigue has been seen in unmarried patients with lower yearly income levels.[78] CRF has been consistently correlated with full-time employment status.[70]

THE OUTCOMES OF FATIGUE

Functional status may be defined as an individual's abilities to meet their basic needs, fulfil usual roles and maintain health and well-being.[79] Functional status is frequently discussed as a key element of nursing practice and a critical outcome criterion. Assessing functional status in patients with CRF can provide information on the individual's functioning in routine occupations and about the individual's well-being. Functional status is a significant concern for patients with cancer, and impairment is often associated with symptoms such as fatigue.[22,80,81]

A high percentage of patients with CRF state that fatigue affects their physical and psychosocial well-being and ability to work, which may lead to a decreased level of their quality of life.[22] Quality of life is dependent upon the interpretation and perception of the individual. As patients with cancer become too tired to participate fully in the roles and activities that make life meaningful, the most important effect of CRF might be in the realm of quality of life.[30]

ASSESSMENT OF CANCER-RELATED FATIGUE

Decisions about managing CRF are based on assessing both the level of sensations and the impact of fatigue on the patient.[82] If interventions are to be implemented, measures must be available to study the effects of the interventions. The goal of a clinical or research-based assessment of fatigue and the ways to measure fatigue are different, but both approaches need instruments that are sensitive to changes in the levels of fatigue.[82] Validated multidimensional instruments provide a more sophisticated way of assessing fatigue, but they are difficult to use in clinical practice because of time limitations and the burden on the patient, among other factors. Fatigue is a symptom influenced by multiple factors that include both biologic and psychosocial domains. When evaluating CRF, the healthcare provider therefore needs to include both subjective and objective data.

Portenoy and Itri[9] suggest the routine use of three questions to help assess the severity of fatigue and its impact over time:

1 Are you experiencing any fatigue?
2 If so, how severe has it been, on average, during the past week?
3 How does the fatigue interfere with your ability to function?

If fatigue is present, it is possible to use a simple 0–10 numeric rating scale, where mild fatigue may be indicated as a score 0–3, moderate fatigue as 4–6 and severe fatigue as 7–10.[8]

These three questions may give the healthcare provider some knowledge of the patient's status. This information may also indicate whether there is need for further investigation and serves as a baseline for future follow-up of the patient's experience of CRF. The 0–10 numeric rating scale, however, only provides a unidimensional assessment of the multidimensional concept of fatigue. Winningham et al[16] suggest that it is also important to get information on the temporal pattern, the exacerbating and relieving factors, the impact of fatigue on day-to-day activities, the meaning of fatigue to the individual and the cultural influences on expression of feelings of fatigue. A patient-held diary can be used to evaluate fatigue and to determine appropriate interventions.[83]

The development of standards and guidelines could encourage a more systematic approach and help to stimulate further research. Data from a comprehensive assessment may suggest plausible hypotheses concerning pathogenesis, which in turn may suggest appropriate strategies. Other characteristics are similarly important: for example, onset, duration, severity, daily pattern, time course, exacerbating and reducing factors and distress associated with fatigue.[34] In the United States, the National Comprehensive Cancer Network (NCCN)[84] proposed in their Fatigue Practice Guidelines an algorithm in which patients are assessed regularly for fatigue using a brief screening instrument. The algorithm includes the following phases: screening, primary evaluation, intervention and re-evaluation. Screening for the presence and severity of CRF should occur at the patient's initial contact with an oncology provider, at appropriate intervals and as clinically indicated. If fatigue is reported during screening, it should be quantified for future comparison. When the screening process reveals moderate or severe levels of CRF, a focused history and a physical examination, including an evaluation of the patient's disease and treatment status and an in-depth fatigue assessment, is recommended. As part of the evaluation, the guidelines identify five common clinical conditions that are often causative elements and should be specifically assessed. The five factors are pain, emotional distress, sleep disturbance, anaemia and hypothyroidism.[8] If any of the five conditions are present, they should be treated as an initial approach to fatigue management. If no primary factor is identified that accounts for the patient's fatigue, a comprehensive assessment is indicated, including a review of systems, undiagnosed or unmanaged co-morbidities, nutritional status and the patient's daily activity patterns and degree of inactivity.[8,85] The NCCN Guidelines provide an overall framework for clinical practice but no outcomes research has been conducted to determine the effectiveness of the guidelines on fatigue in cancer populations.[29]

Instruments to measure cancer-related fatigue

Researchers need measures that maximize both variance and precision. Fatigue may occur as one of several subjects in an instrument that is used for a broader purpose, e.g. in connection with evaluating quality of life. Since fatigue is primarily a subjective symptom, self-report measures are the most commonly described type of instrument for measuring fatigue. There are a number of instruments that were designed specifically to measure fatigue and that are available for clinical testing (Table 30.1).

It is important that research designs include measurement of multiple symptoms simultaneously, in an attempt to define and correlate the constellation of symptoms that may occur with fatigue or may be cofactors in the aetiology of fatigue.[91] Fatigue is considered to be a multidimensional construct, but this is not always reflected in the choice of measurement strate-

gies. Comparisons are hindered by the fact that there has been little standardization of fatigue measurement between studies. Available self-report instruments can be divided into one-dimensional or multidimensional instruments. The response formats of these instruments include yes/no, Likert-type scales and visual analogue scales. Although several instruments have been developed, they generally require further psychometric testing within the cancer population.[92]

When measuring CRF, there are several factors that should be considered. Because CRF fluctuates in severity over time, it must be measured as a state rather than a stable characteristic. Also potential confounding exists in the measurement of CRF because of its close association with other concepts linked to fatigue, e.g. depression, muscle weakness and functional status.[29] Furthermore, instrument reactivity is a critical issue with CRF, because respondent burden can induce fatigue.[93] It is important that research designs include measurement of multiple symptoms simultaneously, in an attempt to define and correlate the constellation of symptoms that may occur with fatigue or may be cofactors in the aetiology of fatigue. These symptom clusters generally include fatigue, difficulty sleeping, pain and emotional distress, especially depression.[94]

MANAGEMENT

As the number of people surviving cancer for extended periods of time continues to increase, the phenomenon of CRF that persists following the completion of treatment needs to be recognized. The development of effective interventions for the treatment of CRF could profoundly affect the lives of many patients with cancer.[95]

Careful assessment of the pattern of fatigue and its onset, duration, intervention and resolution is required if the varied types of fatigue are to be identified and managed successfully. The most effective approach to symptom management is to identify the cause of the distressing symptom and correct it if possible. However, in many patients with cancer, no cause for CRF can be readily identified and the

Table 30.1: Examples of instruments to measure cancer-related fatigue

Instrument	Description	Comment
The revised Piper Fatigue Scale (PFS)[86,87]	PFS covers four subjective dimensions (cognitive, behavioural, sensory and affective dimensions) plus three open questions regarding cause, other symptoms and relief measures. The PFS contains 22 items scored on a numerical scale of 0–10	PFS is probably the most comprehensive method available for use as a research instrument
The Functional Assessment of Cancer Therapy-Fatigue (FACT-F)[80]	The FACT-F is designed to measure fatigue symptoms of cancer patients and consists of the 28 items of the FACT-General to assess health-related quality of life and an additional 13 items to assess fatigue	The length of the entire questionnaire could burden fatigued patients. The fatigue scale is brief, simple and easy to use
The Schwartz Cancer Fatigue Scale[88,89]	This is a 28-item scale with four subscales: physical, emotional, cognitive and temporal. This scale exists also in a revised version, with six items measuring two dimensions: physical and perceptual	The 28-item instrument is simply worded but long
The Multidimensional Fatigue Inventory[90]	The MFI-20 is designed to cover five areas: general fatigue, physical fatigue, reduced activity, reduced motivation and mental fatigue, and consists of 20 items	The instrument is most used in patients receiving radiotherapy
The Brief Fatigue Inventory[4]	The Brief Fatigue Inventory (BFI) comprises nine items measured on a 10-point scale that assesses the severity of fatigue and its effects on the subject in conducting activities of daily living. The tool has a high internal consistency for the total scale (alpha 0.96).	The instrument is short and easy to use but has only a single-dimension measure of fatigue
The Cancer Linear Analog Scale (CLAS), also known as Linear Analog Scale Assessment (LASA)	It includes one or a series of symptoms or outcomes related to symptoms – such as quality of life and ability to perform daily activities. Patients score their perceptions of these symptoms by placing a mark on a 100-mm line to indicate magnitude of the symptom	Easy to use in clinical practice

approach to management is a general one. Interventions can be categorized as non-pharmacological interventions and pharmacological treatment.

Non-pharmacological interventions

Patient education

Research has documented the beneficial effects of providing patients with preparatory knowledge, including sensory information, about their disease and treatment.[96–99] If patients receive valid information about what to anticipate, they are more likely to develop accurate expectations and are less likely to experience the stress that accompanies unforeseen problems: e.g. uninformed patients with cancer often interpret fatigue to mean that their cancer treatment is not working or that their disease is progressing.[8] Cassileth and colleagues[100] studied whether the expectations of the patient prior to the start of treatment affected the experience of side-effects and found that 82% of the patients ($n = 56$) reported fatigue as the most commonly occurring side-effect, but that the expectation of the patient was not proportional to the experience.

A randomized clinical trial[101] compared patients undergoing an initial course of chemotherapy who reported pain and fatigue at baseline and who received conventional care alone ($n = 60$) with those receiving conventional care plus a nursing intervention ($n = 53$) on outcomes reported at 20 weeks. Interviews were conducted at baseline, 10 and 20 weeks. An 18-week, 10-contact nursing intervention utilizing problem-solving approaches to symptom management and improving physical functioning and emotional health was implemented. The study showed that patients who received the intervention reported a significant reduction in the number of symptoms experienced and improved physical and social functioning. Fewer patients in the experimental arm reported both pain and fatigue at 20 weeks. The conclusion from the study was that behavioural interventions targeted to patients with pain and fatigue can reduce symptom burden, and improve the quality of the daily life of patients. These data support the 'value-added' role of nursing interventions for symptom management and improved quality of life during the course of cancer treatment.[101]

With appropriate educational preparation, patients can be prepared for the side-effects and learn management strategies. However, the limited research on educational and preparatory information for patients with cancer has not looked specifically at fatigue as an end point but has demonstrated more positive emotional outcomes and decreased disruption of usual activities.[98,102]

Exercise

For healthy individuals, it is generally accepted that activity is an effective way of reducing fatigue. Exercising regularly provides a number of psychological and physiological advantages in the form of improved cardiovascular and respiratory efficiency, reduction of anxiety and depression, improved quality of life and self-esteem and reduced fatigue. Results from studies show that physical activity generally makes patients with cancer feel better both physically and mentally.[67,103,104] However, contraindications for physical activity may be present in widespread bone metastasis and extreme thrombocytopenia with a risk of bleeding.[15]

In the management of CRF, exercise is the intervention with the most supporting evidence of effectiveness. The theory supporting exercise as a treatment for fatigue proposes that the combined toxic effects of cancer treatment and a decreased level of physical activity during treatment cause a reduction in the capacity for physical performance. When patients need to use greater effort and expend more energy to perform usual activities, fatigue levels increase. Exercise training leads to a reduction in the loss of or even an increase in functional capacity, leading to reduced effort and decreased fatigue.[105] There are reports conducted by different research teams testing the effects of exercise on fatigue during active cancer treatment and additional reports of exercise programmes after cancer treatment. All demonstrated significantly lower levels of fatigue in subjects who exercised when compared to control or comparison groups.[29] Although the results have been consistent across studies, the studies are limited in number, sample sizes are often small and there are methodological limitations associated with most of them. In addition, all studies except one have only included patients with breast cancer. There is limited information about the effectiveness and acceptability of an exercise programme with patients who already suffer from high levels of fatigue.[29]

Rest and sleep

Clinical recommendations for additional rest and sleep have been common advice by healthcare professionals to patients who report CRF[12] and may be the most frequent self-care activity of fatigued patients. The relationship between sleep disturbance and fatigue in patients with cancer has been inadequately investigated.[106] Patients with cancer report significant disruptions in sleep, and the essential issue may be sleep quality rather than quantity.[66] Studies have shown that patients with cancer spend increased time resting and sleeping but the pattern of sleep is often severely disrupted, awakening almost every hour during the sleep period.[107,108] Patients with cancer who try additional rest and sleep to manage CRF do not report it to be particularly effective.[109] The research testing rest or sleep to manage fatigue is in preliminary stages.

Energy conservation

Energy conservation is a frequent treatment recommendation for CRF from care providers. However, currently there is no published evidence available testing this theory in patients with cancer, although at least one multicentre study is in progress. Furthermore, decreasing activity to 'save' energy contributes to deconditioning and decreased activity tolerance. However, using limited energy to perform highly valued activities instead of mundane tasks that can be delegated may increase personal satisfaction and quality of life.

Stress reduction

Studies testing interventions to reduce stress and increase psychosocial support have also demonstrated reductions in fatigue, usually as a component of mood state.[110–112] Because these interventions did not have fatigue as a primary end point, fatigue measures are often limited to a subscale on an instrument to measure emotional distress, and the interventions generally did not attempt to elucidate a mediating mechanism of CRF. It has been proposed that CRF is essentially a response to stress or that emotional state influences perception and reporting of CRF. Although a strong correlation exists between emotional distress and CRF,[67,104,113] the precise relationship is not clearly understood. The specific interventions tested have included support groups, individual counselling and a comprehensive coping strategy.[29]

The research in this field is preliminary and needs further development. Also, the relationship between attentional fatigue and CRF is unclear as no measures of self-reported fatigue levels were used in the studies.

Pharmacological therapy

Cancer-related anaemia is commonly associated with fatigue and decreased quality of life. One area of pharmacological therapy that is well supported by clinical evidence is erythropoietin-alpha in patients with cancer-related anaemia and fatigue.[29] Blood transfusion, the traditional method of treating anaemia, is effective and relatively inexpensive, but is associated with certain risks and is subject to limitations in blood supply. Erythropoietin-alpha therapy provides healthcare providers with an effective alternative to blood transfusion, and trial results suggest that this intervention has a positive effect on patients' quality of life.[114] Three large community-based non-randomized studies and two double-blind randomized clinical trials have shown a clinical benefit with erythropoietin-alpha treatment on cancer-related anaemia and fatigue. In these studies, erythropoietin-alpha reduced the need for transfusions, decreased fatigue levels and improved quality of life in patients receiving chemotherapy.[115–119] Published guidelines support this conclusion.[120] The newer erythropoietic agent darbepoetin alfa has demonstrated similar outcomes with less frequent dosing.[121]

Besides the treatment with erythropoietin, there are few controlled studies investigating pharmacological therapy for CRF or therapy-related fatigue. Megestrol acetate has been described as reducing fatigue to some degree in patients with advanced cancer.[122] Accordingly, prednisone was more effective than flutamide in improving the quality of life, including the level of fatigue, in patients with prostatic cancer.[123] Psychostimulants have been effective in reducing fatigue related to HIV infection[124] and in multiple sclerosis,[125] but there are no data concerning efficacy in CRF. Amifostine has been shown to ameliorate cisplatin-induced toxicity, but there was apparently no effect upon the degree of the therapy-induced fatigue in women with metastatic breast cancer.[126]

CANCER-RELATED THERAPY FROM THE CAREGIVERS' PERSPECTIVE

Patients are often reluctant to report fatigue, and healthcare professionals frequently do not screen for it because they are uncertain about how to treat it.[12] Patients with cancer report that their healthcare professionals fail to recognize and adequately manage their fatigue. Healthcare professionals have come to accept CRF as expected and normal. Magnusson et al[127] carried out a study to determine if oncology nurses perceived that fatigue was a problem for patients with cancer and, if so, its frequency and extent, and if there were any established nursing interventions for the patients.[127] The survey found that the nurses estimated that fatigue was the most common symptom in patients with cancer, that there were few established nursing procedures for patients and that there was a need for educational and assessment tools regarding CRF. The results indicate that it may be difficult to interpret whether and to what extent a patient is suffering from fatigue. In the same study, it was found that fatigue was ranked as the most frequently occurring symptom, although only by 25%, a low figure if it is compared to other similar studies (i.e. Knowles et al[128]). Knowles and colleagues[128] found that while nurses were able to describe a number of discrete components of fatigue, they did not necessarily acknowledge the intensity of the symptom or assess fatigue utilizing a specific assessment tool. The majority of nurses in that study believed further education in this area would be beneficial in helping them to care for these patients. In their study, Miller and Kearney[129] found that knowledge and practice on the part of nurses was poor regarding fatigue assessment and management. However, the nurses demonstrated good understanding of the impact of fatigue on patients with cancer and an appreciation of the importance of the nurse's role in fatigue management. Tiesinga and colleagues[130] reported that nurses, as compared with the patients themselves, are still unable to accurately assess a patient's fatigue (fair agreement), exertion fatigue (fair agreement) and types of fatigue (slight agreement). As a result, CRF is frequently underreported, underdiagnosed and undertreated.[131] A survey that was designed to assess CRF from the perspective of the patient, primary caregiver and oncologist showed that, among other things, the impact of fatigue on a patient with cancer is underestimated by both caregivers and oncologists.[12] This indicates that healthcare professionals still have a low level of knowledge regarding what fatigue is and how it affects a patient with cancer.

CONCLUSION

We want our patients to be in good general condition and to have a high quality of life while at the same time being able to carry out cancer treatment according to plan. The first steps in treating a patient's fatigue are to determine the patient's expectations and to establish realistic goals. This necessitates mutual discussion, with emphasis on individual patients' experience of their situation, the disease, treatment plan and quality of life. Although CRF is the most prevalent symptom reported by patients with cancer, evaluation and management of this distressing side-effect of cancer and cancer treatment has been limited in clinical practice. This limitation is related to many factors, including a lack of understanding of the mechanisms responsible for CRF, a lack of awareness by cancer-care providers of the significance of the problem and a lack of evidence-based interventions to manage CRF.

Patients with cancer suffer from a multitude of symptoms. Effective treatment strategies are available for a number of the common symptoms. The literature states that the fatigue belongs to one of the most distressing symptoms in patients with cancer. Assessment is one key to the recognition and management of cancer-related fatigue. Since fatigue changes over time, evaluations of the experience of fatigue should be done repeatedly in relation to the disease, the cancer therapy and the patient's situation as well as to treatment of fatigue and other symptoms. Patients should be taught that fatigue is an expected effect in connection to treatment and that fatigue may be increased due to other influencing factors. Educating patients also includes helping them choose the most appropriate interventions to manage fatigue.

Passive approaches frequently fail to reduce fatigue in patients with cancer. Alternative approaches based on the growing body of theoretical and research evidence should be adopted. Patients do require guidance in managing CRF. Systematic research programmes based on sound theoretical premises and previous research will contribute to the growing body of evidence to aid future management of this troublesome symptom.[132]

Nurses need to develop and evaluate relief interventions. Nurses play a critical role in maintaining and improving well-being and quality of life of patients at risk for developing fatigue by understanding their experience, risk factors and outcomes. Although specific gaps in knowledge need to be addressed to guide future practice, nurses need to use existing knowledge in the care they are delivering today. All of the interventions proposed for managing cancer treatment-related fatigue are health policy challenges because they represent additions to usual care rather than replacements of existing components of care.[82]

Theories that underlie interventions being tested have not been consistently well explicated, and thus our understanding of mediating mechanisms of CRF is insufficient. Study designs have been limited by lack of control groups, small sample sizes and other threats to validity and reliability. Little research has been conducted with patients with advanced disease or those who are elderly, of low socioeconomic status or ethnically diverse. These patients represent obvious challenges as research subjects, as they are often more debilitated and have many co-morbidities and life demands that make participation in research difficult. In addition, ethnic and cultural diversity is often limited in research studies because valid and reliable instruments are not available in a variety of languages.[29]

A high degree of fatigue prevents patients from returning to work and keeps them from being able to lead a normal life. It is important to clarify further the differences between patients at high risk for this outcome and those at low risk. As the number of people surviving cancer for extended periods of time continues to increase, the phenomenon of symptoms that persist following the completion of treatment need to be recognized. The awareness by healthcare professionals of the significance of this disruptive symptom is increasing. Further research is needed in order to improve current knowledge and create interest for the symptom and bring it into focus. Intervention studies are required to evaluate the best ways for nurses, amongst others, to assist patients to live with and adapt to fatigue.

REFERENCES

1. Griffin AM, Butow PN, Coates AS, et al. On the receiving end. V: Patient perceptions of the side effects of cancer chemotherapy in 1993. Ann Oncol 1996; 7(2):189–195.
2. Sitzia J, Huggins L. Side effects of cyclophosphamide, methotrexate, 5-fluorouracil (CMF) chemotherapy for breast cancer. Cancer Pract 1998; 6(1):13–21.
3. Broeckel JA, Jacobsen PB, Horton J, Balducci L, Lyman GH. Characteristics and correlates of fatigue after adjuvant chemotherapy for breast cancer. J Clin Oncol 1998; 16(5):1689–1696.
4. Mendoza TR, Wang XS, Cleeland CS, et al. The rapid assessment of fatigue severity in cancer patients: use of the Brief Fatigue Inventory. Cancer 1999; 85:1186–1196.
5. Stone P, Richards M, A'Hern R. A study to investigate the prevalence, severity and correlates of fatigue among patients with cancer in comparison with a control group of volunteers without cancer. Ann Oncol 2000; 11:561–567.
6. Ahlberg K. Cancer-related fatigue. Experience and outcomes. Akademisk avhandling 2004. Göteborg University. ISBN: 91-628-5969-2.

7. Gutstein HB. The biologic basis of fatigue. Cancer 2001; 92(6):1678–1683.

8. Mock V, Atkinson A, Barsevick A, et al (chair & panel); National Comprehensive Cancer Network. NCCN Practice Guidelines for Cancer-Related Fatigue. Oncology 2000; 14 (11A):151–161.

9. Portenoy RK, Itri L. Cancer-related fatigue: guidelines for evaluation and management. Oncologist 1999; 4:1–10.

10. Glaus A, Crow R, Hammond S. A qualitative study to explore the concept of fatigue/tiredness in cancer patients and in healthy individuals. Eur J Cancer Care 1996; 5:8–23.

11. Glaus A. Fatigue in patients with cancer: analysis and assessment. Berlin: Springer-Verlag; 1998.

12. Vogelzang N, Breitbart W, Cella D, et al. Patient, caregiver, and oncologist perceptions of cancer-related fatigue: results of a tripart assessment survey. Semin Haematol 1997; 34:4–12.

13. Ream E, Richardson A. Fatigue: a concept analysis. Int J Nurs Stud 1996; 33(5):519–529.

14. Piper B, Lindsey A, Dodd M. Fatigue mechanisms in cancer patients: developing a nursing theory. Oncol Nurs Forum 1987; 14(6):17–23.

15. Aistars J. Fatigue in the cancer patient: a conceptual approach to a clinical problem. Oncol Nurs Forum 1987; 14(6):25–30.

16. Winningham M, Nail L, Barton Burke M, et al. Fatigue and the cancer experience: the state of the knowledge. Oncol Nurs Forum 1994; 21:23–36.

17. Cimprich B. Attentional fatigue following breast cancer surgery. Res Nurs Health 1992; 15:199–207.

18. Cimprich B. Developing an intervention to restore attention in cancer patients. Cancer Nurs 1993; 16:83–92.

19. Cimprich B. Attention and symptom distress in women with and without breast cancer. Nurs Res 2001; 50(2):86–94.

20. Larsson PJ, Carrieri-Kohlman V, Dodd M, et al. A model for symptom management. The University of California, San Francisco School of Nursing Symptom Management Faculty Group. Image: J Nurs Scholarship 1994; 26(4):272–276.

21. Dodd M, Janson S, Facione N, et al. Advancing the science of symptom management. J Adv Nurs 2001; 33(5):668–676.

22. Curt G, Breitbart W, Cella D, et al. Impact of cancer-related fatigue on the lives of patients: new finding from the fatigue coalition. Oncologist 2000; 5:353–360.

23. Glaus A. Assessment of fatigue in cancer and non-cancer patients and in healthy individuals. Support Care Cancer 1993; 1(6):305–315.

24. Lewis G, Wessely S. The epidemiology of fatigue: more questions than answers. J Epidemiol Community Health 1992; 46(2):92–97.

25. Pawlikowska T, Chalder T, Hirsch SR, et al. Population based study of fatigue and psychological distress. BMJ 1994; 308(6931):763–766.

26. Robinson KD, Posner JD. Patterns of self-care needs and interventions related to biologic response modifier therapy: fatigue as a model. Semin Oncol Nurs 1992; 8(4):17–22.

27. Longman AL, Braden CJ, Mishel MH. Side effects burden in women with breast cancer. Cancer Pract 1996; 4:274–280.

28. Jacobsen PB, Hann DM, Azzarello LM, et al. Fatigue in woman receiving adjuvant chemotherapy for breast cancer: characteristics, course and correlates. J Pain Symptom Manage 1999; 22:277–288.

29. Ahlberg K, Ekman T, Gaston-Johansson, Mock V. Evaluation and management of cancer-related fatigue in adults – a review. Lancet 2003; 362:640–650.

30. Ferrell B, Grant M, Dean G, Funk B, Ly J. 'Bone tired': the experience of fatigue and its impact on quality of life. Oncol Nurs Forum 1996; 23:1539–1547.

31. Messias DKH, Yeager KA, Dibble SL, Dodd MJ. Patients' perspective of fatigue while undergoing chemotherapy. Oncol Nurs Forum 1997; 24(1):43–48.

32. Magnusson K, Moller A, Ekamn T, Wallgren A. A qualitative study to explore the experience of fatigue in cancer patients. Eur J Cancer Care 1999; 8:224–232.

33. Heinz L, Fritz E. Anemia in cancer patients. Semin Oncol 1998; 25:2–6.

34. Cella D. Factors influencing quality of life in cancer patients: anemia and fatigue. Semin Oncol 1998; 25(Suppl 7):43–46.

35. Mercadante S, Gebbia V, Marrazzo A, Filosto S. Anaemia in cancer: pathophysiology and treatment. Cancer Treat Rev 2000; 26(4):303–311.

36. Loney M, Chernecky C. Anemia. Oncol Nurs Forum 2000; 27(6):951–962.

37. Cella D, Dobrez D, Glaspy J. Control of cancer-related anemia with erythropoietic agents: a review of evidence for improved quality of life and clinical outcomes. Ann Oncol 2003; 14(4):511–519.

38. Glaus A, Muller S. [Hemoglobin and fatigue in cancer patients: inseparable twins?] Schweiz Med Wochenschr 2000; 130(13): 471–477. [in German]

39. Hickok JT, Morrow GR, McDonald S, et al. Frequency and correlates of fatigue in lung cancer patients receiving radiation therapy: implications for management. J Pain Symptom Manage 1999; 11(6):370–377.

40. Janda M, Gerstner N, Obermair A, et al. Quality of life changes during conformal radiation therapy for prostate carcinoma. Cancer 2000; 89:1322–1328.

41. Jones T, Wadler S, Hupart K. Endrocrine-mediated mechanisms of fatigue during treatment with interferon-alpha. Semin Oncol 1998; 25:54–63.

42. Stasi R, Abriani L, Beccaglia P, Terzoli E, Amadori S. Cancer-related fatigue: evolving concepts in evaluation and treatment. Cancer 2003; 98(9): 1786–1801.

43. Magnan MA, Mood DW. The effects of health state, hemoglobin, global symptom distress, mood disturbance, and treatment site on fatigue onset, duration, and distress in patients receiving radiation therapy. Oncol Nurs Forum 2003; 30(2):E33–9.

44. Smets EM, Visser MR, Willems-Groot AF, et al. Fatigue and radiotherapy: (B) experience in patients 9 months following treatment. Br J Cancer 1998; 78(7):907–912.

45. Furst CJ, Ahsberg E. Dimensions of fatigue during radiotherapy. An application of the Multidimensional Fatigue Inventory. Support Care Cancer 2001 9(5):355–360.

46. Irvine DM, Vincent L, Graydon JE, Bubela N. Fatigue in women with breast cancer receiving radiation therapy. Cancer Nurs 1998; 21(2):127–135.

47. Schwartz AL, Nail LM, Chen S, et al. Fatigue patterns observed in patients receiving chemotherapy and radiotherapy. Cancer Invest 2000; 18(1):11–19.

48. Stone P, Hardy J, Broadley K, et al. Fatigue in advanced cancer: a prospective controlled cross-sectional study. Br J Cancer 1999; 79(9/10):1479–1486.

49. Okuyama T, Tanaka K, Akechi T, et al. Fatigue in ambulatory patients with advanced lung cancer: prevalence, correlated factors and screening. J Pain Symptom Manage 2001; 22(1):554–564.

50. Given CW, Given B, Azzouz F, Kozachik S, Stommel M. Predictors of pain and fatigue in the year following diagnosis among elderly cancer patients. J Pain Symptom Manage 2001; 21(6):456–466.

51. Andrykowski MA, Curran SL, Lightner R. Off-treatment fatigue in breast cancer survivors: a controlled comparison. J Behav Med 1998; 21(1):1–18.

52. Greenberg DB, Gray JL, Mannix CM, Eisenthal S, Carey M. Treatment-related fatigue and serum interleukin-1 levels in patients during external beam irradiation for prostate cancer. J Pain Symptom Manage 1993; 8(4):196–200.

53. Kurzrock R. The role of cytokines in cancer-related fatigue. Cancer 2001; 92:1684–1688.

54. Herskind C, Bamberg M, Rodemann HP. The role of cytokines in the development of normal-tissue reactions after radiotherapy. Strahlenther Onkol 1998; 174:12–15.

55. Anisman J, Baines MC, Berczi I et al. Neuroimmune mechanisms in health and disease.

2. Disease. Can Med Assoc J 1996; 155:1075–1082.

56. Moss RB, Mercandetti A, Vojdani A. TNF-alpha and chronic fatigue syndrome. J Clin Immunol 1999; 19(5):314–316.

57. Inui A. Cancer anorexia-cachexia syndrome: are neuropeptides the key? Cancer Res 1999; 59:4493–4501.

58. Kalman D, Villani LJ. Nutritional aspects of cancer-related fatigue. J Am Diet Assoc 1997; 97(6): 650–654.

59. Ahles TA, Ruckdeschel JC, Blanchard EB. Cancer-related pain – I. Prevalence in an outpatient setting as a function of stage of disease and type of cancer. J Psychosom Res 1984; 28(2):115–119.

60. Miaskowski C, Kragness L, Dibble S, Wallhagen M. Differences in mood states, health status, and caregiver strain between family caregivers of oncology outpatients with and without cancer related pain. J Pain Symptom Manage 1997; 13(3):138–47.

61. Miaskowski C, Lee KA. Pain, fatigue, and sleep disturbances in oncology outpatients receiving radiation therapy for bone metastasis: a pilot study. J Pain Symptom Manage 1999; 17(5):320–332.

62. Kaasa S, Loge JH, Knobel H, Jordhoy MS, Brenne E. Fatigue. Measures and relation to pain. Acta Anaesthesiol Scand 1999; 43(9):939–947.

63. Blesch K, Paice J, Wickham R, et al. Correlates of fatigue in people with breast or lung cancer. Oncol Nurs Forum 1991; 8(1):81–87.

64. Burrows M, Dibble SL, Miaskowski C. Differences in outcomes among patients experiencing different types of cancer-related pain. Oncol Nurs Forum 1998; 25(4):735–741.

65. Ancoli-Israel S, Moore PJ, Jones V. The relationship between fatigue and sleep in cancer patients: a review. Eur J Cancer Care 2001; 10(4):245–255.

66. Berger AM, Farr L. The influence of daytime inactivity and nighttime restlessness on cancer-related fatigue. Oncol Nurs Forum 1999; 26(10):1663–1671.

67. Mock V, Dow KH, Meares C, et al. Effects of exercise on fatigue, physical functioning, and emotional distress during radiation therapy for breast cancer. Oncol Nurs Forum 1997; 24(6):991–1000.

68. Gaston-Johansson F, Fall-Dickson JM, Bakos AB, Kennedy MJ. Fatigue, pain, and depression in pre-autotransplant breast cancer patients. Cancer Pract 1999; 7(5):240–247.

69. Tchekmedyian NS, Kallich J, McDermott A, Fayers P, Erder MH. The relationship between psychologic distress and cancer-related fatigue. Cancer 2003; 98(1):198–203.

70. Akechi T, Kugaya A, Okamura H, Yamawaki S, Uchitomi Y. Fatigue and its associated factors in

ambulatory cancer patients: a preliminary study. J Pain Symptom Manage 1999; 17(1):42–48.

71. Mock V, McCorkle R, Ropka ME, Pickett M, Poniatowski B. Fatigue and physical functioning during breast cancer treatment. Oncol Nurs Forum 2002; 29(2):338.

72. Visser MR, Smets EM. Fatigue, depression and quality of life in cancer patients: how are they related? Support Care Cancer 1998; 6(2):101–108.

73. Chen MK. The epidemiology of self-perceived fatigue among adults. Preventive Medicine 1986; 15(1):74–81.

74. Aapro MS, Cella D, Zagari M. Age, anemia, and fatigue. Semin Oncol 2002; 29(3 Suppl 8):55–59.

75. Schwarz R, Hinz A. Reference data for the quality of life questionnaire EORTC QLQ-C30 in the general German population. Eur J Cancer 2001; 37(11):1345–1351.

76. Liao S, Ferrell BA. Fatigue in an older population. J Am Geriatr Soc 2000; 48(4):426–430.

77. Tiesinga LJ, Dassen TW, Halfens RJ, van den Heuvel WJ. Factors related to fatigue; priority of interventions to reduce or eliminate fatigue and the exploration of a multidisciplinary research model for further study of fatigue. Int J Nurs Stud 1999; 36(4):265–80.

78. Bower J, Ganz P, Desmond K. Fatigue in breast cancer survivors: occurrence, correlates, and impact on quality of life. J Clin Oncol 2000; 18(4):743–753.

79. Leidy NK. Functional status and the forward progress of merry-go-rounds: toward a coherent analytical framework. Nurs Res 1994; 43(4):196–202.

80. Yellen SB, Cella D, Webster K, Blendowski C, Kaplan E. Measuring fatigue and anaemia related symptoms with the Functional Assessment of Cancer Therapy (FACT) measurement system J Pain Symptom Manage 1997; 13(2):63–74.

81. Cella D, Peterman A, Passik S, Jacobsen P, Breitbart W. Progress towards guidelines for the management of fatigue. Oncology 1998; 12:369–377.

82. Nail L. Fatigue in patients with cancer. Oncol Nurs Forum 2002; 29(3):537–544.

83. Richardson A. The health diary: an example of its use as a data collection method. J Adv Nurs 1994; 19:782–791.

84. National Comprehensive Cancer Network Practice Guidelines Cancer-Related Fatigue Panel 2002 Guidelines (Ver 1.2002, March). Rockledge, PA: NCCN.

85. Mock V. Fatigue management: the evidence and the guidelines for practice. Cancer 2001; 92(6):1699–1707.

86. Piper B, Lindsey A. Development of an instrument to measure the subjective dimension of fatigue. In: Funk S, Tornquist E, eds. Key

aspects to comfort. Berlin: Springer; 1989:199–208.

87. Piper BF, Dibble SL, Dodd MJ, et al. The revised Piper Fatigue Scale: psychometric evaluation in women with breast cancer. Oncol Nurs Forum 1998; 25(4):677–684.

88. Schwartz, A. The Schwartz Cancer Fatigue Scale: testing reliability and validity. Oncol Nurs Forum 1998; 25:711–717.

89. Schwartz A, Meek P. Additional construct of validity of the Schwartz Cancer Fatigue Scale. J Nurs Meas 1999; 7(1):35–45.

90. Smets EMA, Garssen B, Bonke B, de Haes JCJM. The multidimensional fatigue inventory (MFI). Psychometric qualities of an instrument to assess fatigue. J Psychosom Res 1995; 39:315–325.

91. Rieger PT. Assessment and epidemiologic issues related to fatigue. Cancer 2001; 92(6):1733–1736.

92. Varricchio CG. Measurement and assessment: What are the issues? In: Winningham ML, Barton-Burke M, eds. Fatigue in cancer: a multidimensional approach. Boston: Jones and Bartlett; 2000:55–68.

93. Meek PM, Nail LM, Barsevick A, et al. Psychometric testing of fatigue instruments for use with cancer patients. Nurs Research 2000; 49:181–190.

94. National Institutes of Health State-of-the-Science Conference; Washington, DC; July 15–17, 2002. Available at: http://consensus.nih.gov on July 17, 2002.

95. Manzullo E, Liu W, Escalante C. Treatment for cancer-related fatigue: an update. Expert Rev Anticancer Ther 2003; 3(1):99–106.

96. Morrow GR, Morrell C. Behavioral treatment for the anticipatory nausea and vomiting induced by cancer chemotherapy. N Engl J Med 1982; 307:1476–1480.

97. Rainey LC. Effects of preparatory patient education for radiation oncology patients. Cancer 1985; 56:1056–1061.

98. Johnson J, Nail L, Lauver D, King K, Keys H. Reducing the negative impact of radiation therapy. Cancer 1988; 61:46–51.

99. Burish TG, Snyder SL, Jenkins RA. Preparing patients for cancer chemotherapy: effect of coping preparation and relaxation interventions. J Consult Clin Psychol 1991; 59:518–525.

100. Cassileth BR, Lusk EJ, Bodenheimer BJ, et al. Chemotherapeutic toxicity – the relationship between patients' pre-treatment expectations and posttreatment results. Am J Clin Oncol 1985; 8(5):419–425.

101. Given B, Given CW, McCorkle R, et al. Pain and fatigue management: results of a nursing randomized clinical trial. Oncol Nurs Forum 2002; 29(6):949–956.

102. Johnson J. Self-regulation theory and coping with physical illness. Res Nurs Health 1999; 22:435–438.

103. MacVicar MG, Winningham ML. Promoting the functional capacity of cancer patients. Cancer Bull 1986; 38:235–239.

104. Mock V, Burke MB, Sheehan PK, et al. A nursing rehabilitation program for women with breast cancer receiving adjuvant chemotherapy. Oncol Nurs Forum 1994; 21(5):899–908.

105. American College of Sports Medicine. ACSM's exercise management for person with chronic diseases and disabilities. Champaign, IL: Human Kinetics; 1997.

106. Lee KA. Sleep and fatigue. Annu Rev Nurs Res 2001; 19:249–273.

107. Berger AM. Patterns of fatigue and activity and rest during adjuvant breast cancer chemotherapy. Oncol Nurs Forum 1998; 25(1):51–62.

108. Young-McCaughan S, Dramiga SA, Yoder LH, et al. Physical and psychological health outcomes in patients with cancer participating in a structured exercise program. Oncol Nurs Forum 2002; 29(2):334.

109. Graydon JE, Bubela N, Irvine D, Vincent L. Fatigue-reducing strategies used by patients receiving treatment for cancer. Cancer Nurs 1995; 18(1):23–28.

110. Forester B, Kornfeld DS, Fleiss JL. Psychotherapy during radiotherapy: effects on emotional and physical distress. Am J Psychiatry 1985; 142(1):22–27.

111. Fawzy FI, Cousins N, Fawzy NW, et al. A structured psychiatric intervention for cancer patients: I. Changes over time in methods of coping and affective disturbance. Arch Gen Psychiatry 1990; 47:720–725.

112. Fawzy NW. A psychoeducational nursing intervention to enhance coping and affective state in newly diagnosed malignant melanoma patients. Cancer Nurs 1995; 18(6):427–438.

113. Mock V, Pickett M, Ropka M, et al. Fatigue and quality of life outcomes of exercise during cancer treatment. Cancer Pract 2001; 9 (3):119–127.

114. Cella D, Bron D. The effect of Epoetin alfa on quality of life in anemic cancer patients. Cancer Pract 1999; 7(4):177–182.

115. Littlewood TJ, Bajetta E, Nortier JWR, et al. Effects of epoetin alfa on hematologic parameters and quality of life in cancer patients receiving nonplatinum chemotherapy: results of a randomized, double-blind, placebo-controlled trial. J Clin Oncol 2001; 19:2865–2874.

116. Demetri G, Kris M, Wade J, Degos L, Cella D. Quality-of-life benefit in chemotherapy patients treated with epoetin alfa is independent of disease response or tumor type: results from a prospective community oncology study. Procrit Study Group. J Clin Oncol 1998; 16:3412–3425.

117. Glaspy J, Bukowski R, Steinberg D, et al. Impact of therapy with epoetin alfa on clinical outcomes in patients with nonmyeloid malignancies during cancer chemotherapy in community oncology practice. J Clin Oncol 1997; 15(3):1218–1234.

118. Gabrilove JL, Cleeland CS, Livingston RB, et al. Clinical evaluation of once-weekly dosing of epoetin alfa in chemotherapy patients: improvements in hemoglobin and quality of life are similar to three-times weekly dosing. J Clin Oncol 2001; 19:2875–2882.

119. Österborg A, Brandberg Y, Molostova V, et al. Randomized double-blind, placebo-controlled trial of recombinant human erythropoietin, epoetin beta, in hematologic malignancies. J Clin Oncol 2002; 20(10):2486–2494.

120. Turner R, Anglin P, Burkes R, et al. Epoetin alfa in cancer patients: evidence-based guidelines. J Pain Symptom Manage 2001; 22(5):954–965.

121. Glaspy JA, Tchekmedyian NS. Darbepoetin alfa administered every 2 weeks alleviates anemia in cancer patients receiving chemotherapy. Oncology (Huntingt) 2002; 16(10):23–29.

122. Bruera E, Macmillan K, Hanson J, et al. A controlled trial of megestrol acetate on appetite, caloric intake, nutritional status, and other symptoms in patients with advanced cancer. Cancer 1995; 66:1279–1282.

123. Fossa SD, Slee PH, Brausi M, et al. Flutamide versus prednisone in patients with prostate cancer symptomatically progressing after androgen-ablative therapy: a phase III study of the European organization for research and treatment of cancer genitourinary group. J Clin Oncology 2001; 19(1):62–71.

124. Breitbart W, Rosenfeld B, Kaim M, Funesti-Esch J. A randomized, double-blind, placebo-controlled trial of psychostimulants for the treatment of fatigue in ambulatory patients with human immunodeficiency virus disease. Arch Intern Med 2001; 161(3):411–420.

125. Weinshenker BG, Penman M, Bass B, et al. A double-blind, randomized crossover trial of pemoline in fatigue associated with multiple sclerosis. Neurology 1992; 42:1468–1471.

126. Gelmon K, Eisenhauer E, Bryce C. Randomized phase II study of high-dose paclitaxel with or without amifostine in patients with metastatic breast cancer. J Clin Oncol 1999; 17:3038–3047.

127. Magnusson K, Karlsson E, Palmblad C, Leitner C, Paulson A. Swedish nurses' estimation of fatigue as a symptom in cancer patients – report of a questionnaire. Eur J Cancer Care 1997; 6(3):186–191.

128. Knowles G, Borthwick D, McNamara S, et al. Survey of nurses assessment of cancer-related fatigue. Eur J Cancer Care 2000; 9:105–113.

673

129. Miller M, Kearney N. Nurses' knowledge and attitudes towards cancer-related fatigue. Eur J Oncol Nurs 2001; 5(4):208–217.

130. Tiesinga LJ, Dijkstra A, Dassen TW, Halfens RJ, van den Heuve WJ. Are nurses able to assess fatigue, exertion fatigue and types of fatigue in residential home patients? Scand J Caring Sci 2002; 16(2):129–136.

131. Mock V. Clinical excellence through evidence-based practice: fatigue management as a model. Oncol Nurs Forum 2003; 30(5):787–796.

132. Ream E, Richardson A. From theory to practice: designing interventions to reduce fatigue in patients with cancer. Oncol Nurs Forum 1999; 26(8):1295–303.

CHAPTER 31

The Impact of Cancer and Cancer Therapy on Sexual and Reproductive Health

ISABEL D WHITE

CHAPTER CONTENTS

Introduction   675

Sexuality in context   676

Sexual expression: the human sexual
response cycle   677

The impact of cancer and its treatment
on sexual expression   678
   The impact of surgery   678
   The impact of chemotherapy   680
   The impact of radiotherapy   682
   The impact of endocrine therapy   683

Impact of cancer therapy on
reproductive health   683
   Contraceptive advice   684

Male fertility and cancer treatment   684
Female fertility and cancer treatment   685
Reproductive technology techniques
in cancer care   687

Psychosexual assessment in cancer care   688
   Levels of psychosexual intervention
   in cancer nursing practice   691
   Specialist interventions for
   psychosexual health in cancer care   691

Future developments in psychosexual
and reproductive health for people
affected by cancer   696

Conclusion   697

References   697

INTRODUCTION

There are a number of developments that have led to increased awareness among healthcare professionals regarding the sexual and fertility concerns of people affected by cancer.

Societal attitudes to sexual and reproductive issues have altered, principally as a result of the second wave sexual revolution of the 1980s, created by the emergence of acquired immunodeficiency syndrome (AIDS) and human immunodeficiency virus (HIV) infection.[1] There was an initial tendency, particularly by Western governments, to call for a return to traditional family values and to attempt to recreate social restrictions around sexual behaviour, including intolerance to sexual diversity.[2] However, one positive outcome from what we now recognize as the AIDS pandemic was that sexual health and sexuality became a legitimate concern for governments, policy makers and leaders in public health.

Associated with the increased prominence of sexual issues in society at large, health professionals in a variety of clinical specialities began to recognize the contribution of sexual and reproductive health to the overall well-being of client groups they encountered in clinical practice.

In cancer care, improved patterns of survival have led to increased expectations regarding the quality of that survival by those affected by cancer and by healthcare professionals. As a result, exploring the impact of cancer and its treatment on sexual and reproductive health have now become legitimate aspects of both contemporary cancer care practice and research.

Although practitioners appear to recognize their responsibilities in relation to the discussion of sexual concerns as part of the process of informed consent, there are still a myriad of barriers to overcome if this domain of practice is to be adequately addressed.[3]

It is beyond the scope of this chapter to address the diverse factors that continue to subvert the provision of appropriate psychosexual care for those affected by cancer across Europe. Heath and White[2] consider the wider social and organizational influences on this marginalized element of healthcare practice, including the consequences of failing to reconstruct the image of nursing from that of a sexualized occupation.[4]

The aim of this chapter is to offer an accessible resource for nurses who provide care and support to those facing the sexual and reproductive consequences of cancer and its treatment.

This chapter will include an exploration of the concept of sexuality; an overview of the physical and psychological impact of cancer and principal treatment modalities on both sexual and reproductive health; issues around psychosexual assessment in cancer care; and a discussion of the role of cancer care professionals and other agencies in the provision of psychosexual care and reproductive technology.

SEXUALITY IN CONTEXT

> What is most essentially human is precisely that our lives, women's and men's, are not just determined by biological necessity but crucially also by human action and vision.[5(p10)]

Sexuality embraces the associated concepts of sexual identity, sexual expression or behaviour and intimacy. It is also closely allied with concepts such as body image or self-concept (see Ch. 32), gender identity, gender roles and relationships.

The concept of sexuality and its subsequent expression cannot be understood in a vacuum, devoid of the socially constructed norms that influence all of us as members of contemporary society. Across Europe there are notable differences in social acceptability and comfort with diversity of sexual orientation and expression, from the apparent liberalism of Scandinavian countries and Holland to the relatively conservative social norms prevalent in Ireland, Italy and the UK.[6]

Medical literature tends to represent sexuality and sexual expression as a physiological behaviour based on some innate biological drive, a view that emanates from influential 20th century sexologists such as Kinsey et al[7,8] and Masters and Johnson.[9]

The challenge to a dominant biological definition of gender and sexuality probably dates from the 1970s, from work by the medical sociologist and philosopher Foucault.[10] He argued that the meaning of sexuality is constantly changing, both culturally and historically, and in contrast to being stable and preordained, is a concept that is multifaceted, diverse and most importantly, socially constructed. Thus, behaviours that appear physically identical may possess different social significance and meaning dependent on how they are understood by different cultures and at different times in history.

The idea that sexuality is socially constructed is an important one for healthcare professionals if they are to understand the stigma and prejudice that often accompanies any dysfunction or disease associated with sexual behaviour. The media portrayal of AIDS provided a powerful example of the way medical facts can be constructed to deliver a moral message about a disease that is still associated with areas of social and sexual behaviour deemed illicit and therefore worthy of moralistic and voyeuristic attention.[11]

A parallel in the field of cancer care may be the way in which some women who develop cervical cancer, particularly at a young age, view themselves as sexually promiscuous and their illness as punishment for sexual indiscretions. Such a moralistic stance may lead to considerable difficulties in the resumption of sexual activity and make the attainment of sexual health a challenging goal.

In Western societies, male and female sexuality are defined and redefined through the language of sexual expression, one that appears mechanistic, male-orientated and heterosexual, emphasizing the powerful male phallus in pursuit of the passive, yet sexually responsive and available, female. Male sexuality is normally represented as phallocentric, associated with power and performance more than its diffuse female counterpart. In contrast, female sexuality is often viewed predominantly in relation to women's reproductive capacities, such that women have become '... victims of their own reproductive anatomy'.[12(p101)]

As will be seen later in this chapter, it is the social meanings of sexual expression and fertility that are challenged and altered through the experience of cancer and its treatment, often requiring greater adjustment than that determined solely by an altered physical or physiological state.

The social construction of sexuality, despite biological drives and hormonal influences, is important both in the way we view sexuality as individuals and for the ways healthcare professionals reconstruct this concept in the context of illness and disability. It follows that any alteration in sexual expression arising from illness or treatment may require patients and their partners to reconstruct the meaning of sex and sexual expression within this revised personal and social context.

The effective sexual and reproductive rehabilitation of the person affected by cancer thus requires an integrated approach that embraces the physical, psychological and social or relationship domains of cancer care.

SEXUAL EXPRESSION: THE HUMAN SEXUAL RESPONSE CYCLE

Cancer impacts on the human sexual response in a myriad of ways, often affecting more than one aspect of sexual expression, potentially creating tension or distress in sexual relationships.[13] In understanding the complexity of human sexuality it is helpful to consider how cancer and its treatment may impact on the four discrete phases of the human sexual response cycle.[9] Figure 31.1 provides an outline of the four-phase model of human sexual response devised by Masters and Johnson[9] following detailed laboratory research into both male and female sexual response.

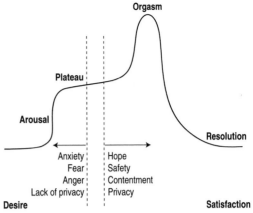

Figure 31.1: Human sexual response cycle. (From Masters and Johnson.[9])

Sexual desire is sometimes referred to as *sexual interest* and is an important initial state of receptiveness or willingness for sexual contact.

A state of sexual interest is partially mediated by hormonal influence, although this relationship appears more direct for men than for women.[6] There are clear gender differences between the manifestation of sexual interest, with men more likely to acknowledge the occurrence of sexual daydreams, fantasies and spontaneous erections associated with both internal and external sexual stimuli. Women may also have spontaneous sexual daydreams but tend to experience them less frequently and mainly demonstrate sexual arousability as a direct result of being approached by a partner for sexual contact.[14,15]

Recent exploration of the female sexual response has suggested that the Masters and Johnson model[9] does not equate with what is encountered clinically or empirically.[15] A composite model of women's sexual response that incorporates physiological, psychological and social factors has been proposed, depicting the complexity of female sexual desire.[15]

Sexual arousal is the phase where the penis becomes erect and the woman experiences vulval and clitoral engorgement and increased sensitivity. In addition, vaginal lubrication occurs and there is a 'ballooning' of the upper third of the vagina in readiness for penile penetration.

Respiratory rate, pulse rate and blood pressure increase and the face and upper body may show signs of flushing due to skin vasodilation.

677

During *orgasm*, both men and women experience a release of sexual tension and extremely enjoyable genital and bodily sensations. The man will ejaculate semen from his urethra and the woman will be aware of multiple rhythmic muscular contractions of the outer third of the vagina, with some women aware of those emanating from the uterus.

In the *resolution phase*, increased cardiorespiratory effort returns to normal and pelvic vasocongestion diminishes rapidly, resulting in a loss of erection and reduction in clitoral engorgement. Both men and women typically experience a sense of relaxation following orgasm and perceive a sense of sexual satisfaction. Whereas women can continue to respond to additional sexual stimulation, thus achieving a series of orgasmic responses, for men there is a refractory period of varying duration, normally dependent on the man's age. In a young man this may be a matter of minutes, whereas in the older man it could be hours or days. During this refractory period, it is not usually possible for a man to attain another full erection in response to sexual stimuli.[6]

As can be seen from this short introduction to the human sexual response cycle, sexual expression is dependent on intact vascular, neural and endocrine pathways in addition to the psychological, interpersonal and social factors that influence the specific behaviours in which any individual or couple choose to engage.

THE IMPACT OF CANCER AND ITS TREATMENT ON SEXUAL EXPRESSION

Literature and research largely focus on the types of cancer and treatments that affect parts of the body normally associated with sexual expression: namely, breast, gynaecological and genitourinary malignancies.

How much more person-centred might our care be if we explored how living with cancer affects an individual's sexuality and reproductive health, rather than focusing narrowly on functional changes arising from illness or therapy?

Serious illness and disability remove a person from their accustomed personal, social and sexual relations, threatening self-esteem and attractiveness at a time when the need for intimacy and belonging may be greatest. The person with cancer may find it difficult to be sexual where there is extreme fatigue, pain, loss of control over bodily functions and temporary or permanent alterations in body image.[16]

The psychological impact of a cancer diagnosis and associated treatment effects can also result in the development of anxiety or depression. Up to 40% of people affected by cancer have moderate or high levels of anxiety, with a similar prevalence of depression.[17] Anxiety, depression and their pharmacological management can cause a variety of sexual difficulties, ranging from loss of sexual interest to erectile dysfunction (ED) and difficulty reaching orgasm.[18,19]

Given the complexity of the human sexual response, the interdependency of its phases and the nature of modern multimodal cancer therapy, it is not surprising that cancer and its treatment often has a significant impact on multiple aspects of sexual expression. Indeed, many sexual difficulties experienced by patients and their partners are compounded by the use of multiple treatment modalities, whether concurrently as in chemoradiation, or in sequence such as radiotherapy as an adjunct to surgery.[20]

For the purpose of this chapter the treatment impact will be discussed according to the phase predominantly affected, although it should be understood that some treatments have a global effect on sexual function, creating an impact on more than one phase simultaneously.

The impact of surgery

Much is written about the impact of both illness and surgery on those experiencing genitourinary or gynaecological malignancies. Furthermore, the association between the female breast and sexual expression has ensured a comprehensive evidence base regarding the psychological and psychosexual impact of breast cancer and related surgery.[21,22] However, it is important not to ignore patients whose surgery affects 'non-sexual' parts of the body such as the cerebral malignancies, maxillofacial surgery for head and neck cancer or the functional difficulties created by endoprosthetic replacement or amputation for upper or lower limb sarcomas.[23,24]

Surgical intervention may have a direct or indirect impact on sexual expression. Following partial glossectomy for carcinoma of the tongue, the patient may have difficulty with speech or eating, with excessive salivation and poor oral seal. Kissing and close intimate contact may prove difficult due to the presence of both deformity and dysfunction. This can have a significant impact on a person's ability to form social and thus sexual relationships.[25]

Limb salvage surgery or amputation is most commonly required in the treatment of soft tissue or bone sarcomas, often occurring in adolescence or young adulthood. This age group have had less time to develop confidence in relation to their body image and sexual attractiveness or may not have had the opportunity to establish an intimate or sexual relationship. As a result they may feel both socially and sexually inept as they face the prospect of attracting a partner with a significant body image or functional deficit.[23]

Patients with a lower limb amputation for cancer may find their balance is adversely affected, necessitating modifications to their normal repertoire of sexual positions or the use of pillows to aid stability. Patients with an upper arm amputation may opt to alter their usual side-lying position to ensure their existing arm is free to caress their partner.[23] Similar adjustments may be necessary for a patient following cranial surgery for a cerebral tumour, where a hemiparesis or hemiplegia may interfere with mobility, balance and dexterity in sexual situations.

Surgical treatment of pelvic malignancies can cause sexual difficulties through a number of mechanisms, including vascular or neural disruption, loss of pelvic structures, adhesions or reduction in hormone production.[26] Tables 31.1 and 31.2 summarize the impact of selected treatments, including surgical interventions, on sexual function.

Hysterectomy for the management of cervical, endometrial or ovarian malignancies can alter the sensation of orgasm due to awareness of the absence of uterine contractions normally associated with orgasm. In radical hysterectomy, the upper third of the vagina is removed, resulting in a shorter vagina that may cause dyspareunia associated with deep penetration.[27] Removal of the ovaries will induce menopause with attendant symptoms of oestrogen depletion, such as vaginal dryness and vulval irritation.[28]

Although carried out far less frequently, pelvic exenteration has an even greater disruption on female sexual expression through loss of the vagina, problems associated with vaginal reconstruction and the negative psychological impact of stoma formation. Vulvectomy can cause narrowing of the vaginal introitus and altered vulval sensitivity, whereas radical excision may result in the clitoris being removed and reduced orgasmic capacity.[29]

Surgical interventions have multiple effects on female sexuality and these physical effects are frequently accompanied by a woman's sense of altered femininity, loss of fertility and anxiety regarding the resumption of sexual relations post-treatment due to fear of pain or postcoital bleeding.[30]

Pelvic surgery for genitourinary or colorectal malignancies also has significant effects on sexual function and satisfaction. Radical prostatectomy is associated with the development of ED in approximately 40–76% of men[31] and although nerve-sparing techniques are available, outcomes remain variable.[32] Where erectile function is preserved, there is always a loss of ejaculation (dry ejaculation), with an altered orgasmic sensation as a consequence. Some men may thus complain of reduced orgasmic intensity or sexual satisfaction following surgery on the prostate gland.

The prevalence of ED after cystectomy is probably closer to 100%.[32] After cystectomy, women may experience both vaginal stenosis and dyspareunia due to resection of the anterior vaginal wall, together with altered orgasmic sensation as a result of loss of the G-spot.

Penile and testicular cancer, while relatively rare and affecting men at opposite ends of the age spectrum, can have both physical and psychological sequelae that adversely affect sexual function. Recent clinical guidelines in the UK advise that the multidisciplinary management of urological cancers should include access to individuals who can provide counselling and information regarding both psychosexual and fertility concerns prior to treatment selection and commencement.[32]

Table 31.1: Female sexual difficulties associated with cancer and its therapy

Treatment	Reduced sexual desire	Reduced vaginal lubrication	Vaginal stenosis or shortening	Painful intercourse	Delayed or absent orgasm
Chemotherapy	++	+++	No	+	+
Endocrine therapy (breast cancer)	+++	++	No	+	+
Pelvic radiotherapy	+++	+++	+++	++	+
Total body irradiation (TBI)	++	++	++	++	+
Radical hysterectomy	+	++	+++	++	+
Bilateral oophorectomy	++	++	No	No	+
Pelvic exenteration	+++	Absent vagina	Absent vagina	Absent vagina	++
Radical vulvectomy	++	+	+	++	+++
Radical cystectomy	+	++	+++	++	++
Abdominoperineal resection	++	+	+	++	+
Breast surgery	++	No	No	No	+
Antidepressants	+++	++	No	++	++
Depression	+++	++	No	+	++
Anxiety	+	++	No	++	+++
Fatigue	+++	No	No	+	++
Pain	+++	No	No	++	+++
Altered self-concept	+++	No	No	No	++

In the management of anorectal cancer, there is a significant risk of ED secondary to nerve damage and even where erections are preserved there may still be ejaculatory disturbance. The new technique of mesorectal excision may help to retain sexual function where careful attention is given to autonomic nerve preservation.[33] Sphincter-sparing surgery, such as coloanal anastomosis, is being performed more commonly now in an attempt to reduce the psychological, functional and psychosexual morbidity associated with stoma formation.[34]

The impact of chemotherapy

Far more is known about the impact of cytotoxic agents on the fertility of patients receiving cancer treatment than is known regarding the effects of specific regimens or single agents on sexual function. As patients often receive

Table 31.2: Male sexual difficulties associated with cancer and its therapy

Treatment	Reduced sexual desire	Erectile dysfunction	Delayed or absent ejaculation	Retrograde ejaculation	Painful ejaculation	Reduced semen volume
Chemotherapy	+	+	+	No	No	No
Endocrine therapy (prostate cancer)	+++	+++	++	No	No	++
Pelvic radiotherapy	+	++	+	No	++	++
Total body irradiation (TBI)	+	+	+	No	+	+
Abdominoperineal resection	+	++	+	No	No	No
Retroperitoneal lymph node dissection (RPLND)	No	+	+	+	No	Loss of ejaculatory force
Radical prostatectomy	+	++	+++ Absent	No	+	+++
Radical cystectomy	+	+++	+++ Absent	No	+	+++
Partial phalectomy	+	++	+	No	No	No
Total phalectomy	++	+++	++	No	No	No
Unilateral orchidectomy	+	+	No	No	No	No
Antidepressants	++	++	+++	No	No	No
Depression	+++	++	++	No	No	No
Anxiety	+	+++	+++	No	No	No
Fatigue	+++	+++	++	No	No	No
Pain	+++	+	++	No	No	No
Altered self-concept	+++	++	+	No	No	No

more than one treatment in sequence or concurrently, as in chemoradiation regimens, it may be difficult to attribute sexual problems to any single causative factor.

Intensive chemotherapy, stem cell and bone marrow transplantation have an impact on both fertility and sexuality that lasts well beyond the acute treatment phase.[35–37] In addition to treatment-related effects, this group of patients may also have to contend with the impact of chronic graft versus host disease, particularly the development of genital lesions.

A number of women experience vaginal dryness during their chemotherapy treatment, often associated with chemotherapy-induced menopause.[38,39] Vaginal dryness may result in dyspareunia or the development of opportunistic vaginal infection such as *Candida*, due to mucosal trauma during immunosuppression. These women often complain of reduced sexual interest and sexual enjoyment due to the concomitant treatment side-effects such as fatigue, nausea or alopecia.

Patients experiencing severe bone marrow suppression should be made aware that their treatment could cause difficulties related to sexual expression. The extreme fatigue associated with systemic treatment has a significant impact on levels of sexual desire and orgasmic capacity. This may be important to explain to the patient and their partner in order to promote couple communication and support. Where patients remain sexually active, they should be made aware of the need for contraception. This issue is discussed in more detail later in the chapter. A barrier method of contraception is advocated (condoms) to reduce the potential risks associated with sexual intercourse causing vaginal or penile infection that may be more severe due to immunosuppression. Patients are also advised to pay particular attention to intimate hygiene, e.g. washing the perineum and genital area after sex. It is generally recommended that patients should refrain from engaging in anal intercourse, as even minor trauma to the rectal mucosa could cause the development of bacteraemia or septicaemia. Anal intercourse should also be avoided where there is severe thrombocytopenia, due to the risk of significant bleeding; like-

wise, vaginal intercourse should be taken gently in order to avoid trauma and potential bleeding.

Cytotoxic agents that cause peripheral neuropathy, such as vincristine, have been implicated in the development of ED following chemotherapy treatment. However, it is often difficult to elicit a direct causal relationship due to the multifactorial nature of ED in these men.

The impact of radiotherapy

The effects of radiotherapy are, as with surgery, predominantly local, with the exception of total body irradiation (TBI), where effects are seen throughout the body.

Pelvic radiotherapy has a direct effect on sexual function due to vascular and nerve damage and to fibrotic changes in tissues as a medium-to long-term effect.

Vascular changes in the penile arteries can be a direct cause of ED, particularly in men who are already experiencing some deterioration in strength and frequency of erections as a result of age or arteriosclerotic changes. ED can also be mediated by damage to the neurovascular bundles. The introduction of conformal radiotherapy and, more recently, prostate brachytherapy that spare the function of the neurovascular bundles may reduce the likelihood of developing ED.[40]

Women receiving pelvic radiotherapy for the management of gynaecological, bladder or anorectal cancers are at risk of the development of vaginal stenosis and vaginal dryness. These effects are seen more severely in those who have received a combination of both external beam radiotherapy and brachytherapy, as frequently occurs in the management of some gynaecological malignancies.[41,42] However, women receiving TBI as part of the management of haematological malignancies may also develop vaginal atrophy and dryness as a result of treatment-induced ovarian failure and should also receive psychosexual assessment and intervention as appropriate.[43]

Women should be told of these potential side-effects and given a set of vaginal dilators to use once the acute radiation reaction has subsided, although we are aware that compliance with regular vaginal dilatation is very poor.[44] Research still has to determine what is the optimal frequency and duration of use for this preventative strategy. Such information, in addition to specific risk factors associated with patient characteristics, stage of disease or volume of tissue irradiated, would also help us to target interventions more appropriately.

The impact of endocrine therapy

In general, healthcare professionals appear to pay scant attention to the sexual and fertility effects of endocrine management of cancer, perhaps because such treatment is more often associated with cancers occurring in later life or with a more advanced stage of illness. Nevertheless, one cannot make assumptions based on either the age of the client or on a diminished need for sexual contact in the presence of advanced disease. As Searle[45] explains: the fact that someone is dying does not remove their need for intimacy; it could even increase such a need, and sexual contact may be part of that expression.

Advanced prostate cancer is frequently treated with antiandrogen therapy, such as cyproterone acetate or luteinizing hormone releasing hormone (LHRH) analogues. These agents deprive malignant cells of testosterone, thus reducing their rate of growth and dissemination. Total androgen blockade can be achieved through a combination of LHRH analogues and cyproterone acetate, blocking both testicular and adrenal sources of androgen production. Most men receiving this therapy will lose sexual desire (73%), together with spontaneous erections (80%).[46] This effect is manifest by loss of early morning and nocturnal erections, as well as the inability to respond to sexual stimulation. Men receiving endocrine therapy may also experience an altered sexual identity or masculinity due to the fatigue and hot flushes experienced as a side-effect. Many men liken these effects to going through a menopause like their female partners.[47,48]

Women may be given antioestrogen therapy such as tamoxifen or an aromatase inhibitor for oestrogen receptor-positive breast cancer, resulting in the induction of a medical menopause. Women experience intense menopausal symptoms that include hot flushes, dry skin, irritability, vaginal dryness and loss of sexual interest.[49] In addition, some women experience greater difficulty in achieving orgasm while receiving endocrine therapy.[50] While these side-effects are normally reversible on cessation of treatment, it is important to recognize the significant disruption they cause to sexual function and satisfaction. Cancer nurses need greater awareness of the support and information needs of patients experiencing psychosexual and body image concerns during endocrine therapy.

IMPACT OF CANCER THERAPY ON REPRODUCTIVE HEALTH

Advances in both the diagnosis and treatment of malignant disease have led to improved long-term survival or cure for a significant number of adults experiencing cancer.[51] Those patients who survive the experience of cancer have rightly adjusted their expectations regarding the quality of survival they might expect. In response, healthcare professionals have accelerated their search for treatment regimens that are less toxic to gonadal tissues, while not compromising rates of long-term disease control or cure.

Reduced fertility or infertility remains a common side-effect of cancer treatment that can cause considerable psychological distress to those affected. Although we assume that this is mainly a concern to younger people with cancer, there are now a significant number of older men who enter subsequent relationships and wish to preserve their reproductive potential where their partner is of childbearing age.

Each of the three main treatment modalities (surgery, chemotherapy and radiotherapy), either alone or in combination, can have an adverse effect on the fertility potential of a person being treated for cancer. It is therefore important that there is good communication between the cancer treatment centre and the fertility unit in order to promote rapid access for patients and their partners for fertility advice and counselling. In addition, funding for fertility treatment should be considered as part of the overall provision of a comprehensive supportive cancer care service,[52] particularly as funding and access to fertility services across Europe is often limited and inconsistent.

Contraceptive advice

Temporary or permanent infertility is not immediate following the first cycle of chemotherapy or the initial fraction of pelvic radiotherapy. It is associated with the increasing total dose of drugs or irradiation through treatment cycles or fractions.[13,53,54]

Both radiotherapy and cytotoxic drugs have a potential teratogenic effect on the embryo, particularly in the first trimester of pregnancy. It is therefore important to make patients aware of the need to avoid pregnancy during treatment through the use of a reliable contraceptive.[55] A barrier contraceptive method such as the condom is most often advocated, as it also provides some protection from infection while the patient is immunocompromised. Where there is a risk of severe bleeding due to thrombocytopenia, medication such as northisterone or an LHRH analogue may be administered to suppress menstruation.

After completion of treatment, patients with an uncertain prognosis may be advised to avoid creating a pregnancy for a minimum of 1 year following cessation of therapy, as this is when disease recurrence is most likely to occur.[55] However, this has to be balanced against the increased incidence of premature menopause in women post-chemotherapy, and so a woman who wishes to conceive may be advised not to delay childbearing.[51]

It is important to have fertility counsellors available for patients and their partners to discuss the implications of reduced fertility, infertility, assisted reproductive techniques and future wishes with regards to childbearing within the context of their overall prognosis or that of their partner. These complex emotional, ethical and at times legal issues do need to be considered as an integral facet of modern cancer treatment.

The role of nurses working in cancer care is to be aware not only of the impact of specific treatments on fertility but also of the services available in their locality and of the routes of referral for patients and their partners to address fertility and assisted reproduction issues.[56] Cancer nurses working at an advanced practice level may engage in infertility counselling as part of their role and therefore need to have a sound understanding of the common individual and couple dynamics that develop as people come to terms with the losses associated with treatment-induced infertility. Interested readers are encouraged to explore the psychological reactions associated with this life crisis and their resolution through specialist texts.[57]

Male fertility and cancer treatment

The *surgical management* of testicular malignancies usually requires unilateral orchidectomy, thus preserving fertility, although it is occasionally necessary to undertake bilateral orchidectomy if both testes are affected. Some centres advocate pre-surgery sperm cryopreservation for all men with testicular malignancies, as orchidectomy has been shown to lower an already compromised sperm count at diagnosis.[55]

Other surgical procedures, such as retroperitoneal lymph node dissection (RPLND) and, more commonly, prostatectomy, can result in ejaculatory disturbance, particularly retrograde ejaculation. These procedures do not actually render the patient infertile but, where normal ejaculation does not occur, it is often possible to retrieve sperm by direct aspiration from the epididymis or through centrifuging a postcoital urine sample.

The impact of *radiotherapy* on male gonadal function may occur at a variety of points along the craniospinal axis, e.g. hypogonadism as a result of cerebral irradiation.

Spermatogenesis is extremely radiosensitive, where doses as low as <0.5 gray (Gy) are sufficient to cause oligospermia, with full recovery usually being seen between 12 and 48 months following treatment. Fractionated radiation causes more damage than a single dose, with fractions of >2.5 Gy likely to produce azoospermia from 1–2 months following radiotherapy, with variable recovery over a time period of 12–30 months for some men and permanent sterility for others.[55,58] Generally, less mature spermatogonia are more sensitive to radiation than spermatocytes and demonstrate a dose-dependent reduction in numbers.[55]

TBI results in permanent azoospermia for most men, particularly if they have previously received chemotherapy regimens containing significant doses of alkylating agents.[55]

Leydig cell function is more resistant to the effects of radiation than spermatogenesis and so testosterone levels are often unaffected. However, doses of around 20–30 Gy can cause Leydig cell dysfunction, resulting in raised luteinizing hormone (LH) and reduced testosterone levels, especially in prepubertal boys.[59]

Where no systemic cancer therapy is indicated, but pelvic radiotherapy is planned, it may be possible to reduce the total dose of radiation to the testes using the technique of either *testicular shielding* or *testicular transposition*. Testicular shielding can reduce the dose of radiation to the gonads to 1–2% of the total dose delivered, although some scatter radiation may still cause adverse effects on overall spermatogenesis. Where there is no disease-related contraindication and radiotherapy is restricted to the inguinopelvic region, testicular transposition may be used to increase the distance between the testicle and the treatment field, thereby reducing the testicular dose.[60]

Male fertility is also readily damaged through the adverse impact of *chemotherapy* on sperm production. Fortunately, testosterone production is usually preserved, as Leydig cell function is relatively resistant to the action of cytotoxic agents.

Cytotoxic drugs cause reduction in or eradication of germ cell numbers in the testes, particularly where spermatogonia are going through the process of differentiation.[55] Agents proven to be gonadotoxic are the same for both male and female patients, with alkylating agents causing the most severe and irreversible damage on a cumulative dose-dependent basis. Box 31.1 provides a summary of the cytotoxic agents most commonly associated with male and female infertility.

As discussed later in this chapter in relation to female patients, there is considerable individual variation in the extent to which men recover fertility and over what time frame. The potential for recovery is affected by the regimen administered, cumulative dosage of gonadotoxic agents, pretreatment semen quality and the duration of follow-up.[55]

Box 31.1

Chemotherapy agents associated with male and female gonadotoxicity

Cytotoxic agent class/name

Alkylating agents:
Busulfan
BiCNU (carmustine)
CCNU (lomustine)
Chlorambucil
Cyclophosphamide
Ifosfamide
L-phenylalanine mustard
Melphalan
Nitrogen mustard

Vinca alkaloids:
Vinblastine

Antimetabolites:
Cytarabine

Platinum agents:
Cisplatin
Carboplatin

Miscellaneous:
Procarbazine

Female fertility and cancer treatment

Surgical management of gynaecological or other pelvic malignancy may result in permanent infertility due to the loss of ovarian and/or uterine function through operative procedures such as total abdominal hysterectomy, bilateral salpingo-oopherectomy, radical cystectomy or pelvic exenteration.

These women not only have to come to terms with permanent loss of their fertility but also, if both ovaries have been removed, to adjust to the impact of a surgically induced menopause.

While women with later-stage malignancies will still have to undergo radical surgical resection to ensure long-term control or cure of their disease, a relatively new surgical procedure, specifically for early-stage invasive cervical cancer, has been developed called radical trachelectomy.

Radical trachelectomy can be offered to premenopausal women who wish to retain their fertility and who have small-volume, early-stage tumours.[61] Radical trachelectomy entails radical excision of the cervix, together with pelvic lymphadenectomy. The most proximal portion of the cervix, uterus and ovaries are retained, a *cerclage* is placed in the remaining portion of cervix with a large permanent suture and the vaginal mucosa is sutured to the circumference of the cervical stump. Insertion of the cervical suture is necessary to ensure a controlled cervical os capable of retaining any subsequent pregnancy.

Radical trachelectomy is still a relatively new procedure, performed as part of ongoing trials in selected treatment centres to ensure careful evaluation of the technique, and so is not yet widely available throughout Europe. In a small UK study (*n* = 30), successful pregnancies have been achieved following this treatment.[61] In selected women with surgically staged 1 epithelial ovarian cancer, *fertility-sparing surgery* is being undertaken using unilateral oophorectomy. Initial studies indicate good levels of subsequent conception (71%) among those trying to conceive and estimated survival rates of 98% at 5-year follow-up.[62–64] However, caution should be exercised in the interpretation of results from such studies, as the sample size tends to be small (*n* ≤ 52) and results may not prove to be as reliable in larger samples or with longer median follow-up.

Radiotherapy-induced infertility can occur as a result of direct irradiation to the pelvis, resulting in ovarian and uterine damage or as a result of damage to the hypothalamic–pituitary axis,[65] as is the case in total body or cranial irradiation. Due to the radiosensitivity of gonadal tissue, ovarian function can be affected by a dose as small as 1–2 Gy of either direct or scatter irradiation. The overall radiation tolerance of the ovary is adversely affected by a woman's increasing age, a higher total radiation dose and larger fraction size.[66]

Ovarian shielding or *unilateral laparascopic ovarian transposition* may be used to reduce the dose to the ovary, with preservation of both fertility and hormone production. Ovarian transposition involves surgery to lift the ovary out of the pelvis suspended on its ligament, with preservation of an intact blood supply and fixating it temporarily in an area outside the treatment field such as in the paracolic gutter. In one small study, this technique reduced the ovarian dose to an average of 1.75 Gy, with 100% preservation of ovarian function at 2-year follow-up among women aged below 40 years.[67] These techniques can only be used where there is no risk of micro metastases in the ovaries being protected.

Pelvic irradiation also causes damage to the uterus, resulting in reduced uterine muscle elasticity, poor vascular supply to the endometrium and reduced uterine size, particularly when the radiotherapy treatment was administered in childhood. As a consequence, a woman who has preserved fertility may be unable to achieve embryo implantation due to endometrial damage or to carry a pregnancy to term due to the adverse effects on uterine volume.[54]

Theoretically, a woman with preserved ovarian function but a damaged or absent uterus could seek a surrogacy arrangement to allow her to produce a child. However, there are substantial legal and ethical considerations that would have to be considered before such steps were taken and these differ according to the laws of the country where the surrogacy arrangement takes place.

Chemotherapy-induced ovarian failure occurs as a result of depletion in the numbers of primordial follicles in the ovary, leading to a premature menopause. The number of primordial follicles is at its peak around 6 months of intrauterine life and declines throughout infancy and childhood to adulthood.[68] Thus, if a woman receives chemotherapy treatment aged 30–40 years old, when her reserve of remaining oocytes is already diminished, she is more likely to become permanently infertile and to enter a treatment-induced early menopause.[69]

Infertility related to cytotoxic therapy is most commonly associated with combination regimens that include alkylating agents, although a number of other agents are associated with reduced fertility, as outlined in Box 31.1. Although accurate information regarding the dose threshold for permanent infertility from these agents is lacking, it is generally accepted that more intensive or high-dose regimens, the use of multiple gonadotoxic agents in combination regimens such as MOPP (nitrogen mustard, Oncovin (vincristine), procarbazine, prednisolone) and the inclusion of adjuvant radiotherapy below the diaphragm increases the risk of permanent ovarian failure.[68–70] Thus, women receiving bone marrow or stem cell transplantation have a very high risk of ovarian failure, with some studies stating this to be 95–99%, particularly where radiation has been used as part of the conditioning regimen.[71]

In the management of malignancies such as Hodgkin's lymphoma, fertility preservation for male and female patients has been improved through the adoption of alternative chemotherapy regimens that reduce or remove the presence of the most gonadotoxic agents without compromising survival rates. Hybrid regimens where alkylating-containing cycles are alternated with those not containing such agents have been used with some success, as well as the adoption of the regimen ABVD (Adriamycin (doxorubicin) (Doxorubin Rapid Dissolution), bleomycin, vinblastine, dacarbazine), resulting in reduced gonadal damage among men and younger women under 30 years old. Ovarian function may recover up to 2–3 years post-treatment in younger women, while women aged 40 years old or older with treatment-induced amenorrhoea are unlikely to recover ovarian function and should be offered hormone replacement therapy (HRT) unless medically contraindicated.[51]

Reproductive technology techniques in cancer care

The range of fertility preservation approaches are more limited for women than for men, with a number of reproductive technologies remaining experimental at the time of writing.

Cryopreservation of sperm

Cryopreservation of sperm (sometimes referred to as sperm banking) remains the most commonly adopted technique for the preservation of male fertility associated with cancer treatment.

Men should be referred for sperm banking before commencement of treatment and 2 ejaculates obtained for storage, preferably at a 2–3 day interval to maximize the quality of the samples obtained. In the UK, it is usual to store sperm samples for an initial period of 10 years,

although this period is renewable until the man reaches the age of 55 years. The semen is stored in 0.5 ml samples taken from a usual 3 ml donation. The outcome of semen cryopreservation is a reported pregnancy rate of 25% with each sample when intrauterine insemination is used.[72]

Even sperm that is of poor quality (low sperm count or motility sometimes associated with testicular, lymphoid and leukaemic malignancies) can result in a fertilization rate of 60% through the use of reproductive techniques such as in vitro fertilization (IVF) with intracytoplasmic sperm injection (ICSI). Thus, only azoospermic semen samples should be rejected for cryopreservation.[73]

If the man is unable to produce a semen sample, it is theoretically possible to obtain sperm for cryopreservation through direct sperm aspiration from the testes, although there are practical considerations in undertaking such a procedure: for example, in relation to the effects of the presenting disease (e.g. thrombocytopenia).[51]

Despite the recent increase in semen samples suitable for cryopreservation, currently in the UK only 1 in 10 samples stored are subsequently used. There are a number of reasons for this low figure. Recent research suggests that 41% of patients discontinued storage because their fertility had recovered, resulting in pregnancy; 37% of patients had died; 14% had regained good sperm quality; and 7% had decided they did not wish to have children.[74]

Cryopreservation of testicular tissue

This technique remains experimental at the time of writing and is reserved for men or boys who are unable to provide a semen sample for cryopreservation of sperm. There is particular interest within paediatric oncology in the potential of this technique to preserve future fertility for boys or adolescents undergoing cancer treatment that will render them sterile. However, there are a number of ethical and legal issues that remain to be resolved quite apart from the technical advances that must be made.[75]

Cryopreservation of embryos

Cryopreservation of embryos is the only established technique for women and requires the presence of a fertile male partner in order to create an embryo. This technique may therefore not be available to those outside a committed relationship. Also, it normally takes up to 1 month to retrieve sufficient suitable eggs after ovulation induction; such a delay may be inadvisable where treatment is considered urgent.[68] While success rates vary between fertility centres, 15–20% conception rates per cycle of IVF are generally reported.[76]

Cryopreservation of oocytes

Cryopreservation of oocytes is as yet not as successful in preserving fertility potential due to the low number of oocytes that survive the freeze–thaw process (25–40%), resulting in a live birth rate of only 1% per thawed oocyte.[70] This is an ongoing area of active research to improve the freeze–thaw technique.

Cryopreservation of ovarian cortex

This procedure is being carried out in some centres by laparoscopic retrieval of ovarian cortex strips or the whole ovary for cryopreservation. Theoretically, it may be possible to mature the follicles following reimplantation of the ovarian tissue into the abdominal or pelvic cavity or forearm of the patient following cessation of treatment, thus restoring ovarian function and fertility. At the time of writing, this procedure remains experimental, with no pregnancies resulting from this technique as yet. There is also concern that reimplanted tissue could harbour viral agents or malignant cells that would also survive the freeze–thaw process.[68]

Gonadotrophin hormone releasing hormone antagonists

The use of gonadotrophin hormone releasing hormone (GnHRH) antagonists to suppress and protect ovarian function has been reported, but as yet without success in preserving adequate numbers of primordial follicles, although research is ongoing.[68]

Egg donation

As one can see, the options available for female patients are both complex and more limited, and some women may wish to consider alternatives such as egg donation or adoption.

Egg donation is the most successful technique for women with chemotherapy-induced infertility, with a success rate of approximately 40% per cycle in the best fertility centres. Donors are normally required to be under 35 years old, whereas the recipient can be up to 50 years old. Despite these advantages, the availability of donors is generally poor, particularly in countries where no payment is made for egg donation. Furthermore, as hormone support is normally provided for the first trimester of any pregnancy, women with oestrogen positive breast cancer may be ill advised to attempt pregnancy using this approach.[72] As discussed previously, women who have had uterine irradiation are also unlikely to sustain a pregnancy to term, including women who have had TBI, due to reduced uterine elasticity and blood flow.

PSYCHOSEXUAL ASSESSMENT IN CANCER CARE

In conducting a comprehensive assessment of sexual difficulties experienced by the person with cancer, it is important to place disease- and treatment-related issues in the context of that person's pre-illness sexuality. As discussed previously, there is considerable diversity in human sexuality and the ways in which sexual behaviours may be expressed. Any assessment must take account of individual patient and couple norms, values and established sexual repertoire if subsequent biomedical and psychological interventions to promote sexual well-being are to be appropriate.

A number of personal and social factors determine the degree of comfort individuals have with regard to sexual issues: this applies to healthcare professionals as well as to the patients or couples they encounter in clinical practice. Such factors are also influential in determining the range or diversity of sexual behaviours an individual considers part of their accepted sexual repertoire at any given point in time. Table 31.3 provides a summary of some of the factors that influence how individuals view their sexual identity, role and sexual behaviour.

There are two principal challenges to health professionals working in cancer care who endeavour to conduct a comprehensive sexual assessment in clinical practice:

Table 31.3: Factors influencing attitudes to and engagement in sexual expression	
Individual/family factors	**Social factors**
Restricted upbringing	Cultural beliefs
Avoidance of discussion of sexual issues in family	Influence of subcultures (gay scene)
Traditional/negative attitudes to sex	Religious influences (virginity, contraception, masturbation, adultery)
Prejudice, e.g. towards sexual diversity	
Lack of prior sexual experience	Gender roles
Negative sexual experiences, e.g. childhood sexual abuse, sexual assault or rape	Sexual stereotyping
Personality: introvert/extrovert	Sexual harassment
Mental and physical illness	Sexual myths
Physical or learning disability	Legal controls regarding sexual behaviour, e.g. age of consent Ageism Impact of media images Environment (lack of privacy)

1 The person with cancer enters a healthcare setting in order to have their cancer treated, not to discuss their sexual health. It is likely that the patient has not had an opportunity to consider any cancer-related alterations in sexual function due to the overwhelming focus on their potential for survival and how to cope with the acute side-effects of treatment.[77]

2 Even prior to treatment commencement, it is almost impossible to obtain a baseline assessment of normal sexual functioning and satisfaction for the patient and their partner. We only encounter patients post-diagnosis, when even the knowledge they have cancer may alter that person's perception of their sexuality and gender identity. Furthermore, many patients will have experienced symptoms that have already modified their sexual frequency or expression, e.g. vaginal discharge/bleeding, unilateral testicular enlargement or intermittent ED associated with prostate cancer.

It is difficult to broach the subject of sexual health when the priority of care is rightly cancer control or cure and effective treatment delivery not the sexual consequences of disease or treatment.

Further challenges are encountered when one considers the changes in cancer service provision from longer inpatient admissions to short stay, outpatient or day-care contexts. This may alter the rapport between the patient, their partner and the health professional, often considered a necessary prerequisite for the discussion of sensitive or intimate personal issues. Particular attention needs to be paid to the clinical environment when embarking upon a discussion of sexual issues to ensure adequate privacy and to reduce the likelihood of interruptions.

Box 31.2 provides a summary of the areas of enquiry covered in a thorough sexual assessment prior to embarking on psychosexual therapy or a specific biomedical intervention.[78] Such an assessment leads to the development of a *formulation* of the sexual problem and incorporates an initial evaluation of specific *predisposing, precipitating and maintaining factors* for the sexual difficulty as experienced by the individual or couple.[78]

In cancer care it is not usually necessary to conduct such an in-depth assessment where there is clear evidence that the sexual difficulty experienced by the patient has arisen as a direct result of cancer or its treatment. The items in Box 31.2 in bold type are the assessment details most likely to be of direct relevance to the multidisciplinary team in reaching a decision regarding both the nature of the patient's sexual difficulty and what is likely to be the most appropriate intervention and/or route of referral.

There are sexual assessment models that lend themselves to direct use in cancer care: one such model is **ALARM** (Box 31.3).[79] Although the **ALARM** model has not been specifically validated for use in a cancer setting, it does provide a clear and familiar structure to guide sexual assessment within the clinical environment.

It is imperative that any sexual assessment undertaken in cancer care takes account of the specific client group and treatments, the nature of sexual difficulties commonly encountered, the skills of personnel conducting the assessment and the resources available within that care context for sexual health interventions or for making an appropriate referral.

While it is recognized that some practitioners may be embarrassed discussing sexual issues with patients, the most useful approach from a patient perspective is for the professional to address their questions in a direct yet sensitive manner. Such a direct approach not only normalizes the patient's sexual life, it legitimizes the patient's sexuality as a recognized aspect of quality of life and recovery from cancer. The use of direct questions also gives the patient a form of words or vocabulary that both can then use to explore specific sexual concerns and likely causes.[80]

Box 31.2

Talking about sex – sexual history taking

- **Nature of presenting sexual difficulty**
- **History of present sexual difficulty**
- Individual sexual development (masturbation, first sexual encounter, sexual orientation)
- Relationship history (including detail of children from previous relationships)
- **Current relationship: nature and duration**
- **Current sexual relationship and impact of current sexual difficulty**
- **History of sexual abuse/sexual trauma**
- Family history (religious, cultural, parental, gender roles, family relationships)
- Individual history (schooling, education, occupation, employment)
- Concurrent life events (marriage, pregnancy, relationship breakdown, bereavement, other losses, redundancy, retirement)
- **Previous physical, mental and sexual health (including prior surgery, medication or therapy/counselling)**
- **Medication history (prescription drugs and social drugs – alcohol, tobacco, cannabis, other recreational drugs or substances)**

Box 31.3

The ALARM model	
Activity	Types of sexual behaviours, form of sexual relationships (heterosexual, homosexual, bisexual)
Libido	Changes from normal level or pattern of sexual desire. How important is this? Is the person satisfied with current situation?
Arousal	Are there any difficulties in attaining or maintaining an erection? Does vaginal lubrication occur normally? Are there emotional or relationship difficulties as a result?
Resolution	Is the nature or intensity of orgasm satisfying? Are there any problems with pain or discomfort during/after intercourse?
Medical history	Are there prior physical or mental problems that need to be explored? What medication (if any) is the person taking? Any concurrent illness?

It remains the responsibility of the healthcare professional to raise the subject of sexual concerns with the patient as an integral part of informed consent for treatment.[81] This must be approached sensitively, individualizing the information giving and support processes. Sensitivity is of particular importance, as the pretreatment period is often a time of considerable anxiety, with the potential for both information overload and difficulty in retaining what has been discussed.

Readers may wish to consult White[82] for a useful summary of ways to overcome or manage the discomfort some practitioners feel when considering this domain of cancer practice.

Levels of psychosexual intervention in cancer nursing practice

There are no accurate statistics for the prevalence of sexual difficulties internationally let alone the prevalence of sexual difficulties encountered among people affected by cancer. From clinical experience it would seem reasonable to assume that while some patients with sexual concerns may still go unrecognized, the majority of those receiving cancer treatment do not require intensive psychosexual intervention. Such assumptions are based on the spectrum of sexual difficulties encountered in the general population and the fact that many individuals and couples appear to resolve their own difficulties with little or no professional assistance.

The **P-LI-SS-IT** model, developed by an American psychosexual therapist, incorporates levels of psychosexual intervention, and has been used extensively within nursing literature both in America and Europe.[83] Although originally intended as a cognitive-behavioural programme to use with those experiencing sexual dysfunction, Annon's model[83] has been adapted to represent the different levels of clinical intervention provided by nurses based on the complexity of sexual difficulty experienced by the patient and on the level of skill and knowledge needed from the nurse. Box 31.4 offers a summary of this model, with examples of the appropriate level of clinical intervention normally available from nurses in cancer care.

Cancer nurses, by virtue of their detailed knowledge of the impact of common cancer therapies and of the psychological responses experienced by patients, together with the judicious use of advanced communication skills, should normally be able to offer the first two levels of intervention in this model. Cancer nurses should aim to create an environment or culture of **P**ermission and be able to offer **L**imited **I**nformation regarding the specific sexual effects of commonly encountered cancer treatments and their management.

As seen in Box 31.4, **S**pecific **S**uggestions are more often the province of clinical nurse specialists, requiring a greater depth of knowledge and advanced clinical assessment, communication and counselling skills in order to address the more complex psychosexual responses patients may have to the effects of both illness and treatment. **I**ntensive **T**herapy remains the province of health or therapy professionals who have undergone additional postgraduate education in psychosexual medicine or therapy. It is this latter level of intervention that is discussed in more detail within the next section of this chapter.

Specialist interventions for psychosexual health in cancer care

As has been discussed in the previous section, many patients will benefit from timely and sensitively delivered information regarding sexual difficulties encountered during or following cancer treatment. Likewise, the routine provision of treatment-specific interventions such as vaginal dilators and advice regarding vaginal lubrication can reduce the likelihood of long-term side-effects that have a detrimental impact on the future sexual health of the patient and her partner.

However, even when patient information and support is available, there may be some patients who would benefit from specialist psychosexual interventions to restore their sexual well-being.

Loss of sexual interest/desire

Although the cause of reduced sexual interest in people with cancer is often multifactorial, where there is evidence of treatment-induced ovarian or testicular failure contributing to the loss of sexual desire, patients may benefit from

Box 31.4

P-LI-SS-IT model in cancer care

Permission:
- Inclusive organizational culture
- Equal opportunity policy enforced regarding sexual orientation of patients/staff
- Intolerance of sexual harassment
- Respect for patient privacy in clinical environment
- Controlled professional disclosure of sensitive information, verbally and in documentation
- Inclusion of questions related to sexual concerns within patient assessment
- Nurse-initiated discussion of sexual concerns
- Provision of patient information leaflets related to sexual issues in clinical environment

Limited **I**nformation:
- Provision of information regarding specific impact of cancer treatment on sexual expression (e.g. loss of sexual desire as result of antiandrogen therapy in prostate cancer treatment, provision of vaginal dilator and lubrication advice for women receiving pelvic radiotherapy)
- Contraceptive advice during chemotherapy
- Awareness of sexual side-effects of commonly encountered drugs (e.g. antihypertensives and erectile dysfunction (ED), antidepressants and loss of sexual desire)
- Rationale for and routes of specialist referral to sexual health services in local area (e.g. ED services, local psychosexual counsellors, infertility counselling and reproductive health services)

Specific **S**uggestions:
- Alternative positions for sexual intercourse for patients with illness or treatment-induced sexual difficulties (e.g. female superior position for women with reduced vaginal length post-Wertheim's hysterectomy or for a man experiencing excessive breathlessness secondary to lung cancer)
- Non-coital sexual expression approaches (mutual masturbation, use of sexual aids) for a couple who can no longer achieve intercourse due to effects of illness/treatment
- Limited knowledge of biomedical interventions or devices for specific sexual difficulties (e.g. sildenafil or vacuum constriction devices for ED)

Intensive **T**herapy
- Provision of psychosexual therapy
- Extensive knowledge and provision of a range of biomedical interventions and devices related to the management of most commonly encountered female and male sexual difficulties

Source: Adapted from Annon.[83]

HRT unless there is a medical contraindication, such as the presence of a hormone-dependent malignancy.[39]

If it is thought that loss of sexual interest is predominantly associated with psychological responses to the effects of illness, such as concurrent depression or altered self-concept, or to treatment-induced fatigue, then the patient may benefit from a short programme of psychosexual therapy (6–10 sessions).

Psychosexual therapy is offered through a variety of publicly funded and private health services and typically follows an adapted cognitive-behavioural approach such as that recommended by Masters and Johnson[84] or Kaplan.[85] Psychosexual therapy addresses the psychological, physical and relationship aspects of the sexual difficulty, working with an individual or couple to promote greater understanding and to enhance communication and sexual adaptation. Most psychosexual therapy programmes incorporate the three components of:

- education/re-education regarding sexual myths and 'normal' sexual expression within the context of health and illness

- behavioural 'tasks' for the individual/couple to perform at home to improve trust and communication and to re-establish or modify their sexual repertoire to adapt to illness- or treatment-induced limitations

- counselling to support the individual/couple through the challenge of overcoming blocks to progress.

Figure 31.2 provides a summary of psychosexual interventions. For a more detailed discussion of psychosexual therapy, readers are advised to consult texts such as Hawton[78] or Crowe and Ridley.[86]

Erectile dysfunction

There are a variety of treatments available for the management of ED, as outlined in Table 31.4. Even when there is clear evidence of organic dysfunction, as in the case of ED arising following radical prostatectomy, there is usually a psychological response of varying intensity to that altered function. It is this psychological response and that of the partner that can be explored and modified through counselling or psychosexual therapy, often combined with a biomedical intervention for the management of organic ED.

Although some older men ask about penile prostheses, such devices are normally considered the last resort when other methods have failed to restore a satisfactory erection. This is because the insertion of semi-rigid or inflatable penile implants requires the removal of both corpora cavernosa, thus removing any significant contribution from the patient's residual erectile function.[87]

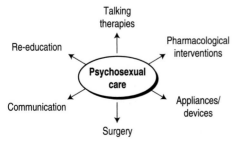

Figure 31.2: Summary of psychosexual interventions.

Vaginal stenosis/vaginal dryness

Vaginal stenosis associated with pelvic radiotherapy, or vaginal shortening associated with Wertheim's hysterectomy, is commonly encountered in clinical practice, although the impact on female sexual functioning remains poorly evaluated in long-term follow-up studies. There is no empirical evidence to confirm the benefit of vaginal dilation, as vaginal toxicity tends to be poorly monitored post-radiotherapy.[88] Limited research and anecdotal evidence from clinical nurse specialists in gynaecological oncology state that women they work with report low levels of compliance with vaginal dilatation advice.[44] The extent to which vaginal dilation prevents the development of vaginal stenosis remains unknown; this is an area for further research. Within Europe, there is no consistency regarding technique or duration of dilatation, and standardization of this intervention would be the first step towards conducting a multicentre trial into the efficacy of vaginal dilation in pelvic radiotherapy care.

Women who experience vaginal dryness, regardless of aetiology, require advice in relation to vaginal lubrication or the use of topical oestrogen. It is recognized that even where HRT has been provided to ameliorate the symptoms of a treatment-induced menopause, many women report that the symptom least likely to respond is that of vaginal dryness. There are a number of vaginal moisturizers and lubricants on the market that can be used, some of which have a more natural and long-lasting lubrication preferred by women. Oestrogen cream remains controversial for women who may be at risk from the theoretical possibility of systemic absorption. Topical oestrogen cream can be useful where vulvo-vaginitis associated with premature menopause has occurred. In severe cases of vaginal stenosis it may be necessary to perform a vaginoplasty to create vaginal patency. However, this situation is best avoided, as there is an increased risk of poor tissue healing due to prior irradiation damage to microcirculation.[89]

Absent vagina due to pelvic exenteration

Vaginal reconstruction can be performed, as mentioned in Table 31.5, and may be considered a priority by some women. Others are

Table 31.4: Interventions for the management of male sexual difficulties in cancer care

Sexual difficulty	Psychosexual intervention
Loss of sexual desire	Testosterone replacement therapy (oral or transdermal patches) Psychosexual therapy
Erectile dysfunction	Oral medication (sildenafil, tadalafil, vardenafil, apomorphine) Alprostadil urethral pellet (MUSE: medicated urethral system for erections) Intracavernosal injection of alprostadil Vacuum constriction devices Penile implants/prostheses (last resort) Psychosexual therapy
Delayed/absent orgasm/ejaculation	Psychosexual therapy Review antidepressants Treat concurrent anxiety Vibrators
Painful ejaculation	Patient/couple education
Decreased semen volume	Rule out persistent underlying cause: e.g. infection, inflammation
Retrograde ejaculation	Patient/couple education
Partial/total penile amputation	Psychosexual therapy Penile reconstruction (if feasible)

either too ill or have concurrent medical problems that make this extensive reconstructive work impossible. Whether or not a neovagina is created, it is often helpful for these women to receive psychosexual therapy to broaden their sexual repertoire and to discover other areas of their bodies from which they can gain sexual sensation and pleasure. The same applies to women who have had their clitoris removed through radical vulvectomy. As there may be some clitoral tissue remaining, the woman can experiment with touch and vibrators to elicit sexual stimulation from her vulval area as well as other erogenous zones in the body.

Dyspareunia

Dyspareunia can be defined as being 'deep' or 'superficial', depending on where in the vulva or vagina the discomfort or pain is felt.[78] Surface discomfort in the vagina or vulva can be alleviated by adequate lubrication, if caused by vaginal dryness, fragile vaginal mucosa or vulvovaginitis. If the vaginal introitus is tight, then gentle dilation may help to stretch the tissues and make penetration more comfortable. If it is caused by loss of support/padding to the vagina or by the development of fibrotic plaques associated with extensive pelvic surgery, then women may benefit from guidance regarding alternative positions for intercourse where the rate and depth of penetration is more under the woman's control. Table 31.5 provides an outline of the management of dyspareunia.

Anorgasmia

The inability to have an orgasm may be associated with high levels of anxiety related to diagnosis, prognosis or treatment. In this situation, psychosexual or general counselling coupled with relaxation exercises may help the woman to relax sufficiently to permit orgasm to occur.[78] In

Table 31.5: Interventions for the management of female sexual difficulties in cancer care

Sexual difficulty	Psychosexual intervention
Reduced sexual desire	Hormone replacement therapy (oral, topical or transdermal patches) Psychosexual therapy
Reduced vaginal lubrication	Topical oestrogen to vagina/vulva Vaginal lubricants
Vaginal stenosis or shortening	Vaginal dilators or vibrators Alternative sexual positions to control rate and depth of penetration (female superior or side-lying)
Painful intercourse	Alternative sexual positions to control rate and depth of penetration (female superior or side-lying) Vaginal lubricants
Delayed or absent orgasm	Psychosexual therapy Review antidepressants Treat concurrent anxiety Clitoral stimulation devices Vibrators
Absent vagina	Surgical creation of neovagina from myocutaneous flaps or segment of colon (if feasible) Psychosexual therapy
Absent clitoris	Identification and development of alternative erogenous zones for orgasm Psychosexual therapy

some instances a small dose of an anxiolytic medication may assist the process and if the woman is receiving antidepressant therapy that is potentially contributing to a lack of orgasm then this medication may be altered or reduced with some effect. Some women benefit from provision of a clitoral stimulation device or vibrator to improve the quality and regularity of orgasm.[78] The management of retarded ejaculation in men adopts similar principles.

Ejaculatory problems

Absent ejaculation as a result of radical prostatectomy can alter orgasmic sensation or quality for a man and can also cause concern regarding the lack of an obvious emission for himself or in relation to his partner's response. Patient education about the anatomical changes resulting from surgery is important in promoting adjustment to this altered function. Some men also benefit from psychosexual counselling in order to explore what this altered orgasmic sensation means to them and to explore alternative erogenous zones and enhanced orgasmic sensations through the use of vibrators.[90]

Painful ejaculation and blood in the ejaculate may be associated with trauma or inflammation of the urethra or prostate gland as a result of prostatic biopsy, surgery (transurethral resection of the prostate or TURP) or radiotherapy. The symptoms usually diminish as tissue healing takes place in the weeks following completion of treatment. Persistence of such a symptom may indicate an underlying infection that requires investigation and treatment.

FUTURE DEVELOPMENTS IN PSYCHOSEXUAL AND REPRODUCTIVE HEALTH FOR PEOPLE AFFECTED BY CANCER

Cancer nursing remains a vibrant and progressive speciality, with opportunities for role and service development as a result of both healthcare policy and treatment advances. As cancer treatment continues to improve and long-term survival becomes a reality for increasing numbers of patients, there is likely to be a corresponding increase in demand for both psychosexual and fertility services in oncology. Thus, it follows that cancer nurses who offer advanced practice interventions in these domains of care will also be in demand.

A question remains over the extent to which advanced clinical nursing roles reflect the dominant biomedical agenda in cancer care as

Table 31.6: Enhancing the evidence base for psychosexual and reproductive practice in cancer care

Psychosexual research	Reproductive research
Prevalence of psychosexual difficulties in different patient groups	Threshold for ovarian failure following chemotherapy or radiotherapy
Defining 'at-risk' individuals/patient groups to target psychosexual interventions Prospective, longitudinal and multicentre studies of psychosexual difficulties in cancer care	Threshold for testicular failure following chemotherapy or radiotherapy
Development of resarch instruments and methodologies that have been validated within a cancer population	Development and evaluation of fertility-sparing treatment regimens in all treatment modalities
Combination of self-report and physiological measurements of sexual function where possible Standardization of sexual dysfunction definitions in research	Development of improved tissue cryopreservation techniques
Comparison of biomedical management of sexual difficulties vs an integrated biomedical and psychosexual therapy approach Integrated treatment toxicity and psychosexual assessment	Development of techniques to detect residual disease in ovarian or testicular tissue grafts
Impact of psychosexual difficulties on relationship dynamic and partners Vaginal toxicity evaluation in pelvic radiotherapy Evaluation of psychosexual therapy techniques within a cancer patient population	Improved follicle culture technology Larger clinical studies of gonadotrophin releasing hormone antagonists for protection of ovarian or testicular function following chemotherapy

opposed to contributing to skilled psychosocial support for patients and their partners. Patient information, counselling and treatment interventions associated with psychosexual and fertility practice remain an important element of psychosocial or supportive cancer care provision.

In England, an ambitious policy agenda, The National Cancer Plan,[91] is driving modernization of cancer services after years of underinvestment. A key feature of this modernization is greater emphasis on the centrally funded provision of supportive cancer care services, with the aim of enhancing patient experience at all stages of the cancer journey.[93]

It is imperative that the management of iatrogenic sexual or reproductive dysfunction is considered a part of mainstream service provision in contemporary cancer care, and associated funding of these services should be included in business plans for cancer centres. A secure funding base can promote standardization of services and create a more integrated approach to the management of both psychosexual and fertility concerns.[93]

From a research perspective, there is a need for improved funding for studies that address the psychosexual and reproductive impact of cancer and its management, particularly in groups that have received limited study to date. Such groups include patients diagnosed with cancers that do not affect parts of the body traditionally associated with sexual expression, such as head and neck cancer, cerebral tumours or haematological malignancies.[92] The psychosexual support and information needs of older men with pelvic malignancies, together with an understanding of the impact on the couple relationship, are also poorly understood. Psychosexual research in other groups suggests that the couple dynamic is important for both adjustment to residual psychosexual difficulties and for compliance with psychological or biomedical interventions.

Improving the quality and quantity of the evidence base for psychosexual and reproductive practice within oncology is central to improved standards in supportive cancer care. To this end, Table 31.6 offers suggestions regarding improvements to the existing evidence base.

CONCLUSION

Future education of cancer nurses must promote an increased awareness of the sexual and reproductive consequences of cancer and its treatment, coupled with improvements in the advanced communication skills necessary to discuss sensitive or emotionally laden aspects of cancer care and patient choice. Some advanced practitioners in cancer care may wish to develop the specialist knowledge and skills associated with infertility counselling or psychosexual therapy in order to boost the scarce resource of psychosocial care provision in Europe.

The majority of people affected by cancer do not need specialist psychosexual interventions: they need a knowledgeable and comfortable practitioner who is able to hear their concerns and to respond in a professional and informed manner.[2,3,13]

REFERENCES

1. Grigg E. Post HIV/AIDS: emergence of a new morality In: Heath H, White I, eds. The challenge of sexuality in health care. Oxford: Blackwell Science; 2002.

2. Heath H, White I. The challenge of sexuality in health care. Oxford: Blackwell Science; 2002.

3. Wells D, ed. Caring for sexuality in health and illness. Edinburgh: Churchill Livingstone; 2000.

4. White ID. Nursing as a sexualised occupation. In: Heath H, White I, eds. The challenge of sexuality in health care. Oxford: Blackwell Science; 2002.

5. Segal L. Sensual uncertainty, or why the clitoris is not enough. In: Crowley H, Himmelweit S, eds. Knowing women: feminism and knowledge. Cambridge: Polity Press; 1992.

6. Bancroft J. Human sexuality and its problems. 2nd edn. Edinburgh: Churchill Livingstone; 1989.

7. Kinsey AC, Pomeroy WB, Martin CF. Sexual behavior in the human male. 1948. Cited in: Bancroft J. Human sexuality and its problems. 2nd edn. Edinburgh: Churchill Livingstone; 1989.

8. Kinsey AC, Pomeroy WB, Martin CF, Gebhard PH. Sexual behavior in the human female. 1953. Cited in: Bancroft J. Human sexuality and its problems. 2nd edn. Edinburgh: Churchill Livingstone; 1989.

9. Masters WH, Johnson VE. Human sexual response. London: Churchill Livingstone; 1966.

10. Foucault M. The history of sexuality: Vol. 1: an introduction. London: Penguin Books; 1979.

11. Wellings K. Perceptions of risk – media treatment of AIDS. In: Aggleton P, Homans H, eds. Social aspects of AIDS. London: The Falmer Press; 1988.

12. Lawler J. Behind the screens: nursing, somology and the problem of the body. Edinburgh: Churchill Livingstone; 1991.

13. Schover L. Sexuality and fertility after cancer. New York: John Wiley and Sons; 1997.

14. Leiblum SR. Reconsidering gender differences in sexual desire: an update. Sexual and Relationship Therapy 2002; 17(1):57–68.

15. Basson R. Biopsychosocial models of women's sexual response: applications to management of 'desire disorders'. Sexual and Relationship Therapy 2003; 18(1):107–115.

16. Kelly D. Male sexuality in theory and practice. Nurs Clin North Am 2004; 39:341–356.

17. Krishnasamy M. Anxiety and depression. In: Corner J, Bailey C, eds. Cancer nursing: care in context. Oxford: Blackwell Science; 2001.

18. Benbow SM, Jagus CE. Sexuality in older women with mental health problems. Sexual and Relationship Therapy 2002; 17(3):261–270.

19. Pesce V, Seidman SN, Roose SP. Depression, antidepressants and sexual functioning in men. Sexual and Relationship Therapy 2002; 17(3):281–287.

20. Juraskova I, Butow P, Robertson R, et al. Post-treatment sexual adjustment following cervical and endometrial cancer: a qualitative insight. Psychooncology 2003; 12:267–279.

21. Hordern A. Intimacy and sexuality for the woman with breast cancer. Cancer Nurs 2000; 23(3):230–236.

22. Wilmoth MC. The aftermath of breast cancer: an altered sexual self. Cancer Nurs 2001; 24(4):278–285.

23. Shell JA, Miller ME. The cancer amputee and sexuality. Orthopaed Nurs 1999; Sept/Oct:53–64.

24. Woodford J. Women's experiences of limb salvage surgery for the treatment of sarcoma. Proc RCN 2nd Biennial Joint Cancer Conference: a journey through cancer: choices and dilemmas, York; 2003.

25. Roberts H. Sexuality expression for people with disfigurement. In: Heath H, White ID, eds. The challenge of sexuality in health care. Oxford: Blackwell Science; 2002.

26. Bruner DW, Boyd CP. Assessing women's sexuality after cancer therapy: checking assumptions with the focus group technique. Cancer Nurs 1999; 21(6):438–447.

27. Katz A. Sexuality after hysterectomy: a review of the literature and discussion of nurse's role. J Adv Nurs 2003; 42(3):297–303.

28. Gotheridge SM, Dresner N. Psychological adjustment to gynecologic cancer. Primary Care Update in Obstet Gynecol 2002; 9(2)80–84.

29. Gossfeld LM, Cullen ML. Sexuality and fertility issues. In: Moore GJ, ed. Women and cancer: a gynecologic oncology nursing perspective. Boston: Jones and Bartlett; 1997.

30. Auchincloss SS. After treatment: psychosocial issues in gynecologic cancer survivorship. Cancer Suppl 1995; 76(10):2117–2124.

31. Potosky AL, Legler J, Albertsen PC, et al. Health outcomes after prostatectomy or radiotherapy for prostate cancer: Results from the Prostate Cancer Outcomes Study. J Natl Cancer Inst 2000; 92(19):1582–1591.

32. National Institute for Clinical Excellence. Improving outcomes in urological cancers: the manual. London: NICE; 2002.

33. Banerjee AK. Sexual dysfunction after surgery for rectal cancer. Lancet 1999; 353:1900–1901.

34. Allal AS, Bieri S, Pelloni A, et al. Sphincter-sparing surgery after preoperative radiotherapy for low rectal cancers: feasibility, oncologic results and quality of life outcomes. Br J Cancer 2000; 82(6):1131–1137.

35. Wingard JR, Curbow B, Baker F, Zabora J, Piantadosi S. Sexual satisfaction in survivors of bone marrow transplantation. Bone Marrow Transplant 1992; 9:185–190.

36. Lesko LM Psychiatric aspects of bone marrow transplantation: Part 2: Life beyond transplant, Psycho-oncology 1993; 2:185–193.

37. Marks DI, Crilley P, Nezu CM, Nezu AM. Sexual dysfunction prior to high-dose chemotherapy and bone marrow transplantation. Bone Marrow Transplant 1996; 17:595–599.

38. Knobf MT. The menopausal symptom experience in young mid-life women with breast cancer. Cancer Nurs 2001; 24(3):201–210.

39. Rogers M, Kristjanson LJ. The impact on sexual functioning of chemotherapy-induced menopause in women with breast cancer. Cancer Nurs 2002; 25(1):57–65.

40. Hamilton AS, Stanford JL, Gilliland FD, et al. Health outcomes after external-beam radiation therapy for clinically localized prostate cancer: results from the Prostate Cancer Outcomes Study. J Clin Oncol 2001; 19(9):2517–2526.

41. Bergmark K, Avall-Lundqvist E, Dickman PW, Henningsohn L, Steineck G. Vaginal changes and sexuality in women with a history of cervical cancer. N Engl J Med 1999; 340(18):1383–1389.

42. Katz A, Njunguna E, Rakowsky E, et al. Early development of vaginal shortening during radiation therapy for endometrial or cervical cancer. Int J Gynecol Cancer 2001; 11:234–235.

43. Schubert MA, Sullivan KM, Schubert MM, et al. Gynecological abnormalities following allogeneic

bone marrow transplantation. Bone Marrow Transplant 1990; 5:425–430.

44. Robinson JW, Faris PD, Scott CB. Psychoeducational group increases vaginal dilation for younger women and reduces sexual fears for women of all ages with gynaecological carcinoma treated with radiotherapy. Int J Radiat Oncol Biol Phys 1999; 44(3):497–506.

45. Searle E. Sexuality and people who are dying. In: Heath H, White ID, eds. The challenge of sexuality in health care. Oxford: Blackwell Science; 2002.

46. Schover LR. Sexual rehabilitation after treatment for prostate cancer. Cancer Suppl 1993; 71(3):1024 –1230.

47. Chen CT, Valicenti RK, Lu J, et al. Does hormonal therapy influence sexual function in men receiving 3D conformal radiation therapy for prostate cancer? Int J Radiat Oncol Biol Phys 2001; 50(3)591–595.

48. Kelly D. In the company of men: embodiment and prostate cancer. Unpublished Doctoral Thesis, Goldsmiths College, University of London; 2002.

49. Kunkel EJ, Chen EI, Okunlola TB. Psychosocial concerns of women with breast cancer. Primary Care Update in Obstet Gynaecol 2002; 9(4):129–134.

50. Berglund G, Nystedt M, Bolund C, Sjoden P, Rutquist L. Effect of endocrine treatment on sexuality in premenopausal breast cancer patients: a prospective randomized study. J Clin Oncol 2001; 19(11):2788–2796.

51. Bahadur G. Fertility issues for cancer patients. Mol Cell Endocrinol 2000; 169:117–122.

52. Wilford H, Hunt J. An overview of sperm cryopreservation services for adolescent cancer patients in the United Kingdom. Eur J Oncol Nurs 2003; 7(1):24–32.

53. Kinsella TJ, Trivette G, Rowland J, et al. Long term follow up of testicular function following radiation therapy for early-stage Hodgkin's disease. J Clin Oncol 1989; 7:718–724.

54. Waring AB, Wallace WH. Subfertility following treatment for childhood cancer. Hosp Med 2000; 61(8):550–557.

55. Giwercman A, Petersen PM. Cancer and male infertility. Baillière's Best Pract Res Clin Endocrinol Metab 2000; 14(3):453–471.

56. Quinn B, Kelly D. Sperm banking and fertility concerns: enhancing practice and the support available to men with cancer. Eur J Oncol Nurs 2000; 4(1):55–58.

57. Read J. Counselling for fertility problems. London: Sage Publications; 1995.

58. Centola GM, Keller JW, Henzler M, Rubin P. Effect of low-dose testicular irradiation on sperm count and fertility in patients with testicular seminoma. J Androl 1994; 15:608–613.

59. Shalet SM. Effect of irradiation treatment on gonadal function in men treated for germ cell cancer. Eur Urol 1993; 23:148–152.

60. Deo SVS, Asthana S, Shukla NK, et al. Fertility preserving testicular transposition in patients undergoing inguino pelvic irradiation. J Surg Oncol 2001; 76:70–72.

61. Shepherd JH, Mould T, Oram DH. Radical trachelectomy in early stage carcinoma of the cervix: outcome as judged by recurrence and fertility rates. Br J Obstet Gynaecol 2001; 108:882–885.

62. Schilder JM, Thompson AM, DePriest PD, et al. Outcome of reproductive age women with stage Ia or Ic invasive epithelial ovarian cancer treated with fertility-sparing therapy. Gynecol Oncol 2002; 87:1–7.

63. Morice P, Wicart-Poque F, Rey A, et al. Results of conservative treatment in epithelial ovarian carcinoma. Cancer 2001; 92: 2412–2418.

64. Brown CL, Dharmendra B, Barakat R. Preserving fertility in patients with epithelial ovarian cancer: the role of conservative surgery in the treatment of early stage disease. Gynecol Oncol 2000; 76:40.

65. Chatterjee R, Goldstone AH. Gonadal damage and effects on fertility in adult patients with haematological malignancy undergoing stem cell transplantation. Bone Marrow Transplant 1996; 17:5–11.

66. White ID, Faithfull S. Sexuality and fertility. In: Faithfull S, Wells M, eds. Supportive care in radiotherapy. Edinburgh: Churchill Livingstone; 2003.

67. Clough KB, Goffinet F, Labib A, et al. Laparoscopic unilateral ovarian transposition prior to irradiation. Cancer 1996; 77(12):2638–2645.

68. Bath LE, Wallace WHB, Critchley HOD. Late effects of the treatment of childhood cancer on the female reproductive system and the potential for fertility preservation. Br J Obstet Gynaecol 2002; 109:107–114.

69. Revel A, Laufer N. Protecting female fertility from cancer therapy. Mol Cell Endocrinol 2002; 187:83–91.

70. Posada MN, Kolp L, Garcia JE. Fertility options for female cancer patients: facts and fiction. Fertil Steril 2001; 75(4):647–653.

71. Mertens AC, Ramsay RK, Kouris S, Neglia JP. Patterns of gonadal dysfunction following bone marrow transplantation. Bone Marrow Transplant 1998; 22:345–350.

72. Denton J. Fertility after cancer care: What are the options? A journey through cancer: choices and dilemmas. RCN 2nd Biennial Joint Cancer Conference and Exhibition, York; 2003.

73 Tournaye H. Storing reproduction for oncological patients: some points for discussion. Mol Cell Endocrinol 2000; 169:133–136.

74. Hallak J, Sharma RK, Thomas AJ, Agarwal A. Why cancer patients request disposal of cryopreserved semen specimens post-therapy: a retrospective study. Fertil Steril 1998; 69:889–893.

75. Bahadur G, Ralph D. Gonadal tissue cryopreservation in boys with paediatric cancers. Hum Reprod 1999; 14(1):11–17.

76. Human Fertilisation and Embryology Authority. Ninth Annual Report 2000:20.

77. Faithfull S. 'Just grin and bear it and hope that it will go away'. Coping with urinary symptoms from pelvic radiotherapy. Eur J Cancer Care 1995; 4:158–165.

78. Hawton K. Sex therapy: a practical guide. Oxford: Oxford Medical Publications; 1985.

79. Andersen BL. How cancer affects sexual functioning. Oncology 1990; 4(6):81–88.

80. Green J. Taking a sexual history. Trends Urol Gynaecol Sexual Health 1999; September/October:31–33.

81. Waterhouse J. Nursing practice related to sexuality: a review and recommendations. Nurs Times Res 1996; 1(6):412–418.

82. White ID. Facilitating sexual expression: challenges for contemporary practice. In: Heath H, White I, eds. The challenge of sexuality in health care. Oxford: Blackwell Science; 2002.

83. Annon J. The P-LI-SS-IT model: a proposed conceptual scheme for behavioural treatment of sexual problems. J Sex Educ Ther 1976; 2:1–15.

84. Masters WH, Johnson VE. Human sexual inadequacy. London: Churchill Livingstone; 1970.

85. Kaplan HS. The new sex therapy. New York: Brunner/Mazel; 1974.

86. Crowe M, Ridley J. Therapy with couples: a behavioural-systems approach to couple relationship and sexual problems. 2nd edn. Oxford: Blackwell Science; 2000.

87. Kirby R, Holmes S, Carson C. Fast facts – erectile dysfunction. 2nd edn. Oxford: Health Press; 1998.

88. Denton AS, Bond SJ, Mathews S, Bentzen SM, Maher EJ. National audit of the management and outcome of carcinoma of the cervix treated with radiotherapy in 1993. Clin Oncol 2000; 12:347–353.

89. Khoo V. Other late effects. In: Faithfull S, Wells M, eds. Supportive care in radiotherapy. Edinburgh: Churchill Livingstone; 2003.

90. Zilbergeld B. The new male sexuality. revised edn. New York: Bantam Books; 1999.

91. Department of Health. The NHS Cancer Plan. London: Department of Health; 2000.

92. Champion A. Male cancer and sexual function. Sexual and Marital Therapy 1996; 11(3)227–244.

93. National Institute for Clinical Excellence (NICE). Improving supportive and palliative care for adults with cancer: the manual. London: NICE; 2004.

CHAPTER 32

Altered Body Image

DIANA HARCOURT AND NICHOLA RUMSEY

CHAPTER CONTENTS

Introduction	701	Information provision	708
Body image and cancer	701	Facilitating patient decision-making	709
		Identifying patients with body image	
Influences upon body image	702	concerns	709
		Nursing care	710
The consequences of an altered body image after cancer	703	Issues in body image research: assessment and tools	711
The effects of specific treatments on body image	704	Issues in the provision of body image care	712
Surgery	704		
Chemotherapy	706	Conclusion	712
Radiotherapy	706		
Hormonal therapy	706	Useful addresses	713
Coping with an altered body image	706	References	713
Body image concerns and the provision of care	707		

INTRODUCTION

This chapter critically evaluates, discusses and summarizes current understanding of the psychosocial effects of an altered body image amongst people with cancer. After defining body image, this chapter then considers whether the impact of cancer may be influenced by sociodemographic or treatment factors. The possible psychosocial consequences of an altered body image are then outlined and the specific impact of surgery, chemotherapy, radiotherapy and drug therapy on body image and appearance are examined. Reconstructive breast surgery and prophylactic mastectomy are then used as examples of current develop-

ments in cancer care that have a direct impact upon body image. The importance of patients' attempts to cope with an altered body image are considered and suggestions are made for ways in which cancer care could be provided to meet their needs, focusing particularly on the role of specialist nurses in this context. Finally, issues inherent in research and the provision of care in this area are examined.

BODY IMAGE AND CANCER

Around one-third of all patients with cancer experience levels of psychological distress that are sufficiently high to warrant further emotional support at some stage during the course of their disease and treatment.[1,2] Whereas most patients' concerns are related to the fear of a potentially life-threatening condition,[3] it is also evident that for many distress is focused around negative feelings towards their body.

Although some cancer-related changes to appearance are temporary (e.g. hair loss) or amenable to change (e.g. reconstructive surgery after mastectomy), others will be permanent (e.g. amputation) and will necessitate continued adjustment and adaptation to an altered body image.[4] Furthermore, emotional distress is caused by changes to appearance which can act as vivid, constant reminders of the cancer and its treatment.[4] Disfiguring changes may be especially difficult to manage in a society that places a strong emphasis upon appearance and in which we are surrounded by media images of healthy, perfect bodies.[5]

Body image is a multifaceted, integral component of the way people view themselves. Grogan[6(p1)] defines body image as 'a person's perceptions, thoughts and feelings about his or her body – incorporating appearance, body size, shape and attractiveness. It is a dynamic construct that changes in response to life experiences and since it includes the personal significance attached to the body, it follows that any changes in appearance can be an emotionally difficult experience. Body image also refers to feelings of integrity and wholeness, concepts that are likely to be threatened by cancer and its treatment.

Price[7] identifies three aspects of body image (body reality, body ideal and body presentation) and emphasizes the importance of coping strategies and social support in determining a person's ability to adapt to any changes in their appearance. This model offers a useful explanation of the experiences of many patients with cancer. Body reality refers to the objective, physical appearance of the body (e.g. height, weight, hair colour): in other words, how the body really is.[7] Cancer treatment may have an obvious impact upon body reality (e.g. patients may have lost their hair, lost or gained weight, be scarred or have lost bodily function as in colostomy or laryngectomy). Body ideal is how the individual thinks their body *should* look and function. The changes to appearance brought

on by cancer treatment are likely to contradict the prevailing Western body ideal as being youthful, fit, slim and attractive[5] with healthy hair, no scarring and being able to function without the need for aids or support. Body presentation refers to the way in which the body is presented to the social world[7,8] and includes clothing and non-verbal behaviour such as posture. In a cancer context, body presentation includes the use of a wig, prosthetics, a colostomy or clothes that might disguise the altered appearance. Such actions reflect, in part, the individual's continued attempts to deal with both their own and other people's reactions to their changed appearance.[7]

Price[7] defines altered body image as 'any significant alteration outside the realms of expected human development'. Certainly, cancer and its treatment have the potential to cause significant alteration that is not a normal part of the developmental process.

INFLUENCES UPON BODY IMAGE

Cancer care that purports to be holistic must recognize and address appearance and body image issues amongst patients with cancer. Researchers have repeatedly tried to identify those factors that may indicate an increased susceptibility to body image problems, since the results would have clear benefits in enabling care to be directed towards those patients deemed more at risk. The results of this research are largely equivocal, since body image is such a personal concept; however, some research suggests that appearance-related issues may, to some extent, be influenced by treatment, age-related or demographic details. For example, younger patients with head and neck cancer have reported higher levels of anxiety prior to disfiguring surgery,[9] and more concerns around body image and sexuality have been reported by younger patients with breast, colon, testicular, female reproductive or lymphatic cancer than by older patients with the same disease.[10] Similarly, a prospective study of 307 patients with breast cancer treated by mastectomy or breast-conserving surgery found those women who had undergone mastectomy reported poorer body image, with younger, married women reporting a less favourable body image than those who were divorced, separated, widowed or never married.[11] However, as King et al[11] stress, it cannot be assumed that older women will necessarily be immune to the possible detrimental impact of mastectomy on body image. Similarly, the possible impact of any other cancer treatment should not be presumed according to age.

Advancing age may bring with it a number of unique problems in dealing with the practicalities of a changed appearance.[10] For example, conditions such as arthritis may compound any difficulties in cleaning or using a stoma or other prosthetic device. At the other end of the spectrum, treatment during adolescence may also present particular challenges because the normal processes of physical, social and sexual development at this time often result in individuals being acutely aware of their body and appearance.[12] A comparison of adolescents who had undergone cancer treatment with age- and gender-matched controls found no significant difference in reported body image between the two groups.[13] However, amongst the cancer group, the authors found that body image perceptions became more negative as the time since treatment increased and those who perceived their cancer to have affected their appearance also reported higher levels of social anxiety and loneliness. It seems appearance issues become more important as the immediate threat of the cancer and its treatment declines, as contact with other patients with cancer and hospital staff reduces and patients start to compare themselves with their healthy peers as opposed to other patients with cancer.

Cultural, religious and ethnic issues may mean that body image is experienced differently by people from diverse backgrounds. Research is needed so that holistic yet appropriate care can be made available to all patients with cancer, but as yet there is a relative dearth of research into the impact of ethnicity on body image concerns. Exceptionally, Spencer et al[3] found that Hispanic women with breast cancer reported elevated concerns about sexuality whereas African-American women indicated lower levels of concern about sexuality

and femininity. Concerns regarding sexual issues were also less common amongst older patients.

THE CONSEQUENCES OF AN ALTERED BODY IMAGE AFTER CANCER

The psychosocial impact of an altered appearance after cancer can be far-reaching and varied. Not only do patients have to contend with a new body image but they must also deal with their feelings towards the loss of their previous looks. Changes to body image might be acutely embarrassing and looking and/or feeling visibly different can have a detrimental impact on quality of life, including reduced self-confidence, low self-esteem, difficulty with social interactions and, ultimately, social withdrawal.[14] An audit of patients with head and neck cancer found that 50% of participants avoided certain activities as a result of their appearance.[15] Some patients are very self-conscious of subtle changes to their appearance that are not immediately obvious to other people.[1] Indeed, research has found that the severity or visibility of a disfigurement does not predict levels of distress.[16] It is therefore important to remember that the patient's own, subjective experience of their body image and appearance may or may not equate with an observer's objective rating. For example, a patient with breast cancer may be very distressed by a lumpectomy scar that her nurse considers to be small and unobtrusive whereas another patient whose mastectomy surgery has resulted in a more obvious and radical change to their appearance might, to the nurse's surprise, be less concerned about appearance issues.

Social situations may prove particularly challenging for those with disfigurements affecting the face or neck. In addition to the increased visibility of these areas, and the problems of effective camouflage, some patients may find it difficult or impossible to use particular facial expressions or find that their speech has been affected following surgery.[16] Piff[17] gives a personal account of her experiences following treatment for head and neck cancer.

In addition to physical problems, including difficulties in eating, speaking and drinking, she reports feeling isolated and rejected as she went through a process of grieving for her previous appearance.

Changes to body image are also likely to have an impact upon feelings of attractiveness, especially when the tumour is located in a part of the body particularly associated with sexuality. For example, studies have reported how treatment for prostate cancer had a negative impact upon patients' sexual relationships and sense of masculinity,[18,19] whereas the impact of breast cancer surgery on women's sense of 'womanliness' and sexuality has been well documented.[20-22] The impact of an altered body image is not necessarily eased by the passage of time. Early research[22] concluded that women undergoing mastectomy only started to report self-image problems several months after surgery because they had been denying the personal impact of the treatment in order to protect their self-esteem.

Research examining the impact of cancer on global self-esteem is equivocal. However, the existing literature does support the notion that specific body self-esteem is generally lower amongst patients with cancer than amongst control groups. This is particularly the case amongst patients for whom disfiguring treatment affects highly visible, prized or socially valued parts of the body such as the face or breast.[23] Indeed, individuals' differing reactions to changes in their appearance may be explained by the extent to which they rely upon appearance as a determinant of their self-esteem.[24] Carver et al[25] examined the extent to which, in 66 patients with early-stage breast cancer, investment in their body image (i.e. the extent to which their self-esteem relied upon their appearance) and sense of body integrity predicted psychological adjustment following surgery. Women who invested highly in their appearance persistently reported higher levels of distress than did those who reported placing less importance on their looks. They also found investment in body integrity did not predict emotional distress but did have a detrimental impact upon feelings of attractiveness, social activities and of 'not feeling oneself anymore'.

Some patients may feel that their body is failing them and out of their control because it no longer functions or looks as expected.[26] Furthermore, some changes to appearance (e.g. weight loss or nausea) might be perceived by the patient as an indicator of cancer recurrence or a symptom of additional cancer, thereby increasing anxiety and cancer-related concerns.[26] Finally, people who look different after treatment must also deal with the reactions (e.g. staring, avoidance), comments and questions from other people.[27] It is not surprising that patients often fear the reaction they will receive and that those who are conscious of their appearance try not to draw attention to themselves, e.g. by avoiding eye contact, social withdrawal or not engaging in conversation.[16] However, these poor social skills tend only to compound the problems associated with social situations. Instead, good social skills can be an effective way of taking control of such difficult situations and are a coping strategy that nurses can teach and encourage amongst their patients (as addressed below).

THE EFFECTS OF SPECIFIC TREATMENTS ON BODY IMAGE

Naturally, patients are distressed and anxious prior to any cancer treatment. It is possible that such anxieties may be exacerbated by concerns about the extent to which the treatment will result in changes to appearance and body image.[9] Surgery, chemotherapy, radiotherapy and drug/hormone therapy have the potential to impact upon appearance in numerous ways, which will now be discussed.

Surgery

It is impossible to predict the precise psychological impact that any particular surgical procedure will have upon a patient. Although less-invasive diagnostic techniques such as fine-needle aspiration (FNA) or ultrasound have in many instances reduced the need for surgical biopsy in order to ascertain or confirm a diagnosis, these innovations can still feel invasive and may have a negative effect upon body image. Likewise, the process of marking the patient with the planned incisions prior to surgery can have a detrimental impact (e.g. as in breast reconstruction procedures when such markings are extensive). In many instances, patients undergo a series of surgical procedures and must contend with successive changes to their appearance. Any surgery has the potential to result in scarring to a greater or lesser degree; radical surgery can also result in loss of function, lymphoedema and the need to rely on prostheses, appliances or people in a way that was not previously necessary. For example, patients with a stoma may be bothered by smell and noise in addition to the appearance of the stoma, the loss of normal functioning and the ensuing impact on daily living. It is commonly assumed that more extensive surgery will have a greater psychological impact on the patient than will less-invasive or mutilating surgery.[16] For example, a body of literature has found that women who undergo lumpectomy report more favourable post-surgical body image and greater satisfaction with their bodies than do patients who have had a mastectomy.[11,21,28] However, a lumpectomy will still result in scarring and, depending on the size and location of the lump that is removed, can have an obvious impact on appearance and body image.[29] Patients with breast cancer who mistakenly believe that a lumpectomy will not change the appearance of their breasts may be disappointed.[20] Amongst patients with malignant melanoma, satisfaction with the cosmetic outcome of surgery has been shown to be unrelated to the length of resection scars:[30] rather, dissatisfaction was related to indentation and a tendency to underestimate the extent of scarring,[30] suggesting that pre-surgical preparation should involve clarification of patients' expectations of scarring after surgery.

Recent years have seen increased recognition of the potential benefits of involving patients in decision-making about treatment, while surgical developments have increased the options available to them (including procedures impacting upon body image). For example, the availability of risk-reducing or 'prophylactic' procedures (e.g. mastectomy or oophorectomy) now offers choice to people with a high risk of developing the disease. These procedures bring with them the possibility of altered body image in the absence of any malignancy, and a body of literature investigating the psychological impact of prophylactic cancer surgery is now emerging.[31–34] As yet, results are equivocal. For example, a prospective study[31] concluded that prophylactic mastectomy may offer psychological benefits without any negative impact upon body image, and a retrospective survey[32] found only minor degrees of body image deterioration, although more than half the participants felt less physically and sexually attractive. However, a small minority of women in Hopwood et al's[32] study did report serious body image concerns and disappointment after surgery. Similarly, Payne et al[33] found that around 5% of their participants expressed regrets about their decision to undergo prophylactic mastectomy. Although relieved that their risk of breast cancer had been reduced, their regrets focused around body image and sexuality issues, specifically surgical complications, dissatisfaction with cosmetic outcome, lack of sensation and disfiguring scarring. A study of long-term follow-up has suggested that one-third of patients reported poorer body image satisfaction after prophylactic breast surgery.[34] Clearly, this literature is in its infancy and needs to be developed further as the number of patients contemplating and undergoing prophylactic surgery increases. Already it is evident that patients contemplating prophylactic surgery warrant specific information regarding the impact of treatment on body image and appropriate support both before and after treatment.

Surgical developments are also increasing patients' options regarding plastic and reconstructive surgery aiming to address the negative impact of their primary cancer treatment. The widespread availability and increasing take-up of reconstructive surgery after mastectomy is testament to the increased recognition of the negative impact of breast loss and to the motivation of patients to restore their pretreatment appearance.[35] Yet again, common assumptions regarding the benefits of reconstructive surgery are not necessarily supported by research evidence. Prospective research[35] has concluded that breast reconstruction is not a universal panacea for the emotional and psychological consequences of mastectomy, and women still felt conscious of an altered body image 1 year after surgery, regardless of whether or not they had elected for breast reconstruction.

Chemotherapy

The personal impact of chemotherapy, including concerns surrounding its impact upon appearance and body image, can be considerable.[36] Patients with breast cancer have reported good general quality of life but poor body image, regardless of the intensity of their chemotherapy.[37] Rapid alopecia and hair loss is often a particularly traumatic experience and can be the most feared side-effect of chemotherapy.[38] Wigs may not be a simple solution, since some patients report that they feel unnatural and emphasize feelings of abnormality.[39] It is possible that the negative impact of chemotherapy may be softened as hair starts to regrow[12] but patients may have to make further adjustment to an altered appearance if it grows back with a different texture and colour. As with other aspects of body image and cancer treatment, the personal impact of hair loss is relatively unresearched[40] and recommendations for the provision of information about alopecia are rarely evidence-based[38] (see Ch. 27).

Chemotherapy can also result in significant changes in weight that can prove particularly difficult to hide or disguise, while feelings of nausea and vomiting can impact upon a patient's sense of body reality.[7] In addition, patients may find Hickman lines and frequent injections both intrusive and threatening to body integrity.

Radiotherapy

Radiotherapy can result in a range of distressing side-effects[41] that have the potential to impact upon body image. Prior to treatment, patients must have their skin marked in order that the rays are directed to the same site with every application. These markings might be perceived as disfiguring, can act as a permanent reminder of the treatment and contribute towards body image concerns. The extreme fatigue commonly associated with radiotherapy treatment may conflict with daily functioning and therefore contribute towards body image problems. This can be particularly distressing for patients seeking evidence of recovery, as fatigue may be interpreted as a symptom of the ongoing presence of cancer. Radiotherapy can result in permanent hair loss, which may be especially distressing for patients undergoing radiotherapy for treatment of a brain tumour if they are left with patches of baldness on the head. Although less frequent than fatigue, some patients do suffer skin reactions to radiotherapy. These can take weeks or months to heal and may result in permanent scarring, yet there is currently a dearth of research into the personal impact of changes to appearance as a result of radiotherapy (see Ref 42 for an overview).

Hormonal therapy

Hormonal therapy may also have a distressing impact on body image. For example, the negative side-effects of tamoxifen for breast cancer may involve menopausal-like symptoms,[4] including weight gain and hot flushes, whereas patients with prostate cancer treated by hormonal therapy have reported feeling more feminine as a result of their treatment.[19]

In summary, all forms of cancer treatment have the potential to detrimentally affect body image. This may be compounded for those patients who undergo a combination of treatments, yet the precise impact of treatment on each individual is difficult to predict. In addition, the impact of changes to body image may be mediated by the success or otherwise of any coping strategies that patients employ.

COPING WITH AN ALTERED BODY IMAGE

Successful coping with an altered body image involves the patient reintegrating their changed appearance into their view of themselves.[9] The ability to cope successfully does not appear to be determined by the extent, location, type or aetiology of a disfigurement.[43] It is important to remember that nurses have a role to play in establishing the extent to which an individual is coping with changes to their appearance and the effectiveness of the strategies being used. Some researchers have tried to identify adaptive and less adaptive ways of coping. Rather than coming out in favour of any one style of coping, the research suggests that the effectiveness of any single strategy will depend on the individual's personal appraisal of the situation, and their previous experience of using a particular way of coping. It appears that people who have a broader repertoire of coping strategies available to them and are flexible in how they attempt to deal with the different aspects of their treatment may cope more effectively than those with a limited and rigid approach.[43]

Strategies may be classified as either problem-focused or emotion-focused, an approach based on Lazarus and Folkman's transactional model of stress and coping.[44] Problem-focused coping attempts to manipulate, control or eliminate the source of stress (e.g. concealing or camouflaging an altered appearance by the use of prosthetics, clothing, wigs, etc.), whereas emotion-focused strategies aim to reduce or manage the emotional aspects of the situation (e.g. trying to avoid thinking about the issue, expressing emotions or distress relating to altered appearance). Alternatively, strategies can be viewed as avoidant (e.g. avoiding social situations, denying the situation) or non-avoidant (e.g. seeking information, positively reappraising the situation).

Patients with cancer often try to deal with the stress of disease and treatment by drawing favourable comparisons between themselves and others deemed less fortunate in order to bolster or protect their self-esteem.[45] Body image problems may become more evident if the patient compares themselves negatively against healthy peers rather than positively against others undergoing more intense cancer treatment.[12] For example, a patient receiving chemotherapy who has not experienced hair loss may make a favourable comparison with someone who is bald as a result of treatment, whereas a patient with breast cancer who undergoes lumpectomy might see herself as more fortunate than a patient who has undergone mastectomy. In contrast, a patient with breast cancer who has undergone both mastectomy and chemotherapy might compare herself negatively against a patient who has been treated by way of lumpectomy and who has not needed adjuvant treatment.

Social support is an essential resource in patients' adaptation to their disease and treatment.[8] As well as demonstrating acceptance of the patient's changed looks, other people may also be a valuable source of information, practical help and emotional support. In these respects, nursing staff can become vital members of a patient's social support network. Some patients may try to cope with their altered body image by seeking surgical or medical intervention to restore their changed appearance. Although this could be construed as trying to avoid or deny the changes, it may also demonstrate the patient's active engagement in trying to manage the impact of the disease. As such, it can be seen as a positive acceptance of the situation and a way of maintaining a sense of control over the treatment and disease, both of which are important factors in the process of adjustment to threatening events.[45] The number and complexity of the factors involved in coping highlight the need for individual assessment, support and care provision.

BODY IMAGE CONCERNS AND THE PROVISION OF CARE

Current cancer care is primarily based on the biomedical model, with the dominant focus on the surgical and medical interventions that are vital in addressing the physical aspects of care. Less attention is paid to eliciting and meeting psychosocial needs. A more comprehensive approach to care recognizes the need to address psychosocial concerns, including those relating to body image and appearance. In addition to the psychosocial benefits, Dropkin[9] suggests there may be practical, medical benefits of helping patients to adjust to their altered appearance since failure to accept an altered body image might contribute to reduced compliance with treatment and increased incidence of infections.

The benefits of including specialist nurses within multidisciplinary cancer teams are widely recognized.[46] As core members of such groups, nurses with advanced and specialist knowledge are in a strong position to ensure that body image issues are considered throughout the course of an individual's care. However, the identification and care of body image problems is not only an issue for specialist nurses. All staff (including nursing support staff, prosthesis-fitting staff) need to be aware of the importance of body image and should avoid making assumptions about an individual's reaction to changes in their appearance or to their likely preference or suitability for disfiguring treatment.[47,48] Despite the potential for specialist nurses to play a key role in the provision of psychosocial support, a recent survey of specialist head and neck cancer nurses found that respondents did not feel sufficiently skilled in offering this care.[49] It seems reasonable to suggest that specialist nurses working with other cancers would also report greater confidence in providing physical as opposed to psychosocial care. The following sections suggest several ways in which nurses might improve the extent to which care meets patient need: for example, through information provision, facilitating decision-making, identifying and referring those patients experiencing body image problems, patient support and education and training.

Information provision

Providing patients with accurate information prior to treatment is recognized good practice[50] and may be effective in helping many patients adjust better to diagnosis and treatment. Routine preparation for treatment should include information about how the patient's appearance may be altered and what, if any, functions will be affected (e.g. colostomy or surgery affecting vocal cords or facial muscles). However, a series of focus groups with patients with head and neck cancer and their families[51] found that patients often perceived the information on such side-effects to be lacking.

Patients are not a homogenous group[52] and the amount, type and form of information desired varies greatly between individuals and over time. Typically, individuals who want extensive, detailed information are likely to become anxious and frustrated if this is not forthcoming, whereas others may be equally distressed if presented with detail that far exceeds their minimal requirements.[53] Time spent exploring patients' individual information needs, concerns about their appearance and attitudes towards their treatment options may be more beneficial than providing uniform, standardized written or visual information, such as photographs.[54] Numerous ways in which patients' information needs might be met have been explored. Ambler et al[55] developed a nurse-led intervention that involved helping the patient to prepare a list of questions that they wanted answered in their consultation. This encouraged health professionals to provide relevant information and to discuss all the patient's concerns, including appearance and body image issues.[56]

Patients may benefit from photographs of the possible outcomes of treatment, yet it is important that they realize there can be no guarantee that their own outcome will be the same as that shown in photographs. Patients offered breast reconstruction have reported that a library of photographs would be a valuable resource, but stressed that these should include patients with different physiques, at different stages in the recovery process and treated by the variety of surgical options available.[35]

Advances in computer technology have the potential to offer innovative means of information provision and support for patients and their families. McGarvey et al[40] describe the use of computer-imaging to enable women to prepare themselves in advance of possible chemotherapy-induced hair loss. Whilst supported by a psychologist, patients viewed a simulation of their hair loss before treatment began in the belief that the opportunity to see this image and to express the emotions that it generates would enable the patient to anticipate and deal more easily with any real hair loss. However, McGarvey et al[40] give anecdotal rather than research evidence for the benefits of this intervention. Such interventions will not suit all patients (some prefer not to anticipate outcomes) and they have considerable resource and staffing implications. Furthermore, patients who have experienced chemotherapy-induced alopecia report that warnings about possible hair loss could not prepare them for the full impact of the loss.[39] Batchelor[38] lists information that should be addressed in both written and verbal form to patients who are at risk of hair loss (see Ch. 27). Again, such information needs to be tailored to meet individual need and to be sensitively given at a time that is appropriate for the patient.

Information about diet and fitness programmes might be useful for patients whose weight has changed, whereas other patients may benefit from advice regarding camouflage make-up. However, make-up might successfully cover a disfigurement to a greater or lesser degree, but will not address patients' anxieties about their appearance. Patients should also be informed of support organizations that offer specific advice and support to those who are troubled by their appearance.

Facilitating patient decision-making

We mentioned earlier that continued developments in surgical and reconstructive techniques have increased the treatment options available to patients. Increased choices have taken place alongside policies encouraging greater patient involvement in decision-making (e.g. the Patients' Charter in the UK[57]) and evidence suggests that many patients with breast cancer benefit psychologically from active involvement in their treatment.[58] However, patients do not necessarily appreciate the responsibility of decision-making and many still prefer a passive role in decisions about their treatment and care.[59]

Deber et al[60] concluded that patients do not wish to be involved in 'problem-solving' tasks (i.e. identifying a 'correct solution' to a medical problem) since this requires an expert knowledge. Rather, they seek participation when choices with different risks and trade-offs are available, and when acting on patient preference is a viable option. Decisions relating to body image and appearance often fit this criterion. For example, a patient may decide whether the more extreme scarring resulting from TRAM (transverse rectus abdominus myocutaneous) flap breast reconstruction is compensated for by the supposed better cosmetic results of successful procedures over alternative techniques.

Decision-making about treatment that may alter appearance can be especially stressful because the outcome is uncertain, initial decisions must often be made soon after the diagnosis of cancer has been given and because decision-making is influenced by a multitude of factors, only some of which are within the patient's control. For example, a study of decision-making about breast reconstruction in patients with breast cancer[61,62] found that the decision was influenced by, amongst other things, the perceived norms within the clinic setting (i.e. information about what 'most' women decide) and the language (e.g. words such as 'disfigured' or 'deformed') used by healthcare professionals to describe the appearance of a mastectomy. Many patients chose not to make decisions about appearance-altering surgery until they were aware of the success or otherwise of their primary cancer treatment. The decision about breast reconstruction can be particularly complicated since it may involve choices about the type of reconstruction, timing of surgery, nipple reconstruction and surgery on the contralateral breast. Further research is needed to investigate ways in which patient decision-making about appearance-altering treatment might be facilitated, particularly for those patients finding it difficult to make such choices. Decision-making aids (e.g. card-sort techniques that enable women to 'sort' the perceived advantages and disadvantages) aim to clarify patient values and to increase perceived confidence in taking part in decision-making[63] without affecting levels of anxiety or satisfaction with either the decision or the decision-making process.[64] This may also reduce the chances of decisional errors[65] and make it easier to provide appropriate information.

Identifying patients with body image concerns

It is important to remember that many patients adjust well to their diagnosis and its treatment without the need for any specialist intervention geared towards improving their psychosocial well-being.[66] Indeed, Dean[2(p391)] commented: 'Women undergoing treatment for breast cancer appear to be remarkably psychologically resilient to the effects of treatment.' However, it is imperative that people who are unable to make this adjustment so easily are identified and supported appropriately.

Routine care should begin with assessment and intervention for concerns about body image both prior to and following treatment:[8] for example, by sensitively ascertaining whether patients are avoiding their altered appearance (e.g. by not looking at themselves in mirrors or avoiding social situations). Specialist nurses are ideally placed to identify any patients who require support for body image concerns, and clear protocols should be established for referrals to a clinical psychologist who is part of the cancer team. Not all patients will want or require support beyond that provided by their family and friends. A study of ratings of support[67] of patients with orofacial cancer confirmed the importance of family and friends and the perceived usefulness of nurses in outpatient clinics and on the ward, but identified problems with the support received from the primary care sector, e.g. GP's, community nurses and from other patients. However, the study did not clarify which aspects of support and care were being met or the nature of the difficulties encountered.

Nursing care

The act of providing nursing care offers a series of opportunities in which appearance-related concerns can be explored and discussed in a sensitive way. Standing in normal, close proximity to the patient, using eye contact and sensitively touching the patient (e.g. when changing dressings or through massage) are ways in which acceptance of the patient's appearance can be demonstrated.[68,69] Seeing the results of surgery for the first time can be a particularly distressing experience for many patients and, however well prepared they may be, it is likely that patients will still experience a degree of shock. Nurses can support the patient by being available to answer questions and to offer any appropriate reassurance about

the extent to which swelling and bruising may subside. Some patients might also appreciate the presence of a supportive member of staff when their partner or family first sees their changed appearance.

Patients who have or are about to undergo appearance-altering treatment may benefit from meeting others with similar personal experience, either through self-help support groups or on a one-to-one basis. Nurses have a role to play in facilitating and maintaining such meetings, which can be beneficial for a number of reasons. First, they give patients the chance to express their feelings and concerns with people who are independent of the patient's immediate support network (members of which are likely also to be distressed by the situation). Secondly, it is an opportunity to exchange information and offer help. For example, patients who will be using a prosthesis after treatment may benefit from meeting other patients who are already coping well with a similar aid. Finally, the process of being supported by and offering support to other patients may instil a sense of purpose at a time when previous roles have been adversely impacted by the treatment and disease.[70]

A review of the usefulness of self-help amongst patients with cancer[71] concluded that fears about possible negative effects of such meetings were unfounded. However, staff must be aware that contact with other patients will not suit everyone. For example, whereas some patients who have undergone mastectomy report that meetings with patients who have previously undergone breast reconstruction were an invaluable resource when making their own decision about reconstructive surgery,[62] others found this unnecessary or even unhelpful since it complicated their choices. There is also a possibility that patients will not get on and that they will be adversely affected by the deteriorating health or death of other patients. Furthermore, it is important to recognize that a 'buddy system' might place unexpected demands upon all participants (e.g. raising unresolved issues in previous patients). Nurses need to explore the suitability of volunteers on a case-by-case basis and be in a position to provide support to all those involved in such a system, as necessary.

Whilst nursing staff may feel ill-equipped to deal with psychosocial and appearance-related issues, a relatively simple 1-day training course and supporting resource pack has been found to significantly improve their perceived ability to meet the specific needs of patients with head and neck cancer, in particular through the promotion of coping strategies to be used in social situations.[49]

Those nurses who are experienced in caring for patients with cancer with an altered appearance can play a role in educating other members of the healthcare team in order that appearance-related issues are recognized and considered at every stage of the patient's cancer journey.

ISSUES IN BODY IMAGE RESEARCH: ASSESSMENT AND TOOLS

Despite examples of good practice in the provision of care for patients with cancer with body image concerns, a number of difficulties remain. A major problem is the need for evidence-based practice, yet research in this area is fraught with difficulties. First, much of the literature concerning altered body image amongst patients with cancer has been written on a comparatively anecdotal basis,[4] using small samples of patients often without any control or comparison groups and at times relying upon ratings of appearance given by third parties rather than by the patients themselves.[72] Furthermore, there is currently no 'gold standard' measure of body image, with the result that a wide range of assessment tools are used, thereby complicating direct comparisons of studies that have employed different definitions and measures of body image. Many of the assessment tools used in this research lack acceptable levels of reliability and validity,[4] although advances are being made in this area. For example, the Body Image Scale[73] has undergone psychometric validation and appears to be a useful, reliable measure of body image for patients with breast cancer.

Another problem is that wholly prospective research is difficult in this area, with the result that much of the research has been retrospec-tive. This is problematic because participants may describe current feelings and concerns about their body image and appearance rather than portray their actual past experience, so both positive and negative experiences may be misrepresented. Furthermore, retrospective analysis is unlikely to identify fluctuations in body image, which are especially relevant given its dynamic nature.[72] Recent events and the context in which assessment takes place are also likely to influence an individual's perceptions of their body and appearance.[74] In summary, research needs to be longitudinal and prospective over the course of diagnosis and treatment if patients are to receive appropriate support and nursing care.

Many aspects of cancer care are researched using randomized controlled trials (RCTs). However, this methodology may not be suitable when investigating body image issues relating to treatments in which patient choice is imperative (e.g. breast reconstruction), since an RCT essentially replaces informed decision-making with chance.[75] A more detailed consideration of current issues inherent in body image research, using breast reconstruction as an example, can be found in an article by Harcourt and Rumsey.[76]

Finally, there is a tendency for body image assessments to be worded in a predominantly negative way, giving little scope to the expression of possible positive attitudes towards appearance and body image.[72] Indeed, further research is needed to investigate factors that might contribute to a positive body image after cancer treatment and to identify those factors that are characteristic of people who adjust well to an altered appearance. Research suggests that the concept of 'resilience' is important in coping with other forms of disfigurement[27] but this warrants further investigation within the field of cancer.

Several other areas of cancer care necessitate further investigation with regards to body image issues. First, there remains a dearth of research into appearance concerns amongst older patients with cancer or those from diverse ethnic backgrounds. Secondly, it is vital that body image research is conducted in tandem with the development and implementation of new surgical procedures, since surgery does not always have the anticipated (or even widely publicized) benefit or impact upon body image and psychological distress.[35] Unfortunately, funding for research in this area can be difficult to acquire since the appearance-related aspects of cancer and its treatment tend not to be a priority for funding bodies.[72]

ISSUES IN THE PROVISION OF BODY IMAGE CARE

It is essential that any comprehensive care package for people with cancer should include appropriate consideration of the impact of changes to the patient's body image and appearance. Particular consideration must be given to the needs of specific groups such as adolescents.[13] However, a number of factors may combine to result in these needs going unmet.

First, it has been suggested that the level of appearance-related concerns amongst people with cancer may be underestimated, since the medical system and health professionals may eschew such issues, thus preventing patients from reporting their concerns for fear of appearing ungrateful, vain or wasting professionals' time.[77] A challenge facing any multidisciplinary cancer team is therefore to develop an ethos in which appearance concerns can be discussed at every stage of the patient's cancer journey. Individuals should not feel stigmatized if they are identified as needing psychological support to deal with changes to their appearance. It is important that there should be adequate time and privacy in busy outpatient departments and hospital wards to facilitate discussion of appearance issues. In many instances, it may be beneficial just to know that psychosocial support is available if needed. Yet, even if such concerns are elicited and care plans do specifically mention body image, staff may not be in a position to provide the specific, individual support and care that the patient needs.[7] Constraints include staff shortages, lack of a suitable hospital-based environment, time pressures within busy clinic settings and, as mentioned previously, a lack of confidence and little guidance in how to deal with such issues.

Furthermore, shorter hospital stays for patients undergoing surgery have reduced the time available for nurses to implement any planned body image care before the patient is discharged.[8] Patients can feel especially vulnerable when they leave the relative security of the hospital ward[51] and the time comes to confront the full impact of their changed appearance. It is therefore imperative that appropriate support for both the patient and their family/carers is made available outside the hospital environment. All members of the multidisciplinary team, but especially nurses, have a key role to play in coordinating such support before discharge. Nurses can also be a source of information about appearance and disfigurement-related support groups, websites and organizations that the patient might find useful.

CONCLUSION

This chapter has highlighted the importance of considering body image and appearance issues at every stage in the patient's cancer journey. Historically, the importance of appearance and body image issues amongst patients with cancer have been assumed and underestimated. Reactions and adjustment to an altered body image are individual and vary over time and do not only result from extensive disfigurement. All patients can be affected by changes to their body image, not only those whose outward appearance has changed. Viewing patients with cancer as a homogenous group with similar body image concerns is therefore short-sighted, problematic and inappropriate.

Too often, care has been provided on the basis of well-meaning intention and assumptions about body image issues, rather than on the basis of research evidence. Future research needs to examine ways of meeting the psychosocial needs of patients with an altered body image and systematically evaluating the impact of developments in treatment upon appearance.

Nurses have a vital role to play in the provision of care that effectively meets patients' psychosocial needs. Although some people cope extremely well with an altered appearance, it is important that appropriate and adequate support and care are available for those who do not make this adjustment so easily. This can be achieved by placing appearance and body image issues higher on the agenda of those responsible for planning and implementing cancer care.

USEFUL ADDRESSES

The following organizations offer support in the UK specifically in relation to issues of appearance and altered body image:

Changing Faces

Changing Faces is a charity that offers help to anyone with concerns about disfigurement and any disfiguring condition.

Changing Faces
1–2 Junction Mews
London W2 1PN
Tel: 020 7706 4232
Website: www.changingfaces.co.uk
Email: info@changingfaces.co.uk

Let's Face It

Let's Face It is a support network for people with facial disfigurement, their families, friends and professionals.

Let's Face It
14 Fallowfield
Yateley
Hampshire GU46 6LW
Tel: 01252 879630

REFERENCES

1. Barraclough J. Cancer and emotion, a practical guide to psycho-oncology. 3rd edn. Chichester: John Wiley and Sons; 1999.
2. Dean C. Psychiatric morbidity following mastectomy: preoperative predictors and types of illness. J Psychosom Res 1987; 31(3):385–392.
3. Spencer SM, Lehman JM, Wynings C, et al. Concerns about breast cancer and relations to psychosocial well-being in a multi-ethnic sample of early-stage patients. Health Psychol 1999; 18(2):159–168.
4. White CA. Body images in oncology. In: Cash TF, Pruzinsky T, eds. Body image: a handbook of theory, research and clinical practice. New York: The Guilford Press; 2002
5. Rumsey N. Historical & anthropological perspectives on appearance. In: Lansdown R, Rumsey N, Bradbury E, Carr T, Partridge J, eds. Visibly different: coping with disfigurement. London: Butterworth-Heinemann; 1997.
6. Grogan S. Body image. London: Routledge; 1999.
7. Price B. Body image: nursing concepts and care. New York: Prentice Hall; 1990.
8. Price B. A model for body-image care. J Adv Nurs 1990; 15:585–593.
9. Dropkin MJ. Body image and quality of life after head and neck cancer surgery. Cancer Pract 1999; 7(6):309–313.
10. Harrison J, Maguire P. Influence of age on psychological adjustment to cancer. Psycho-oncology 1995; 4:33–38.
11. King MT, Kenny P, Shiell A, Hall J, Boyages J. Quality of life three months and one year after first treatment for early stage breast cancer: influence of treatment and patient characteristics. Qual Life Res 2000; 9:789–800.
12. Levine, MP, Smolak L. Body image development in adolescence. In: Cash TF, Pruzinsky T, eds. Body image: a handbook of theory, research and clinical practice. New York: The Guilford Press; 2002.
13. Pendley JS, Dahlquist LM, Dreyer Z. Body image and psychosocial adjustment in adolescent cancer survivors. J Pediatr Psychol 1997; 22(1):29–43.
14. Newell RJ. Altered body image: a fear-avoidance model of psycho-social difficulties following disfigurement. J Adv Nurs 1999; 30:1230–1238.
15. Rumsey N, Clarke A, White P, Wyn-Williams M, Garlick W. Altered body image: appearance-related concerns of people with visible disfigurement. J Adv Nurs 2004; 48(5):443–453.
16. Robinson E. Psychological research on visible differences in adults. In: Lansdown R, Rumsey N, Bradbury E, Carr T, Partridge J, eds. Visibly different: coping with disfigurement. London: Butterworth-Heinemann; 1997.
17. Piff C. Body image: a patient's perspective. Br J Theatre Nurs 1998; 8(1):13–14.
18. Lavery JF, Clarke VA. Prostate cancer: patients' and spouses' coping and marital adjustment. Psychol Health Med 1999; 4(3):289–301.
19. Navon L, Morag A. Advanced prostate cancer patients' relationships with their spouses following hormonal therapy. Eur J Oncol Nurs 2003; 7(2):73–80.
20. Fallowfield L. Breast cancer. London: Routledge; 1991.
21. Mock V. Body image in women treated for breast cancer. Nurs Res 1993; 42 (3):153–157.

22. Polivy J. Psychological effects of mastectomy on a woman's feminine self-concept. J Nerv Ment Dis 1977;164(2):77–87.

23. Katz MR, Rodin G, Devins GM. Self-esteem and cancer: theory and research. Can J Psychiatry 1995; 40:608–615.

24. White CA. Body image dimensions and cancer: a heuristic cognitive behavioural model. Psycho-oncology 2000; 9:183–192.

25. Carver CS, Pozo-Kaderman C, Price AA, et al. Concern about aspects of body image and adjustment to early stage breast cancer. Psychosom Med 1998; 60:168–174.

26. Price B. Living with altered body image: the cancer experience. Br J Nurs 1992; 1(13):641–645.

27. Rumsey N. Body image and congenital conditions with visible differences. In: Cash T, Pruzinsky TF, eds. A handbook of theory, research and clinical practice. New York: The Guilford Press; 2002.

28. Moyer A. Psychological outcomes of breast-conserving surgery versus mastectomy: a meta-analytic review. Health Psychol 1997; 16:284–298.

29. Hall A, Fallowfield L. Psychological outcome of treatment for early breast cancer: a review. Stress Med 1989; 5:167–175.

30. Cassileth BR, Lusk EJ, Tenaglia AN. Patient's perceptions of the cosmetic impact of melanoma resection. Plast Reconstr Surg 1983; 71 (1):73–75.

31. Hatcher MB, Fallowfield L, A'Hern R. The psychosocial impact of bilateral prophylactic mastectomy: prospective study using questionnaires and semi-structured interviews. BMJ 2001; 322(7278):76–79.

32. Hopwood P, Lee A, Shenton A, et al. Clinical follow-up after bilateral risk reducing ('prophylactic') mastectomy: mental health and body image issues. Psychooncology 2000; 9:462–472.

33. Payne DK, Biggs C, Tran KN, Borgen PI, Massie MJ. Women's regrets after bilateral prophylactic mastectomy. Ann Surg Oncol 2000; 7(1):150–154.

34. Frost MH, Schaid DJ, Sellers TA, et al. Long-term satisfaction and psychological and social function following bilateral prophylactic mastectomy. JAMA 2000; 284(3):319–324.

35. Harcourt D, Rumsey N, Ambler N, et al. The psychological impact of mastectomy with or without immediate breast reconstruction: a prospective, multi-centre study. Plast Reconstr Surg 2003; 111(3):1060–1068.

36. Parsaie FA, Golchin M, Asvadi I. A comparison of nurse and patient perceptions of chemotherapy treatment stressors. Cancer Nurs 2000; 23(5):371–374.

37. Makar K, Cumming CE, Lees AW, et al. Sexuality, body image and quality of life after high dose or conventional chemotherapy for metastatic breast cancer. Can J Human Sexuality 1997; 6(1):1–8.

38. Batchelor D. Hair and cancer chemotherapy: consequences and nursing care – a literature study. Eur J Cancer Care 2001; 10:147–163.

39. Williams J, Wood C, Cunningham-Warburton P. A narrative study of chemotherapy-induced alopecia. Oncol Nurs Forum 1999; 26(9):1463–1468.

40. McGarvey EL, Baum LD, Pinkerton RC, Rogers LM. Psychological sequelae and alopecia among women with cancer. Cancer Pract 2001; 9(6):283–289.

41. Irvine L, Jodrell N. The distress associated with cranial irradiation: a comparison of patient and nurse perceptions. Cancer Nurs 1999; 22(2):126–133.

42. Faithfull S. Radiotherapy. In: Corner J, Bailey C, eds. Cancer nursing: care in context. London: Blackwell Science; 2001:222–261.

43. Lansdown R, Rumsey N, Bradbury E, Carr T, Partridge J, eds. Visibly different: coping with disfigurement. London: Butterworth-Heinemann; 1997.

44. Lazarus RS, Folkman S. Stress, appraisal and coping. New York: Springer; 1984.

45. Taylor SE. Adjustment to threatening events: a theory of cognitive adaptation. Am Psychol 1983; 38(3):1161–1173.

46. RCN Cancer Nursing Society. A structure for Cancer Nursing Services. RCN Cancer Nursing Society; 1996.

47. Hopwood P. The assessment of body image in patients with cancer. Eur J Cancer 1993; 29A(2):276–281.

48. Lockhart JS. Nurses' perceptions of head and neck oncology patients after surgery: severity of facial disfigurement and patient gender. ORL Head Neck Nurs 1999; 17(4):12–25.

49. Clarke A, Cooper C. Psychosocial rehabilitation after disfiguring injury or disease: investigating the training needs of specialist nurses. J Adv Nurs 2001; 43(1):18–26.

50. NHS. NHS Cancer Plan: a plan for investment, a plan for reform. London: Department of Health; 2000.

51. Edwards D. Face to face: patient, family and professional perspectives of head and neck cancer care. London: King's Fund;1997.

52. Zabora J, Brintzenhofeszoc K, Curbow B, Hooker C, Piantadosi S. The prevalence of psychological distress by cancer site. Psychooncology 2001;10:19–28.

53. Miller SM. Monitoring versus blunting styles of coping with cancer influence the information patients want and need about their disease. Implications for cancer screening and management. Cancer 1995; 76 (2):167–177.

54. Neill KM, Briefs BA. Factors that influence plastic surgeon's advice about reconstruction to

women with breast cancer. Plast Surg Nurs 1997; 17(2):61–67.

55. Ambler N, Rumsey N, Harcourt D, et al. Specialist nurse counsellor interventions at the time of diagnosis of breast cancer: comparing 'advocacy' with a conventional approach. J Adv Nurs 1999; 29(2):445–453.

56. Barker J, Harcourt D. Breast cancer: giving women a more proactive role. Nurs Times 1998; 94(13):58–59.

57. Secretary of State for Health. The Patients' Charter. London: HMSO; 1995.

58. Morris J, Royle GT. Offering patients a choice of surgery for early breast cancer: a reduction in anxiety and depression in patients and their husbands. Soc Sci Med 1988; 26(6):583–585.

59. Fallowfield LJ, Hall A, Maguire P, Baum M, A'Hern RP. A question of choice: results of a prospective 3 year follow-up study of women with breast cancer. The Breast 1994; 3:202–208.

60. Deber RB, Kraetschmer N, Irvine J. What role do patients wish to play in treatment decision making? Arch Intern Med 1996; 156(13):1414–1420.

61. Harcourt D, Rumsey N. Mastectomy patients' decision-making for or against immediate breast reconstruction. Psychooncology 2004; 139(2):106–115.

62. Harcourt D. The psychosocial implications of recent changes to the provision of care for women with breast cancer: speedier diagnosis & breast reconstruction. Unpublished PhD thesis, University of the West of England, Bristol; 2001.

63. Bunn H, O'Connor AM. Validation of client decision-making instruments in the context of psychiatry. Can J Nurs Res 1996; 28 (3):13–27.

64. O'Connor AM, Rostom A, Fiset V, et al. Decision aids for patients facing health treatment or screening decisions: systematic review. BMJ 1999; 319:731–734.

65. Pierce PF. Decisional control and distress in breast cancer treatment choices. Psychooncology 1999; 8(6 Suppl):67.

66. Watson M. Psychosocial intervention with patients with cancer: a review. Psychol Med 1983; 13:839–846.

67. Broomfield D, Humphris GM, Fisher SE, et al. The orofacial cancer patient's support from the general practitioner, hospital teams, family and friends. J Cancer Educ 1997; 12:229–232.

68. Burgess L. Facing the reality of head and neck cancer. Nurs Stand 1994; 8(32):30–34.

69. Bredin M. Altered self-concept. In: Corner J, Bailey C, eds. Cancer nursing: care in context. London: Blackwell Science; 2001:414–419.

70. Guex P. An introduction to psycho-oncology. London: Routledge: 1994.

71. van den Borne HW, Pruyn JFA, van Dam-de Mey K. Self-help in patients with cancer: a review of studies on the effects of contacts between fellow-patients. Patient Educ Couns 1986; 8:367–385.

72. Rumsey N, Harcourt D. Body image and disfigurement: issues and interventions. Body Image 2004; 1(1):83–97.

73. Hopwood P, Fletcher I, Lee A, Al Ghazal S. A body image scale for use with patients with cancer. Eur J Cancer 2001; 37:189–197.

74. Cash TF, Fleming EC, Alindogan J, Steadman L, Whitehead A. Beyond body image as a trait: the development and validation of the body image states scale. Eating Disorders: The Journal of Treatment and Prevention 2002; 10(2):103–113.

75. Bottomley A. To randomise or not to randomise: methodological pitfalls of the RCT design in psychosocial intervention studies. Eur J Cancer Care 1997; 6:222–230.

76. Harcourt D, Rumsey N. Psychological aspects of breast reconstruction: a review of existing literature. J Adv Nurs 2001; 35(4):477–487.

77. Hopwood P, Maguire P. Body image problems in patients with cancer. Br J Psychiatry 1988; 153(Suppl 2):47–50.

CHAPTER 33

Psychological Care for Patients With Cancer

EILEEN FURLONG AND SINEAD O'TOOLE

CHAPTER CONTENTS

Introduction	717	Management of post-traumatic stress disorder	728
The cancer experience	717	Delirium	728
Hope and meaning for patients with cancer	718	Management of delirium	728
Psychological response to the cancer diagnosis	719	Assessment of psychological distress	729
Coping strategies for patients with cancer	721	Psychotherapeutic interventions	731
Depression	723	Humanistic approaches to psychological distress	732
Prevalence and risk factors	723	Behavioural approaches to psychological distress	733
Symptoms of depression	723	Cognitive approaches to psychological distress	734
Management of depression	725	Psychoanalytic approaches to psychological distress	734
Suicide	725		
Anxiety	725		
Features of anxiety	726		
Management of anxiety	726	Conclusion	734
Post-traumatic stress disorder	727	References	735

INTRODUCTION

The psychological response to cancer is unique for each individual and the response extends to family, friends and healthcare professionals. Psychological care incorporates assessment, identification and prevention of affective disorders, maintenance of hope, management of uncertainty and supporting the patient's ability to adapt and cope with serious illness. The provision of psychological support is an important aspect of care for people with cancer. Cancer nurses are in a unique position to facilitate the adjustment of patients and their families from the time of diagnosis and throughout the disease trajectory. In this chapter the cancer experience,

incorporating the psychological response to cancer, the nature of the disease and treatment, and the relationship between patients and healthcare professionals, is discussed. The coping strategies utilized by patients with cancer are outlined. In addition, the psychosocial sequelae, including depression, anxiety and post-traumatic stress symptoms, are presented with the focus on psychotherapeutic interventions, which nurses may utilize when caring for people with cancer.

THE CANCER EXPERIENCE

Cancer can occur at anytime of a person's life span and the cancer experience has many different manifestations. Therefore, each patient will encounter a variety of physical and psychological challenges. The cancer journey has many routes, in that some people will face a progressive illness and impending death while the majority cope with surviving. Thus, the psychological impact of cancer cannot be the same for all patients, and the psychological needs of patients and their family and friends will also be different. Just as the dosages of chemotherapy and radiation are titrated according to the individual needs of a patient, psychological care needs to take into account many different facets of a patient's life: personality, age, gender, social support, previous experience of illness, health information processing style, physical condition, mood and emotional stability.[1] This diversity of experience and needs provides, for practitioners, one of the most challenging aspects of providing psychological care and, accordingly, this care must be individualized. To maximize the care provided to patients with cancer, the psychological impact of cancer and the associated distress needs to be understood by healthcare professionals.

Psychological distress is a normal reaction to the diagnosis of cancer, as Houldin[2] has indicated, and one of the reasons for this is the mythology that surrounds cancer itself. The meanings with which cancer is imbued have little in common with current scientific facts of the disease. Cancer is no longer considered by the medical community to be a usually fatal disease.[3] It is a curable illness for some people and a chronic condition for many others.[2] However, it is still considered by patients and families to be more frightening than other equally serious diseases. Indeed, as Flanagan and Holmes[4] have indicated, it appears to be especially significant in evoking negative feelings. This means that the people with cancer will need support in overcoming emotional reactions as well as support in tackling the cancer itself. In providing psychological care, the key role of the nurse is to communicate effectively with the patient with cancer. This involves skilfully interacting with patients, which is based on an understanding of what cancer means for the person. Given that distress is to be anticipated as the usual reaction to the crisis of a cancer diagnosis, it is important that patients understand that this distress is normal and adaptive, and that it is not an indication of personal weakness.[1] Early studies[5] suggested that some reactions may be more useful in terms of survival than others. However, there is no consistent evidence to demonstrate that the way in which individuals react to cancer will have any influence on their survival.[6] Supporting people in an individualized way with their distress, and fostering hope and meaning, are central to the provision of psychological care.

Hope and meaning for patients with cancer

There are several observational studies, reported by Scheier and Carver,[7] which indicate that people who have hope and meaning in their lives are more likely to do better when confronted by adversity. It may be that psychotherapeutic interventions that are successful in supporting patients in adjusting to cancer do so because they induce hope and meaning in the person's life.[7] Hope and meaning alter with the changes in a person's cancer journey and there are many opportunities for healthcare professionals to foster reality-based hope and recognize meaning, throughout the illness trajectory. As patients' clinical status changes, they may need help in realigning hope,[1] and some of these strategies will be described in the section on psychotherapeutic interventions. In addition, clinicians' caring presence can influence hope as much as the interventions they employ. Having one's individuality recognized, despite illness and failing health, fosters hope, whereas being subjected to responses that are uncaring, belittling or patronizing threatens hope.[8] How patients are spoken to, as well as what is said, will influence their capacity for hopefulness. The ability of nurses to listen to patients tell their stories will also influence meaning and hope.[9]

The belief that hope is always useful is not universally held. Omar and Rosenbaum[10] offer another perspective on hope and suggest that it may be maladaptive when unrealistic and can lead to mindless sacrifices, to rigid attitudes or behaviours, and the undervaluing of the present. They suggest that patients who cling to unrealistic hope may be unable to engage in anticipatory planning for bad news and their distress will be increased when events are not as they expected. They are unable to engage in what Janis[11] called the work of worry. Houldin[2] suggests that when this is the case, healthcare professionals need to support individuals to let go of hope and allow the work of despair to provide benefit.

Hoping implies looking to the future, whereas some Eastern philosophies indicate that it is only in looking at the present that any of us will find happiness. Supporting individuals with living in the present may be as useful as encouraging them to look to the future. Using mindfulness meditations allows an individual to realize the preciousness of the moment and can facilitate living in the present and foster meaning and hope.[2,12] In a less formal way, people can be helped to live in the present by taking notice of beauty in their surroundings, calling attention to the shape of a flower, the colour of a grandchild's hair, the quality of sunlight or the sound of rain. It is important that healthcare professionals balance hope and living in the present from the first encounter with a patient. Nurses need to take every opportunity to be fully aware of the patient and consciously attend to psychological care: at some times, patients with cancer may need nurses to discuss their cancer treatment; at other times, they may want a break from their disease and may choose to talk about the garden or tell a joke.[12] What is significant is that these interactions are important and part of the work of providing psychological care. Although psychological care may seem more apparent at diagnosis, it is essential throughout the cancer trajectory.

Psychological response to the cancer diagnosis

Cancer is diagnosed in a myriad of different circumstances. Some people will already have a strong suspicion that the tests will reveal cancer or its recurrence, whereas others may be diagnosed following a routine test. A person may awaken one morning feeling perfectly healthy and go to bed that night knowing that they have cancer. Some patients will already be aware of their increased genetic risk and for them the diagnosis may have been anticipated for some time. Despite the circumstances in which it occurs, it is normal that patients and their families experience the diagnosis of cancer as a major life crisis.[2] An early description of the reaction to a cancer diagnosis is as an existential crisis. Weisman and Worden[13] describe the experience as encompassing great distress caused by fear of abandonment, loss of control, intense loneliness and psychological pain. This description has been echoed by subsequent research and clinical work,[1] as well as many personal descriptions.[14]

It is not possible to predict how any one individual will respond to the challenge that the illness presents, as people vary widely in how well or how poorly they adapt to cancer. Nevertheless, there are many factors that influence individual psychological responses to cancer and its treatment.[5,15] The individual influences on response fall into three categories, as outlined below: those associated with the patient, the nature of the disease and treatment and the relationship between the patient with cancer and healthcare professionals.

Influences on psychological response related to the patient

Massie and Holland[16] have described a three-phase response to a diagnosis of cancer or its recurrence. Initially, the response is that of shock, disbelief and denial. The response in the second phase includes feelings of anxiety and depression, anger and guilt. People often lose their appetite and have difficulty concentrating and sleeping. The third phase involves coming to terms with the illness and meeting the demands of treatment. It is important to recognize that these phases are not neatly distinct from each other or that they necessarily occur in this order. There are so many influences on how a person may feel that some people may experience a roller coaster of emotions whereas others may feel detached for the duration of their illness. Therefore, it is important for nurses to remain flexible and open and to consider how the patient with cancer is feeling at this particular time. The first step is to ask the person how they are feeling and listen to the reply.

The task of adapting to cancer in the short and long term is influenced by the developmental stage of the individual, and thus the challenges presented will vary according to the age of the person with cancer.[1] As Holland has indicated, an understanding of the patient's developmental stage and the associated psychological and social tasks facilitate a clearer understanding of the meaning of cancer for that individual.[1] For example, a challenge for a child with cancer may be in maintaining school grades, whereas a challenge for an older person may be in maintaining the role as a family provider. Knowing that forming friendships is an important social task for an adolescent, the nurse might be prompted to ask adolescent patients about their friendships and how the cancer has affected these relationships. This is facilitating a discussion about a topic that is usually very important to most teenagers; however, the challenges of cancer are individual and dynamic and it is important not to assume that nurses know what is worrying patients but that patients are asked about their concerns.

Influences on psychological response related to the disease and treatment

The response of the individual with cancer is influenced by the type, stage, treatment modality and manifestations of the disease. In particular, symptoms such as pain, breathlessness, delirium and functional disability increase the difficulty of coping with the disease.[1] Generally, the stage of the disease will influence how an individual copes: for example, the task of coping with advanced disease is made more difficult by increased symptoms, exhaustion and existential issues.[17] The selected treatment modality or combined modalities has an impact on the psychological response of the patient with cancer. The patient's perception, past experience and knowledge of the treatment plan influences the patient's ability to cope psychologically. A delay in diagnosis may occur because patients do not recognize the disease, or they may ignore the disease in the hope that it will go away. Delay in diagnosis is not only associated with less successful treatment but is also associated with psychological morbidity.[16]

Another significant influence is the site of the disease, particularly those sites associated with special meaning for the individual. Different site-specific cancers may have cultural or sexual meaning for people, resulting in a delay in presentation and an increase in suffering.[16] When visual disfigurement is caused by cancer or its treatment, the toll on the patient is increased.[18] Additional effects of treatment increase the impact on the patient: for example, alopecia, nausea, vomiting, weight gain, fatigue and infertility. Some of these effects will be immediately felt and transient, whereas others will have long-term and permanent effects.[16] The outcome of cancer is not universal, and while some people with cancer will be cured others are almost certain to die from the disease. The prognosis for many patients with cancer falls somewhere between these extremes.[1] It is not usually possible to give an exact prognosis but it is always possible to give guidelines that depend upon the type of cancer and its stage of advancement. It is important to check that the prognosis as understood by the patient and family is the same as that of the clinicians. The subjective belief of the patient will influence their psychological adjustment.[19,20] To provide effective psychological care it is important to provide good-quality physical care. As Ferrell and Dow[21] indicate, the quality of a person's life is affected by physical, social, spiritual and psychological factors: these interlinked facets of a person's life influence how the person will feel. Thus, at any one particular time a patient's happiness or psychological comfort may be influenced more strongly by physical condition than by any psychological factors. Severe stomatitis, for example, may lead a person to question whether they will continue treatment.[22] So, starting with simple questions – 'How are you feeling right now? How can I help? What's causing you the most distress right now?' – may help to indicate the best place to begin to provide care. Sometimes this will be a physical intervention while at other times it will be appropriate to intervene psychologically. Sometimes it is difficult to distinguish between the two: for example, an explanation of a worrying symptom as a physical side-effect of treatment that is likely to be transient may bring psychological relief. Letting a person know that the difficulty in concentration that they are experiencing is more likely to be a transient effect of the chemotherapy than a permanent effect of the cancer.

Influences on psychological response related to healthcare professionals

The relationship that healthcare professionals have with patients exerts a strong influence on the patient's ability to cope.[23] Patients have expressed a need for nurses to develop a human relationship with them in which they can feel affirmed and understood.[23] This means that as nurses interact with patients while caring for them they need to take every opportunity to develop and nurture good relationships. This involves taking the time to talk to patients, to listen to them and to demonstrate the desire to understand the meaning of their suffering.[2] Effective communication with patients is also associated with improved pain control, adherence to treatment regimens and better psychological functioning.[24]

In contrast, non-caring responses from nurses are associated with decreased hope and poorer psychological outcomes.[8,10] Poor communication results in increased anxiety, uncertainty and decreased satisfaction with care.[24] Although skilful communication seems to be easier for some staff members than others, it is an art that can be learned and practised, so that communicating well becomes a natural response.[15] This will not always guarantee trouble-free interactions, but the use of the interventions outlined later in this chapter will facilitate the nurturing and development of good relationships. However, good techniques are not sufficient on their own, as Fagerstrom et al[23] have discovered. The personal characteristics of the nurse are important in that patients express their needs according to how able they perceive the nurse to be in understanding and responding to these needs.[23] In addition, the relationship between patients and healthcare professionals can be permanently influenced by the manner in which the cancer diagnosis was disclosed.[15] Nurses need to develop skills to enhance the relationship at the time of diagnosis to minimize distress. There is a potential for bad news throughout the treatment and beyond. Indeed, worries about

recurrence may last for many years, and some people will continue to need support and contact with the unit in which they were treated. The diagnosis of recurrence usually causes significant stress, which may be more distressing than that caused by the initial diagnosis.[25] Individuals with relapsing or progressing disease may experience renewed anxiety about their ability to cope. The task of managing the disease is made more difficult by many factors, including the increased uncertainty of the patient's future, the disappointment over the failure of the treatment and, guilt related to feelings of personal responsibility for the progression of the cancer.[26] On the other hand, many people with recurrent and advanced cancer adjust, manage to engage in meaningful activities, and function well in their lives.[27] In addition, suffering can continue in the absence of a recurrence of the illness and cure does not necessarily signify the end of psychological distress.[28-31] The patient with cancer, the nature of the disease and the relationship with healthcare professionals all have an impact on the psychological aspect of care. In addition, the coping mechanisms of the patient with cancer will influence the interventions of healthcare professionals.

Coping strategies for patients with cancer

Individuals are likely to use the same coping strategies when confronted with cancer as they use when coping with other crises.[31] Therefore, it is useful to ask about other times of crisis for the family. This is beneficial for many reasons, in that by hearing about previous coping strategies used successfully in the past, similar strategies for a current crisis can be suggested. The term 'coping' is subject to different interpretations.[32] Lazarus and Folkman[32] describe coping as constantly changing cognitive and behavioural efforts to manage specific external and/or internal demands that are appraised as taxing or exceeding the resources of a person.[32] This definition is broad and permits coping to include anything that a person does or thinks, regardless of how well or badly it works. Coping does not imply success, but efforts to resolve a stressful situation.[33] It is not only a reaction to stress; it can also be preventative, by anticipating a stressful situation. According to Ceslowitz,[34] coping may be viewed as a buffer that moderates the impact of stress. It has also been viewed as a continually changing and varying process, which is important, as individuals in stressful situations may use a limited or an inappropriate range of coping strategies.

The literature on coping focuses on two major theoretically based themes of coping: problem-focused and emotion-focused.[32] Problem-focused coping is aimed at reducing the demands of the stressful situation or expanding the resources to deal with it.[35] In problem-focused coping, the person seeks information and tries to cope through problem-solving strategies which may help to regain self-control. Patients who want to know their treatment schedule in detail are likely to be utilizing problem-focused coping. Emotion-focused coping, on the other hand, is a means of regulating tension and the emotional response to the patient.[32] One method of implementing emotion-focused forms of coping consists of the development of cognitive processes which are directed at lessening emotional distress. Strategies to achieve such a goal include avoidance, minimization, distancing, selective attention, positive comparisons and wrestling positive value from negative events.[32] Patients with cancer use emotion-focused coping when they will not talk about the cancer or appear to ignore what is happening with their treatment.

Another benefit of listening to descriptions of past crises is the discovery of the patient's locus of control.[36] The locus of control can be internal or external and can be identified when talking to patients with cancer:[36] for example, does this person usually like to do things for themselves (internal locus of control) or do they usually like to have help to do things (external locus of control)? The nurse can then suggest strategies most likely to be appealing to the individual patient. For example, you may see that a patient is finding radiotherapy administration very difficult and you believe that the patient may find using a distraction or relaxation strategy such as guided imagery helpful. If the person has an internal locus of control, the nurse could introduce the strategy by saying: 'I can show you a technique that you can use while you are having your radiotherapy that will make things easier. It's quick to learn and you can use it yourself at any time; you can even make a tape for yourself'. The underlying message here is that the person does not have to be totally dependent during their radiotherapy session; rather, there is something that they can do for themselves. For a patient with an external locus of control, the nurse could introduce the strategy by saying: 'Would you like us to work on a technique that's easy to learn that will make things more comfortable while you are having radiotherapy. We can make a tape of the guided imagery and then you can have the tape as well as the radiotherapy staff during the radiotherapy sessions'. The underlying message here is that the person does not have to do this alone; rather, there is something that they can bring to the session that will be an added support.

Previous personal experience with cancer will also influence how a patient will cope. Positive outcomes are associated with knowing someone who did well in the past,[16] whereas a previous adverse experience of cancer in the family is associated with increased risk of psychological problems.[3] Being diagnosed with the same illness from which a family member died increases the challenge presented by the illness.[3] Thus, it is important to ask patients and families about the experience of other people that they know with cancer. This is useful because it helps in exploring beliefs and misconceptions about cancer. It also helps to quickly identify people at increased risk of psychological problems.[3] In addition, a previous history of psychiatric illness is associated with increased risk of psychological distress.[16] Patients who have been depressed or anxious in the past are at risk of relapsing when confronted with the crisis of a cancer diagnosis.[15] Also, people with learning difficulties, schizophrenia or Alzheimer's disease may present with a delayed diagnosis as they may not have noticed or spoken about their symptoms.[15] Thus, it is especially important to establish good relationships not only with the patients themselves but also with family members and carers, as social support is essential for these patients.[15]

Social support is believed to be beneficial in helping individuals adjust to stressful life events such as serious physical illness, anxiety and depression.[37] In addition, physical functioning and well-being are enhanced when the individual is supported by family and significant others. However, people with cancer may have difficulty in finding adequate support, as fear and dread may cause family and friends to avoid them.[4] Thus, family and friends may become a source of distress rather than support. This may result in increasing the isolation and suffering of the person with cancer, as lack of support is associated with increased risk of psychological distress.[4]

Most people with cancer cope with the illness and its treatment;[2] however, some people are traumatized by the cancer experience. The most common psychological reactions are depression and anxiety. It is important for nurses to be able to distinguish normal sadness, worry and distraction from depression, anxiety and delirium.

DEPRESSION

Prevalence and risk factors

The expected and normal reaction to being diagnosed and treated for cancer is that of sadness and worry; nevertheless, most patients will manage remarkably well.[2] However, for some individuals the distress is more intense and becomes a clinical depressive disorder.[38] Estimates of the incidence of depression, including major depression and depressive symptoms, range from 0 to 58%.[38] This range in estimated prevalence figures indicates a lack of uniformity in measurement, population and methodology between individual studies. Massie[38] indicates that the clinical rule of thumb is that 25% of patients with cancer at some point during their disease are likely to need evaluation and treatment for depression. Risk factors for developing depression are influenced by the individual, the illness and the treatment. These are presented in Box 33.1.

There are higher incidences of depression reported with different cancers.[38] The reasons

---

Box 33.1

Risk factors for developing depression in patients with cancer

Individual

Family or personal history of depression

Family or personal history of suicide attempts

Family or personal history of addictions (alcohol, drugs)

Lack of supportive/confiding relationships

Conspiracy of silence

Recent bereavement

Loss of independence

Spiritual difficulties

Threat of death

Illness and treatment

Advanced stage of cancer

Poorly controlled pain

Increased physical impairment or discomfort

Concurrent illness that produces depressive symptoms

Metabolic disturbances

Nutritional abnormalities

Endocrine disturbances

Neurological imbalance

Whole brain irradiation

Drugs: antihypertensives, benzodiazepines, corticosteroids, cytotoxics, neuroleptics, as well as hormones and antiviral agents

Source: data from Holland,[1] Houldin[2] and Twycross.[17]

---

for the variations in incidence are not uniform: for example, increased incidence of depression with oropharyngeal cancer may be associated with the changes in speech and facial appearance, whereas the depression associated with pancreatic cancer may be influenced by prognosis or paraneoplastic syndrome. Massie[38] provides an overview of the prevalence of depression in site-specific cancers. Knowledge of the risk factors for developing depression can assist nurses in assessing symptoms that patients with cancer may develop.

Symptoms of depression

It is important to distinguish between a reaction of normal sadness and depression. Depression usually responds to treatment, and untreated depression intensifies other symptoms, leads to social withdrawal and can prevent patients from completing unfinished business.[1,17,39] Carroll[40] notes that patients who are depressed may look physically worse than they are and may be investigated for complications of treatment or advancement of their disease. Depression in people with cancer often goes unnoticed.[41] The distinction between ordinary sadness and depression is not always easy to make, as healthcare workers may assume that the sadness is an appropriate reaction to the diagnosis of cancer. Staff working in the area of cancer care may be unable to recognize the symptoms of depression. They may be unwilling to ask patients about their emotions, as quality of life issues do not have the same urgency, nor are they given the same importance as improvements in disease-free survival.[39] If stigma is associated with mental health problems, then healthcare workers may be reluctant to ask about mood, and patients may not volunteer information. In addition, the recognition of depression can be hampered because both depression and cancer share symptoms such as fatigue, weakness, insomnia, anorexia, loss of libido, as well as difficulties with motivation and concentration. Therefore, depression in patients with cancer is best evaluated using the psychological clinical features, as the somatic signs and symptoms are less useful. If these symptoms of sadness are intense, if they persist and are interfering with daily functioning, then patients should be evaluated for depression.[1,16,17] Mood disorders judged to be secondary to a medical condition are included in a subcategory of the *Diagnostic and Statistical Manual of Mental Disorders, Fourth Edition* (DSMIV).[42] However, in the International Classification of Disease (ICD)[43] they are classified as mood disorders under organic mental conditions.[43] Clinical features of depression are outlined in Box 33.2

Twycross[17] presents a useful way of distinguishing between sadness and depression. He suggests that some features of depression and sadness are shared, whereas other features are indicative of depression rather than normal sadness. The shared features include depressed mood, tearfulness, anxiety, suicidal ideas, tiredness, decreased concentration, loss of interest

---

Box 33.2

Clinical features of depression

Psychological

Dysphoric mood (sad, depressed, anxious), crying, diurnal mood change

Feelings of hopelessness, helplessness, worthless, guilt

Loss of interest and pleasure

Loss of concentration and motivation

Mood incongruent to disease outlook

Suicidal thoughts or plans

Somatic

Insomnia

Anorexia and weight loss

Fatigue

Psychomotor retardation or agitation

Constipation

Loss of libido

Source: data from Massie and Holland[16] Twycross.[17]

---

and anorexia. Those features that are more likely to suggest depression are profound sadness, loss of emotion, irritability, physical anxiety (sweating, tremor, panic attacks), hopelessness (particularly in relation to family and friends), guilt, intractable pain, suicide attempts and requests for euthanasia. He indicates that, when depressed, patients cannot be distracted from their low mood and when talking to patients this inability to be distracted becomes apparent. People with expected levels of sadness often find relief having spoken about their feelings or having cried with someone, and when their mood lifts they may manage to smile again and talk about something else for a while. In contrast, a person who is depressed appears down fairly constantly and gets little relief from talking or crying.[17] In depression, diurnal mood variation is common, with patients feeling worse early in the morning and gradually appearing less depressed during the day. This very low mood is often apparent to nurses when talking to patients in the early hours of the morning, as later in the day when the patient is talking to their doctor their mood may have lightened. The social mask that patients display when interacting with healthcare professionals can hamper the detection of depression. Patients may wish to protect us from their feelings, or may not wish to be seen as moaning all the time. People with cancer may wish to appear stronger than they are feeling, for fear their psychological state will impede their physical treatment.[26]

Management of depression

It has been suggested that depression is managed initially by maintaining good relationships with patients, helping them to normalize their emotions and mobilize support.[1,16] The recommended treatment of major depression is a combination of both psychology and pharmacology. In this chapter, pharmacological management will not be addressed.

Psychological management

Psychotherapeutic interventions that nurses may find useful in practice include those that emphasize past strengths, support previously successful ways of coping and enhance inner resources.[3] Individual and group strategies allow patients an opportunity to discuss their thoughts and feelings. Cognitive and behavioural interventions support patients in reframing the problems more constructively and alter distressing symptoms and their responses to them. Meta-analysis of cognitive-behavioural or psychosocial interventions showed a modest benefit.[2] Psychotherapy can be used alone to treat moderate to severe depression but is usually applied in addition to drug treatments.[44]

SUICIDE

As Barraclough[15] notes, many healthy people believe that they would be tempted to commit suicide if they developed cancer. Holland[1] believes that patients with cancer use the idea of suicide as a protective mechanism, one that will allow them to take control if their suffering becomes unbearable in the future. It is a way of coping with the fear of uncontrollable symptoms and a painful protracted death. In reality, although the incidence of suicide is increased in patients with cancer, where it is

almost twice that of the general population, it is still uncommon.[1,15] However, suicide at home by overdose, when the patient is at an advanced stage of the disease process, is likely to be under-reported.[1]

Risk factors that predict suicide are similar to those predicting depression and include a history of psychiatric illness, prior suicide attempts, prior alcohol or drug abuse, recent loss or bereavement and poorly controlled symptoms including pain, fatigue, depression and hopelessness. Evaluating the risk of suicide begins with establishing a trusting relationship and having a clear understanding of how patients are feeling. It is important to remember that asking about suicidal thoughts does not cause them to happen, and patients are usually relieved to tell someone of their despair.

When patients have suicidal ideation, intent and plan, they must be referred immediately for psychiatric evaluation and treatment. Some people may make a rational decision to commit suicide; however, given time for reflection and more information, they may change their intention as this rational decision may have been based on false premises.[45] Suicidal wishes are often reduced with good control of a patient's symptoms and distress, especially pain and depression.[1,3]

ANXIETY

Anxiety is a normal response to unfamiliar, uncertain, unpredictable and dangerous situations: therefore, it is an appropriate response to a diagnosis of cancer.[3] Usually, this response is time limited in that it is a protective mechanism that allows the individual to prepare for a stressful life event. Anxiety usually occurs with anticipation of test results, at the time of diagnosis, when preparing for treatments or procedures and at transitional points during the illness. It is likely to continue when treatment is finished and may remain with fears of recurrence. The initial management of mild to moderate anxiety is the provision of support and information. Although expected, not all anxiety is normative or easily managed, and excessive or prolonged anxiety will interfere with coping and activities of daily living for some patients. As with depression, the risk factors for developing anxiety disorders are influenced by the individual, the illness and treatment (Box 33.3).

Features of anxiety

Physical symptoms of anxiety vary considerably between people. Many patients have difficulty sleeping or report frightening dreams.[31] Some patients may be afraid to sleep or may be frightened when left alone, whereas others may be consistently tense and cannot be distracted from their worrying. The prevalence and magnitude of the clinical features (Box 33.4) will be determined by the severity of the anxiety.[1] In the DSMIV,[42] acute stress disorder and post-traumatic stress disorder are classified as anxiety disorder, whereas the ICD[43] has a classification of reactions to severe stress and adjustment disorder.[43]

Management of anxiety

The belief that it is reasonable for a patient to worry when they have cancer may present a barrier to appropriate evaluation and treatment.[16] As with depression, the first step is in establishing a trusting relationship with patients and understanding their experience. Nurses are in a privileged position to develop such a relationship because of their constant presence with the patient 24 hours a day. It is important to normalize a patient's response and to provide educational and emotional support. Facilitating the mobilization of social support is also useful. The usual techniques for treating anxiety include a combination of psychological and pharmacological management strategies.[16]

Psychological management

Psychological interventions frequently used by nurses and other healthcare professionals

---

Box 33.3

Risk factors for developing anxiety in patients with cancer

Individual

Exacerbation of pre-existing anxiety disorder
Phobias (cancer, needles, claustrophobia)
Post-traumatic stress disorder
Worry about family or finances
Conflict with family or staff
Thoughts about the past (guilt, regret)
Fear of pain
Fear of dying

Illness and treatment

Frightening and painful procedures
Poorly controlled pain
Abnormal metabolic states (e.g. hypoxia, sepsis, delirium)
Hormone-secreting tumours (e.g. thyroid adenoma or carcinoma, parathyroid adenoma, insulinoma)
Paraneoplastic syndromes (remote CNS effect)
Anxiety-producing drugs (e.g. antiemetic neuroleptics, bronchodilators)
Withdrawal states (e.g. alcohol, benzodiazepines, opioids)
Conditioned anxiety (e.g. anticipatory anxiety, nausea and vomiting with cyclic chemotherapy)

Source: data from Holland[1] and Twycross.[17]

Box 33.4

Clinical features of anxiety

Restlessness
Tense worried expression
Sweating, tremor
Dizziness, nausea
Weakness, exhaustion
Poor concentration and memory
Irritability
Headaches
Palpitations
Sinus tachycardia
Elevated systolic blood pressure
Precordial pain
Hyperventilation
Dyspnoea, feeling of suffocation, air swallowing
Anorexia
Diarrhoea
Polyuria

Source: data from Massie and Holland[16] and Twycross.[17]

include cognitive-behavioural techniques,[6,7,19,26] crisis counselling,[19,26] brief supportive counselling,[19,26] support groups,[6,7,19,26] together with couple and family therapy[19,26] where appropriate. Several behavioural interventions have been found to be helpful, including relaxation techniques[26] and guided imagery.[2] Meditation has also been effective in relieving anxiety.[1,2,12]

POST-TRAUMATIC STRESS DISORDER

Recent studies have indicated that many patients with psychological morbidity may also have post-traumatic stress disorder (PTSD).[46,47] Kwekkeboom and Seng[48] suggest that the diagnosis of PTSD can go unrecognized because the symptoms are not conceptualized within a PTSD framework, and the diagnosis is not made in this population. In 1994, the DSMIV of the American Psychiatric Association revised the definition of the trauma understood to precipitate

PTSD.[42] This revised definition now includes events that involve actual or threatened death or serious injury or other threat to one's physical integrity that evokes intense fear, helplessness or horror.[42] Thus, it is now acknowledged that a diagnosis of cancer can evoke responses that fulfil the criteria for PTSD.[49] Estimates of the incidence of PTSD in people with cancer range from 2.5 to 20%.[47] Again, this range in estimated prevalence figures indicates a lack of uniformity in population and methodology between individual studies.[48–51]

A diagnosis of PTSD is made not just on the experience of trauma but requires the presence of three characteristic symptom clusters (re-experiencing of the traumatic event, avoidance or numbing and hyperarousal), occurring for at least 1 month, and resulting in impaired social or occupational functioning (Table 33.1).[42] For the diagnosis to be made, the patient must have experienced at least one symptom of intrusive re-experiencing, at least three symptoms of avoidance/numbing and at least two symptoms of increased arousal.[42]

Table 33.1: Symptoms of post-traumatic stress disorder

Symptom cluster	Symptom
Intrusive re-experiencing of trauma	Nightmares Flashbacks Unwanted memories that last from a second to hours
Avoidance	Avoiding activities, places or people that trigger memories of the traumatic event Attempting to prevent thinking or talking about the event
Numbing	Feelings of detachment Loss of interest in activities Loss of memory for the traumatic event
Hyperarousal	Feelings of increased vulnerability Need to maintain hypervigilance Difficulty sleeping Irritability Problems with concentrating Exaggerated startle response

Source: data from Kwekkeboom and Seng.[48]

There have been reports of increased risk of physical and behavioural sequelae associated with PTSD.[48] Physical consequences include changes in stress hormone regulation and possible immune function.[52,53] Behavioural consequences include an increased association with substance abuse, eating disorder and risk-taking. Co-morbid conditions include depression, anxiety, panic, phobias, somatization and dissociation.[42] There have been reports of decreased physical, mental, social and spiritual functioning in individuals with PTSD.[50,51]

Management of post-traumatic stress disorder

There is no evidence base that is specific to the treatment of patients with cancer who are experiencing PTSD. However, Kwekkeboom and Seng[48] suggest that therapeutic communication, pain management, education, understanding and advocacy interventions could be appropriate. They emphasize the need to prevent the development of PTSD by providing emotional support and ensuring that procedures are not traumatizing. Mobilizing social support and legitimizing and normalizing the patient's experience are also believed to be helpful.[54] The nurse–patient relationship is central to the prevention of PTSD, as nurses have many opportunities to facilitate therapeutic communication about the traumatic nature of the cancer experience.

DELIRIUM

Delirium has been reported as occurring with the same frequency as anxiety and depression in patients with cancer.[55] Early symptoms of delirium, such as sudden changes in mood and behaviour, are often misdiagnosed as anxiety, anger, depression or psychosis,[56] whereas these manifestations may be changes in the patient's neurological, vascular or metabolic state. Any delay in recognizing delirium will result in a subsequent delay in treatment and will increase the distress of the individual and their family. People with cancer are at increased risk (Table 33.2) of becoming delirious because of the effects of cancer and its treatments.[55,56]

Delirium may become apparent when patients suddenly become disorientated, irritable, uncooperative, agitated or restless. They may become uncharacteristically noisy or aggressive. It is important to distinguish between depression, anxiety, dementia and delirium, so that interventions can be initiated as early as possible.[17] Although dementia and delirium share some common features, their differences allow them to be distinguished from one another.

Dementia has an insidious onset in that the course of the illness is usually progressive and irreversible, with symptoms remaining stable throughout the day. Awareness and alertness remain relatively unaffected. Thinking is impoverished and the patient's speech is usually stereotyped and limited. There is not usually any other physical illness or any drug toxicity.[17] However, dementia may be compounded by delirium.

In contrast, delirium usually has an acute onset that frequently occurs at night (Box 33.5). Symptoms often change throughout the day, with the patient experiencing periods of lucidity during the day while symptoms worsen at night. Awareness is reduced, while alertness can be unusually high or low. Thinking is disorganized and the patient's speech is usually incoherent and rambling. The patient with delirium frequently experiences illusions and hallucinations.[17,55]

Management of delirium

The principal management of delirium is the identification of underlying causes and the treatment of reversible causes. It is important to reassure relatives that delirium is a manifestation of the illness or an effect of the treatment and is usually reversible.[55]

When patients are lucid, they must be given this information also. They must continue to be treated with care and respect and have procedures explained. The presence of a relative or family member and the reduction of unfamiliar stimuli and changes of environment can reduce fears and suspicions. It can be helpful to explore the content of hallucinations, nightmares and illusions, as they can reflect the fears and anxieties of the individual. It is usually very

Table 33.2: Risk factors for developing delirium

Risk factor	Description
Metabolic encephalopathy	Due to vital organ failure – liver, kidney, lung, thyroid, adrenal
Electrolyte imbalance	Sodium, potassium, calcium, glucose
Treatment side-effects	Narcotics, anticholinergics, phenothiazines, antihistamines, chemotherapeutic agents, steroids, radiation therapy
Withdrawal state	Alcohol, nicotine, psychotropic drugs
Haematological abnormalities	Microcytic and macrocytic anaemias, coagulopathies
Nutritional	General malnutrition, thiamine, folic acid, vitamin B_{12}, dehydration
Paraneoplastic syndromes	Remote effects of tumours, hormone-producing tumours
Precipitating factors	Pain Change in environment Depression Anxiety Fatigue Constipation Urinary retention Unfamiliar excessive stimuli Decreased mobility Poor quality of sleep Decreased contact with family and friends

Source: data from Holland,[1] Twycross[17] and Krishnasamy.[55]

distressing for the family and friends of the person who is delirious and therefore there is a need for increased support from the healthcare professionals.[1,17,55]

It may not be possible to correct the underlying cause of the delirium, and the focus will then be on the control of the symptoms of confusion and agitation. Symptoms can be treated if they are causing distress to the patient or the relatives. The individual needs of the patient will determine the drugs used. Knowledge of the psychological impact of cancer on the individual and the family is paramount if effective psychological interventions are to be developed and initiated. There are many assessment tools available that will enable the nurse to devise patient-specific interventions in the delivery of psychological care.

ASSESSMENT OF PSYCHOLOGICAL DISTRESS

Barker[57] believes that assessment is the most important aspect of care and he notes that nurses cannot offer reliable nursing care without valid and effective assessment. Although Barker[57] was speaking about psychiatric nursing, his observations apply as soundly in cancer nursing, particularly in relation to psychosocial needs. In both situations the

Box 33.5

Clinical features of delirium

Early
Change in sleep patterns
Transient periods of disorientation
Unexplained anxiety and sense of dread
Outbursts of anger and increased irritability
Withdrawal from staff and family
Short-term memory problems

Late
Refusing to cooperate with requests
Escalation of angry and aggressive outbursts
Swearing and shouting
Illusions
Hallucinations
Paranoid ideas

Source: data from Holland,[1] Twycross[17] and Krishnasamy.[55]

patients' needs cannot be met until they are identified; this involves considering the whole person and identifying strengths as well as weaknesses. Nurses, because of their relationship with patients and the amount of time spent with patients, are in a unique position to make holistic assessments of psychosocial needs. Early identification of patients who are struggling to cope and prompt referral to mental healthcare professionals are important both for treatment compliance and control of distress.[1]

There are many individual factors that need to be considered when assessing psychosocial needs, including psychological, behavioural and biological functioning as well as ecological factors that include the family, interpersonal and social environments.[57] The cancer nurse is offered opportunities to notice how the patient and family are interacting, and over time to observe changes in this interaction. For example, it is apparent when family members visit less frequently, for shorter periods of time or if they spend the visit speaking to the patient or to one another. The presence or absence of get well cards or family photographs provide information about a patient's support structure and also opportunities to talk with the patient and deepen the nurse–patient relationship. Even when treatment is delivered on an ambulatory care or outpatient basis, nurses have opportunities to notice if the patient arrives alone or is accompanied. In either setting, it is easy to notice if the patient is interacting with others or is withdrawn. Noticing is just the first step in the screening procedure towards assessing patients' needs.

As Kelly[58] noted, the best way to find out what is wrong with patients is to ask them. In asking patients how they are, and in listening carefully to their reply, nurses are not only screening for signs of difficulty, like anxiety or delirium, but are also allowing the patient to express their emotions about the stressful nature of the cancer experience. Thus, assessment and intervention may not be clearly separate entities but may merge somewhat. This informal assessment and integral intervention may occur while a third task is taking place. For example, a nurse caring for a patient's wound may take the opportunity to ask how the patient is coping. In this way, the nurse is gathering information about the patient's physical status (the condition of the wound), as well as psychological status. At the same time, the patient is provided with an opportunity in which negative emotions can be expressed and debriefed. Allowing the expression of emotion acts as a preventative measure against the development of PTSD, by reducing the distress associated with the emotion and reducing the frequency by which intrusive thoughts occur.[48] Therefore, the nurse may be engaged in prevention, assessment and intervention simultaneously. The success of these interactions depends largely on the nature and quality of the relationship between the nurse and the patient. In addition to informal assessment, nurses are increasingly involved in making formal assessments. Talking with the patient can be transformed into a formal assessment by the use of a semi-structured format. Thus, talking with the patient allows the exploration of any problems and provides the cues to introduce other methods of assessment,[57] or to make referrals to other members of the multidisciplinary team.

Increasingly, nurses assess and monitor the individual's psychosocial functioning by utilizing measurement scales. In particular, brief distress scales are used, as patients may not have the energy to complete longer measures.[57,59] It is important to use measures that are valid and reliable in this patient population, so that the somatic symptoms of cancer will not interfere with interpretation. Examples of these measures include the Beck Depression Inventory, the Hospital Anxiety and Depression (HAD) scale, the Brief Symptom Checklist[26] or shortened versions of scales such as the Shortened Version of Profile of Mood Scale.[60] There have been a great many instruments developed to measure distress levels in patients with cancer. Bowling[61] and Gotay and Stern[59] provide excellent reviews of these instruments. The best-developed quality of life measure for use with cancer patients is the scales of the European Organisation for Research and Treatment of Cancer (EORTC).[61,62] As well as assessing site-specific symptoms, it also covers physical, social and psychological functioning. The importance of the judgements or diagnoses made following assessment is emphasized by Barker:[57]

> In some cases a nursing assessment, combined with other forms of medical or psychological assessment, might make the difference between life and death. This could be said of the person who is a suicide risk or the disturbed or disorientated person who might unwittingly be a danger to himself. Having said that, we cannot afford to be glib about the potential value of assessment information.[57]

Having identified the patient's psychological needs, psychotherapeutic interventions can be chosen and initiated. In the same way that assessments can be formal and informal, psychotherapeutic interventions can occur as part of a formal therapy session with specialists in mental health, either nurse specialists, psychiatrists or psychotherapists. Alternatively, nurses can make psychotherapeutic interventions in their everyday interactions with patients. It is important to realize that the term 'informal' does not imply casual or thoughtless; rather, these assessments and interventions need to be performed in a knowledgeable and careful way. Nurses also need to make explicit the possible nature of the relationship with the person with

cancer in order to focus on agreed goals.[63] Using these interventions in a responsive and effective way is facilitated by access to clinical supervision.

PSYCHOTHERAPEUTIC INTERVENTIONS

There are many different approaches to psychotherapy based on different theoretical concepts, each striving to make sense of distress and to promote methods of effective help.[64] Although there are a myriad of different psychotherapies, the principal approaches used in psycho-oncology are humanistic, behavioural, cognitive and psychoanalytic. It is apparent that the outcomes of the interventions made by any healthcare professional, irrespective of the setting, the type of problem or the treatments used, are most strongly influenced by the relationship with the patient. Thus, the most important psychotherapeutic intervention that can be made is the development of a therapeutic relationship with the patient and family. A therapeutic relationship represents a conscious commitment on the part of the nurse to engage with the person's experience of distress.[57,65] Stanley[66] notes that patients with cancer recognize and value nursing presence across the illness continuum. The fostering of a therapeutic relationship is also enhanced by skilful communication strategies and the personal qualities of the nurse. The qualities of warmth, positive regard, respect and interest appear consistently across studies as being correlated with therapeutic outcomes.[55] The appropriate use of humour by nurses has been found to assist in the development of a deeper relationship with patients, with nurses who used humour appearing more human, sensitive and trustworthy.[67]

Therapeutic communication strategies include active listening, confirming responses, the use of metaphors, reframing, clarification and validation. Many texts provide explanations and examples of these skills.[65,68] Skilful communication strategies are an integral part of psychotherapeutic interventions from all theoretical approaches. It is important to have an understanding of the central ideas of the various psychological theories, as they facilitate an appreciation of what may be happening for patients and how they can be helped. The very existence of such a variety of therapeutic modalities is reassuring in its indication that there are many ways to heal. As Camic and Knight[69] indicate:

> ... it is the quality of the relationship between provider and client that begins and sustains the healing process. It is this process of healing – meaning to restore to wholeness and health – that both mystifies and comforts us as clinicians.

Humanistic approaches to psychological distress

The central idea of humanism is the optimistic view that all human beings have a tendency for natural growth and development in a positive direction.[68] There are many different schools of thought that have a humanistic philosophy. Essentially, they all share a phenomenological approach that views individuals as experts in their own lives.[64] They focus on providing an environment that will facilitate the tendency towards positive self-actualization, growth and choice. They seek to explore the individual experience, at the same time acknowledging one's interdependence with others.[70] This approach emphasizes the importance of allowing the person to tell their own story and supporting them in making sense of what is happening to them in their own individual way. This means that each person's story needs to be heard with fresh ears, and the listener needs to demonstrate that they understand what they are being told. Many relationship-building interventions and communications strategies have come from the humanistic tradition, although humanists are more concerned with the process of the therapeutic encounter than techniques. Carl Rogers[71] advocated three essential conditions that facilitate therapeutic interactions:[72] these are empathy with the client, genuineness in the therapist and positive regard. Empathy is the ability to understand the feelings of another person.[73] In attempting to demonstrate empathy it is seldom useful to say to someone that you understand what he or she is going through. What is required is careful listening until the emotions imbuing the story are identified. Then, this insight is offered in a tentative way: for example, saying something like: 'It sounds as if it's the loneliness that's the worst for you. Have I got it right?' In this way you can really demonstrate that you understand what this person is going through. If you have not correctly identified what the person is experiencing you have established that you are trying to understand and in addition you are providing an opportunity for the correct identification of the underlying emotions.[65] In this instance, the person will usually say something like: 'I don't think its loneliness, I think I feel let down by them all.' Then this can be explored. It is imperative to remain tentative, not only because the interpretation of emotional response may be wrong but also because it is important to be descriptive and not prescriptive. There is not one right way to cope with cancer, only this individual's way of coping.[2]

Genuineness in the therapist refers to the therapeutic stance of being yourself while having a real belief in the optimistic humanistic view that people will work things out for themselves.[65] Thus, with your support, patients can come to the best solutions for themselves. Positive regard refers to the ability to establish a relationship in which individuals feel fully accepted and supported as human beings, no matter how undesirable their behaviour may be. Frankl[9] supported the general existential analysis of the meaning of life and death, suffering, work and love. He wrote about the deep human need to find meaning in life, the need to make sense out of what is happening.[9] This need is facilitated by listening to each individual's story and providing support in this quest for meaning. Humanistic interventions are made in both formal and informal settings, in individual and group encounters. Groups have the advantage of providing support and understanding from others who are experiencing cancer and can be a powerful source of affirmation. Considerable research evidence exists on the efficacy of group interventions.[74–76] Humanistic interventions are usually non-directive; this means that the nurse, as humanistic therapist, avoids telling patients what to do. However, nursing care frequently involves being directive and giving explicit instructions to patients; thus, many nurses build therapeutic relationships using humanistic principles but are also directive in their approach.[77,78]

Behavioural approaches to psychological distress

The behavioural approach, with its strong focus on direction, is a popular approach with nurses.[79,80] The central idea of behavioural theory is that all behaviour is learnt, either by association (classical conditioning), by reinforcement (operant conditioning) or by watching others (vicarious learning).[73] From the behaviourists' point of view, problems are caused by maladaptive behaviours that have been learned and conditioned by past experiences. Intervention is focused on stopping the maladaptive behaviour and learning new adaptive behaviours.[26,73,79]

Classical conditioning provides an understanding of phobias, anticipatory nausea, taste aversion and conditioned anxiety. For example, anticipatory nausea occurs when nausea associated with chemotherapy is poorly controlled. Therefore, the chemotherapy becomes associated with nausea so that the patient's thinking about the impending treatment can produce physiological changes that result in the experience of nausea; thus, the patient may vomit before receiving the nausea-producing treatment.[26,72,79,80] Behavioural theories support the role of prevention strategies for chemotherapy-induced nausea and procedure-related anxiety and are outlined in Chapter 20.

Operant conditioning provides an understanding of pain and illness behaviour. If illness behaviour is the only behaviour responded to, then that is the behaviour that will dominate. This means if we only notice (reinforce) what patients cannot do and ignore what they can do, their strengths will diminish. Noticing and reinforcing what patients achieve can increase their sense of self-efficacy.[81,82] For example, a patient may comment that they feel useless during their treatment; they are unable to do anything to help the family coping at home. Noticing that they made telephone calls to thank neighbours who collect the children from school or suggesting that they make one such call or write one thank you card can reinforce a sense of self-efficacy. Vicarious learning, learning by watching others, explains how patients learn from one another and from healthcare professionals; however, Smoyak[83] warns that it is difficult for nurses to role model good self-care unless they are caring of themselves.

Behavioural interventions have been used in the care of patients with cancer with good effect.[26] Many of these techniques, such as relaxation, guided imagery and activities scheduling, are used by nurses in their everyday work with patients.[84] Relaxation training can be used to help cope with fear, anxiety and tension, so that patients can learn to relax in any context that previously would have caused tension. Guided imagery is particularly useful when combined with relaxation; this allows the patient to conjure up an image of a safe or relaxing place for themselves.[26,73] Nurse specialists and health psychologists more often use these interventions in a formal way, or use more complex or lengthy interventions, e.g. systematic desensitization and biofeedback. Systematic desensitization allows an individual to confront a particular fearful situation or stimulus gradually. It is useful when patients have a particular fear, e.g. a fear of needles. There are three steps in desensitization. The first step is to learn a different response to anxiety such as relaxation. The second step is the establishment of an anxiety hierarchy: to do this, the patient outlines a list of situations, ranging from the least to the most frightening for them. Seeing a photograph of a syringe may be the least frightening and having an injection may be the most frightening. The third step is for the patient to practice the new response to anxiety with each frightening situation, starting with the least frightening until they are able to stay relaxed in any situation.[26,73,85] Biofeedback uses machines that monitor the patient's physiological state through lights or sounds. These can allow patients to gain more control over their physiological state, e.g. controlling their heart rate by focusing their attention on this feedback while they relax. This is useful in reducing tension[26,73] and can also be used in chronic pain management.[84] It can be useful for patients to work not only with behavioural responses but also to notice and work with negative thoughts which may be associated with anxiety. This focus on thinking and self-talk as well as behaviour is the focus of cognitive theory.

Cognitive approaches to psychological distress

The central idea of cognitive theory is that the way a person feels or behaves is determined by their thinking and judgement of events. Cognitive therapists are predominantly interested in self-defeating thoughts that contribute to low moods.[73] From this perspective, problems are caused and maintained by thinking errors and unhelpful schema.[73] Intervention is focused on helping people to modify their thinking. This involves identifying and challenging the thinking errors, then changing to realistic and more positive ways of thinking. Thinking errors include all or nothing thinking, selective attention, negative predictions, overgeneralizing, fortune-telling and negative automatic thoughts.[26,73,85]

Nurses often engage in cognitive interventions by supporting patients engaged in reality testing or in making coping cognitive statements. Reframing is a cognitive intervention frequently used by nurses.[85] Moorey and Greer[81] have adapted cognitive therapy for patients with cancer. Their approach allows for more emotional expression and explorations of personal meaning than is usual in traditional cognitive approaches. Nurse specialists and healthcare psychologists more often use these interventions in a formal way, which may include homework assignments. These are individually focused and may involve keeping a diary of thoughts and activities or may involve activities such as writing a letter or making a telephone call.

Psychoanalytic approaches to psychological distress

Psychoanalytic interventions have evolved from the work of Freud in the beginning of the last century.[73] The goal of the therapy is to resolve unconscious conflicts.[73] Psychoanalytic interventions are never made in an informal context, but take place in a formal therapy session with a trained therapist, some of whom are nurses. Although the majority of cancer nurses will not become therapists, knowledge of psychoanalytic theory is essential to understand the manifestations of distress.

A central idea of psychoanalysis is that of an unconscious dimension to the mind, which has complex conflicts and defence mechanisms. These defence mechanisms occur outside the awareness of the individual and act as a protective mechanism against anything which would be anxiety-provoking. Thus, the experience of cancer can provoke responses of which the patient is unaware.[31,86] These defences include suppression, denial, sublimation, reaction formation, regression and projection. Houldin[2] regards denial as a self-protective response used to lower distress in patients with cancer. She further describes it as an important and necessary phase when adapting to the realities of a serious illness.[2] It is not usually appropriate to try to break down these defences, as they exist to protect the individual. In any case, challenging defences usually results in strengthening them and increasing the defensive behaviour. The challenge in cancer nursing practice is not in confronting denial but the avoidance of collusion with its use.[2] Houldin advocates non-confrontational techniques such as providing factual information, using a non-judgemental approach and listening empathetically as helpful interventions.[2]

CONCLUSION

The provision of evidence-based care intended to address the complex psychosocial needs of people with cancer poses an exciting challenge for European cancer nurses. A structured assessment and multidisciplinary approach fosters an objective and supportive environment where patient-specific interventions can be implemented. While the diagnosis of cancer will always provoke a psychosocial response, the nurse can develop skills to support patients and family to minimize their psychosocial distress. Adaptation and positive coping are important outcomes to be evaluated.

The context of caring for people with cancer is evolving as our understanding of the disease process and treatment modalities is developing. In the future, the time spent by nurses in direct patient contact will be reduced, and therefore the establishment of a therapeutic relationship will be further challenged. However, the therapeutic relationship is central to the delivery of psychological care. A further challenge for European nurses is to engage in meaningful research, which will provide an evidence base for effective interventions and ensure people with cancer receive the optimum psychosocial care.

REFERENCES

1. Holland J. Principles of psycho-oncology. In: Holland J, Bast RC, Morton DL, et al, eds. Cancer medicine. 4th edn. Baltimore: Williams and Wilkins; 1997:1327–1343.

2. Houldin A. Patients with cancer: understanding the psychological pain. Philadelphia: Lippincott; 2000.

3. National Institute of Health (NIH). State-of-the-Science Statement. Symptom management in cancer: pain, depression and fatigue. Washington: NIH; 2002.

4. Flanagan J, Holmes S. Social perception of cancer and their impacts: implications for nursing practice arising from the literature. J Adv Nurs 2000; 32(3):740–749.

5. Greer S, Morris T, Pettingale KW. Psychological responses to breast cancer: effect on outcome. Lancet 1979; ii:785–787.

6. Buddeberg C, Buddeberg-Fischer B, Schnyder U. Coping strategies and 10-year outcome in early breast cancer. J Psychosom Res 1997; 43:625–626.

7. Scheier M, Carver C. Adapting to cancer: the importance of hope and purpose. In: Baum A, Anderson BL, eds. Psychosocial interventions for cancer. Washington: American Psychological Association; 2001.

8. Herth K. Fostering hope in terminally ill people. J Adv Nurs 1990; 18:538–548.

9. Frankl V. Man's search for meaning. New York: Washington Square Press; 1984.

10. Omar H, Rosenbaum R. Diseases of hope and the work of despair. Psychotherapy 1997; 34(3):225–232.

11. Janis IL. Psychological stress. New York: Wiley; 1958.

12. Longaker C. Facing death and finding hope. London: Arrow; 1998.

13. Weisman AD, Worden JW. The emotional impact of recurrent cancer. J Psychos Oncol 1986; 3(4):5–16.

14. Wilbour K. Grace and grit. Boston: Shambala; 1991.

15. Barraclough J. Cancer and emotion: a practical guide to psycho-oncology. 3rd edn. Chichester: Wiley; 1999.

16. Massie MJ, Holland J. Overview of normal reactions and prevalence of psychiatric disorders. In: Holland JC, Rowland JH, eds. Handbook of psychooncology: psychological care of the patient with cancer. New York: Oxford University Press; 1989:273–282.

17. Twycross R. Symptom management in advanced cancer. 2nd edn. Oxford: Radcliffe Medical Press; 1997.

18. Salter M, ed. Altered body image: the nurses role. 2nd edn. London: Ballière Tindall; 1997.

19. National Breast Cancer Centre. Psychosocial clinical practice guidelines: information, support and counselling for women with breast cancer. Canberra: National Health and Medical Research Council; 1999.

20. National Breast Cancer Centre. Draft clinical practice guidelines on the psychosocial care of adults with cancer. Canberra: National Health and Medical Research Council; 2002.

21. Ferrell BR, Dow KH. Portraits of cancer survivorship: a glimpse through the eyes of survivors' eyes. Can Pract 1996; 4(2):76–80.

22. Dougherty L, Bailey C. Chemotherapy. In: Corner J Bailey C, eds. Cancer nursing: care in context. Oxford: Blackwell Science; 2001:179–221.

23. Fagerstrom L, Eriksson K, Bergbom EI. The patients' perceived caring needs as a message of suffering. J Adv Nurs 1998; 28(5):978–987.

24. Wilkinson SM, Gambles M, Roberts A. The essence of cancer care: the impact of training on nurses' ability to communicate effectively. J Adv Nurs 2002; 40(6):731–738.

25. Hall A, Fallowfield L, A'Hern R. When breast cancer recurs: a 3 year study of psychological morbidity. Breast J 1996; 2:197–203.

26. Knight SJ. Oncology and hematology. In: Knight SJ, Camic P, eds. Clinical handbook of health psychology. Seattle: Hogrefe and Huber; 1998.

27. Payne SA. A study of quality of life in cancer patients receiving palliative chemotherapy. Soc Sci Med 1992; 35:1505–1509.

28. Lingren CL. Chronic sorrow in long term illness across the life span. In: Miller J, ed. Coping with chronic illness: overcoming powerlessness. 3rd edn. Philadelphia: Davis; 2000;125–144.

29. Dale B. Parenting and chronic illness. In: Altschuler J. Working with chronic illness: a family approach. London: Macmillan; 1997.

30. Altschuler J. Working with chronic illness a family approach. London: Macmillan; 1997.

31. Holland J, Lewis S. The human side of cancer: living with hope, coping with uncertainty. New York; HarperCollins; 2000.

32. Lazarus RS, Folkman S. Stress appraisal and coping. New York: Springer; 1984.

33. Folkman S. An approach to the measurement of coping. J Occup Behav 1982; 3:95–107.

34. Ceslowitz SB. Burnout and coping strategies among hospital staff nurses. J Adv Nurs 1989; 14:553–557.

35. Sarafino EP. Health psychology: biopsychococial interactions. 2nd edn. New York: John Wiley; 1994.

36. Marks DF. Murray M, Evans B, Willig C. Health psychology: theory, research and practice. London: Sage: 2000.

37. Nevelle K. The relationship among uncertainty, social support and psychological distress in adolescents recently diagnosed with cancer. J Pediatr Oncol Nurs 1998; 15:37–46.

38. Massie M. The prevalence of depression in patients with cancer. NIH State of the Science Conference on Symptom Management in Cancer: Pain, Depression and Fatigue. Washington: National Institute of Health; 2002.

39. Greenberg D. Impediments in the management of depression and suggestions for solutions. NIH State of the Science Conference on Symptom Management in Cancer: Pain, Depression and Fatigue. Washington: National Institute of Health; 2002.

40. Carroll S. Psychological support. In: Burnet K, ed. Holistic breast care. London: Baillière Tindall; 2001:152–188.

41. Byers G. Psychiatric care of the cancer patient. Mod Med Ireland 1999; 29(7):45–48.

42. American Psychiatric Association. Diagnostic and statistical manual of mental disorders. 4th edn. Washington: American Psychiatric Press; 1994.

43. World Health Organization. The ICD-10 classification of mental and behavioural disorders. Geneva: World Health Organization; 1992.

44. Fisch MJ. Treatment of depression. NIH State of the Science Conference on Symptom Management in Cancer: Pain, Depression and Fatigue. Washington: National Institute of Health; 2002.

45. Gelder M, Gath D, Mayou R, et al. Oxford textbook of psychiatry. 3rd edn. Oxford: Oxford University Press; 1996.

46. McGrath P. Post traumatic stress and the experience of cancer: a literature review. J Rehabil 1999; 65 (3):17–23.

47. Smith MY, Redd WH, Peyser C, et al . Post traumatic stress disorder in cancer: a review. Psychooncology 1999; 8:521–537.

48. Kwekkeboom K, Seng J. Recognising and responding to post traumatic stress disorder in people with cancer. Oncol Nurs Forum 2002: 29(4):643–650.

49. Alter CL, Pelcovitz D, Axelrod A, et al. Identification of PTSD in cancer survivors. Psychosomatics 1996; 37:137–143.

50. Jacobsen PB, Widows MR, Hann DM, et al. Post traumatic stress disorder symptoms after bone marrow transplantation for breast cancer. Psychosom Med 1998; 60:366–371.

51. Meeske KA, Ruccione K, Globe DR, et al. Post traumatic stress, quality of life, and psychological distress in young adult survivors of childhood cancer. Oncol Nurs Forum 2001; 28:481–489.

52. Friedman M, Schnurr PP. The relationship between trauma posttraumatic stress disorder, and physical health. In: Friedman M, Charney D, Deuch A, eds. Neurobiological and clinical consequences of stress: from normal adaption to posttraumatic stress disorder. Philadelphia: Lippencott-Raven; 1995:507–524.

53. Kimerling R, Calhoun KS, Forehand R, et al. Traumatic stress in HIV infected women. AIDS Educ Prev 1999; 11:321–333.

54. Andrykowski MA, Cordova MC. Factors associated with PTSD symptoms following treatment for breast cancer: test of the Anderson model. J Trauma Stress 1989; 11:189–203.

55. Krishnasamy M. Confusion. In: Corner J, Bailey B, eds. Cancer nursing: care in context. Oxford: Blackwell Science; 2001:435–441.

56. Breitbart W. Psycho-oncology: depression, anxiety, delirium. Semin Oncol 1994; 21:754–769.

57. Barker PJ. Assessment in psychiatric and mental health nursing: in search of the whole person. Cheltenham: Stanley Thornes; 1997.

58. Kelly G. The psychology of personal constructs, Vols 1 and 2. New York: Norton; 1995.

59. Gotay CC, Stern JD. Assessment of psychological functioning in cancer patients. Special Issue: psychosocial resource variables in cancer studies: conceptual and measurement issues. J Psychos Oncol 1995; 13(1–2):123–160.

60. DiLorenzo TA, Bovbjerg DA, Montgomery GH, et al. The application of a shortened version of the profile of mood states in a sample of breast cancer chemotherapy patients. Br J Health Psychol 1999; 4:315–325.

61. Bowling A. Measuring disease: a review of disease-specific quality of life measurement scales. 2nd edn. Buckingham: Open University Press; 2001.

62. European Organisation for Research on Treatment of Cancer (EORTC). Quality of life: methods of measurement and related areas. Proceedings of the 4th Workshop EORTC Study Group on Quality of Life. Odense: Odense University Hospital; 1983.

63. Lanceley A. Therapeutic strategies in health care. In: Corner J, Bailey C, eds. Cancer nursing: care in context. Oxford: Blackwell Science; 2001:120–138.

64. Felthem C. An introduction to counselling and psychotherapy. In: Palmer S, ed. Introduction to counselling and psychotherapy: the essential guide. London: Sage Publications; 2000.

65. Arnold E, Underman Boggs K, eds. Interpersonal relationships: professional communication skills for nurses. 3rd edn. Philadelphia: WB Saunders; 1999.

66. Stanley KJ. The healing power of presence: respite from the fear of abandonment. Oncol Nurs Forum 2002; 29(6):935–940.

67. Johnson P. The use of humor and its influences on spirituality and coping in breast cancer survivors. Oncol Nurs Forum 2002; 29(4):691–695.

68. Egan E. The skilled helper: a systematic approach to effective helping. 5th edn. Belmont: Brooks/Cole; 1994.

69. Camic P, Knight S. Clinical handbook of health psychology: a practical guide to effective interventions: Seattle: Hogrefe and Huber; 1998:6.

70. Hawkins PJ. Hypnosis in counselling and psychotherapy. In: Palmer S, ed. Introduction to counselling and psychotherapy: the essential guide. London: Sage Publications; 2000.

71. Rogers CA. Theory of therapy, personality, and interpersonal relationships, as developed in the client-centered framework. In: Kirschenbaum H, Henderson V, eds. The Carl Rogers reader. London: Constable; 1989.

72. Rungapadiachy DM. Interpersonal communication and psychology for health care professionals: theory and practice. Oxford: Butterworth Heinemann; 1999.

73. Seiser L, Wastell C. Interventions and techniques. Buckingham: Open University Press; 2002.

74. Fawzy FI, Fawzy NH, Hyun CS, et al. Brief coping-orientated therapy for patients with malignant melanoma. In: Spira JL, ed. Group therapy for medically ill patients. New York: Guilford; 1996.

75. Cella DF, Yellen SB. Cancer support groups: the state of the art. Cancer Pract 1993; 1:56–61.

76. Spira JL. Existential group therapy for advanced breast cancer and other life-threatening illnesses. In: Spira JL, ed. Group therapy for medically ill patients. New York: Guilford; 1996.

77. Barker P. The humanistic therapies. Nurs Times 1998; 94(6):52–53.

78. Burnard P. Spiritual distress and nursing response: theoretical considerations and counselling skills. J Adv Nurs 1987; 12:377–382.

79. Barker P. The behavioural therapies. Nurs Times 1998; 94(10):44–46.

80. Redd WH. Advances in behavioural intervention in comprehensive cancer treatment. Support Care Cancer 1994; 2:111–115.

81. Moorey S, Greer S. Pschological therapy for patients with cancer: a new approach. Washington: American Psychiatric Press; 1989.

82. Watson M, Greer S, Blake S, Shrapnel K. Reaction to a diagnosis of breast cancer: relationship between denial, delay and rates of psychological morbidity. Cancer 1984; 53:2008–2012.

83. Smoyak SA. Self-concept in the nurse–client relationship. In: Arnold E, Underman Boggs K, eds. Interpersonal relationships: professional communication skills for nurses. 3rd edn. Philadelphia: WB Saunders; 1999:41–79.

84. Pettinati PM. Meditation, yoga and guided imagery. Holistic Nursing Care 2001; 16(1):47–53.

85. Baum A, Andersen B, eds. Psychosocial intervention and cancer: an introduction. In: Psychosocial interventions for cancer. Washington: American Psychological Association; 2001.

86. Miles M, Morse J. Using the concepts of transference and counterference in the consultation process. J Am Psychiatr Nurse Assoc 1995; 1(2): 42-47.

737

SECTION 6

Care delivery systems

34. Cancer Care and Cancer Nursing 741

35. Intensive Nursing Care of the
    Patient with Cancer 771

36. Rehabilitation and Survivorship 799

37. Palliative Care 821

CHAPTER 34

Cancer Care and Cancer Nursing

MAGGIE GRUNDY

CHAPTER CONTENTS

Introduction	741	The research agenda	754	
		Other sources of evidence	755	
Cancer care in Europe	742	Implementing evidence into practice	755	
Cancer nursing as a speciality	742	Education for cancer nursing practice	757	
		Pre-registration education	757	
The contribution of cancer nursing to		Post-basic education	757	
cancer care	743	Education for advanced cancer practice	758	
		Education for general nurses	759	
Scope of cancer nursing	743	Interprofessional education	759	
		Impact of education on practice	759	
Specialist and advanced cancer nursing		Other issues affecting education	759	
practice	745	Educational delivery	760	
Advanced cancer nursing practice	745			
		Nursing leadership in cancer care	760	
Knowledge for cancer nursing practice	746	Fostering leadership	761	
Development of knowledge	746			
Development of expertise	747	Patient involvement	762	
		Involvement in decisions about care	762	
Caring	747	Involvement in service planning	763	
Patients' and nurses' perceptions		Challenges to patient involvement	763	
of caring	748			
		Impact of information technology on		
Therapeutic nursing	749	cancer care	764	
Nurse–patient relationships	749			
Specific therapeutic actions	750	The future	764	
Use of complementary techniques	751			
Development of new knowledge	751	References	765	

INTRODUCTION

In recent years, advances in cancer treatment and care have extended and improved the lives of people with cancer. Cancer care involves all members of the multidisciplinary team, and cancer nursing is an important and integral aspect of cancer care. As cancer care has developed, the nature and boundaries of cancer nursing have also evolved, with cancer nurses constantly striving to develop their practice. Cancer nursing is required throughout the life span, as cancer affects children, adolescents, adults and the elderly. Individuals have different forms of the disease and receive different treatments; in meeting their needs and those of their families, cancer nurses require specialist knowledge and competence. Education and research are also required to inform practice. This chapter examines the scope of cancer nursing and its contribution to cancer care.

CANCER CARE IN EUROPE

Cancer is a major cause of ill health in Europe, causing almost 20% of deaths.[1] Mortality and morbidity rates for different types of cancer vary between different countries and, as might be expected, cancer care and cancer nursing also vary greatly, with vast differences in the quality of care available in the poorer Eastern European countries and the more affluent Western ones.[2] Furthermore, differences in language and culture and in social and economic problems all influence the provision of care. Dissemination of knowledge on cancer management is also seen to be problematic between different European countries. However, cancer is a public health priority and the European Commission and World Health Organization (WHO) are committed to improving equity of cancer care through:

- providing an integrated service between primary, secondary and tertiary care
- focusing on primary care
- improving the knowledge, training and education of healthcare professionals
- coordinating research between countries
- disseminating research findings.[3–5]

In working towards achieving equity of care, nurses will need to work with colleagues from other disciplines to establish a framework for cancer services in individual countries. This requires nurses to have equal status with other healthcare professionals. Yet, in many European countries nurses are undervalued and their work goes unrecognized.[6] Nurses comprise the largest single body of healthcare professionals in Europe (estimated to be almost 5 million) yet, currently, only about one-third of European countries have nursing representation in central government and their formal power and influence vary.[6] Differences also exist in nurses' roles, the tasks undertaken, training and education, status in society and remuneration.[6,7]

If this situation is to change, education, expert knowledge, political awareness, strong leadership, involvement in policymaking, planning,

decision-making and organization of cancer services will be essential. The potential for cancer nurses to influence and contribute to improving cancer care is enormous, and cancer nurses across Europe must be prepared to take up the challenges presented and work with colleagues to plan the future of cancer care.

CANCER NURSING AS A SPECIALITY

The speciality of cancer nursing has developed in response to a perceived need to improve care and support for people with cancer and their families and increasing recognition that cancer nurses require specialized knowledge and skills.[8] However, nursing specialization is still not recognized in some European countries, particularly in Central and Eastern Europe and the newly independent states (NIS).[2,7,9]

In some countries such as the UK, cancer nursing specialization is well established and innumerable roles have been established. Furthermore, increasing recognition of the importance of cancer prevention is being reflected with the creation of new specialist nursing roles in cancer prevention in several European countries (e.g. Denmark, Finland, Iceland, Italy, Sweden, Switzerland, UK, Israel, Czech Republic, Serbia[7]). New thinking in relation to professional roles and responsibilities has been reported in countries where nursing specialization has not previously been recognized[2] and further increases in cancer nurse specialization are predicted.[10] Currently, cancer nurses with specialist knowledge and expertise remain unequally distributed across Europe. The availability of specialist cancer nursing education and opportunities to develop expertise in the speciality vary both between and within different countries. Cancer nursing mirrors the situation in nursing generally, with nursing shortages in the majority of European countries and the average age of nurses increasing.[7] The creation of specialist roles may therefore be an unrealistic proposition in some countries. Yet, if we are to achieve the European Commission and WHO vision of equity of care, the issues surrounding specialist cancer nurses will need to be addressed. In doing this, human and economic resources and the appropriateness of specialist nurses in cancer care in individual European countries will need consideration.

The speciality of cancer nursing has grown in strength over a relatively short period of time and was one of the first nursing specialities to network at European level.[7,9] This growth can be attributed to the passion, enthusiasm, dedication, motivation, leadership and vision of both individuals and groups of nurses who are committed to improving care for people with cancer, and have managed to create a strong and cohesive voice for cancer nursing. As a group, cancer nurses have achieved much in a short period of time and the future holds great potential for further developing the speciality.

THE CONTRIBUTION OF CANCER NURSING TO CANCER CARE

Effective multidisciplinary working is an essential component of cancer care. Each member of the team has their own specific expertise and role while working with other team members towards achieving common goals. Cancer nurses are frequently viewed as the coordinators of the multidisciplinary team and cancer nursing is an integral part of cancer care. Yet, the specific contribution of nurses to cancer care is frequently hard to articulate, as many aspects of cancer nursing are difficult to describe. The skills of nursing are therefore hidden and invisible and this has major implications for its future.[11]

This inability to articulate aspects of cancer nursing is incongruent with contemporary healthcare policy, which expects that interventions be clearly identified, are based on available evidence and their effectiveness is demonstrated by measuring their impact on patient outcomes. Cancer nursing needs to clarify its major responsibilities and characteristics if it is to be viewed as a profession in its own right rather than being viewed as supportive to medicine. Furthermore, cancer nurses need to be able to articulate the purpose and unique contribution of nursing to cancer care. Cancer nursing is diverse and complex and if nurses are to argue for resources, develop services and have appropriate education

they must be able to both articulate and demonstrate their contribution to multiprofessional cancer care.

Contemporary cancer care services are perceived to be based on a biomedical model. Corner[12] calls for a radical reconstruction of cancer care involving a change in focus from disease, treatment and survival to a more patient-focused and supportive environment based on the needs, problems and everyday experiences of people living with the disease. It is suggested that cancer care is already evolving to have a greater multidisciplinary and collaborative input, with both an individual and primary care focus.[13] However, in Eastern Europe and the NIS, nurses continue to be educated by doctors, and their role is largely confined to that of doctor's assistant, whereas across Europe nurses still tend to operate within a disease- and task-oriented system.[14] Although there is much rhetoric about patient-focused care, there is still a long way to go to achieve the individual supportive focus envisioned by Corner.[12] Yet, this is undoubtedly the way forward for both cancer care and cancer nursing and provides both opportunities and challenges for cancer nursing.

SCOPE OF CANCER NURSING

The scope of cancer nursing is diverse, reflecting the needs of individuals of different ages, with different forms of the disease, receiving different treatments and the different healthcare systems in place in different European countries. The impact of both the disease and its treatment require individuals and their families to make changes to their lifestyles, and cancer nurses require the knowledge and competence to help them achieve this. Cancer nursing incorporates physical, psychological, social and spiritual care and the following elements of cancer nursing have been identified:

- assisting patients and their families to adjust and adapt to life with cancer
- administering cancer treatment and providing supportive care to patients during intensive cancer treatment programmes

743

- preventing and managing the problems caused by cancer and its treatment
- providing physical, psychological and social support and symptom management to individuals with recurrent and advanced disease
- managing cancer care services to ensure optimal care delivery
- researching and evaluating nursing practice in cancer care.[15]

These elements of cancer nursing are mainly concerned with providing optimum care to patients throughout the cancer experience. However, in moving towards a more integrated service between primary, secondary and tertiary care, two additional elements of cancer nursing are identified:

- provision of advice, information and education to other healthcare professionals
- leadership for the development of cancer nursing practice.

Individuals with cancer are cared for in a variety of settings across Europe, including:

- general medical
- surgical
- care of the elderly
- paediatric
- outpatient departments
- rehabilitation
- in the community
- in specialist centres.[9,10]

Throughout their disease and treatment experience, individuals with cancer are likely to be cared for by both specialist cancer nurses and a variety of other healthcare professionals with different levels of knowledge, competence, education and expertise. It is not possible or desirable for all nurses who work with people with cancer to be experts in cancer care, as these patients may only form a small part of many nurses' caseload. However, in improving the quality of care, cancer nurses with expertise, advanced knowledge and competence in cancer care have a vital role in both delivering and directing care and providing advice, information and education to general nurses.

Current healthcare policy advocates a move to concentrating cancer care and treatment in specialist cancer centres staffed by healthcare professionals with expertise in cancer care. However, the demand for cancer treatment and care is increasing, and there is pressure on the demand for beds within these facilities. Difficulties also exist in recruiting healthcare professionals with specialist expertise and knowledge. Most specialist nurses are based in hospital settings or work in defined geographical areas, whereas individuals with cancer spend most of their time at home. Furthermore, many individuals live in remote and rural areas and may not have access to specialist nurses. As cancer care becomes more sophisticated, with shorter and less toxic treatment regimens, more effective management of side-effects and an increased emphasis on ambulatory and community care, specialist centres are becoming increasingly used for short-term and acute episodes of care.

Devising ways of ensuring continuity of care across professional and geographical boundaries is therefore essential. Specialist cancer nurses are likely to play a major part in this: for instance, in working with multidisciplinary colleagues in the development of shared protocols and pathways of care. There are already examples of nursing role development in improving continuity of care. Nurse-led follow-up after cancer treatment has been found to be safe and effective and increases patient satisfaction with care through greater opportunities for psychosocial advice, support and information-giving.[16–18]

A further example of continuity of care is a primary care-based cancer nurse role which incorporates elements of health promotion, links with school nurses and practice nurses to increase awareness of cancer and provides support and assistance to patients and their families while acting as a constant link between the community setting and the hospital.[19] Nurses have a crucial role in the redevelopment and redesign of cancer services, and enormous potential for role development exists, particularly in relatively unexplored areas such as cancer prevention, early detection and screening, genetics and rehabilitation and survivorship.

Cancer is more prevalent in the elderly, with 60% of all cancers occurring in those over the age of 65.[20] With an increasing elderly population, there is a growing interest in identifying and addressing the specific needs of the elderly person with cancer. The elderly are less likely to be invited to participate in clinical trials and more likely to have other co-morbid conditions affecting their functional ability and quality of life. Current assessments used in the context of cancer nursing may therefore be inappropriate for assessing the needs of the elderly with cancer. The elderly may also have increased need for services and family support following treatment.[21] Furthermore, there is a paucity of evidence on treatment effectiveness and the wishes of the elderly in relation to treatment, symptom management and end of life care.[22] Innumerable opportunities therefore exist for developing cancer nursing practice with this particular age group.

SPECIALIST AND ADVANCED CANCER NURSING PRACTICE

It is increasingly acknowledged that different levels of practice exist in cancer care and that these levels of practice equate to different levels of knowledge, expertise and education. The terms 'specialist practice' and 'advanced practice' are now commonly used to describe levels of practice, and much has been written about these terms.[23,24] However, the inconsistent use of role titles such as 'specialist practitioner', 'clinical nurse specialist', 'advanced practitioner' and 'nurse practitioner' has resulted in much overlap between roles and confusion about titles, educational requirements and levels of practice. Furthermore, there is no European consensus on specialist and advanced practitioner roles with specialist and advanced practice developing in an uncoordinated manner across Europe.

Irrespective of title and role, there appears to be general agreement that nurses who are practicing at specialist or advanced level possess knowledge and skill in a particular speciality and have undertaken further education in that area. Both specialist and advanced practitioners are involved in advancing and developing cancer nursing practice. Castledine[25] suggests that advanced practice includes innovations and

discoveries which impact on nursing practice. This definition is congruent with that adopted by an European Oncology Nursing Society (EONS) project working group[26(p228)] who suggest that advanced nursing practice:

> ... aims to adjust the boundaries of health care to impact patient/client outcomes. This is a dynamic innovative process demonstrated in practice and informed by education, scientific research and clinical expertise.

Advanced cancer nursing practice

In recent years, cancer nurses have acquired a reputation for continually expanding the boundaries of their practice and innumerable new roles have been developed. As healthcare professionals strive to improve cancer care and devise new ways of working, a blurring of professional boundaries is occurring. Two models of advanced practice appear to be developing, one which involves advancing nursing practice and the second which involves acting as a substitute doctor.[27] Many nursing role developments incorporate technical and previously medical skills. There is nothing wrong with this, provided the role development benefits patients and upholds the principles of cancer nursing.[8]

Nevertheless, such developments have been criticized. Nursing roles and functions have often changed in response to medical and institutional needs rather than a conscious decision by nurses to advance their practice. Nurses may have been delegated tasks because other healthcare professionals found them tedious or because they are more cost-effective than doctors. Often nurses have taken on these tasks, with little questioning of whether or not they enhance or advance nursing practice or benefit the patient.[28,29] There can be no doubt that such developments expand the boundaries of nursing practice. In developing these roles, nurses will have undertaken some education and developed expertise if technical competencies are required; the role may also have had some impact on patient outcomes. However, there is still the question of whether such a development constitutes advanced nursing practice.

Corner[30] argues that advanced cancer nursing practice requires nursing itself to be taken to a more advanced level, and contends that the concepts of caring and therapeutic nursing are central to cancer nursing.[15,30] Caring and therapeutic nursing are not unique to cancer nursing but become unique when they are combined with a specific body of knowledge and incorporated into the care of cancer patients. A distinct body of knowledge is therefore an essential component of cancer nursing. Means of combining these different components in creative and innovative ways are required to advance cancer nursing itself.

KNOWLEDGE FOR CANCER NURSING PRACTICE

Cancer nurses need different skills and knowledge to function well in a variety of settings and situations.[31] Continuing development of knowledge and skills is also required to keep pace with new developments in cancer treatment and care. Cancer nurses acquire knowledge in different ways and from a variety of different sources. Four different ways of knowing are commonly identified in the literature: empirical, aesthetic, personal and ethical.[32] Although criticisms have been levelled at Carper's work,[33–35] it is still the most widely accepted view of nursing knowledge. Carper's[32] four ways of knowing complement each other and are interrelated (Box 34.1).

Sociopolitical knowledge has also been proposed as a further way of knowing.[40] Sociopolitical knowledge includes social, political and economic factors that affect health and influence nursing roles and health care and would appear to be essential for cancer nurses. Specialization can result in a very narrow focus and, to be effective in leading and influencing care, cancer nurses require knowledge and understanding of the political, professional and cultural agendas affecting health care.

Development of knowledge

Different knowledge is acquired in different ways. Formal education is obviously important for the development of empirical, and to a certain extent, ethical and sociopolitical knowledge, whereas aesthetic and most personal knowledge can only be gained through experience. Ethical and sociopolitical knowledge are also developed

---

Box 34.1

Carper's ways of knowing

Empirical knowledge

Objective, formal scientific knowledge gained from research, textbooks and peer-reviewed journals

Aesthetic knowledge

Subjective knowledge gained through experience and reflection on that experience. Often referred to as the art of nursing, perhaps the most difficult to articulate and describe. Knowing what to do in a situation without conscious deliberation.[36] Sometimes called intuition but not a sixth sense. Based on experience of previous similar situations. Not expressed in language but by actions of the nurse[36]

Personal knowledge

Concerned with understanding of self. Knowledge of own beliefs and values. Involves being open, genuine and authentic with others.[37] An understanding of own personal feelings and reactions to cancer helps the cancer nurse to understand the meanings of patients' actions and reactions and respond.[38] Personal knowing involves reciprocity and engagement with the individual[32]

Ethical knowledge

Formed by knowledge of ethics and morals. Concerned with respect for people as individuals, preserving dignity, and protecting vulnerability. Knowledge of ethical theories and principles applied to complex and difficult situations. Gives insight into alternative modes of action to arrive at decisions to protect best interests of patient.[39] Ethical decisions are made possible by developing relationships with patients and their family.

through experience with people with cancer. Yet, experience alone is not enough to develop expertise. Reflection on that experience to critically examine what is known and create new insights and knowledge is also necessary.[36]

Empirical knowledge is often highly valued in health care, especially with the current emphasis on evidence-based practice. There can be no argument about the need for scientific knowledge in cancer nursing. Knowledge of the disease process, advances in treatments and genetics, mode of action and effects of treatments, symptom management, supportive care and the effectiveness of nursing interventions is essential; however, cancer nursing requires more than empirical knowledge.

Personal and aesthetic knowledge tend to be expressed by actions and behaviour, and these types of knowledge are therefore not always obvious. They are often referred to as 'tacit' or hidden knowledge[41] or the practical know-how that an individual has in a particular situation.[42] These ways of knowing are of immense importance in cancer nursing. Patient experiences are individual, frequently complex, unpredictable and idiosyncratic. Such complex individual situations do not readily lend themselves to off-the-shelf solutions gained from empirical knowledge. Knowledge developed from practice is required in finding solutions to such problems.[43] The development of higher levels of aesthetic and personal knowledge is vital in providing creative and individualized care for patients, and these ways of knowing underpin essential elements of cancer nursing such as caring and therapeutic nursing.[36,38,44–46]

Development of expertise

Expertise in cancer nursing is developed gradually through acquiring and integrating knowledge generated from the different patterns of knowing and the development of practical know-how, which is perceived to be more than just the application of theoretical knowledge.[46] Expert nurses are thought to move from:

- application of rules and abstract principles to the use of past concrete experience
- conscious analysis and rules to use of unconscious reasoning (intuition)

- viewing parts of a situation to perceiving the whole situation
- detached observer to being fully engaged in the situation.[47]

An expert practitioner notices subtle changes in an individual's condition, can identify the relevant issues in a situation and can combine this knowledge with scientific knowledge to inform her actions and interventions.[48] The identification of subtle differences, recognition of previous similar situations and the ability to grasp the relevant aspects of a situation are often referred to as intuition. However, the term 'intuition' does not depict the expert knowledge and clinical judgement that underpins expert nursing intervention.[42] Intuition is based on integrating empirical evidence, ethical issues and knowledge gained from past experiences with many other people in similar situations. Knowledge of past experiences is thought to be linked to established knowledge in an expert practitioner's memory, and assimilated so that its use in problem-solving becomes second nature.[42] The expert practitioner ceases to be aware of what she knows and responds to situations spontaneously.[49] It is this integration of the different ways of knowing in an unconscious way, to inform clinical decision-making in unpredictable situations, that is often referred to as the art of nursing and that informs caring.

CARING

Further exploration of the concept of caring has been advocated as a means of helping to clarify the specific contribution of cancer nursing within the biomedical culture of cancer care.[30] Caring is part of the role of all health-care professionals and Kelly[50] contends that caring should be seen as the central component of health care to which nursing has the most input. Nurses are generally perceived to be more accessible than other healthcare professionals, are seen by patients more frequently and consistently and for longer periods of time[51,52] Nurses are perceived to be easier to speak to than doctors because of their more equal social status with the patient.[53] They are also more involved in personal and bodily care, creating an intimacy with patients that is not shared with other healthcare practitioners[54,55] and making the caring aspect of nursing unique.

Despite the vast literature on care and caring in nursing, in comparison to the biomedical aspects of care, the concept appears to have received relatively little attention within cancer care. This lack of attention is thought to be due to the largely invisible nature of caring. Caring is often regarded as women's work and perceived as not requiring any particular skill or knowledge.[56,57] However, Carper[32] argues that caring is informed by empirical, personal, aesthetic and ethical knowledge and this knowledge distinguishes the caring behaviours of cancer nurses from those of the lay carer. Caring therefore requires cancer nurses to have well-developed knowledge.

In a review of the palliative care literature, Prior[58] found that the skills of caregiving were taken for granted and not considered as topics for research. Prior[58] argues that nurses need to reclaim the caring ethic and demonstrate its worth. Although she is discussing palliative care, the argument is equally applicable to all aspects of cancer care. If the concept of caring is viewed as central to cancer nursing, it is vital that nurses can both identify the caring aspects of their work and the underlying knowledge which informs that care.

The goal of nurse caring is enhancing patient well-being.[45] Given the current economic climate within health care, it is imperative that cancer nurses demonstrate the impact of their caring actions on patient well-being and positive outcomes. However, providing evidence of the importance of caring is not straightforward due to the lack of consensus on what constitutes caring. Caring is a complex, diverse phenomenon and is acknowledged as both a process and an intervention.[59] A vast number of caring attributes have been identified, e.g. compassion, conscience, competence, confidence, commitment, love, empathy, helping, friendship, touching and listening.[60–63] Watson[61] identified 10 carative factors and Leininger[60] developed a taxonomy of 55 caring constructs which are context-specific and culturally dependent. The list of caring attributes is enormous, yet caring remains an elusive concept.

Kyle[64] suggests that the words 'nursing' and 'caring' are used interchangeably, whereas Aranda[11] proposes that all aspects of nursing work which are difficult to describe or articulate are clustered under the term 'caring'. Use of the term 'caring', therefore, does little to help extend our understanding of the complexity of cancer nursing.

Patients' and nurses' perceptions of caring

To date, research findings have generally shown significant disagreement between cancer nurses' and patients' views of the importance of nurses' caring behaviours.[65–70] Nurses have cited affective behaviours such as touching, listening and informational support as most important, whereas patients have been found to value competent clinical expertise as the most important caring behaviour. Carers of cancer patients have also reported competence as the most important aspect of care.[71]

There is no simple explanation for these differences in perception. However, patients' perceptions of their illness and the effect it has on their life and personhood is likely to affect their perception of caring.[35] For most people, cancer, as a life-threatening illness, is likely to significantly affect both their personhood and their life aspirations. Receiving the most appropriate treatment and care would therefore appear to be important. Individuals are unlikely to perceive that this is the case if they do not view healthcare professionals as competent. Competence would therefore appear to be a prerequisite to caring. Cancer nurses can, however, only be competent if they have the knowledge and ability to provide accurate information about the disease and treatment, advise and educate patients and help empower them to self-care. In providing these interventions in a sensitive manner, it is likely that the important affective caring behaviours identified by nurses are incorporated into the more tangible aspects of caring identified by patients.

Patients' and carers' perceptions of their needs and whether they are met will affect the degree to which they perceive particular actions/interventions to be caring acts. Perceptions of caring are also based on health-related criteria and the perceptions of both the caregiver and recipient of care. Caring is clearly a subjective experience and, perhaps like pain, it should be defined as: 'what the patient says it is'. Yet, nurses still need to find ways of measuring caring if they are to claim that the concept is central to cancer nursing. Mitchell et al[72] suggest that patients' perceptions of being cared for should be used as an indicator of quality care and this would appear to be a feasible way of demonstrating the impact of caring interventions on patient outcomes.

Cancer disrupts people's daily lives in many ways and requires adjustment and adaptation. Corner[30] believes that the task for cancer nurses is to make visible the needs and difficulties people have in their daily lives and the ways in which individuals can be helped to cope. She suggests that the concept of therapeutic nursing offers the opportunity to raise the visibility of these needs and difficulties, advances cancer nursing practice and reconstructs the nature of caring.

THERAPEUTIC NURSING

The central premise of therapeutic nursing proposes nursing as a therapy in its own right. Therapeutic nursing promotes adaptation and healing, emphasizes the holistic approach and considers the mind and body inseparable.[73] Over the years, the concept of therapeutic nursing has been incorporated into the theories of many nurses.[74–76] However, it could be argued that within the current healthcare climate, with increased blurring of professional boundaries, restructuring of cancer services and the emphasis on evidence-based practice, therapeutic nursing in cancer care is now more important than ever.

Therapeutic nursing is underpinned by nursing knowledge, personal insight and experiential understanding. McMahon[77] combines the work of Muetzel[78] and Ersser[79] to outline activities in therapeutic nursing:

- The nurse–patient relationship, which incorporates the key elements of partnership, intimacy and reciprocity.

  Both nurse and patient have to give something of themselves for the relationship to be therapeutic.
- Caring and comforting.
- Using evidence-based interventions.
- Patient teaching: providing information and support empowers patients, enabling them to make informed decisions and become active participants in their care while focusing on the promotion of independence and self-care.
- Manipulating the environment (both physical and interpersonal).
- Adopting complementary health practices.

It is intended that these areas should be considered as an integrated whole rather than isolated parts.[77] A further aspect of therapeutic nursing, 'the presentation of the nurse', has been added by Ersser.[80] This has two main characteristics:

1 the *personal qualities* of the nurse, which include being warm, friendly and genuinely concerned about the patient

2 *presence* – being with the patient and able to communicate their physical or psychological presence, mainly non-verbally.

Possessing these personal attributes to a high degree and demonstrating presence are considered to be crucial and integral components of therapeutic nursing and central to positive patient outcomes.[81,82]

Nurse–patient relationships

Knowing the patient

Development of a therapeutic relationship entails becoming involved and engaging with patients and 'knowing the patient' as a unique individual.[83–85] 'Knowing' the patient is regarded as an essential element in clinical judgement, therapeutic decision-making and the provision of ideal care.[84,85] As people with cancer have multiple encounters with nurses over the course of their disease and treatment, there are increased opportunities for getting to know the patient and developing close relationships.

Knowing the patient can only be achieved if the patient's beliefs and the meanings of the impact of the disease and treatment are explored. Having knowledge of how the patient and family perceive their overall situation through the exploration of meaning helps nurses understand patient experiences, subsequently identify and meet their needs and concerns and is a core element of therapeutic cancer nursing.[30,86,87]

Time is a significant component in developing a trusting therapeutic relationship: yet, it is a scarce commodity in today's health services. Time constraints have often prevented nurses from talking to patients about their concerns.[85,87] Several studies have found that speaking to patients and their relatives is frequently done behind the front of physical activity, and therefore the importance of having time to speak to people is not identified as a separate activity, or acknowledged by the organization.[82,85,88] It is essential that cancer nurses identify the time required to develop relationships and articulate these in both workforce planning and in arguments for resources to ensure the provision of quality care.

Involvement with patients

The formation of close emotional nurse–patient relationships is considered inevitable in cancer nursing because of repeated encounters over extended periods of time and the emotional and intimate nature of the circumstances.[88] The terms 'friendliness' and 'friendships' have also been used to describe these relationships.[89,90]

Friendliness encompasses being friendly, smiling, use of humour, responding to the humanity of individuals with interest and warmth, making individuals feel comfortable and helping them through a difficult time. Friendliness is thought to take on more significance when a person is ill.[90] This may be particularly so for individuals with cancer, who may be feeling vulnerable and insecure and for whom a friendly manner may make all the difference.

Friendship appears to indicate a much more intense permanent involvement and is sometimes associated with emotional demands on the nurse and over-involvement.[88–90] Conversely, being a 'professional friend' is considered to increase job satisfaction for cancer

nurses[91] and, in terms of positive outcomes for patients, both friendliness and friendship include relief of tension and alienation.[90] These outcomes may be particularly important for an individual with cancer, as a degree of social stigma is still attached to the word 'cancer'.

Aranda[11] found that nurses who regarded their involvement with patients as a friendship went out of their way to help patients and undertook extraordinary activities to help patients that would be considered above and beyond their professional role. Yet, this involvement made a real difference to the lives of patients and their relatives and it could be argued that this reflects the true nature of a therapeutic relationship rather than over-involvement. Aranda[11] argues that the issue is not about involvement or over-involvement but finding a balance between intimacy/reciprocity and distance in the nurse–patient relationship. A balance between intimacy and distance needs to be reached, and relationships need to be purposeful, with role clarity to reduce emotional demands on nurses.[11,88]

Cancer nursing has not been shown to generate greater stress than other areas of nursing.[92] However, there will inevitably be times when cancer nurses are affected by some of their experiences with patients. These experiences can be used positively in a supportive, supervisory relationship to help individuals to develop and to teach others if support is available in the workplace.[11] Opportunities for discussions with colleagues, supported and structured reflective practice and clinical supervision are essential to maintaining the mental health of all cancer nurses.

Specific therapeutic actions

Nursing is viewed as therapeutic if activities are beneficial to patient outcomes.[52,77] Sharing of professional knowledge has been found to empower patients to become partners in care and promote independence and self-care.[93] All patients have different needs and concerns and, when acting therapeutically, nurses use their clinical judgement to choose the most appropriate intervention from a range of strategies rather than following a recipe or rulebook and applying the same intervention to all individuals with the same condition.[56,91] The range of strategies available to cancer nurses is dependent on their experience and education. Expert cancer nurses have greater ability to interpret, synthesize and apply their knowledge in creative and imaginative ways to produce a personalized package of care for an individual.[45,47,94,95]

There are a growing number of examples of cancer nurses demonstrating innovative, therapeutic approaches to patient care with positive effects on patient outcome. Some recent examples are shown in Table 34.1.

The therapeutic interventions featured in Table 34.1 emphasize the importance of the holistic nature of care, with psychological status impacting on physical symptoms and vice versa. It has been suggested that it is the quality of the therapeutic relationship which creates the conditions for symptom reduction and improved emotional well-being that makes a difference, rather than the intervention itself.[105,106] This so-called placebo effect purports that the perceived effectiveness of an intervention may be due to the time spent with individuals, the attention given to them and the caring attitudes displayed or the actual physical presence of another person which creates the conditions for symptom reduction and enhanced emotional well-being.[56,107]

Other explanations for symptom reduction include:

- anxiety reduction
- expectation on the part of patients that an intervention will change their experience of a symptom
- the suggestion on the part of a trusted healthcare professional that symptoms will improve
- motivation or a desire for a change in the symptom experience on the part of the patient.

Loss of control is often experienced by cancer patients and, as cancer nurses work to empower patients and increase their self-care abilities, patients may perceive an improvement in symptoms because they are able to do something to help themselves.[106]

Use of complementary techniques

The majority of the studies cited in Table 34.1 include use of complementary techniques as part of the nursing intervention. There also appears to be a general trend towards the use of complementary techniques in cancer nursing. A meta-analysis of oncology nursing research in the USA between 1981 and 1990 and two subsequent literature reviews have demonstrated the effectiveness of complementary techniques in reducing pain, anxiety, vomiting, dyspnoea and attentional fatigue.[108–110] (Complementary therapies are discussed further in Ch. 18.)

Use of complementary techniques such as massage, relaxation and distraction may be a means for cancer nurses to demonstrate caring;[56] yet, these techniques are not part of initial nurse education programmes. If such techniques do make a difference to patient outcomes, as suggested in these studies, then it is perhaps time that they were included in initial nurse education. They are certainly techniques that skilled competent cancer nurses appear to require, and consideration should be given to including them in post-registration cancer nursing education.

Development of new knowledge

Promotion of therapeutic nursing is dependent upon developing new knowledge and understanding about nursing and implementing changes in practice required by these.[111] In effect, therapeutic nursing is a means of generating research from practice. Ramprogus[112] contends that the purpose of researching nursing is to improve patient care through developing and advancing practice. He argues that nursing is dynamic and constantly changing and the context in which nurses work is frequently unpredictable, requiring nurses to respond appropriately in interactions with patients. This necessitates research to be undertaken in context and generating knowledge from practice. In this way, practice and knowledge are inextricably linked. Perhaps, the best-known example of such knowledge generation in cancer nursing is the development of a nursing intervention for breathlessness in

Table 34.1: Recent developments in therapeutic nursing

Authors	Intervention	Rationale for intervention	Type of Study
Bredin et al[96]	Improve experience of breathlessness in individuals with lung cancer by detailed assessment, breathing retraining, exploration of the meaning of breathlessness, coping and adaptation strategies, relaxation and distraction	Emotional response to breathlessness inseparable from physical experience. Integrated model of care enables breathlessness to be understood holistically	Randomized controlled trial
Faithfull[97]	Nurse-led care for men receiving radiotherapy for bladder and prostate cancer	Supportive care by specialist nurse will prevent and minimize impact of radiation-induced side-effects	Randomized controlled trial
Bredin[98]	Relaxation and therapeutic massage to help women adjust to changed body image after mastectomy	Embarrassment and fear may prevent women from articulating their feelings about altered body image. Having an empathetic listener may help women to tell their story. Massage may help women adjust to altered body image	Small qualitative study
Gaston-Johansson et al[99]	Comprehensive coping strategy comprised of preparatory information, cognitive behavioural techniques, relaxation and guided imagery	Physical symptoms of fatigue, nausea, pain also have psychological components/effects. Cognitive behavioural therapies help to develop coping skills; relaxation induced by massage reduces subjective perceptions of fatigue and nausea	Randomized controlled trial

Grealish et al[100]	Foot massage to reduce cancer-related pain and nausea	Relaxation induced by massage reduces subjective perceptions of pain and nausea	Quasi-experimental
Herth[101]	Interventions for enhancing hope and therefore improving quality of life in people with first recurrence of cancer	Hope identified as vital for enhancing quality of life	Quasi-experimetal
Fenlon[102] (in progress)	Relaxation training to help women with breast cancer overcome menopausal symptoms	Stress increases flushing. Intervention aims to reduce flushing by reducing stress	Randomized controlled trial
Smith et al[103]	Massage therapy to decrease selected symptoms in patients hospitalized for cancer treatment	Relaxation induced by massage will result in decreased pain, anxiety and symptom distress and improved sleep quality	Quasi-experimental
Barsevick et al[104]	Energy conservation and activity management to reduce cancer treatment-related fatigue	Based on 'Common sense model of illness' that suggests interventions must be individual to the problem and the person. Three-phase individual intervention, including providing information, guidance in devising and implementing an energy conservation and activity management plan, and help with evaluating the effectiveness of the strategies used will help to reduce fatigue	Quasi-experimental

patients with lung cancer.[96,113] This research approach explores individuals' experiences of ill-health in order to inform practice and develop new ways of working. Research generated from practice is immediately relevant to practice. In theory this should overcome one of the major barriers to implementation of research into practice.

However, difficulties have been experienced in implementing therapeutic interventions found to be effective in research into practice.[114] The philosophy of therapeutic nursing proposes that it is the integrated whole, rather than isolated parts, that make a difference. Yet within a busy clinical environment, it is not always easy to implement the integrated whole, and practitioners have been found to take a reductionist approach and adopt individual elements of an intervention. Johnson and Moore[114] identify several reasons for these difficulties, and these are outlined in Table 34.2.

These findings suggest that even when research is generated from practice, it needs to be adapted to be successfully incorporated into practice and to be useful in practice.

THE RESEARCH AGENDA

A sound evidence base for cancer nursing is essential for the delivery of high-quality patient care. In the different countries of Europe, nursing research development varies, as do the number of experienced nurse researchers and university nursing research departments. Nursing research has a longer history and is stronger in Northwestern Europe.[115]

Cancer nursing research is part of the larger picture of nursing research and is affected by the same wider issues. Barriers to research development are well documented: uncoordinated development, lack of strategic planning and direction and variations in funding across the different European countries. Even countries with a strong research background lack sustained and coordinated funding, with a lack of research training for nurses and an inadequate infrastructure.[81,115–117]

Although an enormous number of cancer nursing research studies have been undertaken, there is still little robust evidence to support the effectiveness of specific nursing interventions.[117] Much cancer nursing research is criticized for its methodological limitations. Many studies have small sample sizes, have often been undertaken as part of higher degrees, are isolated studies and are lacking in methodological rigor. They often focus on areas of academic rather than clinical interest and have not been replicated; those that have been replicated often demonstrate variable results.[108,116–118]

The development of structured, strategic programmes of cancer nursing research is vital at international, national and local levels to

Table 34.2: Differences between researchers and practising nurses that affect implementation of therapeutic interventions in everyday practice[114]

Researcher	Practising nurse
Small caseload and can focus on specific intervention(s)	Competing demands on their time Loss of confidence in abilities as cannot focus on one intervention
Motivation, support and protected time	May not have any support or protected time
Required resources available	May not be able to access resources, e.g suitable room, easily
Have necessary skills to implement intervention	May not feel confident that they have the technical or communication skills necessary to undertake the intervention

strengthen the evidence base for cancer nursing, improve patient care and help distinguish the unique contribution of nursing to cancer care. Programmes should include both projects specific to cancer nursing and collaborative, multicentre and multidisciplinary projects with nurses as equal partners with other healthcare professionals, incorporate patients' perceptions of care and remain flexible enough to incorporate unanticipated developments and new areas of investigation.[117-119] Collaborative and multidisciplinary projects are likely to strengthen research initiatives, not least in arguments for funding.

However, developing strategic programmes of research is not enough; programmes must be implemented and adequately funded. A decade ago, a framework for nursing research in cancer care was developed[116] and a number of priority-setting exercises have also been undertaken.[120-124] To date, recommendations from such exercises have not been taken forward, as they have lacked the necessary professional and political impetus.

Nevertheless, priority-setting exercises may help rational planning so that research develops in a coordinated way and scarce resources are directed to the most appropriate areas.[125,126] Browne et al[124] undertook their study as part of the development of a research strategy by EONS and, although it is acknowledged that the results may not be representative of all cancer nurses in Europe, it is currently the best information available. The five top research priorities identified were:

- patient needs related to communication, information and education
- symptom management, particularly pain, nausea and vomiting and fatigue
- experiences of disease and its treatment, particularly psychological experiences
- cancer nursing research issues, such as research facilitation and utilization
- cancer nursing education issues, such as nurses' educational needs.

It is recommended that further priority setting exercises should be undertaken to examine research questions relating to these five priority areas.[124]

A coordinated European programme of cancer research requires priorities to be identified both collectively and for individual countries. As research expertise varies both within and between countries, collaborative partnerships between those with a strong research culture and expertise and others who are developing such a culture will help in building a research infrastructure and developing research expertise.

Collaborative European research is already happening: for example, the EONS-initiated Action on Fatigue programme, focusing on researching and educating European nurses about fatigue, and the WISECARE project (Workflow Information Systems for European Nursing Care), which utilizes information technology in the systematic assessment of selected patient symptoms.[127] Additionally, the International Society of Nurses in Cancer Care[128] has published the 3rd issue of the *Directory of Oncology Nurse Researchers*: available in print and electronic versions, it contains information about nurses from around the world who are involved in cancer nursing research.

However, much remains to be done to build a research infrastructure for cancer nursing. In achieving this, strong political influence and leadership will be essential at both European Union and government levels, as will securing adequate funding for sustained cancer research projects.

Other sources of evidence

It has already been acknowledged that there is a lack of robust research to underpin cancer nursing practice. However, research is not the only source of evidence. Evidence produced from expert opinion, consensus conferences, policy documents and clinical guidelines are recognized as valid forms of evidence and can be used to guide practice. However, to be relevant to practice and impact on patient care, evidence must be implemented into practice.

Implementing evidence into practice

It is unrealistic to expect all cancer nurses in Europe to be involved in undertaking research. However, developing and advancing practice across Europe depends on dissemination of knowledge and incorporating the evidence base, into practice and all cancer nurses should be basing their practice on the available evidence. Dissemination and implementation of evidence into practice can be difficult because of differences in language, culture and resources, and the barriers to dissemination and implementation are well documented:

- not knowing about it
- not having the knowledge of skills to understand, interpret and evaluate research
- lack of authority/support/time/incentive to change practice
- not having anyone to discuss findings with
- not being convinced of their value
- research not being presented in an understandable and accessible form[119,129–131]

Dissemination and utilization of evidence has occurred in an ad hoc manner. Few healthcare organizations identify any one person to be responsible for implementing evidence and it is frequently left to individuals or groups of individuals to access the evidence and then implement it.[132] This situation is slowly changing, but it will still take some time before evidence is disseminated and implemented into practice in a coordinated manner. Information technology is already making a substantial contribution to the dissemination of information and is likely to become increasingly important in the future.

Completion of literature reviews has been advocated as one means of increasing the dissemination of research findings, and the number of systematic reviews of the literature is increasing. Systematic reviews disseminated by the Cochrane Collaboration have made an extremely important and valuable contribution to the healthcare research evidence base.[133] However, these reviews focus on evidence presented within randomized controlled trials and there are few systematic reviews of nursing interventions.

Recognizing the increasing demand for evidence to support practice, a collaborative approach to evaluation of a diverse range of evidence and the implementation of evidence into practice has been developed by the Joanna Briggs Research Institute (JBI), a joint initiative between The University of Adelaide and the Royal Adelaide Hospital.[134] JBI produce systematic reviews with recommendations for practice. The recommendations for practice are evaluated in practice for variability, health outcomes and cost. Health service partners may develop the recommendations further and an evaluation report is presented. Best practice guidelines are then produced.

JBI have a number of paired academic and clinical collaborating centres globally and reviews and best practice statements produced in any of these centres are shared with all other centres. Commitment and support for implementing evidence-based practice is available, increasing the potential for successful implementation. Developing such collaborations is beneficial to building a body of nursing research knowledge, disseminating and implementing research findings. Although differences in culture, language, social and economic resources and organizational structures are challenges to the implementation of such initiatives, the support of a collaborative environment may help to meet these challenges.

Practising nurses require help to implement evidence into practice. Expert cancer nurses have a role in educating their less-experienced colleagues. Helping colleagues become aware of and implement research findings in practice is a vital part of this educational role. This can be done on an individual institutional basis, with groups of expert cancer nurses collaborating to help implement specific research findings.

Supporting practising nurses in developing and changing practice is also an important role for educators. Programmes of education that encourage cancer nurses to develop such skills are invaluable and benefit both the individual nurse and their workplace. Successful implementation of such programmes will also ensure that education is fit for purpose.

Ultimately, implementing evidence into practice should improve patient care. Information on the process of implementing evidence into practice and how this was evaluated also need to be disseminated widely to increase the evidence base. Within the Cancer Services Collaborative programme in England,[135] pilot projects have been set up to implement and evaluate improvements in patient care. Information about these projects has been disseminated throughout the country. This dissemination has allowed people in different geographical areas to incorporate effective practice into their areas while reducing repetition of effort. Similar pan-European projects could increase the dissemination and implementation of best practice.

The WISECARE project[57,127] is a further example of how evidence can be disseminated and implemented in practice. Using information technology (IT), this project has facilitated cancer nurses in centres across Europe to share clinical information on the common patient problems of fatigue, oral care, pain and nausea and vomiting. Debate on best practice was therefore stimulated, encouraging the incorporation of evidence into everyday practice. Such initiatives facilitate the increased implementation of evidence into practice.

EDUCATION FOR CANCER NURSING PRACTICE

Cancer nursing education is required across the spectrum of cancer nursing practice. Additionally, general nurses involved in cancer care have educational needs, and there is a growing emphasis on interprofessional cancer care education. Inequities remain in cancer nursing education across Europe, with some countries providing a range of specialist post-registration courses up to and including masters and doctoral qualifications and others emphasizing learning in the job.[10]

Pre-registration education

Several authors have suggested that nurses are not adequately prepared for caring for those with cancer during initial training.[136,137] In 1995, the Standing Committee of Nurses of the European Union[138] made recommendations about the content of cancer nursing education for pre-registration nursing programmes. Although these recommendations have been incorporated into pre-registration education in most European countries, there is

a paucity of evidence evaluating their impact.[139] All nurses will at some time in their careers be required to care for patients with cancer, and it would appear sensible to ensure that they have sufficient knowledge to provide a satisfactory level of care for these patients on qualification. Further evaluation of the effectiveness of pre-registration education on the ability to care for cancer patients is therefore urgently required.

Post-basic education

The need for improved specialist cancer education for cancer nurses was recognized in the first 'Europe against Cancer' action plan[140] and confirmed in subsequent action plans of the European Commission.[3,4] The development of common training courses in cancer nursing across Europe was also recommended over a decade ago.[141] Subsequently, EONS developed a core curriculum for post-basic education in cancer nursing in 1991[142] and a revised edition in 1999.[26] The revised curriculum suggests that courses in cancer nursing should be practice-driven and dynamic enough to reflect changes in practice in individual countries. In recognizing the diversity of cancer nursing practice and education within Europe, minimum broad standards for educational preparation have been devised. It is anticipated that these standards should be achievable in every member state and prepare nurses to care for people with cancer across a range of different settings. In an attempt to further increase standardization between courses and improve the status of nurses in countries where doctors are normally responsible for cancer nurse education, the core curriculum stipulates that courses must be coordinated by a cancer nurse expert and states a minimum student contact time of 200 hours, including 50 hours in clinical practice.[143]

The core curriculum offers an excellent framework for developing post-basic cancer nurse education. Although it is intended to be a minimum standard, it does not state an academic level for post-basic education. This issue requires to be addressed if standardization of cancer nursing education is to be achieved in Europe. Additionally, the core curriculum has not been universally adopted. Much work has already been undertaken in developing the core curriculum, but further work is required to ensure that the curriculum is accepted and used throughout Europe.

Education for advanced cancer practice

Education for advanced cancer nursing practice is a thorny issue, not least because of the difficulties with recognizing nurse specialization and advanced practice in some European countries. Differences in educational opportunities and educational provision prevent implementation of a common educational framework beyond post-basic education across Europe. Despite these limitations, Knowles et al[144(p229)] found sufficient agreement between seven Western European countries to suggest:

> ... that a programme for advanced practice should be aimed at preparing nurses to facilitate advancing therapeutic nursing practice and develop leadership skills to implement change at strategic level.

Common themes reflecting the processes involved in advancing cancer nursing practice have been identified (Table 34.3) and it is suggested that these processes could be used in developing educational programmes for advanced cancer nursing practice.

Knowles et al[144] acknowledge that developing one advanced practice programme to meet the needs of all European countries would be currently virtually impossible. However, they recommend that educational programmes should be aimed at facilitating cancer nurses to be visionary in their approach, developing leadership skills required at both clinical and strategic levels for advancing practice and improving patient outcomes.

One of the key issues arising from these recommendations is whether any educational programme is capable of producing an advanced practitioner. The components of advanced practice suggest expertise and leadership in practice. This is not the same as undertaking an academic course where specific cancer nursing knowledge or leadership theory are taught. Educational programmes for advanced practice must focus on how individual practitioners use their knowledge and expertise in practice, and such programmes should be process rather than content driven, allowing nurses to focus on issues of importance and relevance to them. Such an approach would encourage and welcome diversity, allowing nurses to be visionary and creative in advancing cancer nursing practice.

Rolfe[145] clearly outlines the constructs of a process-driven course which aims to develop the skills of learning how to learn, critical appraisal and critical self-appraisal and building of knowledge and theory from reflection on action. Content is brought to such a course by the practitioners themselves, based on a reflective philosophy that learning from practice

Table 34.3: Processes involved in advancing cancer nursing practice	
Skills	Expertise, advanced knowledge, leadership, critical reflection, commitment to advancing cancer nursing practice
Processes	Networking, collaboration, facilitates change through reflection, discussion, utilization of research findings and conducting research, sets agenda for change, fosters interdisciplinary working
Outcomes	Creates opportunities to advance cancer nursing practice, develops and empowers staff, facilitates advancing therapeutic nursing, aims to ultimately improve patient outcomes

Source: reproduced with kind permission of publishers from Knowles et al.[144]

means learning about practice. Individual projects undertaken as part of a programme help practitioners to change and adjust the boundaries of their practice and are therefore congruent with the concept of advanced practice.[145] Development of such process driven programmes could help cancer nurses to develop their own practice and develop leadership skills relevant to both their own needs and the development of cancer nursing practice.

Education for general nurses

Much of the care for individuals with cancer is provided by healthcare workers in medical and surgical wards and in their homes, and their need for education in cancer care is increasingly being recognized.[146,147] Education is needed to facilitate recognition of side-effects and early detection of problems to ensure patient safety. Additionally, patients emphasize the importance of staff who are knowledgeable about their condition and treatment.[147] These issues are likely to become more important with a changing focus in the organization of cancer services and an increased emphasis on primary care.

Although the need for education is recognized, meeting the need is more problematic. With competing requests for finite resources, cancer education may be a low priority for community and general nurses. It is therefore crucial that education to meet the needs of these nurses is planned and developed in tandem with any reorganization or redesign of services. In achieving this goal, practitioners and educationalists need to work closely together at local, regional, national and international levels.

Interprofessional education

Changes in healthcare policy across Europe have resulted in an increased demand for teamwork and collaborative working practices. Shared learning between different healthcare disciplines is viewed as a means of facilitating effective teamwork, and effective teamwork is perceived to improve patient outcomes. Furthermore, it is postulated that sharing discipline-specific knowledge between practitioners of different disciplines may encourage practitioners to think in novel ways and, in this way, new knowledge may emerge.[148] However, there is little evidence to support any of these perceptions.[149]

That is not to say that shared learning between disciplines is not valuable, only that more rigorous research is required to support the claims for its effectiveness. Collaborative working is essential in cancer care and sharing learning would appear to be beneficial to patient care. There are already examples of multidisciplinary courses in cancer care, particularly palliative care. However, it is essential to ensure that learning is transferred into practice and the effects on patient outcomes measured.

Impact of education on practice

Few educational programmes have evaluated the impact of education on practice. Measuring the effectiveness of education is not straightforward, as it is difficult to distinguish whether any changes in practice are due to the learning that has occurred from an educational course or other extraneous factors. However, if effort and resources are to be invested in providing cancer nursing education, some evidence of effectiveness is required and evaluation research should be a priority.

Other issues affecting education

Course provision is not sufficient to ensure the education of cancer nurses. Even in countries where specialist courses are available, few nurses undertake post-registration cancer nursing education.[139] The reasons for this are unclear, although difficulties with access to courses, release from the workplace due to staff shortages and increased demands on nurses, funding, motivation, lack of recognition of the value of such education and lack of knowledge about course availability have all been suggested.[139,147]

These issues all require to be addressed if the uptake of educational courses is to be improved and numbers of qualified cancer nurses increased. Linking education and development of competence to a career framework is one means of achieving this; however, coordination and agreement at a national level are required.

Educational delivery

Blunden et al[139] suggest measures such as increasing the flexibility of education, taking education to the practitioner rather than providing education in educational establishments and providing more flexible learning packages such as distance learning may improve the uptake of education. There is merit in all these approaches. However, in taking education to the learner, time away from patient care is still required and the problems of release may not be fully addressed. Creative and relevant work-based learning programmes that facilitate self-directed learning may be a further way of both improving uptake of education and making education relevant to practice and service needs.

Distance education is increasingly being advocated as a means of increasing the flexibility of learning; it can be delivered in different ways and has the potential to reach a greater number of cancer nurses. Participants can access course materials at a time that is convenient to them. Distance education has great potential, although its impact has still to be fully explored and evaluated.

Limitations of distance education

Language is an obvious limitation to distance education, as educational materials may only be available in the language in which they were originally produced. However, it may be possible to use materials which conform to the EONS core curriculum,[26] or a framework for advanced practice, and have these translated and available across Europe.

Distance learning certainly increases flexibility, but the learner still requires time to study and support. Distance learning can be an isolated experience, and motivation and self-discipline are required to complete a programme of learning. Support from both employers and tutors is imperative, and the impact of this on success and completion rates should not be underestimated.

Coordination of education is required on both a national and international basis to improve equity of educational provision and sharing of experiences. The Union Internationale Contre le Cancer (UICC) and the WHO Collaborating Centre for Cancer Education have initiated a pilot that involves offering assistance to medical schools wanting to implement a multidisciplinary cancer care course aimed at general practice.[150] One of the aims of this project is to develop a network of medical schools to share experiences and learn from one another. Development of networks between establishments offering cancer nursing courses could also be considered.

The value of clinical learning is also important in any discussion of educational provision. Sharing practice between countries is a valuable educational experience. Increasing the number and availability of nursing scholarships, allowing practising nurses to visit other countries and explore each other's practice, would also be extremely beneficial, provided that language barriers can be overcome.

It appears that doctors are more adept at organizing international educational provision than nurses. One of the reasons for this may be that doctors are more influential in policymaking arenas. It is suggested that lack of investment in nursing practice, education and research mean that there are few nurses who can take an equal place with their medical colleagues in planning or developing the future of cancer services.[151] This applies equally to educational provision, and highlights yet again the need for nursing leadership in cancer care.

NURSING LEADERSHIP IN CANCER CARE

The issue of nursing leadership has constantly reoccurred throughout this chapter and its importance in shaping the future of cancer care cannot be underestimated. Strong and coherent leadership is imperative in moving cancer nursing forward. It is required both clinically to enhance patient care, and strategically to influence the development of cancer services towards more patient-focused care. Achieving patient-focused care requires a change in the culture of cancer care, and leadership is recognized as key to cultural change.[152]

With strong leadership, cancer nurses could be the key to bringing about cultural change in cancer care. However, culture is notoriously difficult to change, and requires coordination, strength of character, perseverance and coordinated effort. It requires leaders who will not be intimidated by others, and who have the ability to negotiate at the highest level, sound cancer nursing knowledge and confidence. Such leadership is required to ensure that cancer nurses are equal partners with other cancer care professionals. Without this leadership, it is likely that cancer care will continue to be medically dominated and cancer nursing across Europe will remain uncoordinated.[153]

However, nursing does not have a strong history of leadership. Much of the literature on leadership in nursing has focused on clinical nursing leadership rather than on strategic or political leadership. According to Antrobus and Kitson,[154] health policy in the UK has, to date, been formed and imposed with very little input from nursing. They suggest that nurses tend to be informed of strategic decisions and expected to implement them rather than be involved in making these decisions. Although nurses are the largest single group of healthcare professionals in Europe, at strategic and policymaking level there is frequently an imbalance. Frequently, there is only one nurse on a committee with several doctors, and nursing representation and leadership at political and strategic level are therefore lacking. There are no quick fixes to this situation and a long-term view is required to ensure development of leadership in nursing generally, and in cancer nursing specifically.

That is not to say that leaders in cancer nursing do not exist. All cancer nurses will be able to identify individuals who they perceive to be leaders in the speciality. These individuals may be leaders in clinical practice, education, research or management. All cancer nurses have leadership potential and the ability to make a difference. However, the amount that any one person can achieve is limited, and to be able to influence politically, leadership efforts therefore need to be coordinated to create a unified voice and clear direction.[152,154] Cancer nursing already has a strong voice through individuals and the various national and international cancer nursing societies. However, this voice is still not as strong as the voice of other healthcare disciplines with a longer history of political influencing. Cancer nurses need to continue to strengthen their leadership and political influencing abilities to have an equally strong influence on the development of cancer services.

Fostering leadership

The leadership situation in cancer nursing will only change if nurses have the ability and confidence to influence and negotiate with others. The development of future nursing leaders is currently the subject of much attention across Europe. Continual investment is required to develop leaders who will influence and shape policy.[154] It is suggested that development of leadership should have increased attention within pre-registration education.[155] Leadership also requires to be a consistent theme throughout continuing education. However, perhaps more importantly, leadership potential requires to be fostered and supported in practice. Many cancer nurses are passionate about their speciality and improving patient care. They are often overworked and may become demotivated in their constant attempts to improve practice within organizational constraints. Cancer nurses need support and encouragement to develop their leadership role. Colleagues, managers and educationalists all have a role to play in supporting potential leaders and helping them to develop. If we are serious about the development of leadership, this cannot be left to chance. Coordinated efforts are required to identify and support potential future leaders.

There is thought to be little incentive for potential leaders to remain in clinical practice.[154] These authors describe a scenario where all potential leaders are in academic, managerial and political arenas and have limited contact with clinical practice. They suggest that, to avoid this, a reconstruction of the nursing career structure is required so that nurses have opportunities for different experiences: for instance, being able to move in both directions between clinical practice and education or clinical practice and research. It is clearly acknowledged that to develop knowledge and creativity, individuals need to have new opportunities and gain new perspectives so that they can generate new visions for the future. To achieve this, freedom and support away from the demands of 21st century health care are needed.[151,155,156] Providing experiences which allow potential leaders to develop different perspectives while still retaining contact with clinical practice may help to stimulate creativity and vision and ultimately enhance patient care. Such experiences can also be used to develop networks of influential contacts and will aid understanding of the different roles of educationalists, researchers and practitioners, which in turn will help to strengthen and develop a unified voice for cancer nursing.

PATIENT INVOLVEMENT

Patient involvement in health care is becoming increasingly important in the reconfiguration of cancer services in Europe.[157] Yet, historically, cancer services have been organized around the way that health professionals work rather than focusing on patient needs. Patient needs have therefore not always been met. A recent study demonstrated that universal needs (needs important to everyone) were largely met but situational and personal needs, particularly those of carers, were frequently unmet.[158] These authors suggest that cancer services may need to move on from meeting the universal needs of many to meeting individual personal and situational needs. This is particularly pertinent given the emphasis on primary care in contemporary cancer care and the increased involvement of family members and friends in care. Little evidence exists about how lay carers are prepared for their role or the stress that may be generated by undertaking a caring role and how carers can be helped to balance the caring role within their lives.[159] Combined with the view that health care is largely unsatisfactory from a user perspective,[160] focusing on meeting individual personal and situational needs would appear to be a key priority. Greater involvement of patients and their informal carers is being advocated through partnerships with healthcare professionals in choices and decisions about care and treatment, and in the planning, organization, delivery and evaluation of cancer services.

Involvement in decisions about care

Involvement in treatment decisions is thought to lessen the psychological trauma of the cancer experience, increase autonomy and be empowering for patients.[161–163] Additionally, a perception of lack of involvement in decision-making may influence regrets about treatment decisions.[164,165] Both support and information are required to enable individuals to make an informed decision, and patients can only participate in decisions in a meaningful way if they have proper understanding of available options.[159,166,167]

Yet, several recent studies have demonstrated that patients do not receive enough information to enable them to make informed decisions. A large European survey of women with cancer found that before diagnosis women's knowledge of cancer was poor, and they had insufficient information to adequately prepare them for what to expect from treatment.[168] Lack of information about the effects of cancer and its treatment and prognosis, or the advantages and risks of alternative treatment options, have also been reported.[169] The major barrier to participation in decision-making appears to be a deficiency in the written information provided to patients. Patients may find it difficult to remember or retain information given verbally, and this can be further compounded by anxiety and denial.[162]

Even when patients are fully informed, it is extremely difficult for them to make decisions about treatment options as they do not have the professional knowledge and experience of healthcare professionals. Additionally, wanting to be fully informed does not infer that individuals wish to be responsible for the final treatment decision.[170]

Some people may find it overwhelming to have to make decisions about treatment, especially at initial diagnosis and treatment stages, where copious amounts of information may be imparted.[171] Focus groups have found some patients thought it impossible to participate in decision-making about their care.[172] These findings are interesting, as the sample was drawn from adaptation training courses for patients. Involvement in such a voluntary programme suggests that participants were motivated and wanted to be informed and empowered. Yet, the prospect of decision-making about treatments remained difficult for these individuals and the importance of information and support in involving patients in treatment decision-making is emphasized.

Other factors which may affect the desire and extent of involvement in decision-making include age, physical condition and educational and literacy levels. Veronesi et al[168] found that patients under 60 years old who had suffered a relapse and who were very knowledgeable, or who had received higher education, were more likely to want to be involved in decision-making. It is also suggested that those who are less fit may be less able to participate.[173] It is important that cancer nurses are aware of the wishes of individuals in relation to treatment decision-making and ensure that they determine what involvement individuals want rather than make assumptions about their wishes.

People can be involved in and consulted about their care without having to make decisions about treatment options, and being involved may be more important than having treatment choice.[174] It is therefore important that patients receive the information they require in both oral and written forms and have the opportunity to ask questions and discuss issues with healthcare professionals.

Involving patients in their care requires changes in culture and attitudes within the healthcare systems of Europe. Both culture and attitudes are notoriously difficult to change and a conscious effort is required on the part of healthcare professionals to ensure the extent of patient involvement in their care meets with their individual wishes.

Involvement in service planning

The extent to which individuals with cancer or patient representative groups are systematically involved in service planning and monitoring of services is as yet unknown.[175] However, in the future, patient involvement is likely to be required at all levels in the planning of cancer services. Ensuring that those involved are representative of the total patient population presents a number of challenges, and ways of overcoming these require to be carefully thought through.

Challenges to patient involvement

- Requires preparation for role.
- May be a tendency to use the same few articulate people repeatedly over a number of years.
- Retrospective memories of experiences may not be so vivid as previously.
- People with different types of cancer and at different stages of their disease are likely to have different needs.
- Ensuring representativeness between different socioeconomic groups, geographical location, levels of education, numeracy, literacy, gender, race and age.
- Those with less advanced disease are more likely to be involved.[176,177]

These issues all require to be addressed to ensure that service provision is equitable. Progress is already being made: for example, in the UK, the charity Macmillan Cancer Relief, working in conjunction with health services and voluntary cancer support and self-help groups, has been instrumental in developing and supporting a national independent network of cancer service users – 'Cancer Voices'.[178] The aim of this initiative is to empower patients to get their voices heard and help them to shape policies and services at both local and national level. Training and support are provided. Regional networking events are also held to help people communicate and disseminate ideas and experiences.

In a further initiative in Scotland, patient involvement officers are being employed to help increase patient involvement in service planning and evaluating the effectiveness of services from a user perspective. These initiatives are, however, only the start, and much work is still required to ensure that health services across Europe are truly patient-focused. Strategies are required to ensure that cancer patients are systematically and effectively involved in all aspects of cancer care, including organization of services, research and education.[175,179] Evaluation of all initiatives is also required to determine effectiveness. Several recent initiatives use IT as a means of increasing patient involvement and making services more patient-focused.

IMPACT OF INFORMATION TECHNOLOGY ON CANCER CARE

Information technology is becoming increasingly important, both as a communication medium and as a means of involving patients in their care. The full potential of IT in cancer care has yet to be realized, but it is a valuable means of sharing information about patients with all healthcare professionals involved in their care, enables patients to book their own appointments at a time convenient to them and communicates test results faster. Electronic patient records and telemedicine have enormous potential for communication and networking across geographical boundaries. However, this requires compatible information systems and coordination and planning at a strategic level are required to achieve this.

Information technology is also being used to improve patient care. The use of handheld computers has been piloted to assess and manage symptoms for patients receiving chemotherapy.[180] The handheld computer was used to answer questions about symptoms and obtain self-care feedback on how best to manage symptoms dependent on the nature and severity of symptoms entered. Information entered into the computer was sent to the hospital, reviewed by a specialist nurse and individual advice given to patients. The majority of patients in this study had never used a computer before but responded positively, indicating that their symptoms were better managed and the self-care information was helpful. It is anticipated that use of IT in this way will help to improve continuity of care.

In a further initiative, computer touch-screen technology has been found to have a high level of acceptability when used by patients to report psychosocial functioning in an ambulatory cancer clinic.[181] Accuracy and completeness of the data were reported to be excellent and better than pen and paper questionnaires. Although this method requires economic evaluation, it is suggested that once the initial expensive set-up costs have been paid it has the potential to both save money and enhance the data collection process for research and audit purposes.

THE FUTURE

A number of challenges and opportunities exist for cancer nurses across Europe in the 21st century. Cancer is a public health priority, and cancer prevention and screening are likely to become increasingly important. Cancer nurses will be at the forefront of developing and evaluating innovative roles and initiatives. Continuing advances in cancer care and treatment will continue and cancer nursing will need to evolve with these advances. Recent advances in genetics, the identification of genes expressed in specific cancers and the development of specifically targeted therapies with less toxic side-effects will all affect the nature of cancer nursing. Cancer nurses will increasingly be asked for advice about familial cancers and this is a further area for development.

An increasingly elderly population and more people surviving cancer present further challenges and opportunities for the development of cancer nursing. Changes in demographics and organization of health services may result in fewer nurses with cancer nursing education and clinical expertise. This, combined with the emphasis on early discharge and a focus on primary care, means networking and communicating across geographical and organizational boundaries will become increasingly important in ensuring equity of care. The potential for cancer nurses to be instrumental in devising new ways of working is enormous.

Changing the culture of cancer care from a biomedical one to one that is patient-focused is a major challenge for the future and will require coordinated effort from all healthcare professionals. Cancer nurses, with their close contact with patients, have a major role in helping patients to have their voices heard and in ensuring that patients are involved in decisions about their care and the planning and delivery of cancer services.

Coordination of research and education across Europe presents further opportunities for development. Cancer nurses are already at the forefront of research derived from practice, and this will be instrumental in helping to determine the effectiveness of nursing interventions on patient outcomes and demonstrating the unique contribution of nursing to cancer care.

Cancer nursing is a strong nursing speciality. It will only continue to be so if cancer nurses take up the challenges presented, work closely with their multidisciplinary colleagues, value and support the leaders they have and foster new leaders who will take cancer nursing forward into the 21st century.

REFERENCES

1. World Health Organisation. The European Health Report 2002. European Series No. 97. Copenhagen: WHO; 2002.

2. Salvage J, Heijnen S, Nursing and midwifery in Europe. In: Salvage J, Heijnen S, eds. Nursing in Europe: a resource for better health. Copenhagen: WHO Regional Office for Europe; 1997:21–123.

3. European Commission. Action Plan to Combat Cancer (1996–2000). 1996. www.doc http://europa.eu.int/comm/health/ph/progra mmes/cancer/action.htm – consulted 27/10/02.

4. European Commission. Action Plan to Combat Cancer within the framework for Action in the Field of Public Health (1996–2000). Annual Work Programme for 2001 indicating the priorities for action: 2000. www.doc http://europa.eu.int/comm/health/ph/progra mmes/cancer/wrkprog2001_en.pdf – consulted 27/10/02.

5. World Health Organisation. Health21: The Health for all Policy Framework for the WHO European Region, European Health for all Series No. 6. Copenhagen: WHO; 1999

6. Asvall JE. Foreword. In: Salvage J, Heijnen S, eds. Nursing in Europe: a resource for better health. Copenhagen: WHO Regional Office for Europe; 1997:xiii–xiv.

7. Glaus A. The status of cancer nursing – a European perspective. Abstract 1187. Abstract Book ECCO 12. The European Cancer Conference 2003; 1(5):S363

8. Oliver G. Moving oncology nursing forward, an agenda for the 21st century. The Robert Tiffany Annual Nursing Lecture, 14 June 1999. Eur J Cancer Care 1999; 8(4):192–197.

9. Kremar CR. Cancer nursing as a speciality. In: Kearney N, Richardson A, Di Guilio P, eds. Cancer nursing practice: a textbook for the specialist nurse. Edinburgh: Churchill Livingstone; 2001:1–17.

10. Ferguson A, Kearney N. Towards a European framework for cancer nursing services In: Kearney N, Richardson A, Di Guilio P, eds. Cancer nursing practice: a textbook for the specialist nurse. Edinburgh: Churchill Livingstone; 2001:179–196.

11. Aranda S. Silent voices, hidden practices: exploring undiscovered aspects of cancer nursing. Int J Palliat Nurs 2001; 7(4):178–185

12. Corner J. Inaugural lecture. Nursing and the counter culture for cancer. Eur J Cancer Care 1997; 6(3):174–181.

13. Yarbro CH. Cancer nursing into the millenium. The Robert Tiffany Annual Lecture, Royal Marsden Hospital. Eur J Cancer Care 1998; 7(2):77–84.

14. Fawcett-Henesy A. Speaking out ... a new World Health Organization European region health policy document ... sets out the agenda for improving the public's health across the 51 WHO European member states. Nurs Times 1998; 94(23):23.

15. Corner J. The scope of cancer nursing. In: Horwich A, ed. Oncology: a multidisciplinary approach. London: Chapman and Hall; 1995.

16. Guerrero D. A nurse-led service. Nurs Stand. 1994; 9(6):21–23.

17. Campbell J, German L, Lane C. Radiotherapy outpatient review: a nurse-led clinic. Nurs Stand 1999; 13(22):39–44.

18. Moore S, Corner J, Haviland J, et al. Nurse led follow up and conventional medical follow up in management of patients with lung cancer: randomised trial. BMJ 2002; 325(7373):1145–1147.

19. Dawson T. A cancer nurse in a primary care setting. Eur J Oncol Nurs 1999; 3(4):251–252.

20. Monfardini S. Cancer in the elderly: facts and figures in Europe. Abstract 1126. Abstract Book ECCO 12. The European Cancer Conference 2003; 1(5):S340.

21. Bailey C, Corner J, Addington-Hall J, Kumar D, Haviland J. Older patients' experiences of colorectal cancer: functional status and service use following treatment. Abstract 1105. Abstract Book ECCO 12. The European Cancer Conference 2003; 1(5):S333.

22. Kearney N, Chouliara Z, Miller M, Molassiotis A. Older people with cancer: issues in clinical practice and research. Abstract 1110. Abstract Book ECCO 12. The European Cancer Conference 2003; 1(5):S335.

23. Castledine G, McGee P. Advanced and specialist nursing practice. Oxford: Blackwell Science; 1998.

24. Rolfe G, Fulbrook P, eds. Advanced nursing practice. Oxford: Butterworth-Heinemann; 1998.

25. Castledine G. Developments in the role of the advanced nursing practitioner: a personal

perspective. In: Rolfe G, Fulbrook P, eds. Advanced nursing practice. Oxford: Butterworth-Heinemann; 1998:3–7.

26. European Oncology Nursing Society. A core curriculum for a post-basic course in cancer nursing. 2nd edn. Prepared for the Europe Against Cancer Programme. Brussels: Commission of the European Communities; 1999.

27. Manley K. A conceptual framework for advanced practice: an action research project operationalizing an advanced practitioner/consultant nurse role. In: Rolfe G, Fulbrook P, eds. Advanced nursing practice. Oxford: Butterworth-Heinemann; 1998:118–135.

28. Muff J. Of images and ideals: a look at socialisation and sexism in nursing. In: Jones AH, ed. Images of nursing: perspectives from history, art and literature. Philadelphia: University of Pennsylvania Press; 1988:197–220.

29. MacAlister L. Why do nurses agree to take on doctors' roles? Br J Nurs 1995; 4(21): 1238–1239.

30. Corner J. Beyond survival rates and side-effects: cancer nursing as therapy. Cancer Nurs 1997; 20(1):3–11.

31. Richardson A. Cancer nursing – a changing and vital role [editorial]. Eur J Oncol Nurs 1999; 3(4):203–204.

32. Carper B. Fundamental patterns of knowing in nursing. Adv Nurs Sci 1978; 1:13–23.

33. Boykin A, Parker ME, Schoenhofer SO. Aesthetic knowing grounded in an explicit conception of nursing. Nurs Sci Q 1994; 7(4):158–161.

34. Wainwright P. Towards an aesthetics of nursing. J Adv Nurs 2000; 32(3):750–756.

35. Edwards SD. Philosophy of nursing: an introduction. Basingstoke: Palgrave; 2001.

36. Chinn PL, Kramer MK.Theory and nursing: a systematic approach. 4th edn. St. Louis: Mosby; 1995.

37. Fawcett J, Watson J, Neuman B, Walker PH, Fitzpatrick JJ. On nursing theories and evidence. J Nurs Scholarsh 2001; 33(2):115–119.

38. Jacobs LA. Personal knowing in cancer nursing. Nurs Forum 1998; 33(4):23–28.

39. Clarke D. Beyond the theory–practice gap: the contribution of theory in nursing. In: Clarke D, Flanagan J, Kendrick K, eds. Advancing nursing practice in cancer and palliative care. Basingstoke: Palgrave Macmillan; 2002:43–64.

40. White J. Patterns of knowing: review, critique, and update. Adv Nurs Sci 1995; 17(4):73–86.

41. Polanyi M. The tacit dimension. New York: Doubleday & Co; 1967. Cited in Schon DA. The reflective practitioner: how professionals think in action. London: Temple Smith; 1983.

42. Hampton D. Expertise: the true essence of nursing art. Adv Nurs Sci 1994; 17:15–24.

43. Schon DA. The reflective practitioner: how professionals think in action. London: Temple Smith; 1983.

44. Benner P, Wrubel J. The primacy of caring. Menlo Park, California: Addison Wesley; 1989.

45. Swanson KM. Nursing as informed caring for the well-being of others. Image J Nurs Sch 1993; 25(4):352–357.

46. Benner PA, Tanner CA, Chesla CA. Expertise in nursing practice: caring clinical judgement and ethics. New York: Springer; 1996.

47. Benner PA. From novice to expert: excellence and power in clinical nursing practice. Menlo Park, California: Addison Wesley; 1984.

48. Benner PA, Tanner CA, Chesla CA. Becoming an expert nurse. Am J Nurs 1997; 97(6):16BBB, 16DDD.

49. Carlsson G, Drew N, Dahlberg K, Lutzen K. Uncovering tacit knowledge. Nurs Philos 2002; 3:144–151.

50. Kelly D. Caring and cancer nursing: framing the reality using selected social science theory. J Adv Nurs 1998; 28(4):728–736.

51. Ersser SJ. Nursing as a therapeutic activity: an ethnography. Aldershot: Avebury; 1987.

52. Costain Schou K, Hewison J. Experiencing cancer. Buckingham: Open University Press; 1999

53. Fawcett-Henesy A.. Nurse practitioners: the South Thames RHA experience. Nurs Times 1995; 91(12):40–41.

54. Lawler J. Behind the screens: nursing, somology and the problem of the body. London: Churchill Livingstone; 1991.

55. Lawton J. The dying process: patient's experiences of palliative care. London: Routledge; 2000.

56. Barker P. Reflections on caring as a virtue ethic within an evidence-based culture. Int J Nurs Stud 2000; 37:329–336.

57. Kearney N. Classifying nursing care to improve patient outcomes: the example of WISECARE. NT Res 2001; 6(4):47–56.

58. Prior D. Caring in palliative nursing: competency or complacency? Int J Palliat Nurs 2001; 7(7):339–344.

59. Watson J. Postmodern nursing and beyond. Edinburgh: Churchill Livingstone; 1999.

60. Leininger M. Leininger's theory of nursing: cultural care, diversity and universality. Nurs Sci Q 1988; 1:152–160.

61. Watson J. Nursing: human science and human care, a theory of nursing. New York: National League for Nurses; 1988.

62. Dunlop MJ. Is a science of caring possible? J Adv Nurs 1986; 11(6):661–670.

63. Roach MS. The call to consciousness: compassion in today's health world. In: Gaut DA, Leininger MM, eds. Caring the compassionate healer. New York: National League for Nursing Press; 1991:7–17.

64. Kyle J. The concept of caring: a review of the literature. J Adv Nurs 1995; 21(3):506–514.

65. Larson PJ. Important nurse caring behaviours perceived by patients with cancer. Oncol Nurs Forum 1984; 11(6):46–50.

66. Larson PJ. Cancer nurses' perceptions of caring. Cancer Nurs 1986; 9:86–91.

67. Larsson G, Peterson, VW, Lampic C, von Essen L, Sjoden PO. Cancer patient and staff ratings of the importance of caring behaviours and their relations to patient anxiety and depression. J Adv Nurs 1998; 27(4):855–864.

68. von Essen L, Sjoden PO. Patients and staff perceptions of caring: review and replication. J Adv Nurs 1991; 16(11):1363–1374.

69. Widmark-Petersson V , von Essen L, Lindeman E, Sjoden PO. Cancer patient and staff perceptions of caring vs cinical care. Scand J Caring Sci 1996; 10:227–233.

70. Widmark-Petersson V, von Essen L, Sjoden P. Perceptions of caring among patients with cancer and their staff. Cancer Nurs 2000; 23(1):32–39.

71. Eriksson E. Caring for cancer patients: relatives' assessments of received care. Eur J Cancer Care 2001; 10(1):48–55.

72. Mitchell P, Heinrich J, Moritz P, Hinshaw A. Measurement into practice: summary and recommendations. Med Care 1997; 35(Suppl):NS124–NS127.

73. McMahon R, Pearson A, eds. Nursing as therapy. 2nd edn. Cheltenham: Stanley Thornes; 1998.

74. Henderson V. The nature of nursing. New York: Macmillan; 1966.

75. Orem D. Nursing concepts of practice. 3rd edn. New York: McGraw-Hill; 1985.

76. Roper N, Logan WW, Tierney AJ. The elements of nursing. 2nd edn. Edinburgh: Churchill Livingstone; 1985.

77. McMahon R. Therapeutic nursing: theory, issues and practice. In: McMahon R, Pearson A, eds. Nursing as therapy. 2nd edn. Cheltenham: Stanley Thornes; 1998:1–20.

78. Muetzel PA.Therapeutic nursing. In: Pearson A, ed. Primary nursing: nursing in the Burford and Oxford Nursing Development Units. Beckenham: Croom Helm; 1998.

79. Ersser SJ. Nursing beds and nursing therapy. In: Pearson A, ed. Primary nursing: nursing in the Burford and Oxford Nursing Development Units. Beckenham: Croom Helm; 1998.

80. Ersser SJ. The presentation of the nurse: a neglected dimension in the therapeutic nurse–patient relationship. In: McMahon R, Pearson A, eds. Nursing as therapy. 2nd edn. Cheltenham: Stanley Thornes; 1998:37–63.

81. Luker KA. Research and configuration of nursing services. J Adv Nurs 1997; 6:259–267.

82. Bertero C. Caring for and about cancer patients: identifying the meaning of the phenomenon "caring" through narratives. Cancer Nurs 1999; 22(6):414–420.

83. May C. Affective neutrality and involvement in nurse–patient relationships: perceptions of appropriate behaviour among nurses in acute medical and surgical wards. J Adv Nurs 1991; 16:552–558.

84. Radwin L. 'Knowing the patient': a review of the research on an emerging concept. J Adv Nurs 1996; 23(6):1142–1146.

85. Luker KA, Austin L, Caress A. Hallet CE. The importance of 'knowing the patient': community nurses' constructions of quality in providing palliative care. J Adv Nurs 2000; 31(4):775–782.

86. Appleton C. The art of nursing: the experience of patients and nurses. J Adv Nurs 1993; 18:892–899.

87. Richer MC, Ezer H. Understanding beliefs and meanings in the experience of cancer: a concept analysis. J Adv Nurs 2000; 32(5):1108–1115.

88. Roberts D, Snowball J. Psychosocial care in oncology nursing: a study of social knowledge. J Clin Nurs 1999; 8(1):39–47.

89. Turner M. Involvement or over-involvement? Using grounded theory to explore the complexities of nurse–patient relationships. Eur J Oncol Nurs 1999; 3(3):153–160.

90. Geanellos R. Exploring the therapeutic potential of friendliness and friendship in nurse–client relationships. Contemp Nurse 2000; 12:235–245.

91. Trygstad L. Professional friends: the inclusion of the personal into the professional. Cancer Nurs 1986; 9(6):326–332.

92. Corner J. Nurses' experiences of cancer. Eur J Cancer Care 2002; 11(3):193–199.

93. Radwin L. Oncology patients' perceptions of quality nursing care. Res Nurs Health 2000; 23:179–190.

94. Tanner CA, Benner P, Chesla C, Gordon DR. The phenomenology of knowing the patient. Image J Nurs Sch 1993, 25(4):273–280.

95. Kitson A. The essence of nursing. Nurs Stand 1999; 13(23):42–46.

96. Bredin M, Corner J, Krishnasamy M, et al. Multicentre randomised controlled trial of nursing intervention for breathlessness in patients with lung cancer. BMJ 1999; 318(7188):901–904.

97. Faithfull S. Randomized trial, a method of comparisons: a study of supportive care in radiotherapy nursing. Eur J Oncol Nurs 1999; 3(3):176–184.

98. Bredin M. Mastectomy, body image and therapeutic massage: a qualitative study of women's experience. J Adv Nurs 1999; 29(5):1113–1120.

99. Gaston-Johansson F, Fall-Dickson JM, Nanda J, et al. The effectiveness of the comprehensive coping strategy program on clinical outcomes in breast cancer autologous bone marrow transplantation. Cancer Nurs 2000; 23(4):277–285.

100. Grealish L, Lomasney A, Whiteman B. Foot massage: a nursing intervention to modify the distressing symptoms of pain and nausea in patients hospitalised with cancer. Cancer Nurs 2000; 23(3):237–243.

101. Herth K. Enhancing hope in people with a first recurrence of cancer. J Adv Nurs 2000; 32(6):1431–1441.

102. Fenlon D. Research notes. Nurs Stand 2002; 16(38):24.

103. Smith MC, Kemp J, Hemphill L, Vojir CP. Outcomes of therapeutic massage for hospitalized cancer patients. J Nurs Scholarsh 2002; 34(3):257–262.

104. Barsevick A, Whitmer K, Sweeney C, Nail L. A pilot study examining energy conservation for cancer treatment-related fatigue. Cancer Nurs 2002; 25(5):333–341.

105. Wall M, Wheeler S. Benefits of the placebo effect in the therapeutic relationship. Complement Ther Nurs Midwifery 1996; 2(6):160–163.

106. Kwekkeboom K. The placebo effect in symptom management. Oncol Nurs Forum 1997; 24(8):1393–1399.

107. Penson J. Complementary therapies: making a difference in palliative care. Complement Ther Nurs Midwifery 1998; 4:77–81.

108. Smith MC, Stullenbarger E. An integrative review and meta-analysis of oncology nursing research: 1981–1990. Cancer Nurs 1995; 18(3):167–179.

109. Wallace K. Analysis of recent literature concerning relaxation and imagery interventions for cancer pain. Cancer Nurs 1997; 20(2):79–88.

110. Pan CX, Morrison S, Ness J, Fugh-Berman A, Leipzig RM. Complementary and alternative medicine in the management of pain, dyspnoea and nausea and vomiting near the end of life: a systematic review. J Pain Symptom Manage 2000; 20(5):374–387.

111. Pearson A. Taking up the challenge: the future for therapeutic nursing. In: McMahon R, Pearson A, eds. Nursing as therapy. 2nd edn. Cheltenham: Stanley Thornes; 1998:245–260.

112. Ramprogus V. Eliciting nursing knowledge from practice: the dualism of nursing. Nurse Res 2003; 10(1):52–64.

113. Corner J, Plant H, A'Hern R, Bailey C. Non pharmacological intervention for breathlessness in lung cancer., Palliat Med 1996; 10(4):299–305.

114. Johnson M, Moore S. Research into practice: the reality of implementing a non-pharmacological breathlessness intervention into clinical practice. Eur J Oncol Nurs 2003; 7(1):33–38.

115. Tierney A. Nursing research in Europe. Int Nurs Rev 1998; 45(1):15–19.

116. Corner J. A framework for cancer nursing research. Eur J Cancer Care 1993; 2:112–116.

117. Richardson A, Miller M, Potter H. Developing, delivering and evaluating cancer nursing services: building the evidence base. Nurs Times Res 2001; 6(4):726–735.

118. Kearney N. Seventh Robert Tiffany Annual Nursing Lecture. Cancer nursing in the UK: practice, policy or just pretending. Eur J Oncol Nurs 2002; 6(4):205–212.

119. Hunt J. Research into practice: the foundation for evidence-based care. Cancer Nurs 2001; 24(2):78–87.

120. Cawley N. Webber J. Research priorities in palliative care. Int J Palliat Nurs 1995; 1(2):101–113.

121. Wengstrom Y, Häggmark C. Assessing nursing problems of importance for the development of nursing care in a radiation therapy department. Cancer Nurs 1998; 21(1): 50–56.

122. Daniels L, Ascough A. Developing a strategy for cancer nursing research: identifying priorities. Eur J Oncol Nurs 1999; 3(3):161–169.

123. Rustøen T, Schjølberg TK. Cancer nursing research priorities: a Norwegian perspective. Cancer Nurs 2000; 23(5):375–381.

124. Browne N, Robinson L, Richardson A. A Delphi study on the research priorities of European oncology nurses. Eur J Oncol Nurs 2002; 6(3):133–144.

125. Oberst MT. Priorities in cancer nursing research. Cancer Nurs 1978; 1(2):281–290.

126. Daly J, Chang EM, Bell PF. Clinical nursing research priorities in Australian critical care: a pilot. J Adv Nurs 1996; 23(1):145–151.

127. Kearney N, Miller M, Sermeus W, Hoy D, Vanhaecht K. Collaboration in cancer nursing practice. J Clin Nurs 2000; 9(3):429–435.

128. International Society of Nurses in Cancer Care. Directory of oncology nurse researchers. 3rd issue. 2002 (www.isncc.org/publications/index.htm) consulted 14/9/03.

129. Hunt J. Indicators for nursing practice: the use of research findings. J Adv Nurs 1981; 6:189–194.

130. Hunt J. Barriers to research utilization. J Adv Nurs 1996; 23(3):423–425.

131. Rutledge DN, Ropka M, Greene PE, Nail L, Mooney KH. Barriers to research utilization for oncology staff nurses and nurse managers/clinical nurse managers. Oncol Nurs Forum 1998; 25(3):497–506.

132. Sitzia J. Barriers to research utilization: the clinical setting and the nurses themselves. Eur J Oncol Nurs 2001; 5(3):154–164.

133. The Cochrane Collaboration. 2003. www.cochrane.org. Site last updated 23/10/03. Consulted 29/10/03.

134. Joanna Briggs Institute. 2003. www.joannabriggs.edu.au/about/home.php. Site last updated 23/10/03. Consulted 29/10/03.

135. NHS Modernisation Agency, Cancer Services Collaborative. 2003.

www.modern.nhs.uk/scripts/default.asp?site_id=26&id=5620 undated. Consulted 29/10/03.

136. Corner J, Wilson-Barnett J. The newly registered nurse and the cancer patient: an educational evaluation. Int J Nurs Stud 1992; 29(2):177–190.

137. Ferguson A. Evaluating the purpose and benefits of continuing education in nursing and the implications for the provision of continuing education for cancer nurses. J Adv Nurs 1994; 19:640–646.

138. Standing Committee of Nurses of the European Union. Report: workshop on cancer nursing in basic nurse education. Brussels: Standing Committee of Nurses of the European Union; 1995.

139. Blunden G, Langton H, Hek G. Professional education for the cancer care nurse in England and Wales: a review of the evidence base. Eur J Cancer Care 2001; 10(3):179–182.

140. Commission of the European Communities. Europe against cancer programme: proposal for a plan of action 1987–1989 (Com 86/717 final). Brussels, 1986.

141. Commission of the European Communities. Advisory Committee on training in nursing; report and recommendations on training in cancer. Brussels; 1988.

142. European Oncology Nursing Society. A core curriculum for a post-basic course in cancer nursing. Revised edn. Prepared for the Europe Against Cancer Programme. Brussels: Commission of the European Communities; 1991.

143. Redmond K, Kearney N, Collins R, et al. The EONS core curriculum revision project. Eur J Oncol Nurs 2001; 5(1):26–31.

144. Knowles G, Kearney N, Webb P. The development of a conceptual framework for advancing cancer nursing practice in Europe. Eur J Oncol Nurs 2000; 4(4):219–226.

145. Rolfe G. Education for the advanced practitioner. In: Rolfe G, Fulbrook P, eds. Advanced nursing practice. Oxford: Butterworth-Heinemann; 1998:271–280.

146. Boal E, Hodgson D, Banks-Howe J, Husband G. A cultural change in cancer education and training. Eur J Cancer Care 2000; 9(1):30–35.

147. Ward J, Wood C. Education and training of healthcare staff: the barriers to its success. Eur J Cancer Care 2000; 9(2):80–85.

148. Hammick M, Robertshaw H. Interprofessional work in cancer care: towards team work through interprofessional education. J Radiother Pract 1999; 1:27–34.

149. Cooper H, Carlisle C, Gibbs T, Watkins C. Developing an evidence base for interdisciplinary learning: a systematic review. J Adv Nurs 2001; 35(2):228–237.

150. Haagedoorn EML, De Vries J, Robinson E. The UICC/WHO-CCCE Cancer Education Project: a different approach. J Cancer Educ 2000; 15(4):204–208.

151. Corner J. Academia, cancer nursing and a new decade. Eur J Cancer Nurs 2001; 10(3):164–165.

152. Manley K. Organisational culture and consultant nurse outcomes: Part 1: Organisational culture. Nurs Stand 2000; 14(36):34–38.

153. Molassiotis A. Quo vantis: cancer nursing in Europe [editorial]. Eur J Oncol Nurs 2003; 7(1):1–2.

154. Antrobus S, Kitson A. Nursing leadership influencing and shaping health policy and nursing practice. J Adv Nurs 1999; 29(3):746–753.

155. Cook MJ. The attributes of effective clinical leaders. Nurs Stand 2001; 15(35):33–36.

156. Mullally S. Leadership and politics (LPNS Lecture). Nurs Manage 2001; 8(4):21–27.

157. Tritter JQ, Calnan M. Cancer as a chronic illness? Reconsidering categorization and exploring experience. Eur J Cancer Care 2002; 11(3):161–165.

158. Soothill K, Morris SM, Thomas C, et al. The universal, situational and personal needs of cancer patients and their main carers. Eur J Oncol Nurs 2003; 7(1):5–13.

159. Post-White J. Wind behind our sails: empowering our patients and ourselves. Oncol Nurs Forum 1998; 25(6):1011–1017.

160. National Cancer Alliance. Patient-centred services? What patients say. Oxford: National Cancer Alliance; 1996.

161. Luker KA, Beaver K, Leinster SJ, Owens RG. Information needs and sources of information for women with breast cancer: a follow up study. J Adv Nurs 1996; 23:487–495.

162. Davison B, Degner L. Empowerment of men newly diagnosed with prostate cancer. Cancer Nurs 1997; 20(3):187–196.

163. Tomori C, Angelos P, Bennett CL. Communication: from paternalism to shared decision making. Oncol News Int 2001; 10(2):28–32.

164. Clark JA, Wray NP, Ashton CM. Living with treatment decisions: regrets and quality of life among men treated for metastatic prostate cancer. J Clin Oncol 2001; 19(1):72–80.

165. McVea KL, Minier WC, Johnson Palensky JE. Low-income women with early stage breast cancer: physician and patient decision making styles. Psycho-oncology 2001; 10:137–146.

166. McKillop WJ, Stewart WE, Ginsberg AD, Stewart SS. Cancer patients' perceptions of their disease and its treatment. Br J Cancer 1988; 3(5):355–726.

167. Hinds C, Streater A, Mood D. Functions and preferred methods of receiving information related to radiotherapy. Cancer Nurs 1995; 18(5):374–384.

168. Veronesi U, von Kleist S. Redmond K. Costa A. Delvaux N. Freilich G. Glaus A. Hudson T. McVie JG, Macnamara C, et al, and the CAWAC Study Group. Caring about Women and Cancer (CAWAC): a European survey of the perspectives and experiences of women with female cancers. Eur J Oncol Nurs 1999; 3(4):240–250.

169. Sainio C, Eriksson E. Keeping cancer patients informed: a challenge for nursing. Eur J Oncol Nurs 2003; 7(1):39–49.

170. Hack TF, Degner LF, Dyck DG. Relationship between preferences for decisional control and illness information among women with breast cancer: a quantitative and qualitative analysis. Soc Sci Med 1994; 39(2):279–289.

171. Huizinga G, Sleijfer D, van de Wiel HB, Van der Graff, WTA. Decision-making process in patients before entering phase III cancer clinical trials: a pilot study. Cancer Nurs 1999; 22(2):119–125.

172. Sainio C, Eriksson E, Sirkka L. Patient participation in decision making about care: the cancer patient's point of view. Cancer Nurs 2001; 24(3):172–179.

173. Thornton H. Patient perspectives on involvement in cancer research in the UK. Eur J Cancer Care 2002; 11(3):205–209.

174. Gatterellari M, Butow PN, Tattersall MHN. Sharing decisions in cancer care. Soc Sci Med 2001; 52:1865–1878.

175. Flanagan J. Public participation in the design of educational programmes for cancer nurses: a case report. Eur J Cancer Care 1999; 8(2):107–112.

176. Moynihan C. Men, women, gender and cancer. Eur J Cancer Care 2002; 11(3):166–172.

177. Taylor K. Researching the experience of kidney cancer patients. Eur J Cancer Care 2002; 11(3):200–204.

178. Cancer Voices (undated) www.cancerlink.org/voices Consulted 1/11/03.

179. Maslin-Prothero S. Developing User Involvement in Research, Journal of Clinical Nursing, 2003, 12, (3), 412-421

180. Kearney N, Muir L, Miller M, et al. Using handheld computers to support patients receiving chemotherapy. Abstract 1206. Abstract Book ECCO 12. The European Cancer Conference 2003; 1(5):S368–369.

181. Allenby A, Matthews J, Beresford J, McLachlan SA. The application of computer touch-screen technology in screening for psychosocial distress in an ambulatory oncology setting. Eur J Cancer Care 2002; 11(4):245–253.

CHAPTER 35

Intensive Nursing Care of the Patient with Cancer

SHELLEY DOLAN

CHAPTER CONTENTS

Introduction	771
Critical illness categories most commonly admitted to critical care	772
The sepsis syndrome	772
Disseminated intravascular coagulation	776
Acute respiratory failure	778
Acute renal failure	781
Tumour lysis syndrome	782
Haemodynamic instability	783
Assessment and monitoring	783

The postoperative care of people with cancer in the intensive therapy unit	785
Essential care following major surgery for cancer	786
Pain assessment and management	786
Deep vein thrombosis prophylaxis	788
Postoperative nausea and vomiting	788
End of life care in the intensive therapy unit	789
Conclusion	790
References	790

INTRODUCTION

As treatments for people with cancer become more complex, and people live longer, the support they require increases. For some cancer patients the nature of their disease or its treatment may necessitate acute support and even warrant admission to a critical care unit (CCU). This chapter therefore illustrates the nursing care provided to the cancer patient who is critically ill. For the purposes of this chapter, a critical illness is defined as an acute event resulting in the need for much greater nursing and multidisciplinary care and technological support. An important additional factor is that at the outset there must be the possibility of a recovery from this acute event.

People with cancer become critically ill for many reasons, but these can be divided into two major groups:

- those that are electively admitted to a CCU following major surgery, e.g. an oesophago-gastrectomy for adenocarcinoma
- those whose critical illness is a sudden event as a result of disease or their anticancer treatment such as severe sepsis following immune suppression.

People with cancer may also be affected by any acute event, such as a myocardial infarction, major trauma, burns, status epilepticus, status asthmaticus or pulmonary embolus. However, in this chapter only those conditions that are particularly prevalent in the person with cancer, or those that become more common, such as pulmonary embolus, are discussed. In the following sections the most common categories of critical illness will be described, together with their cause, treatment and relevant priorities for nursing care. Critical illness is a complex and dynamic phenomenon and the patient is often affected by several toxicities at once; however, for clarity each will be described separately.

The nursing care of the cancer patient who is critically ill is a wonderful challenge, combining the best features of cancer and critical care nursing. It is an opportunity to use the therapeutic skills of nursing assessment, monitoring and care together with an advanced knowledge and application in the fields of cancer and critical care. One of the key components to advanced nursing practice in critical care is the ability to work well collaboratively in a multidisciplinary team; this is particularly necessary in the care of critically ill cancer patients, where the complex needs of a chronic illness and the application of multimodality therapy necessitates a team approach.[1]

Critical care in many countries is not now confined within the walls of the intensive therapy unit (ITU). Having learnt from colleagues in Australia,[2] many ITU nurses and doctors are involved in critical care outreach teams.[3,4] These teams work to identify patients who are at risk of deteriorating, either to avert admissions to the ITU, or to effect early transfer to the ITU.[5] These teams are also key to ensuring safe and effective transfer of patients leaving the ITU for general wards, and in the coaching and teaching of junior doctors and nurses on general wards.[6] Several teams in the UK have also taken the care of the patient further by providing follow-up care clinics for patients who have been critically ill.[7–9]

CRITICAL ILLNESS CATEGORIES MOST COMMONLY ADMITTED TO CRITICAL CARE

The sepsis syndrome

One of the most common complications facing the person being treated for cancer is the sepsis syndrome. Although sepsis and severe sepsis do occur in the healthy population, occurrence is directly correlated with age, chronic disease, co-morbidities and, most importantly, any disease or treatment that renders the person susceptible to infection.[10]

Sepsis and severe sepsis are stages of a complex clinical syndrome that remains a major challenge for all multidisciplinary teams working with critically ill patients with cancer. Despite many clinical trials and advances in intensive care, the mortality rate for sepsis syndrome remains high. Incidence is projected to increase as we treat more vulnerable patients who are immune suppressed (through therapy or disease) and an increasingly aged population.

Epidemiology of sepsis

The incidence of sepsis worldwide is increasing, with severe sepsis remaining the highest cause of death in patients admitted to non-coronary intensive care units (ICUs).[11–13] Sepsis is also the 13th leading cause of death among all hospitalized patients, with an estimated annual incidence in the United States of approximately 750,000 cases per annum. The associated mortality rates in these hospitalized patients have been shown to be between 30 and 50%.[14–22] Although there is, as yet, no national or international register of the incidence of sepsis in cancer patients, all are susceptible to sepsis and its sequelae for the reasons shown in Table 35.1.

Some cancer patients are more vulnerable to infection because their cancer is in the bone marrow and therefore directly affects the body's immune response; these cancers are often known as the liquid cancers (leukaemia, lymphoma, myeloma). The definitive treatment for these cancers is to ablate the bone marrow before replacing it with allogeneic (from another person) or autologous (from the self) stem cells or bone marrow. There are also some cancer patients with solid tumours, e.g teratoma, who may need to receive the same marrow ablative chemotherapy. The mortality rate for these patients who develop sepsis and then severe sepsis is between 65 and 85%.[23,24] In patients such as those with leukaemia, sepsis is the major reason for transplant-associated deaths in the first 6 weeks of therapy.[10] It is therefore essential that those working with these people endeavour to try and reduce the incidence of sepsis and mortality rates.

Sepsis is the systemic response to severe infection in the body. The sequelae of sepsis, such as generalized inflammatory response, fibrinolysis,

Table 35.1: The risks of infection and sepsis for the person with cancer

Characteristic	Reason for greater risk of sepsis
Repeated hospitalization	Increase in nosocomial (hospital-acquired) infections
Repeated invasive therapy, utilizing short- or long-term central venous access devices (CVAD)	Increased exposure to CVAD-associated infections
Bone marrow suppression because of disease infiltration of the marrow – liquid cancers or metastatic disease involving the bone	Bone marrow suppression results in pancytopenia, with a resultant lowering of the white blood cell count, the platelet count and the red cell count. White cells are the body's first and most important response to infection
Bone marrow suppression as a result of treatment either chemo or radiotherapy	The resultant neutropenia (reduction in the absolute neutrophil count (ANC)) renders the body exquisitely susceptible to infections, particularly opportunistic infections in the immunosuppressed host
Malnutrition associated with disease or treatment	Poor immunity and resistance to infection
A predominantly older population who are more likely to have co-morbid conditions	Generally frail health more likely to be less resistant to infections
Increased exposure to transfused blood and its components, either as a result of repeated surgery or the disease and chemo/radiotherapy	The transfusion of donated blood and its components such as platelets, clotting factors and fibrinogen carry the risk of transmitting donor infections

and procoagulation, shock and organ dysfunction can be seen as progressive stages of the same illness.[11] Historically, there have been various terms used for these stages of sepsis, such as bacteraemia, septicaemia and septic shock. In an attempt to reduce confusion and introduce agreed definitions, in 1991 the American College of Chest Physicians and Society of Critical Care Medicine convened a consensus conference[25] (see Table 35.2). These definitions are now more than 10 years old, with an update expected in late 2004 to early 2005; however, they are widely used across Europe, the United States and Australasia.

Inflammation is an essential part of the body's response to infection, with the host mounting and then down-regulating the inflammatory response. A healthy endothelium is essential for the maintenance of the equilibrium between coagulation and fibrinolysis. In sepsis, the regulatory function of the endothelium fails and the balance of activation and down-regulation is lost.[26] An excessively high level of the pro-inflammatory cytokines are released, leading to systemic endothelial damage. In response to these pro-inflammatory mediators, excessive anti-inflammatory mediators are also released, resulting in immune suppression, which then leads to the onset of secondary infections. Hence, the sequelae of sepsis: endothelial damage, inflammatory changes, alterations to coagulation, fibrinolysis and immune suppression.[11,27–30]

As the sepsis syndrome develops, the following clinical picture develops:

- excessive vasodilation
- hypoperfusion

Table 35.2: Definitions for sepsis and organ failure

Terminology	Definition
Infection	Microbial phenomenon characterized by an inflammatory response to the presence of microorganisms or the invasion of normally sterile host tissue by those organisms
Bacteraemia	Presence of viable bacteria in the blood
Systemic inflammatory response syndrome (SIRS)	The systemic inflammatory response to a wide variety of severe clinical insults, manifested by two or more of the following conditions: (1) temperature >38°C or <36°C; (2) heart rate >90 beats/min; (3) respiratory rate >20 breaths/min or $PaCO_2$ <32 mmHg; and (4) WBC count >12000/mm³, <4000/mm³ or >10% immature (band) forms
Sepsis	The systemic inflammatory response to infection. In association with infection, manifestations of sepsis are the same as those previously defined for SIRS. It should be determined whether they are a part of the direct systemic response to the presence of an infectious process and represent an acute alteration from baseline in the absence of other known causes for such abnormalities
Severe sepsis	Sepsis associated with organ dysfunction, hypoperfusion or hypotension. Hypoperfusion and perfusion abnormalities may include, but are not limited to, lactic acidosis, oliguria or an acute alteration in mental status
Septic shock	A subset of severe sepsis and defined as sepsis-induced hypotension despite adequate fluid resuscitation along with the presence of perfusion abnormalities that may include, but are not limited to, lactic acidosis, oliguria or an acute alteration in mental status. Patients receiving inotropic or vasopressor agents may no longer be hypotensive by the time they manifest hypoperfusion abnormalities or organ dysfunction, yet they would still be considered to have septic shock
Multi-organ-dysfunction syndrome (MODS)	Presence of altered organ function in an acutely ill patient such that homeostasis cannot be maintained without intervention

Source: American College of Chest Physicians/Society of Critical Care (ACCP/SCCM), 1992.[25]

- generalized tissue damage
- inappropriate cytokine response
- coagulopathy
- microthrombi formation.

In patients with severe sepsis, because of the developing procoagulant state, thromboses develop in the microvasculature, leading to organ failure.[31]

Microbiological causes of sepsis

Approximately 60% of patients with sepsis have a microbiologically confirmed infection.[32] Where the infection can be identified, the most likely site is the lungs (46%), followed by the abdominopelvic region (15%) and then the urinary tract (10%).[33] An infection from almost any type of microorganism can result in sepsis, with the clinical progression of sepsis syndrome being similar, regardless of the cause.[32,34] Gram-negative bacteria have been thought to be the most common organism to be associated with sepsis syndrome, but the cases associated with Gram-positive bacterial infection are increasing.[34,35] Although the way that the inflammatory process is initiated differs in Gram-negative and Gram-positive bacterial infections, there is a final common pathway that results in similar severity of illness and mortality.

In Gram-negative bacterial infections, the most important product associated with sepsis is endotoxin, a lipopolysaccharide (LPS) that is a major part of the Gram-negative bacteria's cell wall.[36] Following infection, LPS interacts with CD14 (a cell surface receptor) expressed by white blood cells. LPS then activates both the classical and alternative complement pathways.[37]

In Gram-positive bacterial infections it is lipoteichoic acid that activates the CD14 receptor on white blood cells. Gram-positive bacteria also have other toxins that employ a range of toxic mechanisms.[34,37]

Other microorganisms such as fungi are also associated with sepsis syndrome, with *Candida* being most common and associated with a high mortality rate.[38] Other studies in certain vulnerable groups have identified *Aspergillus* as the most common organism associated with sepsis.[39,40]

Finally, nosocomial infection and drug-resistant infections are a growing problem in ICUs. Pittet and Wenzel's study in 1995 showed that ICU patients were more at risk from nosocomial infections than other hospital patients.[15] Nosocomial pathogens such as methicillin-resistant *Staphyloccus aureus* (MRSA) and vancomycin-resistant *Enterococcus* (VRE) may be multiresistant to drug therapy and thus pose a major challenge in ICU.[41]

Diagnosis of sepsis

Sepsis in cancer patients, especially those receiving marrow ablative chemotherapy or immediately following surgery, must always be suspected. A careful clinical history and examination of the patient is essential. The major clinical signs of sepsis are shown in Table 35.3, but there may be few clinical signs of change. It is therefore essential that the cancer nurse

and the whole team have an awareness of the vulnerability of the person with cancer to severe sepsis.

An essential part of the care of patients with sepsis is establishing the diagnosis early by undertaking microbiological examination of any fluids, or areas of the body known to be commonly involved in sepsis. All fluids such as sputum, urine, blood, swabs from wounds, throat, axilla, groin, stool specimen are sent for microbiological examination regularly, usually every 48 hours, or as dictated by the patient's condition, and particularly if an infection is suspected. However, many of these cultures, e.g. blood cultures, take 48 hours to incubate and this is too long clinically in the care of cancer patients. Attention is therefore being focused on finding other indicators of infection.

Table 35.3: Major clinical signs of sepsis

Organ system	Dysfunction
Pulmonary	Tachypnoea (>20 breaths/min) Dyspnoea Basal consolidation Cyanosis or other colour change
Cardiovascular	Tachycardia (>90 beats/min) Decreased blood pressure Raised or lowered temperature
Central nervous system	Changes in mental state – irritability, lack of concentration, sleepy
Haematological	Rashes (purpura fulminans), echymoses
Gastrointestinal	Abdominal rebound/ tenderness Jaundice
Renal	Oliguria Loin tenderness Pyuria Decreased creatinine clearance

Clinical management of sepsis syndrome

The essential management of a patient with sepsis will always include the following measures:

- oxygen support – adequate tissue oxygenation
- cardiovascular support
- the rapid and effective treatment of infection – may include surgical debridement or other intervention
- monitoring and supportive care of all organs
- antimicrobial therapy directed by a microbiologist.

Over the last 15 years there have been many attempts to find specific treatments to interrupt or control the inflammatory and procoagulant process associated with sepsis. Manipulation of the immune response with various monoclonal antibodies has not been shown to alter the outcome and reduce mortality rates.[42,43] Two studies which have demonstrated significant reductions in expected mortality are treatment with recombinant activated protein C, which has an effect on haemostasis,[19] and the monitoring and control of blood sugars.[44] It is clear that early identification and careful monitoring of people with cancer and sepsis and good communication with the relevant CCU are essential.

Disseminated intravascular coagulation

Disseminated intravascular coagulation (DIC) is an acquired disorder that follows major insult or injury to the body, the strongest association being with sepsis.[45,46] All cancer patients are susceptible to sepsis, and therefore DIC; however, particular cancers, such as acute promyelocytic leukaemia (AML-M3), and solid tumours, particularly of the pancreas and prostate, are specifically linked with DIC. Other causes of DIC that may affect the person with cancer are:

- trauma, including major surgery/major blood loss
- obstetric complications – amniotic embolism, abruption placentae

- vascular disorders – giant haemangioma, aortic aneurysm
- reactions to toxins – snake venom, drugs, amphetamines
- immune reactions – anaphylaxis, haemolytic transfusion reaction, transplant rejection.[45,47,48]

Definition of disseminated intravascular coagulation

DIC at its most severe is a catastrophic combination of widespread thrombotic formation combined with a systemic haemorrhagic syndrome.[47] The widespread activation of coagulation that leads to the formation of fibrin and then thrombotic occlusion of small, mid-size and occasionally large blood vessels leads to hypoxia and organ damage. In addition, the consumption of platelets, clotting factors and inhibitors, resulting from disseminated thrombus formation, can lead to severe bleeding.[49] Clinical presentation of this condition varies between severe bleeding and the signs of acute organ failure, such as renal failure.[50]

The pathogenesis of disseminated intravascular coagulation

In response to the conditions listed above, the coagulation system is triggered by the generation of thrombin within the systemic circulation.[49] At the same time there is suppression of anticoagulation mechanisms and impaired removal of fibrin.[50] These changes are caused by damage to the endothelium and the generation of several proinflammatory cytokines, with tumour necrosis factor alpha (TNF-α) being mainly involved in the dysregulation of anticoagulation and fibrinolysis, and interleukin-6 (IL-6) being involved in the activation of coagulation. In patients with DIC, none of the three most important anticoagulant mechanisms (antithrombin III, protein C and S, and tissue factor–pathway inhibitor) are able to function optimally. Therefore people with DIC have deposition of fibrin in the microvasculature and it cannot be removed because fibrinolysis is depressed. This results in decreased perfusion to the resultant organs.[45]

Diagnosis of disseminated intravascular coagulation

For nurses caring for the patient with cancer there should always be a high index of suspicion of DIC, particularly when caring for patients with severe sepsis, patients that have sustained a major blood loss or patients that have the associated malignant conditions of AML-M3, pancreatic or prostate cancer. The clinical presentation of DIC varies: the patient may be asymptomatic or there may be severe haemorrhage, or thrombosis and organ failure.[49] Bleeding is the most common presentation, sometimes to be found at puncture sites around intravenous or intra-arterial cannulae, or from wounds. Commonly, bleeding will be seen in the patient's skin as petechiae, purpura and haematomas, or in the form of haematuria, haemoptysis, gastrointestinal bleeding or occasionally intracranial haemorrhage.[49,51–53] The diagnosis will be confirmed by a combination of laboratory tests, as listed in Table 35.4. It is important to recognize that serial laboratory findings are more useful in the diagnosis than one result. It is also essential to look at the global clotting tests rather than one part of the clotting cascade, as there are several reasons for the person with cancer to have a low platelet count or changes in their clotting.[50]

The treatment of disseminated intravascular coagulation

As DIC is a secondary condition, it is essential to treat the condition that has led to its development. Aggressive reversal of the damage caused by conditions such as sepsis or major surgery is essential. Treatment strategies for DIC are supportive therapy, replacement of clotting factors and platelets and, finally, arrest of coagulation by using heparin or another thrombin inhibitor.[49] Other than DIC associated with AML-M3, the following strategies will apply.

Supportive therapy

The supportive therapy of patients with DIC includes the correction of electrolyte abnormalities, control and if possible normalization of acidosis and reversal of hypovolaemia and hypoxia.

Replacement therapy

Replacement therapy in DIC is essential if the patient is bleeding or if any surgical or invasive procedure is planned. Replacement will be with fresh frozen plasma (FFP) at a dose of 10–15 ml/kg. If the FFP does not raise the patient's fibrinogen level above 0.5 g/L, then cryoprecipitate can be used. Platelets should be replaced if the level is below $20 \times 10^9/L$, or if the patient is actively bleeding or is going to undergo invasive procedures when the count is less than $50 \times 10^9/L$.[49]

Anticoagulant therapy

The use of anticoagulant therapy in DIC is controversial, and as yet unsupported by robust prospective research studies. However, small experimental studies have demonstrated that heparin is probably useful in those cancer patients with clinically overt thromboembolism

Table 35.4: Laboratory tests used to confirm disseminated intravascular coagulation (DIC)

Laboratory finding	Normal value	Result in DIC
Platelet count	150,000–450,000/mm³	Markedly decreased
Prothrombin time	10–13 seconds	Increased
Activated partial thromboplastin time	20–32 seconds	Increased
Fibrin degradation products	<0.25 mg/L	Markedly increased
Fibrinogen	1.7–4.0 g/L	Normal or decreased
Antithrombin III	0.20–0.45 mg/ml	Markedly decreased
Protein C	60–150% inhibition	Markedly decreased

or with purpura fulminans. Low doses of heparin, at 5–10 U/kg/h, are usually infused continuously; low molecular weight heparin has also been tried.[45,49] Some work has been undertaken looking at other anticoagulant and antifibrinolytic drugs, such as activated protein C,[54,55] aprotinin and tissue plasminogen activator (tPA).[49,56] Although there is little evidence so far, early results appear promising.

Treatment of disseminated intravascular coagulation associated with AML-M3

In AML-M3 there is a specific treatment pathway for DIC. AML-M3 accounts for about 25% of cases of promyelocytic leukaemia.[57,58] About 8% of patients with acute leukaemia develop DIC, but most patients with AML-M3 will have some laboratory or clinical evidence of the syndrome. In AML-M3, the granules of the malignant promyelocytes release tissue factor and procoagulant.[48,62] AML-M3 has a good prognosis provided the associated DIC can be well managed; the use of all-trans-retinoic acid (ATRA) has improved the remission rates to higher than 90%.[59–62] ATRA has a major impact on the haemostatic system, by aiding the promyelocytes to develop into mature cells, and also has a direct effect on the TF synthesis of abnormal or dying malignant cells.[48,62] However, the pattern of coagulopathy can differ between patients with AML-M3, especially in those patients whose DIC is complicated by sepsis; therefore, although ATRA has a major role in the treatment of AML-M3. so too will the other supportive and replacement strategies described above.[63]

Acute respiratory failure

Sixty per cent of people with cancer admitted as an emergency to a CCU are admitted with acute respiratory failure.[64,65] A high percentage will have respiratory failure associated with infection.[66] Other causes of respiratory failure in the person with cancer are shown in Table 35.5.

Acute respiratory failure is diagnosed by a combination of clinical history and clinical findings, including:

- respiratory rate usually elevated > 30 breaths/min
- worsening serial chest X-rays
- lowered tissue oxygen saturation <90% on 60% inspired oxygen
- worsening arterial blood gases
- worsening respiratory pattern
- increased work of breathing.

Treatment of acute respiratory failure depends to some extent on the cause and severity of the failure, but it is also essential to make treat-

Table 35.5: Causes of acute respiratory failure in the person with cancer

Cause	Reference and date
Major bleeding	65, 2002 67, 2000 68, 1998 69, 1996 70, 1994 71, 1987
Chemotherapy-induced lung injury, e.g. bleomycin	72, 2003 73, 2002 74, 1997
Radiotherapy-induced lung injury	75, 2000 76, 1987
Pleural effusions	
Adult respiratory distress syndrome	77, 2003 78, 2003 79, 2003 80, 2002 81, 2002 82, 2002
Postoperative complications	77, 2003 83, 2001 84, 2000 82, 2002
Massive or multiple pulmonary emboli	85, 2001 86, 2000 87, 2000 88, 2000 89, 2000 90, 1991

ment decisions following a multidisciplinary discussion about the patient's likelihood of recovery. It is essential, where there is time, to ensure that the intensive care and the cancer care teams discuss together the patient's previous performance status, type and stage of disease and whether the respiratory failure is a preterminal event or a stage in an acute illness where the patient has a chance of meaningful recovery. Where possible, the patient should be a part of this discussion.

If it is felt that the patient is not suitable for endotracheal intubation and mechanical ventilation, some thought should be given to whether they can best be cared for outside of the ITU with support from the ITU team. The patient's respiratory effort in this situation may be eased by the use of low-dose opioids and/or sedative agents such as midazolam; they may also benefit from the application of oxygen therapy with or without continuous positive airways pressure (CPAP) or BiPAP via a face mask.

If, however, after multidisciplinary review of the patient and discussion with the patient themselves, it is decided that ITU therapy is appropriate, there should be no delay in transfer and treatment. It is important to recognize that a cancer diagnosis alone does not mean that mechanical ventilation is futile. Several studies have demonstrated that people with cancer do benefit: the key is careful selection, and all patients referred to the ITU team for ventilatory support are reviewed individually.[64,91-95]

The principles of caring for a patient in respiratory failure in the ITU are directed at achieving the following:

- optimum gaseous exchange
- optimum delivery of oxygen to the tissues
- protective strategies to avoid lung deterioration or further damage to the lungs
- protective strategies to avoid other organ damage, particularly renal damage
- care to ensure optimum weaning strategies to facilitate timely weaning in an emotionally supportive manner for the patient and their family

- care to protect patients from their environment while they are sedated
- care of the patient's family.

As the cause of respiratory failure in many cancer patients admitted to an ITU is infection, or infection superimposed on another condition such as pneumonitis, aggressive investigation and treatment of the infective cause is imperative. The following strategies are used to identify the infective organism:

- clinical history
- sputum samples for microbiological assay
- serial chest X-rays
- bronchoalveolar lavage
- computed tomography (CT) scans
- magnetic resonance imaging (MRI) scans.

It is essential to target antimicrobial therapy for two main reasons: effective control of the infective organisms; limitation of the damage suffered by the kidneys exposed to antimicrobial drugs.

The principles of mechanical ventilation

The overall aim of mechanical ventilation is to improve oxygenation and gaseous exchange, either prophylactically following surgery or in response to acute respiratory failure. Mechanical ventilation can be provided in several ways; the most common method in cancer patients who are critically ill is a type of positive pressure ventilation. Other techniques of mechanical ventilation and conditions most likely to be treated by that type of ventilation are listed in Table 35.6.

Mechanical ventilation is an important part of the treatment of acute respiratory failure. However, there are several disadvantages associated with mechanical ventilation:

- depression of the cardiovascular system
- ventilator-induced lung injury
- barotrauma
- pneumothorax
- nosocomial pneumonia
- gastrointestinal problems such as 'paralytic ileus'
- water retention

779

Table 35.6: Types of mechanical ventilation

Type of ventilation	Characteristics	Typical condition treated by this type of ventilation
Negative pressure ventilation	First described in 1920 and used extensively during the polio epidemic. Tank ventilators, 'Iron Lung' Cuirass Ventilator. Patient's thorax is enclosed by a tight shell or tank and a negative pressure is exerted during which the patient's chest expands and air enters the lungs. The patient does not have an endotracheal tube	Polio, muscular dystrophy, sleep apnoea syndrome (can affect the person with cancer)
Intermittent positive pressure ventilation (IPPV)	Between 1980 and 1990 this was the most common type of ventilation used in an ITU. The lungs are intermittently inflated by applying positive pressure through either an endotracheal or tracheostomy tube	All elective mechanical ventilation: for example, for respiratory failure or prophylactically following major surgery or trauma
Synchronized intermittent mandatory ventilation (SIMV)	Since the mid 1990s this mode has largely replaced IPPV. Its advantages are that it synchronizes ventilator breaths with the patients and is therefore more 'natural' and causes less cardiovascular depression and the risk of barotrauma is reduced[96]	All elective mechanical ventilation as above, but especially used to facilitate patients being weaned from ventilation, with mechanical breaths gradually reduced as the patient becomes stronger
Pressure support ventilation (PSV)	Used since early 1990, this technique utilizes a constant pre-set positive pressure that is triggered by the patient's spontaneous inspiratory effort. PSV is a more comfortable mode of ventilation and can reduce the work of breathing	PSV is often used with SIMV in the process of weaning a patient from mechanical ventilation. Particularly useful where ventilator-induced lung injury is likely
Biphasic ventilation (BiPAP)	Originally designed as a weaning technique, BiPAP allows spontaneous breathing at a low and high pressure during each cycle[97]	
High-frequency jet ventilation (HFJV)	Described and used in research and in the clinical ITU setting since early 1990. The technique involves the injection of gas at a rate of between 60 and 1000 breaths/min. These breaths are very small and can be delivered through a small-bore cannula inserted into the centre of an endotracheal tube. The theoretical advantages of HFJV are associated with low airway pressures and therefore less risks of haemodynamic compromise, barotrauma and ventilator-induced lung injury. There are, however, problems associated with hypercapnia, iatrogenic injuries and mechanical difficulties in achieving adequate humidification. Large studies have failed to demonstrate a major advantage[98–100]	Used for the treatment of patients with severe acute lung injury (ALI) such as acute respiratory distress syndrome (ARDS) where the lung compliance is severely reduced. Used much less commonly than other modes of ventilation

Table 35.6: Types of mechanical ventilation—cont'd

Type of ventilation	Characteristics	Typical condition treated by this type of ventilation
Extracorporeal methods Extracorporeal membrane oxygenation (ECMO)	Specialist intervention in a cardiothoracic setting using a circuit and artificial lung[101]	Specialist intervention used as a last resort in neonates or adults who have not responded to conventional ventilation
Non-invasive ventilation Continuous positive pressure ventilation (CPAP) and BiPAP	Used in the spontaneously breathing patient via an endotracheal tube or tracheostomy, or via a face mask. Can improve lung mechanics; the work of breathing is decreased, the respiratory rate falls and oxygenation improves. Haemodynamic depression is minimal and the incidence of barotrauma is less than with the invasive methods	Used in the weaning of patients from mechanical ventilation. Used prophylactically to improve breathing postoperatively. Increasingly used as an alternative to mechanical ventilation in acute respiratory failure. Can be used by the patient at home who has chronic respiratory or neurological deficits, e.g. with sleep apnoea[96,102,103]

- local problems associated with the endotracheal tube
- separation from society – sedated
- exposure and vulnerability to the environment.

One of the most important roles for the nurse working with people with cancer in an ITU is to be aware of the dangers, outlined in Table 35.6, to constantly monitor the patient and act to minimize the risks. The person with cancer is more vulnerable than the patient without a chronic disease, and particular care will need to be taken with tissue integrity and the risk of infection. It is also important to remember that unlike other patients in an ITU the cancer patient often has to face more treatment, repeated surgery for example, and it is therefore very important that they receive the most sensitive care to minimize distress and the impact of the admission.

For many patients the process of being weaned from mechanical ventilation can be lengthy, frightening and hard work for the patient and family. This process may be improved by using one of the nurse-led weaning protocols developed by critical care nurses. These nurse-led protocols seek to ensure that the patient has an individualized care plan to work towards as they strive for independence from their ventilator. Individualized rehabilitation plans are a method of ensuring optimal care and a tool for involving the patient and their family.[104,105] Continued respiratory monitoring, support and physiotherapy are essential to achieve optimum recovery. The process can be greatly helped by the addition of a CCU outreach team on the ward, in conjunction with expert physiotherapy.

Acute renal failure

The person with cancer is exquisitely susceptible to acute renal failure, either as a single organ failure or in combination with other organs, particularly the lungs. Once the person with cancer has developed two organ failures, their likelihood of survival is severely reduced. In many instances renal failure is preventable, and part of the key role for cancer nurses and CCU outreach teams is to be alert to the patient at particular risk, and to undertake early steps to prevent its occurrence. The person with cancer may have developed renal failure as the result of a discreet injury, but once critically ill, the cause is often multifactorial, occurring as a result of the combination of several factors, such as:

- the disease itself – myeloma, renal cell cancer, solid tumours of the kidney
- severe sepsis
- nephrotoxic anticancer chemotherapy
- nephrotoxic drug therapy – antimicrobial therapy
- critical illness – reduced mean arterial pressure, dehydration
- tumour lysis syndrome.

The dangers of severe sepsis have been outlined previously, but it is important to emphasize the resultant dangers for all organs from the systemic effects of sepsis and the antimicrobial agents used to treat infection. Cancer and critical care nurses are used to monitoring patients carefully for the blood levels of aminoglycosides such as gentamycin, vancomycin and amikacin, but it is important to remember that most drugs are filtered through the kidneys. It is therefore imperative in the ITU setting that drug prescriptions are constantly revised and healthcare professionals are alert to the damage caused to kidneys already vulnerable to damage.

If the cancer patient develops acute renal failure, overall recovery of the patient will depend on the cause and whether any other organ is affected. If the kidneys are affected following severe sepsis or in the presence of respiratory failure, mortality rates are very high, rising to 85–95%, depending on the stage of their cancer. Renal protective therapy is therefore essential in the management of the person with cancer.

Monitoring and support for the cardiovascular system and general perfusion are discussed later, as haemodynamic instability is common to all critically ill patients and the kidneys are particularly vulnerable to a lowered mean arterial pressure and lack of perfusion. One danger that is, however, particular to the person with cancer in the ITU is tumour lysis syndrome; this will therefore be discussed in detail.

Tumour lysis syndrome

Tumour lysis syndrome (TLS) is described as a laboratory or clinical syndrome that can cause life-threatening complications and death, occurring as a result of the metabolic and electrolyte abnormalities that result from the rapid tumour breakdown. The clinical syndrome is described here. TLS starts soon after the beginning of treatment, most typically following chemotherapy, but it can occur following radiotherapy.[106–110] TLS has also been recorded in the person with a haemato-oncology malignancy following the administration of steroid therapy.[111–113] It is, however, more commonly seen in bulky disease that rapidly proliferates and is highly treatment-sensitive[114] and most commonly associated with Burkitt's lymphoma, teratoma, high white cell count leukaemia and myeloma. It also occurs less commonly in small cell lung cancer, breast cancer and neuroblastoma.[107,109,110]

The syndrome is characterized by the release of intracellular products into the circulation following the rapid breakdown of tumour cells. This breakdown of cells leads to the development of severe hyperuricaemia, hyperphosphataemia, hypocalcaemia, hyperkalaemia, acute renal failure and metabolic acidosis.[107] The kidney damage is caused by obstruction of the distal tubules and collecting ducts due to the deposition of uric acid crystals.[109] Untreated rapidly rising potassium levels can cause life-threatening cardiac arrhythmias and death.[110]

Nursing treatment of TLS is firstly concentrated on identifying high-risk patients and then trying to prevent TLS. Nursing management of patients at risk should include the following:

- accurate and frequent monitoring of the 24-hour fluid and electrolyte balance
- optimum hydration and the maintenance of a urine output of at least 3 L/24 hours
- if the urine output falls, the use of inotropic and/or diuretic therapy in the presence of optimum hydration

- allopurinol, orally or intravenously 500 mg/m² daily, inhibits xanthine oxidase, which is an enzyme that catalyses the conversion of hypoxanthine and xanthine to uric acid

- azetazolamide, 250 mg intravenously, to increase the excretion of uric acid through the kidneys

- the use of a recombinant urate oxidase protein rasburicase converts uric acid into the soluble compound allantoin and has been shown to control hyperuricemia faster and more reliably than allopurinol.[115–119]

If severe TLS develops, despite the above measures, initial rises in potassium may be controlled with calcium gluconate administered enterally or the administration of a dextrose and insulin intravenous infusion. However, if the patient's urine output can no longer be maintained in the presence of a rapidly worsening electrolyte and metabolic imbalance, renal replacement therapy will have to be instituted immediately.

The dialytic method of choice for TLS is a continuous filtration method to compensate for the continuing lysis of cells.

HAEMODYNAMIC INSTABILITY

At some time during their stay in an ITU all cancer patients will undergo some degree of haemodynamic instability. This instability may be severe and life-threatening, e.g. when associated with severe sepsis or severe bleeding, or it may be moderate and transient, as experienced by the postoperative patient who needs extra colloid hydration. The clinical manifestations of haemodynamic instability are listed in Table 35.7.

Assessment and monitoring

As with much nursing care in the ITU, the key to optimum patient safety is the nurse's knowledge and awareness, accompanied by careful assessment and monitoring with timely reac-

---

Table 35.7: Clinical manifestations of haemodynamic instability

Cardiovascular change	Normal values	Causes for change
Lowered mean arterial pressure (MAP)	Individual to the patient; typically for an adult, normal value is >70 mmHg	Sepsis, severe sepsis Bleeding Post-anaesthesia Lowered circulating fluid volume, dehydration Opioid therapy via epidural or intravenous route, sedation infusions Alteration to cardiac output – cardiac arrhythmia, myocardial infarction. Invasive mechanical ventilation, especially with high levels of positive end-expiratory pressure (PEEP)
Raised MAP	Individual to patient ,but generally normal value is <90 mmHg	Pain, agitation, fear, reaction to drugs, cerebral irritation, severe raised intracranial pressure, atheroscleroma
Hypothermia	<36°C	Severe sepsis, cardiovascular shock, post-anaesthesia, continuous renal replacement therapy
Hyperthermia	>38°C	Infection, severe sepsis, rare reaction to anaesthesia – malignant hyperpyrexia

783

(continues)

Table 35.7: Clinical manifestations of haemodynamic instability—cont'd

Cardiovascular change	Normal values	Causes for change
Raised heart rate – tachycardia	>100 beats/min	Infection, severe sepsis, severe bleeding, pain, fear, agitation, electrolyte imbalance – hypo/hyperkalaemia, hypomagnesaemia, hypo/hypercalcaemia Cardiac instability – myocardial infarction, cardiac arrhythmias Acid–base imbalance
Decreased heart rate – bradycardia	<60 beats/min	Severe raised intracranial pressure, myocardial instability or myocardial infarction (typically inferior infarction), heart conduction defect – heart block 1st, 2nd or 3rd degree, drug effect – overdose of opioid or sedation
Raised central venous pressure (CVP)	Normal CVP = 3–5 cmH$_2$O	Overhydration with fluid, congestive cardiac failure, pulmonary hypertension; it is important to ensure the lumen of CVP catheter is not blocked
Lowered CVP	<3 cmH$_2$O	Loss of intravascular fluid – bleeding, dehydration, combination of anaesthesia and epidural therapy, invasive mechanical ventilation especially with high levels of PEEP
Raised systemic vascular resistance (SVR)	Normal level 800–1500 dyne/s/cm^{-5}	Left ventricular failure
Lowered SVR	<800 dyne/s/cm^{-5}	Shock, severe sepsis, overdose of drugs designed to reduce the afterload of the heart such as nitroprusside, hydralazine, and captopril[120]
Cardiac output (CO)	Calculated by multiplying the stroke volume (SV) by the heart rate (HR): CO = SV × HR	The stroke volume is the volume of blood ejected by the ventricle in a single contraction (heart beat). Stroke volume is determined by three interdependent variables: preload, afterload and myocardial contractility[96]
Pulmonary artery wedge pressure (PAWP)	Normal value 4–12 mmHg	PAWP provides an estimation of pulmonary venous and left atrial pressure. PAWP is monitored intermittently in critically ill patients to monitor left heart filling pressure and the intravascular volume[96]

tions when changes occur. When assessing the individual's haemodynamic stability, a key value is the person's pre-morbid status, e.g. their 'normal' blood pressure.[96] In order to make an assessment, the ITU nurse therefore needs to have access to the patient's pre-ITU records, including electrocardiogram (ECG) and cardiovascular records. It is then essential that all patients admitted to an ITU have baseline recordings of their cardiovascular status to allow a comparison should their parameters change. The following measurements are essential for all patients admitted to an ITU:

- Attachment to a cardiac monitor to facilitate the continuous recording of cardiac rate and rhythm.

- Arterial blood pressure (ABP), and mean arterial pressure (MAP) – in the critically ill patient this is measured directly via a cannula that has been introduced into an artery. The typical site would be into the radial artery or, failing this, the femoral artery. This cannula is then connected to a transducer and the cardiac monitor, providing a continuous record of the blood pressure and MAP, but also providing a route via a three-way tap to blood for arterial blood gas measurement for the assessment of oxygenation and acid–base balance.

- Central venous pressure (CVP) is monitored directly, utilizing the central venous catheter connected to a transducer and the cardiac monitor.

- A 12-lead ECG.

- Temperature – the gold standard for the critically ill is blood temperature measured via a pulmonary artery catheter (PAC); however, only a few cancer patients in the ITU will have a PAC, and temperature will therefore often be recorded, especially in those patients who are intubated, via a tympanic thermometer. This does, however, require care in its use to minimize error.[121]

The following cardiovascular assessments may be required where the patient's cardiovascular status is unstable, to titrate inotropic therapy, as an aid to diagnosis or to provide prognostic information:[120,122]

- Invasive cardiac monitoring, including cardiac output (CO) pulmonary artery pressure (PAP), pulmonary artery wedge pressure (PAWP) and systemic vascular resistance (SVR). These measurements are obtained either by using a direct method and introducing a catheter directly into the pulmonary artery, or by an indirect method using a derived calculation such as the lithium injection dilution cardiac output method (LIDCO) which utilizes the CVP and arterial cannula.[123] As the person with cancer in an ITU is exquisitely susceptible both to sepsis and bleeding, the insertion of a catheter directly into the pulmonary artery needs to be justified against the risk.[120,124,125]

In addition to the above measurements, further assessments of cardiovascular function may include the use of the following:

- X-ray and or CT scan to assess the heart size

- echocardiogram – to assess the function of the heart and vessels

- ultrasound to assess cardiac size and the presence of effusions

- specific blood tests to assess cardiac health – such as cardiac enzymes creatinine phosphokinase (CPK), CKMB and tropinin I.

THE POSTOPERATIVE CARE OF PEOPLE WITH CANCER IN THE INTENSIVE THERAPY UNIT

Within the constraints of this chapter, there is not space to describe in detail the postoperative nursing care undertaken in intensive care for people with cancer. It is important to recognize, however, that much of the care provided in the postoperative period is generic, and therefore the following sections will concentrate on the essentials for care in the postoperative period. Many people having surgery for cancer will not need to be admitted to an ITU; there are, however, certain operations that will commonly warrant admission to an ITU, and for some patients it will be their concomitant health problems, preoperative performance status or an unexpected event during surgery such as major blood loss or cardiac instability that necessitate their admission. Table 35.8 lists operations for cancer that commonly necessitate admission to an ITU with both medical and nursing references.

Table 35.8: Operations for cancer that commonly necessitate admission to an intensive therapy unit

Operation	Type of cancer/tumour	Relevant literature
Neurosurgical procedures	Primary brain tumour, spinal tumours	126–129
Complex major head and neck surgery	Squamous cell tumours of the face, tongue, oral cavity, eye, neck	130–135
Gastrointestinal surgery – oesophago-gastrectomy, pancreato-duodenectomy	Adenocarcinoma, squamous cell cancer	136–142
Cardiothoracic surgery and lung surgery	Small cell and large cell lung cancer, thymoma, melanoma or sarcoma affecting the heart	143–148
Complex major gynaeoncology surgery – pelvic exenteration, Wertheim's hysterectomy	Cancer of the cervix, uterus and gynaecological structures.	149–154
Complex major genitourinary surgery – pelvic clearance, reconstruction surgery such as Mitrofanoff	Bladder and urinary tree cancers, para-aortic lymph node dissections associated with teratoma	155–161
Complex major sarcoma, melanoma surgery – hind quarter amputations	Sarcoma and melanoma	162–167

Essential care following major surgery for cancer

Many people admitted to an ITU following complex major surgery will require mechanical support with their breathing, undergo periods of haemodynamic instability and sepsis and require care as outlined previously. Other key nursing care areas include assessment and management of pain and nausea, deep vein thrombosis prophylaxis and mobilization.

Pain assessment and management

People who are critically ill following major surgery for cancer experience moderate to severe pain for many reasons. Experience reveals that pain can be caused by the following, often in combination: the surgical incision itself; the therapeutic drainage tubes, particularly chest drains; and therapeutic interventions.[168,169] Pain assessment and therapy are integral to good care in the ITU and poor pain management has been shown to cause complications and hinder recovery.[170,171] A key principle of safe critical care is early mobilization. Patients are aided into their bedside chairs the day following even the most major surgery; it is therefore essential that the patient's pain is well-assessed and managed for humane reasons and also to ensure that the patient can achieve good compliance with chest physiotherapy and early mobilization.[172–174] Early mobilization and chest physiotherapy are essential to minimize the risks of respiratory deterioration and deep vein thrombosis (DVT).[175] Indeed, high pain scores have been shown to be significantly associated with a higher morbidity.[176]

Frequent pain assessment is essential and, if conscious, the patient should be a partner in this assessment. Before proceeding to pain assessment, it is important to note that many patients in the ITU will be unconscious through illness or sedation, and the practice of most clinicians in the ITU is to administer background analgesia, usually an opioid with a short half-life such as fentanyl, in a continuous infusion intravenously. This continuous infusion ensures that the patient who cannot communicate is not suffering pain and also that when awakening the patient's pain can be effectively managed.[177]

Pain assessment

To achieve a meaningful assessment of a patient's pain in any setting, it is important to recognize the multiple dimensions of pain:

- intensity
- distress
- quality
- behaviours
- analgesics.[169]

Puntillo et al's[169] research investigating the pain of adults in the ITU found that a heightened awareness of pain and distress associated with procedures such as turning, endotracheal suction and wound care were important in pain assessment. Other researchers have sought to identify preoperative predictors of those patients who will experience high levels of postoperative pain. Caumo et al, in 2002, found that moderate to intense acute postoperative pain was experienced by patients who had the following preoperative characteristics: ASA III, the presence of moderate to intense preoperative pain, chronic pain, high-trait anxiety and depressive moods.[178]

In the care of the critically ill patient, it may be that pain assessment is often focused on being aware of and looking for the behavioural signs of pain such as grimacing, rigidity, wincing, shutting eyes and frowning. Where patients can comply verbally with pain assessment, then questions about the intensity and quality of pain, both at rest and on movement, are important. A 10 cm visual analogue scale is thought to be the most appropriate and most easily used, or one of the dedicated tools developed for use in the ITU.[179-183] Having chosen a method of pain assessment, it is essential that this assessment is used regularly and is also used to evaluate the efficacy of pain management strategies.

Pain management

The goals for pain management in the critically ill person with cancer are to achieve comfort and facilitate weaning from ventilation, turning and positioning, compliance with chest physiotherapy and mobilization. It is important to remember that a percentage of patients in the cancer ITU will have been receiving large doses of opioids preoperatively and their opioid needs postoperatively may therefore be higher. Many patients in the ITU are unable to use medications via the enteral route and the intravenous or epidural route is therefore preferred. However, where the patient's bowel function has recovered, analgesia or co-analgesia can be administered via a nasogastric or percutaneous enterogastromy tube.

Where the patient has undergone major intra-abdominal, intrapelvic or lower limb surgery, the gold standard pain strategy is to use a combination of opioid and local anaesthetic such as fentanyl and bupivacaine 1% via an epidural catheter.[172,174,175,184,185] There are also several studies showing an advantage in using patient-controlled epidural analgesia (PCEA).[186-188] The advantages of using the epidural route are effective pain management with fewer side-effects such as reduced gastric motility, nausea and vomiting and sedation, especially when the epidural catheter is located in the appropriate spinal segment to ensure optimum pain control.[189] There are, however, disadvantages, including the risk of infection, malplacement of the catheter and inadequate pain control, and the rare risk of an epidural haematoma.[190] It is also important to recognize that some patients with cancer who undergo major surgery cannot have an epidural catheter inserted, e.g. those who have had previous spinal surgery or have spinal disease, or patients with changes in clotting such as individuals with chronic lymphocytic leukaemia undergoing a splenectomy.

Other commonly used routes for analgesic therapy in the ITU are a continuous opioid infusion such as morphine or fentanyl intravenously, or a patient-controlled analgesia (PCA) intravenous infusion of an opioid. While in the ITU, the patient's respiratory, cardiovascular and sedation status can be closely monitored and the dangers of respiratory depression or sedation avoided. PCA with a background infusion is therefore safe in this setting.

Deep vein thrombosis prophylaxis

Deep vein thrombosis and pulmonary embolus (PE) are major causes of morbidity, with PE carrying a 3-month mortality rate found to be as high as 17%.[191,192] Surgery, cancer and immobility are three of the main causes of DVT, and therefore PE awareness and effective prophylaxis are an important part of the intensive care management of all patients with cancer.[193–195] It should also be noted that long-term catheter use in the patient with cancer carries a risk variously reported between 2 and 40% of thromboembolic complications.[196,197] As more people with cancer receive multimodality treatment, the likelihood of cancer patients in the ITU having several of these risk factors is increased, e.g. patients with gynaecological and upper gastrointestinal cancer with long-term venous access devices undergoing complex major surgery.[198]

The three key components of care are the use of prophylactic anticoagulant, graduated compression stockings (TEDs) or intermittent compression devices and early mobilization. In high-risk patients, such as the patient with cancer with several risk factors, a combination of these preventative measures has been shown to be effective in minimizing the incidence of DVT and PE.[199–201]

Anticoagulant prophylaxis has improved over the last 10 years, with the development of the low molecular weight heparins (LMWHs). Several studies have illustrated improved patient outcomes with the routine prophylactic use of LMWHs, with reduced incidence of thrombosis and no increase in bleeding.[202–205] LMWHs are administered subcutaneously and, together with intermittent compression devices, have been well tolerated by cancer patients.[206]

Postoperative nausea and vomiting

The incidence of postoperative nausea and vomiting (PONV) remains high in all patients recovering from surgery, with figures quoted between 20 and 30%.[207–209] PONV is a serious complication of surgery, as it completely alters the patient's postoperative comfort, and can also lead to serious physical deterioration as the result of aspiration, fluid and electrolyte imbalance, dehydration, loss of integrity of surgical wounds and problems with mobilization. As with pain assessment, it is important that the nurse caring for the person who has undergone cancer surgery is aware of the pre-, peri- and postoperative risk factors for PONV.[208,209,210–213]

Preoperative risks

- Age – adults >55 years old.
- Gender – women before the menopause are 2–3 times more likely than men; after the menopause, equivalent incidence with men
- Weight – obesity increases likelihood of PONV.
- Stomach contents – adequate preoperative fasting reduces the risk, whereas starvation increases the risk. In emergency surgery, where elective fasting is impossible, the risk is increased.
- Previous history of PONV.
- Previous experience of motion sickness.

Perioperative risks

- Laparascopic surgery – abdominal distension (due to instillation of carbon dioxide).
- Middle ear, ophthalmic and otolaryngology surgery.
- Longer surgery – related to longer period of anaesthesia.[214,215]

Postoperative risks

- Pain.
- Hypotension.
- Opioid analgesia.
- Mobilization – early mobilization is associated with a greater risk.
- Start of oral/enteral intake.

The management of postoperative nausea and vomiting

The management of PONV should be centred on a multimodal approach to reducing risk factors. Various authors/institutions have designed guidelines to ensure this comprehensive approach to the management of PONV.[216–219] The efficacy of using a risk assessment model and targeting therapy for high-risk groups has also been demonstrated.[220,221]

Key factors in the effective management of PONV are:

- pre- and postoperative fluid hydration
- effective relief of pain
- pre- and postoperative strategies for the relief of anxiety such as education, relaxation techniques, distraction, therapeutic touch and acupressure
- planned pharmacological interventions using one of the 5-HT$_3$ (5-hydroxytryptamine type 3) antagonists plus or minus another co-antiemetic such as the steroid dexamethasone, depending on the patient's risk factor profile.[218–220,222–225]

Finally, there are a small percentage of patients who despite careful assessment and multi-modality therapy still experience severe and prolonged nausea. It is the author's experience that much can be gained from the involvement of the palliative care team, who have a wealth of experience in symptom management and a definite place in the multidisciplinary care of the critically ill cancer patient.

END OF LIFE CARE IN THE INTENSIVE THERAPY UNIT

Even if the correct decisions are made regarding admission to the ITU, it is inevitable that deaths will occur. The mortality rate for cancer patients being admitted to an ITU depends largely on the disease, generally being much higher in the haemato-oncology population than in the postoperative solid tumour population. With mortality rates as high as 60–85% in haemato-oncology patients, it is imperative that end of life care in an ITU is a collaborative and caring process. All members of the multidisciplinary team need to feel as though they are part of the decision-making process.[226] When decisions such as withdrawal of treatment or Not For attempted Resuscitation (NFaR) are being discussed it is imperative that nurses feel they can initiate or become part of such discussions. If the patient is conscious, it may be possible to involve them in these discussions, but this must be assessed and managed by nurses or doctors who are experienced in this aspect of care.[227]

For the family of a patient in the ITU, the fear and dread associated with sitting day by day and watching a loved one cannot be overemphasized. Qualitative research and the experience of clinical staff in the ITU demonstrate that one of the most essential aspects of the relationship between clinical staff and the family is the building of trust. It is therefore essential that from the very beginning of this relationship frequent update and information meetings take place. During these conversations nurses need to work very hard at truth-telling; it takes experience and courage to be clear and honest when a family are desperate for you to provide good news. It is the author's experience that a family need to have hope, but that this can coexist with truthful conversations about the severity of an illness and the possibility of death. It is essential that the nurse in the ITU develops a sense of presence and a therapeutic relationship with patients and their families. Families can also derive much comfort and pleasure from the ordinariness of human interaction with the team on the ITU, enjoying a humorous banter or hearing about the nurse's family, social occasions or study.[228]

If a patient's condition is deteriorating or not improving despite maximum support, the ITU team may need to discuss either withdrawal of care or a NFaR decision. For the family and the clinical team, this decision will be much easier to embrace if there is a truthful and collaborative collegiate culture on a ITU. For the family, decisions such as these should never come as a shock but should always be part of a communication continuum. Although the distress and pain are not lessened, the family are already partners in the decision-making. A change in the rationale for care from curative to palliative does not mean a lack of care but a change in emphasis for patient, family and staff. It is absolutely imperative that this end of life care is of the highest standard using evidence-based care in terms of symptom management and any therapy used.[226,229–231] Individual families will have different wishes regarding their presence, the support/presence of religious leaders and the amount/type of information that they wish to receive. The experienced nurse will ensure that these areas are discussed, so that the patients' and families' wishes are known and respected as much as is possible.

An important adjunct to any clinical team on an ITU is the palliative care team; this is perhaps especially so in the cancer ITU. Doctors and nurses from the palliative care team have much knowledge and skill that is useful for the total care of the ITU patient, both during their acute care and towards the end of life.[232,233] The importance of the other members of the multidisciplinary team should always be recognized and nursing leadership should develop everyone's awareness of the vital roles that each discipline gives to the care of the person with cancer in the ITU.

CONCLUSION

As people with cancer live longer and undergo major multimodality therapy for their disease, there will be a continued need for admissions to ICUs. Nurses have a unique role in shaping the patient and their family's experience in the ITU. It is important to remember that people with cancer may make repeated visits to an ITU, requiring repeated complex major surgery for recurrence, or as another episode of sepsis develops following chemotherapy. It is therefore essential that practice is aimed not only at cure but also at care in an ITU. Cancer care adds another dimension to intensive care, requiring nurses to expand their knowledge and skills in diverse areas ranging from haematological toxicities to complex pain management. It also requires a different approach to care with cancer patients and their families being increasingly knowledgeable about their condition and presenting a challenge for the nurse who is unfamiliar with the rigors of chemotherapy, or the daily request for information about the neutrophil or platelet count. It is essential therefore that those of us who

work in intensive care open our doors and welcome the multidisciplinary teams who work daily with cancer patients. Caring for people with cancer who are critically ill is a complex challenge and it is essential to work in partnership with the referring cancer teams, pain management teams, microbiologists, palliative care teams and the specialist nurses who have often developed a relationship with the patient. As different teams work in partnership, they will learn from each other and as professional silos and barriers are traversed, truly person-centred cancer care may be achieved in the ICU.

Acknowledgement

I would like to thank Natalie Pattison for help with the literature search.

REFERENCES

1. Kaplow R. Special nursing considerations. Crit Care Clin 2001; 17(3):769–789.
2. Hillman K. Critical care without walls. Curr Opin Crit Care 2002; 8(6):594–599.
3. Goldhill D, McGinley A. Outreach critical care. Anaesthesia 2002; 57(2):183, 833–834.
4. Department of Health. Comprehensive critical care: a review of adult critical care services. London: Department of Health; 2000.
5. Leary T, Ridley S. Impact of an outreach team on re-admissions to a critical care unit. Anaesthesia 2003; 58(4):328–332.
6. Pittard A. Out of our reach? Assessing the impact of introducing a critical care outreach service. Anaesthesia 2003; 58(9):882–885.
7. Jones C, Humphris G, Griffiths R. Psychological morbidity following critical illness – the rationale for care after intensive care. Clin Intensive Care 1998; 9(5):199–205.
8. Waldmann C. Setting up a doctor-led clinic. In: Griffiths R, Jones C, eds. Intensive care aftercare. Oxford: Butterworth-Heinemann; 2002.
9. Griffiths R, Jones C, eds. Intensive care aftercare. Oxford: Butterworth-Heinemann; 2002.
10. Williamson EC, Millar MR, Steward CG, et al. Infections in adults undergoing unrelated donor bone marrow transplantation. Br J Haematol 1999; 104(3):560–568.
11. Bone RC, Grodzin CJ, Balk RA. Sepsis: a new hypothesis for pathogenesis of the disease process. Chest 1997; 112(1):235–243.
12. Sands KE, Bates DW, Lanken PN, et al. Epidemiology of sepsis syndrome in 8 academic medical centers. JAMA 1997; 278(3):234–240.
13. Edbrooke DL, Hibbert CL, Kingsley JM, et al. The patient-related costs of care for sepsis

patients in a United Kingdom adult general intensive care unit. Crit Care Med 1999; 27(9):1760–1767.

14. Rangel-Frausto MS, Pittet D, Costigan M, et al. The natural history of the systemic inflammatory response syndrome (SIRS). A prospective study, JAMA 1995; 273:117–123.

15. Pittet D, Wenzel RP. Nosocomial blood stream infections. Secular trends in rates, mortality and contribution to total hospital deaths. Arch Intern Med 1995; 155:1177–1184.

16. Friedman G, Silva E, Vincent JL. Has the mortality of septic shock changes with time? Crit Care Med 1998; 26:2078–2086.

17. Linde-Zwirble WT, Angus DC, Carcillo J, et al. Age-specific incidence and outcome of sepsis in the US. Crit Care Med 1999; 27(Suppl 1):A33.

18. Angus DC, Linde-Zwirble WT, Lidicker J, et al. Epidemiology of severe sepsis in the United States: analysis of incidence, outcome, and associated costs of care. Crit Care Med 2001; 29:1303–1310.

19. Bernard GR, Vincent JL, Laterre PF. Efficacy and safety of recombinant human activated protein C for severe sepsis. N Engl J Med 2001; 344(10):699–708.

20. Goldfrad C, Padkin AJ, Young JD. Admissions with severe sepsis: ICU and hospital resource use in England, Wales and Northern Ireland. Intensive Care Med 2001; 27(Suppl 2):S252.

21. Padkin A, Rowan K, Black N. Using high quality clinical databases to complement the results of randomised controlled trials: the case of recombinant human activated protein C. BMJ 2001; 323(7318):923–926.

22. Young JD, Goldfrad C, Padkin AJ. Hospital mortality for ICU admissions with severe sepsis in England, Wales and Northern Ireland. Intensive Care Med 2001; 27 (Suppl 2):S242.

23. Groeger JS. Critical care of the cancer patient. St. Louis: Mosby Year Book; 1991.

24. Chernecky CC, Berger BJ. Advanced and critical care oncology nursing. Philadelphia: WB Saunders; 1998.

25. American College of Chest Physicians/Society of Critical Care Medicine Consensus Conference. Definitions for sepsis and multiple organ failure, and guidelines for the use of innovative therapies in sepsis. Crit Care Med 1992; 20:864–874.

26. Bellingan G. Inflammatory cell activation in sepsis. Br Med Bull 1999; 55(1):12–29.

27. Levi M, Ten Cate H, Vand der Poll T, et al. Pathogenesis of disseminated intravascular coagulation in sepsis. JAMA 1993; 270(8):975–979.

28. Kidokoro A, Iba T, Fukunaga M, et al Alterations in coagulation and fibrinolysis during sepsis. Shock 1996; 5(3):223–228.

29. Gando S, Nanzaki S, Sasaki S, et al. Activation of the extrinsic coagulation pathway in patients with severe sepsis and septic shock. Crit Care Med 1998; 26(12):2005–2009.

30. Vervloet MG, Thijs LG, Hack CE. Derangements of coagulation and fibrinolysis in critically ill patients with sepsis and septic shock. Semin Thromb Hemost 1998; 24(1):33–44.

31. Esmon C. The protein C pathway. Crit Care Med 2000; 28(Suppl):S44–48.

32. Cohen J, Abraham E. Microbiologic findings and correlations with serum tumour necrosis factor-alpha in patients with severe sepsis and septic shock. J Infect Dis 1999; 180:116–121.

33. Bernard GR, Wheeler AP, Russell JA. The effects of ibuprofen on the physiology and survival of patients with sepsis. N Engl J Med 1997; 336:912–918.

34. Opal SM, Cohen J. Clinical gram-positive sepsis: does it fundamentally differ from gram-negative bacterial sepsis? Crit Care Med 1999; 27(8):1608–1616.

35. Brun-Buisson C, Doyon F, Carlet J. Incidence, risk factors, and outcome of severe sepsis and septic shock in adults. JAMA 1995; 274:968–974.

36. Morrison DC, Ryan JL. Endotoxins and disease mechanisms. Ann Rev Med 1987; 38:417–432.

37. Noursadeghi M, Cohen J. Immunopathogenesis of severe sepsis. J R Coll Physicians Lond 2000; 34(5):432–436.

38. Warren HS. Understanding sepsis: new findings, new theories. 37th Annual Meeting of the Infectious Disease Society of America; 1999:18–21.

39. Rosen MJ, Clayton K, Schneider RF, et al. Intensive care of patients with HIV infection: utilisation, critical illnesses, and outcomes. Pulmonary Complications of HIV Infection Study Group, Am J Respir Crit Care Med 1997; 155(1):67–71.

40. Ewig S, Paar WD, Pakos E, et al. [Nosocomial ventilator-associated pneumonias caused by *Aspergillus fumigatus* in non-immunosuppressed, non-neutropenic patients.] Pneumologie 1998; 52(2):85–90. [in German]

41. House of Lords Select Committee on Science and Technology. Resistance to antibiotics and other antimicrobial agents. HL 7th report session. London: HMSO; 1998:paper 81-1, 56.

42. Zeni F, Freeman B, Natanson C. Anti-inflammatory therapies to treat sepsis and septic shock: a reassessment. Crit Care Med 1997; 25(7):1095–1100.

43. Abraham E, Anzueto A, Gutierrez G, et al. Double-blind randomised controlled trial of monoclonal antibody to human tumour necrosis factor in treatment of septic shock. Lancet 1998; 351:929–933.

44. Van Den Berghe G. Beyond diabetes: saving lives with insulin in the ICU. Int J Obes Relat Metab Disord 2002; 26(Suppl 3):S3–8.

45. Levi M, Cate HT. Disseminated intravascular coagulation. N Engl J Med 1999; 341(8):586–592.

46. Stephan F, Hollande J, Richard O, et al. Thrombocytopenia in a surgical ICU, Chest 1999; 115(5):1363–1370.

47. Bick RL. Syndromes of disseminated intravascular coagulation in obstetrics, pregnancy, and gynaecology. Haematol Oncol Clin N Am 2000; 14(5):999–1045.

48. Dolan S. Haemorrhagic problems. In: Grundy M, ed. Nursing in haematological oncology. London: Baillière Tindall; 2000:201–210.

49. Rocha E, Paramo JA, Montes R, Panizo C. Acute generalized, widespread bleeding. Diagnosis and management. Haematologica 1998; 83:1024–1037.

50. Levi M, de Jonge E. Current management of disseminated intravascular coagulation; 2000. www.hosppract.com/issues/2000/08/celevi.htm

51. Baglin T. Disseminated intravascular coagulation: diagnosis and treatment. BMJ 1996; 312:683–687.

52. Marder VJ, Feinstein DI, Francis CW, et al. Consumptive thrombohemorrhagic disorders. In: Colman RW, Hirsh J, Marder VJ, Salzman EW, eds. Hemostasis and thrombosis: basic principles and clinical practice. 3rd edn. Philadelphia: Lippincott; 1994:1023–1063.

53. Bick RL. Disseminated intravascular coagulation. Objective criteria for diagnosis and management. Med Clin N Am 1994; 78:511–543.

54. Okajima K, Imamura H, Koga S, et al. Treatment of patients with disseminated intravascular coagulation by protein C. Am J Hematol 1990; 33:277–278.

55. Gerson WT, Dickerman JD, Bowill EG, et al. Severe acquired protein C deficiency in purpura fulminans associated with disseminated intravascular coagulation: treatment with protein C concentrate. Pediatrics 1993; 91:418–422.

56. Paloma MJ, Paramo JA, Rocha E. Endotoxin-induced intravascular coagulation in rabbits: effect of tissue plasminogen activator vs. urokinase on PAI generation, fibrin deposits, and mortality. Thromb Haemost 1995; 74:1578–1582.

57. Bennett JM, Catovsky D, Daniel MT, et al. A variant form of hypergranular promyelocytic leukaemia (M3). Br J Haematol 1980; 44:169–170.

58. Bassan R, Battista R, Viero P, et al. Short-term treatment for adult hypergranular and microgranular acute promyelocytic leukaemia. Leukaemia 1995; 9:238.

59. Warrell RP, de The H, Wang Z-Y, et al. Acute promyelocytic leukaemia. N Engl J Med 1993; 329:177–181.

60. Fenaux P, Le Deley MC, Catsaigne S, et al. Effect of all-trans retinoic acid in newly diagnosed acute promyelocytic leukaemia. Results of a multicenter leukaemia trial. Blood 1993; 82:3241–3249.

61. Grignani F, Fagioli M, Alcalay M, et al. Acute promyelocytic leukaemia from genetics to treatment. Blood 1994; 83:10–25.

62. Barbui T, Finazzi G, Falanga A. The impact of all-trans-retinoic acid on the coagulopathy of acutepromyelocytic leukaemia. Blood 1998; 91(9):3093–3102.

63. Higuchi T, Shimizu T, Mori H, et al. Coagulation patterns of disseminated intravascular coagulation in acute promyelocytic leukaemia. Haematol Oncol 1997; 15:209–217.

64. Hilbert G, Gruson D, Vargas F, et al. Noninvasive ventilation in immunosuppressed patients with pulmonary infiltrates, fever and acute respiratory failure. N Engl J Med 2001; 344(7):481–487.

65. Ripamonti C, Fusco F. Respiratory problems in advanced cancer. Support Care Cancer 2002; 10:204–216.

66. Hicks KL, Chemaly RF, Kontoyiannis DP. Common community respiratory viruses in patients with cancer: more than just "common colds". Cancer 2003; 97(10):2576–2587.

67. Jean-Baptiste E. Clinical assessment and management of massive hemoptysis. Crit Care Med 2000; 28:1642–1647.

68. Lipchik RJ. Hemoptysis. In: Berger AM, Portenoy RK, Weissman DE, eds. Principles and practice of supportive oncology, Vol. 24. Philadelphia: Lippincott-Raven; 1998:309–314.

69. Coliche GL. Hemoptysis. Three questions that can direct management. Postgrad Med 1996; 100:227–236.

70. Cahill BC, Ingbar DH. Massive hemoptysis: assessment and management. Clin Chest Med 1994; 15:147–130.

71. Corey R, Hla KM. Major and massive hemoptysis: reassessment of conservative management. Am J Med Sci 1987; 294:301–309.

72. Kirch C, Blot F, Fizazi K, et al Acute respiratory distress syndrome after chemotherapy for lung metastases from non-seminomatous germ-cell tumours. Support Care Cancer 2003; 11:575–580.

73. Read WL, Mortimer JE, Picus J. Severe interstitial pneumonia associated with docetaxel administration. Cancer 2002; 94(3):847–853.

74. Kouroukis C, Hings I. Respiratory failure following vinorelbine tartrate infusion in a patient with non-small cell lung cancer. Chest 1997; 112(3):846–848.

75. Fujita J, Bandoh S, Ohtsuki Y, et al The role of anti-epithelial cell antibodies in the pathogenesis of bilateral radiation pneumonitis caused by unilateral thoracic irradiation. Respir Med 2000; 94(9):875–880.

76. Mah K, Van Dyk J, Keane T, Poon PY. Acute radiation-induced pulmonary damage: a clinical study on the response to fractionated radiation therapy. Int J Radiat Oncol Biol Phys 1987; 13(2):179–188.

77. Hagry O, Coosemans W, De Leyn P. Effects of preoperative chemoradiotherapy on postsurgical morbidity and mortality in cT3-4 +/− cM1 lymph cancer of the oesophagus and gastro-oesophageal junction. Eur J Cardiothorac Surg 2003; 24(2):179–186; discussion 186.

78. Kumar P, Goldstraw P, Yamada K. Pulmonary fibrosis and lung cancer: risk and benefit analysis of pulmonary resection. J Thorac Cardiovasc Surg 2003; 125(6):1321–1327.

79. Yazar S, Eser B, Yalcin S, Sahin I. A case of pulmonary microsporidiasis in an acute myeloblastic leukemia (AML) -M3 patient. Yonsei Med J 2003; 44(1):146–149.

80. Sabria-Trias J, Bonnaud F, Sioniac M. Severe interstitial pneumonitis related to gemcitabine. Review des Maladie Respiratoires 2002; 19(5 Pt 1):645–647.

81. Mannaerts GH, Van Zundert AA, Meeusen VC. Anaesthesia for advanced rectal cancer patients treated with combined major resections and intraoperative radiotherapy. Eur J Anaesthesiol 2002; 19(10):742–748.

82. Stamatis G, Djuric D, Eberhardt W. Postoperative morbidity and mortality after induction chemoradiotherapy for locally advanced lung cancer: an analysis of 350 operated patients. Eur J Cardiothorac Surg 2002; 22(2):292–297.

83. Murata K, Kubota T. Impairment of chest wall mechanics and increased chest wall work of breathing cause postoperative respiratory failure in patients who have undergone radical esophagectomy. J Anesthesia 2001; 15:125–131.

84. Nomori H, Horio H, Suemasu K. Assisted pressure control ventilation via a mini-tracheostomy tube for postoperative respiratory management of lung cancer patients. Respir Med 2000; 94:214–220.

85. Roberts JR, Eustis C, Devore R, et al Induction chemotherapy increases perioperative complications in patients undergoing resection for non-small cell lung cancer. Ann Thorac Surg 2001; 72(3):885–888.

86. Yamaura K, Higashi M, Akiyoshi K, et al. Pulmonary lipiodol embolism during transcatheter arterial chemoembolization for hepatoblastoma under general anaesthesia. Eur J Anaesthesiol 2000;, 17(11):704–708.

87. Koskinas J, Betrosian A, Kafiri G, et al Combined hepatocellular-cholangiocarcinoma presented with massive pulmonary embolism. Hepatogastroenterology 2000; 47(34):1125–1128.

88. Schenk JF, Berg G, Morsdorf S, et al. Heparin-induced thrombocytopenia: a critical risk/benefit analysis of patients in intensive care treated with R-hirudin. Clin Appl Thromb Hemost 2000; 6 (3):151–156.

89. Meyer G, Sanchez O. Acute circulatory failure caused by primary pulmonary hypertension or pulmonary embolism. Review des Maladies Respiratoires 2000; 17(1):51–65.

90. Papadakis MA, Mangione CM, Lee KK, et al. Treatable abdominal pathologic conditions and unsuspected malignant neoplasms at autopsy in veterans who received mechanical ventilation. JAMA 1991; 265(7):885–887.

91. Vallot F, Paesmans M, Berghmans T, et al Leucopenia is an independent predictor in cancer patients requiring invasive mechanical ventilation: a prognostic factor analysis in a series of 168 patients. Support Care Cancer 2003; 11:236–241.

92. Basheer Y, Khassawneh MD, White P, et al. Outcome from mechanical ventilation after autologous peripheral blood stem cell transplantation. Chest 2002; 121(1):185–188.

93. Azoulay E, Alberti C, Bornstain C, et al. Improved survival in cancer patients requiring mechanical ventilatory support: impact of non-invasive mechanical ventilatory support. Crit Care Med 2001; 29(3):519–525.

94. Azoulay E, Moreau D, Alberti C, et al. Predictors of short-term mortality in critically ill patients with solid malignancies. Intensive Care Med 2000; 26:1817–1823.

95. Kongskaard UE, Meidell NK. Mechanical ventilation in critically ill cancer patients: outcome and utilisation of resources. Support Care Cancer 1999; 7:95–99.

96. Hinds CJ, Watson D. Intensive care: a concise textbook. London: WB Saunders; 1999.

97. Kiehl M, Schiele C, Stenzinger W. Volume-controlled versus biphasic positive airway pressure ventilation in leukopenic patients with severe respiratory failure. Crit Care Med 1996; 24(5):780–784.

98. Patel A, Randhawa N, Semenov RA. Transtracheal high-frequency jet ventilation and iatrogenic injury. Br J Anaesthesia 2001; 87(6):870–875.

99. Ong EL. A case of pulmonary haemorrhage following jet ventilation for vocal cord surgery. Ann Acad Med Singapore 2002; 31(4):531–534.

100. MacIntyre NR. High-frequency jet ventilation. Respir Care Clin N Am 2001; 7(4):599–610.

101. Wright J, Doyle P, Yoshihara G. Mechanical ventilation: current uses and advances. In: Clochesy JM, Breu C, et al, eds. Critical care nursing. 2nd edn. Philadelphia: WB Saunders; 1996:262–288.

102. Ram F, Picot J, Lightowler J, Wedzicha J. Non-invasive positive pressure ventilation for treatment of respiratory failure due to exacerbations of chronic obstructive pulmonary disease. Cochrane Database Syst Rev 2004; 3:CD004104.

103. Meert AP, Close L, Berghmans T. Noninvasive ventilation: application to the cancer patient admitted to the intensive care unit. Support Care Cancer 2003; 11:56–59.

104. Crocker C. Nurse-led weaning from ventilatory and respiratory support. Intensive Crit Care Nurs 2002; 18(5):272–279.

105. Price AM. Nurse-led weaning from mechanical ventilation: where's the evidence? Intensive Crit Care Nurs 2001; 17(3):167–176.

106. Hande KR, Garrow GC. Acute tumour lysis syndrome in patients with high-grade non-Hodgkin's lymphoma. Am J Med 1993; 94(2):133–139.

107. Kalemkerian GP, Darwish B, Varterasian ML. Tumour lysis syndrome in small cell carcinoma and other solid tumours. Am J Med 1997; 103(5):363–367.

108. Robison J. Tumour lysis syndrome. In: Chernecky CC, Berger BJ, eds. Advanced and critical care oncology nursing: managing primary complications. Philadelphia: WB Saunders; 1998:637–659.

109. Akasheh MS, Chang CP, Vesole DH. Acute tumour lysis syndrome: a case in AL amyloidosis. Br J Haematol 1999; 107(2):386–387.

110. Fassas ABT, Desikan KR, Siegel D, et al. Tumour lysis syndrome complicating high-dose treatment in patients with multiple myeloma. Br J Haematol 1999; 105(4–11):938–941.

111. Tiley C, Grimwade D, Findlay M, et al. Tumour lysis following hydrocortisone prior to a blood product transfusion in T-cell acute lymphoblastic leukaemia. Leuk Lymphoma 1992; 8(1–2):143–146.

112. Lerza R, Botta M, Barsotti B, et al. Dexamethazone-induced acute tumor lysis syndrome in a T-cell malignant lymphoma. Leuk Lymphoma 2002; 43(5):1129–1132.

113. Yang SS, Chau T, Dai MS, Lin SH. Steroid-induced tumor lysis syndrome in a patient with preleukemia. Clin Nephrol 2003; 59(3):201–205.

114. O'Regan S, Carson S, Chesney RW, Drummond KN. Electrolyte and acid–base disturbances in the management of leukaemia. Blood 1977; 49:345–353.

115. Mahmoud HH, Leverger G. Patte C, Harvey E, Lascombes F. Advances in the management of malignancy-associated hyperuricaemia. Br J Cancer 1998; 77(4):18–20.

116. Larson RA, Daley GQ, Schiffer CA. Treatment by design in leukaemia, a meeting report. Philadelphia, Pennsylvania, December 2002. Leukemia 2002; 17(12):2358–2382.

117. Holdsworth MT, Nguyen P. Role of i.v. allopurinol and rasburicase in tumor lysis syndrome. Am J Health Syst Pharm 2003; 60 (21):2213–2222 .

118. Coiffier B, Mounier N, Bologna S, et al Efficacy and safety of rasburicase (recombinant urate oxidase) for the prevention and treatment of hyperuricemia during induction chemotherapy of aggressive non-Hodgkin's lymphoma: results of the GRAAL1 (Groupe d'Etude des Lymphomes de l'Adulte Trial on Rasburicase Activity in Adult Lymphoma) study. J Clin Oncol 2003; 21(23):4402–4406.

119. Bosly A, Sonet A, Pinkerton CR. Rasburicase (recombinant urate oxidase) for the management of hyperuricemia in patients with cancer: report of an international compassionate use study. Cancer 2003; 98(5):1048–1054.

120. Miller LR. Hemodynamic monitoring. In: Clochesy JM, Breu C, Cardin S, Whittaker AA, Rudy EB, eds. Critical care nursing. 2nd edn. Philadelphia: WB Saunders; 1996.

121. Giuliano KK, Scott SS, Elliot S, Giuliano AJ. Temperature measurement in critically ill orally intubated adults: a comparison of pulmonary artery core, tympanic, and oral methods. Crit Care Med 2001; 27(10):2188–2193.

122. Bridges EJ, Woods SL. Pulmonary artery pressure measurements: state of the art. Heart Lung 1993; 22:99–111.

123. Jonas MM, Tanser SJ. Lithium dilution measurement of cardiac output and arterial pulse waveform analysis: an indicator dilution calibrated beat-by-beat system for continuous estimation of cardiac output. Curr Opin Crit Care 2002; 8(3):257–261.

124. Sakka SG, Reinhart K, Wegscheider K, Meier-Hellmann A. Is the placement of a pulmonary artery catheter still justified solely for the measurement of cardiac output? J Cardiothorac Vasc Anesthiol 2000; 14(2):119–124.

125. Chen YY, Yen DH, Yang YG. Comparison between replacement at 4 days and 7 days of the infection rate for pulmonary artery catheters in an intensive care unit. Crit Care Med 2003; 31(5):1353–1358.

126. Martin AJ, Fisher C, Igbaseimokumo U, et al. Solitary fibrous tumours of the meninges: case series and literature review. J Neuro-Oncol 2001; 54(1):57–69.

127. Quinn JA, DeAngelis M. Neurologic emergencies in the cancer patient. Semin Oncol 2000; 27(3):311–321.

128. McKinley, BA. Parmley, CL, Tonneson, AS. Standardised Management of Intracranial Pressure: A Preliminary Clinical Trial, Trauma 1999, 46 (2), 271–279.

129. Guerrero D, ed. Neuro-oncology for nurses. London: Whurr Publishers; 1998.

130. Vural E. Surgical reconstruction in patients with cancer of the head and neck. Curr Oncol Rep 2004; 6(2):133–140.

131. Tomicic J, Wanebo HJ. Mucosal melanomas. Surg Clin N Am 2003; 83(2):237–252.

132. Urken ML. Advances in head and neck reconstruction. Laryngoscope 2003; 113(9):1473–1476.

133. Strome SE, Weinman EC. Advanced larynx cancer. Curr Trea Options Oncol 2002; 3(1):11–20.

134. Orgill R, Krempl GA, Medina JE. Acute pain management following laryngectomy. Arch Otolaryngol Head Neck Surg 2002; 128(7):829–832.

135. Downey RJ, Friedlander P, Groeger J. Critical care for the severely ill head and neck patient. Crit Care Med 1999; 27(1):95–97.

136. Varadarajulu S, Wallace MB. Applications of endoscopic ultrasonography in pancreatic cancer. Cancer Control 2004; 11(1):15–22.

137. Neal JM, Wilcox RT, Allen HW. Near-total esophagectomy: the influence of standardised multimodel management and intraoperative fluid restriction. Reg Anesth Pain Med 2003; 28(4):328–334.

138. Lin JW, Leach SD. Current treatment of gastric cancer: is adjuvant therapy of benefit? Adv Surg 2003; 37:95–121.

139. Rullier E, Laurent C. Advances in surgical treatment of rectal cancer. Minerva Chirurgica 2003; 58(4):459–457.

140. Fong Y. Hepatic colorectal metastasis: current surgical therapy, selection criteria for hepatectomy, and role for adjuvant therapy. Adv Surg 2000; 34:351–381.

141. Guillem JG, Cohen AM. Treatment options for mid- and low-rectal cancers. Adv Surg 2000; 34:43–66.

142. Siewert JR, Sendler A. The current management of gastric cancer. Adv Surg 1999; 33:69–93.

143. Lee LS, Singhal S, Brinster CJ, et al. Current management of esophageal leiomyoma. J Am Coll Surg 2004; 198(1):136–146.

144. Birim O, Zuydendorp HM, Maat AP, et al. Lung resection for non-small-cell lung cancer in patients older than 70: mortality, morbidity, and late survival compared with the general population. Ann Thorac Surg 2003; 76(6):1796–1801.

145. Ghosh S, Sujendran V, Alexiou C, Beggs L, Beggs D. Long term results of surgery versus continuous hyperfractionated accelerated radiotherapy (CHART) in patients aged >70 years with stage 1 non-small cell lung cancer. Eur J Cardiothorac Surg 2003; 24(6):1002–1007.

146. Margolis M, Alexander P, Trachiotis GD. Percutaneous endoscopic gastrostomy before multimodality therapy in patients with esophageal cancer. Ann Thorac Surg 2003; 76(5):1694–1697

147. Reed CE, Harpole DH, Posther KE. Results of the American College of Surgeons Oncology Group Z0050 trial: the utility of positron emission tomography in staging potentially operable non-small cell lung cancer. J Thorac Cardiovasc Surg 2003; 126(6):1943–1951.

148. Patel NA, Keenan RJ, Medich DS, et al. The presence of colorectal hepatic metastases does not preclude pulmonary metastasectomy. Am Surg 2003; 69(12):1047–53; discussion 1053.

149. Goldberg JM, Piver MS, Hempling RE. Improvements in pelvic exenteration: factors responsible for reducing morbidity and mortality. Ann Surg Oncol 1998; 5(5):399–406.

150. Cirese E, Larciprete G. Emergency pelvic packing to control intraoperative bleeding after a Piver type-3 procedure. An unusual way to control gynaecological hemorrhage. Eur J Gynaecol Oncol 2003; 24(1):99–100.

151. Querleu D, Leblanc E. Laparoscopic surgery for gynaecological oncology. Curr Opin Obstet Gynecol 2003; 15(4):309–314.

152. Ryan M, Stainton MC, Jaconelli C. The experience of lower limb lymphedema for women after treatment for gynecologic cancer. Oncol Nurs Forum 2003; 30(3):417–423.

153. Wong L, Rao S, Barton DP. Transvaginal tamponade for intra-operative pelvic haemorrhage in gynaecological oncology patients. Br J Obstet Gynaecol 2003; 110(7):707–709.

154. Mirhashemi R, Janicek MF, Schoell WM. Critical care issues in cervical cancer management. Semin Surg Oncol 1999; 16(3):267–274.

155. Harris MJ. Radical perineal prostatectomy: cost efficient, outcome effective, minimally invasive prostate cancer management. Eur Urol 2003; 44(3):303–308.

156. Chung SY, Meldrum K, Docimo SG. Laparoscopic assisted reconstructive surgery: a 7-year experience. J Urol 2004; 171(1):372–375.

157. Master VA, Meng MV, Grossfeld GD. Treatment and outcome of invasive bladder cancer in patients after renal transplantation. J Urol 2004; 171(3):1085–1088.

158. Michaelson MD, Shipley WU, Heney NM. Selective bladder preservation for muscle-invasive transitional cell carcinoma of the urinary bladder. Br J Cancer 2004; 90(3):578–581.

159. Peyromaure M, Guerin F, Debre B. Surgical management of infiltrating bladder cancer in elderly patients. Eur Urol 2004; 45(2):147–153; discussion 154.

160. Revelo MP, Cookson MS, Chang SS. Incidence and location of prostate and urothelial carcinoma in prostates from cystoprostatectomies: implications for possible apical sparing surgery. J Urol 2004; 171(2 Pt 1):646–651.

161. McKiernan JM, Motzer RJ, Bajorin DF. Reoperative retroperitoneal surgery for nonseminomatous germ cell tumor: clinical presentation, patterns of recurrence, and outcome. Urology 2003; 62(4):732–736.

162. Enneking WF, Spanier SS, Goodman MA. A system for the surgical staging of musculoskeletal sarcoma. Clin Orthop 2003; 415:4–18.

163. Ballo MT, Lee AK. Current results of brachytherapy for soft tissue sarcoma. Curr Opin Oncol 2003; 15(4):313–318.

164. Clark MA, Thomas JM. Major amputation for soft-tissue sarcoma. Br J Surg 2003; 90(1):102–107.

165. Kotz R, Dominkus M, Zettl T, et al. Advances in bone tumour treatment in 30 years with respect to survival and limb salvage. A single institution experience. Int Orthop 2002; 26(4):197–202. Epub 2002 Jun 13.

166. Singer S, Demetri GD, Baldini EH, et al. Management of soft-tissue sarcomas: an overview and update. Lancet Oncol 2000; 1:75–85.

167. Balch CM. Randomized surgical trials involving elective node dissection for melanoma. Adv Surg 1999; 32:255–70.

168. Nelson JE, Meier DE, Erwin JO, et al. Self-reported symptom experience of critically ill cancer patients receiving intensive care. Crit Care Med 2001; 29(2):277–282.

169. Puntillo KA, White C, Morris AB, et al. Patient's perceptions and responses to procedural pain: results form the Thunder Project II. Am J Crit Care 2001; 10:238–251.

170. Kroll W, List WF. Pain treatment in the ICU: intravenous, regional or both? Eur J Anaesthesiol 1997; Suppl 15:49–52.

171. Graf C, Puntillo K. Pain in the older adult in the intensive care unit. Crit Care Clin 2003; 19(4):749–770.

172. Tsui SL, Law S, Fok M, et al Postoperative analgesia reduces mortality and morbidity after oesophagectomy. Am J Surg 1997; 173:472–478.

173. Waterman H, Leatherbarrow B, Slater R, et al. Post-operative pain, nausea and vomiting: qualitative perspectives from telephone interviews. J Adv Nurs 1999; 29(3):690–696.

174. Brodner G, Van Aken H, Hertle L, et al. Multimodal perioperative management – combining thoracic epidural analgesia, forced mobilisation, and oral nutrition – reduces hormonal and metabolic stress and improves convalescence after major urologic surgery. Anaesth Analges 2001; 92:1594–1600.

175. Wu CL, Anderson GF, Herbert R, et al. Effect of postoperative epidural analgesia on morbidity and mortality following total hip replacement surgery in medicare patients. Reg Anesth Pain Med 2003; 28:271–278.

176. Puntillo KA. Pain assessment and management in the critically ill: wizardry or science? Am J Crit Care 2003; 12(4):310–316.

177. Society of Critical Care Medicine practice parameters for systemic intravenous analgesia and sedation for adult patients in the intensive care unit. Anaheim, CA: Society of Critical Care Medicine; 1995.

178. Caumo W, Schmidt AP, Schneider CN. Preoperative predictors of moderate to intense acute postoperative pain in patients undergoing abdominal surgery. Acta Anaesthesiol Scand 2002; 46(10):1265–1271.

179. Jenkinson C, Carroll D, Egerton M. Comparison of the sensitivity to change of long and short form pain measures. Qual Life Res 1995; 4(4):353–357.

180. Gaston-Johansson F. Measurement of pain: the psychometric properties of the Pain-O-Meter, a simple, inexpensive pain assessment tool that could change health care practices. J Pain Symp Manage 1996; 12(3):172–181.

181. Kelly AM. Setting the benchmark for research in the management of acute pain in emergency departments. Emerg Med 2001, 13(1):57–60.

182. Blenkharn A, Faughnan S, Morgan A. Developing a pain assessment tool for use by nurses in an adult intensive care unit. Intensive Crit Care Nurs 2002; 18(6):332–341.

183. Majani G, Tiengo M, Giardini A. Relationship between MPQ and VAS in 962 patients. A rationale for their use. Minerva Anestesiologie 2003; 69(1–2):67–73.

184. Liu SS, Carpenter RL, Mackey DC, et al. Effects of perioperative analgesic technique on rate of recovery after colon surgery. Anaesthesiology 1995; 8(3):757–765.

185. Mahon SV, Berry PD, Jackson M. Thoracic epidural infusions for post-thoracotomy pain: a comparison of fentanyl-bupivacaine mixtures vs. fentanyl alone. Anaesthesia 1999; 54(7):641–646.

186. Neal JM, Wilcox RT, Allen HW. Near-total esophagectomy: the influence of standardized multimodal management and intraoperative fluid restriction. Reg Anesth Pain Med 2003; 28(4):328–334.

187. Weinbroum AA, Bender B, Bickels J. Preoperative and postoperative dextromethorphan provides sustained reduction in postoperative pain and patient-controlled epidural analgesia requirement: a randomized, placebo-controlled, double-blind study in lower-body bone malignancy-operated patients. Cancer 2003; 97(9):2334–2340.

188. Standl T, Burmeister MA, Ohnesorge H. Patient-controlled epidural analgesia reduces analgesic requirements compared to continuous epidural infusion after major abdominal surgery. Can J Anaesth 2003; 50(3):258–264.

189. Wulf H, Winckler K, Maier C. Pharmacokinetics and protein binding of bupivacaine in postoperative epidural analgesia. Acta Anaesthesiol Scand 1988; 32(7):530–534.

190. Ng JM, Goh MH. Problems related to epidural analgesia for postoperative pain control. Ann Acad Med Singapore 2002; 31(4):509–515.

191. Anderson FA, Wheeler HB, Goldberg RJ, et al. A population-based perspective of the hospital incidence and case-fatality rates of deep vein thrombosis and pulmonary embolism. The Worcester DVT Study. Arch Intern Med 1991; 151:933–938.

192. Kim V, Spandorfer J. Epidemiology of venous thromboembolic disease. Emerg Med Clin North Am 2001; 19:839–859.

193. Goldhaber SA, Tapson VF & DVT Free Steering Committee. A prospective registry of 5,451 patients with ultrasound-confirmed deep vein thrombosis. Am J Cardiol 2004; 93(2):259–262.

194. Kearon C. Duration of venous thromboembolism prophylaxis after surgery. Chest 2003; 124(6 Suppl):386S–392S.

195. Lee AY, Levine MN, Baker RI et al. Randomized Comparison of Low-Molecular-Weight Heparin versus Oral Anticoagulant Therapy for the Prevention of Recurrent Venous Thromboembolism in Patients with Cancer (CLOT) Investigators. Low-molecular-weight heparin versus a coumarin for the prevention of recurrent venous thromboembolism in patients with cancer. N Engl J Med 2003; 349(2):146–153.

196. Bona RD. Central line thrombosis in patients with cancer. Curr Opin Pulm Med 2003; 9(5):362–366.

197. Verso M, Agnelli G. Venous thromboembolism associated with long-term use of central venous catheters in cancer patients. J Clin Oncol 2003; 21(19):3665–3675.

198. Estes JM, Rocconi R, Straughn JM. Complications of indwelling venous access devices in patients with gynecologic malignancies. Gynecol Oncol 2003; 91(3):591–595.

199. Lowry JC. Thromboembolic disease and thromboprophylaxis in oral and maxillofacial surgery: experience and practice. Br J Oral Maxillofacial Surg 1995; 33(2):101–106.

200. Samama MM. [Prevention of venous thromboembolic disease.] Rev Prat 1996; 46(10):1245–1253. [in French]

201. Goldhaber SZ, Dunn K, Gerhard-Herman M. Low rate of venous thromboembolism after craniotomy for brain tumor using multimodality prophylaxis. Chest 2002; 122(6):33–37.

202. Lee AY. The role of low-molecular-weight heparins in the prevention and treatment of venous thromboembolism in cancer patients. Curr Opin Pulm Med 2003; 9(5):351–355.

203. Kakkar AK. An expanding role for antithrombotic therapy in cancer patients. Cancer Treat Rev 2003; 29(Suppl 2):23–26.

204. Levine MN. Can we optimise treatment of thrombosis? Cancer Treat Rev 2003; 29(Suppl 2):19–22.

205. Klerk CPW, Smorenburg SM, Buller HR. Thrombosis prophylaxis in patient populations with a central venous catheter. Arch Internal Med 2003; 163:1913–1921.

206. Maxwell GL, Synan I, Hayes RP. Preference and compliance in postoperative thromboembolism prophylaxis among gynecologic oncology patients. Obstet Gynecol 2002; 100(3):451–455.

207. Thompson HJ. The management of post-operative nausea and vomiting. J Adv Nurs 1999; 29(5):1130–1136.

208. Ku CM, Ong BC. Postoperative nausea and vomiting: a review of current literature. Singapore Med J 2003; 44(7):366–374.

209. Habib AS, Gan TJ. Pharmacotherapy of postoperative nausea and vomiting. Expert Opin Pharmacother 2003; 4(4):457–473.

210. Tate S, Cook H. Postoperative nausea and vomiting. 1: Physiology and aetiology. Br J Nurs 1996; 12–25;5(16):962, 964, 966 passim.

211. Everett LL. Can the risk of postoperative nausea and vomiting be identified and lowered during the preoperative assessment? Int Anesthesiol Clin 2002; 40(2):47–62.

212. Nelson TP. Postoperative nausea and vomiting: understanding the enigma. J Perianesth Nurs 2002; 17(3):178–87; quiz 187–189.

213. Biedler A, Wermelt J, Kunitz O. A risk adapted approach reduces the overall institutional incidence of postoperative nausea and vomiting, Can J Anaesth 2004; 51(1):13–19.

214. Broomhead CJ. Reducing the incidence of postoperative nausea and vomiting. Br J Hosp Med 1995; 53(10):511–512.

215. Larsson S, Lundberg D. A prospective survey of postoperative nausea and vomiting with special regard to incidence and relations to patient characteristics, anesthetic routines and surgical procedures. Acta Anaesthesiol Scand 1995; 39(4):539–545.

216. Golembiewski JA, O'Brien D. A systematic approach to the management of postoperative nausea and vomiting. J Perianesthiol Nurs 2002; 17(6):364–376.

217. Jolley S. Managing post-operative nausea and vomiting. Nurs Stand 2001; 15(40):47–52; quiz 53–55.

218. Gan TJ, Meyer T, Apfel CC. Consensus guidelines for managing postoperative nausea and vomiting. Anesth Analg 2003; 97(1):62–71.

219. Ali SZ, Taguchi A, Holtmann B. Effect of supplemental pre-operative fluid on postoperative nausea and vomiting. Anaesthesia 2003; 58(8):780–784.

220. Ku CM, Ong BC. Postoperative nausea and vomiting: a review of current literature. Singapore Med J 2003; 44(7):366–374.

221. Cameron D, Gan TJ. Management of postoperative nausea and vomiting in ambulatory surgery. Anesthesiol Clin North Am 2003; 21(2):347–365.

222. Alkaissi A, Evertsson K, Johnsson VA. P6 acupressure may relieve nausea and vomiting after gynecological surgery: an effectiveness study in 410 women. Can J Anaesth 2002; 49(10):1034–1039.

223. Moretti EW, Robertson KM, El-Moalem H. Intraoperative colloid administration reduces postoperative nausea and vomiting and improves

postoperative outcomes compared with crystalloid administration. Anesth Analg 2003; 96(2):611–617.

224. Paech MJ, Rucklidge MW, Banks SL. The efficacy and cost-effectiveness of prophylactic 5-hydroxytryptamine3 receptor antagonists: tropisetron, ondansetron and dolasetron. Anaesth Intensive Care 2003; 31(1):11–17.

225. Henzi I, Walder B, Tramer MR. Dexamethasone for the prevention of postoperative nausea and vomiting: a quantitative systematic review. Anesth Analg 2000; 90(1):186–194.

226. Ciccarello GP. Strategies to improve end-of-life care in the intensive care unit. Dimens Crit Care Nurs 2003; 22(5):216–222.

227. Resuscitation Council UK, British Medical Association & The Royal College of Nursing. Decisions relating to cardiopulmonary resuscitation: a joint statement from the British Medical Association, The Resuscitation Council UK & The Royal College of Nursing. Resuscitation Council UK, 2001.

228. Benner P, Hooper-Kyriakidis P, Stannard D. Clinical wisdom and interventions in critical care. Philadelphia: WB Saunders; 1999.

229. Seymour JE. Facing death: critical moments death and dying in intensive care. Buckingham, UK: Open University Press; 2001.

230. Hawryluck LA, Harvey WR, Lemieux-Charles L. Consensus guidelines on analgesia and sedation in dying intensive care unit patients. BMC Med Ethics 2002; 3(1):3.

231. Rubenfeld GD, Curtis JR. Improving care for patients dying in the intensive care unit. Clin Chest Med 2003;, 24(4):763–773.

232. Hurst S, Whitmer M. Palliative care services. Dimens Crit Care Nurs 2003;, 22(1):35–38.

233. Campbell ML, Guzman JA. Impact of a proactive approach to improve end-of-life care in a medical ICU. Chest 2003; 123(1):266–271.

CHAPTER 36

Rehabilitation and Survivorship

MARY WELLS AND SHEILA MACBRIDE

CHAPTER CONTENTS

Introduction	799	Rehabilitation and survivorship: transitions	812
The history of rehabilitation and survivorship	800	Making rehabilitation and survivorship a reality: the role of the nurse	812
What is rehabilitation?	800	Reshaping care for survivors of cancer	816
The goals of rehabilitation	801	Useful websites	816
Living with cancer	802	Conclusion	816
Physical rehabilitation and survival	802		
Psychological rehabilitation and survival	803	Useful websites	817
Support, rehabilitation and survival	809	References	817
Existential rehabilitation and survival	811		

INTRODUCTION

As survival rates continue to improve and more and more people are living with cancer, rehabilitation and survivorship become increasingly important issues for cancer nurses. The concepts of rehabilitation and survivorship originate from the United States, and are founded on the recognition that patients who are treated for cancer do not automatically 'recover' once treatment is complete. Even when patients are effectively 'cured', profound physical, psychosocial and spiritual changes may result from the experience of having cancer, and it may be very difficult for 'normal' life to resume. The traditional medical endpoint of survival is measured in terms of 1- or 5-year survival after diagnosis, but this reflects only a small part of what survival from cancer is really about. The scope of cancer nursing provides an opportunity to address the quality, rather than just the quantity, of patients' survival.

The quality of a patient's survival is probably largely dependent on the quality of his or her rehabilitation, yet the focus of care is often on safe and timely diagnosis and treatment, rather than on the problems that are caused by the cancer or its management. As Mullan[1(p273)] states:

> It is as if we have invented sophisticated techniques to save people from drowning but once they have been pulled from the water, we leave them to cough and splutter on their own in the belief we have done all we can.

It is not enough to provide effective therapies and supportive care while patients are on treatment; we must also address patients' needs for getting on with life once treatment is over. This chapter will discuss the concepts of rehabilitation and survivorship, using current evidence to support the integration of rehabilitative care into the daily work of cancer nurses, with the aim of enhancing the quality of patients' survival.

THE HISTORY OF REHABILITATION AND SURVIVORSHIP

Since the 1960s, rehabilitation has been recognized as a key component of care programmes for patients recovering from myocardial infarction, stroke, head or spinal cord injury, amputation and other physical or neurological disability. Rehabilitation medicine has, over the last 20 years, become a speciality in its own right across Europe. However, the place of rehabilitation in cancer care has been much slower to gain recognition. Research and service developments in cancer rehabilitation started in the USA during the 1970s, and continued in Germany.[2,3] Other European countries such as the Netherlands and the UK did not, until fairly recently, explicitly support the concept of rehabilitation within cancer care, and offered few dedicated rehabilitative services for patients recovering from cancer. Richard Wells,[4] who founded the first cancer rehabilitation centre in the UK, acknowledged that most Western hospitals were probably providing some aspects of rehabilitation, but pointed out that different practitioners were working in isolation and, as a result, rehabilitative care was extremely fragmented. Fortunately, there is an increasing recognition of the importance of rehabilitation within cancer care in the 21st century, but there is still a need to promote rehabilitative care as a *central* focus of cancer nursing, rather than as an afterthought.

The concept of survivorship began to take shape in the USA in the 1980s, in response to the failure of most definitions of cancer survival to include patients' *experiences* of surviving cancer. Initially, research focused on survival as an outcome of therapy and looked at the long-term side-effects of treatments, particularly in patients with lymphoma or testicular cancer. Psychologists then began to explore the psychological effects of survival, identifying groups who were more likely to be 'at risk' for poor adjustment back into 'normal' lifestyles, such as those with previous psychological or psychiatric difficulties, alcohol and drug addicts, and those with poor social support.[5]

At the same time, a group of healthcare professionals who had also 'survived' cancer led the development of a US consumer movement, The National Coalition for Cancer Survivors (NCCS; see Useful websites section), which has effectively challenged conventional definitions of survivorship.[1,6] Leigh[6] pointed out that patients and their professional carers may hold very different views of survival and that the 'quality of survival is in the eye of the beholder'. Although the focus of cancer 'survival' continues to be on the length of time a patient survives after diagnosis, or on the duration of the period in which a patient is 'disease-free', there is increasing recognition that *quality* of life is equally important.[7]

Although there is no European equivalent to the NCCS, the language of '5-year survival' and 'disease response' has also been challenged this side of the Atlantic. Corner[8] suggests that we need to look beyond survival rates and side-effects, and cautions that even the concept of quality of life has been reduced to a series of reductionist 'measures'. It is certainly time to look beyond conventional definitions of survivorship and rehabilitation, towards an approach which is about *living with cancer*.

WHAT IS REHABILITATION?

The Oncology Nursing Society[9] defines rehabilitation as 'a process by which individuals, within their environments, are assisted to achieve optimal functioning within the limits imposed by cancer'. Other definitions refer to the restoration of a patient to as normal a functional state as possible[10] or suggest that the goal of rehabilitation is to enable people to function at their maximum level in terms of physical, mental, emotional, social or economic potential.[11] These definitions recognize that optimal or normal functioning has to be considered within the context of the individual's cancer diagnosis, but they fail to explicitly acknowledge the patient's place at the centre of the rehabilitative process. Wells[4(p507)] points out that:

In delivering rehabilitation services, the ultimate goal is to ensure that control remains where it rightly belongs – with the patient. Rehabilitation is not about doing things to people but rather enabling a return to what they were or as near as possible to what they were, reintegrated with loved ones, and physically, psychologically and socially stable.

Given that most people would acknowledge that life is never the same following a diagnosis of cancer, it is interesting that several authors refer to restoring or returning to what was before. Perhaps a more useful way of conceptualizing rehabilitation is offered by Veach et al,[12(p118)] who suggest that rehabilitation 'is a time of reorganisation, often requiring a reinvention of the patient and family'. It seems that the key to rehabilitation must be to understand *who* the person was prior to diagnosis, *how* and *why* things have changed as a result of having cancer

and *where the person would like to be*. Within this context, it is possible to set goals that are both realistic and patient-centred. In 1984, Kenneth Calman[13] hypothesized that quality of life in cancer patients represents the difference between the hopes and expectations of an individual and the actual experience of their present situation. Perhaps it is the role of rehabilitation to lessen the gap between these two realities.

THE GOALS OF REHABILITATION

Several authors have attempted to categorize the goals of rehabilitation (Table 36.1). Some make a distinction between the rehabilitation of patients who are cured of their disease and those who are in a palliative phase. Others describe the aims of rehabilitation in terms of the focus on particular activities within the

Table 36.1: The goals of rehabilitation

Dietz (1981)[84]	Wells (1990)[4]	Strobel (2002)[57]
Preventative – to reduce morbidity or improve physical functioning e.g. postoperative physiotherapy after radical neck dissection	Life expectancy is good – no residual disfigurement or disability e.g. healthy eating after curative bowel surgery	Somatic – control or reduction in symptoms, improvement in function or movement e.g. management of bowel dysfunction after rectal surgery
Restorative – to control or eliminate residual disability after cure e.g. education and support for the management of a limb prosthesis after amputation for sarcoma	Life expectancy is good – but some physical or psychological disability or disfigurement e.g. assessment and management of body image	Functional – development of other functions in order to compensate for limitations e.g. development of oesophageal speech after laryngectomy
Supportive – to lessen disability for those with ongoing disease e.g. goal-setting for activities of daily living	Life expectancy is shortened – future is uncertain e.g. nursing intervention for the management of breathlessness	Psychosocial – reintegration into family/work/social life, restoration of health and quality of life e.g. vocational rehabilitation
Palliative – to maximize quality of life in those with advanced disease e.g. management of pain		Educative – information and education about disease, management of symptoms or prostheses e.g. importance of skin care for affected limb after axilliary surgery

rehabilitative approach. These models are useful in that they help to clarify the context in which rehabilitation takes place, and to determine specific areas of need. However, by separating the goals of rehabilitation into different components, they also imply that patients needs fit neatly into a particular box, and this may not be the case.

It may be helpful to consider each of these models of rehabilitation within an overall framework of 'living with cancer'. Both survival and rehabilitation have tended to be seen in terms of time, functional recovery or resumption of normal life. Although these aspects of living with cancer are vitally important, it is essential that healthcare professionals also fully address quality of life from the patient's perspective. There are many tools that measure quality of life using a structured approach, such as the EORTC[14] and FACT[15] questionnaires. These ask patients to rate aspects of emotional, social, physical and functional well-being, and include symptoms that relate specifically to their type of disease. Although these tools can provide extremely useful information about the extent to which a patient is affected by the particular issues specified, they do not tell us what has most impact on the individual and his family. For example, a quality of life questionnaire may pick up the existence of bowel symptoms in a patient who has undergone surgery, but cannot elicit the extent to which a patient has had to change their life as a result. Questionnaire categories do not generally reflect how such a patient may have had to alter the way they live, travel to work, dress, keep fit, enjoy sexual relationships, etc., after the formation of a stoma, removal of a breast or commencement of continuous infusional chemotherapy.

Although useful in large-scale research studies, prescribed quality of life tools are unable to assess, in sufficient detail, the problems that are most distressing for patients on a day-to-day basis. In recent years, quality of life instruments have been designed to enable patients to specify what is most important to them. Such tools are more responsive to the less obvious but legitimate concerns of individual patients. Because they provide a means of assessing patients' own priorities of what matters most, and what is most troublesome, they have a great deal of potential in routine clinical practice, and lend themselves ideally to the assessment and management of rehabilitative needs.

An example of such a tool is the Patient-Generated Index (PGI):[16] first, patients are asked to specify the five most important areas of their life which are affected by their illness (cancer); secondly, patients must state the degree to which each of these areas are troublesome, on a scale of 0–10, from not at all to the worst imaginable; thirdly, patients are asked to 'spend' 14 points on these areas, allocating points to those aspects that are most important to their sense of quality of life. So, a patient might decide to spend *all* his points in one particular area which is of primary importance, or might divide his points fairly equally between the five areas. The level of information generated from this type of tool could provide exactly the information necessary to plan truly patient-focused rehabilitative care, as it enables healthcare professionals to address the most important aspects of that person's life.

LIVING WITH CANCER

Cancer turns life upside down and the process of resuming some kind of 'normal' life during and after cancer treatment can be extremely challenging. Although the concept of quality of life captures many of the physical, functional, emotional and social aspects of life, less attention has been given to the existential components of living with cancer which are so important.[17] Cohen et al[17] suggest that framing quality of life in terms of physical symptoms, psychological symptoms, existential well-being and support is of more relevance to people who are living with a life-threatening illness. We have chosen to highlight issues of rehabilitation and survivorship in terms of these four key areas, although it must be acknowledged that none exists in isolation (Fig. 36.1).

Physical rehabilitation and survival

The physical effects of cancer and its treatment can interfere fundamentally with the individual's ability to get on with normal life. The basis

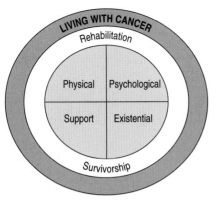

Figure 36.1: Living with cancer framework.

of rehabilitation lies in understanding the potential impact of such effects on physical and psychosocial functioning and quality of life in its widest sense. It is absolutely vital that these issues are considered as early as possible, so that there is adequate time to address patients needs. Table 36.2 illustrates the extent to which the physical consequences of cancer and cancer therapy can affect patients' quality of life and ability to function, and highlights specific needs for rehabilitation in a number of different patient groups. Common themes appear in all patient groups, including the assessment and management of altered body image, psychological support, symptom management, sexual function, activities of daily living, mobility, fatigue management, nutrition, bladder or bowel control and communication. These themes can be applied to other groups of individuals not specified in the table, such as patients with sarcoma who undergo amputation or major plastic surgery, or patients with cancers of the orbit, who may suffer blindness and disfigurement. In addition, it must be remembered that survivors of cancer constantly live with the potential that they may develop late effects of cancer treatments, recurrence, or even second malignancies, all of which can compromise quality of life, health and survival.

There is increasing evidence that rehabilitation programmes, which include some of the strategies listed in Table 36.2, can have a real impact on functioning and quality of life. Kirshblum et al[18] review a number of studies which illustrate that patients with brain tumours benefit from inpatient rehabilitation as much as patients with traumatic brain injury or stroke, although the available time frames for interventions are usually shorter. Rehabilitation programmes have also been found to improve the physical and mental functioning of extremely vulnerable groups such as elderly palliative care patients with asthenia (physical and mental fatigue in advanced cancer).[19] Despite these encouraging findings, there are very few designated centres for cancer rehabilitation in the UK and many parts of Europe. Instead, rehabilitative care may be concentrated in areas where particular therapists practice, such as lymphoedema management. In contrast, rehabilitation programmes for patients with stroke, cardiac disease, pulmonary disease and traumatic injury are generally more widely available, and are considered integral to the overall service.

Psychological rehabilitation and survival

It is important to acknowledge that symptoms that reflect a complex interrelationship between physical, social and psychological factors also occur in the context of a life-threatening illness. Cancer changes lives, removes all sense of control, introduces uncertainty and often takes away the sense of self-identity and confidence which makes people feel like themselves. As Diamond[20(p191)] explains:

> When I told people that I was not myself I meant it almost literally: in the mirror I was somebody else. Precisely, I was a little old man whom I imagined to be called Albert or Norman or George.

Because the sense of self is so diminished, and is often accompanied by unpleasant symptoms, fatigue and communication problems, many patients withdraw from their usual activities or find it difficult to resume work, social or family roles and responsibilities. A 66-year-old man with cancer of the tongue explained why he had given up being on the committee for his local parish council:

> I dribble at the corner of my mouth and this upsets me, I've never quite got full control, the whole thing makes me feel that I'm not functioning properly … . I don't want to get into one of these things and not be able to do it properly[21]

Table 36.2: Physical functioning, quality of life and rehabilitative care in different patient groups

Type of cancer	Impact of cancer or cancer treatments on functioning and quality of life	Rehabilitative care strategies
Brain and spinal cord[18,68,69]	Loss of autonomy and independence Cognitive impairment	Early recognition and treatment of depression and anxiety Patient and family education Psychological support for patient and family
	Vocational and social problems	Vocationally based community integration
	Risk of seizures	Consideration of side-effects of medication (e.g. antiepileptic drugs) Prophylactic antiepileptic drugs (although evidence of efficacy is lacking)
	Compromised safety/risk of injury	Risk management and support, e.g. falls, blood sugar monitoring
	Steroid-induced myopathy, gastric ulceration, diabetes Altered body image	
	Weakness	Multidisciplinary assessment and intervention by doctor, nurse, occupational therapist, physiotherapist, psychologist, dietitian, social worker, speech therapist
	Reduced mobility/paresis/plegia Difficulties with communication and speech	
	Difficulty with activities of daily living	Goal-setting and support/aids for activities of daily living Home assessment and adaptation
	Excess weight gain	Nutritional advice and support
	Consequences of immobility, e.g. deep vein thrombosis	Skin care to minimize complications of reduced mobility Maintenance of physical activity
	Fatigue and somnolence	Assessment, exercise and rest, nutritional care, information
	Symptoms of raised intercranial pressure, e.g. headache, nausea and vomiting	Symptom management, particularly pain and nausea/vomiting
	Impaired bladder and bowel function	Bowel and bladder retraining/continence care as appropriate

	Problems	Management
Breast[69-72]	Loss or change in size and shape of breast(s)	Assessment and management of body image changes
	Body image problems	Psychological support
		Reconstructive surgery
		Prostheses fitting
		Advice/support about clothing and swimwear
	Reduced arm mobility	Physiotherapy and arm exercises
	Shoulder stiffness	
	Pain	Pain assessment and management
	Brachial plexus injury causing weakness and numbness in upper limbs	Skin care for affected limb
	Infection and cellulitis in affected limb	Monitoring of complications and early intervention
	Lymphoedema	Symptom management
		Hosiery and bandaging if lymphoedema
		Manual lymph drainage if lymphoedema
	Risk of cardiomyopathy, pericardial damage, coronary artery damage, valvular damage due to late effects of chemotherapy and radiotherapy	Monitoring of complications and early intervention
	Sexual difficulties	Management of hormonal problems, assessment and psychological support
Head and neck[72-75]	Altered body image and disfigurement	Assessment and management of body image changes
		Psychological support
	Reduced shoulder and neck mobility, particularly after neck dissection	Physiotherapy for shoulder mobility, airway maintenance
	Communication and speech difficulties	Assessment and intervention from multidisciplinary team, specifically including speech therapy for swallowing, speech and development of oesophageal speech in laryngectomies;
	Eating difficulties	Dietetic intervention for weight loss and eating difficulties
	Risk of aspiration and airway problems	Close monitoring. Education and support for airway maintenance

(continues)

Table 36.2: Physical functioning, quality of life and rehabilitative care in different patient groups—cont'd

Type of cancer	Impact of cancer or cancer treatments on functioning and quality of life	Rehabilitative care strategies
	Potential reliance on tracheostomy	Social support
	Loss of social life	Support and intervention for smoking and alcohol cessation
	Need to address alcohol and smoking dependence in many individuals	
	Pain – visceral and neuropathic	Pain and symptom assessment and management
	Dry mouth	Oral and dental assessment and care
	Mucositis	Symptom management
	Risk of osteoradionecrosis	Early intervention from dental hygienists and dentists
		Pain management
Haematological malignancies, particularly bone marrow transplantation[23,76,77]	Pancytopenia	Risk management and careful monitoring/prompt treatment of complications
	Risk of graft versus host disease	
	Haemorrhage	
	Pulmonary fibrosis	
	Cardiac damage	
	Neutropenia and infection	Patient education
	Weakness and fatigue	Fatigue management
	Mucositis	Oral care, skin care
	Nausea and vomiting	Monitoring and review of medications and side-effects
	Diarrhoea	Symptom assessment and management
	Pain	
	Weight loss and nutritional difficulties	Nutritional support
	Sensory, motor and cognitive impairment	Cognitive assessment
	Boredom and frustration	Psychological support
	Protracted periods of hospitalization and isolation	Occupational therapy
	Reduced mobility	Exercise maintenance and physiotherapy
	Altered body image	Assessment and management of body image changes, sexual problems
	Infertility and sexual difficulties	

Cancer type	Problems	Interventions
Gynaecological malignancies – surgery, radiotherapy, chemotherapy[78,79]	Altered body image Sexual difficulties Infertility Early menopause Lymphoedema of lower limbs Altered bowel/urinary function Fatigue	Psychological support Sexual rehabilitation (assessment, counselling, symptom management, medication) Education and support following plastic surgery e.g. neo-vagina formation Assessment and management of body image changes Education and support for vaginal dilatation, lubrication Fertility conservation or cryopreservation if possible Infertility counselling and/or information about surrogacy Management of lymphoedema (skin care, hosiery and bandaging, manual lymph drainage) Bladder or bowel retraining/management of incontinence Stoma care and education (if applicable) Symptom management Management of hormonal problems
Gastrointestinal cancers – surgery, radiotherapy, chemotherapy[75,80]	Dysphagia Pain Eating difficulties Malabsorption Dumping syndrome Altered bowel habits – diarrhoea, constipation Incontinence and urgency – urinary and faecal Stoma formation Reduced liver function/hepatic failure Fatigue Altered body image Sexual difficulties	Symptom management Nutritional support and advice Bowel or bladder retraining/management of faecal and urinary incontinence Stoma care and education Monitoring liver function and malabsorption Fatigue management Psychological support Assessment and management of body image changes Sexual rehabilitation (assessment, counselling, symptom management, medication)

(continues)

Table 36.2: Physical functioning, quality of life and rehabilitative care in different patient groups—cont'd

Type of cancer	Impact of cancer or cancer treatments on functioning and quality of life	Rehabilitative care strategies
Genitourinary[78,79,81]	Altered urinary function – incontinence, urgency, frequency, nocturia	Patient education Psychological support Bladder retraining Management of incontinence
	Fatigue	Symptom management
	Impotence/sexual and hormonal problems	Sexual rehabilitation (assessment, counselling, symptom management, medication)
	Altered body image	Education and support following plastic surgery e.g. penile implant
	Infertility	Infertility counselling/fertility preservation where possible
	Poor renal function	Monitoring and management of renal function
Lung[82,83]	Reduced independence in activities of daily living	Occupational therapy and physiotherapy for maintenance of activities in daily living and goal-setting
	Breathlessness, fatigue, pain	Management of symptoms Nursing intervention for the management of breathlessness
	Fibrosis	Early detection of complications
	Pneumonitis	
	Weight loss	Nutritional support and advice
	Rapidly deteriorating health	Early involvement of palliative care specialists

Cancer and its treatment (in particular chemotherapy or cranial irradiation) may also interfere with cognitive function. Many patients are extremely frustrated and distressed by loss of short-term memory, confusion or inability to concentrate following cancer treatment. Changes in cognitive function or personality are also very difficult for family members to witness. Seaton[22] describes watching his intelligent wife (who had advanced breast cancer and brain metastases) become disinhibited, reliant on nurses to tell her the date and dependent on notes written on her hand to orientate her to what was happening. Sadly, healthcare professionals often pay little attention, in everyday practice, to the debilitating effects of cancer on people's ability to think, process and retain information and maintain their sense of self.

The disruption caused by cancer evokes a range of psychological responses (Table 36.3), some of which may be defined as psychological disorders.[23] It is clear that the psychological impact of cancer is felt way beyond the completion of treatment. Anxiety and depression have been found to persist for many years,[24] and some individuals find it hard to make sense of this when they are objectively 'cured' and feel they have no reason to feel depressed.[25] Many survivors of cancer continue to live with the fear of recurrence and death, despite having been cured. A small study[26] illustrated the distress experienced by survivors of cancer during 'flashback phenomena', in which they repeatedly recalled aspects of their life as a 'cancer patient'. When expectations and fears have focused on the possibility of death, it can be difficult for a person to come to terms with recovery, particularly when exposed to other patients who appear not to have been so lucky. Naysmith et al[27] describe this phenomena of 'survivor guilt', which is known to many soldiers who survive war.

A survey of cancer survivors in the USA illustrates that the psychological well-being of many survivors of cancer is worse than their functional, social or physical well-being.[28] Ronson and Body[23] suggest that psychosocial issues must be addressed early if effective rehabilitation is to take place. Strategies may include identifying coping strategies or helping patients to rehearse how they might cope with different situations; adapting to changes in relationships, roles or expectations; managing uncertainty, anxiety and depression; dealing with distress; communicating; and dealing with sexuality or altered body image.

Support, rehabilitation and survival

A diagnosis of cancer can have a profound impact on a person's usual support network, either because he or she withdraws from it or because the relationships within it change. As Dow et al[29] explain, it is possible to lose faith not only in one's own body, but also in one's family and friends. Seigel and Christ[5] point out that patterns of friendship can change, particularly when friends and indeed family do not understand why feelings of low mood persist after completion of treatment, believing that the challenge is over and expecting life to revert to 'normal'.

Mullan[1] explains that the challenge is never 'over' and that it is artificial to frame survival in terms of chronological dates. Instead, he proposes that there are phases of 'acute survival' (at the time of diagnosis), 'extended survival' (when treatment is over) and 'permanent survival'. He describes[1(p272)] this as a time of:

> . . . kinship and continuum with the previous seasons of survival. There is no moment of cure but rather an evolution from the phase of extended survival into a period when the activity of the disease or the likelihood of its return is sufficiently small that the cancer can now be considered permanently arrested.

It is clear that the support of others who have experienced cancer can be extremely important during the phases of extended and permanent survival, as contact with healthcare professionals may diminish after the end of treatment. Diamond[20(p8)] refers to a sense of being part of a 'community'. He explains:

> My suspicion is that once you've had that diagnosis it stays with you for good. Like lapsed religion it may not be at the front of your mind all the time but it is yawning away there at the back, just waiting for those moments when it needs to come forward and remind you that you are part of that community which touched death and touches it

Table 36.3: Psychological responses[23]

Psychological responses	Individuals affected	Manifestations and potential sequelae
Post-traumatic stress disorder	Survivors of childhood cancer, parents of survivors, adult patients. Studies suggest between 14% and 39% affected	Re-living previous trauma, sleep disturbances, concentration problems. May require cognitive behavioural psychotherapy
Fear of recurrence	May affect nearly all patients with cancer at some stage in their illness	Anxiety, fear, vulnerability. May be affected by the quality of social support available to the patient or family
Treatment-related body image disturbances	Any patient, although research concentrates on post-surgical patients with breast and head and neck cancer	Distress about appearance, self-consciousness, discomfort about wearing certain clothes, avoidance of social situations
Psychosexual functioning	Particularly patients who have undergone surgery, radiotherapy or chemotherapy for gynaecological, urological and breast cancer. Also those on hormonal therapy	Infertility, vaginal stenosis and shortening, vaginal dryness, erectile dysfunction, dyspareunia, amenorrhoea, emotional distress
Cognitive problems	Patients with brain tumours, those undergoing cranial irradiation, total body irradiation or high-dose chemotherapy (particularly bone marrow transplant patients)	Difficulties with concentration, memory, relationships, professional performance, information processing, everyday activities, language, mood
Ambivalence about discontinuing treatment	All patients, particularly those whose treatment has been a prolonged experience	Difficulty moving on, adjusting into 'normal' life again
Conditioned responses such as anticipatory nausea and vomiting	Patients on emetogenic chemotherapy regimens, particularly cisplatin	Acute anxiety, nausea, vomiting on sight or smell of anything which reminds patient of the chemotherapy

still, the community which has seen a doctor look at his boots and say I'm sorry, but . . . .

The growth of support groups, cancer support and information centres and the World Wide Web has extended this community across traditional boundaries. The experience of surviving cancer is, however, different for each person, and the extent to which each person accesses support is extremely individual.

Effective rehabilitation requires attention to patients' needs for different types of support and the support network within which they operate. Some individuals seek out and benefit from informational support, whereby information about their disease, its management and possible self-care strategies helps them to make sense of their situation and regain some sense of control. Some patients find it easier to accept instrumental support, whereby practical assistance, financial help or provision of transport, meals or aids to activities of daily living may be perceived as most supportive. Other patients appear to need and respond to emotional support more readily than any other form of support. Many patients require help to identify possible sources of support, or to learn how to ask for support.[30] Nurses can be instrumental in facilitating support from resources known to the patient (e.g. family and friends) as well as those which are unknown (e.g. support groups, financial assistance, information sources, community services).

One crucial aspect of rehabilitation, which is often neglected, is that of helping patients resume a working life after cancer. Employment and insurance difficulties have received a great deal of attention in the USA, where several authors have highlighted discrimination against people with cancer, ranging from problems obtaining work to failure to achieve promotion or redundancy.[31-33] Difficulties arise partly because of the emotional or physical consequences of cancer on the individuals themselves (whose confidence and motivation is often affected), and partly because of ignorance, prejudice or fear on the part of their employers. These problems often occur in a context of existing financial difficulty (because of time off work during treatment or the 'hidden' expenses of cancer, such as travelling, food, prescriptions). Many patients also experience difficulties obtaining health or holiday insurance, and at the very least, are forced to pay high premiums. Insurance companies may insist on detailed correspondence and regular medical review, both of which can serve as explicit reminders of the risk of disease recurrence.[33]

Mundy et al[32] suggest that there is a need to integrate vocational rehabilitation into the discharge planning process for people with cancer. They emphasize the need for closer and more effective links between health and social care in hospitals and the community, recognizing that nurses and social workers have a key role to play in this vital aspect of rehabilitation. In the USA, a Cancer Survivors Bill of Rights exists to promote equality for people with cancer in terms of employment and insurance issues. This Bill of Rights states that survivors are entitled to:

1 the right to lifelong medical care
2 the pursuit of happiness
3 the right to equal job opportunities
4 the right to receive adequate health care insurance.[34]

Although issues of medical insurance are less relevant in European countries with National Health Services, patients' rights in terms of job opportunities are universal, yet there is no such code within Europe.

Existential rehabilitation and survival

Existential concerns also play a major part in the quality of patients' survival. Dirksen's[35] study of survivors of malignant melanoma illustrates the search for meaning that often accompanies survival. The search to explain 'Why me?' appears to continue beyond diagnosis, often for the rest of life. Being able to make some sense of the situation is an integral part of adapting to the changes that have occurred as a result of cancer and its treatment. Luker et al[36] point out that it is very important to understand the meanings individuals ascribe to their illness and the language and metaphors they use, in order to identify maladaptive coping strategies and to ensure appropriate ongoing support and recovery.

Many people talk about life *before* and *after* cancer. Breaden[37] describes the difficulties many women experience in regaining a sense of time and believing in the future. In another study[29] one participant illustrates the impact this has on 'normal' activities:

> For about a year, I refused to buy clothes, as I wasn't sure that I'd live long enough to use them. One day, I realised that I felt normal. This was about 18 months after diagnosis. I decided to get some new clothes and become a survivor.

Dow et al[29] believe that control is the sense of perspective an individual gains during survivorship, whereby the cancer is respected and acknowledged as part of the individual's background but no longer dominates every waking thought. Molassiotis[38] also proposes that survivorship is a dynamic process, evolving as time since diagnosis and treatment lengthens.

Many survivors talk about the positive effects of experiencing cancer, including the 'second chance' at life and the ability to focus on and seek out those things that are most important. Others discuss the benefits of giving something back, perhaps by volunteering to help in support groups[29] or by fundraising for cancer charities. The experience of cancer often leads to a re-evaluation of life, as priorities and values change and existential concerns become very much more prominent. Many patients find that having cancer enhances their sense of purpose or meaning in life, renews their spiritual faith and improves their relationships.[39]

Existential rehabilitation addresses spiritual needs of finding meaning in the situation, finding new roles and relationships and integrating back into a meaningful existence. Cohen et al[17] propose that other existential concerns include coping with isolation and dealing with death and dying. Assessing what is most important to patients, discussing the meaning of symptoms or experiences and helping patients to 'tell their stories' can facilitate a focus on existential concerns. O'Connor and Wicker[39] suggest a number of questions, which may help survivors to make sense of what is happening to them. These include asking about what gives patients hope and a sense of purpose in their lives, what helps them to live with having had cancer and what is important in their lives.

REHABILITATION AND SURVIVORSHIP: TRANSITIONS

Historically, the concepts of rehabilitation and survivorship have been linked to the completion of active treatment or to the end of an 'acute' illness. One of the possible reasons cancer rehabilitation services have been slow to develop is that cancer is neither an acute event nor a typical chronic illness. Cancer is often characterized by a series of acute events, within the context of a life-threatening illness, which may be associated with a fluctuating picture of symptoms, functional difficulties and psychological problems. In reality, patients with cancer do not have a clear 'end' to their illness or treatment, and it is artificial to consider rehabilitation or survivorship as a sequential stage in their journey: instead, both must be seen as dynamic processes that need to be addressed *throughout* the patient's experience.

The end of treatment can, however, be a particularly difficult time, full of ambiguity. Maher[40] applies Durkheim's concept of 'anomie'[a] to this experience, suggesting that many individuals feel ambivalent about completing treatment and have difficulty resuming a 'future orientation' in the midst of fears about recurrence and the challenges of disability. As Frank[41(p132)] said of his experience of recovering from treatment for cancer, there is a suspension of consciousness 'between the insulated world of illness and the healthy mainstream'.

Nicholson and Wells[30] suggest that completing cancer treatment is associated with a number of transitions, defined as 'the passage or movement from one state to the other'.[42(p119)] These transitions may be psychological, physical, social or spiritual. Veach et al[12] describe the transition for patients and families as a shift from the 'long haul' of active treatment to a state of limbo in which it is easy to become immobilized by feelings of loss of control. It is at this time that support for rehabilitation may be particularly important, to ensure that the experience of cancer can be integrated into the rest of the person's life. However, the threat of cancer is always there and 'survivors' continue to live 'under the sword of Damocles'.[12]

Veach et al[12] illustrate that the needs of individuals and families during these transitions may differ considerably, depending on the stage of the family life cycle (Table 36.4). Unfortunately, little research has been done to chart the experience of close family members,[43] particularly once treatment is finished.

MAKING REHABILITATION AND SURVIVORSHIP A REALITY: THE ROLE OF THE NURSE

Oncology nurses play a pivotal role in rehabilitation and survivorship. As Wells[4] pointed

---

[a] Durkheim suggests that particular societies define what is normal for their society and that a lack of social norms or conflict between them leads to a moral lawlessness, known as 'anomie'. Durkheim E. The rules of sociological method, tr Halls WD, ed. London: Stephen Lukes; 1982.

Table 36.4: Rehabilitation and the family life cycle during times of transition and limbo

Stage of life	Life cycle tasks	Issues for rehabilitation
Single young adult	Establishing self in the world of work; forming intimate relationships	Confidence, self-image, future career and relationships, body image, sexuality, independence (particularly financial and social)
Newly forming couple	Negotiating roles; balancing power; determining responsibilities; accepting new members into the family	Expectations of self and partner, sexual concerns, body image, fertility, disruption to future plans and boundaries
Family with young children	Changing roles; becoming parents; parents becoming grandparents	Ability to fulfil own expectations of parental role, fears for young children and partner (particularly in relation to recurrence and death), physical and emotional strength for childcare and daily activities, financial worries, appearance, separation from children during periods of hospitalization, hopes for children's future
Family with adolescents	Creating flexible boundaries; adapting to external influences	Tension between adolescents needs for loosening of boundaries and patient's needs for support and assistance, importance of social appearances for adolescent
Family with young adult children who may be leaving home	Creating new boundaries; reassessing life and friendships; addressing midlife concerns	Uncertainty for parents and children, disruption to established roles and relationships, self-doubt, loss, balance between young adult's needs for independence and patient's needs for support and familiarity
Family in later life	Adapting to changes in roles, responsibilities and relationships	Disruption to plans for retirement, financial concerns, lack of purpose and self-worth, stress on carers, potential or actual physical disability in the context of later life

Source: © 2002. From: Cancer and the family life cycle: a practitioner's guide by Veach T, Nicholas D, Barton M. Reproduced by permission of Routledge/Taylor & Francis Books, Inc.

out: 'nursing more than any other health care profession, is an integrative discipline'. Nurses are in a position to assess patients' needs for rehabilitation and to coordinate care, communicate with members of the multiprofessional team, and provide information, education and physical, practical and psychosocial support to patients and their families.

Waters[44] illustrates the role of the nurse in rehabilitation by the use of a mnemonic:

Risk taker
Enabler
Healer
Achiever
Befriender
Imagination (use of)
Love (giver of moderated)
Independence (facilitator of)
Treatment (giver of)
Adviser
Teacher
Intimate care (giver of)
Organizer
Nurturer

Nurses are in a unique position in that they are involved in the care of patients with cancer at all stages of the cancer journey. Nurses provide supportive care and education, assess symptoms and psychological and social needs and have led many initiatives concerned with improving the quality of rehabilitation and survivorship.[45] Even when specific rehabilitation programmes do not exist, nurses play a key coordinating role within the multidisciplinary team, and are able to support the patient and family's position at the centre of this team (Fig. 36.2).

Effective rehabilitation requires investment and commitment within healthcare teams and organizations. The shortage of acute beds for cancer patients in most hospitals and the emphasis on treatment and speedy discharge almost certainly reduces the opportunity to address rehabilitative needs comprehensively. Lack of funding for allied health professionals such as occupational therapists, physiotherapists and dietitians can also be a major barrier to rehabilitation. In addition, poor assessment and a lack of understanding about the potential contribution of allied health professionals can restrict the number of appropriate referrals and the effectiveness of multidisciplinary team-working.[46,47]

It is essential that nurses maximize the potential of multidisciplinary teams and refocus care towards issues of rehabilitation and survivorship from the point of diagnosis or admission to hospital. In order to do this, nurses need to be better equipped to meet patients needs for rehabilitation and survivorship. A recent US survey has concluded that rehabilitation and survivorship issues are insufficiently addressed in published work and that healthcare professionals receive inadequate training and education in these vital aspects of care.[45] UK authors have also highlighted that nurses may need training and support to address issues of social and psychological rehabilitation.[48] This survey of 79 nurses working in areas of head and neck or burns and plastic surgery found that nurses rated their skills as significantly weaker in dealing with aspects such as social interaction, eating in public, taking the initiative or sexual issues. Nurses were much more comfortable with physical aspects of rehabilitation such as managing pain, dealing with tracheostomies or applying pressure garments. The study demonstrated that the provision of a short training programme and resource manual resulted in statistically significant improvements in the perceived skills and confidence of head and neck nurses towards social rehabilitation. Pilot work also suggested that benefits to nurses are transferable to patients who value learning skills for coping with social situations.

The training programme provided for nurses in this study involved considerable input from a lay-led organization in the UK, called Changing Faces. There is no doubt that the potential contribution of voluntary, lay-led and professional charities towards rehabilitation is huge. Information and support centres for patients with cancer, such as the Maggie's Centres (see Useful websites section) in the UK, often run 'living with cancer' programmes (which address issues of nutrition, appearance, relaxation, support, information-seeking, self-help activities, coping strategies and complementary therapies). Gertrude Grahn's work has been influential in the development of such programmes across Europe, and has illustrated that supportive education initiatives can promote positive coping strategies and improve confidence.[49-51]

One of the challenges for healthcare professionals who are organizing such programmes is

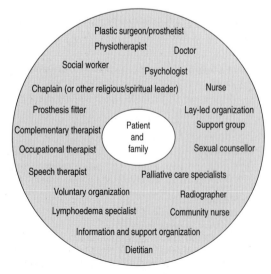

Figure 36.2: The multiprofessional team in rehabilitation.

to facilitate and enable patients from all backgrounds and disease types to attend. There is evidence to suggest that middle class white females are more likely to participate in support groups,[52] and it is possible that this extends to rehabilitation programmes. However, programmes specifically designed for men with cancer can be successful, particularly when activity-orientated interventions are employed.[53] Interest in group participation may be affected by age, sex, level of education, encouragement from medical doctors, beliefs in the usefulness of the group and level of social support outside the group.[54] The extent to which patients perceive they are affected by physical and psychological problems may also be influential. Berglund et al[54] studied participants and non-participants in a randomized trial of a rehabilitation programme for patients with cancer. They found that patients who chose to participate in the trial had higher levels of symptoms, anxiety, depression, cognitive problems, fatigue and other problems than those who chose not to take part. Participants were significantly more likely to be female and have breast cancer, but after adjustment for gender, differences remained. The intervention group (who participated in the rehabilitation programme) had improved 'problem' levels in terms of information, physical strength and fighting spirit during the first year after the intervention, compared with non-participants. Improvements in fatigue, quality of life and other factors also occurred, but these were most likely to be attributed to improvements over time, rather than directly to the intervention. Interestingly, the intervention appeared to have no effect on anxiety, depression, worry, helplessness or anxious preoccupation. The baseline scores of non-participants were lower in all these areas, and remained lower than the scores of participants, 1 year after the programme.

The findings of this study indicate that patients who take part in rehabilitation programmes may well be different from those who do not, and that, despite perceived improvements in well-being, patients' underlying psychological characteristics and coping styles may be difficult to change. This is an interesting finding, given that many psychological interventions are designed to enhance particular coping mechanisms that may prolong survival.[55] A systematic review of the literature concludes that psychological coping styles do not play an important part in survival from or recurrence of cancer, and that patients should not feel pressurized into adopting such styles.[55] However, it must be acknowledged that patients themselves attach importance to self-care and positive thinking, and that such strategies should be facilitated where appropriate.[56]

It is clear that successful rehabilitation programmes must incorporate a wide range of activities for patients with different coping styles, physical symptoms, functional problems and social situations. Fundamental elements of rehabilitation include assessment, education, symptom management, goal-setting and reintegration. Strobel[57] describes a rehabilitation programme that incorporates aspects of physical and psychosocial support and therapy as well as information and training to help people to live with cancer. Physical components of the programme include exercise, physiotherapy, 'medical' support from healthcare professionals (such as symptom management) and manual lymph drainage (for lymphoedema). Psychosocial components include intervention from a psychologist, relaxation and visualization, art therapy and occupational therapy. Information and training courses address all aspects of living with cancer, including diet, prosthesis management and prevention of physical and psychological problems. Strobel[57] states that such a programme can improve symptoms, functional problems, well-being, sleep, strength and energy, and integration into work.

Resources for patients also exist to facilitate survivorship, although these are most well developed in the USA. The best known example is the Cancer Survivor Toolbox (see Useful websites section); a self-advocacy training programme developed by the National Coalition for Cancer Survivorship, the Association of Oncology Social Work and the Oncology Nursing Society (see Useful websites) section. Available in audiocassette form in English and Spanish, the training programme addresses five key aspects of survivorship and is designed to help survivors of cancer develop skills in communication, information-seeking, problem-solving, decision-making and negotiating. A survey of 569 patients and 833 healthcare professionals in the USA[58] found that most did not feel that people with cancer possessed skills of self-advocacy. The authors piloted the Cancer Survival Toolbox with 35 patients of mixed sex, race and diagnosis and elicited feedback. Comments from these survivors illustrated that the training programme had helped them to feel more in control, to participate in decisions and discussions with their doctors and to deal with difficult situations.

RESHAPING CARE FOR SURVIVORS OF CANCER

If rehabilitation and survivorship are to be integrated more effectively, there is a need to reshape the services we provide. Not only must we consider patients' *future* quality of life at the point of diagnosis and throughout treatment but we must also address, more effectively, the needs of patients after treatment is complete. The end of treatment naturally coincides with the cessation of intense monitoring and support provided by the treatment centre. At this time, patients are usually 'discharged' into follow-up, and may not have contact with a healthcare professional for several weeks or months until they, or the health professional, perceives a 'reason' to initiate contact. Evidence suggests that follow-up clinics do not necessarily coincide with problems experienced by patients, and that routine investigations may not be a useful means of detecting recurrence or improving survival.[59,60] Qualitative studies illustrate that patients who have completed treatment may be less likely to seek support, help or advice because they feel their 'share of attention has been used up'[61] and that their concerns are unimportant and less legitimate than those of patients still on treatment.[62]

It has been suggested that this hospital- and physician-centred tradition should be replaced by what patients themselves want and expect from follow-up care.[63] One survivor of testicular cancer described the follow-up clinic as 'psychologically meaningless, a relapse searching conveyor belt'.[64] Certainly, there is little opportunity within most busy follow-up clinics to address psychological, support or existential concerns in any depth. In any case, many patients underplay what they see as insignificant symptoms or concerns because they want everything to be all right.[62] It is vitally important that patients' appearances of being 'well' do not mislead healthcare professionals into believing that they have no needs for support.[25,65]

It is clear that many patients gain particular reassurance from the follow-up clinic, despite experiencing considerable worry during the week before their hospital appointment.[66] Alternative methods of follow-up, which aim to provide the reassurance of being monitored within a more supportive and flexible patient-centred model of care, have recently been evaluated. Nurse-led follow-up has been shown to be as effective as medical follow-up in terms of survival and symptom management, and is associated with greater patient satisfaction.[67] It appears that nurse-led services can be more responsive to patients' needs and can improve communication and coordination between primary and secondary care, thus reducing the number of hospital appointments and even the probability of dying in hospital.[67]

CONCLUSION

Integrating rehabilitation and survivorship issues into everyday practice is essential to the delivery of high-quality care for patients with cancer. Cancer changes people's lives, and cancer nurses are in a unique position to assess the changes that are most difficult, support patients through these changes and contribute to improving quality of life *as it is defined by patients themselves*. Regaining some sort of normality during and after the experience of cancer is extremely challenging. It is vital that nurses address the physical, psychological, support and existential concerns and needs of patients throughout this experience so that effective rehabilitation takes place and the *quality* as well as quantity of survival is as near as possible to what the patient would like it to be.

As the cancer population increases and improvements in treatment and toxicity management continue, the focus of cancer care is shifting towards the needs of patients who are *living with cancer*. Nurses must start to incorporate the goals of rehabilitation and survivorship more effectively into their work and to fully acknowledge the patient's experience of cancer within the context of the rest of their life. Nurses have a responsibility to look beyond patients' immediate needs and to consider the *future* impact of cancer and its treatment on quality of life. Strengthening our focus on rehabilitation and survivorship issues in practice, education and research provides the basis for ensuring that this happens.

USEFUL WEBSITES

http://www.cansearch.org/ National Coalition for Cancer Survivorship
http://www.cansearch.org/programs/tool-box.htm The Cancer Survival Toolbox
http://www.ons.org Oncology Nursing Society
http://www.cancerbacup.org BACUP 'What now?: Adjusting to life after cancer'
http://www.maggiescentres.org Maggie's Cancer Caring Centres UK

REFERENCES

1. Mullan F. Seasons of survival: reflections of a physician with cancer. N Engl J Med 1985;313(4):270–273.
2. DeLisa JA. A history of cancer rehabilitation. Cancer Suppl 2001; 92(4):970–974.
3. van Harten WH, Van Noort O, Warmerdam R, Hendricks H, Seidel E. Assessment of rehabilitation needs in cancer patients. Int J Rehabil Res 1998; 21:247–257.
4. Wells RJ. Rehabilitation: making the most of time. Oncol Nurs Forum 1990; 17(4):503–507.
5. Seigel K, Christ G. Hodgkins disease survivorship: psychological consequences. In: Lacher M, Redman J, eds. Hodgkin's disease: The consequences of survival. Philadelphia: Febiger; 1990:383–399.
6. Leigh SA. Cancer rehabilitation: a consumer perspective. Semin Oncol Nurs 1992; 8(3):164–166.
7. Zerbrack B. Cancer survivors and quality of life: a critical review of the literature. Oncol Nurs Forum 2000 ;27(9):1395–1401.
8. Corner J. Beyond survival rates and side-effects: cancer nursing as therapy. Cancer Nurs 1997; 20(1):3–11.
9. Mayer D, O'Connor L. Rehabilitation of persons with cancer: an ONS position statement. Oncol Nurs Forum 1989; 16(3):433.
10. Gunn AE. Cancer rehabilitation. New York: Raven Press; 1984.
11. Dudas S, Carlson C. Cancer rehabilitation. Oncol Nurs Forum 1988; 15:183–188.
12. Veach T, Nicholas D, Barton M. Cancer and the family life cycle: a practitioner's guide. New York: Brunner-Routledge; 2002.
13. Calman KC. Quality of life in cancer patients – an hypothesis. J Med Ethics 1984; 10(3):124–127.
14. Aaronson H, Ahmedzai S, Bergman B, et al. The European Organization for Research and Treatment of Cancer QLQ-C30: a quality of life instrument for use in international clinical trials in oncology. J Natl Cancer Inst 1993; 85:365–376.
15. Cella D, Tulsky D, Gray G, et al. The functional assessment of cancer therapy (FACT) scale: development and validation of the general measure. J Clin Oncol 1993; 11(3):570–579.
16. Ruta D, Garratt A, Leng M, Russell I, MacDonald L. A new approach to the measurement of quality of life. The Patient-Generated Index. Med Care 1994; 32(11):1109–1126.
17. Cohen S, Mount B, Thomas J, Mount L. Existential wellbeing is an important determinant of quality of life. Cancer 1996; 77(3):576–586.
18. Kirshblum S, O'Dell MW, Ho C, Barr K. Rehabilitation of persons with central nervous system tumors. Am Cancer Soc 2001; 92(4):1029–1038.
19. Scialla S, Cole R, Scialla T, Bednarz L, Scheerer J. Rehabilitation for elderly patients with cancer asthenia: making a transition to palliative care. Palliat Med 2000; 14(2):121–127.
20. Diamond J. C. Because cowards get cancer too. London: Vermilion; 1998.
21. Wells M. The impact of radiotherapy to the head and neck: a qualitative study of patients after completion of treatment. MSc thesis. London; 1995.
22. Seaton M. After words. In: Picardie R, ed. Before I say goodbye. London: Penguin; 1998.
23. Ronson A, Body J. Psychosocial rehabilitation of cancer patients after curative therapy. Support Care Cancer 2002; 10:281–291.
24. Loge J, Abrahamsen A, Ekeberg O, Hannisdal E, Kaasa S. Psychological distress after cancer cure: a survey of 459 Hodgkin's disease survivors. Br J Cancer 1997; 76(6):791–796.
25. Loescher LJ, Clark L, Atwood JR, Leigh S, Lamb G. The impact of the cancer experience on long-term survivors. Oncol Nurs Forum 1990; 17(2):223–229.
26. Wallwork L, Richardson A. Beyond cancer: changes, problems and needs expressed by

adult lymphoma survivors attending an out-patients clinic. Eur J Cancer Care 1994; 3(3):122–132.

27. Naysmith A, Hinton J, Meredith R, Marks M, Berry R. Surviving malignant disease: psychological and family aspects. Br J Hosp Med 1983; 30:22–27.

28. Ferrell BR, Dow KH, Leigh S, Ly L, Gulasekaram P. Quality of life in long-term cancer survivors. Oncol Nurs Forum 1995; 22:915–922.

29. Dow KH, Ferrell BR, Haberman MR, Easton L. The meaning of quality of life in cancer survivorship. Oncol Nurs Forum 1999; 26 (3):519–528.

30. Nicholson C, Wells M. After treatment is over. In: Faithfull S, Wells M, eds. Supportive care in radiotherapy. Edinburgh: Churchill Livingstone; 2003:60–70.

31. Hoffman B. Cancer survivors at work: job problems and illegal discrimination. Oncol Nurs Forum 1989; 16(1):39–43.

32. Mundy R, Moore S, Mundy G. A missing link: rehabilitation counseling for persons with cancer. J Rehabil 2001; April/May/June:47–49.

33. Spelten ER, Sprangers MAG, Verbeek JHAM. Factors reported to influence the return to work of cancer survivors: a literature review. Psycho-oncology 2002; 11(2):124–131.

34. Silverberg E, Lubera J. Cancer survivors' bill of rights. Cancer 1998; 3:32.

35. Dirksen S. Search for meaning in long-term cancer survivors. J Adv Nurs 1995; 21:628–633.

36. Luker KA, Beaver K, Leinster SJ, Owens RG. Meaning of illness for women with breast cancer. J Adv Nurs 1996; 23:1194–1201.

37. Breaden K. Cancer and beyond: the question of survivorship. J Adv Nurs 1997; 26:978–984.

38. Molassiotis A. Psychological transitions in the long-term survivors of bone marrow transplantation. Eur J Cancer Care 1997; 6(2):100–107.

39. O'Connor A, Wicker C. Clinical commentary: promoting meaning in the lives of cancer survivors. Semin Oncol Nurs 1995; 11:68–72.

40. Maher E. Anomic aspects of recovery from cancer. Soc Sci Med 1982; 16(8):907–912.

41. Frank A. At the will of the body. Reflections on illness. Boston: Houghton Mifflin; 1991.

42. Schumacker K, Meleis A. Transitions: a central concept in nursing. Image J Nurs Scholarship 1994; 26(2):119–127.

43. Mellon S, Northouse LL. Family survivorship and quality of life following a cancer diagnosis. Res Nurs Health 2001; 24:446–459.

44. Waters K. The role of nursing in rehabilitation care. Sci Pract 1987; 5(3):17–21.

45. Ferrell BR, Virani R, Smith S, Juarez G. The role of oncology nursing to ensure quality care for cancer survivors: a report commissioned by the National Cancer Policy Board and Institute of Medicine. Oncol Nurs Forum 2003; 30(1):E1–E11.

46. Soderback I, Paulsson EH. A needs assessment for referral to occupational therapy. Cancer Nurs 1997; 20(4):267–273.

47. Fulton C. Physiotherapists in cancer care. A framework for rehabilitation of patients. Physiotherapy 1994; 80(12):830–834.

48. Clarke A, Cooper C. Psychosocial rehabilitation after disfiguring injury or disease: investigating the training needs of specialist nurses. J Adv Nurs 2001; 34(1):18–26.

49. Grahn G. 'Learning to cope' – an intervention in cancer care. Support Care Cancer 1993; 1:266–271.

50. Grahn G. Coping with the cancer experience 1. Eur J Cancer Care 1996; 5:176–181.

51. Grahn G. Coping with the cancer experience 2. Eur J Cancer Care 1996; 5:182–187.

52. Taylor S. Social support, support groups and the cancer patient. J Consult Clin Psychol 1986; 54:608–615.

53. Adamsen L, Ramsussen J, Pederson L. 'Brothers in arms': how men with cancer experience a sense of comradeship through group intervention which combines physical activity with information relay. J Clin Nurs 2001;10(4):528–537.

54. Berglund G, Bolund C, Gustafsson U, Sjoden P. Is the wish to participate in a cancer rehabilitation program an indicator of the need? Comparisons of participants and non-participants in a randomized study? Psycho-oncology 1997; 6:35–46.

55. Petticrew M, Bell R, Hunter D. Influence of psychological coping on survival and recurrence in people with cancer: systematic review. BMJ 2002; 325(7372):1066.

56. Vass A. Website of the week: coping with cancer. BMJ 2002; 325:1120.

57. Strobel ES. Physical and psychosocial rehabilitation of cancer patients. Front Radiat Ther Oncol 2002; 37:38–42.

58. Walsh-Burke K, Marcusen C. Self-advocacy training for cancer survivors. The Cancer Survival Toolbox. Cancer Pract 1999; 7(6):297–301.

59. Brada M. Is there a need to follow-up cancer patients? Eur J Cancer 1995; 31A(5):655–657.

60. Impact of follow-up testing on survival and health-related quality of life in breast cancer patients. A multicenter randomized controlled trial. The GIVIO Investigators. JAMA 1994; 271(20):1587–1592.

61. Bury M. The sociology of chronic illness: a review of research and prospects. Sociol Health Illness 1991; 13(4):451–468.

62. Wells M. The hidden experience of radiotherapy to the head and neck: a qualitative study of patients after completion of treatment. J Adv Nurs 1998; 28(4):840–848.

63. Brada M. Is there a need to follow-up cancer patients? Eur J Cancer Care 1995; 31A:655–657.

64. Johansson S, Steineck G, Hursti T, et al. Aspects of patient care: interviews with relapse-free testicular cancer patients in Stockholm. Cancer Nurs 1992; 15(1):54–60.

65. Ferrell BR, Grant M, Funk B, Otis-Green S, Garcia N. Quality of life in breast cancer survivors: implications for developing support services. Oncol Nurs Forum 1998; 25(5):887–895.

66. MacBride SK, Whyte F. Attendance at cancer follow-up clinic: does it increase anxiety or provide reassurance for men successfully treated for testicular cancer. Cancer Nurs 1999; 22(6):448–455.

67. Moore S, Corner J, Haviland J, et al. Nurse-led follow-up and conventional medical follow-up in management of patients with lung cancer: randomised trial. BMJ 2002; 325:1145–1147.

68. Guerrero D, ed. Neuro-oncology for nurses. London: Whurr; 1998.

69. Khoo V, Faithfull S. Late toxicity:neurological and brachial plexus injury. In: Faithfull S, Wells M, eds. Supportive care in radiotherapy. Edinburgh: Churchill Livingstone; 2003:268–286.

70. Williams A. Lymphoedema. In: Faithfull S, Wells M, eds. Supportive care in radiotherapy. Edinburgh: Churchill Livingstone; 2003:287–302.

71. Khoo V. Other late effects. In: Faithfull S, Wells M, eds. Supportive care in radiotherapy. Edinburgh: Churchill Livingstone; 2003:348–371.

72. Dryden H. Body image. Faithfull S, Wells M, eds. Supportive care in radiotherapy. Edinburgh: Churchill Livingstone; 2003:320–336.

73. Feber T. Head and neck oncology nursing. London: Whurr; 2000.

74. Wells M. Oropharyngeal effects. In: Faithfull S, Wells M, eds. Supportive care in radiotherapy. Edinburgh: Churchill Livingstone; 2003:182–203.

75. Ireland J, Wells M. The effects of radiotherapy on nutritional status. In: Faithfull S, Wells M, eds. Supportive care in radiotherapy. Edinburgh: Churchill Livingstone; 2003:204–226.

76. Grundy M, Bratt-Wyton R, eds. Nursing in haematological oncology. Edinburgh: Ballière Tindall; 2000.

77. Gillis TA, Donovan ES. Rehabilitation following bone marrow transplantation. Am Cancer Soc 2001; 92(4):998–1007.

78. White I, Faithfull S. Sexuality and fertility. In: Faithfull S, Wells M, eds. Supportive care in radiotherapy. Edinburgh: Churchill Livingstone; 2003:303–319.

79. McKee AL, Schover LR. Sexuality rehabilitation. Cancer 2001; 92(4):1008–1012.

80. Faithfull S. Gastrointestinal effects of radiotherapy. In: Faithfull S, Wells M, eds. Supportive care in radiotherapy. Edinburgh: Churchill Livingstone; 2003:247–267.

81. Faithfull S. Urinary symptoms and radiotherapy. In: Faithfull S, Wells M, eds. Supportive care in radiotherapy. Edinburgh: Churchill Livingstone; 2003:227–246.

82. Corner J, Plant H, A'Hern R, Bailey C. Non-pharmacological interventions for breathlessness in lung cancer. Palliat Med 1996; 10:299–305.

83. Wells M. Pain and breathing problems. In: Faithfull S, Wells M, eds. Supportive care in radiotherapy. Edinburgh: Churchill Livingstone; 2003:160–181.

84. Dietz JH. Rehabilitation oncology. New York: John Wiley and Sons; 1981.

CHAPTER 37

Palliative Care

SALLY MIRANDO

CHAPTER CONTENTS

Introduction	821
Development of palliative care	821
Definitions and principles of palliative care and supportive care	822
Supportive care	823
Access to palliative care	824
Locations and delivery of care	824
Specialist palliative care services	824
Specialist palliative interventions	825
Role of the nurse	825
Key characteristics of the role	825
Core competencies	827
Specialist nursing	827
Patient and family care	828

General assessment	828
Symptom assessment	830
Fostering hope	833
Multicultural views of hope	833
Quality of life	837
Family care	839
Care of the dying	840
Diagnosing dying	841
Common issues in the dying phase	841
Emergency situations at the end of life	843
Future challenges in palliative care	844
References	844

INTRODUCTION

Palliative care is a comparatively new speciality, yet is now acknowledged as an essential component of modern health care by a growing number of European countries. Although there is great diversity in palliative care provision across Europe, which relates in part to differences in health policy as well as variations in preferences for particular models of care, palliative care is increasingly being established within the formal structures of government healthcare systems.

This chapter outlines the development of the speciality, the principles underpinning palliative care and the role of the nurse in the provision of palliative care. The importance of systematic and impeccable assessment of symptoms and quality of life, the care of those who will die from cancer and care in an emergency situation at the end of life are also examined.

DEVELOPMENT OF PALLIATIVE CARE

The development of palliative care is closely linked to the rise of the hospice movement, which followed the opening of St Christopher's Hospice in London in 1967 by Cicely Saunders.[1] The movement sought to humanize the care of the dying and provided a radical approach to the impersonal, medicalized, technological management of death reported to be occurring in hospitals at the time.[2] This was done in a number of ways: firstly, through the development of the concept of total pain and the belief that an individual's physical, emotional, social and spiritual concerns are inextricably twined, each potentially contributing to a 'total pain' experience; secondly, hospice philosophy gave emphasis to highly personalized care rather than cure, achievement of a good quality of life and the creation of an environment that as far as possible mirrored home. Importantly, it recognized the needs of family and friends and in doing so promoted the importance of support before and after the death of the patient. Clark[3,4] suggests that palliative care is a major innovation in modern health care, as it has retrieved an area of care previously neglected by health professionals.

Over the last 30 years palliative care has proliferated worldwide. Today, it is delivered in a variety of settings: inpatient facilities, home care services, day care and hospital consultancy services, staffed by multiprofessional teams of doctors, nurses, physiotherapists, occupational therapists, chaplains, dieticians, social workers and volunteers. Although the fundamental principles are the same,[5,6] their implementation has been adapted to suit a variety of demographic, cultural and policy factors.[7] For example, in Spain 80% of deaths take place in hospital. Increasing female participation in the workforce and a low birth rate has resulted in an emphasis on hospital palliative care. In Sweden, a government report in 1979 rejected the opening of hospices as the solution to improving care of the dying in preference for care at home and consulting teams. In Belgium, Royal decrees have set a comprehensive framework for the development of palliative care throughout the country where home care is seen as the most important focus, supported by health policy that incorporates a palliative aspect within general health care.[8]

DEFINITIONS AND PRINCIPLES OF PALLIATIVE CARE AND SUPPORTIVE CARE

Palliative care is:

. . . an approach that improves the quality of life of patients and their families facing the problems associated with life-threatening illness, through the prevention and relief of suffering by means of early identification and impeccable assessment and treatment of pain and other problems, physical, psychosocial and spiritual.[6]

Palliative care is based on the following principles:

Palliative care:

- Provides relief from pain and other distressing symptoms;
- Affirms life and regards dying as a normal process;
- Intends neither to hasten or postpone death;
- Integrates the psychological and spiritual aspects of patient care;
- Offers a support system to help patients live as actively as possible until death;
- Offers a support system to help the family cope during the patient's illness and in their own bereavement;
- Uses a team approach to address the needs of patients and their families, including bereavement counselling, if indicated;
- Will enhance quality of life, and may also positively influence the course of illness;
- Is applicable early in the course of illness, in conjunction with other therapeutics that are intended to prolong life, such as chemotherapy or radiation therapy, and includes those investigations needed to better understand and manage distressing clinical complications.[6]

Figure 37.1 shows the essential components that underpin the successful delivery of palliative care.

There is now wide recognition that if palliative care is applied as early as possible in the course of any chronic life-threatening illness the quality of life and also length of life may be positively affected through mediation of the cytokine-stress reaction associated with symptoms.[6]

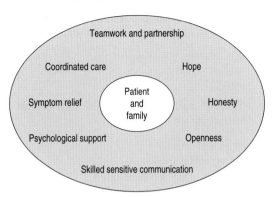

Figure 37.1: The essential components of palliative care. (Adapted from Twycross 2003[9] with permission of Radcliffe Medical Press.)

Box 37.1

The core elements and domains of supportive care[12]

Self-help and support
User involvement
Information-giving
Psychological support
Symptom control
Social support
Rehabilitation
Complementary therapies
Spiritual support
Palliative care
End-of-life care
Services for families and bereavement care

Supportive care

In the context of cancer care, supportive care has emerged as a term to represent a range of care that is provided in addition to curative treatments for cancer patients. It is often used in conjunction with palliative care to describe essential good care that helps the patient and family cope with cancer and its treatment from pre-diagnosis to cure or after death. It is given equal priority alongside diagnosis and treatment as the principles and domains of patient and family care are similar at all stages of the cancer journey. The European Oncology Nursing Society Core Curriculum for a Post-registration Course in Cancer Nursing[10] utilize the term and in England the National Health Service Cancer Plan[11] makes a commitment to develop a supportive and palliative care strategy. As part of this strategy, evidence-based guidance was published in 2004 by The National Institute for Clinical Excellence (NICE).[12] NICE is part of the UK National Health Service (NHS), and its role is to provide patients, health professionals and the public with authoritative, robust and reliable guidance on current 'best practice'.

Although palliative care has a variable foundation in European health policy, the supportive care needs of patients and families at all stages of the cancer journey are increasingly acknowledged: this, coupled with a growing ageing population, many of whom will live with many forms of chronic life-limiting illness, including cancer, is likely to lead to greater integration of palliative and supportive care in the future (Box 37.1).

Unlike palliative care, supportive care is not a distinct specialty and is informed by theories, models, frameworks and evidence from a wide variety of sources. However, as with palliative care, it is the responsibility of all health and social care professionals, whether a generalist or specialist, whatever the stage of disease or care setting. Figure 37.2 illustrates the relationship between treatment, supportive care and palliative care.

Services that contribute to the supportive and palliative care of patients and families include:

- specialist palliative care services
- specialist psychological and psychiatric services
- social care services
- rehabilitation services
- specialist pain services
- complementary therapy services
- palliative interventions, e.g. radiotherapy, surgery
- information, advice and resource centres (National Council for Hospice and Specialist Palliative Care Services (NCHSPCS))[13]

From this brief overview it can be seen that palliative care is one component of supportive care and, as such, should be available to all cancer patients. It exists alongside other forms

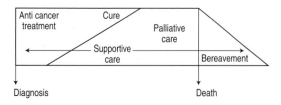

Figure 37.2: The relationship between supportive care and palliative care. (Adapted from: Continuum of Care, World Health Organisation (WHO), 2002,[6] with permission of WHO).

of care and may take greater or lesser importance, depending on the stage of the disease and the preferences and concerns of the patient. Palliative care is particularly important when a person's cancer is no longer curable. At this time, investigations and treatments can become increasingly inappropriate and should only be used when benefits outweigh burdens. Although palliative care acknowledges that cure is no longer possible, as Wilkinson[14] states, this 'does not signify defeat, but demands a change in perspective – a shift from dying from a terminal illness to living with a life-threatening illness'.

Access to palliative care

While one of the precepts of palliative care is the promotion of equitable access, there can be considerable difficulties with access to services. This is due to a variety of reasons, including reluctance on the part of professionals to involve specialist palliative care services because they believe it infers inevitable death and for the patients, families and public the reliance on medical intervention to delay death at all costs.[15,16] However, palliative care is an exercise in health prevention – prevention of suffering through the prompt diagnosis and skilful management of physical symptoms and psychosocial and spiritual concerns, at the earliest possible moment.

Locations and delivery of care

There is a move worldwide to ensure that each WHO member state establishes a national policy and programme for pain relief and palliative care. This is to ensure that:

- each country incorporates palliative care into existing healthcare systems
- minimum standards for pain relief and palliative care are adopted by all levels of care
- health workers are trained in cancer pain relief and palliative care
- specialist support is available
- programmes for home support and primary care are developed
- opioids, especially oral morphine, are accessible and available.[6]

Throughout the world, palliative care is developing in a variety of ways[17] and home-based care is generally promoted as the best way of achieving good-quality care.[6] In essence, palliative care is delivered by two distinct groups of staff:

1. All professional carers who are involved in caring for people with life-threatening illnesses.
2. Specialist palliative care services.

Specialist palliative care services

Specialist palliative care (SPC) is provided by practitioners who have specialist qualifications and experience in the care of palliative care patients and their families. These practitioners might work in the community, hospital or hospice service and often belong to a multiprofessional SPC team. They may provide advice in an advisory capacity or can assume responsibility for the patient's and family care. A range of services may be offered from home care, medical and nursing consultations, outpatient clinics, day care, inpatient care, bereavement support, education and research. Studies in the UK confirm that intervention from SPC improves symptom control.[18–20] SPC involvement is particularly relevant for patients with complex and difficult symptoms and care needs. Referral is particularly recommended for:

- patients with symptoms that are difficult to control (e.g. when no relief has been achieved within 48 hours)
- patients with numerous symptoms

- patients with rapidly progressive disease
- psychosocial, spiritual distress
- complex end of life problems
- young patients, or patients with young children in the family
- where reassurance of a second opinion is sought.[21]

Specialist palliative interventions

Specialist palliative interventions are non-curative treatments aimed specifically at modifying the illness. They are usually performed by specialists in oncology or surgery (e.g. brachytherapy for bleeding, insertion of a stent for dysphagia, radiotherapy for superior vena cava obstruction and spinal cord compression, prophylactic orthopaedic pinning of a bone at risk of fracture from a bone secondary).

ROLE OF THE NURSE

Nurses are often inadequately prepared for dealing with those facing death and the inadequacies of what nurses do when a patient is dying were first highlighted in sociological studies by Glaser and Strauss,[22,23] Strauss and Glaser[24] and Sudnow.[25] Quint,[26] a coresearcher in the team at the time, went on to publish further work about nursing the dying, and her work remains relevant today. These accounts have been substantiated by more systematic studies,[27,28] and there is evidence that nurses continue to find caring for dying people stressful, experiencing feelings of inadequacy, particularly with symptom control.[29–32] A more recent phenomenological study[33] of 28 qualified nurses highlights that nurses also found difficulty talking with dying patients and their families and felt unskilled and unprepared for this aspect of their role. These practitioners perceived that observing expert practitioners, seeking advice and obtaining feedback on their own performance would help them develop confidence and competence.

As there is strong evidence to suggest that nurses are inadequately prepared for caring for palliative care patients, it may be helpful to consider the key characteristics of the role of the nurse in palliative care. Nurses can match these against their own level of skill, knowledge and competence and begin to understand strengths and weaknesses in their practice. Suggestions of how competence can be developed are outlined in the 'specialist nursing' section of this chapter.

Key characteristics of the role

The role of the nurse in palliative care has been defined in a variety of ways. Table 37.1 summarizes the main studies conducted with nurses, whereas Table 37.2 lists studies that have explored patients' perspectives.

Cancer as a life-threatening disease has implications for the physical, psychological, social and spiritual well-being of both the individual and their family. Above all, fostering an environment that allows the patient and family to retain a sense of control and dignity is the foundation of good palliative nursing and, for this, the human qualities of compassion, empathy, being able to provide comfort, combined with knowledge, experience, good communication skills and a confidence to 'be with' those facing the devastating impact of life-threatening illness are essential.[50] In particular, the ability to provide comfort which Penson[51] suggests involves more than the relief of pain and symptoms is the cornerstone of palliative nursing. Comfort has been defined as a key concept in palliative nursing[52] and has also been highlighted in two studies aimed at exploring palliative care professionals' perceptions of good and bad deaths.[53,54] These studies of palliative care professionals in the United Kingdom and Australian nurses, respectively, emphasize the particular importance of comfort during the dying phase.

In practice, comfort may be conveyed through listening, acceptance, touch and attendance to the fine details of physical care and appearance. In summary, several important concepts in palliative nursing can be identified from this brief review and are shown in Box 37.2.

Table 37.1: Studies exploring nurses' perspectives of the nursing role in palliative care

Main role descriptors	Author
Supportive	Heslin and Bramwell[34]
Valuing, connecting, doing for, preserving integrity, finding meaning, empowering	Davies and O'Berle[35,36]
Intense caring, continuous knowing, continuous giving	Dobratz[37]
Hope	Herth;[38,39] Herth and Cutcliffe[40]
Providing comfort. Responding to anger, colleagues and the family. Enhancing the quality of life and personal growth. Responding during the death scene	Degner et al[41]
Biomedical, social–therapeutic and informal	Hunt[42]
Developing an empathic, supportive relationship	Raudonis[43]
Assessing needs, listening, establishing empathy, eliciting and giving information, recognizing situations requiring referral, representing patient and family needs to others	Webber[44]
A systematic integrated approach to comfort (for palliative care patients in the intensive care setting)	McClement and Degner;[45] Stroud[46]

Source: adapted from Johnston 1999,[47] with permission of Churchill Livingstone.

Table 37.2: Studies exploring patients' perspectives of the nursing role in palliative care

Patients' perspectives	Author
24-hour accessibility Effective communication Clinical competence Non-judgemental attitude	Hull[48]
Reciprocal sharing in the context of caring and acceptance Being acknowledged as an individual and a person of value	Raudonis[43]
Personal interactions and qualities: reliable, honest, genuine, caring, understanding Professional interactions and qualities: knowledgeable, decisive, advisor, practical help, liaison, symptom relief	Richardson[49]

Key concepts in palliative nursing

Caring
Comfort
Hope
Dignity
Support
Genuineness
Empathy and listening
Quality of life
Relieving suffering
Knowing the individual and their family
Teamwork
Clinical competence

Core competencies

Considering the literature, qualified nurses delivering palliative care should be able to:

- Plan care, based on the patient and family's values, preferences, goals and needs.

- Encourage and maintain a patient's independence amidst uncertainty and an ever-changing progressive illness.

- Take account of cultural and spiritual diversity and how this may affect the experience of illness, symptom and end of life experience.

- Assess and relieve symptoms that affect quality of life.

- Assess, provide and facilitate the provision of psychosocial spiritual care.

- Assess and provide hope-giving care.

- Promote open and honest dialogue, elicit concerns and give a suitable level of information for the individual.

- Provide comfort.

- Represent the patient and family needs to others.

- Recognize the dying phase and put in place an appropriate plan of care.

- Provide sensitive support during bereavement and undertake a bereavement risk assessment if indicated.

- Have knowledge of local bereavement services.

- Recognize situations requiring referral for specialist advice.

- Work as a team, recognizing each member's expertise and value.

- Understand self and own attitudes to death and dying and the need for self-care.

Specialist nursing

Nurse specialists take on a number of indirect and direct care roles that encompass clinical practice, education, management, research and clinical leadership.[55,56] They can play an important part in the delivery of high-quality care to those with palliative care needs and particularly if able to develop practice from a personal to organizational level. Whereas there continues to be debate on the level of education and specialist experience required for such roles, Box 37.3 outlines the recommended competencies for specialist nursing in palliative care set by the Royal College of Nursing (RCN) in the UK.[57]

Competencies may be developed through a variety of training and development methods, including formal teaching, distance learning, action learning, learning contracts, portfolio, case review, coaching, skilled instruction, delegation, job rotation, secondment and acting up, clinical supervision and feedback.[58] These may involve self, peer, manager and educational assessment mechanisms. The development of clinical competencies in palliative care will enable nurses to advance the speciality in Europe, enhance and manage their own career pathway and deliver a model of excellence in palliative nursing.

Although there are issues with recognition of specialist nurses in Europe, development of competence and career pathways in palliative care is likely to include a balance of clinical experience and competency as well as academic requirements. Academic courses in palliative care are developing and the core curriculum in palliative nursing published by the International Society of Nurses in Cancer Care (ISNCC) may be of help to nurses in Europe.[59]

Box 37.3

Core elements of competency in specialist palliative nursing

Communication

Screen for psychological distress and deliver psychological interventions using a specific counselling or therapeutic model (such as anxiety management, problem solving) and guide others to improve skills.

Teach communication skills.

Quality assurance

Lead and support quality initiatives such as reflective practice, audit, risk assessment and analysis of significant events.

Develop standards, protocols and policies to support practice development and the delivery of a high standard of palliative nursing care.

Clinical practice

Rapidly synthesize complex clinical information to inform diagnosis and decision-making.

Explore, support and lead approaches to complex case management.

Education

Consistently draw on research and literature to influence the practice of self and others.

Use a variety of approaches to education, e.g. reflective diary, self-assessment, observation and critical analysis of practice, portfolio, supervision, education sessions, contributing and leading policy groups.

Management and leadership

Use audit, evaluation and research to influence palliative care at local, regional and national level.

Use networking and influencing skills to raise the profile of palliative care.

Research and development

Proactively disseminate and implement research findings.

Promote an environment where continuous enquiry is valued as a means to improve practice.

Support and lead research, evaluating results to change practice.

Grief, loss and bereavement

Use advanced counselling skills with patients and carers experiencing loss.

Be able to identify abnormal grief and loss, assess risk and refer to other services if needed.

Act as a supervisor and mentor to staff. Advice the bereaved on future care options.

Source: adapted from Royal College of Nursing 2002,[57] with permission of RCN.

PATIENT AND FAMILY CARE

General assessment

An effective palliative nursing assessment involves a systematic approach to identification of problems and sources of concern and distress to the patient and family. It is the key to establishing an appropriate care plan aimed at addressing the issues affecting quality of life.

Assessment can be carried out in three stages, is underpinned by certain principles and must follow a holistic framework. Stages of assessment include:

1 A careful review of the medical notes. A great deal of valuable information and time can be saved if nurses read the medical notes thoroughly before stage 2.

2 A brief interview with the patient and rapid appraisal of the clinical situation. In circumstances where a patient has distressing symptoms, such as pain, breathlessness, vomiting, haemorrhage or airway obstruction, immediate action will

be required. During stage 2, ideally, the patient is seen alone, as people can withhold information if they are seen with a relative or friend.[60]

3 A comprehensive focused assessment.[61]

Principles of assessment[62]

The principles of assessment are:

- establishing a relationship of trust
- identifying the patient's and family's needs
- prioritizing problems
- incorporating a multiprofessional approach
- making a nursing diagnosis.

Establishing a trusting relationship with the patient and family is essential and requires nurses to ask open questions and actively listen and believe what the patient tells us. The following quotations from palliative care patients who were asked what were the most important aspects of a nurse's care in the palliative care situation illustrate this point:

> They talk to you, they listen to you they don't just walk away.
> You just want people to just 'be there', just to listen, and you want to feel they are listening, not just stood there, just *be* there for me.[63]

Also, how devastating poor care can be:

> I felt as if staff wanted to get rid of me because I was ill, no one seemed to want to listen to me.
> It's nice to just talk to people and not for people to go cold and go away, or to just stand there then there's no warmth or care.[63]

Medical experts emphasize that during a medical assessment interview, in which a physician mostly listens and gently guides the patient's story, the physician can accurately diagnose the patient's problems 70–80% of the time.[64] There is no reason why this should not be applicable to nurses, but unfortunately there is evidence that nurses' and doctors' interpretation of a patient's experience can be affected by their own culture, social circumstances, ethnic background and beliefs.[60,65]

An open question such as, 'If I were to ask you how you are feeling today what would you like to say?', can give patients' permission to reveal their concerns and problems. While there are risks attached to this question, as the patient may ask difficult questions or present us with very challenging problems, this is the heart of good palliative care. Only if we do this, will we begin the process of 'knowing the patient',[66] which will help us to plan care based on the patient and family's values, preferences, goals and needs, and begin to gain understanding of cultural and spiritual diversity and how this may affect this patient's experience of illness, symptoms and end of life experience. It may also indicate whether your team can meet the patient and families needs or if you need to involve the additional expertise of SPC service.

Framework for assessment

The definition of palliative care highlights the holistic nature of the approach to care. It therefore follows that assessment is framed around the domains of physical, psychological, social and spiritual well-being. Many nursing models adopt a holistic approach to assessment, and these will not be presented here. However, at this point it may be helpful to consider assessment tools. With regard to palliative care patients, a tool should:

- help assess patient *and* family needs
- provide a holistic framework which can identify and assess the physical, psychological, social and spiritual needs of patients
- help identify the patient's coping strategies, culture, value and belief system and insight into their current situation
- help discover the future goals, hopes and aspirations of the patient
- help identify the patient and family's preferred place of care
- help identify other members of the interdisciplinary team (community, hospital and hospice) who may be involved in the patient and family's care

Many palliative care patients will present with complex problems, and making a good assessment and handling difficult situations are challenges to us all. This can make us want to use our power as health professionals to keep control of the situation by using blocking techniques, and closing patients down.[67] Communication issues such as these are comprehensively reviewed in Chapter 33 and therefore are not addressed here; however, poor communication such as this, has been shown to result in a flawed assessment, poor symptom control and compliance and unmet need on the part of the patient.[68-70]

Symptom assessment

Prevalence

Relief of distressing symptoms forms an important contribution to improving the quality of life of patients with advanced cancer and many patients can have multiple problems. Several studies have been undertaken to establish the prevalence of symptoms[71-73] and, while pain is often reported, others such as fatigue, anorexia, anxiety and sleeplessness have high prevalence but are not often given serious attention by medical and nursing staff. In the context of palliative care, symptoms often act as an ever-present negative reminder of advancing disease and can have a major impact on the ability to enjoy and participate in everyday activities.[74] Symptom experience can also focus attention on multiple losses, changing social and family role and confrontation with dying and death. Despite this high prevalence, there is evidence that symptoms are poorly controlled.[75-77] Reasons for this include inadequate assessment on the part of the professional, poor communication and information leading to poor compliance and a reliance on patients to raise concerns.[68-70,78] In a study by Heaven and Maguire,[78] nurses were able to identify less than 40% of patients' concerns and Aranda et al[79] found nurses reluctant to use a systematic approach to symptom assessment. Other factors include disinclination on the part of the patient to disclose symptoms for fear of being hospitalized, needing medication or acknowledging a worsening condition, and selective disclosure (e.g. people are generally more willing to discuss physical problems than psychological ones).[80] All symptoms are made worse by insomnia, exhaustion, anxiety, helplessness, hopelessness and depression, likewise the person's emotional state; meaning given to the illness and cultural background will also affect the perception and experience of symptoms.[9]

A validated assessment tool, the Symptoms and Concerns checklist, was used to determine the prevalence and severity of symptoms and concerns at a large cancer centre in London, UK.[81-83] Patients were asked to rate how much of a problem each item had been in the previous week, using a 0–3 scale (0 = 'not at all', 1 = 'a little', 2 = 'quite a bit', 3 = 'very much').[82] Table 37.3 shows the proportion of patients reporting checklist ratings of 1, 2 or 3 and the proportion reporting ratings of 2 or 3.

Feeling tired/weak/lacking energy (fatigue) was the most common problem reported by 79% of the sample: 43% rated this item as 2 or 3; 50% or more reported concerns about the future, being unable to do things, feeling tense/worried/fearful, pain, low mood/depression and mouth/taste problems; 20% or more rated these items 2 or 3. Of the six items reported by more than 50% of the sample, four were psychosocial rather than physical. The number and severity of items reported was influenced by tumour type, gender and disease status, with the highest number of symptoms and concerns reported by women, patients with lung cancer, followed by those with brain tumours; the lowest by those with lymphoma and urological cancer. The study revealed a high level of unmet physical and psychological needs, with improvements needed in symptom assessment, symptom control and timely referral to SPC.[82]

Oncologists valued symptom control expertise and community liaison provided by the SPC and the study recommended that this should be met by greater collaboration between oncologists and specialists in palliative care. In practical terms, this could be achieved through placing staff from a community SPC team in oncology outpatient clinics.

Symptom assessment tools

Symptom assessment tools provide frameworks for the systematic approach to the identification

Table 37.3: Frequency of symptoms and concerns reported by the whole sample (*n* = 480)[82]

Checklist items	Patients rating item as 1, 2 or 3 *n* (%)	Patients rating item as 2 or 3 *n* (%)
Group A		
Pain	253 (53)	103 (22)
Mouth/taste (e.g. dry/sore mouth)	240 (50)	113 (24)
Sleep	234 (49)	113 (24)
Change in appetite/weight	220 (46)	102 (21)
Constipation	160 (33)	58 (12)
Feeling/being sick	111 (23)	41 (9)
Other items		
Feeling tense/worried/fearful	267 (56)	99 (21)
Feeling low in mood/depressed	247 (51)	98 (20)
Feeling angry	144 (30)	66 (14)
Feeling weak/tired/lacking energy	379 (79)	207 (43)
Not being able to do the things you usually do	271 (57)	161 (34)
Worries or concerns about the future	273 (57)	155 (32)
Concentrating/remembering	236 (49)	100 (21)
Feeling short of breath	216 (45)	86 (18)
Worries/concerns about the important people in your life	211 (44)	100 (21)
Appearance	161 (34)	69 (14)
Caring for self	156 (33)	86 (18)
Finance	132 (28)	71 (15)
Anything to do with your treatment/side-effects/care	131 (27)	57 (12)
Lack of information about illness/treatment	125 (26)	48 (10)
Bladder/urinary	118 (25)	56 (12)
Relationships with important people in your life	115 (24)	59 (12)
The way in which doctors/nurses communicate with you	94 (20)	52 (11)
Diarrhoea	83 (17)	26 (6)
Work	77 (16)	42 (9)
Swallowing	75 (16)	37 (8)
Sexual relationship	71 (15)	43 (9)
Lack of support from others	61 (13)	31 (7)
Spiritual/religious issues	27 (6)	13 (3)

Note: patients often have several symptoms.
Source: from Lidstone et al 2003[82] with permission of Hodder Arnold.

and assessment of symptoms. Some are also designed to evaluate and monitor care and interventions. The 29-item Symptoms and Concerns Checklist reported in the previous section provides evidence of the acceptability of this particular tool in the outpatient population of a large cancer centre in the UK, with 98% completion by the sample.[82] Table 37.4 provides other examples of symptom assessment checklists and tools.

Table 37.4: Symptom assessment questionnaires and palliative care outcome tools	
Name and author	**Overview and comment**
Rotterdam symptom checklist De Haes et al[84]	34 symptoms, including physical and psychosocial. Developed with patients. High sensitivity but no spiritual questions. Length of questionnaire may not be suitable for weak and very ill patients
Edmonton symptom assessment tool Bruera et al[85]	9 physical and psychological symptoms using a visual analogue scale. Developed in North America for use in a hospice but transferable to other settings. Scores are entered on a chart; therefore useful for audit and evaluation
Palliative Care Assessment Tool (PACA) Ellershaw et al[18]	Evaluates 5 symptoms (pain, anorexia, nausea, insomnia and constipation) using a 4-point scale and semi-structured interview. A useful tool to evaluate interventions and symptom experience
Support Team Assessment Tool (STAS) Higginson[86]	17 items. Developed and tested as an outcome measure for palliative care services. Easy to use. Aimed at professionals. Moderate correlation between patient and professional questioning the reliability of proxy reporting
Patient-evaluated problem score (PEPS) Rathbone et al[87]	Patients are asked to list and rate problems as mild, moderate or severe affecting their quality of life – whether physical, emotional, social or spiritual. A patient-centred tool found to be helpful in the hospital setting
Palliative Care Outcome Scale POS (Version 1) Patients Outcome Scale POS (Version 2) Hearn and Higginson;[89] Aspinal et al[90]	Patient and staff questionnaires. 12 questions scoring 0–4 covering pain, symptom control, anxiety, family anxiety, information, support, depression, self-worth, wasted time and personal affairs. Version 1 has validity in home, hospital and hospice settings. Version 2 includes a question on depression. Results can be plotted on a chart to log assessments
Pain and symptom assessment record (PSAR) Bouvette M et al[91]	Developed by Canadian nurses. Implemented in 12 settings and adjusted following evaluation. Forms a useful addition to the nursing record. 5 sections: pain assessment (including body chart, quality and numerical descriptors), symptom assessment, sedation, patient satisfaction and action taken. No psychosocial, spiritual component or family care. Aimed at nurses; therefore proxy-rated. Plans include formatting for patient use
VOICES questionnaire (Views of Informal Carers Evaluation of Services) Addington-Hall et al[92]	A survey instrument used with the bereaved to evaluate care of the dying in the last year of life in all care settings. 56 core questions with component parts totalling over 150 questions. Lengthy but comprehensive

General principles of symptom assessment

While symptom assessment tools can be useful, the successful management of symptoms requires regular systematic and impeccable assessment. The principles suggested by Twycross[9] underpin the use of any checklist or tool and are detailed in Table 37.5.

Case Study 37.1 illustrates the interrelated nature of seven symptoms in one person – anxiety, breathlessness, insomnia, anorexia, pain, nausea and constipation.

In conclusion, patients with advanced cancer often report a complex array of concerns and symptoms and there is evidence of high levels of unmet need, physical and emotional. Despite improvements in symptom control currently being a prime aim of palliative care, there is no universal acceptance of what constitutes a suitable symptom assessment tool. In general, the principles of symptom assessment will apply whatever the stage of the disease, and symptom assessment tools can be useful, particularly if used as an instrument to guide discussion with patients and to monitor care, treatment and interventions. Although the nature of palliative care contributes to difficulties in collecting and interpreting data in this area, these barriers should not prevent the nurse including symptom assessment tools as part of the routine monitoring and evaluation of care.

However, a flexible sensitive approach is required at all stages of the care pathway as not all people will be able to use these, especially if distressed, very weak or with poor cognitive function or fluctuating levels of consciousness. What will always remain important is regular impeccable skilled assessment that pays attention to direct patient feedback.

FOSTERING HOPE

The time of assessment, especially the first, provides the nurse with a unique opportunity to identify problems affecting quality of life and to understand what the patient and family hope for during this episode of care and in the future. One of the most important aspects of a relationship between a nurse and a palliative care patient is the ability to foster hope and promote autonomy and choice: all of these have been shown to help people cope and adapt to their illness more effectively.[95] Hockley[96] also suggests that nurses are in a powerful position to generate hope.

Hope is defined in the *Oxford Dictionary* as 'a feeling of expectation and desire'. The critical role that hope plays in human life takes on special meaning as death nears[97] and the ability to hope will be constantly challenged as multiple losses are experienced as the disease progresses.[98] Hope can become a significant coping strategy for some people in a close relationship, in that evidence of hope in one person can maintain a sense of hopefulness in the other.[38–40] On some occasions hope can appear to be strong within a patient and may manifest as unrealistic ideas and goals for the future; while some may perceive this as problematic, the patient may be choosing to use hope as a form of denial and as a rational and vital coping mechanism. According to Russell,[99] denial can offer terminally ill people protection from the threat of disintegration that might occur if all hope is destroyed. He saw denial as a buffer against hopelessness. Maintaining a sense of hope is also one way of helping patients to achieve and maintain quality of life. This will be explored in the following sections.

Multicultural views of hope

Over the past three decades our understanding of hope has increased, but the majority of the studies are ethnically homogenous and may not reflect the experience of hope in all cultures.[98] Ersek[98] suggests that the three issues outlined in Table 37.6 may have an impact on views of hope.

It must be stressed that the above are only theories but may help nurses to be open to the unique and varied responses to coping with a terminal illness that they will see in practice. More research needs to be done on hope in multicultural groups to inform our understanding and the range of care and support interventions that may help individuals. Research does suggest that if clinicians are 'fully there' physically and psychosocially, they place themselves in a position to be used as instruments through which hope can be assessed, administered and fostered.[40]

Table 37.5: Principles of symptom assessment

Evaluation. The 'TSRQP' symptom assessment framework is an adaptation of a model by Estes[93]	Explanation	Management	Monitoring	Attention to detail
Timing and cause – Is the symptom new, recent or long-standing. Is it there all the time or does it come and go? How long does it last? What is the cause of the symptom and underlying pathological mechanism? e.g. vomiting from hypercalcaemia and bowel obstruction require different treatments	A clear explanation of the treatment plan will help the person gain a sense of control and security.[94] If omitted, this can undermine the person's self-esteem, and make the symptom seem more frightening, thereby increasing its negative effect. A clear rationale behind treatment may also improve compliance	Correct the correctable: e.g. lowering serum calcium for hypercalcaemia, bronchodilator therapy for breathlessness caused by bronchospasm, aqueous cream for pruritus	Review frequently. Symptoms of frail patients with advanced disease can change frequently and require repeated evaluation. This may mean several times a day	Do not underestimate the therapeutic power of attention to detail in palliative care. This helps people feel less isolated and provides a sense of being 'understood' and 'heard'. Nurses need to constantly ask 'what is happening and why' as well as 'what can I do today that will make a difference to you'
Severity – How severe is it? What is the impact on the person's life?		Use of non-drug treatments and alternative therapies: e.g. an anxious patient who is frightened of dying may find discussing their fears and relaxation therapy more helpful than medication	Complete symptom relief is often unrealistic in advanced cancer and will need to be balanced against the person's wishes: e.g. a desire to stay alert, tolerate some pain and be up and about rather than change analgesics, or in the case of bowel obstruction, the antimuscarinic side-effects and a desire to eat may result in compromise and acceptance of vomiting once or twice a day rather than complete relief	

Region – Is the symptom local or general? e.g. weakness in the legs may indicate a new diagnosis of spinal cord compression, somatic pain is more localized than visceral and may indicate bone metastases	Prophylactic prescribing – persistent symptoms should be treated with regular therapy. As-needed medication means the person has to wait for symptom relief and is the cause of much unrelieved distress
Quality – What exactly is it like? What words does the person use to describe the symptom? Words such as 'frightening' and 'unbearable' indicate the degree of distress caused by the symptom	Provide written advice and write drug regimens in table form for the person and family to work from. This will support compliance.
Provoke – What makes it better or worse? What has been tried and failed? e.g. sedation of an agitated patient with a full bladder when catheterization would be more helpful	Refer to a specialist palliative care service in complex situations
Never say 'nothing more can be done': this could lead to hopelessness and it is surprising how much can be achieved with imagination, persistence, a positive attitude and involving specialist palliative care

Mr Smith has the symptom of breathlessness. He has lung cancer and has had one previous chest aspiration for a pleural effusion. He is 54 years old, self-employed and has been married to Mary for 30 years. They have two children. The eldest son lives in America and they have 'lost touch'. The youngest child, Ann, is due to get married in 6 months' time. Mr Smith says 'I'll be happy if I live long enough to see her married'. Until recently, Mr Smith was fit and well. The diagnosis of lung cancer was made 6 weeks ago. His mother and aunt both died from breast cancer and he recalls his mother dying in 'terrible pain and unable to breath'. He has never been in hospital before until the diagnosis was made. He seems reluctant to ask for help.

Breathlessness

Worsening breathlessness

Panic

Worry about family

Fear of suffocating or choking

Fear of dying

Increased anxiety

Loss of sleep, exhaustion

Lack of understanding about reason for breathlessness

What do you think is on Mr Smith's mind?
What do you think Mr Smith may want from the healthcare team?
Consider all the component parts of this gentleman's symptom experience. Good symptom control requires attention to all of these interrelated factors.

Mr Smith may want to know:
What is causing the breathlessness?
What can be done to improve things?

His treatment options.
The choices he can make.

He might also want:
To know how long his prognosis might be and where he would like to be cared for
To talk about telling his family and rearranging his daughter's wedding
To know what might happen next and reassurance that he will not suffocate or die in terrible pain
To talk about his life.

Mr Smith's breathlessness is partially relieved following a pleural aspiration but he develops pain in his scapula and requires regular opiate analgesics. He is unable to sleep. A regular laxative has not been prescribed. During a conversation he tells you that he is constipated. He remains reluctant to ask for help, is nursed in a four-bedded area and movement provokes the pain. Consider the possible interrelated components to this symptom:

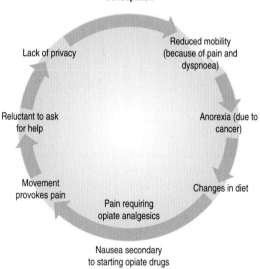

Constipation

Lack of privacy

Reduced mobility (because of pain and dyspnoea)

Reluctant to ask for help

Anorexia (due to cancer)

Movement provokes pain

Changes in diet

Pain requiring opiate analgesics

Nausea secondary to starting opiate drugs

Although some of these aspects require attention from a doctor, the nurse will have a crucial role in this man's care. This encompasses eliciting concerns, answering questions, accurate assessment, planning, implementation and evaluation of treatment, administering medication proactively and on time, providing support to Mr Smith and his family, maintaining and preserving dignity, coordinating care and involving the doctor and other members of the team at appropriate times.

Table 37.6: Issues impacting on hope

Issue	Identified as:
1. Time orientation	Some cultural groups are future-orientated. People look ahead and make short- and long-term plans. These people may appear more hopeful than present-orientated people and set more future-orientated goals. It is possible that hope could be used as a form of denial. Present-orientated people live very much for today, and may be better able to sustain hope at the end of life as the ability to make long-term plans for the future-orientated people is hindered by the uncertainty of a life-threatening diagnosis
2. Truth-telling	The value of truth-telling may affect hope. Informed consent and patient autonomy are impossible without full disclosure. However, truth-telling is not universally viewed as helpful or desirable. Some cultures believe that patients should be protected from information they perceive to be harmful, particularly as it could threaten hope and the patient will 'give up'. Truth-telling may also been seen as rude and disrespectful in some cultures. For some too much information may affect the ability to cope, as demonstrated by the following patient: "I don't want to know too much otherwise I can't get on with my life and have hope in the future" [63]
3. Beliefs in control	Some cultures view death as an inherent part of life. They may accept death as an inevitable part of life and may adopt a passive sick role. These people may be viewed as less hopeful than people from other cultures who manifest a 'fighting spirit'

In Table 37.7 nursing interventions that can influence hope in palliative care are presented.[38–40,96]

QUALITY OF LIFE

Maintaining a level of hope is one way of helping patients to achieve and maintain quality of life. Quality of life is a descriptive term that refers to people's physical, emotional, social and spiritual well-being, and their ability to function in the ordinary tasks of living.[100] Whereas quality of life appears to be strongly linked to normality, and an ability to function normally, in palliative care the concept of normality is challenged in that many patients with major physical and psychological limitations have reported a high degree of overall quality of life.[101,102] Kaasa and Loge[103] suggest this fits in well with the 'gap' theory proposed by Calman.[104] This is described as the inverse relationship between an individual's expectations and their perceptions of a given situation, where the smaller the gap the better the quality of life.

Although some argue that formal assessment of quality of life via scoring systems is crucial for the evaluation of outcomes of care in palliative care,[105,106] there is abundant recognition that measuring the quality of life in individuals with palliative care needs is extremely problematic, not least because of short survival and often poor cognitive condition of dying patients.[107,108] However, although the concept appears to be controversial, possibly because it invites us to mix facts and values and may not capture those aspects of patients' quality of life that are important to them, nurses, by virtue of their close and sustained contact with patients, are able to play a crucial role in helping patients achieve the best possible quality of life.

This can be achieved in three ways:

Table 37.7: Influence of nursing interventions on hope

Hope-decreasing factors	Hope-increasing factors
Unrelieved pain and other symptoms	Pain and symptom relief. Providing physical and emotional comfort so that there is energy for hope
Feeling devalued	Encouraging autonomy and a sense of control over daily activities
Abandonment and isolation	Actively listening and being 'fully there'
Lack of direction/goals	Providing encouragement, support and assistance to establishing or refocusing realistic expectations and aims
	Planning care based on the individual's and family's values, preferences, goals and needs
	Affirming the individual's and family's sense of self-worth and value
	Using appropriate humour and light heartedness
	Supporting reminiscing (present and past joys and successes)
	Encouraging positive self-talk
	Encouraging aesthetic uplifting experiences
	Facilitating religious/spiritual experiences/practice
	Assisting the individual in finding meaning in the situation
	Assisting the individual to keep a journal/tape to record thoughts and feelings/create a memory box/memory book/drawing
	Fostering family/friend relationships
	Provide assistance to develop phone/email/chat room support system
	Providing accurate and an appropriate level and amount of information about the illness and treatment

- promoting and maintaining autonomy, choice and independence
- symptom relief and attention to detail (e.g. impeccable assessment of symptoms, giving medication strictly on time, flexible visiting, attention to enhancing physical appearance, improving the environment, e.g. placing their bed by a window)
- listening to patients, to understand what will help or improve their quality of life, and articulating this to the wider healthcare team.

Perhaps what is most apparent when considering quality of life scores is that they only measure selected aspects and are unable to capture the unique and individual experience of cancer.[109] Despite these concerns, Sahlberg-Blom et al[102] report that several individuals expressed happiness and satisfaction during the last month of their life despite having a low quality of life score. A recent study of 255 patients who were designated 'do not resuscitate' found that 48% of the patients rated their quality of life as good, whereas physicians relied on their assumptions about the patients' quality of life and rated it good for only 9%.[110] What appears to be important is that if a quality of life measure provides a means of monitoring the effect of therapeutic interventions and care and enhances communication it could help to ensure that efforts *are* directed towards patients actual needs and problems as defined by them and not those perceived by medical and nursing staff.

Several quality of life instruments are available,[111,112] but few have been developed with palliative care patients. Kaasa and Loge[103] reviewed palliative care-specific instruments and concluded that many had been developed for use in research but may not be suited for daily clinical use. Cohen and Leis[113] have tried to address this factor, and reported on a qualitative study of 60 Canadian individuals with advanced and progressive cancer who were asked what was important to their quality of life. These individuals identified five broad domains:

1 The individual's own state, including physical, cognitive and psychological.

2 Quality of palliative care (feeling secure, cared for, treated with respect, continuity of care, spiritual care, availability of staff).

3 Physical environment (being in the right place; i.e. home/hospital, pleasant surroundings, access to the outdoors, nature and weather).

4 Relationships (support, communication, change in role, being a burden, growing closer to loved ones).

5 Outlook (existential well-being/spirituality/facing death, hope, coping with uncertainty, control, being able to find some joy in life).

As a result of this study, the authors adjusted the McGill Quality of Life Questionnaire to incorporate the content found to be important to individuals in the study. It is now called Quality of Life in Life-Threatening Illness – Patient Version or QOLLTI-P. The next phase of the research will test this version.

A French study[107] used a version of the European Organization for Research and Treatment of Cancer (EORTC) QLQ-C30 questionnaire[114] and interviews with palliative care cancer patients to gain deeper understanding of quality of life from the individual's perspective. These authors found that information came to light in the interviews that was not covered in the questionnaire and, likewise, issues were addressed in the questionnaires that were not raised during the interview. Individuals did not find a questionnaire burdensome, but also expressed a need to talk. The authors concluded that a quality of life tool could be beneficial when used as a discussion tool with individuals. As one of the prime aims of palliative care is to improve and maintain quality of life, it is appropriate to assess quality of life at the following critical points on the pathway of care:

- at diagnosis
- at the beginning of treatment
- during post-treatment phase
- at disease recurrence
- during the dying phase.

While quality of life in palliative care is difficult to evaluate, quality of life tools can make a useful contribution to understanding.[106]

FAMILY CARE

Cancer affects the whole family system, and families of those receiving palliative care can be profoundly affected by the experience. Many will have to contend with multiple issues, including the physical demands of practical care, emotional strain, change in role and responsibilities, adjustment to work or career schedules and matters of personal and sexual intimacy. Finally, many will be confronted with fear, uncertainty and existential questions regarding the meaning of life, death and suffering. The following four bereaved relatives express the reality of being a carer: '*mentally extremely difficult to keep that "brave face" for 24 hours a day, 7 days a week*', '*terrifying and traumatic*', '*utterly exhausting*' and an '*unforgettable experience, a great leveller. It helps you prioritize your life*'.[115]

The World Health Organizations' definition of palliative care strongly promotes the family, and it is important that the family's needs are addressed and they have access to sufficient levels of practical and emotional support to allow them to perform the role of carer. Whereas the care of the family of those receiving palliative care is clearly important, many nurses feel ill-equipped or that they do not have time to devote to this type of care. What is evident though is that when families receive adequate information and support from the time of diagnosis, they have less needs, cope better and have more confidence in healthcare staff.[116,117] Those whose needs are not met are more likely to experience fatigue, insomnia, weight loss and vulnerability to infections.[118]

Kristjanson et al[119] advise that family care requires nurses to:

1 Define the family (i.e. a broad definition to include committed heterosexual or same sex partners, birth and adoption and others who have strong emotional bonds with the person).

2 Understand the potential needs of the family.

3 Have knowledge of useful interventions (Table 37.8)

CARE OF THE DYING

A good death has always been important to all cultures.[120,121] But what does a good death look like and how high a priority is it in current European health care? If death is seen as a defeat, then it will not have high priority. But if a good death is seen as the culmination of good care and a good life, then it must have priority. What is clear is that each of us will have a different view on what constitutes a good death – 'one size does not fit all' – and we will all want to be different in dying as in living. Perhaps the most important aspect to understanding the good death is one in which I make my own choices about my last days and months and a bad death is one in which I have no autonomy.[122]

In order to die well though, dying must be recognized and appropriate care and support put in place. Smith[123] suggests that the diagnosis of dying is one of the most crucial that a

Table 37.8: Family care interventions in palliative care

Potential need of the family	Nursing intervention
Patient comfort	Explanation, education and ideas of how to keep the patient comfortable
	Teach how to use equipment and how to handle and move the patient safely and comfortably
Information	Provide local information, advice and support
	24-hour helpline numbers and clarity on who to call if worried or in an emergency
	If appropriate, family members should be invited to accompany patients during clinical consultations and be involved in discussions about treatment and care
	Explain signs of impending death and what to do at the time of death if at home
Emotional support	Given the opportunity to have their needs and preferences for support and information assessed separately to those of patients
	Time given to listen to how they are feeling
	Maintaining hope strategies
Practical help	Help families identify their practical help needs
	Arrange practical assistance early (do not assume family members want to be responsible for providing personal hygiene care for the patient regardless of how devoted they are. Many do not want to take on this responsibility or know how to)
	Identify the need for respite care at an early stage

Source: adapted from Kristjanson et al[119] with permission of Radcliffe Medical Press.

doctor can make. While many people may concur with this sentiment, Glare et al[124] found that doctors consistently overestimate the time people with advanced cancer have left to live. They concluded that this may affect a person's prospects of achieving a good death, particularly as discussions regarding stopping treatment, resuscitation and preferred place of care may begin too late. Although the diagnosis of dying can be difficult to make, the signs are often not recognized because a culture of 'cure' exists and few have been trained to care for dying patients and therefore feel helpless.[125] This results in the continuation of invasive procedures, investigations and treatments right up to the point of death and at the expense of the comfort of the patient.[126] Use of active treatments that could prolong life in far advanced cancer requires two considerations:

1 Will they affect quality of life? If so, is this acceptable to the person?

2 Will they lengthen suffering? If so, is this acceptable?

Patients' views on how their illness, life and death should be managed is of key ethical importance and relies on the team communicating well, providing information and understanding what the person wants.

Diagnosing dying

Usually, the dying phase (that is having hours or days to live) for cancer patients is preceded by a gradual deterioration in functional status. For a few it can be abrupt – e.g. massive haemorrhage. Recognizing key signs and symptoms of dying are important clinical skills and nurses, by virtue of their sustained and frequent contact, may be the first to notice these. If the nurse suspects a patient may be dying, he or she must prompt a clinical review. Once dying has been diagnosed, the team can refocus care appropriately. Box 37.4 outlines the key signs and symptoms of dying.

The observation that many people dying from cancer die peacefully has been detailed in studies.[128–132] However, there is abundant evidence that many do not die peacefully and some will have distressing symptoms, many of which can be attributed to organic brain dis-

---

Box 37.4

Key signs and symptoms of dying[127]

Patients who are dying are often:	
Profoundly weak	Having difficulty swallowing
Gaunt	Breathing in abnormal patterns
Drowsy	Unable to concentrate
Disorientated	Having skin colour and temperature changes due to reducing peripheral perfusion

---

ease consequent to metabolic disorder related to multi-organ failure.[132,133]

In the UK, evidence regarding variance in the care of the dying provided strong impetus for one palliative care team to create a care pathway.[126,134–136] Care pathways are multiprofessional documents that replace existing medical and nursing records for a specific episode of care.[137] In this instance, the document provides a clear plan of care developed from best practice in the hospice setting. The document has been widely implemented in the UK and can be used in any care setting: although some[138] warn that we must guard against standardizing care of the dying to a set of boxes to be ticked and there is value in people simply being given space to die well, unstructured and in their own way, this care pathway has led to measurable outcomes and the production of data for audit and research.[136] What remains salient is for innovation and individualized care to exist *alongside* the framework of the care pathway. The care pathway provides a plan of care aimed at attaining specific goals, which are outlined in Box 37.5.

Common issues in the dying phase

The following issues are commonly encountered as the patient is nearing death:

* *Continuation of drugs* – as patients become weaker, many experience difficulty swallowing, and all non-essential medication should be stopped. Drugs that should be continued include opioids, anxiolytics and antiemetics, as symptoms will require continuing control.[126,136]

Box 37.5

Goals of care for patients who are dying

Comfort measures

Goal 1 – Current medication assessed and non-essentials discontinued.

Goal 2 – As-required drugs written up according to protocol (for pain, agitation, respiratory tract secretions, nausea and vomiting).

Goal 3 – Discontinue inappropriate interventions (blood tests, antibiotics, intravenous fluids, turning regimens, vital signs); document not for resuscitation.

Psychological and insight issues

Goal 4 – Ability to communicate assessed (translator as needed).

Goal 5 – Insight into condition assessed.

Religious and spiritual support

Goal 6 – Religious, cultural and spiritual needs assessed with patient and family.

Communication with family and others

Goal 7 – Identify how family or other people involved are to be informed of patient's impending death.

Goal 8 – Family or other people involved given relevant hospital information (if at home – details of who to contact for help and advice).

Communication with community healthcare team

Goal 9 – General practitioner is aware of patient's condition.

Summary

Goal 10 – Plan of care explained and discussed with patient and family.

Goal 11 – Family or other people involved express understanding of plan of care.

Source: adapted from Ellershaw and Ward[126] with permission of BMJ Publishing Group.

Ideally, drugs should be converted to the subcutaneous route and given as a continuous infusion.

- *Continuing artificial fluids* – evidence suggests this provides limited benefit and can, in most cases, be stopped.[139]

- *Excess respiratory tract secretions* – evidence recommends giving an antimuscarinic agent subcutaneously and repositioning.[140] This symptom can get worse if not treated and is a cause of distress to relatives.[140] Suction appears to be of limited help and can be very distressing.

- *Agitation/confusion/terminal restlessness* – this can occur as a result of fear, psychological and spiritual concerns, hypotension, hypoxia, organic brain disease and biochemical disturbance. Exclude any obvious cause for the distress (e.g. a wet bed or full bladder), reassure the patient and family and establish a low-stimulation environment. Medication may be needed if the patient is very distressed. A benzodiazepine, such as midazolam, or an antipsychotic, such as haloperidol, may be helpful and a continued supportive calm nursing presence.

- *Nursing care* – patients will need regular nursing attention to ensure comfort. This may mean at least every 2 hours and should include sustained emotional support to the patient and their family. Particular attention should be paid to prompt control of pain, agitation, respiratory tract secretions, mouth care and continence needs. Invasive measures for bowel care are seldom needed, but a source of agitation is often caused by a full bladder and retention of urine.[126,136] Catheterization in these instances will be required. Routine ritualistic turning is not required near to death and can cause restlessness and disturbance pain.[132]

- *Insight into the situation* – it is suggested that the patient and family's insight is explored sensitively and questions answered appropriately. It is strongly recommended that the family are told that the patient is dying and will die.[126,136] This will allow time to prepare, to say their goodbyes, to ask questions, to stay with the patient and to contact relevant people. Involving the family in care at the end of life should also be offered. For example, mouth care and sponging the face and hands. The level and depth of involvement in care is highly individual. Some may desire a shared responsibility for care, whereas others will prefer to hand over all aspects of care to professional staff.

- *Spiritual/cultural care* – sensitivity to the patient's cultural, spiritual and religious background is essential at the end of life and formal traditions may need to be observed before and after death.

Emergency situations at the end of life

The following are considered to constitute emergencies at the end of life: stridor, pain, haemorrhage, confusion and seizure.[141] Hypercalcaemia, spinal cord compression and superior vena cava syndrome are also potential clinical emergencies in palliative care and may occur before the dying phase.

Emergency situations at the end of life are, fortunately, rare and many can be anticipated. For example, ulcerated neck and facial tumours or previous haemoptysis or haematemesis may predict haemorrhage, bone metastases predict pathological fracture, enlarging upper airway tumour predicts stridor and previous hypercalcaemia predicts confusion.[141] Some symptoms are preventable: e.g. a patient with a brain tumour who can no longer take corticosteroids or anticonvulsant therapy may have a seizure unless anticonvulsant therapy is maintained. In these circumstances, continuous subcutaneous infusion of midazolam (starting 30 mg in 24 hours) or rectal administration of diazepam (10 mg) will be required.[141]

The majority of emergencies in the last 48 hours of life are irreversible and treatment must be aimed at rapid relief of distress. Faull and Hirsch[94] suggest the following management plan for haemorrhage or other acute terminal emergency situations:

- Anticipate, plan and prepare management of the event. Ensure clear written instructions in the nursing and medical notes and that all members of the healthcare team know what to do.

- Drugs should be available for immediate administration by nursing staff without additional consultation with doctors. Useful drugs are injections of midazolam (5–10 mg if no previous exposure to a benzodiazepine), diazepam 10–20 mg rectally and parenteral morphine.

- Ensure plentiful supply of dark or green towels to reduce the visual impact of massive blood loss.

- Prepare the family and patient appropriately. Many patients need to know that help will be immediately available in an emergency. Families cope better if they have a plan and know what to do or who to contact.

- Be aware that these events can be frightening, distressing and memorable for everyone, including staff.

- Stay with the patient. Most events of this nature cause death within minutes and the most important thing is to stay calm and comfort the patient.

During the last hours and days of life, people experience increasing weakness, loss of interest in food and drink, have difficulty swallowing and can become drowsy. In general, this phase can be anticipated, but occasionally deterioration may be sudden and unexpected. The care of patients and families at this time requires the healthcare team to focus attention on symptom control, comfort and support and to adopt a sensitive but structured approach to care. Ensuring the comfort of all dying patients is vital; likewise, consideration to their wishes over place of care, their need for religious ritual or prayer and sustained support to their family is also crucial.

FUTURE CHALLENGES IN PALLIATIVE CARE

Although there is an overall 5-year survival rate of nearly 50% in developed countries, the majority of cancer patients will need palliative care at some point during their cancer journey. The WHO estimate the proportion requiring palliative care is at least 80% worldwide, with most cancers diagnosed when already advanced and incurable.[6] This reality combined with advances in medicine and an overall trend towards increased survival and an ageing population, means that millions will live for longer with complex health and social care needs. Accordingly, access to palliative care will be a vital and critical need, and palliative care as a speciality will be challenged by increasingly complex multiple disease and symptom management, especially in older people. Consequently, imaginative solutions to the sustained support to individuals living with life-threatening conditions such as cancer will challenge government healthcare systems.

Nurses are in an ideal position to take on leadership roles in the development of palliative care and to develop solutions to these challenges. Success will depend on a solid foundation of knowledge, skill and competence and on a political understanding and activity aimed at developing national palliative care policies and standards to guarantee assimilation into all European healthcare systems.

REFERENCES

Note: the National Council for Hospice and Specialist Palliative Care Services has changed its title to the National Council for Palliative Care.

1. Clark D, Seymour J. Reflections on palliative care. Facing Death Series. Buckingham: Open University Press; 1999.
2. Lawton J. The dying process. Patient's experiences of palliative care. London: Routledge; 2000.
3. Clark D. Recent developments in palliative care policy and practice. Physiotherapy 1994; 8(12): 854–855.
4. Clark D. Between hope and acceptance: the medicalisation of dying. BMJ 2002; 324: 905–907.
5. World Health Organisation. Cancer pain relief and palliative care. Report of a WHO Expert Committee. Geneva: WHO; 1990.
6. World Health Organisation. National cancer control programmes: policies and guidelines. Geneva: WHO; 2002.
7. Broadley K. Teamwork and a multidisciplinary approach. Eur J Palliat Care 1997; 4(3):76.
8. Clark D, Ten Have H, Janssens R. Common threads? Palliative care service developments in seven European countries. Palliat Med 2000; 14:479–490.
9. Twycross R. Introducing palliative care. 4th edn. Abingdon: Radcliffe Medical Press; 2003.
10. European Oncology Nursing Society. Core curriculum for a post-registration course in cancer nursing. 2nd edn. EONS; 1999.
11. Department of Health. The NHS Cancer Plan: a plan for investment, a plan for reform. London: Department of Health; 2000.
12. National Institute for Clinical Excellence. Guidance on cancer services: improving supportive and palliative care for adults with cancer. London: National Institute for Clinical Excellence; 2004.
13. National Council for Hospice and Specialist Palliative Care Services. Definitions of supportive and palliative care. A consultation paper. London: NCHSPCS; 2002.
14. Wilkinson K. The concept of hope in life-threatening illness. Prof Nurse 1996; 11(10):659–661.
15. Illich I. Limits to medicine. Medical nemesis: the expropriation of health. Harmondsworth: Penguin; 1976.
16. O'Connor M, Aranda S, eds. Palliative care nursing. Abingdon: Radcliffe Medical Press; 2003.
17. Doyle D. The provision of palliative care. In: Doyle D, Hanks G, MacDonald N, eds. Oxford textbook of palliative medicine. 2nd edn. Oxford: Oxford University Press; 1998.
18. Ellershaw JE, Peat SJ, Boys LC. Assessing the effectiveness of a hospital palliative care team. Palliat Med 1995; 9:145–152.
19. Beynon T, Richards M, Ledger S, Grant J, Ward P. Palliative care assessment tool. Palliat Med 1997; 11:57–58.
20. Jack B, Hillier V, Williams A, Oldham J. Hospital based palliative care teams improve the symptoms of cancer patients. Palliat Med 2003; 17: 498–502.
21. Back IN. Palliative medicine handbook. Cardiff: BPM Books; 2001. www.pallmed.net (accessed 21 May 2005).
22. Glaser BG, Strauss A. Awareness of dying. New York: Aldine Publishing Company; 1965.

23. Glaser BG, Strauss A. Time for dying. New York: Aldine Publishing Company; 1968.

24. Strauss A, Glaser B. Anguish – a case history of a dying trajectory. California: The Sociological Press; 1970.

25. Sudnow D. Passing on: the social organisation of dying. Eaglewood Cliffs, New Jersey: Prentice-Hall; 1967.

26. Quint JC. The nurse and the dying patient. New York: Macmillan; 1967.

27. Bram PJ, Katz L. A study of burnout in nurses working in hospice and hospital oncology settings. Oncol Nurs Forum 1989; 16(4):555–560.

28. Alexander DA, Ritchie E. Stressors and difficulties in dealing with the terminal patient. J Palliat Care 1990; (6):28–33.

29. Hockley J. Caring for the dying in acute hospitals. Nurs Times 1989; 85(39):47–50.

30. Copp G, Dunn V. Frequent and difficult problems perceived by nurses caring for the dying in community, hospice and acute care settings. Palliat Med 1993; 7(1):19–25.

31. Corner J. The nursing perspective. In: Doyle D, Hanks G, MacDonald N, eds. Oxford textbook of palliative medicine. Oxford: Oxford University Press; 1993.

32. Copp G. Palliative care nursing education – a review of research findings. J Adv Nurs 1994; (3):552–557.

33. Hopkinson JB. Facilitating the development of clinical skills in caring for dying people in hospital. Nurse Educ Today 2001; 21:632–639.

34. Heslin K, Bramwell L. The supportive role of the staff nurse in the hospital palliative care situation. J Palliat Care 1989; 5:20–26.

35. Davies B, O'Berle K. Dimension of the supportive role of the nurse in palliative care. Oncol Nurs Forum 1990; 17:87–94.

36. Davies B, O'Berle K. Support and caring – exploring the concepts. Oncol Nurs Forum 1992; 19: 763–767.

37. Dobratz MC. Hospice nursing: present perspectives and future directives. Cancer Nurs 1990; 13:116–122.

38. Herth K. Fostering hope in terminally ill people. J Adv Nurs 1990; 15:1250–1259.

39. Herth K. Hope in the family caregiver of terminally ill people. J Adv Nurs 1993; 18:538–548.

40. Herth K, Cutcliffe JR. The concept of hope in nursing 3: hope and palliative care nursing. Br J Nurs 2002; 11(14):977–983.

41. Degner L, Gow CM, Thompson LA. Critical nursing behaviours in care for the dying. Cancer Nurs 1991; 14: 246–253.

42. Hunt M. Being friendly and informal: reflected in nurses', terminally ill patients' and relatives' conversations at home. J Adv Nurs 1991; 16:929–938.

43. Raudonis BM. The meaning and impact of empathic relationships in hospice nursing. Cancer Nurs 1993; 16:304–309.

44. Webber J. The evolving role of the Macmillan nurse. London: Cancer Relief Macmillan Fund; 1993.

45. McClement SE, Degner LF. Expert nursing behaviours in care of the dying adult in the intensive care unit. Heart Lung 1995; 24:408–419.

46. Stroud R. The withdrawal of life support in adult intensive care: an evaluative review of the literature. Nurs Crit Care 2002; 7(4):176–184.

47. Johnston B. Overview of nursing developments in palliative care. In: Lugton J, Kindlen M, eds. Palliative care: the nursing role. Edinburgh: Churchill Livingstone; 1999.

48. Hull MM. Hospice nurses' caring support for caregiving families. Cancer Nurs 1991; 14(2):63–70.

49. Richardson J. Health promotion in palliative care: the patients' perception of therapeutic interaction with the palliative nurse in the primary setting. J Adv Nurs 2002; 40(4):432–440.

50. Ferrell BR, Coyle N. Textbook of palliative nursing. New York: Oxford University Press; 2001.

51. Penson J. A hope is not a promise: fostering hope within palliative care. Int J Palliat Nurs 2000; 6(2):94–98.

52. Seymour J. What's in a name? A concept analysis of key terms in palliative care nursing. In: Payne S, Seymour J, Ingleton C, eds. Palliative care nursing, principles and evidence for practice. Maidenhead: Open University Press; 2004.

53. Low J, Payne S. The good and bad death perceptions of health professionals working in palliative care. Eur J Cancer Care 1996; 5:237–241.

54. Kristjanson LJ, McPhee I, Pickstock S, et al. Palliative care nurses' perceptions of good and bad deaths and care expectations: a qualitative analysis. Eur J Palliat Care Nurs 2001; 7(3):129–139.

55. Hamric A, Spross J. The clinical nurse specialist in theory and practice. Philadelphia: WB Saunders; 1989.

56. Bamford O, Gibson F. The clinical nurse specialist role: key role components identified. Manag Clin Nurs 1998; 2:105–109.

57. Royal College of Nursing. A framework for nurses working in specialist palliative care. Competencies Project. London: Royal College of Nursing; 2002.

58. Weightman J. Competencies in action. London: The Institute of Personnel and Development; 1994.

59. International Society of Nurses in Cancer Care (ISNCC). A core curriculum for palliative nursing. Macclesfield: ISNCC; 2002.

845

60. Maguire P. Barriers to psychological care of the dying. BMJ 1985; 291(6510):1711–1713.

61. Lyke EM. Assessing for nursing diagnosis. Philadelphia: JB Lippincott; 1992.

62. Pearce C, Lugton J. Holistic assessment of patients' and relatives needs. In Lugton J, Kindlen M, eds. Palliative care. The nursing role. London: Churchill Livingstone; 1999.

63. Mirando S. Palliative care needs assessment of Herefordshire, UK. "What sort of care is helpful and important to you?" Views of palliative care patients and their carers on their perceived needs. Unpublished research; 2003.

64. Cassell EJ, Coulehan JL, Putnam SM. Making good interview skills better. Patient Care 1989; 3:145–166.

65. Davis AJ. Compassion, suffering, morality: ethical dilemmas in caring. Nurs Law Ethics 1981; 2(5):1–2,6,8.

66. Benner P, Tanner CA, Chesla CA. Expertise in nursing practice: caring, clinical judgement and ethics. New York: Springer; 1996.

67. Faulkner A, Maguire P. Talking to cancer patients and their relatives. Oxford: Oxford University Press; 1994.

68. Koffman J, Higginson IJ. Accounts of carers' satisfaction with health care at the end of life: a comparison of first generation black Caribbean's and white patients with advanced disease. Palliat Med 2001; 15:337–345.

69. Davies E, Higginson IJ. Communication, information and support for adults with malignant cerebral glioma: a systematic review. Supp Care Cancer 2003; 11:21–29.

70. Edmonds P, Rogers A. "If only someone had told me": a review of the care of patients dying in hospital. Clin Med 2003; 3:149–152.

71. Hockley J, Dunlop R, Davies RJ. Survey of distressing symptoms in dying patients and their families in hospital and the response to a symptom control team. BMJ 1988; 296:1715–1717.

72. Bruera E. Research into symptoms other than pain. In: Doyle D, Hanks G, MacDonald N, eds. Oxford textbook of palliative medicine. 2nd edn. Oxford: Oxford University Press; 1993.

73. Addington-Hall JM, McCarthy M. Dying from cancer: results of a national population-based investigation. Palliat Med 1995; 9:295–305.

74. Aranda S. Framework for symptom assessment. In: O'Connor M, Aranda S, eds. Palliative care nursing. Abingdon: Radcliffe Medical Press; 2003.

75. Cleeland C, Gonin R, Hatfield A, et al. Pain and its treatment in out-patients with metastatic disease. N Engl J Med 1994; 330:592–595.

76. Higginson IJ, Priest P, McCarthy M. Are bereaved family members a valid proxy for a patient's assessment of dying? Soc Sci Med 1994; 38:553–557.

77. Larue F, Colleau S, Brasseur L, Cleeland C. Multicenter study of cancer pain and its treatment in France. BMJ 1995; 301:1034–1037.

78. Heaven CM, Maguire P. Training hospice nurses to elicit patient concerns. J Adv Nurs 1996; 23:280–286.

79. Aranda S, Kissane D, Long C. Quality in community-based palliative care (QUIC-PC) QUIC-PC Project Report – stage 3. Melbourne: Centre for Palliative Care; 2000.

80. Heaven CM, Maguire P. Disclosure of concern by hospice patients and their identification by nurses. Palliat Med 1997; 11:283–290.

81. Butters E, Pearce S, Ramirez A, et al. A new screening checklist for advanced cancer: the process of content development. J Palliat Care 1998; 14:124.

82. Lidstone V, Butters E, Seed PT, et al. Symptoms and concerns amongst cancer outpatients: identifying the need for specialist palliative care. Palliat Med 2003; 17:588–595.

83. Butters E, Pearce S, Ramirez A, et al. Assessing symptoms and concerns in patients with advanced cancer: the development of a checklist for use in clinical practice. Palliat Med submitted for publication.

84. De Haes JC, van Knippenberg FCE, Neijt JP. Measuring psychological and physical distress in cancer patients: structure and application of the Rotterdam symptom checklist. Br J Cancer Care 1990; 62:1034–1038.

85. Bruera E, Kuehn N, Miller M, Selmar P, Macmillan K. The Edmonton symptom assessment chart (ESAS): a simple method for the assessment of palliative care patients. J Palliat Care 1991; 7:6–9.

86. Higginson IJ. Clinical audit in palliative care. Oxford: Radcliffe Medical Press; 1993.

87. Rathbone GV, Horsley S, Goacher J. A self evaluated assessment suitable for seriously ill hospice patients. Palliat Med 1994; 8:29–34.

88. Farrer K. Research and audit: demonstrating quality. In: Lugton J, Kindlen M, eds. Palliative care: the nursing role. London: Churchill Livingstone; 1999.

89. Hearn J, Higginson IJ. On behalf of the Palliative Care Audit Project Advisory Group. Development and validation of a core outcome measure for palliative care: the palliative care outcome scale. Qual Healthcare 1999; 8(4):219–227

90. Aspinal F, Hughes R, Higginson IJ, et al. A user's guide to the palliative care outcome scale. London: Palliative Care and Policy Publications; 2002. www.kcl.ac.uk/depsta/palliative/pos/aboutpos.html (accessed 21 May 2005).

91. Bouvette M, Fothergill-Bourbonnais F, Perreault A. Pain and symptom assessment record (PSAR). J Adv Nurs 2002; 40(6):685–700.

92. Addington-Hall JM, Walker L, Karlsen S, et al. A randomised controlled trial of postal versus interviewer administration of a questionnaire measuring satisfaction with and use of services received in the year before death. J Epidemiol Commun Health 1998; 52:802–807.

93. Estes MRZ. Health assessment and physical examination. New York: Delmar; 1998.

94. Faull C, Hirsch C. Symptom management in palliative care. Prof Nurse 2000; 16(1) 840–843.

95. Rideout E, Montemuro RN. Hope, morale and adaptation in patients with chronic heart failure. J Adv Nurs 1986; 11:429–438.

96. Hockley J. The concept of hope and the will to live. Palliat Med 1993; 7:181–186.

97. Scanlon C. Creating a vision of hope: the challenge of palliative care. Oncol Nurs Forum 1989; 16(4):491–496.

98. Ersek M. The meaning of hope in the dying. In: Ferrell BR, Coyle N, eds. Textbook of palliative nursing. New York: Oxford University Press; 2001.

99. Russell G. The role of denial in clinical practice. J Adv Nurs 1993; 18:938–940.

100. Bowling A. Measuring disease. A review of disease specific quality of life measurement scales. Buckingham: Open University Press; 2001.

101. Hjermstad M, Holte H, Evenson S, Fayers P, Kaasa S. Do patients who are treated with stem cell transplantation have a health-related quality of life comparable to the general population after one year? Bone Marrow Transplant 1999; 24:911–918.

102. Sahlberg-Blom E, Ternestedt BM, Johansson JE. Is good quality of life possible at the end of life? An explorative study of the experiences of a group of cancer patients in two different care cultures. J Clin Nurs 2001; 10:550–562.

103. Kaasa S, Loge JH. Quality of life in palliative care: principles and practice. Palliat Med 2003; 17:11–20.

104. Calman KC. Quality of life in cancer patients – an hypothesis. J Med Ethics 1984; 10:124–127.

105. Paci E, Miccinesi G, Toscani F, et al. Quality of life and outcome in palliative care. J Pain Symptom Manage 2001; 21(3):179–188.

106. Salek S, Pratheepawanit N, Finlay I, et al. The use of quality of life instruments in palliative care. Eur J Palliat Care 2002; 9(2):52–56.

107. Poussin G, Manes-Gallo MC, Monti R, et al. Can we talk of quality of life before death? Eur J Palliat Care 2000; 7(6):218–220.

108. Koller M, Lorenz W. Quality of life: a deconstruction for clinicians. J R Soc Med 2002; 95(10):481–488.

109. Cohen SR, Mount BM. Quality of life in terminal illness: defining and measuring subjective well-being in the dying. J Palliat Care 1992; 8:40–45.

110. Junod Perron N, Morabia A, de Torrente A. Quality of life of Do-Not-Resuscitate (DNR) patients: how good are physicians in assessing DNR patients' quality of life? Swiss Med Wkly 2002; 132(39–40):562–565.

111. Donnelly S, Walsh D. Quality of life assessment in advanced cancer. Palliat Med 1996; 10:275–283.

112. Hearn J, Higginson IJ. Outcome measures in palliative care for advanced cancer patients: a review. J Public Health Med 1997; 19(2):193–197.

113. Cohen SR, Leis A. What determines the quality of life in terminally ill cancer patients from their own perspective? J Palliat Care 2002;18(1):48–58.

114. Aaronson NK, Ahmedzai S, Bergman B, et al. The European Organisation for Research and Treatment of Cancer QLQ-C30: a quality of life instrument for use in international clinical trials in oncology. J Natl Cancer Inst 1993; 85(5):365–375.

115. Mirando S. Views of informal carers evaluation of services – use of the VOICES questionnaire to evaluate palliative care services and inform a needs assessment. Unpublished research; 2003.

116. Thorne SE, Robinson CA. Reciprocal trust in health care relationships. J Adv Nurs 1988; 13:782–789.

117. Stetz KM, Hanson WK. Alterations in perceptions of care giving demands in advanced cancer during and after the experience. Hospice J 1992; 8:21–34.

118. Ramirez A, Addington-Hall J, Richards M. ABC of palliative care. The carers. BMJ 1998; 316(7126):208–211.

119. Kristjanson L, Hudson P, Oldham L. Working with families. In: O'Connor M, Aranda S. eds. Palliative care nursing. Abingdon: Radcliffe Medical Press; 2003:271–283

120. Seale C. Changing patterns of death and dying. Soc Sci Med 2000; 51:917–930.

121. Clark J. Patient centred death. BMJ 2003; 327:174–175.

122. Walter T. Historical and cultural variants on the good death. BMJ 2003; 327:218–220.

123. Smith R. Death, come closer. Editors choice. BMJ 2003; 327:172.

124. Glare P, Virik K, Jones M, et al. A systematic review of physicians' survival predictions in terminally ill cancer patients. BMJ 2003; 326:195–198.

125. Higgs R. The diagnosis of dying. J R Coll Phys London 2000; 33(2):110–112.

126. Ellershaw JE, Ward C. Care of the dying patient: the last hours of life. BMJ 2003; 326:30–34.

127. Faull C, Woof R. Palliative care: an Oxford core text. Oxford: Oxford University Press; 2002.

128. Parkes CM. Home or hospital? Terminal care as seen by surviving spouses. J R Coll Gen Pract 1978; 28:19–30.

129. Keane WG, Gould JH, Millard PH. Death in practice. J R Coll Gen Pract 1983; 1:347–351.

130. Wilkes E. Dying now. Lancet 1984; 1(8383):950–952.

131. Saunders C. Pain and impending death. In: Wall PD, Melzack R, eds. Textbook of pain. 2nd edn. Edinburgh: Churchill Livingstone; 1989:624–631.

847

132. Lichter I, Hunt E. The last 48 hours of life. J Palliat Care 1990; 6(4):7–15.

133. Mills M, Davies TO, Macrae WA. Care of dying patients in hospital. BMJ 1994; 309:583–586.

134. Ellershaw J, Foster A, Murphy D, et al. Developing an integrated care pathway for the dying patient. Eur J Palliat Care 1997; 4(6):203–207.

135. Ellershaw JE, Smith C, Overill S, et al. Care of the dying: setting standards for symptom control in the last 48 hours of life. J Pain Symptom Manage 2001; 21:12–17.

136. Ellershaw J, Wilkinson S. Care of the dying. A pathway to excellence. Oxford: Oxford University Press; 2003.

137. Campbell H, Hotchkiss R, Bradford N, Porteous M. Integrated care pathways. BMJ 1998; 316:133–137.

138. Kelly D. A commentary on 'Integrated care pathways for the last two days of life'. Int J Palliat Nurs 2003; 9(1):39–40.

139. Joint Working Party between the National Council for Hospice and Specialist Palliative Care Services and the Ethics Committee of the Association for Palliative Medicine of Great Britain and Ireland. Ethical decision making in palliative care: artificial hydration for people who are terminally ill. J Eur Assoc Palliat Care 1997; 4:203–207.

140. Bennet M, Lucas V, Brennan M, et al. Using anti-muscarinic drugs in the management of death rattle: evidence-based guidelines for palliative care. Palliat Med 2002; 16:369–374.

141. Adam J. ABC of palliative care. The last 48 hours. BMJ 1997; 315:1600–1603.

INDEX

Italic page numbers indicate in-depth treatment

A

Acupuncture *see* Complementary medicine
Acute renal failure *see* Intensive nursing care
Acute respiratory failure *see* Intensive nursing care
Adverse drug reactions *see* Side effects
Age/ageing
  cancer treatment experience, 219
  pain (control), 469
Alcohol consumption
  cancer prevention, 148
Alopecia
  biological therapy, 606
  chemotherapy, 603-605
  hair anatomy/physiology, 602
  hair growth, 602-603
  hormone therapy, 606
  introduction, 601
  nursing care, 611-614
  patterns
    complete hair loss, 605
    incomplete hair loss, 605-606
    hair growth, 606
  prevention
    biological measures, 608-609
    hypothermia, 607-608
    mechanical, 606
  psychological aspects, 609-611
    body image, 610
    self-esteem, 610
    sexuality, 611
  radiotherapy, 606
  self-care
    head shaving, 612-613
    scalp protection, 612
    teaching/information, 611-612
    wig wearing, 613
  supporting programmes, 614
Alternative medicine *see* Complementary medicine
Anorexia/Cachexia *see also* Malnutrition
  contributing factors
    local effects, 636
    psychological, 636
    systemic effects, 636
    treatment effects, 636-637
  incidence, 635
  introduction, 619
  lipid mobilizing factor, 637-639
  metabolic alterations
    energy expenditure, 637
    humoral responses, 637
    inflammation, 637-638
  pathway modulations, 639
  protein mobilizing factor, 637
Apoptosis
  immunology, 125
  cell cycle, 79-80
Ascites
  malignant effusions, 620-624

B

Biological therapy
  administration, 325
  angiogenesis inhibitors, 299-300, 312
  assessment, 324-325
  biotechnology, 306
  coordination of care, 326
  definition, 303
  drug development, 307
  gene therapy, 300, 312-315
    gene immunotherapy, 314
    gene marking, 313
    multi-drug resistance gene, 313
    suicide gene, 313-314
    toxicity, 314
  history, 304-305
  immunotherapy
    cytokines, 307-310, 326
    monoclonal antibodies, 309-311, 326-327
    vaccines, 311-312
  introduction, 303
  nausea and vomiting, 423
  nursing care, 314-326
  premedication, 326
  preparation/safety, 325
  radioimmunotherapy, 327

Biological therapy (*Continued*)
rationale, 305-306
side effects
alopecia, 606
characteristics, 317-322
interferon alpha, 323-324
nausea and vomiting, 423
patterns, 316
skin reactions, 538
toxicity mechanisms, 316
Body image alteration
assessment, 711-712
chemotherapy, 706
consequences, 703-704
coping, 706-707
hormone therapy, 706
influences, 702-703
introduction, 701-702
nursing care, 710-712
patient decision making, 709
patient identification, 709-710
patient information, 708-709
radiotherapy, 706
surgery, 704-706
Bone marrow failure *see* **Haematological support**
Bone marrow transplantation
complications, 340
donor issues, 333-334
follow-up care, 347-348
haemopoietic stem cells
allografts, 331-332, 337
autografts, 331-332
harvesting/cryopreservation
bone marrow, 334, 336
cord blood collection, 335-336
donor lymphocyte infusion, 335
high dose treatment, 335-337
peripheral stem cells, 334-336
history, 330
immunity/vaccination, 348
introduction, 329
multiprofessional team, 346
nursing, 339-340
principles, 330-331
psychological aspects, 345-346
rehabilitation, 348-349
side effects
anaemia, 343
cataracts, 347
electrolyte imbalance, 344-345
fertility, 347
gastrointestinal toxicity, 345
graft versus host disease, 343-344
hepatic toxicity, 345
immunosuppression, 340-342
mucositis, 345
physical symptoms, 347
renal failure, 344-345
secondary malignancies, 347
thrombocytopenia, 343

veno-occlusive disease, 345
tissue typing, 332-333
transplant process
engraftment period, 339
pre transplant, 337-339
Breast cancer
body image alteration, 702
cancer screening
BSE and CBE, 173-176
clinical features, 241
decision making, 242
diagnosis, 241
hormone therapy
adjuvant therapy, 355
aromatase inhibitors, 357
gonadotrophins, 357
males, 356
metastasis, 355
oestrogen receptor modulators, 358
prevention, 355-356
principles, 356-357
side effects, *361-373*
summary, 359
use of, 354-355
lymphoedema, 560
mammography, 174-176, 183-184, 242
neoadjuvant downstaging, 242
pathology, 100
principles, 241
staging, 241
surgery, 241-247
palliative, 247
primary cancer, 243
reconstruction, 244-247
regional nodes, 244
Breathlessness
assessment, 511-512
breathing retraining, 515-517
causes, 508
chemotherapy, 512-513
complementary therapies, 521-522
drug therapy
anxiolytics, 513-514
corticosteroids, 514
morphine, 513
oxygen, 514
saline, 514
experience, 509-510
impact on nurses, 522
introduction, 507
mechanisms, 508-509
non-drug therapy, 514-522
other symptoms, 522
panic/anxiety management, 517-519
planning/pacing activities, 519
prevalence, 508
radiotherapy, 512-513
relaxation script, 519
supporting caregivers, 522
therapeutic relationship, 515

C

Cachexia *see* **Anorexia/Cachexia**
Calgary family assessment model
  cancer care, 25
Cancer
  alopecia, *601-614*
  complementary therapy, *381-396*
  anorexia/malnutrition, *633-651*
  biological therapy, *303-327*
  body image alteration, *701-713*
  bone marrow transplantation, *329-349*
  breathlessness, *507-523*
  causation belief, 5-6
  chemotherapy, *283-300*
  constipation, *482-490*
  decision making, *195-211*
  diarrhoea, *490-502*
  early detection, *167-188*
  epidemiology, 55-69
  fatigue, *657-669*
  genetic basis, 73-92
  haematological support, *403-414*
  health behaviour, *3-16*
  hormone therapy, *353-375*
  immunology, *126-129*
  internet/media, 6-8
  lymphoedema, *559-570*
  malignant effusions, *619-629*
  nausea and vomiting, *415-432*
  oral complications, *575-596*
  pain, *439-472*
  palliative care, *821-844*
  pathology, *97-113*
  prevention, *133-160*
  psychological care, *717-735*
  radiotherapy, *265-280*
  rehabilitation, *799-817*
  risk communication, 6-8
  sexuality, *675-697*
  skin/wound care, *527-553*
  surgery, *233-261*
  treatment experience, *213-229*
Cancer care *see* **Nursing/Cancer care**
Cancer screening
  breast cancer, 172-176, 183-184
  cervix cancer, 177-179
  colorectal cancer, 179-181, 184-185
  decision making, 171-172
  diagnostic methods, *183-188*
  effectiveness of programmes, 168-169
  ethical aspects, 170-171
  lead-time bias, 169
  length-time bias, 169-170
  lung cancer, 182-183
  opportunistic, 168
  ovarian cancer, 175-177
  population aspects, 170-171
  prostate cancer, 179-182, 185-187
  recruitment and follow-up, 172
  registries, 170

  surveillance, 171
  tumour markers, 187-188
Cancer treatment experience
  accessing treatment, 218-219
  age, 219
  assessment methods, 227-229
  biomedical perspective, 214
  clinical trials, 220
  costs and benefits, 219-220
  decision making, 219
  environment, 221
  follow-up, 226
  language, 221-222
  nurse-led care delivery, 226-227
  palliative care, 226
  prior experiences, 218
  psycho-oncology perspective, 214-215
  quality of care, 224
  quality of life, 215-217, 222-225
  recurrence, 226
Cervix cancer
  cancer screening, 177-179
Chemotherapy
  administration, *287-291*
    intraarterial, 291
    intramuscular, 290
    intraperitoneal, 291
    intrapleural, 291
    intrathecal, 290-291
    intravenous, 290
    intravesical, 291
    oral, 291
    safety, 292-293
    subcutaneous, 290
  body image alteration, 706
  breathlessness, 512-513
  classification
    alkylating agents, 285-286
    anthracyclines, 286
    antimetabolites, 286
    cytotoxic antibiotics, 286
    mitotic inhibitors, 286
    topoisomerase inhibitors, 286-287
  constipation, 484
  diarrhoea, 494
  goals of treatment, 284
  gonadotoxicity, 684-687
  innovations, 298
  introduction, 283-284
  mitosis, 284-285
  new agents
    antiangiogenic agents, 299-300
    Glivec, 299
    Herceptin, 299
  nursing, *292-298*
  oral complications, 576
  patient assessment, 291-292
  patient education, 293-294
  patient support, 297-298
  pharmacology, 284-287

Chemotherapy (*Continued*)
  risk assessment, 287-288
  sexuality, 680-687
  side effects
    alopecia, 602-605
    dermatological toxicity, 296, 532-537
    fatigue, 297
    flu-like symptoms, 297
    gastrointestinal toxicity, 296
    haematological toxicity, 293-295
    hand/foot syndrome, 297
    nausea and vomiting, 419-422
    neurological toxicity, 295
    organ toxicity, 296
    renal/bladder toxicity, 295
Children
  pain (control), 467-468
Cigarette smoking *see* **Tobacco use**
Classification
  cancer epidemiology, *56-62*
  cancer, 99-103
  constipation, 483
  cytotoxic agents, 285-287
  decision making, 196
  malnutrition, 642
  pain, 444-446
Colorectal cancer
  adjuvant therapy, 259
  cancer screening, 179-181
    barium enema, 185
    colonoscopy, 184
    faecal occult blood test, 184
    sigmoidoscopy, 184
  diagnosis, 254
  multidisciplinary approach, 255
  pathology, 98, 110, 258-259
  perioperative care, 258
  principles, 254
  rehabilitation, 260
  staging, 254
  surgery, 256-260
    innovations, 260-261
    metastasis, 258
    palliative, 260
    prophylactive, 259
Complementary medicine
  access, 383
  benefit for caretakers, 392
  body-mind interventions
    autogenic training, 385
    imagery, 385
    psychoneuroimmunology, 385
  conventional practice, 395
  definitions, 381-382
  effectiveness, 384-392
  energy therapies, 391
  herbs, 391
  homeopathy, 391
  nausea and vomiting, 431
  popularity, 382-383
  reasons for use, 383-384

  regulation
    legal aspects, 393
    managerial aspects, 393
    professional aspects, 393
    self-regulation, 392
    supervision, 393-394
    support, 394
  touch and bodywork
    massage, 386-391
    reflexology, 386-391
Constipation
  aetiology, 483
  assessment
    nursing, 485
  chemotherapy, 484
  classification, 483
  definition, 482
  drug therapy, 488-490
  holistic care, 486
  introduction, 481
  non-drug therapy, 487-488
  normal function, 482
  palliative care, 484-485
  planning and implementation, 486
  radiotherapy, 484
  surgery, 484
Coping *see* **Psychosocial/Cultural aspects**
Culture *see* **Psychosocial/Cultural aspects**

D

Decision making
  breast cancer, 242
  cancer treatment experience, 219
  classification, 196
  decision aids, 208-209
  definition, 195
  ethical approach, 202
  future, 210
  inputs
    language, 203-204
    preferences, 204-205
  logical approach, 198-202
    computers, 201-202
    decision analysis, 198-199
    evidence-based, 199-201
  models, 207-208
  nursing, 209-210
  outcome assessment
    perspective, 207
  pragmatic approach, 202
  psychological approach, 196-198
  quality assessment
    clinical environment, 206
  use of research, 208
Diarrhoea
  assessment
    examination, 496
    further tests, 496
    history, 495
    symptoms, 496
  causes

cancer type, 492
chemotherapy, 494
infection, 494-495
nutrition, 495
radiotherapy, 494
surgery, 492-494
classification, 491
introduction, 481, 490-491
normal function, 482
outcome of nursing, 502
quality of life, 502
severity, 491
treatment
anal plug, 502
biofeedback, 501
bowel retraining, 501
diet, 499-500
drug therapy, 497-499
flow chart, 498
perianal adhesive pouch, 502
surgery, 499
types, 491
Diet *see* **Nutrition**
Disseminated intravascular coagulation *see* **Intensive nursing care**

E

Early detection *see* **Cancer screening**
Emesis *see* **Nausea and vomiting**
Endometrium cancer
hormone therapy, 361
Epidemiology
bias, chance and confounding, 66-67
causes
alcohol, 68
diet, 68
gene-environment interaction, 67
infections, 69
inherited cancer, 67
obesity, 68
tobacco, 67-68
classification, 56-62
descriptive studies, 66
experimental studies, 66
exposure effect, 62-63
grade and stage, 56
incidence, 56-58
Europe, 60-62
worldwide, 60
leading causes of death, 58-59
limitations, 58
malignant pleural effusions, 624-625
mortality rate, 58
observational studies
case control, 65
cohorts, 64-65
pain, 440-441
prevalence, 58
Ethical aspects
cancer prevention, 155
cancer screening, 170-171

decision making, 202
genetic tests, 152-154
haematological support, 411-412
Ethnicity
pain (control), 468

F

Family caregiving
assessment, 24-25
dimensions, 22-23
education, 29
experiences, 23-24
multicultural aspects, 28-30
nurse as mediator, 24
nursing interventions, 26-27
patient empowerment, 30-35
skill and role, 22
Fatigue
aetiology, 660
assessment, 663-665
caregiver's perspective, 668-669
concept, 658-659
demography, 662
drug therapy, 667-668
function, 659
incidence, 659
introduction, 657
non-drug therapy
energy conservation, 667
exercise, 666
patient education, 666
rest and sleep, 667
stress reduction, 667
outcomes, 663
patient perspective, 659-660
physical activity, 662
physiological factors
anaemia, 660
anorexia, 661
cancer therapy, 660-661
cytokines, 661
insomnia, 662
pain, 661
tumour burden, 661
psychosocial factors, 662
theoretical models, 658-659

G

Gastric cancer *see* **Oesophageal/Gastric cancer**
Genetics
cancer development, 86-87
carcinogenesis
chemical, 88-89
hormones, 91
infection/inflammation, 91-92
ionizing radiation, 89-91
physical, 89
ultraviolet radiation, 91
cell cycle
apoptosis, 79-80
differentiation, 79

Genetics (*Continued*)
    meiosis, 78
    mitosis, 77-78
    regulation, 78-79
  counseling, 155-156
  DNA-RNA-protein
    DNA repair, 76-77
    DNA replication, 76
    DNA structure, 74
    DNA transcription, 75
    genome, 74-75
    RNA processing, 75-76
    translation, 76
  family history, 150
  gene therapy, 300, 312-315
  genetic tests, 152-154
  hereditary cancer syndromes, 152-153
  hereditary predisposition, 87-88
  mutations
    deletion, 81
    epigenetic events, 81-82
    gene amplification, 81-83
    point, 80-81, 83
    translocation, 81, 83
  oncogenes, 82-84
  screening indications, 151
  tumour suppressor genes, 83-86
Graft versus host disease
  diarrhoea, 493-494
  nursing care, 539

H

Haematological support
  anaemia, 404
  erythropenia, 404
  ethical aspects, 411-412
  introduction, 403-404
  leucopenia, 404-405
  new approaches
    coagulation factors, 413
    community care, 413
    donor granulocytes, 413
    erythropoietin, 412
    haematopoietic growth factors, 412
  nursing care
    bone marrow suppression, 410
    fluid balance, 411
    infection control, 410
    psychological support, 411
  pancytopenia, 405
  thrombocytopenia, 405
  transfusions
    albumin, 407
    complications/reactions, 408-409
    fresh frozen plasma, 406-407
    gamma irradiation, 408
    HLA-selected platelets, 408
    immunoglobulins
      major ABO incompatibility, 407
      minor ABO incompatibility, 407
    infections, 408-409
    patient information, 409-410
    platelets, 406
    red cells, 405-406
    safety, 409
  venous thromboembolism, 405
Hair *see* **Alopecia**
Hand-foot syndrome
  nursing care, 538
Health behaviour
  cancer causation, 5-6
  concepts, 3-16
  healthcare professionals, 15-16
  internet/media, 6-8
  meaning, coping and adaptation, 13-14
  moral responsibility, 8-9
  social cognition models, 9-13
Health promotion
  role of nurses, 138-139
Homeopathy *see* **Complementary medicine**
Hormone therapy
  alopecia, 606
  body image alteration, 706
  breast cancer, *354-359, 361-373*
    side effects
      body image changes, 371
      drugs for hot flushes, 367-368
      health maintenance, 370-371
      hormone replacement therapy, 366-367
      hot flushes, 365
      menopause, 363-366
      natural progesteron, 368-369
      other therapies
      phytoestrogens, 368
      sexuality, 372
      thromboembolism, 373
      tumour flare, 372-373
      vaginal bleeding, 373
      vaginal dryness, 372
      weight gain, 371
  endometrium cancer, 361
  introduction, 353-354
  principles, 354
  prostate cancer, *358-362, 373-375*
    side effects
      body image changes, 373
      gynaecomastia, 375
      hot flushes, 374
      nausea/vomiting, 375
      sexuality, 374
      tumour flare, 375
  sexuality, *680-683*
  skin reactions, 537
  thyroid cancer, 361

I

Immunology
  acquired immunity
    antibodies, 119-120
    antigenic determinants, 118
    antigens, 118
    B lymphocytes, 119

major histocompatibility complex, 118-119
antibody mediated immunity
  antigen presentation, 123-124
  B lymphocytes, 123
  dendritic cells, 123
  macrophages, 123
  T lymphocytes
    cytotoxic cells, 122
    helper cells, 122
    receptor, 122
apoptosis, 125
bone marrow transplantation, 348
cancer
  antibodies, 127
  cytokines, 128
  macrophages, 128
  NK cells, 128
  T lymphocytes, 127
  tumour antigens, 126-127
  tumour tolerance, 128-129
cytokines, 124
heat shock proteins, 124-125
immune response, 125-129
immunotherapy, *307-312, 327*
innate immunity
  antimicrobial proteins, 117
  complement, 117
  inflammation, 116
  natural killer cells, 117
  phagocytosis, 116-117
  physical and chemical barriers, 116
lymphocyte memory, 124
Integrated model of cancer care
  complementary medicine, 384
Intensive nursing care *see also* **Nursing/Cancer care**
acute renal failure, 781-782
acute respiratory failure
  aetiology, 778
  diagnosis, 778
  mechanical ventilation, 779-781
  treatment, 778-779
disseminated intravascular coagulation
  AML-m3
  anticoagulant, 777-778
  definition, 776
  diagnosis, 777
  pathogenesis, 776
  treatment
    replacement, 777
    supportive, 777
end of life care, 789-790
haemodynamic instability
  assessment, 783-785
  clinical features, 783-784
  monitoring, 783-785
introduction, 771-772
postoperative care, 785-789
  deep vein thrombosis, 788
  major surgery, 786
  nausea/vomiting, 788-789
  pain assessment, 786-787

pain management, 787
sepsis
  clinical features, 775
  definitions, 774
  diagnosis, 775
  epidemiology, 772-774
  microbiology, 774-775
  multi-organ dysfunction, 774
  risk assessment, 773
  treatment, 776
tumour lysis syndrome, 782-783

L

Lung cancer
  cancer screening, 182-183
  malignant pleural effusions, *624-629*
  pathology, 100
Lymphoedema
  altered sensation, 563
  assessment, 562
  breast cancer, 560
  complex decongestive therapy, 565
  compression therapy, 566-567
  differential diagnosis, 561-562
  emotional cost, 563-564
  exercise and movement, 568
  functional ability, 563
  incidence, 560
  infection, 567
  introduction, 559
  lymphatic drainage, 568-569
  multi-layer bandaging, 566
  orthopaedic problems, 563
  pain, 562-563
  pathophysiology, 560
  patient's experience, 562-565
  prevalence, 560
  quality of life, 564
  skin hygiene, 567
  surgery, 560

M

Malignant effusions
  anatomy/physiology, 619-620
  ascites
    aetiology, 620-621
    incidence/prevalence, 621-622
    natural history, 620
    obstruction of vessels, 621
    symptoms, 622
    therapies
      diuretics, 623
      indwelling catheter, 623
      intraperitoneal therapy, 624
      paracentesis, 622
      peritoneovenous shunts, 624
    tumours, 621
  introduction, 619
  pleural effusions
    aetiology, 624
    diagnosis, 625-626

Malignant effusions (*Continued*)
  epidemiology, 624-625
  pathophysiology, 625
  therapies
    pleurectomy, 628
    pleurodesis, 627
    pleuroperitoneal shunting, 628
    sclerosis, 627
    tube drainage, 627
    tunneled catheter, 628
Malnutrition *see also* **Anorexia/Cachexia**
  consequences, 639-640
  nutritional assessment
    body composition, 642
    classification, 642
    dietary history, 641
    laboratory measurements, 642-643
    medical history, 640-641
    physical examination, 641
    psychosocial history, 641
    weight changes, 641
  nutritional support
    diet, 645-647
    drug therapies, 647-648
    eicosapentaenoic acid, 648
    enteral/parenteral nutrition, 647
    fish oil, 648
    guidelines, 649
    non-drug therapies, 648-649
    patient counseling, 645-647
  progression, 639
  quality of life, 649-650
  risk assessment
    oncology screening tool, 643-644
    other tools, 644
    patient-generated, 643
Matrix metalloprotease
  invasive growth, 109-110
Menstruation *see* **Sexuality**
Multi-organ dysfunction *see* **Intensive nursing care**

N

Nausea and vomiting
  advanced cancer, 424
  complementary medicine, 431
  anticipatory, 423-424
  antiemetic drugs, 425
  assessment, 424-425
  biological therapy, 423
  chemotherapy, 419-422
    patient factors, 421-422
  definitions, 416-417
  diet, 430
  introduction, 415
  mechanisms, 417-419
  psychological/behaviour techniques, 428-430
  quality of life, 431-432
  radiotherapy, 422-423
  significance, 415-416
  surgery, 423, 788-789

  treatment failure, 428-429
Nursing/Cancer care *see also* **Intensive nursing care**
  and **Cancer treatment experience**
  advanced practice, 745-746
  alopecia, *601-614*
  complementary medicine, 392
  anorexia/malnutrition, *633-651*
  biological therapy, *314-326*
  body image alteration, 710-712
  bone marrow transplantation, 339-340
  breathlessness, *507-523*
  cancer treatment experience
    nurse-led care delivery, 226-227
  chemotherapy, *292-298*
  complementary techniques, 751
  constipation, *482-490*
  contribution, 743
  decision making, *195-211*
  development of new knowledge, 751-754
  diarrhoea, *490-502*
  education
    advanced cancer, 758-759
    delivery, 760
    general nurses, 759
    impact on practice, 759
    interprofessional, 759
    other issues, 759
    post-basic registration, 757-758
    preregistration, 757
  Europe, 742
  family caregiving, *21-35*
  fatigue, 668-669
  future, 764-765
  haematological support, *403-414*
  health promotion, 138-139
  information technology, 764
  integrated model, 384
  introduction, 741
  knowledge
    development, 746-747
    expertise, 747
  leadership
    fostering, 761-762
  lymphoedema, *559-570*
  malignant effusions, *619-629*
  nausea and vomiting, *415-432*
  nurse–patient relation
    involvement, 750
    knowing the patient, 749-750
  oral complications, *575-596*
  pain, *439-472*
  palliative care, 825
  patient involvement
    care decisions, 762-763
    challenges, 763
    service planning, 763
  patients'/nurses' perceptions, 748-749
  prevention, 138-139
  psychological care, *717-735*
  radiotherapy, *272-276*, 532

rehabilitation, *802*
research, 754-757
   implementing into practice, 755-757
   other evidence sources, 755
scope, 743-745
sexuality, *675-697*
skin/wound care, *538-539*, 544, *550-554*
smoking cessation, 143
social and cultural aspects, *37-49*
speciality, 743
specific therapeutic actions, 750-751
therapeutic nursing, *749-754*
tobacco use, 143
treatment experience, *213-229*

Nutrition *see also* **Malnutrition**
cancer epidemiology, 68
cancer prevention, 143-148
diarrhoea, 495
nausea and vomiting, 430
oral mucositis, 589
xerostomia, 594

O

Obesity
cancer epidemiology, 68
cancer prevention, 147

Oesophageal/Gastric cancer
diagnosis, 247
multidisciplinary approach, 249, 252
neoadjuvant therapy, 249
pathology, 252-253
presentation, 247
rehabilitation, 253-254
staging, 247
surgery
   curative, 249-250
   palliative, 252
   prophylactive, 252
   supportive care, 250-252

Oral complications
introduction, 575
mucositis
   anti-inflammatory therapy, 583
   antiseptic therapy, 583
   assessment, 579-582
   clinical features, 577-579
   diet, 589
   mechanism, 576-577
   multidisciplinary approaches, 580, 584
   oral care, 580-588
      mouthwashes, 587-588
   prevention, 580, 583
   supportive care, 588-589
prevalence, 577
risk factors, 579
taste dysfunctions, 594-595
types, 575-576
xerostomia
   assessment, 590-591
   clinical features, 590

dental caries prevention, 594
food selection, 594
mechanism, 590
nutrition, 594
oral infection prevention, 594
saliva replacement, 591
saliva stimulation, 593

Ovarian cancer
cancer screening
   CA 125, 187-188
   Pap test, 177
   recommendations, 178-179

P

Pain (relief)
adjuvant analgesics, 457-459
algorithms, 466
assessment, 449-452, 786-787
   McGill pain questionnaire, 450
   Memorial pain assessment card, 451
   pain diaries, 451
   pain-arch model, 451-452
   Wisconsin brief pain questionnaire, 451
behaviour, 465
biofeedback, 462
causal therapy, 453
causes, 444-446
classification, 444-446
critical pathways, 466
definition, 440
distracting techniques, 461
educational interventions
   families/caregivers, 470-471
   nurses, 469-470
   patients, 470-471
environmental factors, 463-464
epidemiology, 440-441
evaluation, 464-465
focusing techniques, 461
guidelines, 466
hypnosis, 462
imagery, 461
introduction, 439-440
invasive interventions, 458-460
lymphoedema, 562-563
mechanisms, 442-443
models, 441-442
multiple dimensions, 447-448, 452
neurobiology, 443-444
non-opioid analgesics, 454-455
nurse–patient relationship, 460
opioids, 455-457
patient counseling, 462
patient education, 461, 470-471
physical interventions
   acupuncture, 463
   electric energy, 463
   massage, 463
   relaxation, 462
   skin stimulation, 462

Pain (relief) (*Continued*)
    temperature, 462
    prevention, 453
    prophylactic therapy, 453
    quality assurance, 465-466
    quality improvement, 467
    risk groups
        children, 467-468
        elderly, 468
        ethnic groups, 468
        mental disease, 468-469
    spiritual intervention, 461
    standards, 466
    therapeutic touch, 460
    treatment, 452-472, 787-788
    types
        neuropathic, 444-445
        nociceptive, 444-445
    uncontrolled, 448-449
Palliative care
    access, 824
    assessment
        framework, 829
        general, 828
        principles, 829
        symptoms
            general principles, 834
            prevalence, 830
            tools, 830-832
    cancer treatment experience, 219
    constipation, 484-485
    definition, 822-823
    delivery, 824
    development, 821-822
    dying
        common issues, 841-843
        diagnosis, 841
        emergencies, 843
        goals of care, 842
    fostering hope
        multicultural aspects, 833-837
        nursing interventions, 838
    future challenges, 844
    introduction, 821
    locations, 824
    patient/family care, 828-833, 839-840
    quality of life, 837-839
    role of nurse
        core competencies, 827-828
        key aspects, 825-827
        specialist nursing, 827
    specialist services, 824-825
    supportive care, 823-824
Pathology
    cell growth regulation
        cell cycle, 105
        persistent disturbances, 103-104
        reversible disturbances, 103
        tumour dynamics, 105-106
    circulating tumour cells, 110-111

    classification
        cells and stroma, 102
        clinical relevance, 102
        epithelial tumours, 99-101
        mesenchymale tumours, 101
        mixed tumours, 101
        other tumours, 101-102
    colorectal cancer, 98, 110, 258-259
    invasive growth, 108-110
    lymphoedema, 560
    malignant effusions, 625
    metastasis
        patterns, 111-112
    morphology
        benign tumours, 98
        borderline tumours, 99
        malignant tumours, 98
    oesophageal/gastric cancer, 252-253
    skin cancer, 105
    stromal response
        angiogenesis, 106-107
        tumour stroma, 107
    thyroid cancer, 100
Patient empowerment
    definition, 30-31
    future areas, 35
    interventions
        coping skills, 33
        health education, 33
        stress management, 33
    self care, 34-35
    strategies, 31-32
Peritoneal cavity *see* **Malignant effusions**
Prevention
    alcohol consumption, 148
    chemoprevention, *156-158*
        smoking, 158-159
    counseling, 155-156
    family history, 150-151
    genetic tests, *152-155*
        ethical/legal aspects, 155
        psychosocial aspects, 154
    hereditary cancer syndromes, 152-153
    menstruation/reproduction, 148
    nutrition, *143-148*
        cooking methods, 146
        energy and fat intake, 146-147
        vegetables/fruits/fibres, 145
        vitamins/minerals/nutrients, 145-146
    obesity, 147
    physical exercise, 147-148
    principles
        prevention of suffering, 136
        primary prevention, 134-135
        secondary prevention, 135
        tertiary prevention, 136
    prophylactic surgery, 158
    risk assesment models, 149-150
    risk factors, 148-149
    role of nurses, 138-139

screening, 151-152, *167-188*
social/political issues, 136-138
tobacco use, *139-143*
Prostate cancer
cancer screening, 179-182, 185-187
prostate specific antigen, 187
hormone therapy
antiandrogens, 360-361
gonadotrophins, 360
orchidectomy, 360
other drugs, 361
principles, 360
side effects, 373-375
summary, 362
use of, 358
pathology, 103
Psychosocial/Cultural aspects
adaptation, 41-43, 721-723
alopecia, 609-611
anxiety
clinical features, 726
psychotherapy, 726
risk factors, 726
assessment of distress, 729-731
attitudes towards dying/death, 40-41
body image alteration, *702-713*
bone marrow transplantation, 333, 345-346
cancer care, *37-49*
cancer prevention, 136-138
cancer treatment experience, 214
chemotherapy, 297-298
chronic illness, 37-38
constipation, 485
coping, 41-43, 721-723
decision making, 196-198
delirium
risk factors, 729
symptoms, 728-729
treatment, 728-729
depression
prevalence, 723
psychotherapy, 725
risk factors, 723
symptoms, 723-725
diarrhea, 490
disease/treatment related, 720
family caretaking, 28-30
fatigue, 660-662
genetic tests, 154
haematological support, 411-412
health behaviour, 9-13
health care professionals, 721
hope and meaning, 44-45, 718-719
illness communication, 46-48
illness understanding, 38-39
introduction, 717
meaning, 41-43, 721-723
nausea and vomiting, 428-430
patient related, 719-720
patient stories, 47-48

post-traumatic stress disorder
symptoms, 727
treatment, 728
prevention, 136-138
psychotherapy, 725-726, 731-734
behaviour approaches, 733
cognitive approaches, 734
humanistic approaches, 732-733
psychoanalytical approaches, 734
recovering, 39-40
rehabilitation, 802
sexuality, *688-697*
spirituality, 45-46
suicide, 725

Q
Quality of care
cancer treatment experience, 224
decision making, 206
Quality of life
cancer treatment experience, 215-217, 222-225
diarrhoea, 502
lymphoedema, 564
malnutrition/anorexia, 649-650
nausea and vomiting, 431-432
palliative care, 837-839
rehabilitation, 803-805

R
Radiotherapy
administration, 266-268
body image alteration, 706
breathlessness, 512-513
constipation, 484
diarrhoea, 494
introduction, 265-266
oral complications, 576
patient information, 274
redistribution of cells, 271
repair of radiation damage, 269-270
repopulation of cells, 270-271
sexuality, 680-683
side effects, 276-279
alopecia, 606
lymphoedema, 560
nausea and vomiting, 422-423
skin reactions, 529-532
treatment duration, 272
treatment planning, 272-274
treatment process, 274-276
tumour reoxygenation, 271-272
Rehabilitation
bone marrow transplantation, 348-349
colorectal cancer, 260
definition, 800-801
existential aspects, 811-812
family life cycle, 813
goals, 801-802
history, 800
introduction, 799

Rehabilitation (*Continued*)
  nursing care, 802
  oesophageal/gastric cancer, 253-254
  physical aspects, *802-809*
  psychological aspects, *803-810*
  reshaping care, 816
  role of nurse, *812-816*
  support, 809-811
  transitions, 812
Reproduction *see also* **Sexuality**
  cancer prevention, 148

S

Sepsis *see* **Intensive nursing care**
Sexuality
  alopecia, 611
  chemotherapy, *680-687*
  context, 676-677
  cryopreservation
    embryos, 687-688
    oocytes, 688
    ovarian cortex, 688
    sperm, 687
    testicular tissue, 687
  hormone therapy, 680-683
    side effects, 372-373
  introduction, 675-676
  psychosexual aspects
    assessment, 688-691
    interventions
      absent vagina, 693
      anorgasmia, 694-695
      dyspareunia, 694
      ejaculatory problems, 695
      erectile dysfunction, 693
      loss of desire, 691-693
      vaginal stenosis/dryness, 693
    future developments, 696-697
  radiotherapy, 680-683
  reproduction
    contraception, 684
    egg donation, 688
    female fertility, 685-687
    male fertility, 684-685
  sexual response cycle, 677-678
  surgery, 678-680
Side effects *see also* **Nausea and vomiting**
  analgesics, 454-457
  biological therapy, *316-324*, 423, 538, 606
  bone marrow transplantation, 340-345
  chemotherapy, 293-297, 419-422, 532-537,
    602-605
  constipation drugs, 488-490
  hormone therapy, *361-375*, 537
  radiotherapy, 276-279, 522-523, 530-532, 560, 606
Skin (care) *see also* **Wound (care)**
  biological therapies
    skin reactions, 538
  chemotherapy
    skin reactions, 532-537

  hormonal therapies
    skin reactions, 537
  introduction, 527
  nursing care
    graft versus host disease, 539
    hand-foot syndrome, 538
    hypersensitivity, 538
    pruritus, 538
    sweating, 538
  radiotherapy
    acute skin reactions, 530
    chronic skin reactions, 532
    nursing care, 532
  structure and function
    accessory structures, 529
    dermis, 529
    epidermis, 528
    protection, 529
    subcutaneous layer, 529
Skin cancer
  pathology, 105
Smoking *see* **Tobacco use**
Social aspects *see* **Psychosocial/Cultural aspects**
Suicide
  psychosocial aspects, 725
Supportive care *see* **Palliative care**
Surgery
  body image alteration, 704-706
  breast cancer, *241-247*
  changing practice, 234-235
  colorectal cancer, *254-260*
  constipation, 484
  diarrhoea, *492-494*
  intraoperative care, 237
  lymphoedema, 560
  nausea and vomiting, 423
  oesophageal/gastric cancer, *247-254*
  pain control, 235
  postoperative care, 238
  preoperative care, 236-237
  principles, 239-241
  prophylactic surgery, 235
  reconstructive surgery, 235
  role, 233-234
  sexuality, 678-680
  specialization, 235
Survivorship *see* **Rehabilitation**

T

Therapeutic nursing *see* **Nursing/Cancer care**
Thyroid cancer
  hormone therapy, 361
  pathology, 100
Tobacco use
  cancer epidemiology, 67-68
  cancer prevention, 139-143
  chemoprevention, 158-159
  smoking cessation
    nursing strategy, 143

Treatment *see* Cancer treatment experience
Tumour lysis syndrome *see* Intensive nursing care

W

Wound (care) *see also* **Skin (care)**
   assessment, 542-543
   dressings, 543-546
   extravasation wounds
      nursing care, 544
   fistula
      nursing care, 553
   fungating wounds
      aetiology, 548
      cosmetics, 550

      nursing care, 550
      symptom management, 551
   healing process
      cancer effects, 542
      moist wounds, 541
      normal wounds, 540
   stomas
      appliances, 552
      complications, 552
      indications, 550
      siting, 552
      types, 550
   surgical wounds
      nursing care, 544